MW00973700

SLEEP AND BREATHING IN CHILDREN

LUNG BIOLOGY IN HEALTH AND DISEASE

Executive Editor

Claude Lenfant
Director, National Heart, Lung and Blood Institute
National Institutes of Health
Bethesda, Maryland

1. Immunologic and Infectious Reactions in the Lung, *edited by C. H. Kirkpatrick and H. Y. Reynolds*
2. The Biochemical Basis of Pulmonary Function, *edited by R. G. Crystal*
3. Bioengineering Aspects of the Lung, *edited by J. B. West*
4. Metabolic Functions of the Lung, *edited by Y. S. Bakhle and J. R. Vane*
5. Respiratory Defense Mechanisms (in two parts), *edited by J. D. Brain, D. F. Proctor, and L. M. Reid*
6. Development of the Lung, *edited by W. A. Hodson*
7. Lung Water and Solute Exchange, *edited by N. C. Staub*
8. Extrapulmonary Manifestations of Respiratory Disease, *edited by E. D. Robin*
9. Chronic Obstructive Pulmonary Disease, *edited by T. L. Petty*
10. Pathogenesis and Therapy of Lung Cancer, *edited by C. C. Harris*
11. Genetic Determinants of Pulmonary Disease, *edited by S. D. Litwin*
12. The Lung in the Transition Between Health and Disease, *edited by P. T. Macklem and S. Permutt*
13. Evolution of Respiratory Processes: A Comparative Approach, *edited by S. C. Wood and C. Lenfant*
14. Pulmonary Vascular Diseases, *edited by K. M. Moser*
15. Physiology and Pharmacology of the Airways, *edited by J. A. Nadel*
16. Diagnostic Techniques in Pulmonary Disease (in two parts), *edited by M. A. Sackner*
17. Regulation of Breathing (in two parts), *edited by T. F. Hornbein*
18. Occupational Lung Diseases: Research Approaches and Methods, *edited by H. Weill and M. Turner-Warwick*
19. Immunopharmacology of the Lung, *edited by H. H. Newball*
20. Sarcoidosis and Other Granulomatous Diseases of the Lung, *edited by B. L. Fanburg*
21. Sleep and Breathing, *edited by N. A. Saunders and C. E. Sullivan*
22. *Pneumocystis carinii* Pneumonia: Pathogenesis, Diagnosis, and Treatment, *edited by L. S. Young*
23. Pulmonary Nuclear Medicine: Techniques in Diagnosis of Lung Disease, *edited by H. L. Atkins*
24. Acute Respiratory Failure, *edited by W. M. Zapol and K. J. Falke*
25. Gas Mixing and Distribution in the Lung, *edited by L. A. Engel and M. Paiva*

26. High-Frequency Ventilation in Intensive Care and During Surgery, *edited by G. Carlon and W. S. Howland*
27. Pulmonary Development: Transition from Intrauterine to Extrauterine Life, *edited by G. H. Nelson*
28. Chronic Obstructive Pulmonary Disease: Second Edition, *edited by T. L. Petty*
29. The Thorax (in two parts), *edited by C. Roussos and P. T. Macklem*
30. The Pleura in Health and Disease, *edited by J. Chrétien, J. Bignon, and A. Hirsch*
31. Drug Therapy for Asthma: Research and Clinical Practice, *edited by J. W. Jenne and S. Murphy*
32. Pulmonary Endothelium in Health and Disease, *edited by U. S. Ryan*
33. The Airways: Neural Control in Health and Disease, *edited by M. A. Kaliner and P. J. Barnes*
34. Pathophysiology and Treatment of Inhalation Injuries, *edited by J. Loke*
35. Respiratory Function of the Upper Airway, *edited by O. P. Mathew and G. Sant'Ambrogio*
36. Chronic Obstructive Pulmonary Disease: A Behavioral Perspective, *edited by A. J. McSweeny and I. Grant*
37. Biology of Lung Cancer: Diagnosis and Treatment, *edited by S. T. Rosen, J. L. Mulshine, F. Cuttitta, and P. G. Abrams*
38. Pulmonary Vascular Physiology and Pathophysiology, *edited by E. K. Weir and J. T. Reeves*
39. Comparative Pulmonary Physiology: Current Concepts, *edited by S. C. Wood*
40. Respiratory Physiology: An Analytical Approach, *edited by H. K. Chang and M. Paiva*
41. Lung Cell Biology, *edited by D. Massaro*
42. Heart–Lung Interactions in Health and Disease, *edited by S. M. Scharf and S. S. Cassidy*
43. Clinical Epidemiology of Chronic Obstructive Pulmonary Disease, *edited by M. J. Hensley and N. A. Saunders*
44. Surgical Pathology of Lung Neoplasms, *edited by A. M. Marchevsky*
45. The Lung in Rheumatic Diseases, *edited by G. W. Cannon and G. A. Zimmerman*
46. Diagnostic Imaging of the Lung, *edited by C. E. Putman*
47. Models of Lung Disease: Microscopy and Structural Methods, *edited by J. Gil*
48. Electron Microscopy of the Lung, *edited by D. E. Schraufnagel*
49. Asthma: Its Pathology and Treatment, *edited by M. A. Kaliner, P. J. Barnes, and C. G. A. Persson*
50. Acute Respiratory Failure: Second Edition, *edited by W. M. Zapol and F. Lemaire*
51. Lung Disease in the Tropics, *edited by O. P. Sharma*
52. Exercise: Pulmonary Physiology and Pathophysiology, *edited by B. J. Whipp and K. Wasserman*
53. Developmental Neurobiology of Breathing, *edited by G. G. Haddad and J. P. Farber*
54. Mediators of Pulmonary Inflammation, *edited by M. A. Bray and W. H. Anderson*
55. The Airway Epithelium, *edited by S. G. Farmer and D. Hay*

56. Physiological Adaptations in Vertebrates: Respiration, Circulation, and Metabolism, *edited by S. C. Wood, R. E. Weber, A. R. Hargens, and R. W. Millard*
57. The Bronchial Circulation, *edited by J. Butler*
58. Lung Cancer Differentiation: Implications for Diagnosis and Treatment, *edited by S. D. Bernal and P. J. Hesketh*
59. Pulmonary Complications of Systemic Disease, *edited by J. F. Murray*
60. Lung Vascular Injury: Molecular and Cellular Response, *edited by A. Johnson and T. J. Ferro*
61. Cytokines of the Lung, *edited by J. Kelley*
62. The Mast Cell in Health and Disease, *edited by M. A. Kaliner and D. D. Metcalfe*
63. Pulmonary Disease in the Elderly Patient, *edited by D. A. Mahler*
64. Cystic Fibrosis, *edited by P. B. Davis*
65. Signal Transduction in Lung Cells, *edited by J. S. Brody, D. M. Center, and V. A. Tkachuk*
66. Tuberculosis: A Comprehensive International Approach, *edited by L. B. Reichman and E. S. Hershfield*
67. Pharmacology of the Respiratory Tract: Experimental and Clinical Research, *edited by K. F. Chung and P. J. Barnes*
68. Prevention of Respiratory Diseases, *edited by A. Hirsch, M. Goldberg, J.-P. Martin, and R. Masse*
69. *Pneumocystis carinii* Pneumonia: Second Edition, *edited by P. D. Walzer*
70. Fluid and Solute Transport in the Airspaces of the Lungs, *edited by R. M. Effros and H. K. Chang*
71. Sleep and Breathing: Second Edition, *edited by N. A. Saunders and C. E. Sullivan*
72. Airway Secretion: Physiological Bases for the Control of Mucous Hypersecretion, *edited by T. Takishima and S. Shimura*
73. Sarcoidosis and Other Granulomatous Disorders, *edited by D. G. James*
74. Epidemiology of Lung Cancer, *edited by J. M. Samet*
75. Pulmonary Embolism, *edited by M. Morpurgo*
76. Sports and Exercise Medicine, *edited by S. C. Wood and R. C. Roach*
77. Endotoxin and the Lungs, *edited by K. L. Brigham*
78. The Mesothelial Cell and Mesothelioma, *edited by M.-C. Jaurand and J. Bignon*
79. Regulation of Breathing: Second Edition, *edited by J. A. Dempsey and A. I. Pack*
80. Pulmonary Fibrosis, *edited by S. Hin. Phan and R. S. Thrall*
81. Long-Term Oxygen Therapy: Scientific Basis and Clinical Application, *edited by W. J. O'Donohue, Jr.*
82. Ventral Brainstem Mechanisms and Control of Respiration and Blood Pressure, *edited by C. O. Trouth, R. M. Millis, H. F. Kiwull-Schöne, and M. E. Schläfke*
83. A History of Breathing Physiology, *edited by D. F. Proctor*
84. Surfactant Therapy for Lung Disease, *edited by B. Robertson and H. W. Taeusch*
85. The Thorax: Second Edition, Revised and Expanded (in three parts), *edited by C. Roussos*

86. Severe Asthma: Pathogenesis and Clinical Management, *edited by S. J. Szefler and D. Y. M. Leung*
87. *Mycobacterium avium*–Complex Infection: Progress in Research and Treatment, *edited by J. A. Korvick and C. A. Benson*
88. Alpha 1–Antitrypsin Deficiency: Biology • Pathogenesis • Clinical Manifestations • Therapy, *edited by R. G. Crystal*
89. Adhesion Molecules and the Lung, *edited by P. A. Ward and J. C. Fantone*
90. Respiratory Sensation, *edited by L. Adams and A. Guz*
91. Pulmonary Rehabilitation, *edited by A. P. Fishman*
92. Acute Respiratory Failure in Chronic Obstructive Pulmonary Disease, *edited by J.-P. Derenne, W. A. Whitelaw, and T. Similowski*
93. Environmental Impact on the Airways: From Injury to Repair, *edited by J. Chrétien and D. Dusser*
94. Inhalation Aerosols: Physical and Biological Basis for Therapy, *edited by A. J. Hickey*
95. Tissue Oxygen Deprivation: From Molecular to Integrated Function, *edited by G. G. Haddad and G. Lister*
96. The Genetics of Asthma, *edited by S. B. Liggett and D. A. Meyers*
97. Inhaled Glucocorticoids in Asthma: Mechanisms and Clinical Actions, *edited by R. P. Schleimer, W. W. Busse, and P. M. O'Byrne*
98. Nitric Oxide and the Lung, *edited by W. M. Zapol and K. D. Bloch*
99. Primary Pulmonary Hypertension, *edited by L. J. Rubin and S. Rich*
100. Lung Growth and Development, *edited by J. A. McDonald*
101. Parasitic Lung Diseases, *edited by A. A. F. Mahmoud*
102. Lung Macrophages and Dendritic Cells in Health and Disease, *edited by M. F. Lipscomb and S. W. Russell*
103. Pulmonary and Cardiac Imaging, *edited by C. Chiles and C. E. Putman*
104. Gene Therapy for Diseases of the Lung, *edited by K. L. Brigham*
105. Oxygen, Gene Expression, and Cellular Function, *edited by L. Biadasz Clerch and D. J. Massaro*
106. Beta$_2$-Agonists in Asthma Treatment, *edited by R. Pauwels and P. M. O'Byrne*
107. Inhalation Delivery of Therapeutic Peptides and Proteins, *edited by A. L. Adjei and P. K. Gupta*
108. Asthma in the Elderly, *edited by R. A. Barbee and J. W. Bloom*
109. Treatment of the Hospitalized Cystic Fibrosis Patient, *edited by D. M. Orenstein and R. C. Stern*
110. Asthma and Immunological Diseases in Pregnancy and Early Infancy, *edited by M. Schatz, R. S. Zeiger, and H. N. Claman*
111. Dyspnea, *edited by D. A. Mahler*
112. Proinflammatory and Antiinflammatory Peptides, *edited by S. I. Said*
113. Self-Management of Asthma, *edited by H. Kotses and A. Harver*
114. Eicosanoids, Aspirin, and Asthma, *edited by A. Szczeklik, R. J. Gryglewski, and J. R. Vane*
115. Fatal Asthma, *edited by A. L. Sheffer*
116. Pulmonary Edema, *edited by M. A. Matthay and D. H. Ingbar*
117. Inflammatory Mechanisms in Asthma, *edited by S. T. Holgate and W. W. Busse*
118. Physiological Basis of Ventilatory Support, *edited by J. J. Marini and A. S. Slutsky*

119. Human Immunodeficiency Virus and the Lung, *edited by M. J. Rosen and J. M. Beck*
120. Five-Lipoxygenase Products in Asthma, *edited by J. M. Drazen, S.-E. Dahlén, and T. H. Lee*
121. Complexity in Structure and Function of the Lung, *edited by M. P. Hlastala and H. T. Robertson*
122. Biology of Lung Cancer, *edited by M. A. Kane and P. A. Bunn, Jr.*
123. Rhinitis: Mechanisms and Management, *edited by R. M. Naclerio, S. R. Durham, and N. Mygind*
124. Lung Tumors: Fundamental Biology and Clinical Management, *edited by C. Brambilla and E. Brambilla*
125. Interleukin-5: From Molecule to Drug Target for Asthma, *edited by C. J. Sanderson*
126. Pediatric Asthma, *edited by S. Murphy and H. W. Kelly*
127. Viral Infections of the Respiratory Tract, *edited by R. Dolin and P. F. Wright*
128. Air Pollutants and the Respiratory Tract, *edited by D. L. Swift and W. M. Foster*
129. Gastroesophageal Reflux Disease and Airway Disease, *edited by M. R. Stein*
130. Exercise-Induced Asthma, *edited by E. R. McFadden, Jr.*
131. LAM and Other Diseases Characterized by Smooth Muscle Proliferation, *edited by J. Moss*
132. The Lung at Depth, *edited by C. E. G. Lundgren and J. N. Miller*
133. Regulation of Sleep and Circadian Rhythms, *edited by F. W. Turek and P. C. Zee*
134. Anticholinergic Agents in the Upper and Lower Airways, *edited by S. L. Spector*
135. Control of Breathing in Health and Disease, *edited by M. D. Altose and Y. Kawakami*
136. Immunotherapy in Asthma, *edited by J. Bousquet and H. Yssel*
137. Chronic Lung Disease in Early Infancy, *edited by R. D. Bland and J. J. Coalson*
138. Asthma's Impact on Society: The Social and Economic Burden, *edited by K. B. Weiss, A. S. Buist, and S. D. Sullivan*
139. New and Exploratory Therapeutic Agents for Asthma, *edited by M. Yeadon and Z. Diamant*
140. Multimodality Treatment of Lung Cancer, *edited by A. T. Skarin*
141. Cytokines in Pulmonary Disease: Infection and Inflammation, *edited by S. Nelson and T. R. Martin*
142. Diagnostic Pulmonary Pathology, *edited by P. T. Cagle*
143. Particle–Lung Interactions, *edited by P. Gehr and J. Heyder*
144. Tuberculosis: A Comprehensive International Approach, Second Edition, Revised and Expanded, *edited by L. B. Reichman and E. S. Hershfield*
145. Combination Therapy for Asthma and Chronic Obstructive Pulmonary Disease, *edited by R. J. Martin and M. Kraft*
146. Sleep Apnea: Implications in Cardiovascular and Cerebrovascular Disease, *edited by T. D. Bradley and J. S. Floras*
147. Sleep and Breathing in Children: A Developmental Approach, *edited by G. M. Loughlin, J. L. Carroll, and C. L. Marcus*

ADDITIONAL VOLUMES IN PREPARATION

Pulmonary and Peripheral Gas Exchange in Health and Disease, *edited by J. Roca, R. Rodriguez-Roisen, and P. Wagner*

Environmental Asthma, *edited by R. K. Bush*

Nosocomial Pneumonia, *edited by W. R. Jarvis and O. Tablan*

Fetal Origins of Cardiovascular and Lung Disease, *edited by D. J. P. Barker*

Lung Surfactants: Basic Science and Clinical Applications, *edited by R. H. Notter*

Long-Term Mechanical Ventilation, *edited by N. S. Hill*

Airway Remodeling, *edited by P. Howarth, J. Wilson, J. Bousquet, and R. Pauwels*

Asthma and Respiratory Infections, *edited by D. P. Skoner*

SLEEP AND BREATHING IN CHILDREN

A Developmental Approach

Edited by

Gerald M. Loughlin
John L. Carroll
Carole L. Marcus

Johns Hopkins University School of Medicine
Baltimore, Maryland

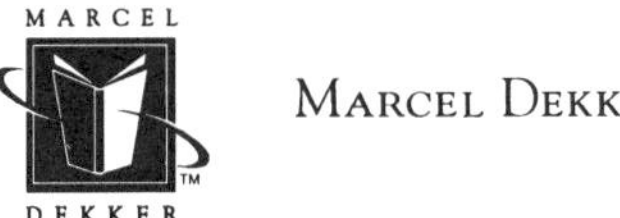

MARCEL DEKKER, INC. NEW YORK • BASEL

ISBN: 0-8247-0300-6

This book is printed on acid-free paper.

Headquarters
Marcel Dekker, Inc.
270 Madison Avenue, New York, NY 10016
tel: 212-696-9000; fax: 212-685-4540

Eastern Hemisphere Distribution
Marcel Dekker AG
Hutgasse 4, Postfach 812, CH-4001 Basel, Switzerland
tel: 41-61-261-8482; fax: 41-61-261-8896

World Wide Web
http://www.dekker.com

The publisher offers discounts on this book when ordered in bulk quantities. For more information, write to Special Sales/Professional Marketing at the headquarters address above.

Current printing (last digit):
10 9 8 7 6 5 4 3 2 1

PRINTED IN THE UNITED STATES OF AMERICA

INTRODUCTION

In some areas of physiology, the transition from life before birth to life after birth is relatively well known. Examples are circulation—that is, heart function—and respiration. In contrast, circadian rhythmicity before and after birth is really not fully understood. Furthermore, the changes that occur in a physiological function such as sleep during the hours, days, and years following birth are enormous. Thus, it should be no surprise that if something disturbs the processes regulating and coordinating these changes, the consequences can be major, if not tragic. SIDS is clearly one of the most striking examples.

In the normal course of events and changes during neonatal, infant, adolescent, and all stages of adult life, it appears that overall human function and performance are best if the rhythmicity between sleep and wakefulness is in phase with the environment. To be sure, this is quite a challenge!

Following birth, the pattern of sleep and wakefulness changes quickly and drastically from very short bouts of sleep and wakefulness to a pattern that recognizes day and night a few months later. Undoubtedly, the "pacemaker" controlling this changing rhythmicity must be well regulated.

But sleep is not all. Tied to it is the respiratory pattern, which, in a way, is a mirror image of the sleep pattern. That is, if the sleep pattern is altered, the breathing pattern will be too. Conversely, if breathing is disrupted by illness or other circumstance, so will sleep. This is a complex interplay, indeed, that has immediate, but also later, consequences.

Sleep and Breathing in Children, is much more than just a description of that interplay from the first hours after birth to adolescence. It is a preparation for the voyage through adult life, as the patterns developed early on will have an influence for years to come.

The field of sleep research and the medicine of sleep is relatively new. Few textbooks of medicine, if any at all, even talk about sleep. Yet, during the past one or two decades, we have seen significant evidence of increasing interest. However, the focus has been on the role of sleep in health and disease of the adult. Insufficient knowledge about the patterns of sleep, their ontogeny, and their dysfunction in earlier life has limited our understanding of the processes in later years. This book remedies that situation.

The pediatric sleep research and sleep disorders center of the Johns Hopkins University School of Medicine is one of the leaders in this field. It was therefore a great honor when Drs. Gerald Loughlin, John Carroll and Carole Marcus gave the Lung Biology in Health and Disease series the opportunity to publish this volume. In addition, the contributors they engaged in this enterprise are themselves pioneers in their areas of expertise, leading to a unique and truly landmark volume.

As the Executive Editor of this series, I want to express my deep appreciation to all the contributors to this monograph, but I know their greatest reward will be that so many young—and old—patients will benefit from their work.

Claude Lenfant, M.D.
Bethesda, Maryland

PREFACE

Publication in the prestigious Lung Biology in Health and Disease series of a volume devoted to the topics of sleep and breathing during sleep in children represents a coming of age for pediatric sleep medicine. Although considerable attention has been focused on sleep disorders in adults, we know far less about these same topics in regard to children. And yet there is tremendous value to the entire field of sleep medicine and sleep research in an improved understanding and broader awareness of the unique aspects of sleep and breathing during sleep in children.

In contrast to the more static conditions in adults, both of these processes are subject to powerful developmental influences as a child passes from infancy through adolescence. This interaction is made even more complex by the effect that sleep, and the breathing that occurs during sleep, has on the growth, development, behavior, and intellectual performance of a child. Knowledge of these interrelationships and the feedback loop that links them is essential for those involved in caring for children. Yet, despite its importance to both the care of well children and management of children with sleep disorders, our understanding of pediatric sleep physiology and the effects of development are limited. If this lack of knowledge were not sufficient reason to focus more attention on children, the potential link between clinical sleep-related disorders in children and similar conditions in adults adds further impetus. Does the snoring child become the adult with obstructive sleep apnea? Perhaps prevention of a significant public health problem in adults may have its foundation in the ability to identify and treat a high-risk population of children.

My co-editors and I would like to acknowledge the vision of Claude Lenfant in recognizing the need for a comprehensive discussion of the topic. We are also grateful to our outstanding group of international contributors. This group includes not only clinicians and sleep researchers, but also an anthropologist, who offers a thought-provoking perspective on the cultural influences that affect the clinical practice of sleep medicine as well as the design and interpretation of current and past pediatric sleep research and clinical practice. We challenged them to be creative, to give us a fresh look at their topics, and to think in terms of developmental biology and physiology.

They have exceeded our expectations and have created a unique work in the field of pediatric sleep medicine. We would also like to acknowledge the peerless editorial assistance of Kathie Bukowski. Her organizational skills, attention to detail, and patience were invaluable in the preparation of this edition

Gerald M. Loughlin
John L. Carroll
Carole L. Marcus

CONTRIBUTORS

Nabeel Jawad Ali, D.M., F.R.C.P. Department of Respiratory Medicine, Kings Mill Hospital, Nottinghamshire, England

Richard P. Allen, Ph.D. Assistant Professor, Department of Neurology, Johns Hopkins University, Baltimore, Maryland

Raanan Arens, M.D. Assistant Professor, Department of Pediatrics, University of Pennsylvania School of Medicine, and The Children's Hospital of Philadelphia, Philadelphia, Pennsylvania

Peter Blair, Ph.D. Medical Statistician, Institute of Child Health, Royal Hospital for Sick Children, University of Bristol, Bristol, England

Carol J. Blaisdell, M.D. Assistant Professor, Department of Pediatrics, Johns Hopkins University School of Medicine, Baltimore, Maryland

Carlos E. Blanco, M.D., Ph.D. Professor, Department of Pediatrics, University Hospital Maastricht, Maastricht, The Netherlands

Lee J. Brooks, M.D. Associate Professor of Pediatrics, Robert Wood Johnson Medical School, University of Medicine and Dentistry of New Jersey, and Head, Pediatric Pulmonary Division, and Director, Family Sleep Center, The Children's Regional Hospital at Cooper Hospital/University Medical Center, Camden, New Jersey

Robert T. Brouillette, M.D. Professor and Head, Divisions of Respiratory and Newborn Medicine, Department of Pediatrics, McGill University Health Center, and Montreal Children's Hospital, Montreal, Quebec, Canada

John L. Carroll, M.D. Associate Professor, Department of Pediatrics, and Director, The Johns Hopkins Children's Center, Johns Hopkins University School of Medicine, Baltimore, Maryland

Marie-Josephe Challamel, M.D. Explorations Neurologiques, INSERM Centre Hospitalier Lyon-Sud, Pierre-Bénite, France

Lilia Curzi-Dascalova, M.D., Ph.D. INSERM Hôpital Robert Debré, Paris, France

Ronald E. Dahl, M.D. Associate Professor, Department of Child and Adolescent Psychiatry, University of Pittsburgh Medical Center, Pittsburgh, Pennsylvania

Bernard Dan, M.D. Head, Department of Neurology, University Hospital for Children Queen Fabiola, Brussels, Belgium

David F. Donnelly, Ph.D. Associate Professor, Department of Pediatrics, Yale University School of Medicine, New Haven, Connecticut

Nalton F. Ferraro, D.M.D., M.D. Surgeon, Department of Plastic Surgery/Oral Maxillofacial Surgery, Children's Hospital, Boston, Massachusetts

Peter J. Fleming, M.B., Ph.D., F.R.C.P., F.R.C.P.(C), F.R.C.P.H. Professor, Faculty of Medicine, and Head, Institute of Child Health, Royal Hospital for Sick Children, University of Bristol, Bristol, England

Patricia Franco, M.D. Neuropediatrician, Pediatric Sleep Unit, Erasmus Hospital, Brussels, Belgium

Claude Gaultier, M.D., Ph.D. Professor, Department of Physiology, University of Paris VII, and Hôpital Robert Debré, Paris, France

Deborah C. Givan, M.D. Clinical Professor, Section of Pediatric Pulmonology and Critical Care Medicine, Department of Pediatrics, Indiana University School of Medicine, and James Whitcomb Riley Hospital for Children, Indianapolis, Indiana

David Gozal, M.D. Professor, Department of Pediatrics, Kosair Children's Hospital Research Institute, University of Louisville School of Medicine, Louisville, Kentucky

Jose Groswasser, M.D. Sleep and Development Unit, University Hospital for Children Queen Fabiola, Brussels, Belgium

Ronald R. Grunstein, M.D.(Syd), Ph.D.(Goth), M.B.B.S., F.R.A.C.P. Clinical Associate Professor, Department of Medicine, University of Sydney, Sydney, Australia

Christian Guilleminault, M.D. Professor, Stanford Sleep Disorders Center, Stanford University, Stanford, California

Mark A. Hanson, D.Phil., Cert.Ed. Professor, Department of Obstetrics and Gynecology, University College London, London, England

Ronald M. Harper, Ph.D. Professor, Department of Neurobiology, School of Medicine, University of California at Los Angeles, Los Angeles, California

Shiroh Isono, M.D. Assistant Professor, Department of Anesthesiology, Chiba University School of Medicine, Chiba, Japan

Sheila V. Jacob, M.D., F.R.C.P.(C) Assistant Professor, Department of Pediatrics, and Director, Children's Sleep Program, Robert Wood Johnson Medical School, University of Medicine and Dentistry of New Jersey, New Brunswick, New Jersey

André Kahn, M.D., Ph.D. Professor and Chairman, Department of Pediatrics, Free University of Brussels, and University Hospital for Children Queen Fabiola, Brussels, Belgium

Ineko Kato, M.D. Instructor, Department of Pediatrics, Nagoya City University Medical School, Nagoya, Japan

Thomas G. Keens, M.D. Professor, Departments of Pediatrics, Physiology, and Biophysics, University of Southern California Keck School of Medicine; Division of Pediatric Pulmonology, Children's Hospital Los Angeles; Visiting Professor of Pediatrics, UCLA School of Medicine; and Pediatric Pulmonary Division, Mattel Children's Hospital at UCLA, Los Angeles, California

Igor A. Kelmanson, M.D., Ph.D. Professor, Department of Pediatrics No. 3, St. Petersburg State Pediatric Medical Academy, St. Petersburg, Russia

James S. Kemp, M.D. Associate Professor, Pulmonary Division, Department of Pediatrics, St. Louis University School of Medicine, St. Louis, Missouri

Suresh Kotagal, M.D. Senior Associate Consultant, Department of Neurology, and Sleep Disorders Center, Mayo Clinic, Rochester, Minnesota

Prem Kumar, B.Sc., D.Phil. Department of Physiology, University of Birmingham School of Medicine, Birmingham, England

Gerald M. Loughlin, M.D. Professor and Director, Eudowood Division of Pediatric Respiratory Sciences, Department of Pediatrics, and Vice Chairman for Clinical Affairs, Johns Hopkins University School of Medicine, Baltimore, Maryland

Mark W. Mahowald, M.D. Director, Minnesota Regional Sleep Disorders Center, Department of Neurology, Hennepin County Medical Center, Minneapolis, Minnesota

Carole L. Marcus, M.B.B.Ch. Associate Professor, Department of Pediatrics, and Medical Director, Pediatric Sleep Laboratory, Eudowood Division of Pediatric Respiratory Sciences, Johns Hopkins University School of Medicine, Baltimore, Maryland

James J. McKenna, Ph.D. Professor, Department of Anthropology, and Director, Mother-Baby Behavioral Sleep Laboratory, University of Notre Dame, Notre Dame, Indiana

Angela Morielli, R.R.T., M.B.A. Supervisor, Sleep Laboratory, Department of Pediatrics, McGill University Health Center, and Montreal Children's Hospital, Montreal, Quebec, Canada

Rafael Pelayo, M.D. Acting Assistant Professor, Stanford Sleep Disorders Center, Stanford University, Stanford, California

Henrique Rigatto, M.D. Professor, Section of Neonatology, Department of Pediatrics, and Director, Newborn Research, University of Manitoba, Winnipeg, Manitoba, Canada

Carol Lynn Rosen, M.D. Associate Professor, Department of Pediatrics, Case Western Reserve University, and Rainbow Babies & Children's Hospital, University Hospitals of Cleveland, Cleveland, Ohio

Gerald M. Rosen, M.D., M.P.H. Assistant Professor, Department of Pediatrics, University of Minnesota, and Department of Neurology, Minnesota Regional Sleep Disorders Center, Hennepin County Medical Center, Minneapolis, Minnesota

Avi Sadeh, D.Sc. Senior Lecturer, Department of Psychology, Tel Aviv University, Ramat Aviv, Israel

Martin P. Samuels, M.D., F.R.C.P., F.R.C.P.C.H. Senior Lecturer, Academic Department of Pediatrics, Keele University, and Consultant Pediatrician, North Staffordshire Hospital, Staffordshire, England

Andrew Sawczenko, B.M., M.R.C.P., M.R.C.P.C.H. Institute of Child Health, Royal Hospital for Sick Children, University of Bristol, Bristol, England

Sonia Scaillet, M.D. (M.Sc.) Research Assistant in Pediatrics, Children's Sleep Unit, University Hospital for Children Queen Fabiola, Brussels, Belgium

Mark S. Scher, M.D. Professor, Department of Pediatrics, Case Western Reserve University, and Chief, Division of Pediatric Neurology, and Director of Pediatric Sleep and Epilepsy Programs, Rainbow Babies & Children's Hospital, University Hospitals of Cleveland, Cleveland, Ohio

Judith M. Sondheimer, M.D. Professor, Department of Pediatrics, and Chief, Pediatric Gastroenterology, Hepatology, and Nutrition, University of Colorado Health Sciences Center, and The Children's Hospital, Denver, Colorado

John R. Stradling, M.D., F.R.C.P.(U.K.) Professor of Respiratory Medicine, Osler Chest Unit, Oxford University, and Churchill Hospital, Oxford, England

Stephanie V. Trentacoste, B.A. Department of Psychology, College of the Holy Cross, Worcester, Massachusetts

Sally L. Davidson Ward, M.D. Associate Professor, Division of Pediatric Pulmonology, Department of Pediatrics, University of Southern California Keck School of Medicine, and Children's Hospital Los Angeles, Los Angeles, California

Karen A. Waters, Ph.D., M.B.B.S., F.R.A.C.P. Department of Respiratory Medicine, The New Children's Hospital, Parramatta, New South Wales, Australia

Debra E. Weese-Mayer, M.D. Professor, Department of Pediatrics, Rush University, and Chief, Pediatric Respiratory Medicine, Rush Children's Hospital at Rush-Presbyterian-St. Luke's Medical Center, Chicago, Illinois

Amy R. Wolfson, Ph.D. Associate Professor, Department of Psychology, College of the Holy Cross, Worcester, Massachusetts

Marco Zucconi, M.D. Sleep Disorders Center, Department of Neurology, San Raffaele Institute, University of Milan, Milan, Italy

CONTENTS

Part One

SLEEP

1

Neurophysiological Basis of Sleep Development

LILIA CURZI-DASCALOVA

INSERM Hôpital Robert-Debré
Paris, France

MARIE-JOSEPHE CHALLAMEL

INSERM Centre Hospitalier Lyon-Sud
Pierre-Bénite, France

I. Introduction

Since the landmark descriptions of cyclic modifications of respiratory, motor, and electroencephalographic (EEG) behavior in sleeping infants (1,2), it has been well known that vital functions are modulated by states of vigilance. The concept of states has made it possible to group movements and physiological parameters into definable entities, whose gradual organization during nervous system maturation can be studied (3). The emergence of behavioral states (namely sleep-wake states) in infants is one of the remarkable achievements of the central nervous system (CNS) and a good indicator of normal or abnormal development (Refs. 4 and 5 and their references).

This chapter is limited to a general discussion of the developmental aspects of the neurophysiological basis of sleep. Autonomic functions (respiration and cardiovascular control), development of the rest-activity cycle, thermoregulation, and endocrine factors, which are all closely linked to states, are discussed in other chapters. After briefly reviewing the CNS structures involved in the control of sleep-wake, we discuss available data on wakefulness and the development of sleep states from the fetal period to early childhood. Behavioral states are constellations of physiological and behavioral variables that are stable over time and occur repeatedly, not only in a given infant but also in all infants (6). Consequently, changes in these variables as state development progresses can be discussed only in reference to age-specific modulations in sleep parameter concordance. The main milestones of maturational changes in behavioral states are relatively well known, but there is little information on certain aspects of state development, including the ontogenesis of circadian cycles and of homeostatic processes. Developmental studies of sleep-wake patterns are of the utmost importance. They contribute to the understanding of CNS maturation and function and may provide answers to many fundamental but still unsettled questions regarding the functional roles(s) of sleep.

II. General Principles of the Development of Sleep–Wake Neural Control: Animal Studies

Sleep onset is a coordinated process involving simultaneous or quasisimultaneous changes in sensory, motor, autonomic, hormonal, and cerebral processes. Sleep onset is strongly dependent on circadian and ultradian oscillations. However, as summarized by McGinty and Szymusiac (7), 1) none of the changes occurring with sleep are exclusively coupled to sleep and 2) sleep is controlled by mutually inhibitory or excitatory interactions between arousing or activating systems on the one hand and hypnogenic or deactivating systems on the other hand. The main three behavioral states—namely, wakefulness, slow-wave (SWS) or non-rapid-eye movement sleep (NREM), and paradoxical or rapid-eye-movement (REM) sleep—all obey these principles, although they are known to be each controlled by specific mechanisms. Sleep and waking states are produced by the activity of excitatory and inhibitory neurons located in several brainstem and forebrain centers, which are organized into "systems" or "networks," each of which is responsible for controlling a given state. Figure 1 shows the main brain centers involved in sleep–wake regulation.

Neurochemical mechanisms underlie the neuron and receptor functions involved in sleep. Monoaminergic systems play a role in sleep state control, most notably in the phasic events of REM sleep (10–13), as well as in several complex regulatory processes that modulate functions linked to sleep, such as thermoregulation, learning, feeding, etc. Recent work has demonstrated that many neurons and glial cells produce, transport, release, and respond to a host of biochemicals that change the patterns of neuronal electrical activity and may also induce sleep. During the last 20 years, several "sleep factors" have been identified (8,9,14), of which some are described below, under "Sleep Development During Early Ontogenesis."

In general, the occurrence of each sleep state involves two neuronal networks. One, the *executive* network, is responsible for sleep phenomenology (each state-characteristic phenomenon may depend on a specific network). The other, called the *permissive* network, triggers sleep (refs. in 15). Wakefulness depends on a complex system involving at least 10 brain structures, including a permissive network that inhibits sleep. Sleep onset has been described as a blockade of waking by an antiwake network that synthesizes hypnogenic factors (refs. in 9, 16, and 17).

REM and NREM sleep have been unambiguously identified in mammals and birds (refs. in 7).

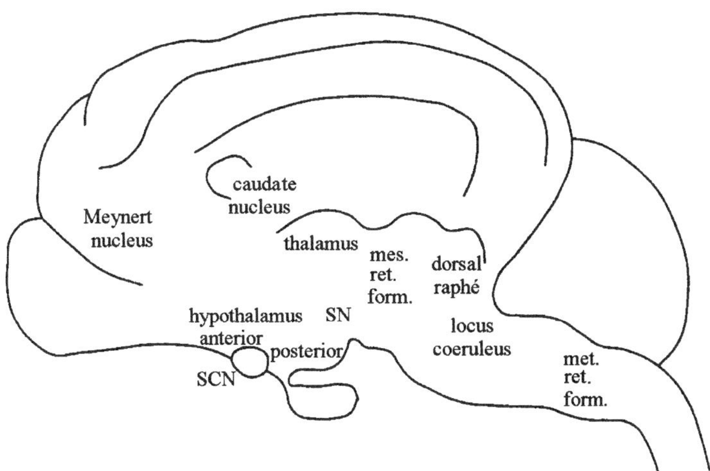

Figure 1 Diagram of the main brain structures involved in behavioral states control. (Adapted from Refs. 8 and 9.)

A. REM Sleep

REM sleep, also called *paradoxical* sleep, is the first sleep pattern to appear during ontogenesis, and is also the best studied sleep pattern. REM sleep can be understood as the result of interactions between an executive network and a permissive network (15).

Converging data suggest that reticular neurons in the pons and spinal cord play a key role in REM sleep regulation. Jouvet and coworkers devised a model in which the executive REM system includes REM-on neurons specific for each of the REM parameters (11,15). In adult humans and animals, REM sleep is associated with muscular atony, ponto-geniculo-occipital (PGO) spikes, rapid eye movements, small facial movements, and cortical activation with paradoxical wakefulness-like EEG. The REM-on system would work as a pacemaker if it were isolated—i.e., it is continuously active when the inhibitory systems are not functional. Cessation of aminergic REM-off system firing lifts the inhibition of REM-on neurons, thus permitting the REM-on executive system to function. REM sleep is characterized by augmented metabolism and oxygen consumption, and its duration may depend on the size of available energy stores (13).

B. NREM Sleep

Like REM sleep, NREM sleep may involve an executive system and a permissive system. Activity of the executive NREM sleep system is identified based on only two criteria: sleep spindles and slow high-voltage EEG activity. Sleep spindles are produced mainly by the thalamic reticular nucleus. Slow, synchronized electrical activity has been found at various cortical and subcortical levels; however, the slow waves characteristic of NREM sleep are strongly dependent on the integrity of the neocortex (18) and result from pyramidal cell hyperpolarization. The isolated thalamic reticular nucleus continues to exhibit rhythmic oscillations, suggesting that it acts as a pacemaker subject to inhibitory influences from the "permissive" system (19). The inhibitory slow-wave sleep (SWS) system includes neurons responsive to acetylcholine (mesenchephalo-pontine nuclei and basal forebrain), histamine (posterior hypothalamus), and noradrenaline (locus ceruleus). Many aspects of the SWS system are under thermoregulatory control. SWS is characterized by a decrease in general metabolism and body temperature accompanied by augmented synthesis of brain proteins and replenishment of energetic reserves to prepare for subsequent waking and REM sleep (11).

C. Promotion of Waking and Sleep Onset

Wakefulness is mainly characterized by cerebral activity desynchronization and by motor activity. While no single cell group seems indispensable to the maintenance of an activated EEG pattern, several cell groups distributed from the medulla to the basal forebrain participate in the control of arousal (details and refs. in 13 and 20). Waking results from the conjunction of sleep inhibition and generalized neuronal activation. Sleep inhibition seems to be produced by systems specific to each of the states. The waking network is activated by endogenous and exogenous stimuli. Several structures possibly involved in sleep-promoting mechanisms have been described in the lower brainstem, magnocellular basal forebrain, and preoptic/anterior hypothalamus. An antiwaking system is probably located in the anterior hypothalamus, an area also involved in the control of many vital functions (thermoregulation, reproduction, etc.). The antiwaking system may integrate information about the general condition of the body and the size of energy stores; sleep onset may be a preventive mechanism influenced by circadian rhythms controlled by biological clock(s).

Advances in biochemical techniques made during the last 20 years have led to intensive research, whose results support the hypothesis that the awake brain produces substances that induce sleep (ref. in 14). Several such substances have been identified (see Chap. 6).

Several models of the process involved in sleep regulation have been developed. Two of these models can be applied to the development of sleep characteristics during early human ontogenesis. The two-process model constructed by Achermann et al. (21) based on EEG slow-wave activity emphasizes interactions between circadian (C) and homeostatic (S) processes, and discussed below under the heading "Development of the Homeostatic Process S." Figure 2 is a diagram of the model of sleep–wake cycle development, which includes four categories: pacemakers for slow-wave, NREM and REM sleep; a waking system that inhibits the two main sleep states; an antiwaking system; and the biological clock that controls circadian rhythms (9,13).

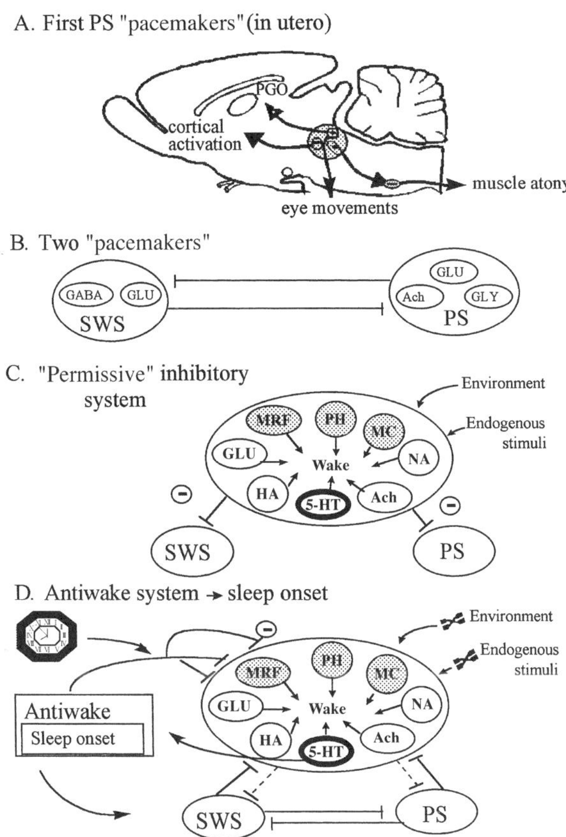

Figure 2 Development of the sleep–wake cycle. (Adapted from Refs. 9 and 13.) The three main brain structures involved in sleep regulation are indicated by closed circles: MRF = mesencephalic reticular formation; PH = posterior hypothalamus; MC = medullary nucleus magnocelluraris. The main known neuromediators are indicated by open circles. Ach = acetylcholine; GLU = glutamate; GLY = glycine; GABA = gamma-aminobutyric acid; HA = histamine; 5-HT = serotonin; NA = noradrenaline. A. Paradoxical (PS) REM sleep, which is dependent on the brain structures that mature earliest, is functional very early during ontogenesis (at least with regard to eye movements and muscle atony). PGO = ponto-geniculo-occipital spikes. B. The SWS/NREM and the PS/REM systems work as mutually regulating pacemakers when the "permissive" systems are not functional. There is ample evidence that the main neurotransmitters involved in pacemaker activity are GLU, GLY, and GABA. This mode of operation may explain the earliest step of sleep states differentiation, before the waking state is recognizable. C. The waking system is the last system to mature. It can inhibit (−) both the PS/REM and the SWS/NREM pacemaker. It is activated by exogenous (environmental), endogenous (autonomic), and emotional stimuli. The main brain structures and neuromediators involved in the maintenance of wakefulness are indicated. D. Sleep onset results from several factors that release sleep pacemakers by blocking the waking system: (a) a decrease or discontinuation (X) of exogenous and endogenous activation; (b) stimulation by 5-HT of the antiwaking system of the hypothalamus under the influence of the circadian biological clock.

III. Sleep Development During Early Ontogenesis: Animal Studies

States are defined by the cyclic concordance of certain specific patterns of physiological variables, including cerebral electrical activity (EEG), motor activity, autonomic functions, and behavior. The neural structure underlying each of these variables must reach a certain degree of development before the corresponding state can appear. Behavioral states are present before birth (ref. in 22). Data on the degree of prenatal morphological development of the main cerebral structures (Fig. 1) involved in sleep control are scant and very fragmentary. A number of neurochemical substances or biochemicals known as sleep factors have been studied as indicators of brain development in various species. To our knowledge, potential correlations with prenatal behavioral states have not yet been investigated. Most of the data reviewed below concern the early postnatal period, and some may be relevant to state development at a later stage. In general, active, REM sleep has been more extensively studied than quiet, NREM sleep.

A. Development of Brain Structures Involved in Sleep Control

Relationships between the maturation of structures and that of functions are complex and nonlinear. However, information on the degree of brain maturation may help to elucidate the complex development of sleep phenomena.

In macaque monkeys, the *neurons* in the cerebral cortex and in all other cerebral structures except the cerebellum and hippocampus are present before E100 (E = days of gestation) of the 165-day gestational period. The neurons in the locus ceruleus, raphe nuclei, and basal forebrain nuclei are generated before E50. However, *axon* overproduction and elimination continue until birth, and *synapse* density continues to increase (in the cortex) between birth and 2 months of age (with a peak between 2 and 4 months). Synapse density declines during the next 3 years, and the total number of neurons (in the visual cortex) is 16% higher in newborn than in adult animals. In humans, the cerebral cortex neurons are produced between E40 and E125 of the 265-day gestation (refs. in 23 and 24), and studies of the visual cortex have found that synapse density peaks between 8 and 12 months after birth, reaching a level about 60% greater than that in adults (25). Cortical neurons are generated from E14 to E20 in rats (21 days of gestation) and from E30 and E57 in cats (65 days of gestation). Thus, generation of cortical neurons occurs at an earlier gestational age in primates than in rodents and cats (ref. in 24).

Although the development of the cholinergic and monoaminergic *neurotransmitters* involved in sleep control begins prenatally, it continues in a significant measure during the first postnatal months in all the species studied. Developmental time curves for neurotransmitters vary from one neurotransmitter to the next and from one brain region to the next. Receptor concentrations sometimes increase at a rate that exceeds the capacity of the neurons to produce their neurotransmitters. The regions that mature earliest are usually the medulla and pons, followed by the midbrain, thalamus, and hypothalamus, and then by the cerebral cortex and striatum (26). This pattern reflects the earlier neurogenesis of the caudal as opposed to the rostral part of the brain.

Data have been reported on the ontogenesis in the brain of *neuropeptides* that may be sleep factors. *Somatostatin* (SRIF), known to promote REM sleep (27), is detectable in the macaque cortex at E120—i.e., after completion of neuron generation and migration. SRIF levels increase prenatally, reaching a peak around birth; in adults they are only 15% to 30% of the level at birth. Similar increases between E100 and near term have been observed in baboons, but there was no subsequent decline during adulthood. *Vasoactive intestinal peptide* (VIP) enhances both NREM and REM sleep in rats and selectively increases REM sleep in cats. This neuropeptide, which is widely distributed in the nervous system of mammalians, influences cell division, neuronal survival, and neurodifferentiation (ref. in 28). VIP is detectable in the cortex of primates on E120, and its levels increase 4- to 11-fold between E120 and near term; in adults, VIP levels in the various cortical regions are only 50% to 9% of those found at birth (24). *Cholecystokinin* (CCK-8) may promote NREM sleep, especially postprandial sleep. In the human brain, high levels of CCK have been found in several cortical areas, in the hypothalamus, and in the cerebellum. In the cortex of nonhuman primates, CKK immunoreactive cells colocalized with GABA cells. In macaques, CKK is detectable at E120 and increases sharply until E165, then decreases in adulthood. In rat cortex, CKK concentrations seem to increase gradually during ontogenesis. *Delta-sleep-inducing-peptide* (DSIP) has been detected in fetal guinea pig hypothalamus at E38 (ref. in 24). *Neuropeptide Y* (NPY), which is known to produce behavioral signs of sedation and significant EEG synchronization (29), is also one of the most abundant peptides in the cerebral cortex of mammalians. NPY levels in baboon visual cortex have been studied throughout ontogenesis and found to increase gradually between E100 and adulthood. In contrast, the number of NPY immunopositive cells decreased in macaque visual cortex between E110 and adulthood (ref. in 24). All these substances act as neurotransmitters or neuromodulators in the developing brain and have been studied chiefly in the cortex. The fact that they are all detectable during embryonic life carries the possibility that they may be functional before birth. However, no data on correlations between neurotransmitter ontogenesis and intrauterine fetal behavior have been reported to date.

B. Development of Behavioral States in Animals

Several studies done starting in the early 1960s found that newborn animals exhibited a number of different behavioral states which were first identified based on the intensity and the pattern of motor activity (30). Behavior observation and polysomnographic recording in chronically implanted kittens and rat pups showed that three main behavioral states were recognizable during the first few days of life. These states were designated as 1) wakefulness (defined by moving and eating behavior), 2) quiet sleep (short periods of quiescence), and 3) active, paradoxical sleep or *sommeil sismique* (32) characterized by neck muscle atony, rapid eye movements, and generalized myoclonic twitches. In these species, characterized by marked immaturity at birth, EEG findings were similar in all three states (31–33). In contrast, in guinea pigs and sheep, whose brains are relatively mature at birth, the characteristics of the three main states, including EEG patterns, were similar during the first days of life and in adulthood (32,34). Active and quiet sleep—defined based on concordance of the electrocorticogram, electro-oculogram (EOG), and nuchal electromyogram (EMG)—were found in preterm lambs born at 133 to 135 days of gestation. Compared to full-term lambs (147 days of gestation), the preterm lambs spent more time in active sleep (35).

Distinct behavioral states have been described in chronically implanted fetuses. In a study using rest-activity and heart rate evaluation, Belich et al. (36) documented cyclic occurrence of three states in rabbit fetuses beyond 25 days of gestation. REM and NREM states were found in lambs between 120 and 140 days of gestation [normal length of gestation, 150 days (37,38)]. In guinea pig fetuses, Astic et al. (39) recorded paradoxical sleep beyond 41 days of gestation, with a peak at 50 days of gestation—i.e., at the time of first appearance of SWS. Paradoxical sleep then decreased until birth (65 days of gestation), while SWS increased. The timing of the fetal sleep cycle was not correlated with that of the maternal sleep cycle. Two distinct EEG states have been described in baboon fetuses recorded from 143 to 153 days of gestation (normal length of gestation, 175 to 185 days). State 1 (quiet sleep) was distinguishable from state 2 (active sleep) based on the presence of tracé alternant. Epoch duration was shorter in state 1 than in state 2, and a smaller percentage of time was spent in state 1 than in state 2 (40).

The rate of age-related modifications in states depends on the degree of maturation at birth. In rats and cats, establishment of adult-like EEG characteristics of quiet sleep occurs around the third week of life and may be facilitated by weaning (32,41).

REM sleep occupies a larger proportion of time in newborns than in adults. During the first days of life, REM sleep contributes most of the total sleep time in animals with very immature brains at birth (e.g., rats) versus 15% to 20% in guinea pigs. The amount of REM sleep declines during the first 3 weeks of life (ref. in 42). However, at 3 weeks of age, the amount of REM sleep in kittens, rat pups, and guinea pig pups remains twice that in adult animals (32). REM sleep in rats continues to decline between 23 and 40 days of age (43). A number of hypotheses on the functional role of REM sleep in brain maturation are discussed below, under "The Functional Role of Sleep States During Development."

In spite of the presence of two of the main REM system characteristics (muscle atony and rapid eye movements), but not typical EEG findings, there are data in the literature that suggest that active (AS) and quiet sleep (QS) during the first few weeks of life may not be the exact counterparts of REM and NREM sleep in adulthood. Adrien et al. (44) demonstrated that electrolytic lesions of the anterior raphe nuclei in 4- to 6-day-old rat pups did not modify NREM or REM sleep. In contrast, identical lesions in 3- to 5-week-old rats produced relative insomnia, which was more severe for REM than for NREM sleep. The same group (45) investigated the impact of early postnatal impairment of the monoaminergic systems on sleep ontogenesis. In rat pups and kittens, both catecholaminergic (CA) and serotoninergic (5-HT) cell bodies are present at birth, whereas the corresponding pathways and terminals achieve maturation only at 2 months of age. Bilateral lesions of the anterior raphe nuclei (5-HT system) and of the locus ceruleus and nucleus subceruleus (CA system) had no disruptive effects on sleep when performed during the first days of life. When the same lesions were produced later, after 3 weeks of age (i.e., when sleep characteristics were almost mature), they induced partial or complete insomnia, and a similar effect was observed in adult animals. The authors concluded that monoaminergic systems are not involved in sleep control at birth in cats and rats. Three hypotheses have been put forward to explain these data. 1) The few (10%) remaining terminals may be sufficient to trigger and maintain NREM sleep and, to some extent, REM sleep; 2) sleep maturation in immature mammals may occur via nonmonoaminergic mechanisms; and 3) AS may be different from adult REM sleep, including in terms of its underlying mechanisms (44,45). The last hypothesis received support from a study by Frank et al. (46) demonstrating that zimelidine (a monoamine uptake inhibitor) and atropine suppressed AS in rats by 14 days postnatal age but not at 11 days postnatal age; in contrast, desipramine, another monoamine uptake inhibitor, significantly suppressed AS at all ages. Work by Brown (47) on the effect of muramyl peptides on sleep suggested between-species differences in sleep mechanisms in immature mammals. Muramyl peptides (MPs) are bacteria-derived sleep factors that may stimulate SWS. In young rabbits, muramyl dipeptide increased QS at the expense of AS. The same substance given twice daily during the first 14 postnatal days did not affect amounts of quiet or active sleep in rat pups. These data are difficult to interpret because the complexity of REM sleep, which is not aminergic per se but involves networks controlled by monoaminergic systems (13). Interestingly, starting very early during human ontogenesis, the control of vital functions during AS is very similar to that during REM sleep in adults (48 and its references).

In conclusion, the first steps of the differentiation of behavioral states seem dependent on the degree of brain maturation; in several species characterized by greater brain maturity at birth, concordance of REM and NREM state characteristics may be established during fetal life or during the first few days after birth. The mechanisms involved in regulation of the main states during early ontogenesis in animals remain controversial.

IV. Development of Behavioral States During Human Ontogenesis

A. Fetal Life

Perception of cyclic fetal movements, an experience that evokes a strong emotional response in many mothers, is one of oldest criteria for assessing fetal well-being. Historically, the gathering of knowledge on fetal behavior has been dependent on advances in techniques used to study fetuses and in the understanding of behavioral states. Prechtl (22) has described the history of fetal states assessment in great detail. Advances in real-time ultrasonography made since 1980 have made it possible to demonstrate that the human fetus exhibits behavioral states similar to those of neonates. Estimates of the time of first appearance of behavioral states in utero have varied according to the parameter and states scoring method used. Using continuous observation and fetal heart rate recording, Prechtl and coworkers defined four fetal behavioral states: State 1F, characterized by a slower regular heart beat, with startles but no eye movements; State 2F, with an irregular heartbeat, eye movements, and occasional gross body movements; State 3F, with a fast regular heart rate and eye movements but no body movements, and State 4F, with a fast irregular heart rate, eye movements, and continual body movements (22). The first studies by Prechtl and coworkers found evidence of behavioral state development in human fetuses between 36 and 38 weeks gestational age (GA) (49). However, Visser et al. (50) reported correlations among heart rate, eye movement, and gross body movement patterns in normal fetuses at 30 to 32 weeks GA. In a study involving simultaneous use of three real-time ultrasound scanners, Okai et al. (51) documented stable periods of REM and NREM of more than three minutes' duration between 28 and 31 weeks GA and also found a strong correlation between the occurrence of rapid eye movements and breathing movements after 27 weeks GA.

Fetal behavior is characterized by state specific patterns of complex motor activity (ref. in 22) and by "breathing" movements that occur mainly during 2F REM sleep. Interestingly, thoracic and abdominal fetal respiratory movements usually occur out of phase during state 2F, a characteristic also found during AS in newborns (48 and 52 and their references).

Fetal states are independent of maternal behavioral states (53).

Groom et al. (54) studied 30 low-risk fetuses at 38 to 40 weeks GA and again at about 2 weeks postnatal age. Behavioral states were assigned similarly based on the HR pattern and the presence or absence of eye and gross body movements. The proportions of active, quiet, and indeterminate sleep were virtually identical in fetuses and neonates.

Studies involving monitoring of fetal EEG activity and heart rate variability recording in healthy fetuses during normal labor demonstrated two alternating sleep states identical to those observed in newborns (55,56).

In conclusion, most recent data show that differentiated behavioral states appear in utero early during the third trimester of gestation. Fetal states are similar to those observed in newborns of the same gestational age, as far as criteria possible to monitor in fetuses are considered (see discussion of sleep in premature and full-term newborns below).

B. Early Postnatal Ontogenesis: From Premature to Full-Term Newborns

The pioneers of behavioral state studies in newborns—including Roffwarg (57), Dreyfus-Brisac (58), Monod (59), Parmelee (60), Prechtl (61), Wolff (62), and Anders and coworkers (63)—argued from the outset that specific terms were needed to designate states in newborns because EEG and behavioral characteristics differed between adults and newborns. They agreed to distinguish two major sleep states in early infancy: the AS (state 2) and the QS (state 1), to which they subsequently added undifferentiated (indeterminate) sleep based on results of polysomnography studies. As befitted careful neurophysiologists, they defined the main state-related modifications of various parameters and used combinations of several of these parameters to define states. Thus, whereas the classification of sleep states in adults was developed solely on the basis of EEG patterns (64), polygraphic recording became the "gold standard" for state classification and developmental physiology studies in neonates. However, attempts at state classification based on a single parameter (movement or heart rate) have been made (65).

Successful polysomnography in newborns requires that a number of technical criteria be met (5): 1) the person in charge of the recording must have some training in neonatal care; 2) the data should be interpreted by a person conversant with age-related EEG characteristics in premature and full-term newborns (for details and references, see refs. 5, 66, and 67); 3) piezoelectric transducers rather than EOG should be used for the detection of eye movement because of the very low amplitude of retinocorneal electrical potential differences in neonates (Fig. 3, refs. in 5); 4) chin EMG recording may be unsuccessful because of the possibility of low amplitude activity at this level; and 5) extremely lightweight transducers should be used for the detection of leg movement. Use of recording methods that are not suited to newborns causes errors in the identification of sleep states. When the technician is experienced in neonatal polysomnography, the baby usually falls asleep before the end of electrode placement.

Sleep state scoring data are dependent on a number of methodological factors, including 1) the nature of the variables chosen for state definition (Fig. 4); 2) whether or not the characteristics of these variables are quantified or scored based on their general "gestalt" aspect (example: what is regular versus irregular breathing?); 3) the minimum duration used to define the state; 4) the predefined duration of parameter discrepancies that can be kept within the ongoing state (state smoothing); 5) the criteria used to define onset of a given state; and 6) the criteria used to define termination of a given state.

Although scoring is done epoch by epoch, stability of concordance between parameters throughout successive epochs of the major states (wakefulness and crying, active sleep, quiet sleep) is required before a recording period can be assigned to a given state. Onset of a major state is defined as presence of the corresponding constellation of state-specific criteria for 1 min (68,69), 3 min (61,65), or 4 min (refs. in 3). Discrepancies among parameters lasting less than 60 sec are included within the state (5,68,70), whereas a longer-lasting discrepancy (>60 sec) or occurrence of a constellation specific for another state defines termination of the state. Periods with discrepancies between the main states criteria are scored as undifferentiated or indeterminate or ambiguous sleep. *Transitional sleep* (68) is the term used to designate periods of transition from one main state to another; its duration can be less than 60

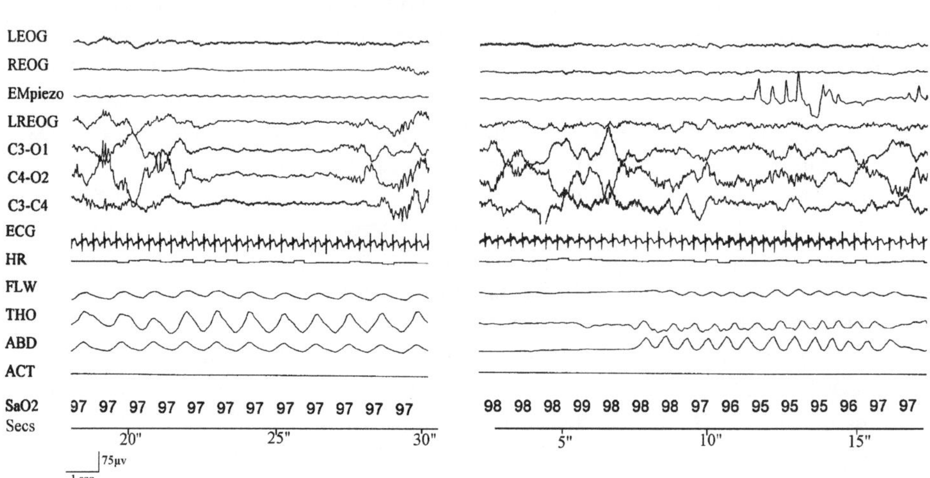

Figure 3 Polygraphic (digitized) recording of a 34 weeks conceptional age (CA) normal premature infant. Gestational age: 32 weeks, 2 days; Postnatal age: 12 days; Conceptional age: 34 weeks. LEOG = left electro-oculogram, the left canthus being referred to the left mastoid electrode; REOG = right electro-oculogram, the right canthus being referred to the right mastoid electrode; EMpiezo = eye movements recorded by a sheet piezoelectrical transducer attached to one of the upper eyelids; LREOG = electro-oculogram, the left canthus being referred to the right canthus electrode; C3-O1, C4-O2, and C3-C4: ECG = electrocardiogram; bipolar EEG recordings; HR = heart rate determined by instantaneous automatic RR intervals measurement; FLW = left and right nostril and mouth airflow detected using thermistors; THO, ABD = thoracic and abdominal respiratory movements detected using strain gauges; ACT = piezoactimetry (no body movements in these examples); SaO_2 in percentage; Secs: time in seconds. On the left: 12 sec of quiet sleep (QS) characterized by discontinuous EEG activity and no eye movements; thoracic and abdominal respiratory movements are in phase. On the right: 17 sec of active sleep (AS) characterized by continuous EEG activity and rapid eye movements detected only by observation and the piezotransducer; note the brief central respiratory pause and the out-of-phase thoracic and abdominal respiratory movements. For details on methods of recording and analysis of sleep states in newborns, see Ref. 5.

sec. Table 1 summarizes the main and secondary criteria used to define active and quiet sleep in newborns.

In addition to the consensual AS versus QS concept (63), many authors use the classification developed in the late 1960s by Prechtl and coworkers in full-term newborns. This classification, which does not use the EEG pattern as a state criterion, distinguishes five behavioral states (6,61), as follows: state 1, eyes closed, regular respiration, no movements; state 2, eyes closed, irregular respiration, no gross movements; state 3, eyes open, no gross movements; state 4, eyes open, gross movements, no crying; state 5, eyes open or closed, crying.

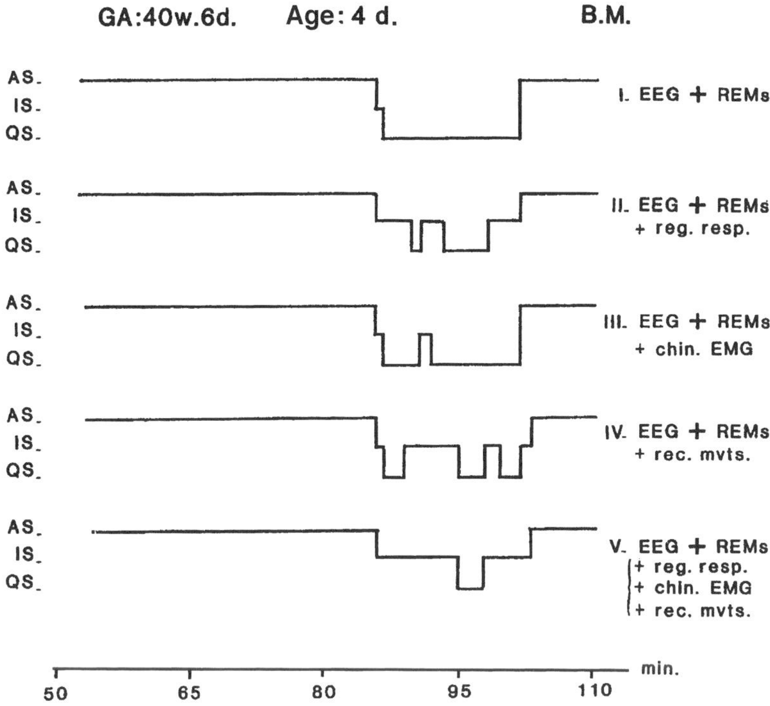

Figure 4 Hypnograms in a normal full-term newborn (65-min sleep period) scored using combinations of state criteria. The amount of active sleep, AS, (defined on the basis of EEG and eye movement criteria only, scoring I) was virtually unchanged when additional criteria were used (regular versus irregular respiration for scoring II; present versus absent chin EMG for scoring III, present versus absent body movements for scoring IV, concordance of all five criteria for scoring V). In contrast, in comparison with scoring I, use of additional criteria resulted in a reduction in quiet sleep (QS) due to periods with irregular respiration (scoring II), inhibited EMG (scoring III), or presence of body movements (scoring IV); the reduction in quiet sleep in favor of indeterminate sleep (IS) was striking when concordance of all five criteria was required (scoring V). (Adapted from Ref. 5.)

The basic procedure for recording and scoring behavioral states is the same whether a chart polygraph or a computerized data acquisition system is used. For references on the computerized method for state parameter analysis in newborns, see Sher's studies (71) and Chapter 2 in this book.

Periods of active and quiet sleep of more than 3 min duration defined on the basis of concordance of EEG and REM criteria exist in neurologically normal premature newborns of more than 27 (70) or 28 weeks GA (72), although marked inter- and intraindividual differences occur. In premature babies, AS and QS sleep is char-

Table 1 Summary of the Major Variables (A) and Ancillary Variables (B) Used for Sleep State Scoring at Various Conceptional Ages*

A. Major variables for sleep state scoring

	CA in weeks					
	27–34		35–36		37–41	
State	AS	QS	AS	QS	AS	QS
EEG	Cont: $\Delta \pm \Theta$, or Δ, or semidiscontinuous	Discontinuous	Cont: $\Delta + \Theta$, or Δ	Discontinuous or semidiscontinuous	Continuous: Θ, or $\Delta + \Theta$, or Δ	Tracé alternant
Eye movements	+	−	++	−	+++	−

B. Other variables

	CA in weeks							
	31–34[†]		35–36		37–38		39–41	
State	AS	QS	AS	QS	AS	QS	AS	QS
Respiratory rate[†]	Irregular	Regular or irregular	Irregular	Regular or irregular	Irregular	Regular or irregular	Irregular	Regular or irregular
Tonic chin EMG[‡]	−	+ or − (20%)	−	+ or − (20%)	−	+ or − (20%)	−	+ or − (20%)
Body movements[‡]	+++ (20%)	++ (5.2%)	+++ (22%)	++ (7%)	+++ (22%)	++ (10%)	++ (14%)	+ (3%)

*Some authors (61) used variable/nonvariable heart rate as a state criterion; however no quantified data are available.
[†]No quantitative data available for infants younger than 31 weeks CA.
[‡]In parentheses: percent of 20 sec spent with this parameter.
CA = conceptional age; AS = active sleep; QS = quiet sleep; cont. = continuous EEG trace; discontinuous = discontinuous EEG trace; Δ = delta EEG activity; Θ = theta EEG activity. The number of pluses is a relative indication of eye or body movement density. Note that about 20% of quiet sleep is spent with inhibited tonic chin EMG. Body movements decrease in amount with age. For irregular respiration definition and amount, see Ref. 5.
Source: Ref. 5.

acterized by striking differences in EEG activity (continuous in active sleep versus discontinuous in quiet sleep (Fig. 3) and rapid eye movements (present in AS and absent in QS). Over time, slow-wave burst duration increases slightly and the amplitude of background EEG activity between the slow-wave bursts on discontinuous tracings steps up significantly, finally producing the *tracé alternant* pattern characteristic of QS near normal term (66,73). During the first few weeks of life, the *tracé alternant* pattern is replaced by a slow-wave high-voltage pattern (refs. in 74 and 75).

Between 27 and 34 weeks GA, indeterminate sleep (IS) contributes a mean of 30% of the total sleep time. IS is defined on the basis of discordance between the two main criteria defining AS and QS sleep. IS diminishes significantly at 35 to 36 weeks GA and then remains stable until term (69). Beyond 31 to 34 weeks GA, a significantly larger percentage of time is spent in AS than in QS (69,70). Near term, 55% to 65% of the sleep time is spent in AS versus about 20% in QS.

The durations of sleep states can vary widely across successive sleep cycles in a given infant. In contrast to adults, premature and full-term newborns fall asleep in AS. The first AS period following a period of wakefulness is usually characterized by a shorter duration and a slower EEG pattern as compared with the next AS period occurring after a QS period. Sleep cycles, defined as an AS and a QS period with the interpolated IS period, are shorter before 35 weeks GA, with a mean duration of 45 to 50 min according to the study. From 35 to 36 weeks GA to term, the sleep cycle duration is about 55 to 65 min (Fig. 5), similar to that observed during the first months of life (69,76–77). In general, our recent unpublished observations suggest that the main maturation-related modifications previously described at 35 to 36 weeks GA may in fact occur somewhat earlier, around 33 to 34 weeks GA.

Artificial ventilation per se does not modify sleep structure in premature babies who are neurologically normal and clinically stable (70,79). Sleep organization in premature babies reaching normal term (71,80) and in full-term small-for-gestational-age newborns (81) does not differ from that observed in full-term controls.

In general, both in the literature and in our own experience, sleep-state differentiation was documented earlier during ontogenesis in studies performed after the 1980s (70,79,82–83) than in those done previously (61,84–85). This is probably ascribable to the improvements made in neonatal care in industrialized countries during the last few decades.

In conclusion, differentiated AS and QS are observed starting at 27 weeks GA in neurologically normal and clinically stable premature infants. Until 34 weeks GA, about 30% of the sleep time is spent in IS. Beyond 35 and 36 weeks GA, IS decreases significantly and sleep structure becomes very similar to that observed during the first month of postterm life. Thus, 27 weeks and 35 to 36 weeks GA appear as turning points in the ontogenesis of human sleep.

Knowledge of early state differentiation is important because 1) a number of physiological parameters are correlated to sleep states in young babies (48) and 2) a number of abnormalities in newborns occur primarily in one or the other of the two main sleep states (respiratory events are more common during AS, whereas EEG abnormalities are more readily detected during QS).

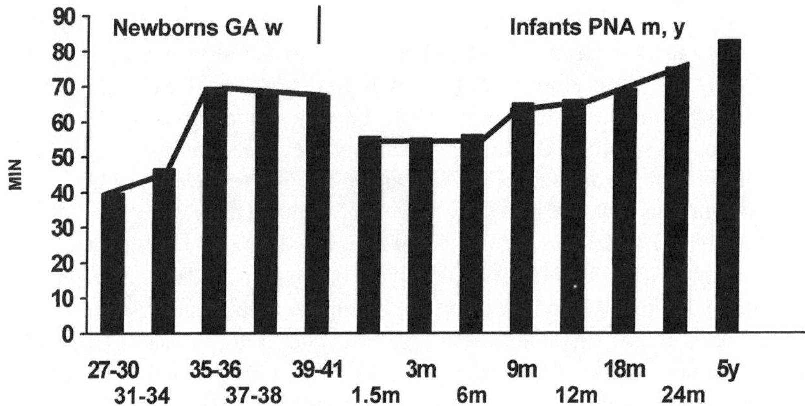

Figure 5 Mean duration of the sleep cycle in minutes at different ages. Data from different laboratories are connected by a dark line. On the left, daytime sleep in newborns from 27 to 41 weeks gestational age (GA). (Adapted from Refs. 69 and 70.) On the right, nighttime sleep in infants from 1.5 to 24 months (m) of postnatal age (adapted from Refs. 4 and 76) and in children aged about five years (y) (adapted from Refs. 4, 77, and 78).

C. The First 2 Years of Life

Sleep maturation from the neonatal period through early childhood is characterized by considerable changes in EEG activity, in the quality of sleep states, and in the percentage and temporal organization of the various states of vigilance. Almost all of these modifications occur during the first 2 years of life.

The First 6 Months of Life

The main stages in EEG development during sleep can be summarized as follows:

1. Disappearance of *tracé alternant* between 3 and 6 weeks (74,75,86).
2. Appearance of spindles between 6 and 9 weeks postterm. The rapid development of sleep spindles during the first 3 months of infancy (87–89) probably reflects developmental changes in thalamocortical structures (90) and also in dendrite myelination and growth (see refs. in 89). The appearance of well defined K complexes toward the end of this period (91) may be associated with a maturational advance in the processing of information, since Halasz et al. (92) suggested that the short period following a K complex may be a microstate during which information-processing capabilities are enhanced.
3. Beginning of differentiation of stages 1, 2, and 3–4 in quiet sleep between 1½ months and 3 months (93–95).

The development of sleep structure (Figs. 6 and 7) during the first 6 months of life is very well known and has been the focus of numerous studies aimed at gathering information relevant to sudden infant death syndrome (SIDS) (95–103). After the first month of life, sleep patterns undergo dramatic changes, consisting of a significant decrease in active sleep from 60% at term to about 34% at 3 months and 31% at 6 months (Fig. 6), with a concomitant increase in quiet sleep from about 49% at 3 months to 55% at 6 months (69,70,77,102).

Using the criteria developed by Rechtschaffen and Kales (64) and adapted for children by Guilleminault and Souquet (94), we identified a stable stage 2 during quiet sleep (77,95) starting at 3 months of age or sometimes as early as 1½ months. The percentage of total sleep time spent in stage 2 increased sharply over time (Fig. 7). Before 6 months of age, stage 2 is present only at the beginning of NREM sleep (93).

From 6 Months to 2 Years

Very few studies have been done in children aged 6 months to 2 years (Figs. 6 and 7) (77,99,101,104). Louis et al. (77) found a significant decrease in REM sleep resulting from a significant decrease in the number of REM sleep episodes, with no change in their duration. This phase of life is characterized by high stability of nocturnal SWS (Fig. 7). Sleep onset no longer occurs in REM sleep after the age of 6 months. Sleep

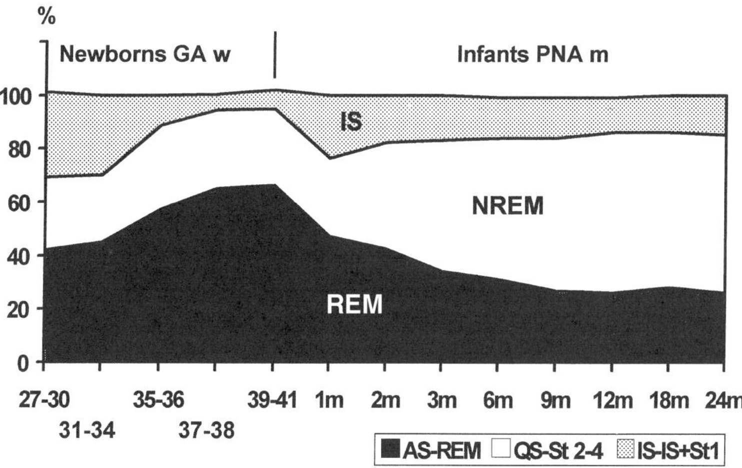

Figure 6 Percentage of the total sleep time spent in active, REM sleep; quiet, NREM sleep; and indeterminate sleep (IS). On the left, daytime sleep in newborns from 27 to 41 weeks gestational age (GA). (Adapted from Refs. 69 and 70.) On the right, nighttime sleep in infants from 1 to 24 months of postnatal age. (Adapted from Ref. 102 for 1- to 6-month-old infants and from Ref. 77 for 9- to 24-month-old infants.) The data on NREM sleep from the study by Louis et al. (77) include the amount of states 2 to 4, and the data on IS are the sum of IS and state 1, according to the state scoring system developed by Retchtschaffen and Kales (64). Abbreviations are the same as in Figure 4.

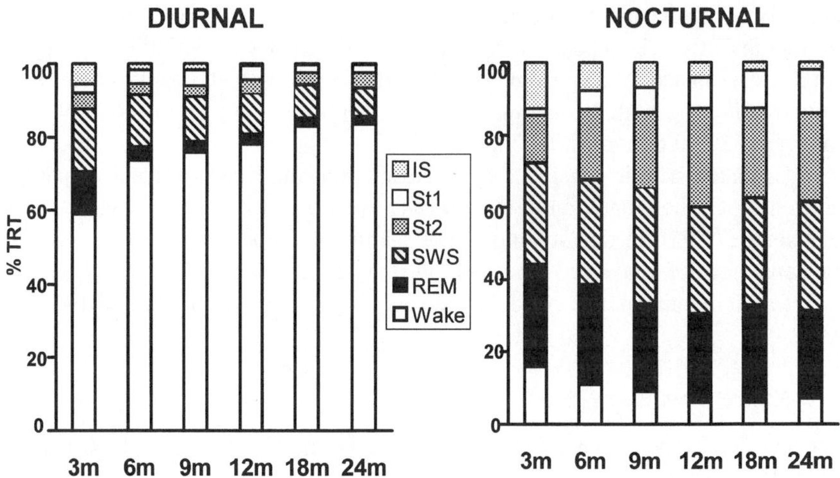

Figure 7 Evolution with age of the different behavioral stages as percentages of total 24-hr home recordings. (Adapted from Ref. 77.) Diurnal and nocturnal periods were defined based on the light-off and light-on times given by the parents. Note that waking and REM sleep are negatively correlated, especially during the daytime.

changes occur earlier in the diurnal part than during the nocturnal part of the 24-hr cycle (Fig. 7).

D. From 2 to 6 Years

Polygraphic studies of sleep between 2 and 6 years are few in number and involved very small numbers of subjects (78,105–107). None used a longitudinal design. Comparisons are difficult due to differences in scoring methods and environmental conditions.

The main developmental steps during this period can be briefly described as follows: 1) REM sleep decreases to adult levels or even lower because naps are eliminated; also, the latency of nocturnal REM sleep increases to 180 min and SWS increases during the first third of the night. 2) Sleep cycle duration increases to the adult value (about 90 min). 3) Phase shift decreases.

These changes are related not only to physiological development but also to the change in SWS distribution due to elimination of daytime naps.

V. Development of Sleep–Wake Rhythms

In neonates, sleep and wakefulness follow a clear-cut ultradian rhythm of about 4 hr (108). This rhythm is endogenous and independent of feeding patterns (109). Within this ultradian rhythm, REM/AS and NREM/QS states recur cyclically. Sleep cycles are measured from the beginning of one to the beginning of the next REM or NREM period (refs. in 5 and 77). Sleep cycle duration is 40 to 45 min in very premature babies and 50 to 60 min beyond 35 weeks GA; it remains stable until 12 months postnatal age and then increases gradually, reaching adult values before 6 years of age (Fig. 5).

The circadian pacemaker is probably already functional during the last months of fetal life. Mirmiran et al. (110) found evidence of a circadian rhythm of about 25 hr for body temperature and the rest-activity cycle in preterm infants of 28 to 34 weeks GA. McMillen et al. (111) demonstrated that preterm infants as young as 35 weeks GA were entrainable to the light–dark cycle.

A circadian rhythm of about 25 hr emerges during the first few weeks of life (112,113). By 1 month of age, periods of sleep are longer during the night, and a period of prolonged wakefulness begins to occur in the early evening hours. By 3 to 4 months of age, entrainment of sleep and wakefulness to the 24-hr cycle is apparent (112,114–116). Figure 8 clearly illustrates this phenomenon at 3 months: the longest sleep periods are not randomly distributed over the 24 hr as they were at a younger age and are present only during the night. By 6 months of age, an unbroken period of sleep longer than 7 hr occurs during the night (117). The longest periods of sleep and wakefulness occur at fixed times of the day, and the longest sleep period generally occurs immediately after the longest waking period (Fig. 8) (116).

Circadian rhythms for heart rate, body movements, body temperature, cortisol, and melatonin also appear during the first few months of life, and their amplitude increases significantly starting at 3 months of age (118–121). Some of these rhythms probably play an important role in the development of the sleep–wake cycle and probably also influence the maturation of sleep states (121,122).

Ultradian and circadian rhythms and sleep states characteristics are genetically determined, although environmental time cues play a key role in their synchronization over the 24 hr (123) starting during the first few weeks of life (111–124).

Many studies have investigated sleep duration and nighttime arousals from infancy through adolescence. They relied mainly on responses to questionnaires and results of actigraphic tracings (108,125–132). The total amount of sleep was found to decrease from a mean of about 16 to 17 hr during the neonatal period to 14 to 15 hr by 6 months, 13 hr by 2 years, 9 hr by 10 years, and 7 to 8 hr at the end of adolescence. Interindividual variability exceeds 2 hr, whereas intraindividual variability is small (125). Differences exist across ethnic groups; for example, epidemiological studies have shown that Italian children sleep much less than children from Switzerland or England (refs. in 132), probably because the later bedtime in Italy leads to a decrease in nocturnal sleep duration that is not compensated for by an increase in diurnal sleep (132). The decrease in sleep duration seen during the first 6 months of life is due to a decrease in daytime sleep (Fig. 7) (77). After 6 years of age, the decline in sleep duration is due to a later bedtime with a fixed morning awakening time.

Night sleep consolidation, also known as "settling," has been defined as unbroken sleep from midnight to 5 A.M. (117,133). Most infants settle between 3 and 6 months of age, but Moore and Ucko (134) and Anders (117) have shown that many

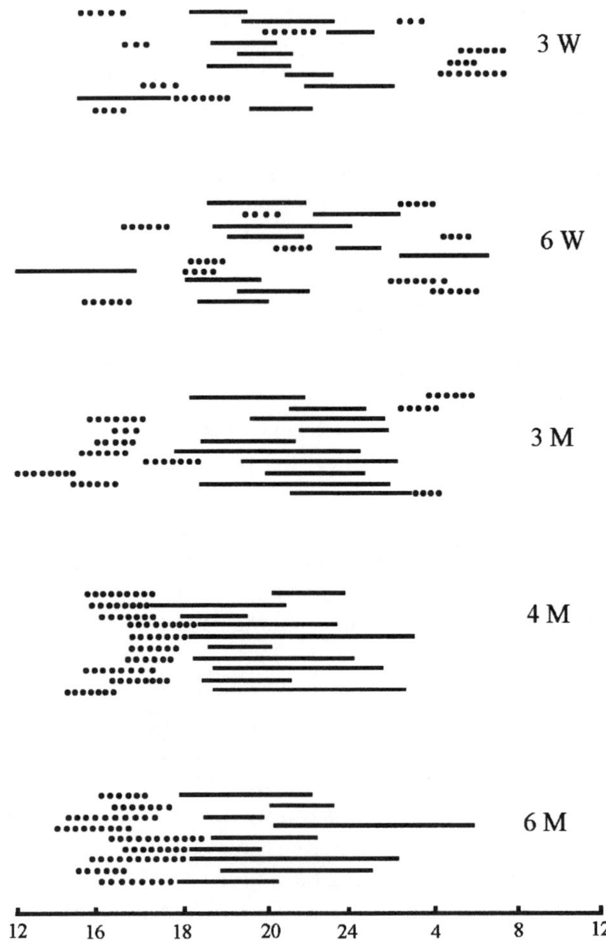

Figure 8 Development of consolidated sleep-wake periods: distribution over 24 hr of the longest waking period (dotted line) and longest sleep period (solid line) in 10 infants recorded at 3 weeks, 6 weeks, 3 months, 4 months, and 6 months of age. (Adapted from Ref. 116.)

children who settle at the usual age experience an increase in nighttime awakenings starting at 9 months of age. This increase is probably due not only to social and environmental factors but also, to some extent, to biological factors. Louis et al. (77) also found a transient increase in the number of awakenings at the age of 9 months.

Nighttime arousals are normal in infants and young children. Epidemiological studies have revealed that these sleep disruptions are very common, affecting 20% to 40% of 1- to 2-year-olds (135). These physiological awakenings occur chiefly during REM sleep (136). They decline sharply in frequency after 6 months of age and become concentrated within the period between midnight and 5 A.M. as SWS increases during the first part of the night. The virtual disappearance of these nighttime awakenings after the age of 3 years is probably a result of the lengthening of the sleep cycle and large increase in SWS during the first part of the night seen at this age.

The organization of both SWS and REM sleep over the 24 hr is established by the age of 1 year (77,101,137,138).

VI. Development of the Homeostatic "Process S"

Experiments involving manipulation of sleep—such as sleep deprivation, sleep extension, or shifting of sleep—demonstrated that non-REM sleep, and more specifically the intensity of slow wave activity (SWA) and the quantity of its SWS component, were largely dependent on the duration of the prior period of wakefulness in adult humans (21,139,140). This suggests the existence of a homeostatic process, designated *process S*, that becomes more active as the duration of prior wakefulness increases and less active as the duration of sleep increases. In adults—i.e., when process S is mature—SWA is abundant immediately after sleep onset and recurs during each cycle with decreasing intensity from one cycle to the next (16).

Process S has not been studied in children for several reasons: recording durations are too short or do not include a diurnal period, and automatic analysis of delta activity over periods equal to 24-hr have not been performed.

In infants, SWS becomes predominant during the first part of the night starting at 3 months of age. Harper et al. (96), Hoppenbrouwers et al. (97), Coons et al. (98), and Louis et al. (77) reported that SWS in infants aged 5 to 12 months is predominant in the first part of the night. Salzarulo et al. (144), Schechtman et al. (143), and Bes et al. (142) reported that the amount of SWA is largest during the first NREM sleep episode after sleep onset and decreases significantly over the sleep period. However, if the first cycle is excluded, this decrease is no longer evident: SWA recurs mainly during alternate REM/NREM cycles throughout the night rather than during consecutive cycles as in adults (138,145). The results of these night studies suggest the emergence of the homeostatic process S (144), which is also supported by the fact that, starting at 6 months of age, the longest sleeping period generally follows the longest waking period (Fig. 8) (116).

VII. The Functional Role of Sleep States During Development

None of the many hypotheses put forward to explain the functional role of sleep have been confirmed as yet. Some of these hypotheses, especially those on REM sleep, have received strong support from data gathered during studies of the developmental characteristics of sleep.

NREM sleep (especially stages 3 and 4), which is enhanced during childhood, is associated with energy maintenance, an increase in the synthesis of proteins (used during subsequent paradoxical sleep to ensure proper synapse function), cell mitosis, and most notably release of growth hormone (146,147). We are not aware of any data on the functional role of NREM sleep in infants and children.

The most important presumptive functions of REM sleep—including CNS maturation and differentiation (57), genetic programming (148–150), and consolidation of memory and learning (151,152)—are crucial during early development.

There is an extremely high percentage of REM sleep during the prenatal and neonatal period (Fig. 6). REM sleep is characterized by a very high level of CNS activation. Cerebral blood flow, which is a good marker of neuronal activity, is similar or even greater during REM sleep than during wakefulness in adult humans (153,154). In infants beyond 36 weeks GA, cerebral blood flow is higher during AS than during QS and wakefulness (155,156), whereas in younger premature infants it has been found to be lower during REM sleep than during quiet sleep (157).

All the physiological and behavioral parameters that characterize REM sleep are present at 35 to 36 weeks or perhaps even earlier (refs. in 48 and 69).

In adults, relationships have been described between the frequency of rapid eye movements, their pattern of occurrence, and the degree of mental activity during REM sleep. The frequency of rapid eye movements seems to increase during the first 6 months of life, and the pattern of their occurrence seems to become more complex during the first year of life (158,159).

Our discussion is limited to the hypotheses that are directly linked to cognitive and neurological processes—i.e., consolidation of memory and learning, the maturational hypothesis of Roffwarg et al. (57), and the hypothesis of endogenous genetic programming developed by Jouvet (148,149).

VIII. Consolidation of Memory and Learning During Sleep

In animals, studies of consolidation of memory and learning during sleep have relied mainly on REM sleep analysis (160–162). The main findings from these studies can be described briefly as follows:

REM sleep deprivation disrupts learning of complex or new tasks.

Only successful learning is accompanied by an increase in REM sleep.

The first REM sleep episode that immediately follows a learning process is the one that shows the greatest modifications in quality and quantity, suggesting that it makes the largest contribution to learning consolidation.

The increase in REM sleep is due primarily to an increase in the number of episodes rather than to an increase in their duration.

The results of two studies in human infants have provided data on the last three points mentioned above. Dittrichova et al. (163) showed that the REM sleep episodes following a period of wakefulness had a higher frequency of rapid eye movements than those following a period of quiet sleep. In another study, Paul and Dittrichova (164) found an increase in REM sleep after a learning process in infants. A strong word of caution regarding the interpretation of these results should be added, because of the very short duration of REM sleep following periods of wakefulness and of the usual distribution of rapid eye movements throughout REM sleep (progressive increase in eye movement density during the first minutes of an active sleep period, personal unpublished data.)

The high proportion of REM sleep during the first months of life as well as the large number of REM sleep periods and the linkage between wakefulness and REM sleep support a role for REM sleep in memory consolidation and learning in young infants (165).

IX. The Maturational Hypothesis of Roffwarg and Coworkers

Roffwarg and associates (57) put forward two hypotheses regarding the physiological significance of the high proportion and rapid decrease of REM sleep in early life. First, the immature nervous system of small babies may be unable to inhibit REM sleep centers (Fig. 2) (9,13), and the decrease in REM sleep seen with increasing age may reflect CNS maturation. This hypothesis may explain why "undifferentiated active sleep" is so abundant in fetuses and very premature infants before 30 weeks of GA; this type of sleep may be comparable to the "active" sleep of immature mammals (32,44,45).

The second hypothesis postulates that the developing nervous system needs stimulation in order to grow and mature and that the functional role of REM sleep may be to provide endogenous stimuli to the developing nervous system. Under this hypothesis, the decrease in REM sleep during ontogenesis reflects a reduced need for REM sleep once CNS maturation is complete. A study by Denenberg and Thoman (166) provided support for this hypothesis by showing that alert inactivity, which is the only waking state in which neonates are aware of their environment, is negatively correlated with REM sleep during the first few months of life. Louis et al. (77) reported that the significant decrease in REM sleep during the first few months of life was especially strong between 3 and 6 months and was more pronounced during the diurnal part of the 24-hr cycle—i.e., during the part characterized by longer and longer periods of wakefulness (Fig. 7).

Efforts to produce REM sleep deprivation have consistently failed in human neonates (167), developing monkeys (168), rats aged less than 1 week, and rat fetuses (169). REM sleep deprivation cannot be achieved in human or monkey neonates without causing complete sleep deprivation and without affecting behaviors essential for survival, such as regulation of body temperature and feeding. This suggests that REM sleep plays a major role in fetuses and neonates.

Several experiments in young mammals lend support to the maturation hypothesis of Roffwarg et al. (57). Oksenberg (170) showed that REM sleep deprivation worsened the effects of monocular vision deprivation in kittens. Lesions of the PGO pathways in kittens (171–173), which eliminate the phasic activities of REM sleep, suggest that the impulses provided by PGO waves may have an important effect on the morphological and electrophysiological maturation of the lateral geniculate nucleus. Oksenberg et al. (170) suggested that REM sleep–generated discharges may also "protect" the CNS against excessive plasticity changes. Finally, Mirmiran et al. (174) demonstrated that REM sleep deprivation obtained using pharmacological substances such as clonidine or clomipramine in rats aged 1 to 3 weeks was followed in adulthood by increased anxiety, deficient sexual performance, and disturbances in the sleep-wake pattern. Subsequent measurements of regional brain weights showed significant reductions for the cerebral cortex and medulla oblongata. Data obtained during studies of clonidine-induced REM sleep deprivation in rat pups suggest that REM sleep deprivation during early development can inhibit the growth response of the brain to environmental stimuli later in life (42,175).

These results obtained using pharmacological methods do not allow us to rule out a possible role of cerebral monoamines independent from REM sleep deprivation. If they are confirmed, they may indicate that REM sleep plays a role in the *engram* of epigenetic stimuli.

X. The Endogenous Genetic Programming Hypothesis Developed by Jouvet

Jouvet (148) held that REM sleep in fetuses and neonates triggers genetically programmed behavioral patterns. Sastre and Jouvet (149) showed that when the neural systems responsible for postural atony during paradoxical sleep were destroyed, sleeping cats periodically displayed specific sets of activities such as orienting, rage, or grooming activities, which Jouvet called "oneiric" behaviors. He postulated that genetic programming of the brain occurred during paradoxical sleep and maintained, facilitated, or induced the system of neurons responsible for these innate behaviors.

XI. A Contribution to the Function of REM Sleep (Personal Study)

The purpose of this study was to investigate hypotheses about the functional role of REM sleep during ontogenesis. It was based on an analysis of facial expression during sleep in neonates (165,176).

Twelve healthy, full-term neonates and three infants with brain malformations were videotaped and polygraphically recorded for an unbroken period of 3 hr. First, we analyzed smiling, frowning, and expressions indicating sadness in all healthy and abnormal infants. In a second study, we analyzed all the facial expressions observed in one of the healthy neonates.

In the first study, 383 smiles were analyzed. All but 6 occurred during REM sleep. Neonatal smiling during sleep was similar to adult smiling; it was an organized behavior and was more marked on the left side of the face. The study of rapid eye movements showed that the density of rapid eye movements occurring in bursts was positively correlated with both the density and the duration of smiles. The finding that the smiles were more marked on the left side of the face was in keeping with the well-known role of the right hemisphere in the production of emotional expression and communication. The asymmetry of smiles in healthy neonates also provided support for cortical mediation.

In the second study, 1469 different facial muscular action units in a single infant were analyzed. All the facial expressions observed in adults were present in this neonate, but only those expressions that were related to emotions were seen during REM sleep.

A separate study of facial expressions in two hydrocephalic children suggested that the production of emotion-related expressions during REM sleep involves the cortex, in particular the somatotopic area.

These data from neonates lend some support to the hypotheses of Roffwarg and Jouvet (57,150) that REM sleep may support a form of genetic programming for emotional behavior patterns. The positive correlation we found between frowning, which can be considered to denote a negative emotion, and smiling suggests that this endogenous programming of the motor pathway of emotional expressions is not specific.

XII. Summary

1. Behavioral states are constellations of physiological and behavioral variables—such as cerebral electrical activity (EEG), motor activity, autonomic functions, and behavior—that are stable and occur repeatedly over time. The main states are 1) wakefulness; 2) SWS or NREM sleep, or quiet sleep (QS) in early ontogenesis; and 3) paradoxical or REM sleep, or active sleep (AS) in early ontogenesis. All these states are produced by active excitatory and inhibitory neuronal discharges in a number of brainstem and forebrain centers organized in “systems” or “networks,” each of which controls a given state. Neurochemical mechanisms underlie the neuronal and receptor functions involved in sleep.
2. The first steps of behavioral states differentiation depend on the degree of brain maturation. Active, REM sleep characteristics are the first and waking characteristics the last to appear during early ontogenesis. In several species characterized by greater brain maturity at birth, REM and NREM states parameters may be concordant during fetal life and the first days of postnatal life. The mechanisms underlying regulation of the main states during early animal ontogenesis remain controversial.
3. Most recent data suggest that differentiated behavioral states are present in humans in utero from the beginning of the third trimester of gestation, and that they are similar to those of newborns of the same gestational age.
4. Differentiated AS and QS are observed starting at 27 weeks GA in neurologically normal and clinically stabilized premature infants. The main steps

of the development of the sleep–wake cycle and of sleep structure are shown in Table 2; they are closely interrelated.

5. Adult sleep is regulated via two processes, a chronobiological process called process C and a homeostatic process called process S. In human neonates, sleep and wakefulness follow an ultradian rhythm of about 4 hr. Circadian rhythmicity emerges during the very first weeks of life. Entrainment of sleep and wakefulness to a 24-hr cycle, which occurs between 2 and 4 months, is dependent on time cues. Emergence of circadian rhythmicity probably plays a key role in the ontogenesis of sleep structure and in the consolidation of nocturnal sleep. The homeostatic component begins to emerge at 6 months of age. The two processes are probably closely linked from the first months of life.
6. Near normal term in humans, sleep is characterized by stable periods of quiet sleep, a very high percentage of active sleep, and sleep onset in active sleep; active sleep is the equivalent during the very early phases of life of REM sleep. The sleep cycle in neonates is of short duration and lengthens to adult values between 2 and 6 years of age.
7. Beyond the first month of life, sleep patterns change dramatically: AS/REM sleep decreases significantly; at the same time, QS/NREM sleep increases and differentiates into stages 1, 2, and 3–4. Sleep onset no longer occurs in REM sleep after 6 months of age. Sleep changes occur at an earlier age during the diurnal than the nocturnal part of the 24-hr cycle. For both SWS and REM sleep, the nocturnal temporal organization is estab-

Table 2 Main Steps in Sleep–Wake Maturation

Sleep–Wake Cycle	Sleep Structure
Ultradian rhythm during the fetal period and first days of life	Emergence of AS/QS at 27 weeks gestational age AS increases, IS decreases; cycle duration increases (40–45 to 55–60 min) at 34–35 weeks gestational age
Emergence of circadian rhythmicity during the first weeks of life (free running cycle of 25 hr)	Emergence of sleep spindles between 1.5 and 3 months Significant decrease in REMS with concomitant increase in NREMS; emergence of stages 1, 2, and 3–4 between 2 and 3 months
Entrainment to a 24-hr cycle after 3 months	Disappearance of REM sleep onset from 9 months
Consolidation of nocturnal sleep from 6 months of age	Nyctohemeral organization of SWS and REMS between 9 and 12 months
Disappearance of naps between 3 and 6 years of life	Lengthening of the sleep cycle to adult level between 2 and 6 years

lished by the age of 1 year. Between the age of 2 and 6 years, the disappearance of naps is associated with substantial reorganization of nocturnal sleep characterized by a significant increase in SWS during the first part of the night and by an increase in REM sleep latency of up to 3 hr.

The understanding of sleep disturbances in childhood requires a good working knowledge of the development of state organization, since the problem is often age-specific and also closely linked to the mechanisms underlying the ontogenesis of the sleep-wake cycle and of sleep structure.

Although many hypotheses have been put forward, the functional role of sleep is still unknown. The principal hypotheses, especially those concerning REM sleep, are strongly supported by findings from the studies of the developmental characteristics of sleep.

References

1. Denissova MP, Figurin NL. [Periodic phenomena during sleep in infants]. In (Russian): [News in Nervous System Reflexology and Physiology] 1926; 2:338–345.
2. Aserinsky E, Kleitman N. A motility cycle in sleeping infants as manifested by ocular and gross bodily activity. J Appl Physiol 1955; 8:11–18.
3. Parmelee AH, Garbanati JA. Clinical neurobehavioral aspects of state organisation in newborn infants. In: Yabuuchi H, Watanabe K, Okada S, eds. Neonatal Brain and Behaviour. Nagoya, Japan: University of Nagoya Press, 1987:131–144.
4. Challamel MJ. Development of sleep and wakefulness in humans. In: Meisami E, Timiras PS, eds. Handbook of Human Growth and Developmental Biology. Boca Raton, FL: CRC Press, 1988:269–284.
5. Curzi-Dascalova IL, Mirmiran M. Manual of Methods for Recording and Analysing Sleep-Wakefulness States in Preterm and Full-Term Infants. Paris: INSERM, 1996.
6. Prechtl HFR, O'Brien MJ. Behavioral states of the full-term newborn: the emergence of a concept. In: Stratton P, ed. Psychobiology of the Human Newborn. Wiley, 1982:53–73.
7. McGinty D, Szymusiac R. Neurobiology of sleep. In: Saunders NA, Sullivan CE, eds. Sleep and Breathing. New York: Marcel Dekker, 1994:1–26.
8. Adrien J. Neurobiologie du cycle veille-sommeil. In: Billard M, ed. Le sommeil normal et pathologique. Troubles du sommeil et de l'èveil. Paris: Masson, 1994:27–38.
9. Valatx JL. Sommeils et insomnies. Pour la Science 1998; 243:80–87.
10. Jouvet M. Biogenic amines and the states of sleep. Science 1969; 163:32–41.
11. Jouvet M. Paradoxical sleep mechanisms. Sleep 1994; 17:S77–S83.
12. Lydic R, Baghdoyan HA. The neurobiology of rapid-eye-movement sleep. In: Saunders NA, Sullivan CE, eds. Sleep and Breathing. New York: Marcel Dekker, 1994:47–77.
13. Valatx JL. Régulation du cycle veille/sommeil. In: Benoit O, Foret J, eds. Le sommeil humain. Paris: Masson, 1995:25–37.
14. Krueger JM, Obal F Jr. Sleep factors. In: Saunders NA, Sullivan CE, eds. Sleep and Breathing. New York: Marcel Dekker, 1994:79–112.
15. Sakai K. Executive mechanisms of paradoxical sleep. Arch Ital Biol 1988; 126: 239–257.
16. Borbély AA. A two process model of sleep regulation. Hum Neurobiol 1982; 1:195–204.

17. Cespuglio R, Marinesco S, Baubet V, Bonnet C, El Kafi B. Evidence for a sleep-promoting influence of stress. Adv Neuroimmunol 1995; 5:145–154.
18. Jouvet M, Michel F. Recherche sur l'activité électrique cérébrale au cours du sommeil. C R Soc Biol 1958; 152:1167–1170.
19. Steriade M, Buszacki G. Parallel activation of thalamic and cortical neurons by brainstem and basal forebrain cholinergic systems. In: Steriade M, Biesold D, eds. Brain Cholinergic Systems. Oxford: Oxford University Press, 1990:33–62.
20. Szymusiac R, McGinty D. Brainstem and forebrain regulation of sleep onset and slow-wave sleep. In: Saunders NA, Sullivan CE, eds. Sleep and Breathing. New York: Marcel Dekker, 1994:27–45.
21. Achermann P, Borbély AA. Simulation of human sleep: ultradian dynamics of electroencephalographic slow-wave activity. J Biol Rhythms 1990; 5:141–157.
22. Prechtl HFR. Assessment of fetal neurological function and development. In: Levene MI, Bennett MJ, Jonathan P, eds. Fetal and Neonatal Neurology and Neurosurgery. Edinburgh and London: Churchill Livingstone, 1988:35–40.
23. Rakic P. Neuronal migration in primate telencephalon. Postgrad Med J 1978; 54:25–40.
24. Hahashi M. Ontogeny of some neuropeptides in the primate brain. Prog Neurobiol 1992; 38:231–260.
25. Huttenlocher PR, de Courten C, Garey LJ, Van der Loos H. Synaptogenesis in human visual cortex-evidence for synapse elimination during normal development. Neurosci Lett 1982; 33:247–252.
26. Semba K. Development of central cholinergic neurons. In: Björklund A, Hökfelt T, Tohyama M, eds. Handbook of Chemical Neuro-Anatomy. Vol 10. Ontogeny of Transmiters and Peptides in the CNS. The Netherlands: Elsevier Science, 1992:35–62.
27. Danguir J. Intracerebroventricular infusion of somatostatin selectively increases paradoxical sleep in rats. Brain Res 1986; 367:26–30.
28. Gressens P, Paindaveine B, Hill JM, Brenneman DE, Evrard P. Growth factor of VIP during early brain development. In: Neuropeptides in Development and Aging. Ann NY Acad Sci 1997; 814:152–160.
29. Zini I, Pich EM, Fuxe K, Lenzi PL, Agnati LF, Harfstrand A, Mutt V, Tatemoto K, Moscara M. Action of centraly administered neuropeptide Y and EEG activity in different rat strains and different phases of their circadian cycle. Acta Physiol Scand 1984; 122:71–77.
30. Corner M. Spontaneous motor rhythms in early life-phenomenological and neurophysiological aspects. In: Corner MA, ed. Maturation of the Nervous System. Prog Brain Res 1978; 48:349–364.
31. Valatx JL, Jouvet D, Jouvet M. Evolution électroencéphalographique des différents états de sommeil chez le chaton. Electroencephalogr Clin Neurophysiol 1964; 7:218–233.
32. Jouvet-Monnier D, Astic L, Lacote D. Ontogenesis of the states of sleep in rat, cat and guinea pig during the first postnatal month. Dev Psychobiol 1969; 2:216–239.
33. Garma L, Verley R. Ontogenèse des états de veille et de sommeil chez les mammifères. Rev Neuropsychiat Infant 1969; 17:487–504.
34. Jouvet D, Valatx JL. Etude polygraphique du sommeil chez l'agneau. CR Soc Biol 1962; 156:1411–1414.
35. Walker AM, De Preu ND. Preterm birth in lambs: sleep patterns and cardiorespiratory changes. J Dev Physiol. 1991; 16:139–145.
36. Belich AI, Nazarova LA. The development of the rest-activity cycle in rabbit foetus. J Evol Bioch Physiol 1988; 24:217–222.

37. Ruckebush Y, Gaujoux M, Eghbali B. Sleep cycles and kinesis in the foetal lamb. Electroencephalogr Clin Neurophysiol 1977; 42:226–237.
38. Gauwerky J, Wernicke K, Boos R, Kubli F. Heart rate variability, breathing and body movements in normoxic fetal lambs. J Perinat Med 1982; 10 (suppl 2):111–112.
39. Astic L, Sastre JP, Brandon AM. Polygraphic study of vigilance states in the guinea-pig fetus. Physiol Behav 1973; 11:647–654.
40. Stark RI, Haiken J, Nordli D, Myers MM. Characterization of electroencephalographic state in fetal baboons. Am J Physiol 1991; 26:R496–R500.
41. Hoppenbrouwers T, Sterman MB. Development of sleep state patterns in the kitten. Exp Neurol 1975; 49:822–838.
42. Mirmiran M, van Someren E. The importance of REM sleep for brain maturation. J Sleep Res 1993; 2:188–192.
43. Alföldi P, Tobler I, Borbély AA. Sleep regulation in rats during early development. Am J Physiol 1990; 27:R634–R644.
44. Adrien J, Bourgoin S, Hamon M. Midbrain raphe lesion in the newborn rat: I. Neurophysiological aspect of sleep. Brain Res 1977; 127:99–110.
45. Adrien J. Ontogenesis of some sleep regulations: early postnatal impairment of the monoaminergic systems. In: Corner MA, ed. Maturation of the Nervous System. Prog Brain Res 1978; 48:393–403.
46. Franc M, Page J, Heller HC. The effect of REM sleep-inhibiting drugs in neonatal rats: evidence for a distinction between neonatal active sleep and REM sleep. Brain Res 1997; 778:64–72.
47. Brown R. Muramyl peptides and the function of sleep. Behav Brain Res 1995; 69: 85–90.
48. Curzi-Dascalova L. Physiological correlates of sleep development in premature and full-term newborns. Clin Neurophysiol 1992; 22:151–166.
49. Nijhuis J, Martin C, Prechtl H, Bots R. The implication of fetal behavioural states for perinatal monitoring. Europ J Obstetr Gynecol Reprod Biol 1983; 15:433–436.
50. Visser GHA, Poelmann-Weesies G, Cohen TMN, Bekedam DJ. Fetal behavior at 30–32 weeks of gestation. Pediatr Res 1987; 22:655–658.
51. Okai T, Kozuma S, Shinozuka N, Kuwabara Y, Mizuno M. A study on the development of sleep-wakefulness cycle in the human foetus. Early Hum Dev 1992; 29:391–396.
52. Curzi-Dascalova L. Phase relationships between thoracic and abdominal respiratory movements during sleep in 31–38 week CA normal infants: comparison with full-term (39–41 weeks) newborns. Neuropediatrics 1982; 13(suppl):15–20.
53. Hoppenbrouwers T, Ugartechea JC, Combs D, Hodgman JE, Harper RM, Sterman MB. Studies of maternal-fetal interaction during the last trimester of pregnancy: ontogenesis of the basic rest-activity cycle. Exp Neurol 1978; 61:136–153.
54. Groom LJ, Swiber MJ, Atterbury JL, Bentz LS, Holland SB. Similarity and differences in behavioral state organization during sleep periods in perinatal infant before and after birth. Child Dev 1997; 68:1–11.
55. Challamel MJ, Revol M, Bremond A, Fargier P. Electroencéphalogramme foetal au cours du travail: modifications physiologiques des états de vigilance. Rev Fr Gynecol 1975; 70:235–239.
56. Rosen MG, Dierker LJ, Hertz RH, Sorokin Y, Timortritdch IE. Fetal behavioral states and fetal evaluation. Clin Obstet Gynecol 1979; 22:605–611.
57. Roffwarg HP, Muzio JN, Dement WC. Ontogenetic development of human sleep-dream cycle. Science 1966; 152:604–619.

58. Dreyfus-Brisac C. Ontogenesis of sleep in human prematures after 32 weeks of conceptional age. Dev Psychobiol 1970; 3:91–121.
59. Monod N, Dreyfus-Brisac C, Morel-Kahn F, Pajot N. Les premières étapes de l'orgaisation du sommeil chez le prématuré et le nouveau-né à terme. Rev Neurol 1964; 110: 304–305.
60. Parmelee AH, Wenner WH, Akiyama Y, Schultz M, Stern E. Sleep states in premature infants. Dev Med Child Neurol 1967; 9:70–77.
61. Prechtl HFR, Akiyama Y, Zinkin P, Grant DK. Polygraphic studies in the full-term newborns: 1. Technical aspects and qualitative analysis. In: Bax M, MacKeith RC, eds. Studies in Infancy. Clin Dev Med 1968; 27:1–21.
62. Wolff P, Ferber R. The development of behaviour in human infants, premature and newborn. Annu Rev Neurosci 1979; 2:291–307.
63. Anders T, Emde R, Parmelee A, eds. A Manual of Standardized Terminology, Techniques and Criteria for Scoring of States of Sleep and Wakefulness in Newborn Infants. Los Angeles: UCLA Brain Information Service, MINDS Neurological Information Network, 1971.
64. Rechtschaffen A, Kales A, eds. A Manual of Standardized Terminology, Techniques and Scoring System for Sleep Stages of Human Subjects. Washington DC: Public Health Service, U.S. Government Printing Office, 1968.
65. Thoman EB, McDowell K. Sleep cycling in infants during the earliest postnatal weeks. Physiol Behav 1989; 45:217–522.
66. Dreyfus-Brisac C. Neonatal electroencephalography. In: Scarpelli EM, Cosmi EV, eds. Review of Perinatal Medicine. Vol. 3. New York: Raven Press, 1979:397–472.
67. Stockard-Pope JE, Werner SS, Bickford RG. Atlas of Neonatal Electroencephalography, 2d ed. New York: Raven Press, 1992.
68. Monod N, Curzi-Dascalova L. Les états transitionnels de sommeil chez le nouveau-né è terme. Rev EEG Neurophysiol 1973; 3:87–96.
69. Curzi-Dascalova L, Peirano P, Morel-Kahn F. Development of sleep states in normal premature and full-term newborns. Dev Psychobiol 1988; 21:431–444.
70. Curzi-Dascalova L, Figueroa JM, Eiselt M, Christova E, Virassami A, d'Allest AM, Guimaraes H, Gaultier Cl, Dehan M. Sleep state organization in premature infants of less than 35 weeks' gestational age. Pediatr Res 1993; 34:624–628.
71. Scher MS. Normal electrographic-polysomnographic patterns in preterm and full-term infants. Semin Pediatr Neurol 1996; 3:2–12.
72. Karch D, Rothe R, Jurisch R, Heldt-Hildebrandt R, Lübbesmier A, Lemburg P. Behavioural changes and bioelectric brain maturation of preterm and full-term newborn infants: a polygraphic study. Dev Med Child Neurol 1982; 24:30–47.
73. Eiselt M, Schendel M, Witte H, Dörschel J, Curzi-Dascalova L, d'Allest AM, Zwiener U. Quantitative analysis of discontinuous EEG in premature and full-term newborns during quiet sleep. Electroencephalogr Clin Neurophysiol 1997; 103:528–534.
74. Curzi-Dascalova L. EEG de veille et de sommeil du nourrisson normal avant 6 mois d'âge. Rev EEG Neurophysiol 1977; 7:316–326.
75. Ellingson RJ, Peters JF. Development of EEG and daytime sleep patterns in low risk premature infants during the first year of life: longitudinal observation. Electroencephalogr Clin Neurophysiol 1980; 50:165–171.
76. Borghese IF, Minard KL, Thomas EB. Sleep rhythmicity in premature infants: implication for developmental status. Sleep 1995; 18:523–530.

77. Louis J, Cannard C, Bastuji H, Challamel MJ. Sleep ontogenesis revisited: a longitdinal 24-h home polygraphic study on 15 normal infants during the first two years of life. Sleep 1997; 20:323–333.
78. Kahn E, Fisher C, Edwards A, Davis DM. 24 hour sleep patterns: a comparison between 2 to 3 years old and 4 to 6 years old children. Arch Gen Psychiatry 1973; 29:380–385.
79. Karch D, Rohmer K, Lemburg P. Prognostic significance of polygraphic recordings in newborn infants on ventilation. Dev Med Child Neurol 1984; 26:358–368.
80. Curzi-Dascalova L, Peirano P, Morel-Kahn F, Lebrun F. Developmental aspect of sleep in premature and full-term infants. In: Yabuuci H, Watanabe K, Okada S, eds. Neonatal Brain and Behaviour. Nagoya, Japan: University of Nagoya Press, 1987:167–182.
81. Curzi-Dascalova L, Peirano P. Sleep states organization in small-for-gestational-age human neonates. Brain Dysfunc 1989; 2:45–54.
82. Dittrichova J, Paul K. Development of behavioural states in very premature infants. Arch Nerv Sup (Praha) 1983; 25:187–188.
83. Stefanski M, Schulze K, Bateman D, Kairam R, Pedley TA, Masterson J, James LS. A scoring system of sleep and wakefulness in term and preterm infants. Pediatr Res 1984; 18:58–62.
84. Stern E, Parmelee AH, Harris MA. Sleep states periodicity in premature and young infants. Dev Psychobiol 1972; 6:357–365.
85. Lombroso CT. Neonatal polygraphy in full-term and premature infants: a review of normal and abnormal findings. J Clin Neurophysiol 1985; 2:105–155.
86. Dittrichova J. Development of sleep in infancy. In: Robinson RJ, ed. Brain and Early Behaviour. London: Academic Press, 1969:193–201.
87. Metcalf DR. EEG sleep spindle ontogenesis. Neuropädiatrie 1970; 1:428–433.
88. Louis J, Zhang JX, Revol M, Debilly G, Challamel MJ. Ontogenesis of nocturnal organization of sleep spindles: a longitudinal study during the first 6 months of life. Electroencephalogr Clin Neurophysiol 1992; 83:289–296.
89. Hughes JR. Development of sleep spindles in the first year of life. Clin Electroencephalogr 1996; 37:107–115.
90. Steriade M, Deschênes M, Domich L, Mulle C. Abolition of spindle oscillation in thalamic neurons disconnected from nucleus reticularis thalami. J Neurophysiol 1985; 54: 1473–1497.
91. Samson-Dollfus D, Nogues B, Verdure-Poussin A, Malleville F. Electroencephalogramme de sommeil de l'enfant normal entre 5 mois et 3 ans. Rev Electroenceph Clin Neurophysiol 1977; 7:335–345.
92. Halasz P, Rajna P, Pal I, Kundra O, Vargha M, Balogh A, Kemeny A. K-complexes and micro-arousals as functions of sleep process. In: Koella WP, Levin P, eds. Sleep 1976. Basel: Karger, 1977:292–294.
93. Sterman MB, Harper RM, Havens B, Hoppenbrouwers T, McGinty DJ, Hodgman JE. Quantitative analysis of infant EEG development during quiet sleep. Electroencephalogr Clin Neurophysiol 1977; 43:371–385.
94. Guilleminault C, Souquet M. Sleep states and related pathology. In Korobkin R, Guilleminault C, eds. Advance in perinatal neurology. New York: SP Medical and Scientific Books, 1979:225–247.
95. Challamel MJ, Debilly G, Leszczynski MC, Revol M. Sleep state development in near-miss sudden death infants. In: Harper RM, Hoffman HJ, eds. Sudden Infant Death Syndrome: Risk Factors and Basic Mechanisms. New York: PMA Publishing, 1988:423–434.

96. Harper RM, Leake B, Miyahara L, Hoppenbrouwers T, Sterman MB, Hodgman JE. Temporal sequencing in sleep and waking states during the first 6 months of life. Exp Neurol 1981; 72:294–307.
97. Hoppenbrouwers T, Hodgman J, Harper RH, Sterman MB. Temporal distribution of sleep states, somatic and autonomic activity during the first half year of life. Sleep 1982; 5:131–144.
98. Coons S, Guilleminault C. Development of sleep-wake patterns and non rapid eye-movement sleep stages during the first 6 months of life in normal infants. Pediatrics 1982; 69:793–798.
99. Navelet Y, Benoit O, Bouard G. Nocturnal sleep organization during the first months of life. Electroencephalogr Clin Neurophysiol 1982; 54:71–78.
100. Hoppenbrouwers T. Sleep in infants. In: Guilleminault C, ed. Sleep and Its Disorders in Children. New York: Raven Press, 1987:1–16.
101. Fagioli I, Salzarulo P. Sleep states development in the first year of life assessed through 24-hour recordings. Early Hum Dev 1982; 6:215–228.
102. Hoppenbrouwers T, Hodgman J, Arakawa K, Geidel SA, Sterman MB. Sleep and waking states in infancy normative studies. Sleep 1988; 11:387–401.
103. Vecchierini-Blineau MF, Nogues B, Colin J. Awake periods during sleep in infants: a comparison between control and near-miss infants. In: Koella WP, Obal F, Schultz H, Visser P, eds. Sleep 1986. Stuttgart and New York: Gustav Fisher-Verlag, 1988:435–437.
104. Kohler WC, Dean Coddington R, Agnew HW. Sleep patterns in 2 year old children. J Pediatr 1968; 72:228–233.
105. Roffwarg HP, Dement W, Fisher C. Preliminary observation of the sleep dream pattern in neonates, infants, and adults. In: Hormes E, ed. Monographs on Child Psychiatry, New York: Pergamon Press, 1964:60–72.
106. Feinberg I, Korsko RL, Heller N. EEG sleep pattern as a function of normal and pathological aging in man. J Psychiatr Rev 1967; 5:107–144.
107. Navelet Y, D'Allest AM. Organisation du sommeil au cours de la croissance. In: Gaultier C, ed. Pathologie respiratoire du sommeil du nourrisson et de l'enfant. Paris: Vigot, 1989:23–32.
108. Parmelee AH, Wenner WH, Schulz HR. Infant sleep patterns: from birth to 16 weeks of age. J Pediatr 1964; 65:576–582.
109. Salzarulo P. Sleep patterns in infants under continuous feeding from birth. Electroencephalogr Clin Neurophysiol 1980; 49:330–336.
110. Mirmiran M, Kok JH, de Kleine MJK, Koppe, JG, Overdijik J, Witting W. Circadian rhythms in preterm infants: a preliminary study. Early Hum Dev 1990; 23:139–146.
111. McMillen IC, Kok JS, Adamson TM, Deayton JM, Nowak R. Development of circadian sleep-wake rhythms in preterm and full term infants. Pediatr Res 1991; 29:381–384.
112. Kleitman N, Engelmann TG. Sleep characteristics of infants. J Appl Physiol 1953; 6:269–282.
113. Tomioka K, Tomioka F. Development of circadian and ultradian rhythms of premature and full-term infants. J Interdiscipl Cycle Res 1991; 22:71–80.
114. Hellbrugge T. The development of circadian sleep wakefulness rhythmicity of three infants. In: Scheving LE, Halberg F, Pauly JE, eds. Chronobiology. Stuttgart: Thieme, 1974:339–341.
115. Meier-Koll A, Hall U, Hellwig U, Kott G, Meier-Koll VA. Biological oscillator system

and development of sleep-waking behavior during early infancy. Chronobiologia 1978; 5:425–440.

116. Coons S. Development of sleep and wakefulness during the first 6 months of life in normal infants. In: Guilleminault C, ed. Sleep and Its Disorders in Children. New York: Raven Press, 1987:17–27.
117. Anders TF, Halpern LF, Hua J. Sleeping through the night: a developmental perspective. Pediatrics 1992; 90:554–560.
118. Lodemore M, Petersen SA, Wailoo MP. Development of nighttime temperature rhythms over the first 6 months of life. Arch Dis Child 1991; 66:521–524.
119. Glotzbach SF, Dale ME, Boeddiker M, Ariagno RL. Biological rhythmicity in normal infants during the first 3 months of life. Pediatrics 1994; 94:482–488.
120. Weinert D, Sitka U, Minors DS, Waterhouse JM. The development of circadian rhythmicity in neonates. Early Hum Dev 1994; 36:117–126.
121. Sadeh A. Sleep and melatonin in infants: a preliminary study. Sleep 1997; 20: 185–191.
122. Spangler G. The emergence of adrenocortical circadian function in newborns and infants and its relationship to sleep, feeding and maternal adrenocortical activity. Early Hum Dev 1991; 25:197–208.
123. Ferber R, Boyle MP. Persistence of free-running sleep-wake rhythm in a one year old girl. Sleep Res 1983; 12:364.
124. Martin du Pan R. Some clinical applications of our knowledge of the evolution of the circadian rhythm in infants. In: Schewing LF, Halberg DF, Pauly JE, eds. Chronobiology. Stuttgart: Thieme, 1974:342–347.
125. Klackenberg G. Sleep behaviour studied longitudinally. Acta Paediatr Scand 1982; 71:501–506.
126. Beltrami AU, Hertzig ME. Sleep and bedtime behavior in pre-school-aged children. Pediatrics 1983; 71:153–158.
127. Koch P, Soussignan R, Montagner H. New data on the sleep-wake rhythm of children aged from 2½ to 4½ years. Acta Paediatr Scand 1984; 73:667–673.
128. Ferber R. Solve Your Child's Sleep Problems. New York: Simon & Schuster, 1985.
129. Sadeh A, Lavie P, Scher A, Tirosh E, Epstein R. Actigraphic home monitoring in sleep disturbed and control infants and young children: a new method for pediatric assessment of sleep wake patterns. Pediatrics 1991; 87:494–499.
130. Ardura J, Andres J, Aldana J, Revilla MA. Development of sleep-wakefulness rhythm in premature babies. Acta Paediatr 1995; 84:484–489.
131. Weissbluth M. Naps in children: 6 month-7 years. Sleep 1995; 18:82–87.
132. Ottaviano F, Giannotti F, Cortesi O, Bruni O, Ottaviano C. Sleep characteristics in healthy children from birth to 6 years of age in the urban area of Rome. Sleep 1996; 19:1–3.
133. Anders TF. Night-waking in infants during the first year of life. Pediatrics 1979; 63:860.
134. Moore T, Ucko LE. Night waking in early infancy. Arch Dis Child 1957; 32:333–342.
135. Adair R, Bauchner H, Philip B, Levenson S, Zucherman B. Night waking during infancy: the role of parental presence at bedtime. Pediatrics 1991; 87:500–503.
136. Schulz H, Massetani R, Fagioli I, Salzarulo P. Spontaneous awakening from sleep in infants. Electroencephalogr Clin Neurophysiol 1985; 61:267–271.
137. Schulz H, Salzarulo P, Fagioli I, Massetani R. REM latency: development in the first year of life. Electroencephalogr Clin Neurophysiol 1983; 56:316–322.
138. Bes F, Schulz H, Navelet Y, Salzarulo P. The distribution of slow wave sleep across the night: a comparison for infants, children and adults. Sleep 1991; 14:5–12.

139. Borbély AA, Baumann F, Brandeis D, Strauch I, Lehmann D. Sleep deprivation effect on sleep stages and EEG power density in man. Electroencephalogr Clin Neurophysiol 1981; 51:483–493.
140. Feinberg I, March JD. Observation on delta homeostasis, the one-stimulus model of NREM-REM alternation and the neurobiologic implications of experimental dream studies. Behav Brain Res 1995; 69:97–108.
141. Bes F, Baroncini P, Dugovic C, Fagioli I, Schulz H, Franc B, Salzarulo P. Time course of EEG activity during night sleep in the first year of life based on automatic analysis. Electroencephalogr Clin Neurophysiol 1988; 69:501–507.
142. Bes F, Fagioli I, Peirano P, Schulz H, Salzarulo P. Trend in EEG synchronisation across nonREM sleep in infants. Sleep 1994; 17:323–328.
143. Schechtman VL, Harper RK, Harper RM. Distribution of slow-wave EEG activity across the night in developing infants. Sleep 1994; 17:316–322.
144. Salzarulo P, Fagioli I. Postnatal development of sleep organization in man: speculations on the emergence of the "S process." Neurophysiol Clin 1992; 22:107–115.
145. Fagioli I, Bes F, Peirano P, Salzarulo P. Dynamics of EEG background activity level within quiet sleep in successive cycle in infants. Electroenceph Clin Neurophysiol 1995; 94:6–11.
146. Oswald I. Sleep as a restorative process: human clues. Prog Brain Res 1980; 50:279–287.
147. Adam K, Oswald I. Protein synthesis, bodily renewal and the sleep-wake cycle. Clin Sci 1983; 65:561–567.
148. Jouvet M. Does a genetic programming of the brain occur during paradoxical sleep? Cerebral correlation of conscious experience. In: Buser PA, Rougeul-Buser A, eds. Symposium INSERM. Amsterdam: Elsevier, 1978; 6:256.
149. Sastre JP, Jouvet M. Le comportement onirique du chat. Physiol Behav 1978; 22:979–989.
150. Jouvet M. Programmation génétique itérative et sommeil paradoxal. Confrontations psychiatriques 1986; 27:153–181.
151. Horne JA, McGrath MJ. The consolidation hypothesis for REM sleep function and other confounding factors: a review. Biol Psychol 1984; 18:165–184.
152. Cipolli C. Sleep, dreams and memory: an overview. J Sleep Res 1995; 4:2–9.
153. Sawaya R, Ingvar D. Cerebral blood flow and metabolism in sleep. Acta Neurol Scand 1989; 80:481–491.
154. Madsen PL, Vostrup S. Cerebral blood flow and metabolism during sleep. Cerebrovasc Brain Metab Rev 1991; 3:281–296.
155. Rahilly PM. Effects of sleep state and feeding on cranial blood flow in the human neonate. Arch Dis Child 1980; 55:265–270.
156. Mukhtar AL, Cowan FM, Sothers JK. Cranial blood flow and blood pressure changes during sleep in the human neonate. Early Hum Dev 1982; 6:59–64.
157. Greisen G, Hellström-Vestas L, Lou H, Rosen I, Svenningsen N. Sleep-waking shifts and cerebral blood flow in stable pre-term infants. Pediatr Res 1985; 19:1156–1159.
158. Dittrichova J, Paul K, Pavlikova E. Rapid eye movements in paradoxical sleep in infants. Neuropaediatrie 1972; 3:248–257.
159. Ktonas PY, Bes FW, Rigoard MT, Wong C, Mallart R, Salzarulo P. Developmental changes in the clustering pattern of sleep rapid eye movement activity during the first year of life: a Markov-process approach. Electroenceph Clin Neurophysiol 1990; 75:136–140.

160. Fishbein W, Gutwein BM. Paradoxical sleep and memory storage process. Behav Biol 1977; 19:425–464.
161. Smith C. Sleep states and learning: a review of the animal literature. Neurosci Behav Rev 1985; 9:157–168.
162. Dujardin K, Guerrien A, Leconte P. Review: sleep, brain activation and cognition. Physiol Behav 1990; 47:1271–1278.
163. Dittrichova J, Paul K, Vondracek J. Le développement de l'endormissement au cours des premiers mois de la vie chez l'homme. Rev EEG Neurophysiol 1981; 11:17–22.
164. Paul K, Dittrichova J. Sleep patterns following learning in infants. In: Levin P, Koella V, eds. Sleep 74. New York: Karger, 1975:388–390.
165. Challamel MJ. Fonction du sommeil paradoxal et ontogenese. Neurophysiol Clin 1992; 22:117–132.
166. Denenberg VH, Thoman EB. Evidence for a functional role for active (REM) sleep in infancy. Sleep 1981; 4:185–191.
167. Anders TF, Roffwarg HP. The effect of selective interruption and deprivation of sleep in the human newborn. Dev Psychobiol 1973; 6:77–90.
168. Berger RJ, Meier GW. The effect of selective deprivation of states of sleep in the developing monkey. Psychophysiology 1966; 2:354–371.
169. Valatx JL, Nowaczyck T. Essai de suppression pharmacologique du sommeil paradoxal chez le rat nouveau-né. Rev EEG Neurophysiol 1977; 7:269–272.
170. Oksenberg A, Shaffery JP, Marks GA, Speciale SG, Mihailoff G, Roffwarg HP. Rapid eye movement sleep deprivation in kittens amplifies LGN cell-size disparity induced by monocular deprivation. Brain Res Dev Brain Res 1996; 97:51–61.
171. Davenne D, Frégnac Y, Imbert M, Adrien J. Lesion of the PGO pathways in the kitten. II. Impairement of the lateral geniculate nucleus. Brain Res 1989; 485:267–277.
172. Marks GA, Shaffery JP, Oksenberg A, Speciale SG, Roffwarg HP. A functional role for REM sleep in brain maturation. Behav Brain Res 1995; 69:1–11.
173. Pompeiano O, Pompeiano M, Corvaja N. Effects of sleep deprivation on the postnatal development of visual-deprived cells in the cat's lateral geniculate nucleus. Arch Ital Biol 1995; 143:121–140.
174. Mirmiran M, Van De Poll NE, Corner MA, Van Oyen HG, Bour HL. Suppression of active sleep by chronic treatment with chlorimipramine during early post-natal development: effects upon adult brain and behavior in the rat. Brain Res 1981; 204:129–146.
175. Mirmiran M, Sholtens J, Van de Poll NE, Uyglings HBM, Van Der Gutgen J, Boer J. Effects of experimental suppression of active (REM) sleep during early development upon adult brain and behavior in the rat. Brain Res 1983; 7:277–286.
176. Challamel MJ, Lahlou S, Revol M, Jouvet M. Sleep and smiling in neonate: a new approach. In: Koella WP, Ruther E, Schulz H, eds. Sleep 84. Stuttgart: Gustav Fisher Verlag, 1985:290–292.

2

Ontogeny of EEG Sleep from the Neonatal Through Infancy Periods

MARK S. SCHER

Case Western Reserve University
and Rainbow Babies & Children's Hospital
University Hospitals of Cleveland
Cleveland, Ohio

I. Introduction

Electrographic and polygraphic recordings of newborns and infants have been performed for almost half a century. Pioneering studies by multiple researchers worldwide offer neurophysiological information concerning the developing central nervous system (1–8). Earlier investigations predated the creation of the modern neonatal intensive care unit; however, these seminal works described for the first time electrographic patterns and physiological behaviors that define rudimentary state of the preterm neonate. Given the higher rate of neonatal mortality, particularly among premature infants, the clinical neurophysiologist had a more limited consultative role in the neurological care of the sick neonate. With the creation of the modern-day tertiary care neonatal intensive care unit, sophisticated medical care—including technological improvements in physiological recordings—now offer the neurological consultant a more active role in neonatal neurophysiological assessments for medical care.

The decline in neonatal morbidity and mortality has concentrated renewed attention on the infant's neurological performance both during the acute and convalescent periods in the days to weeks after birth. Given the immature clinical repertoire of the newborn and infant as well as limited access to neonates in a busy neonatal intensive care unit (NICU). Electrocardiographic (EEG)-polygraphic studies extend the clinician's abilities to document functional brain maturation as well as the presence and severity of encephalopathic states. Neonatal survivors also require close supervision during infancy as successive stages in brain maturation occur.

Maturation of infant behavior requires careful study of both waking and sleep behaviors. Using neurophysiological monitoring to assess functional brain maturation during infancy, the clinician possesses a powerful probe to evaluate different pediatric populations who are at risk for developmental delay or specific dysfunctional performance during sleep or wakefulness.

II. Caveats Concerning Neurophysiological Interpretation of State

A number of caveats will help the neurophysiologist to understand the application of sleep interpretation from the neonatal through infancy periods. Maturational changes of EEG-polygraphic patterns emerge at successively older postconceptional ages: the neurophysiological maturity of a neonate can be estimated within 2 weeks for the preterm infant and 1 week for the full-term infant, reflecting the postconceptional age of the infant independent of birthweight or postnatal age. Temporal coincidence or concordance among physiological behaviors emerge with increasing maturity, similar to fetal behavioral states. Significant reorganization of state occurs at 30, 36, and 48 weeks postconception. Finally, serial neurophysiological studies rather than a single recording more accurately document normal ontogeny or the evolution of encephalopathic changes reflective of a brain disorder. Subsequent developmental stages also occur during infancy, with sleep reorganization after 3, 9, and 12 months of age.

The clinician needs to develop a confident style of neurophysiological pattern recognition and clinical correlation by repetitive experiences with a wide variety of EEG-polygraphic recordings. Before an accurate interpretation can be imparted to the referring clinician, knowledge of the child's post-conceptional age as well as the range of behavioral phenomena displayed during the recording are needed; this requires close communication between the electrodiagnostic technologist and the neurophysiologist.

A. General Comments on Recording Techniques and Instrumentation for Neonates and Infants

Appropriate recording techniques will yield high-quality EEG-polygraphic studies. The neurophysiologist should apply a minimum of 10 EEG electrodes in addition to a full complement of noncerebral polygraphic electrodes, given that specific regional and hemispheric electrographic patterns need to be correlated with other noncerebral physiological behaviors. Placement of electrodes by either paste or collodion must be achieved with ease and efficiency by the technologist, who is always cognizant of the fragile state of the neonate within the busy NICU environment. While double interelectrode distances may be required for the infant of less than 36 weeks estimated gestational age (EGA), to better visualize electrographic patterns, a complete set of EEG electrodes will be required for monitoring the full-term newborn and older infant.

Adjustments in sensitivity, paper speed, and filter settings will facilitate electrographic/polysomnographic interpretation. Sensitivity settings should begin with standard 7 μV/mm but may need to be periodically adjusted during the recording. Lower-frequency filter settings are preferred between 0.25 and 0.5 for neonatal recordings to avoid the elimination of commonly occurring slow-frequency wave forms. Slower paper speeds (such as 15 mm/sec) will permit easier visualization of slowly recurring normal features, such as EEG discontinuity and asynchrony or abnormal features such as seizures and periodic discharges. Adjustment to a lower filter settings of 1 Hz and a paper speed of 30 mm/sec may be preferred, for infants after 6 to 8 weeks of age.

Motility, cardiorespiratory function, and eye movements are essential noncerebral physiological behaviors to record. Noncerebral physiological observations are relevant for both state identification as well as corroboration of a clinical observation that may have prompted the request for the study. Sources of artifact are also more readily identified and eliminated with the consistent use of noncerebral channels, supplemented by the technologist's comments.

Frequent and accurate annotations by the technologist throughout the study are strongly advised. Eye opening and eye closure as well as repositioning of the patient's head are common annotations that are essential for proper interpretation. Information from the medical record regarding the child's gestational and postconceptional ages should be recorded by the technologist for the physician's use, as well as states of arousal, medications and medical procedures. Skull defects, vital signs, and pertinent laboratory studies should all be described, since certain factors may affect neurophysiological interpretation.

III. Maturation of Electrographic Patterns in the Neonate

A number of principles should be applied by the neurophysiologist for an accurate interpretation of a neonatal EEG-sleep study. It is essential that the neurophysiologist be able to interpret expected age-appropriate neurophysiological patterns before attempting to recognize features (10). Changes in EEG-polygraphic patterns occur for neonates at increasing postconceptional ages (PCAs) up to term and into early infancy. PCA is calculated simply as the infant's estimated gestational age at birth plus the number of weeks of postnatal life (i.e., estimated gestational age at birth plus postnatal age equals PCA in weeks). The neurophysiologist should approximate the electrical maturity of the preterm infant within 2 weeks of other estimates of maturity and 1 week for a term infant. Preterm neonates recorded at PCAs up to term will express EEG patterns similar to those of a child born at that comparable level of maturity;

subtle differences may also be present because of functional brain adaptation to prematurity, as discussed further on.

Two studies exemplify how neurophysiological estimates of gestational maturity can be achieved by pattern recognition of EEG-sleep recordings for either healthy or sick preterm cohorts (11,12). Such neurophysiological estimates of maturity were offered, even without accurate clinical examination criteria, fetal sonographic data, or other obstetrical information regarding gestational maturity; for both the healthy or sick preterm groups, assessment of neurophysiological gestational maturity was as accurate as clinical and/or anatomic estimates. Such neurophysiological information may be essential in problematic situations where gestational maturity is not accurately assessed by other methods. This is particularly true in dealing with high-risk pregnancies where accurate information with respect to gestational maturity may not be available, symptomatic infants who are too medically ill to permit assessment of postural tone or levels of arousal, or infants too premature to exhibit postural tone, primitive reflexes, or behavioral alterations during state transition to allow an accurate estimation of brain maturity.

Regional and hemispheric electrographic patterns for the preterm and fullterm neonate are initially discussed below, emphasizing major features at successively older PCAs. Specific aspects of temporal, spatial and state organization of EEG-polygraphic recordings are subsequently highlighted, but this brief review should be supplemented by more detailed discussions in standard texts (1,4,6–8).

A. EEG Discontinuity

Alternating segments of EEG activity and inactivity (i.e., quiescence) commonly occur in preterm neonates and have been described as EEG or trace discontinuity (13). For the child of less than 30 weeks PCA, neonatal recordings consist of predominantly discontinuous EEG patterns. Varying durations of interburst intervals define this quiescence and have been described by various authors (14–18). For the healthy preterm infant, an interburst interval should follow the "30-20 rule": an interburst interval should not exceed 30 sec in duration on multiple occasions for the child of less than 30 weeks EGA. As the child matures beyond 30 weeks PCA, the interburst interval should be less than 20 sec in duration. Longer periods of EEG continuity interrupt quiescent intervals after 28 weeks PCA.

For the preterm infant of less than 30 weeks PCA, electrographic activities predominate in the vertex and the central and occipital regions; bitemporal attenuation is commonly observed and reflects underdeveloped frontal and temporal regions of the brain at that level of brain maturity (Fig. 1, panel 1).

B. Synchrony/Asynchrony

The electrophysiological description known as asynchrony (19) refers to similarly appearing waveforms of EEG activity in homologous head regions (e.g., left and right temporal regions) that are separated by at least 1.5 sec in time. Preterm neonates express varying degrees of physiological asynchrony. While the infant less than 30

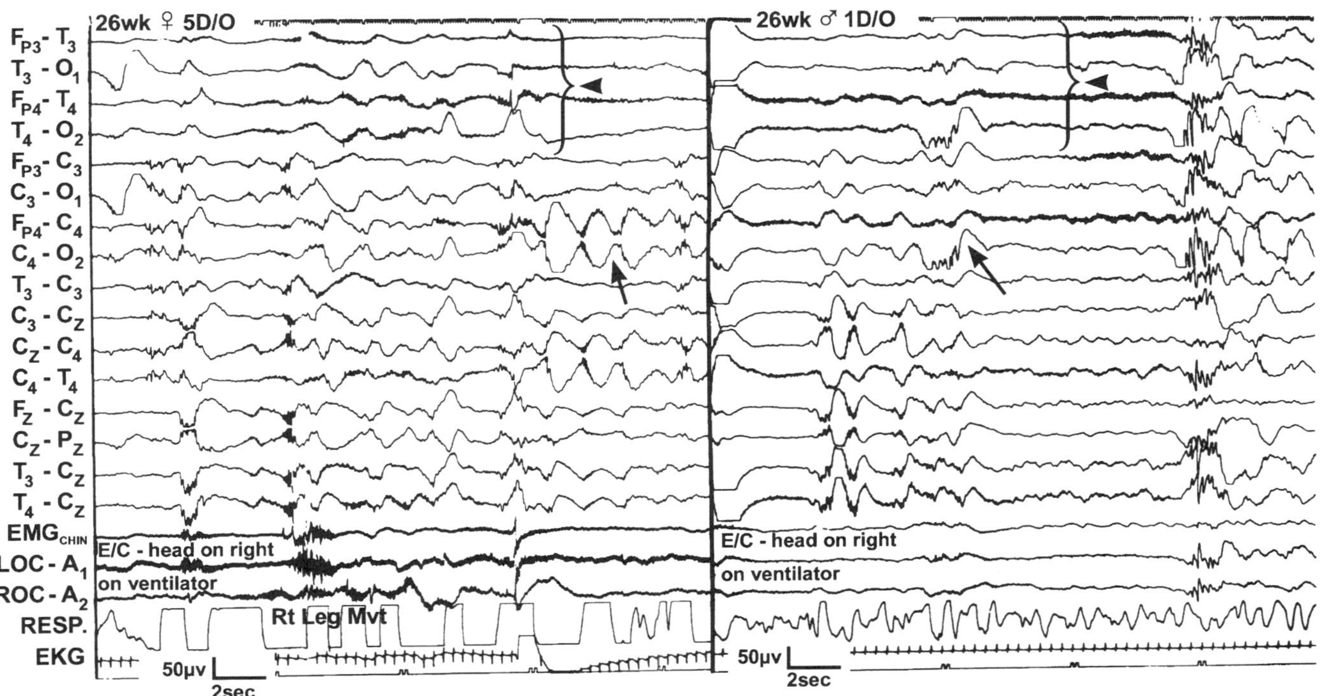

Figure 1 Segments of EEGs of two preterm infants, a less than 26-week PCA 5-day-old and 26-week PCA 1-day-old respectively. Note, the prominent bitemporal attenuation (arrowheads, both panels), the rhythmic delta with superimposed delta brushes in the central regions (first panel, arrow), and the hypersynchronous burst in the second panel. Isolated occipital delta with superimposed occipital theta are also noted in the second panel (arrow).

weeks PCA commonly exhibits "hypersynchrony" because of its extreme cortical immaturity (Fig. 1, panel 2), physiological asynchrony emerges after 30 weeks PCA and persists until 36 weeks PCA. Asynchrony in the child at 30 to 32 weeks may be as much as 50% of the discontinuous portion of the sleep cycle, but after 36 weeks PCA the occurrence of asynchrony rapidly drops to zero percent when the infant's age reaches term.

C. Delta Brush Patterns

An admixture of fast and slow rhythms appears in the preterm EEG record as morphologically discrete waveforms identified with preterm neonates at varying PCAs (Figs. 1, 3, 4, 5). Random or briefly rhythmic 0.3- to 1.5-Hz delta activity of 50 to 250 μV is associated with a superimposed rhythm of low- to moderate-amplitude faster frequencies of 10 to 20 Hz. Historically, different authors have described these complexes as spindle delta bursts, brushes, spindle-like fast waves, and ripples of prematurity. For infants of less than 28 weeks PCA, delta brush patterns are seen in the central and midline locations with only occasional expression in the occipital regions (Fig. 1). After 28 weeks PCA, brushes appear more abundantly in the occipital followed by the temporal regions (Figs. 3, 4, 5). Brushes can be asynchronous or asymmetrical, while at other times they may be symmetrical (Fig. 5). By term PCA, brush patterns are occasionally noted during the non-rapid-eye-movement (NREM) quiet sleep or transitional sleep segments. Persistent expression or attenuation of brush rhythms in one region or hemisphere may reflect structural lesions.

D. Occipital Theta/Alpha Rhythms

Other patterns that can help estimate gestational maturity are the monorhythmic alpha and theta activities located in the occipital region of neonates less than 28 weeks PCA, commonly referred to as the STOP rhythm (20). This pattern usually persists for 6 to 10 sec, can be asynchronous or asymmetrical, but may also be synchronous (Fig. 2). Such a pattern, together with midline/central brushes, is an electrographic feature associated with extremely premature infants.

E. Temporal Theta Rhythm

A third useful developmental marker that estimates brain maturity is the burst of rhythmic 4.5- to 6-Hz activities noted in the midtemporal regions (Fig. 3, panel 1; Fig. 4). Temporal theta bursts are rarely apparent in infants less than 28 weeks PCA but become maximally expressed between 28 and 32 weeks PCA. Historically, this feature has been described as a "temporal sawtooth wave" (14), with amplitudes ranging from 20 to 200 μV. After 32 weeks PCA, its incidence rapidly diminishes (21).

F. Delta Wave Patterns

Rhythmic runs of delta activity can also help estimate the gestational maturity of the asymptomatic preterm neonate. Delta patterns in the central midline location are pre-

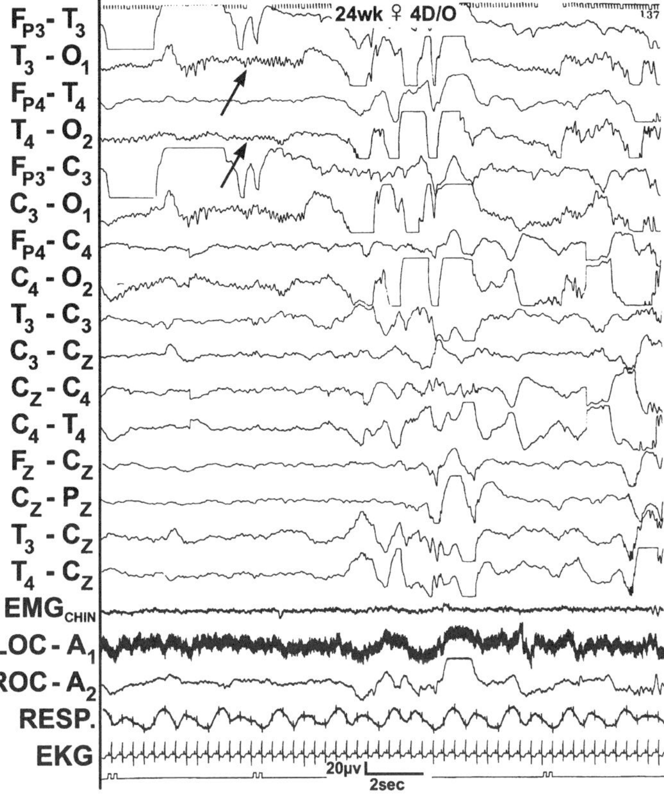

Figure 2 An EEG segment of a 24-week PCA 4-day-old female with prolonged occipital theta alpha that is asymmetrical in amplitude (arrows), characteristic of the STOP rhythm.

dominant for the infant of less than 28 weeks gestation, together with bitemporal attenuation, as previously described (Fig. 1). Other delta rhythms occur in the temporal and occipital locations, particularly after 28 weeks of gestation. Between 30 and 34 weeks PCA, temporal and occipital delta rhythms become quite prominent and rhythmic, with durations that may range from 30 sec to 1 min (Figs. 2 and 3).

G. Midline Theta/Alpha Activity

A recently described waveform phenomenon (22) appears on recordings of both preterm and full-term infants, particularly during transitional or quiet sleep segments. This commonly observed pattern is sharply contoured and usually of low to moderate amplitude (Fig. 6) in the alpha or theta ranges. While it is morphologically similar to a sleep spindle, classical spindles do not appear in the central regions until 2 to 4 months of age (23).

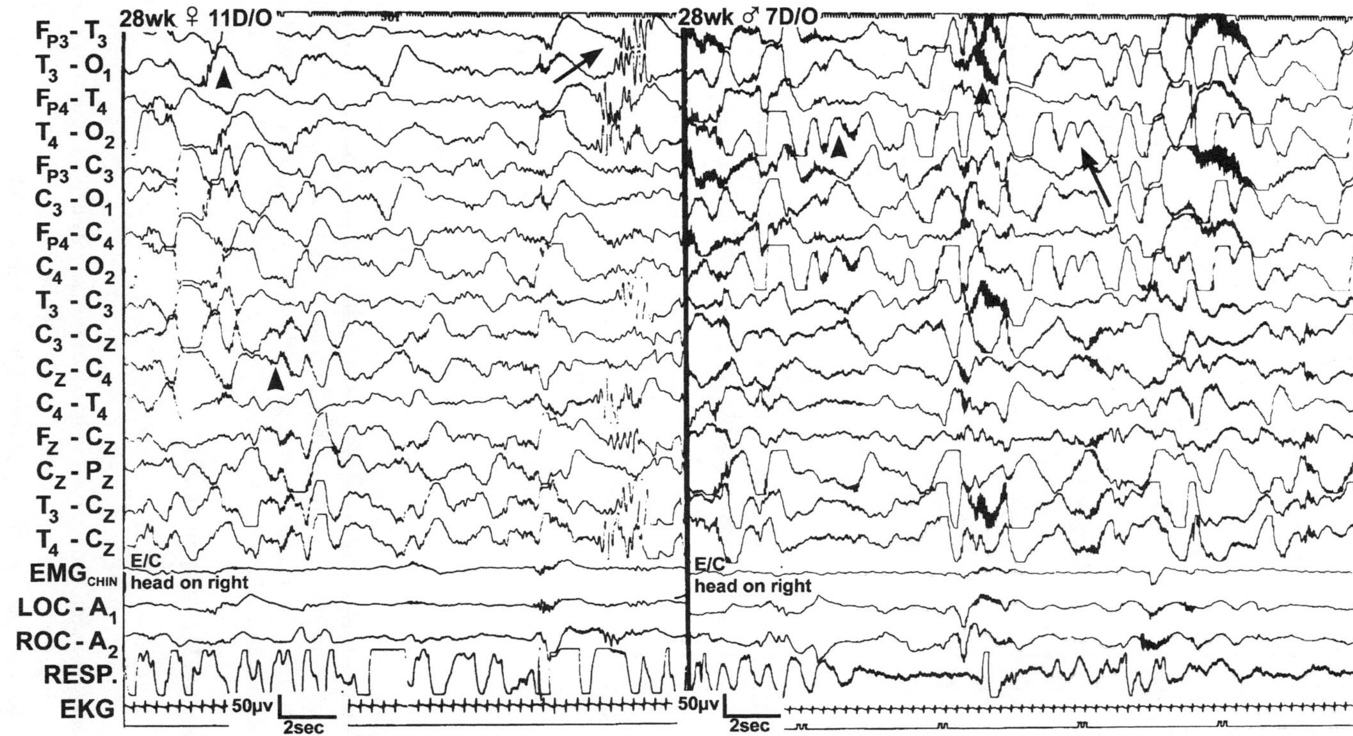

Figure 3 Segments of EEGs of two preterm infants approximately 29 weeks PCA, depicting abundant delta in multiple head regions as well as temporal theta activity (first panel, arrow), temporo-occipital, vertex, and central brush patterns, first and second panels (arrowheads), and rhythmic occipital delta (second panel, arrow).

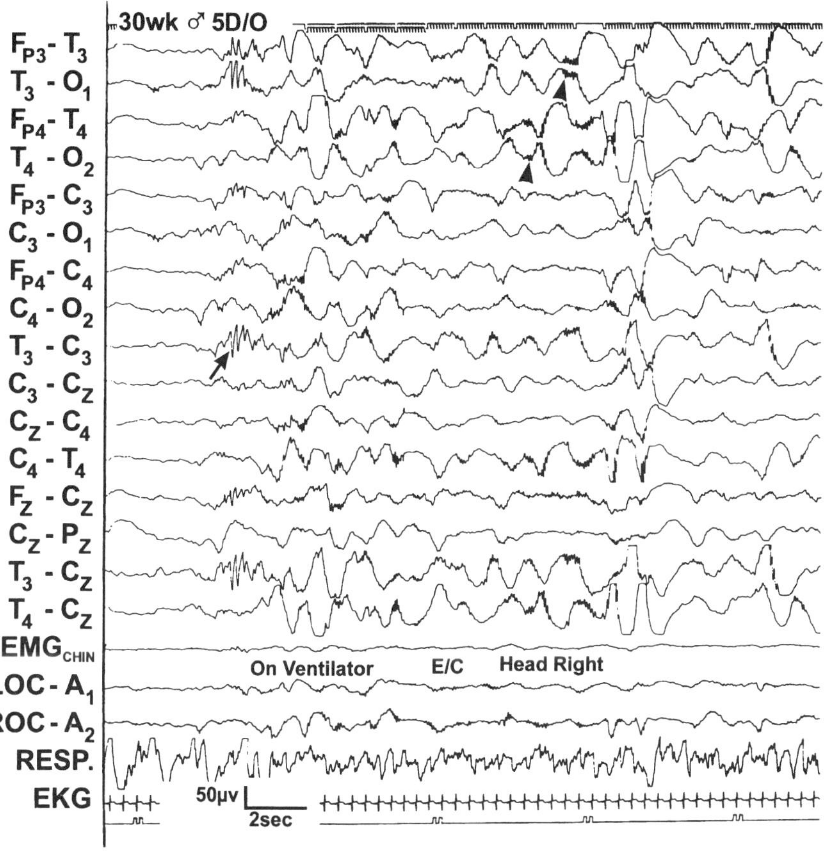

Figure 4 An EEG segment of a nearly 30-week PCA 5-day-old male, depicting the onset of continuous EEG segment with a left temporal theta burst (arrow), prominent delta, and superimposed delta brushes in the temporal regions (arrowheads). Note that the temporal delta is more rhythmic than in Figure 3.

While it may appear sharply contoured, this age-appropriate electrographic rhythm does not reflect a pathological or encephalopathic state.

IV. Maturation of Noncerebral Physiological Behaviors That Define State in the Preterm Infant

State transitions in preterm infants less than 36 weeks PCA are not as easily identified as in the term infant. Sleep reorganization is expected to occur at or around 36 weeks PCA, which is similar to the age in utero when coalescence of physiological

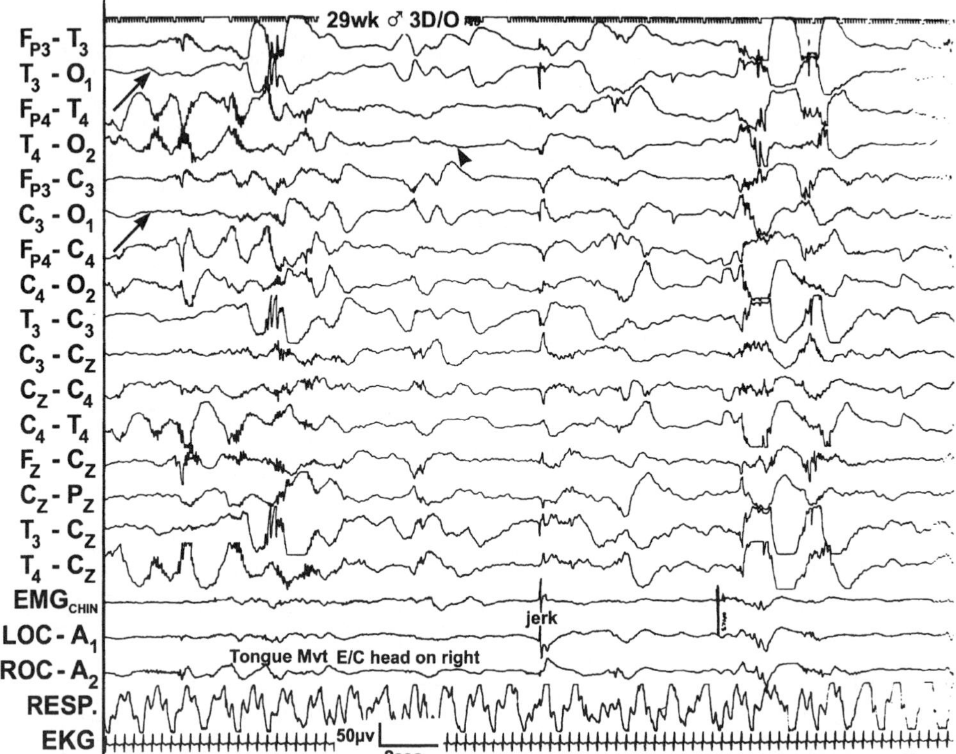

Figure 5 An EEG segment of a 29-week PCA 3-day-old male with a shifting asymmetry between the left temporal-central region (arrows) and the right temporal region (arrowhead), characteristic of physiological interhemispheric asynchrony. Also note the prominent temporal theta and brushes as well as diffuse delta slowing during this discontinuous portion of the EEG.

behavior is documented on abdominal sonography of fetal behavior. As a rule, state organization in the preterm infant is rudimentary and underdeveloped (24,25). The following summary serves as an introduction to a discussion of specific physiological behaviors that highlight state differentiation in the preterm infant at increasing PCAs.

Rapid eye movements represent one of the main identifying features of rudimentary active sleep in the preterm infant. This eye-movement phenomenon becomes more consistently time-locked to continuous EEG activities as early as 30 to 31 weeks gestation (24). Using fetal sonography (29), fetal eye movements during active sleep have also been documented. REM activity is not a random rhythm and does occur in a predictable interval despite brain immaturity (26). Various classes of REM have

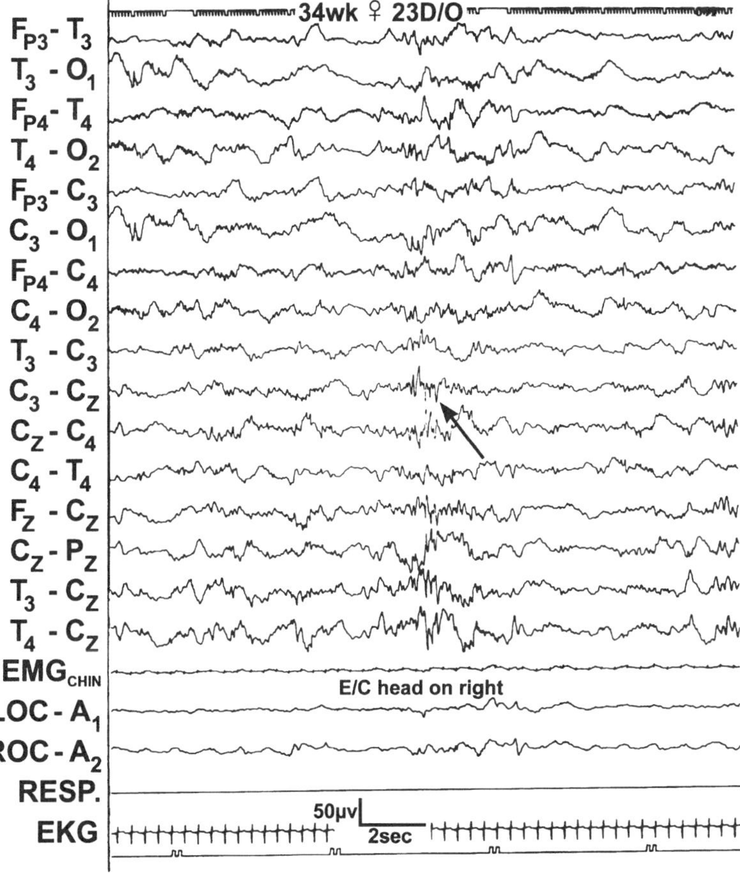

Figure 6 An EEG segment for a 34-week PCA 23-day-old female with a prominent vertex and parasagittal burst of theta/alpha activity (arrow). Note the rare delta brushes and absent temporal theta at a PCA of 37 weeks.

been described during different states of sleep in the neonate, and the number and types of REM movements evolve with brain maturation (27,28). A recent study of multiple physiological behaviors during the sleep in the preterm infant correlated the occurrence of REM with more continuous EEG tracings, while they correlated negatively with discontinuous EEG segments (30) in preterm infants as early as 30 weeks PCA.

Motility patterns are also an integral part of state definition for the neonate but-differ between the preterm and fullterm infants. Different motility patterns emerge at increasing postconceptional ages, both for the fetus as well as the extrauterine-reared neonate (31,32). Myoclonic and whole-body movements predominate for the preterm infant (33,34), while smaller, slower segmental body movements are seen in the full-term neonate. State-specific decreases in the number of small and large body movements have been correlated with increasing EEG discontinuity in preterm infants (30), while increased head and facial movements are associated only with active sleep between 30 and 36 weeks PCA.

Maturational changes in cardiorespiratory behavior have also been studied in the preterm infant. Periodic breathing and respiratory pauses are physiological events that commonly occur in preterm infants (35,36). Using spectral analyses, decreased variability of cardiorespiratory behavior during quiet sleep is seen at increasing PCAs (37). However, EEG measures appear to be stronger indicators of state transitions than noncerebral measures, such as cardiorespiratory behavior. In a recent study of multiple sleep behaviors in the preterm infant less than 36 weeks PCA, rapid eye movements rather than cardiorespiratory, motility, and temperature changes predictably varied with EEG changes, suggesting that specific brain regions coalesce physiologically with EEG activities before other neuronal systems do so (38).

V. Assessment of State Organization in the Full-Term Infant

Extensive information has been published over the last half-century with respect to the functional significance of the relatively short ultradian sleep rhythm in the neonate (39). For older infants, the human sleep cycle is an ultradian period with an interval of 75 to 90 min. The full-term neonate expresses an ultradian cycle that is approximating 30 to 70 min. in duration (40). Sleep segments that comprise the neonatal sleep cycle also differ from those of older individuals when EEG and polysomnographic behaviors are compared. Two active and two quiet sleep segments as well as transitional or indeterminate sleep segments have been described. Arousal periods, defined as reactivity, occur both within and between the sleep segments. Indeterminate or transitional sleep as well as the arousal phenomena are important expressions of sleep continuity in the immature brain.

State definitions in the term infant traditionally require the temporal coalescence of specific physiological behaviors. Based on visual analyses, comparisons between cerebral and noncerebral behaviors are temporally observed to determine state for either adults or children (41). Visual interpretations of EEG-sleep states are also easily identified for the full-term neonate (8). Active or REM sleep for the full-term neonate is traditionally associated with the coalescence of rapid eye movements, increased variability of cardiorespiratory rates, low muscle tone in the context of low-voltage or mixed-frequency continuous EEG patterns, and the abundance of body movements. Conversely, quiet or non-REM sleep is associated with the absence of rapid eye movements, fewer body movements, higher muscle tone, and decreased variability in respiratory rates in the context of continuous high-voltage slow or discontinuous EEG patterns. The patterns described above are not expressed until after

36 weeks PCA, but are no longer seen beyond 46 to 48 weeks PCA. Typically, the ultradian sleep cycle begins as active sleep after sleep onset in over 50% of newborns. This initial active sleep segment is a mixed frequency EEG segment which represents 25% to 30% of the total sleep cycle (Fig. 7). This active sleep segment is then followed by a brief period of high-voltage, slow quiet sleep that is approximately 3% to 5% of the sleep cycle (Fig. 8). Subsequently, a discontinuous quiet sleep period (historically described as a *tracé alternant* pattern) now represents approximately 25% of the sleep cycle of the neonate (Fig. 9). Finally, a post–quiet sleep active sleep segment known as *low-voltage irregular* makes up approximately 15% of the cycle (Fig. 10). Transitional or indeterminate sleep represents between 10% to 15% of the sleep cycle. While the child does not yet express a strong diurnal or circadian rhythmicity of sleep, wakefulness is distributed over a 24-hr period; as many as 6 to 8 hr of waking sleep over a 24-hr period in the neonate may occur.

Two biorhythmic processes define the temporal organization of sleep in the neonate: a weak circadian sleep wave rhythm is present, and a stronger ultradian REM and non-REM rhythm is also active (42). Both biorhythms evolve with increasing age. Internal "biological clocks" become better organized around environmental cues, such as the light/dark cycle, temperature, noise, and social interaction (43). For the normal full-term neonate, sleep alternates with waking states in a 3- to 4-hr cycle during both night and day. This has historically been referred to as the basic rest/activity cycle (BRAC).

Within the first month or two of life after birth for the full-term infant, reorganization of the sleep–wake state begins, particularly with a more dominant diurnal effect to environmental cues. Circadian rhythmicity of body temperature and heart rate is noted in approximately 50% of preterm infants at 29 to 35 weeks PCA (44). Yet stronger ultradian rhythms over a 3- to 4-hr duration correspond to social intervention such as feeding (41). Increases in body movement activities as well as heart rate and decreases in rectal and skin temperatures are noted during interventions, reflecting changes in the infant's microenvironment and the infant–caretaker interaction. The length of the ultradian EEG sleep cycle increases with maturing PCA, demonstrating a positive correlation between cycle length and increasing PCA (30).

VI. Sleep Ontogenesis: State Maturation from Fetal Through Infancy Periods

Reasons for the continuity in the expression of state from the fetal through neonatal ages prior to 46 weeks EGA remains obscure, but may reflect the need for physiological homeostasis during the transition from intrauterine to extrauterine environments. Recent work with fetal baboons has documented similar coalescence among EEG patterns and noncerebral behaviors within the intrauterine environment for primate species similar to humans (45). These same relationships are expressed by preterm neonates in an extrauterine environment. Physiological interrelationships

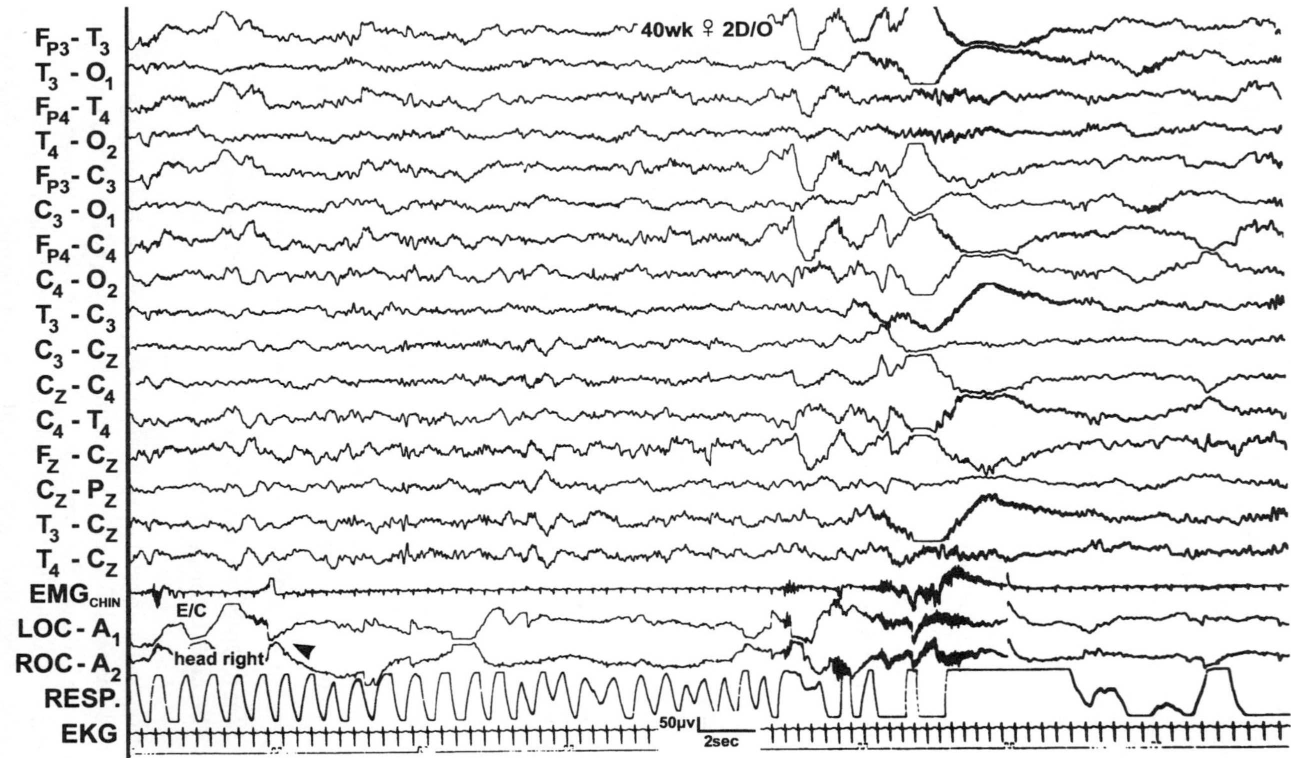

Figure 7 An EEG segment for a 40-week PCA 2-day-old female, depicting mixed-frequency active sleep characterized by continuous EEG, body movements, rapid eye movements (arrowhead), and irregular respirations and heart rate. Note the onset of a spontaneous arousal coincident with a temporary flattening of the EEG background.

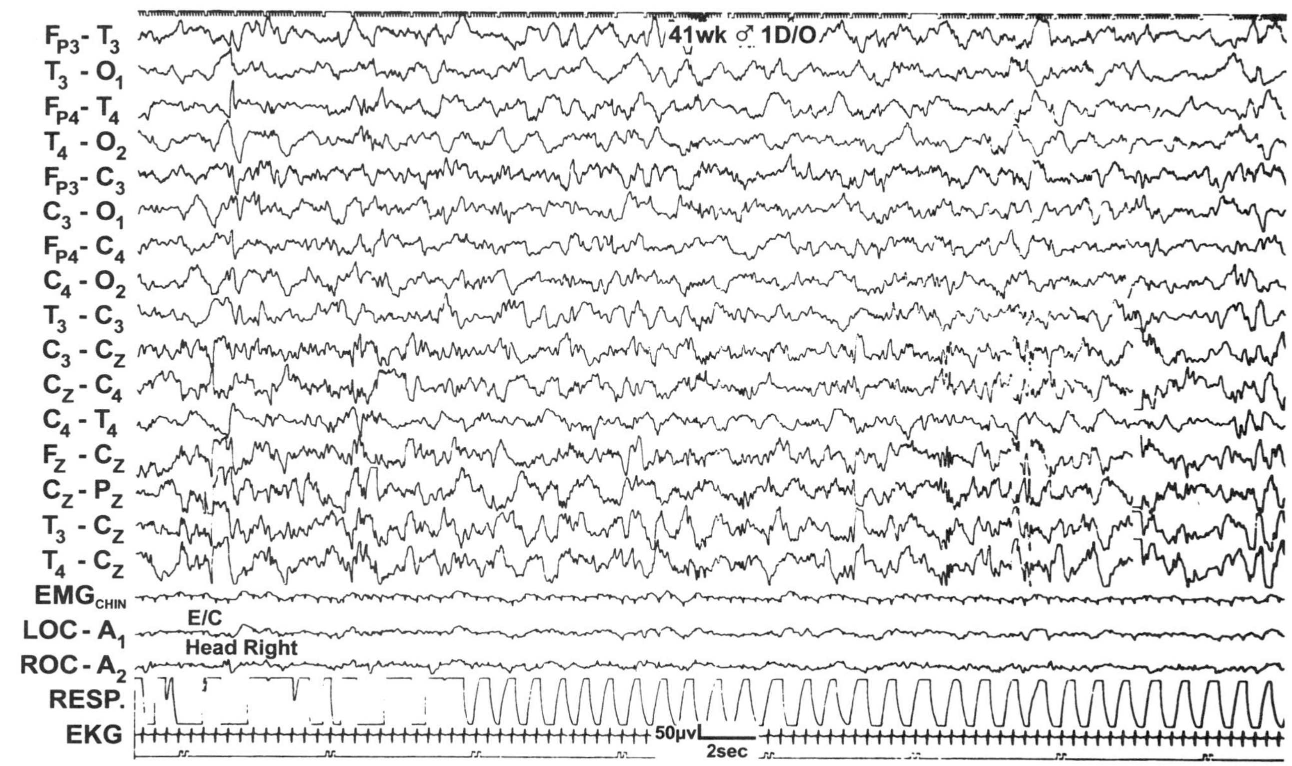

Figure 8 An EEG segment of a 40-week 1-day-old female that documents high-voltage, slow, quiet sleep. Regular respirations and the absence of rapid eye movements are noted.

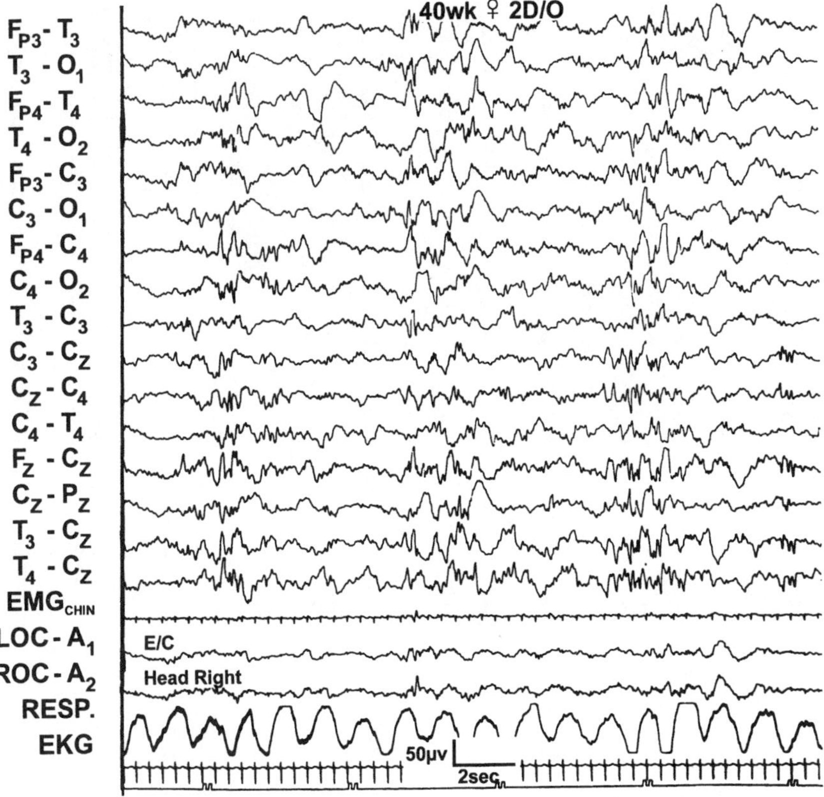

Figure 9 An EEG segment for a 40-week PCA 15-day-old female documenting a discontinuous trace alternant, quiet sleep segment.

that define fetal/neonatal sleep states persist well past the child's expected birthday; however, beyond 6 to 8 weeks of age, infants express sleep rhythms that slowly evolve toward adult sleep rhythms by the second year of life. Following the coalescence of cerebral and noncerebral components of state from fetal through neonatal ages, sleep state reorganization continues after 46 to 48 weeks PCA, with the emergence of more adult-like sleep behaviors.

Specific aspects of reorganization of sleep occur after 46 to 48 weeks EGA, but emerge gradually over the first 2 years of life. Lengthening of the overall sleep cycle as well as reorganization of sleep architecture occurs, gradual reductions in REM sleep percentage are noted, and non-REM sleep becomes more abundant. Rather than a sleep-onset active or REM period, a non-REM sleep segment appears after sleep onset. Non-REM sleep stages I to IV are not fully developed until later during infancy. High-voltage delta slow non-REM sleep becomes the predominant electro-

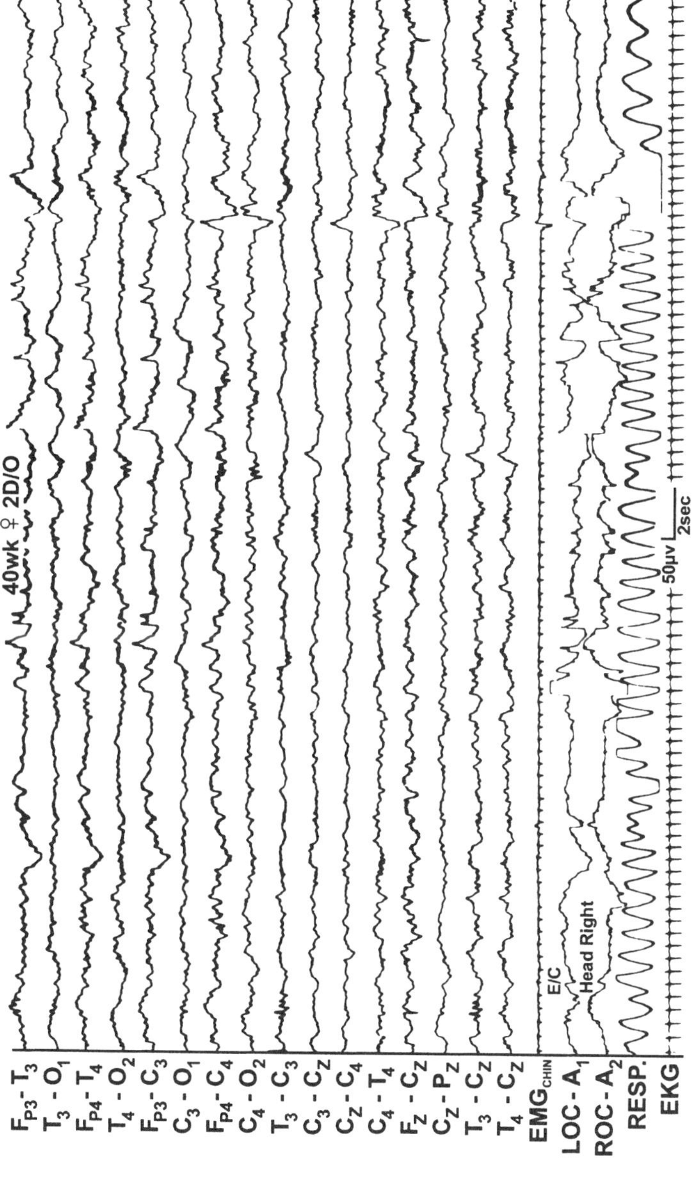

Figure 10 An EEG segment for a 40-week, 2-day-old female, documenting a low-voltage irregular active sleep segment. Note prominent sucking and REMs.

graphic expression of this segment of the sleep cycle, unlike the brief high-voltage slow segment during the neonatal sleep cycle. Decreases in arousals and in body and REM movements are also noted as the child matures past 46 to 48 weeks PCA.

During the first 3 months of life, rapid maturation of electrical activities in the brain occurs, such as the disappearance of *tracé alternant*, the emergence of sleep spindle activity, and the emergence of "adult-type" delta wave activity (46–49). Using quantitative assessments of spectral EEG, increases in theta frequencies by 9 months of age (50,51), herald the emergence of the S1 and S2 segments of the non-REM sleep segment, codified for adult subjects by Rechtschaffen and Kales sleep state criteria (41). There is also a continual decrease in total sleep time, REM sleep, and indeterminate sleep, along with concomitant increases in waking time and quiet sleep, particularly stages I and II non-REM sleep.

Recently, sleep organization for 15 normal infants was studied in their homes during six 24-hr sleeping periods (52). Sleep staging was scored according to adult criteria (41) with modifications for children by Guillenminault (53). While this study reconfirmed earlier reported changes in percentages of total sleep time, REM, non-REM, indeterminate sleep, and wakefulness, the authors also showed age and day/night effects on sleep ontogenesis. Modifications with age were more precocious and more pronounced for the diurnal part of the 24-hr cycle, especially as regards REM sleep. For the nocturnal part of the 24-hour cycle, there was a significant increase in sleep efficiency during the REM period after 12 months of age. The authors went on to demonstrate that the total sleep duration and the number of awakenings decreased. These authors point to the high stability of the percentage of slow-wave sleep during the first 2 years of life. Until 12 months of age, the stage II/REM sleep ratio equals 1 and sleep changes occur earlier during the diurnal part of the 24-hr cycle. These examples of sleep ontogeny highlight the developmental neurophysiological changes that occur within central nervous system's structures responsible for sleep maturation and mechanism. They also underscore the importance of the establishment of a circadian rhythm after 3 months of age, prior to the maturation of nocturnal sleep organization. Those brain structures responsible for circadian cycling predate other regions that are responsible for generation of S2 sleep and the decrease in REM sleep. Nine months of age is also an important developmental age for sleep maturation. During the night, a significant decrease in REM sleep and an increase in S2 sleep occurs after this age. This is also an important time when frontal brain myelination dendritic growth and synaptogenesis occurs, probably with greater interaction between brainstem and thalamocortical structures (54).

In summary, sleep ontogenesis during infancy evolves into adult sleep organization during the first 2 years of life. Circadian rhythms appear after 3 months of age, followed by an adult ultradian sleep cycle after 6 to 9 months of age. There is lengthening of this ultradian sleep cycle after 12 months of age. These maturational processes reflect developmental changes within multiple brain regions responsible for sleep initiation and maintenance.

VII. Brain Adaptation to Stress as Reflected in Sleep Reorganization

Endogenous or exogenous factors may alter the ontogenesis of specific physiological behaviors during sleep. This is exemplified by recent neurophysiological studies that describe differences between preterm and fullterm infants at matched term PCAs concerning sleep architecture, continuity, phasic and spectral phenomena, and cardiorespiratory and temperature behaviors (40,55–58). Unlike that of the full-term infant, the sleep of the preterm infant adapts to an extrauterine environment by expressing a one-third longer sleep cycle, a greater percentage of quiet sleep, fewer movements, and shorter arousals. Preterm infants also exhibit higher rectal temperatures over the ultradian cycle, with less change from non-REM to REM segments. Greater cardiorespiratory irregularity is noted during quiet sleep, and lower spectral EEG energies are observed during specific sleep segments. These differences reflect the effects of prematurity on brain maturation; adaptation of brain function for the preterm infant in an extrauterine environment represents the response of physiological dysmaturity to biological and/or environmental stresses (59). Dysmature EEG sleep measures also predict neurodevelopmental performance for neonates with clinical risk factors other than prematurity, such as prenatal substance exposure (60), chronic lung disease (61), or general medical complications (62). Documentation of the persistence or resolution of dysmature sleep behaviors during infancy needs to be addressed.

VIII. Computer-Assisted Analyses of EEG Sleep Organization

Relationships among multiple physiological processes are certainly less developed in the preterm infant. State transitions are more difficult to recognize, particularly over short recording intervals. Even with longer recording times, less well developed associations among physiological variables may not be obvious by visual analysis. Automated systems for EEG sleep analyses can complement visual inspection (63) (Fig. 11). Computer analyses better characterize relationships among electrographic and polysomnographic components over extended recording intervals and better detect rudimentary sleep behaviors. Recent reports have combined computer and visual analyses of neonatal EEG recordings through infancy to ascertain which physiological relationships best represent state expression; spectral EEG energies and REM best define maturational trends compared with other measures in the preterm infant (37–40). Conversely, other noncerebral measures such as cardiorespiratory, motility, and temperature changes predict maturational trends and state transitions less accurately. Computer algorithms may detect diurnal or nocturnal rhythmicities more accurately than visual inspection (63).

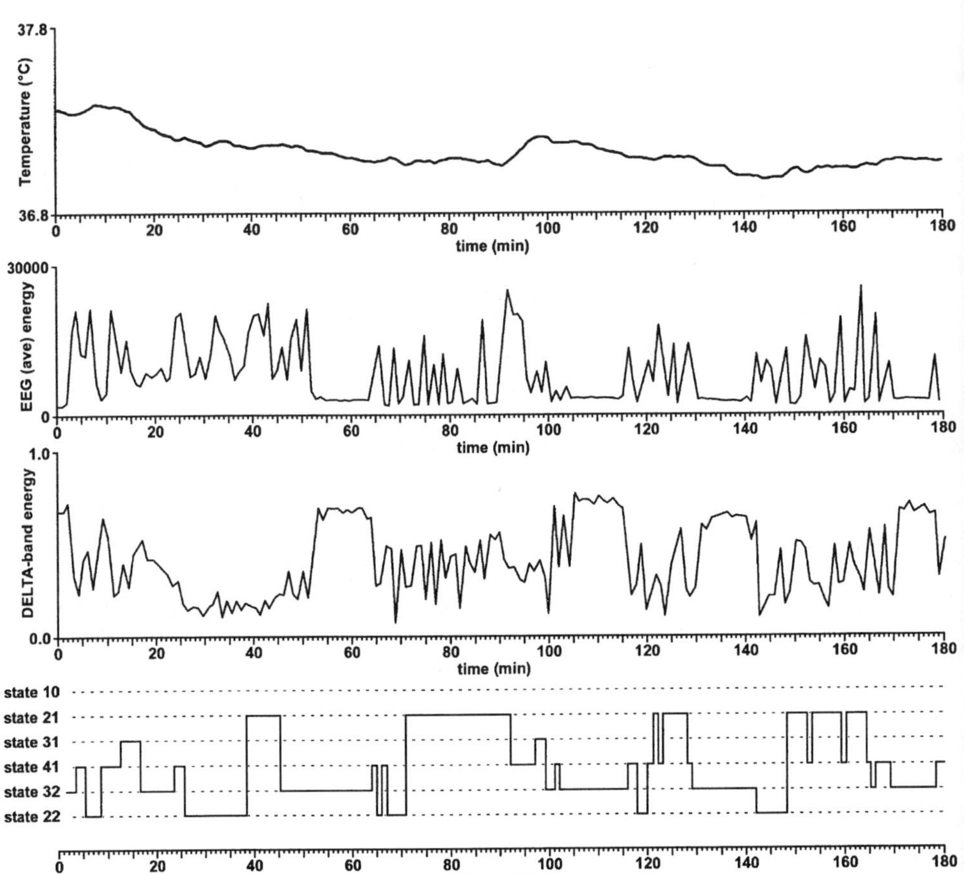

Figure 11 A 3-hr summary of physiological behaviors, constituting neonatal sleep at full-term, in the lower tracing: state 10 awake, state 21 mixed frequency active sleep, state 31 high-voltage slow quiet sleep, state 41 indeterminate sleep, state 32 tracé alternant quiet sleep, state 22 low-voltage irregular active sleep. Spectral delta and total EEG energies in the second and third panels illustrate changes in these values, depending on the segment of the neonatal sleep cycle. Note the minimum total EEG energy and maximum delta energy during tracé alternant quiet sleep. The top panel illustrates a slower multiple-hour temperature rhythm, which changes over multiple sleep cycles.

IX. Summary

Serial neonatal and infant EEG-polysomnographic studies document the ontogeny of cerebral and noncerebral physiological behaviors, based on visual inspection or spectral analyses. EEG patterns and other physiological relationships serve as templates for normal brain maturation and help distinguish intrauterine from extrauterine development. Such strategies will ultimately improve our diagnostic skills for the care of the high-risk fetus, neonate, and infant.

The EEG sleep study remains the only bedside neurodiagnostic procedure that provides a continuous record of cerebral function over long periods of time. While other advanced methods of anatomical or functional inquiry—such as cranial sonography and magnetic resonance imaging—report brief snapshots of cerebral anatomy, neurophysiological studies provide a functional perspective into brain ontogeny. Sleep ontogenesis in asymptomatic neonates and infants documents expected brain maturation, making it possible to better anticipate deviations from these biologically programmed processes under stressful and/or pathological conditions.

Acknowledgments

Supported in part by NS01110, NS26793, NS34508, and NR01894.

References

1. Anders T, Ende R, Parmelee A. A Manual of Standardized Terminology, Technique, and Criteria for Scoring of States of Sleep and Wakefulness in Newborn Infants. UCLA Brain Information Service. Los Angeles: NINDS, Neurological Information Network, 1971.
2. Parmelee AH, Stern R. Development of states in infants. In: Clemente DC, Purpurer DP, Mayer EE, eds. Sleep and the Maturing Nervous System. New York: Academic Press, 1972:199–228.
3. Ellingson RJ. Studies of the electrical activity of the developing human brain. In: Himwich WA, ed. The Developing Brain-Progress in Brain Research. Amsterdam: Elsevier, 1964:26–53.
4. Dreyfus-Brisac C. Neonatal electroencephalography. In: Scarpelli EM, Cosmie EV, eds. Reviews in Perinatal Medicine, Vol. III. New York: Raven Press, 1979:397–430.
5. Prechtl HFR. The behavioral states of the newborn infant. Brain Res 1974; 76:185–212.
6. Lombroso CT. Neonatal electroencephalography. In: Niedermeyer E, Lopez-Desilva F, eds. Electroencephalography, Basic Principles, Clinical Applications in Related Fields. Baltimore and Munich: Urban and Schwarzenberg, 1989:599–637.
7. Hrachovy RA, Mizrahi EM, Kellaway P. Electroencephalography of the newborn. In: Daly DD, Pedley TA, eds. Current Practice of Clinical Electroencephalography, 2d ed. New York: Raven Press, 1990:201–242.
8. Pope JJ, Werner SJ, Bickford RG. Atlas of Neonatal Electroencephalography. New York: Raven Press, 1992.
9. Ajmone-Marsan C ed. American Electroencephalographic Society Guidelines in EEG and Evoked Potentials. J Clin Neurophysiol, 1986; 3(suppl 1):1–152.
10. Scher MS. Neonatal encephalopathies as classified by EEG-sleep criteria: severity and timing based on clinical/pathologic correlations. Pediatr Neurol 1994; 11:189–200.
11. Scher MS, Martin J, Steppe DA, Banks DL. Comparative estimates of neonatal gestational maturity by electrographic and fetal ultrasonographic criteria. Pediatr Neurol 1994; 11:214–218.

12. Scher MS, Barmada A. Estimation of gestational age by electrographic, clinical and anatomical criteria. Pediatr Neurol 1987; 3:256–262.
13. Dreyfus-Brisac C. Sleep ontogenesis in early human prematurity from 24 to 27 weeks of conceptional age. Dev Psychobiol 1968; 1:162–169.
14. Benda GI, Engel RCH, Zhang Y. Prolonged inactive phases during the discontinuous pattern of prematurity in the electroencephalogram of very-low-birthweight infants. Electroencephalogr Clin Neurophysiol 1989; 72:189–197.
15. Connell JA, Oozeer R, Dubowitz V. Continuous 4-channel EEG monitoring: guide to interpretation with normal values in preterm infants. Neuropediatrics 1987; 18: 138–145.
16. Hughes JR, Fino J, Gagnon L. Periods of activity and quiescence in the premature EEG. Neuropediatrics 1983; 14:66–72.
17. Hughes JR, Fino JJ, Hart LA. Premature temporal theta. Electroencephalogr Clin Neurophysiol 1987; 67:7–15.
18. Eyre JA, Nanei S, Wilkinson AR. Quantification of changes in normal neonatal EEGs with gestation from continuous five-day recordings. Dev Med Child Neurol 1988; 30: 599–607.
19. Lombroso CT. Neonatal polygraphy in full-term and preterm infants: a review of normal and abnormal findings. J Clin Neurophysiol 1985; 2:105–155.
20. Hughes JR, Miller JK, Fino JJ, Hughes CA. The sharp theta rhythm on the occipital areas of prematures (STOP): a newly described waveform. Clin Electroencephalogr 1990; 21: 77–87.
21. Scher MS, Bova JM, Dokianakis SG, Steppe DA. Positive temporal sharp waves on EEG recordings of healthy neonates: a benign pattern of dysmaturity in preterm infants at postconceptional term ages. Electroencephalogr Clin Neurophys 1994; 90:173–178.
22. Hayakawa F, Watanabe K, Hakamada S, Kuno K, Aso K. FZ theta/alpha bursts: a transient EEG pattern in healthy newborns. Electroencephalogr Clin Neurophysiol 1987; 67: 27–31.
23. Lenard, HC. Sleep studies in infancy: facts, concepts, and significances. Acta Paediatr Scand 1970; 59:572–581.
24. Curzi-Dascalova L, Peirano P, Morel-Kahn Inserm F. Development of sleep states in normal premature and full-term newborns. Dev Psychobiol 1988; 21:431–444.
25. Curzi-Dascalova L, Figueroa JM, Eiselt M, Christova E, Virassamy A, D'Allest AM, Guimaraes H, Gaultier C, Dehan M. Sleep state organization in premature infants of less than 35 weeks' gestational age. Pediatr Res 1998; 34:624–628.
26. Dittrichová J, Paul K, Pavliková E. Rapid eye movements in paradoxical sleep in infants. Neuropaediatrie 1972; 3:248–257.
27. Ersyukova II. Oculomotor activity and autonomic indices of newborn infants during paradoxical sleep. Hum Physiol 1980; 6:57–64.
28. Lynch JA, Aserinsky E. Developmental changes of oculomotor characteristics in infants when awake and in the active state of sleep. Behav Brain Res 1986; 20:175–183.
29. Prechtl HFR, Nijhuis JG. Eye movements in the human fetus and newborn. Behav Brain Res 1983; 10:119–124.
30. Scher MS, Steppe DA, Dokianakis SG, Guthrie RD. Maturation of phasic and continuity measures during sleep in preterm neonates. Pediatr Res 1994; 36:732–737.
31. Robertson SS. Intrinsic temporal patterning in the spontaneous movement of awake neonates. Child Dev 1982; 53:1016–1021.

32. Robertson SS. Human cyclic motility: Fetal-newborn continuities and newborn state differences. Dev Psychobiol 1987; 20:425–442.
33. Fukumoto M, Mochizuki N, Takeishi M, Nomura Y, Segawa M. Studies of body movements during night sleep in infancy. Brain Dev 1981; 3:37–43.
34. Prechtl HFR, Fargel JW, Weinmann HM, Backter HH. Postures, motility and respiration of low risk preterm infants. Dev Med Child Neurol 1979; 21:3–27.
35. Martin RJ, Miller MJ, Carlo WA. Pathogenesis of apnea in preterm infants. J Pediatr 1986; 109:733–741.
36. Glotzbach SF, Tansey PA, Baldwin RB, Ariango RL. Periodic breathing cycle duration in preterm infants. Pediatr Res 1989; 25:258–261.
37. Scher MS, Steppe DA, Banks DL, Guthrie RD, Sclabassi RJ. Maturational trends of EEG-sleep measures in the healthy preterm neonate. Pediatr Neurol 1995; 12:314–322.
38. Scher MS, Dokianakis SG, Steppe DA, Banks D, Sclabassi RJ. Computer classification of state in healthy preterm neonates. Sleep 1997; 20:132–141.
39. Hildebrandt G. Functional significance of ultradian rhythms and reactive periodicity. J Interdiscip Cycle Res 1986; 17:307–319.
40. Scher MS, Steppe DA, Dahl RE, Asthana S, Guthrie RD. Comparison of EEG-sleep measures in healthy full-term and preterm infants at matched conceptional ages. Sleep 1992; 15:442–448.
41. Rechtschaffen A, Kales A, eds. A Manual of Standardized Terminology, Techniques and Scoring System for Sleep Stages of Human Subjects. Los Angeles: Brain Research Institute/Brain Information Services, University of California, 1968.
42. Glotzbach SF, Edgar DM, Ariagno RL. Biological rhythmicity in preterm infants prior to discharge from neonatal intensive care. Pediatrics 1995; 95:231–237.
43. Anders TF, Sadeh A, Appareddy V. Normal sleep in neonates and children. In: Ferber R, Kryger M, eds. Principles and Practice of Sleep Medicine in the Child. Philadelphia, Saunders, 1995.
44. Mirimiran M, Kok JH. Circadian rhythm in early human development. Early Hum Dev 1991; 262:121–128.
45. Myers MM, Schulze KF, Fifer WP, Stark RI. Methods for quantifying state-specific patterns of EEG activity in Fetal baboons and immature human infants. In: LeCanuet J, Fifer WP, Krasnesor NA, Smotherman R, eds. Fetal Development: A Psychological Perspective. Hillsdale, NJ: Erlbaum, 1995:35–49.
46. Curzi-Dascalova L. EEG de veille et de sommeil du nourisson normal avant 6 mois d'age. Rev EEG Neurophysiol 1977; 7:316–326.
47. Ellingson RJ. The EEGs of prematures and full-term newborns. In: Klass DW, Daly DD, eds. Current Practice of Clinical Electroencephalography. New York: Raven Press, 1979: 149–177.
48. Louis J, Zhang JX, Revol M, Debilly G, Challamel MJ. Ontogenesis of nocturnal organization of sleep spindles: a longitudinal study during the first 6 months of life. Electroencephalogr Clin Neurophysiol 1992; 83:289–296.
49. Schechtman VL, Harper RK, Harper RM. Distribution of slow-wave EEG activity across the night in developing infants. Sleep 1994; 17:316–322.
50. Sterman MP, Harper RM, Havens B, Hoppenbrouwers T, McGinty DJ, Hodgman JE. Quantitative analysis of infant EEG development during quiet sleep. Electroencephalogr Clin Neurophysiol 1977; 43:371–385.

51. Samson-Dollfus D, Nogues B, Menard JF, Bertoli-Lefever I, Geffroy D. Delta, theta, alpha and beta power spectrum of sleep electroencephalogram in infants aged two to eleven months. Sleep 1983; 6:376–383.
52. Louis J, Cannard C, Bastus, H, Challamel M. Sleep Ontogenesis revisited: a longitudinal 24-hour home polygraphic study on 15 normal infants during the first two years of life. Sleep 1997; 20:323–333.
53. Guilleminault C, Souquet M. Sleep states and related pathology. In: Korobkin R, Guilleminault C, eds. Advances in perinatal neurology. New York: SP Medical and Scientific Books 1979;225–247.
54. Van der Knaap MS, Valk J. MR Imaging of the various stages of normal myelination during the first year of life. Neuroradiology 1990; 31:459–470.
55. Scher MS, Sun M, Steppe DA, Banks DL, Guthrie RD, Sclabassi RJ. Comparisons of EEG sleep state-specific spectral values between healthy full-term and preterm infants at comparable postconceptional ages. Sleep 1994; 17:47–51.
56. Scher MS, Dokianakis SG, Sun M, Steppe DA, Guthrie RD, Sclabassi RJ. Rectal temperature changes during sleep state transitions in fullterm and preterm neonates at postconceptional term ages. Pediatr Neurol 1994; 10:191–194.
57. Scher MS, Steppe DA, Dokianakis SG, Sun M, Guthrie RD, Sclabassi RJ. Cardiorespiratory behavior during sleep in fullterm and preterm neonates at comparable postconceptional term ages. Pediatr Res 1994; 36:738–744.
58. Scher MS, Sun M, Steppe DA, Guthrie RD, Sclabassi RJ. Comparisons of EEG spectral and correlation measures between healthy term and preterm infants. Pediat Neurol 1994; 10:104–108.
59. Scher MS. Neurophysiological assessment of brain function and maturation: II. A measure of brain dysmaturity in healthy preterm neonates. Pediatr Neurol 1997; 16:287–295.
60. Scher MS, Richardson GA, Coble PA, Day NL, Stoffer DS. The effects of prenatal alcohol and marijuana exposure: disturbances in neonatal sleep cycling and arousal. Pediatr Res 1988; 24:101–105.
61. Hahn JS, Tharp BR. The dysmature EEG pattern in infants with bronchopulmonary dysplasia and its prognostic implications. Electroencephalogr Clin Neurophysiol 1990; 75:106–113.
62. Beckwith L, Parmelee AH Jr. EEG patterns of preterm infants, home environment, and later IQ. Child Dev 1986; 57:777–789.
63. Scher MS, Sun M, Hatzilabrou GM, Greenberg N, Cebulka G, Sclabassi R. Computer analyses of EEG sleep in the neonate: methodological considerations. J Clin Neurophysiol 1990; 7:417–441.

3

Maturation of Normal Sleep Patterns from Childhood Through Adolescence

AVI SADEH

Tel Aviv University
Ramat Aviv, Israel

I. Introduction

The evolution of normal sleep patterns in children is one of the most fascinating maturational processes that attracts the attention of parents and professionals involved in child-care and developmental research. Although many aspects of this maturational process are visible to the interested observer, some of them require special methods of peeking into the "night life" of the child.

Sleep plays a major role in children's well-being. Sleep is strongly influenced by the child's health status, psychological stress, and family issues as well as by multiple aspects of his or her culture and environment. Also, children's sleep patterns affect their well-being within the same wide range of health and psychosocial phenomena.

This chapter contains a brief description of the maturation of sleep-wake patterns in normal children and adolescents and a discussion of the factors influencing and influenced by the evolving sleep patterns of the child.

II. Consolidation of Nocturnal Sleep

Full-term newborns spend an average daily amount of about 16 hr in sleep. Their sleep is distributed around the clock, day and night, across a number of sleep episodes (five to six on average) with relatively short intervals of wakefulness between them (1–3).

Interestingly, significant variability in sleep consolidation exists already in newborns, where the longest continuous sleep episode ranges between 50 and 300 min (3). Although it may appear to the observer that newborns' sleep is evenly distributed across the day and night, studies have shown that sleep is more concentrated in the nighttime hours than in daytime hours (3,4). During the first year of life, a rapid maturational process leads to a clear preference to sleep during the night and the consolidation of a prolonged nighttime sleep episode, also referred to as "sleeping through the night," is achieved by most infants during this period (2,5–7). This maturational process is influenced by multiple biological and psychosocial factors. From the biological perspective, it has been suggested that the synchronization of the sleep-wake cycle with the light–dark cycle is mediated by the secretion of the pineal hormone melatonin, which rises in the dark hours and drops in response to light exposure. It has been shown that maturation of the melatonin secretion occurs during the first 6 months of life (8), a period that corresponds with the accelerated process of sleep consolidation during the night. Furthermore, a significant association between melatonin secretion patterns and sleep-wake patterns has been demonstrated in 6- to 8-month-old infants, suggesting that the two systems are indeed interrelated (9). In this study, sleep onset was associated with measures of melatonin secretion levels during the evening hours and sleep fragmentation was associated with inappropriate peak time of melatonin secretion. The relationship between the sleep–wake cycle and melatonin secretion patterns has also been demonstrated in older children (10). In blind children, disrupted sleep patterns have been associated with deviate melatonin secretion patterns (11). It has also been shown that exogenous melatonin administration may normalize sleep in blind children (12) and in some neurologically impaired children with severe sleep disruptions (13). However, a failure to achieve favorable therapeutic effects with melatonin has also been reported (14).

Beyond these melatonin-related and possibly other underlying biological mechanisms, the infant is exposed to many environmental cues and psychosocial pressures that favor sleeping during the night and wakefulness during the day. Some of these psychosocial influences are described in Chapter 5.

Another way to describe the maturation of the sleep-wake system is to address the changes in daytime napping. As sleep consolidates during the night and the need for sleep decreases, daytime sleep gradually disappears. A recent longitudinal study of naps in children from 6 months to 7 years of age indicates that the percentage of children who nap, the number of napping episodes, and the time spent in naps decreases with age (15). In this study, most infants were napping two (83.7%) or three (16.3%) times per day at 6 months of age. By 3 years of age, all the children were napping only once a day. Napping disappeared almost completely at 7 years of age. No gender differences were found with regard to the napping habits of the children.

Interestingly, napping often reappears during adolescence as teenagers compensate on a sporadic basis for their accumulated sleep debt, due to their exaggerated curtailment of nighttime sleep (see below).

The process of nighttime sleep consolidation is associated with night-waking problems that are the most prevalent sleep complaints of early childhood. Studies have shown that most infants learn to "sleep through the night" during the first year of life (2,5–7). However, surveys indicate that 20% to 30% of young children suffer from night-waking problems (16–20). Using actigraphy (activity-based monitoring), it has been shown that, on average, normal infants wake up about twice per night, but they usually quickly soothe themselves back to sleep with or without parental intervention (21). In contrast, sleep-disturbed infants wake up about four times per night and usually require significant parental help to resume sleep. The maturational trend of sleep consolidation continues throughout early childhood, and some of these night-waking problems may be spontaneously resolved. Surveys based on parental reports usually find that these problems improve with age. For instance, in a study of 2889 Italian infants and children, Ottaviano et al. found that the prevalence of night-waking problems decreases from a range above 34% during the first 2 years of life to 13.4 in 4- to 6-year-olds (22). However, recent studies suggest that night-waking problems are persistent and may turn into a chronic sleep problem if not treated (23–28).

The prevalence of night-waking problems in older children and adolescents is still unclear. Although surveys suggest that the problem is less frequent compared to that of early childhood (26,29,30), there are data to suggest that subjective reports underestimate this phenomenon in older children, since they are less likely to require parental intervention (31). A recent survey of sleep problems in school-age children reported night-waking problems in 6.5% (29). In a second survey of preadolescents, "poor sleep" was reported in 14% (32). In an EEG study, it was found that children between 6 and 11 years of age had an average of one to three brief night wakings (33). Unfortunately there are no systematic naturalistic studies of night-waking problems using objective measures in older children. A recent naturalistic study that used actigraphic monitoring to assess sleep in normal school-aged children found that they woke up more than twice per night on average, and that 18% of these children could be characterized as "poor sleepers" based on their fragmented sleep patterns (34).

III. Sleep Onset and Duration

Another conspicuous maturational process is the significant reduction in sleep duration across development. The most dramatic changes occur during the first 3 years of life, but a slow monotonic decrease in sleep duration continues through adolescence. From an average of 16 hr of sleep per day as a newborn to an average of 7 to 8 hr as a young adult, the ratio between sleep and wake hours is virtually reversed. However, these age-group means do not reflect the entire picture. The individual differences in sleep duration or sleep needs are striking and preclude simple answers to questions such as how much sleep is appropriate for a child at a certain age. For example, it has been shown that in newborns, during their first 48-hours in the nursery, sleep duration ranges between 10 and 22 hr per day (3).

Another way to look at this issue is to address the duration of sleep during nighttime hours. It has been reported, that by 1 year of age, the longest sleep period reaches

8 to 9 hr (6). The longest sleep period grows to about 10 hr per night at 5 years of age and remains quite stable until puberty, at which point it continues to decline. During this 5- to 10-year period, although there is relative stability in the nighttime sleep duration, there is a decline in the overall 24-hr sleep period, which is mainly due to the decrease in daytime napping.

The issues of sleep onset time and sleep onset difficulties are among the factors determining sleep duration. There are conflicting reports with regard to what maturation does to sleep latency during early and middle childhood. One study reported a trend of a gradual increase with age in the time taken to fall asleep (35). Another study reported a steady, significant decrease in sleep latency from early infancy to 6 years of age (22). When sleep latency over 30 min long was considered as the criterion, the percentages of children meeting this criterion dropped from 13.7% during the first few months of age to 2.2% within the age range of 4 to 6 years. It has been estimated that 10% to 15% of children 1 to 8 years of age have difficulties going to bed or falling asleep (16,26,36).

For most children, child-care, school, or parental requirements and demands determine morning rise time. In contrast, sleep onset time is much more negotiable and is determined by the child's physiological needs and by multiple psychosocial factors of both child and family. Therefore, the maturational trend of reduced sleep duration is primarily determined by the tendency to delay sleep onset. This delay of sleep onset could result from biobehavioral factors associated with the sleep-phase shift or from psychosocial factors ranging from separation difficulties and fears in early childhood to social incentives and academic and work demands in later development (e.g., interaction with parents, siblings or peers, TV, the Internet, work, etc.)

From a psychosocial perspective, it is clear that at around 2 to 3 years of age the child is becoming increasingly aware of and involved in the social life of the family. Sleep rituals are extended, and settling problems become more prevalent. Between 3 and 5 years, nighttime fears and nightmares also increase in prevalence and may complicate going to bed, which is associated with darkness and separation from the parents and family social life (20,38). The pervasive belief is that children's fears subside when they reach school age (the "latency period"). However, Kahn and colleagues reported nighttime fears in as many as 15% of their large sample of preadolescents (32). These fears were associated with difficulties in initiating sleep (i.e., increased sleep latency). In this age group, the bedtime struggles are often associated with the evolving tendency of the child to delay sleep and with parental difficulties in limit setting.

In adolescence, the delay of the sleep phase appears to accelerate. Carskadon and colleagues have demonstrated that the phase shift (a tendency to delay sleep onset and morning rise time) that characterizes adolescence is associated with the pubertal status of the youngster (38,39). They suggested that this is a biobehavioral process that is influenced not only by the psychosocial demands of adolescence but also by underlying biological mechanisms.

Furthermore, Carskadon and others have convincingly demonstrated that the continued reduction of sleep time in adolescence—which in this age group results mainly from delayed sleep onset—leading to chronic sleep debt and an accompanied increase in daytime sleepiness (40–43). Surveys indicate a rising prevalence of direct subjective complaints of fatigue and daytime sleepiness during adolescence (40–45). In a recent study, as many as 63% of the teenagers reported a need for more sleep during weekdays (45). In addition to the subjective reports, compelling evidence comes from studies showing that during school days, adolescents sleep significantly less than on free days (42–47). It appears that school start time plays a major role in restricting sleep due to the delayed sleep onset (42,47). In a recent study, Carskadon and colleagues investigated the transition from ninth to tenth grade, which resulted in an earlier school start time (47), associated with earlier rise time. No change occurred in sleep onset time, and consequently the adolescents slept less. This transition was associated with a delayed dim-light saliva melatonin onset phase, shorter sleep latencies on the Multiple Sleep Latency Test (MSLT), and intrusions of REM sleep episodes into the MSLT. The results of this study suggest that earlier school start time with the resultant earlier rise time is associated with increased signs of sleep deprivation and daytime sleepiness. Thus, it appears that the only way adolescents can compensate for their accumulated sleep debt during school days is by increasing their sleep duration on non-school nights. Another line of evidence for the direct manifestation of this cumulative sleep debt is the growing daytime sleepiness that characterizes adolescents, as documented objectively by the MSLT. It has been shown that adolescents' increased sleepiness is similar to the clinical level of sleepiness presented by patients with severe sleep disorders (40,41).

The normal sleep-phase delay that occurs in adolescents can turn to an exaggerated and dysfunctional pattern that is clinically labeled as the *delayed sleep-phase syndrome*, characterized by an inability to fall asleep before the very late hours of the night (or the early hours of the morning), with the associated inability to rise for normal activities at a reasonable morning hour (48). It has been shown that the emergence of this syndrome is often associated with the adolescent period (49,50).

IV. Sleep State Organization

The maturational changes in sleep structure are subtler than those discussed thus far and require special observation or recording methods for detection. Interestingly, REM sleep was discovered during infant observation and was the breakthrough finding that led to the establishment of the field of sleep research. This finding is not surprising, since among the unique characteristics of infant sleep are the facts that: (1) young infants either fall asleep directly with the onset of REM sleep or with a very short REM latency compared to older children or adults and (2) infants spend a high proportion of their sleep time in REM sleep. These two unique features are the ones that undergo the most prominent maturational processes (see also Chap. 2).

Roffwarg and colleagues (51) published the earliest systematic scientific inquiry of the ontogenesis of sleep structure in 1966. Since then, a limited number of polysomnographic studies have contributed to our knowledge of the normal maturation of sleep organization in children and adolescents (33,52–61). As indicated by Kahn and colleagues (52), the methods used by different laboratories differ in many aspects; therefore, the results do not always overlap. Nevertheless, consistent maturational processes have been identified and are reported in the following subsections.

A. REM-NREM Sleep Distribution

During their earlier months of life, infants spend around 50% of their sleep time in REM sleep (almost 8 hr per day). By the time they are 1 year old, they spend only around 30% of their sleep time in REM sleep, and this proportion decreases only slightly during the next few years to the adult proportion of 20% to 25%. Indeed, the major component of the outstanding decrease in sleep duration from 16 hr in the newborn period to 7 to 8 hr in adults is the reduction in REM sleep. As stated earlier, newborns experience an immediate onset of REM sleep when they fall asleep, but this tendency changes quickly during the first few months as quiet sleep becomes more dominant during the early phases of sleep. There is scientific support for the hypothesis that REM sleep is so predominant in infancy because it facilitates information processing and brain maturation of the human infant, whose brain is small at birth in comparison to its mature size (51,62). It is important to note that during the early childhood period (ages 2 to 5 years), most children nap during the day, and their state distribution might be affected by their napping sleep structure (51,53–56). For instance, it has been suggested that the lower amount of NREM sleep in infants in comparison to older children results from the fact that they spend much more time in NREM sleep during their naps.

Dahl and colleagues have reported a significant association between REM sleep parameters and reproductive hormones in school-age children during their pubertal development (57). Higher levels of reproductive hormones were associated with shorter REM latency, lower REM activity, and lower REM density.

In addition to the maturational changes in REM-NREM sleep, the distribution of the NREM sleep stages also undergoes a significant developmental process. The differentiation of slow-wave sleep stages 3 and 4 becomes possible during the second half of the first year of life (52). During the school years, stage 4 NREM sleep appears to decrease from 18% in 6- to 7-year-olds to 14% in 11-year-olds. This reduction is accompanied by an increase in NREM stage 2 (33). Similar findings have recently been reported by Acebo et al. (61). It has been reported that during adolescence, slow-wave sleep decreases in a linear progression across the Tanner stages (52). Bes and colleagues (60) have compared the distribution of slow-wave sleep (SWS) across the night in infants (aged between 20 weeks and 1 year), children (1 to 6 years of age) and adults (20 to 36 years). They found that SWS reached its peak in all age groups during the first NREM sleep episode. Following the first NREM episode, SWS percent decreased across the night in the children and the adults but not in the infants.

Another maturational tendency observed in this study was the transition from a recurrence of SWS in *alternate* REM-NREM cycles in infants to a recurrence of SWS in *consecutive* REM-NREM cycles.

B. REM-NREM Cycle

The REM-NREM state cycle also undergoes maturational changes. Since different studies use different criteria, the reports are somewhat discrepant, although the trends are similar (52). In newborns and very young infants, the cycle lasts approximately 40 to 60 min. In one study, it was reported that by 2 years of age, the cycle increases to 75 min and continues to increase to an average of 84 min in 5-year-olds. Another study reported an increase of the cycle from 40 min at 2 years of age to 60 min at 5 years of age (53). The length of the REM-NREM cycle continues to increase gradually until it reaches the 90- to 100-minute adult-like cycle during adolescence. Another important aspect that should be noted is that in early infancy, the EEG distinction between REM and NREM sleep is not as sharp as in older children and adults. This is demonstrated by the relatively large proportion of sleep scored as "indeterminate" or "transitional" in infancy.

Bes and colleagues have shown that when REM recurrence times are considered in the assessment of the sleep cycle, there is a clear peak of recurrence time in infants, children, and adults (60). This peak recurrence time increases from about 50 min in infants to almost 100 min in adults. However, when SWS recurrence is considered, there is no clear peak in infants or children; only in adults there is a peak recurrence time of about 100 min. This pattern appears to result from the fact that infants and children often skip SWS in their NREM sleep episodes.

V. Factors Influencing Children's Sleep

The literature on the multiple factors influencing children's sleep is quite extensive and we can only highlight some of the solid findings and directions emanating from this research field. For some phenomena the cause and effect between sleep and associated child or environmental characteristics is unclear. For convenience, these factors are divided into medical and psychosocial factors, although such a clear distinction does not always exist, particularly in children.

A. Medical Factors

Sleep is very sensitive to the medical and physiological status of the child. Any common flu or congestion of the upper airways can lead directly to severe disruptions of sleep. Other, more serious and chronic common medical problems of infancy and childhood have been associated with poor sleep. For instance, in early childhood, allergy to cow's milk (63), an esophageal reflux (64,65), colic (66), atopic dermatitis (67,68), otitis media (69), headaches (70), and neurological disorders (69), are among the conditions that may exert negative effects on sleep. Asthma is another very common childhood disorder that has been repeatedly associated with poor sleep and increased sleepiness (71–73). Furthermore, blindness (74–77) and pervasive developmental disorders and other neurological impairments have also been associated with severe sleep disorders in children (78).

B. Psychosocial Factors

The early environment of the child appears to have a significant influence on the child's developing sleep-wake patterns. During infancy and early childhood, parental personality and psychopathology (particularly maternal), interaction style, and bedtime practices have been associated with infants' and toddlers' sleep patterns and sleep disruptions (see refs. 20, and 79 to 82 for recent reviews). A comprehensive review of parental and cultural influences on children sleep is presented in Chapter 5.

Children's sleep is also very vulnerable to psychosocial stressors (see Refs. 83 and 84 for reviews). There is a growing body of literature suggesting that children's sleep is directly affected by a variety of stressors ranging from minor stressors—sleeping in a sleep laboratory, also known as "the first-night effect"—to extreme ones such as trauma and abuse.

A review of the literature suggests that there are two modes by which children adapt to stressors: one mode has been defined as the "turn-on" response and the other, the "shut-off" response. The turn-on response is observed usually under circumstances of acute external stress or threat that lead infants and children to become hyperalert and vigilant, a physiological state that is incompatible with extended, consolidated sleep. This response is manifest in difficulty initiating and maintaining sleep (e.g., inability to relax and fall asleep, multiple night wakings). The shut-off response is usually seen under conditions of chronic and/or uncontrollable stress. Under these circumstances, the child often appears to turn away from the stressful environment and to spend more time in sleep, which is deeper and characterized by an elevated arousal threshold.

Sleep is closely linked to the child's emotional status and psychopathology. The cause-and-effect relationship between these phenomena is quite complex, since sleep characteristics can modulate the emotional regulation of the child and vice versa (85). The relationship between sleep and psychopathology is discussed in Chapter 17.

C. Gender Differences

The issue of gender differences in children's sleep and sleep maturation is still a very confusing research topic due to many conflicting and inconsistent reports in the literature. It is beyond the scope of this chapter to extensively review this topic and only a few examples based on objective measures of sleep are presented here.

An actigraphic sleep-wake study of more than 200 newborns during their first 48 hr of life did not reveal any significant gender differences (3). A study of 9- to 24-month-old infants using the same methodology revealed significant gender differences, with boys presenting a higher proportion of active sleep than girls (21).

An earlier EEG study of children 6 to 12 years of age reported a different gender difference: boys 10 years of age and older had a higher percentage of stage 3 sleep and a higher delta ratio than girls (33). Carskadon and colleagues have reported higher absolute amounts and percentages of SWS in boys than in girls (58).

Based on a longitudinal EEG study of children during their pubertal development, Dahl and colleagues found significant gender differences (57). Girls spent less time in REM sleep; they also had lower REM activity and lower REM density. The authors also reported a significant age-by-sex interaction for bedtime and sleep onset time. Interestingly, Acebo and colleagues (61) also reported age-by-sex interactions for SWS measures, suggesting that there may be distinct maturational trajectories for boys and girls.

In a naturalistic actigraphic study of school-age children (34), significant gender differences were found on measures of true sleep time (excluding all wakefulness after sleep onset time) and percent of quiet sleep (motionless sleep). In a recent study of adolescent sleep using actigraphic measures, it was found that girls spent more time than boys in sleep during school and nonschool nights. However, in a laboratory study of children 9.7 to 16.8 years of age, it was found that boys spent more time in bed than girls (61).

It is difficult to depict a clear gender-related picture from the pattern of results described above. It appears that gender differences vary with age, and thus the differences appear or disappear in various studies. It is also possible that some findings on gender differences are related to psychosocial factors associated with the methods of the study. For instance, it is possible that girls and boys have different emotional reactions to the issues associated with coming to and sleeping in a sleep laboratory. Such possible differential emotional reactions may lead to variations found on the sleep measures. A close inspection of the differential "first-night effect" seen in boys and girls in the data reported by Carskadon et al. (58) lends some support to this hypothesis.

VI. Maturation of Sleep and Cognitive Function in Children

Beyond the complex relationships between sleep and emotional regulation and psychopathology in children, sleep is also closely associated with cognitive functioning, learning, and attention. The sleep–wake system is a biobehavioral system that lends itself to scientific investigation from the earliest stages of life, and the principles of its organization, which are well documented, may shed light on other brain systems the maturation of which is behaviorally manifest only in later phases of development. Therefore, it appears that it is particularly important to understand the relationships between the developing sleep-wake systems and the maturation of other neurobehavioral systems.

Insufficient sleep and sleep disruptions have been associated with compromised neurobehavioral functioning in numerous studies in adults. It is surprising how limited the work on this topic in children is, where the maturation of sleep parallels and is interrelated to the maturation of brain systems responsible for information processing, response inhibition and modulation, attention, and regulation of motivational systems.

A number of studies have associated infant sleep-wake patterns with neurobehavioral development (86–90). For instance, Scher et al. demonstrated that EEG sleep measures of newborns can predict mental and motor maturation as measured by Bayley mental scores at 12 and 24 months of age (90). Lower Bayley mental scores were associated with higher spectral EEG correlations, lower spectral EEG energies in the beta frequency ranges, fewer arousals per minute, lower rapid eye movements per minute, and shorter sleep latencies from awake state to active sleep. Because of the small number of children studied in these "prediction" studies, it is difficult to conclude if the early organization of the sleep-wake system is indeed a predictor of later neurobehavioral organization. Nevertheless, these studies suggest that this is an important area for future systematic investigation. Additional support comes from other studies in infants that have demonstrated a concomitant relationship between inadequate sleep and short attention span or attention problems in infants (91,92).

In older children, severe sleep disruption has been associated with attention and cognitive problems (93–96). Sleep disruptions have often been implicated in attention deficit hyperactivity disorder (ADHD), and it has been repeatedly suggested that ADHD-like symptoms could result from insufficient or disordered sleep and the resultant decrease in arousal level (see ref. 97 for review). Recent studies have shown that inattention and other ADHD-like symptoms are among the common correlates of sleep-related problems such as sleep apnea (95), periodic leg movements (96), and snoring (94). In a recent intervention study, it was demonstrated that children suffering from sleep-disordered breathing improve their academic achievement following surgical intervention of tonsillectomy and adenoidectomy (98). In normal children, early school start time and shortened sleep duration correlated with subjective complaints of sleepiness and attention problems at school (43). Similarly, in adolescents, irregular sleep patterns, delayed sleep onset, and shorter sleep time have been associated with poor academic performance (42).

In a recent study of school-aged children based on an actigraphic assessment of sleep patterns and computerized neuropsychological tests, Sadeh and colleagues reported a significant correlation between fragmented sleep and poor performance on specific attention and learning tasks (99). Furthermore, a subsequent study demonstrated that extending or restricting the sleep of school-aged children by 30 to 60 min for three consecutive nights has direct positive or negative effects (respectively) on their neurobehavioral functioning (99).

Finally, Randazzo et al. studied the effects of acute sleep restriction on cognitive functioning in 16 children 10 to 14 years of age (100). The sleep-restricted children had shorter sleep latencies the following morning in comparison to the nonrestricted children. Adverse effects of the sleep restriction were found on the cognitive measures of verbal creativity (i.e., fluency, flexibility) and the Wisconsin Card Sorting Test. No effects were found on less complex cognitive functions. The authors concluded that higher cognitive functions in children are vulnerable to sleep restriction of one night, whereas other cognitive functions can be maintained with no detected impairments.

In sum, it appears that the close ties between the evolving sleep–wake system and the neurobehavioral maturation of the child gradually unfold and suggest that inappropriate or disturbed sleep patterns may adversely affect the maturing brain and the concurrent neurobehavioral functioning of the child. These findings reemphasize the critical role of sleep in child development.

VII. Summary and Conclusions

The maturation of sleep–wake patterns during child development consists of a complex dynamic of change and balance. Although sleep time dramatically decreases with age, the relationships among various components of sleep also change to meet what seems to be the changing needs of the maturing brain. These maturational processes appear to be influenced by multiple biological and psychosocial factors. Specific sleep disorders appear to be age-specific or at least to peak in prevalence concomitantly with age-specific maturational trends (e.g., night wakings in infancy or phase delay in adolescents).

Because the maturation of the sleep–wake system is an ongoing process and, at specific periods, a very rapid and dramatic phenomenon, a knowledge of normal sleep development is essential to any evaluation and understanding of clinical phenomena.

The maturation of the sleep–wake system exerts significant influences on the psychosocial and neurobehavioral functioning of the child. Thus, the early identification and treatment of childhood sleep disorders or inappropriate sleep patterns is essential for the child's well-being.

Finally, although the focus of this chapter is not on methodological issues, it is important to note that the representation of many of the maturational and clinical sleep phenomena depends on the instruments used to measure them (82,101,102). For instance, it has been demonstrated that parents are reliable informants of their infant's sleep schedule but do poorly when sleep quality measures are involved (i.e., night wakings) (103). It is therefore important that the evaluation of information on sleep phenomena include critical consideration of the appropriateness of the instruments used to obtain this information.

References

1. Hoppenbrouwers T. Sleep in infants. In: Guilleminault C, ed. Sleep and Its Disorders in Children. New York: Raven Press, 1987:1–15.
2. Coons S. Development of sleep and wakefulness during the first 6 months of life. In: Guilleminault C, ed. Sleep and Its Disorders in Children. New York: Raven Press, 1987:17–27.

3. Sadeh A, Dark I, Vohr BR. Newborns' sleep-wake patterns: the role of maternal, delivery and infant factors. Early Hum Dev 1996; 44:113–126.
4. Freudigman KA, Thoman E. Ultradian and diurnal cyclicity in the sleep states of newborn infants during the first two postnatal days. Early Hum Dev 1994; 30:67–80.
5. Anders TF, Halpern LF, Hua J. Sleeping through the night: a developmental perspective. Pediatrics 1992; 90:554–560.
6. Anders TF, Keener M. Developmental course of nighttime sleep-wake patterns in full-term and premature infants during the first year of life. Sleep 1985; 8:173–192.
7. Bernal J. Night waking in infants during the first fourteen months. Dev Med Child Neurol 1973: 15:760–769.
8. Kennaway DJ, Stamp GE, Goble FC. Development of melatonin production in infants and the impact of prematurity. J Clin Endocrinol Metab 1992; 75:367–369.
9. Sadeh A. Melatonin and sleep in infants: a preliminary study. Sleep 1997; 20:185–191.
10. Cavallo A. The pineal gland and human beings: relevance to pediatrics. J Pediatr 1993; 123:843–851.
11. Tzischinsky O, Shlitner A, Lavie G. The association between the nocturnal sleep gate and nocturnal onset of urinary 6-sulfatoxymelatonin. J Biol Rhythms 1993; 8: 199–209.
12. Espezel H, Jan JE, ODonnell ME, Milner R. The use of melatonin to treat sleep-wake-rhythm disorders in children who are visually impaired. J Visual Impairment Blindness 1996; 90:43–50.
13. Jan GE, Espezel H, Appleton RE. The treatment of sleep disorders with melatonin. Dev Med Child Neurol 1994; 37:97–107.
14. Camfield P, Gordon K, Dooley J, Camfield C. Melatonin appears ineffective in children with intellectual deficits and fragmented sleep: Six "N of 1" trials. J Child Neurol 1996; 11:341–343.
15. Weissbluth, M. Naps in children: 6 months–7 years. Sleep 1995; 18:82–87.
16. Jenkins S, Bax M, Hart H. Behavior problems in preschool children. J Child Psychol Psychiatry 1980; 21:5–17.
17. Johnson M. Infant and toddler sleep: a telephone survey of parents in one community. J Dev Behav Pediatr 1991; 12:108–114.
18. Moore T, Ucko L. Night waking in early infancy: Part 1. Arch Dis Child 1957; 32: 333–342.
19. Richman N. Surveys of sleep disorders in children in a general population. In: Guilleminault C, ed. Sleep and Its Disorders in Children. New York: Raven Press, 1987:115–127.
20. Sadeh A, Anders TY. Infant sleep problems: origins, assessment, intervention. Infant Mental Health J 1993; 14:17–34.
21. Sadeh A, Lavie P, Scher A, Tirosh E, Epstein R. Actigraphic home monitoring of sleep-disturbed and control infants and young children: a new method for pediatric assessment of sleep-wake patterns. Pediatrics 1991; 87:494–499.
22. Ottaviano S, Giannotti F, Cortesi F, Bruni O, Ottaviano C. Sleep characteristics in healthy children from birth to 6 years of age in the urban area of Rome. Sleep 1996; 19:1–3.
23. Hauri P, Olmstead E. Childhood-onset insomnia. Sleep 1980; 3:59–65.
24. Kateria S, Swanson M, Trevarthin G. Persistence of sleep disturbances in preschool children. J Pediatr 1987; 110:642–646.
25. Monroe L. Psychological and physiological differences between good and poor sleepers. J Abnorm Psychol 1967; 72:255–264.

26. Richman N, Stevenson J, Graham P. Preschool To School: A Behavioral Study. London: Academic Press, 1982.
27. Salzarulo P, Chevalier A. Sleep problems in children and their relationships with early disturbances of the waking-sleeping rhythms. Sleep 1983; 6:47–51.
28. Zuckerman B, Stevenson J, Baily V. Sleep problems in early childhood: predictive factors and behavior correlates. Pediatrics 1987; 80:664–671.
29. Blader JC, Koplewicz HC, Abikoff H, Foley C. Sleep problems of elementary school children: a community survey. Arch Pediatr Adolesc Med 1997; 151:473–480.
30. Rona RJ, Gulliford MC, Chinn S. Disturbed sleep: effects of sociocultural factors and illness. Arch Dis Child 1998; 78:20–25.
31. Anders TY, Carskadon MA, Dement WC, Harvey K. Sleep habits of children and the identification of pathologically sleepy children. Child Psychiatry Hum Dev 1978; 9:56–62.
32. Kahn A, Van de Merckt C, Rebuffat E, Mozin MJ, Sottiaux M, Blum D, Hennart P. Sleep problems in healthy preadolescents. Pediatrics 1989; 84:542–546.
33. Coble PA, Kupfer D, Reynolds CF, Houck P. EEG sleep of healthy children 6 to 12 years of age. In Guilleminault C, ed. Sleep and Its Disorders in Children. New York: Raven Press, 1987:29–41.
34. Gruber R, Sadeh A, Raviv A. Sleep of school-age children: objective and subjective measures. Sleep Res 1997; 26:158.
35. Beltramini A, Hertzig M. Sleep and bedtime behavior in preschool-aged children. Pediatrics 1983; 71:153–158.
36. Richman N. A community survey of characteristics of one- to two-year-olds with sleep disruptions. J Am Acad Child Psychiatry 1981; 20:281–291.
37. Terr L. Nightmares in children. In Guilleminault C, ed. Sleep and Its Disorders in Children. New York: Raven Press, 1987:231–242.
38. Carskadon MA, Viera C, Acebo C. Association between puberty and delayed phase preference. Sleep 1993; 16:258–262.
39. Carskadon MA, Acebo C, Richardson GS, Tate BA, Seifer R. Long-nights protocol: access to circadian parameters in adolescents. J Biol Rhythms 1997; 12:278–289.
40. Carskadon MA. Patterns of sleep and sleepiness in adolescents. Pediatrician 1990; 17: 5–12.
41. Carskadon MA, Dement WC. Sleepiness in the normal adolescent. In: Guilleminault C, ed. Sleep and Its Disorders in Children. New York: Raven Press, 1987:53–66.
42. Wolfson A, Carskadon M. Sleep schedules and daytime functioning in adolescents. Child Dev 1998; 69:875–887.
43. Epstein R, Chillag N, Lavie P. Starting times of school: effects on daytime functioning of fifth-grade children in Israel. Sleep 1988; 21:250–256.
44. Tynjala J, Kannas L, Levalahti E. Perceived tiredness among adolescents and its association with sleep habits and use of psychoactive substances. J Sleep Res 1997; 6: 189–198.
45. Mercer PW, Merritt SL, Cowell JM. Differences in sleep need among adolescents. J Adolesc Health 1998: 23:259–263.
46. Manbar R, Bootzin RR, Acebo C, Carskadon MA. The effects of regularizing sleep-wake schedule on daytime sleepiness. Sleep 1996; 19:432–441.
47. Carskadon MA, Wolfson AR, Acebo C, Tzischinsky O, Seifer R. Adolescent sleep patterns, circadian timing, and sleepiness at a transition to early school days. Sleep 1998; 21:871–881.

48. Weitzman ED, Czeisler CA, Coleman RM, Spielman AJ, Zimmerman JC, Dement WC. Delayed sleep phase syndrome, a chronobiological disorder with sleep-onset insomnia. Arch Gen Psychiatry 1981; 38:737–746.
49. Alvarez B, Dahlitz MJ, Vignau J, Parkes JD. The delayed sleep phase syndrome: clinical and investigative findings in 14 subjects. J Neurol Neurosurg Psychiatry 1992; 55: 665–670.
50. Thorpy MJ, Korman E, Spielman AJ, Glovinsky PB. Delayed sleep phase syndrome in adolescents. J Adolesc Health Care 1988; 9:222–227.
51. Roffwarg H, Muzio J, Dement W. Ontogenetic development of the human sleep-dream cycle. Science 1966; 152:604.
52. Kahn A, Dan B, Groswasser J, Franco P, Sottiaux M. Normal sleep architecture in infants and children. J Clin Neuropsychol 1996; 13:184–197.
53. Kahn E, Fisher C, Edwards A. Twenty-four hour sleep patterns: comparison between 2- to 3-year old and 4- to 6-year-old children. Arch Gen Psychiatry 1973; 29:380.
54. Maron L, Rechtschaffen A, Wolpert E. Sleep cycle during napping. Arch Gen Psychiatry 1996; 11:503.
55. Webb W, Agnew H. Sleep cycling within 24-hour periods. J Exp Psychol 1967; 74:158.
56. Ross JJ. Sleep patterns in pre-adolescent children: an EEG-EOG study. Pediatrics 1968; 42:324–335.
57. Dahl R, Trubnick L, Al-Shabbout, Ryan N. Normal maturation of sleep: a longitudinal EEG study in children. Sleep Res 1997; 26:155.
58. Carskadon MA, Keenan S, Dement WC. Nighttime sleep and daytime sleep tendency in preadolescents. In: Guilleminault C, ed. Sleep and Its Disorders in Children, New York: Raven Press, 1987: 43–52.
59. Carskadon MA, Orav EJ, Dement WC. Evolution of sleep and daytime sleepiness in adolescents. In Guilleminault C, Lugaresi E, eds. Sleep/Wake Disorders: Natural History, Epidemiology, and Long-Term Evaluation. New York: Raven Press, 1983: 201–216.
60. Bes F, Schulz H, Navelet Y, Salzarulo P. The distribution of slow-wave sleep across the night: a comparison for infants, children and adults. Sleep 1991; 14:5–12.
61. Acebo C, Millman RP, Rosenberg C, Cavallo A, Carskadon MA. Sleep, breathing, and cephalometrics in older children and young adults: Part I—normative values. Chest 1996; 109:664–672.
62. Zapelin H. Mammalian sleep. In MH Kryger, T Roth and WC Dement Principles and Practice of Sleep Medicine, 2d ed. London: Saunders, 1994:69–80.
63. Kahn A, Mozin M, Rebuffat E, Sottiaux M, Muller MF. Milk intolerance in children with persistent sleeplessness: a prospective double-blind crossover evaluation. Pediatrics 1989; 84:595–603.
64. Kahn A, Rebuffat E, Sottiaux M, Dufour D, Cadranel S, Reiterer F. Arousals induced by proximal esophageal reflux in infants. Sleep 1991; 14:39–42.
65. Ghaem M, Armstrong KL, Trocki O, Cleghorn GJ, Patrick MK, Shepherd RW. The sleep patterns of infants and young children with gastro-oesophageal reflux. J Paediatr Child Health 1998; 34;160–163.
66. Weissbluth M. Colic. In: Ferber R, Kryger M, eds. Principles and Practice of Sleep Medicine in the Child. Philadelphia: Saunders, 1995:75–78.
67. Reid P, Lewisjones MS. Sleep difficulties and their management in preschoolers with atopic eczema. Clin Exp Dermatol 1995; 20:38–41.

68. Stores G, Burrows A, Crawford C. Physiological sleep disturbances in children with atopic dermatitis: a case control study. Pediatr Dermatol 1998; 15:264–268.
69. Sheldon HS, Spire JP, Levy HB. Pediatric Sleep Medicine. Philadelphia: Saunders, 1992.
70. Bruni O, Favrizi P, Ottaviano S, Cortesi F, Giannotti F, Guidetti V. Prevalence of sleep disorders in childhood and adolescence with headache: a case-control study. Cephalalgia 1997; 17:492–498.
71. Madge PJ, Nisbet L, McColl JH, Vallance A, Paton JY, Beattie JO. Home nebuliser use in children with asthma in two Scottish Health Board Areas. Scott Med J 1995; 40:141–143.
72. Kales A, Kales JD, Sly RM, Scharf MB, Tand TL, Preston TA. Sleep patterns of asthmatic children: all night EEG studies. J Allergy 1970; 46:300–308.
73. Sadeh A, Horowitz I, Wolach-Benodis L, Wolach B. Sleep and pulmonary function in children with well-controlled, stable asthma. Sleep 1998; 21:379–384.
74. Okawa M, Nanami T, Wada S, Shimizu T, Hishikawa Y, Sasa H, Nagamine H, Takahashi K. Four congenitally blind children with circadian sleep-wake rhythm disorder. Sleep 1987; 10:101–110.
75. Sadeh A, Klitzke M, Anders TF, Acebo C. Sleep and aggressive behavior in a blind retarded adolescent: a concomitant schedule disorder? J Am Acad Child Adolesc Psychiatry 1995; 34:820–824.
76. Tzischinsky O, Skene D, Epstein R, Lavie P. Circadian rhythms in 6-sulfatoxymelatonin and nocturnal sleep in blind children. Chronobiol Int 1991; 8:168–175.
77. Palm L, Blennow G, Wetterberg L. Long-term melatonin treatment in blind children and young adults with circadian sleep-wake disturbances. Dev Med Child Neurol 1997; 39:319–325.
78. Okawa M, Sasaki H. Sleep disorders in mentally retarded and brain-impaired children. In: Guilleminault C, ed. Sleep and Its Disorders in Children. New York: Raven Press, 1987:269–290.
79. Mindell JA. Sleep disorders in children. Health Psychol 1993; 12:151–162.
80. Wolfson A. Sleeping patterns of children and adolescents: developmental trends, disruptions and adaptations. Psychiatr Clin North Am 1996; 5:685–700.
81. Anders TF, Eiben LA. Pediatric sleep disorders: a review of the past 10 years. J Am Acad Child Adolesc Psychiatry 1997; 36:9–20.
82. Sadeh A, Gruber R. Sleep Disorders. In: Bellack AS, Hersen M, eds. Comprehensive Clinical Psychology. New York: Pergamon, 1998:629–653.
83. Sadeh A. Stress, trauma and sleep in children. Psychiatr Clin North Am 1996; 5:685–700.
84. Sadeh A, Gruber R. Stress and sleep in adolescence: a clinical-developmental perspective. In: Carskadon MA, ed. Adolescent Sleep Patterns: Biological, Social, and Psychological Influences. New York: Cambridge University Press. In press.
85. Dahl RE. The regulation of sleep and arousal: development and psychopathology. Dev Psychopathol 1996; 8:3–27.
86. Thoman EB. Sleeping and waking in infants: A functional perspective. Neurosci Biobehav Rev 1989; 14:93107.
87. Thoman EB. Sleep and wake behaviors in the neonates: consistencies and consequences. Merrill-Palmer Q 1975; 21:295–314.
88. Freudigman KA, Thoman E. Infant sleep during the first postnatal day: an opportunity for assessment of vulnerability. Pediatrics 1993; 92:373–379.

89. Thoman EB, Denenberg VH, Sievel J, Zeidner LP, Becker P. State organization in neonates: developmental inconsistency indicates risk for developmental dysfunction. Neuropediatrics 1981; 12:45–54.
90. Scher MS, Steppe DA, Banks DL. Prediction of lower developmental performances of healthy neonates by neonatal EEG-sleep measures. Pediatr Neurol 1996; 14:137–144.
91. Sadeh A, Lavie P, Scher A. Maternal perceptions of temperament of sleep-disturbed toddlers. Early Educ Dev 1994; 5:311–322.
92. Weissbluth M, Liu K. Sleep patterns, attention span and infant temperament. J Dev Behav Pediatr 1983; 4:34–36.
93. Dahl RE. The impact of inadequate sleep on children's daytime cognitive function. Semin Pediatr Neurol 1996; 3:44–50.
94. Chervin RD, Dillon JE, Bassetti C, Ganoczy DA, Pituch KJ. Symptoms of sleep disorders, inattention, and hyperactivity in children. Sleep 1997; 20:1185–1192.
95. Hansen DE, Vandenberg B. Neuropsychological features and differential diagnosis of sleep apnea syndrome in children. J Clin Child Psychol 1997; 26:304–310.
96. Picchietti DL, Walters AS. Restless legs syndrome and periodic limb movement disorder in children and adolescents: comorbidity with attention-deficit hyperactivity disorder. Psychiatr Clin North Am 1996; 5:729–751.
97. Corkum P, Tannock R, Moldofsky H. Sleep disturbances in children with attention-deficit/hyperactivity disorder. J Am Acad Child Adolesc Psychiatry 1998; 37:637–646.
98. Gozal D. Sleep-disordered breathing and school performance in children. Pediatrics 1998; 102:616–620.
99. Sadeh A, Raviv A, Gruber R. Sleep and neurobehavioral functioning in school children. Paper presented at the 14th Congress of the European Sleep Research Society, Madrid, September, 1998.
100. Randazzo AC, Muehlbach MJ, Schweitzer PK, Walsh JK. Cognitive function following acute sleep restriction in children ages 10–14. Sleep 1998; 15;861–868.
101. Thoman EB, Acebo C. Monitoring of sleep in neonate and young children. In: Ferber R, Kryger M, eds. Principles and Practice of Sleep Medicine in the Child. Philadelphia: Saunders, 1995:55–68.
102. Ferber R. Clinical assessment of child and adolescent sleep disorders. Psychiatr Clin North Am 1996; 5:569–579.
103. Sadeh A. Evaluating night-wakings in sleep-disturbed infants: a methodological study of parental reports and actigraphy. Sleep 1996; 19:757–762.

4

Maturation of the Arousal Response

SALLY L. DAVIDSON WARD

University of Southern California
Keck School of Medicine and
Childrens Hospital Los Angeles
Los Angeles, California

THOMAS G. KEENS

University of Southern California
Keck School of Medicine
Childrens Hospital Los Angeles
UCLA School of Medicine and
Mattel Children's Hospital at UCLA
Los Angeles, California

I. Introduction

Arousal from sleep is an important defense mechanism against danger-signaling stimuli during sleep (1). This has an important role in protection from potential respiratory dangers during sleep. Arousal from sleep commonly occurs during obstructive apnea in adults with obstructive sleep apnea syndrome (OSAS), and it is associated with increasing upper airway skeletal muscle tone and reestablishment of airway patency (2). It has been suggested that absent arousal in response to hypoxia and/or hypercapnia may put infants at risk for sudden infant death syndrome (SIDS) (3). Similarly, absent arousal in response to hypoxia and hypercapnia has been described in children with serious disorders of ventilatory control (4). Thus arousal is an important physiological defense against potentially dangerous situations during sleep. However, the development of arousal responses, specifically to respiratory stimuli, is poorly understood. This chapter reviews spontaneous, sensory, and respiratory arousal responses in infants, children, and adults and what is known about the maturation and development of these responses.

II. Characteristics and Definition of Arousal

Arousal responses may take the form of a relatively brief electromyographic (EMG) increase, a sleep state transition, a brief period of electroencephalographic (EEG) desynchronization, or frank awakening (5). In healthy adults studied with acoustic stimuli, EMG increases were most common (24%), followed by movement arousals (19%), sleep stage shifts (19%), EEG speeding (17%), alpha events (13%), and awakenings (2%) (6). Large, transient increases in systemic blood pressure, heart rate, and ventilation occur in association with arousal from sleep, supporting the notion that awakening from sleep leads to sympathetic nervous system activation (7). These changes are out of proportion to need and may represent an epiphenomenon of the effort required to transition from sleep to wakefulness. Alternately, these responses may be protective, in that they prepare the individual to face the real or potential danger that initiated the arousal from sleep (7).

The neuroanatomical basis of the arousal response is not localized to a specific nucleus but rather projects in the midline from the pons caudally to the pyramidal tracts and includes the posterior hypothalamus, subthalamus, and basal forebrain (8). In the generation of an arousal response, the reticular activating system receives collateral input from visceral, somatic, or other sensory systems. After integration, the reticular activating system transmits information via long ascending projections into the forebrain, with resulting cortical activation (8).

A standardized approach to identifying and scoring arousals has been made available only recently. In 1992, the American Sleep Disorders Association (ASDA) published a set of scoring rules for EEG arousals (9). They recommended that an arousal be scored in non–rapid-eye-movement (NREM) sleep when there is "an abrupt shift in EEG frequency, which may include theta, alpha, and/or frequencies greater than 16 Hz, but not spindles" lasting for at least 3 sec (9). To be scored as an arousal, the change in EEG frequency must follow at least 10 sec of continuous sleep. An arousal from REM sleep also requires an increase in the amplitude of the EMG (9). Increases in EMG amplitude in either NREM or REM sleep not accompanied by EEG changes do not constitute an arousal. If these guidelines are broadly adopted by the research community, they will increase the ability to compare results from different studies. This will be of considerable importance in the understanding of the maturation of the arousal response where, of necessity, much information is derived from cross-sectional studies performed at different ages. These rules were not designed specifically for infants but probably have applicability to all age groups.

Arousals may occur spontaneously during sleep, or they may occur in response to sensory or respiratory stimuli. Of course, when studying induced arousals, one must always consider the possibility that spontaneous arousals may occur coincidentally with a stimulus. Arousal thresholds for sensory and respiratory stimuli can be determined by laboratory testing, and they are often used to assess which groups of subjects or which conditions are associated with more difficulty in waking from sleep. A decreased arousal threshold to a stimulus means that there is increased arousal responsiveness, and vice versa. Such techniques are used to compare groups of subjects, states, different ages, or different environmental conditions.

III. State and Sleep History Influences on Arousal

Arousal thresholds are affected by sleep state. In adult animals, an arousal response to hypoxia occurs at a lower oxygen saturation during REM compared to NREM. Newborn animals also awaken at a lower oxygen saturation during REM sleep compared to NREM (10). Thus, animal studies have suggested that it is more difficult to arouse from sleep during REM sleep than during NREM sleep.

Arousal thresholds are affected by sleep fragmentation. Although habituation may play a role in the progressive difficulty in arousing subjects in response to a repetitive stimulus, increases in the arousal threshold may also be caused by an accelerating need for sleep. The frequent arousals and sleep fragmentation may cause excessive daytime sleepiness in adults with OSAS because of an increased pressure to sleep. The impact of frequent arousals on daytime function appears to depend on their type, number, nocturnal distribution, and chronicity (12). Increased daytime sleepiness can even result from partial arousal responses in adults, as evidenced by studies of acoustic stimulation during sleep that elicited increases in blood pressure without evidence of EEG arousal (13). Thus, both complete and partial arousals, if they occur frequently enough, are capable of causing excessive daytime somnolence.

Sleep deprivation affects respiratory behaviors during sleep in adults with OSAS, including blunting of hypoxic and hypercapnic ventilatory responses and increased number of obstructive apneas (14). Sleep deprivation also decreases arousability in adult dogs (15). Thomas and coworkers evaluated the affects of sleep deprivation on spontaneous and induced arousal responses in healthy 3-month-old infants (16). They found no differences in spontaneous awakenings or movement arousals following sleep deprivation. Induced arousals were studied by auditory and photic stimuli, and they were also not affected by sleep deprivation (16). However, sleep deprivation increased the proportion of quiet sleep, altered the respiratory pattern, and increased peripheral chemoreceptor responses (16). Thus, sleep fragmentation has more of an effect of decreasing arousal in adults than in infants, but it can affect respiratory patterns, ventilatory responses, and sleep architecture in infants.

IV. Environmental Influences on Arousal in Infants

The infant prenatal environment has an impact on arousal patterns and responses. Tirosh and coworkers demonstrated a decreased incidence of arousal responses from quiet sleep following obstructive apneas in 2-day-old healthy term infants born to mothers who smoked cigarettes during pregnancy (17). Newborns of smoking mothers have also been reported to awaken less frequently in response to auditory stimuli (18). Finally, infants of smoking mothers were less likely to arouse in response to hypoxic challenges, although arousal to hypercapnia was not affected (19). These findings taken together suggest that there may be a generalized arousal deficit in infants of mothers who smoke. Prenatal smoking significantly increases the risk of dying from SIDS. Similarly, Davidson Ward and coworkers found abnormal hypoxic arousal responses and increased arousal thresholds to hypercapnia in infants of cocaine-abusing mothers (20). It is not known if these prenatal effects on arousal responsiveness persist beyond infancy.

The infant sleep environment has been shown to affect sleep architecture and the incidence of spontaneous arousals. For example, maternal bed sharing reduced stages 3 to 4 NREM sleep and increased awakenings and transient arousals in infants (21). In addition, there was considerable overlap between infant and maternal arousals during bed sharing, with infant arousals most commonly preceding those of the mother (21).

Infants who sleep in the prone position are at increased risk of dying from SIDS (24). The pathophysiological mechanisms responsible for the increased risk of SIDS in the prone position are not known. However, some researchers believe that infants may suffer asphyxial rebreathing in a face-down position. Infant behavior, including arousal responses, following a change in body position from side to prone during sleep, have been evaluated by Skadberg and Markestad (25). They studied infants at 2.5 and 5.0 months of age during both quiet and active sleep. Infants were initially placed in the side position and then were abruptly moved to the prone position. The ability of the infant to move from the face-down position was then evaluated. About two-thirds of the infants did not move from the face-down position on at least one occasion (25). Infants who were successful in moving their face to the side did so only after considerable effort, with vigorous body movements and grunting, although not crying. There were no differences in responses according to age or sleep states (25). This study suggests that, in some circumstances, infants may arouse in response to a stimulus—i.e., face down position—yet not manage to rescue themselves from potential danger (25).

Behavioral components of the arousal response in infancy were evaluated by Lijowska and colleagues during rebreathing caused by infant bedding, during hypercapnia, and during spontaneous arousals (26). They described four stereotypical behaviors: 1) sighs or augmented breaths; 2) startles; 3) thrashing limb movements; and 4) full behavioral arousal with eye opening and crying (26). The behaviors always occurred in the same order, with a sigh accompanied by a startle, then thrashing, and then full arousal. Incomplete sequences were common. As inspired carbon dioxide tension increased, either by asphyxial rebreathing or by exposure to a gas mixture with elevated CO_2, arousal sequences persisted and became more complete until the bed covers were removed or the baby was completely awake (26). The authors hypothesized that this sequence of behaviors is an airway defense reflex. The arousal sequence occurred in both the supine and prone positions. When the infant was prone, the motor activity occasionally resulted in the face-down position with an actual increase in inspired CO_2concentration, supporting the investigators' conclusion that this series of behaviors is a reflex sequence rather than a learned behavior. The infants studied ranged in age from 2 weeks to 6 months, and no maturational differences were noted in the behavioral response (26).

Thus, the environment influences arousal responses in infants. Some of these induced arousals show maturational patterns and some do not. When maturational patterns are observed, they often reveal more difficulty in arousing at 2 to 4 months of age—a developmental window of vulnerability for SIDS.

V. Arousal Response to Sensory Stimuli

Fetal well-being is often assessed by testing responses to acoustic stimulation. A heart rate acceleration of 15 beats per minute above baseline, lasting for 15 sec, was used as the endpoint in a study of more than 700 fetuses who were products of high-risk pregnancies (27). Only 2% of the tests failed to produce the desired response. These tests were not controlled for fetal state, and the heart rate acceleration was not the equivalent of an EEG arousal or complete behavioral awakening. However, this suggests that the arousal response to sound is a part of normal fetal behavior and that arousal to sound may be relatively common in the fetus.

Auditory arousal thresholds have been studied in 97 normal infants at a mean age of about 10 weeks (28). Arousal responses were tested during an overnight polysomnogram in quiet sleep, after the first cycle of sleep was completed. Approximately 70% of the infants aroused in response to an auditory stimulus with maximum sound level to 120 dB (28). The infants who aroused were significantly older than those who failed to arouse. Auditory arousal thresholds also fell with increasing age (28). These findings suggest an increase in arousal responsiveness to sound with increasing age.

Scant longitudinal information is available regarding arousal responses in infancy. However two longitudinal studies of arousal responses in infancy have been performed by Newman and coworkers (22,23). In one study, they evaluated responses to a vibrotactile stimulus during quiet and active sleep in a group of infants at 1 and 2 weeks of age and monthly from 1 to 6 months of age (22). Arousal was defined as a change in heart or respiratory rate, EEG desynchronization, or an increase in EMG amplitude. Arousal to a vibrotactile stimulus occurred less than 50% of the time in quiet sleep, irrespective of the intensity or frequency of the stimulus, and it was not affected by age (22). However, in active sleep, although variations in stimulus intensity or frequency had no impact, arousal responsiveness changed with age (22). Infants were more likely to arouse between 2 weeks and 2 months of age. Arousal responses from active sleep decreased significantly at 3 months of age and then returned to previous levels by 4 months (22). The other study evaluated responses to partial nasal occlusion during sleep (23). The investigators concluded that arousal was more easily elicited in active sleep than quiet sleep (23); they also found that failure to arouse was more common at 2 months of age than at older or younger ages (23). These findings have important implications for SIDS, which is more common between 1 and 4 months of age, a time of life referred to as a "developmental window of vulnerability."

Like infants, normal children may be very difficult to awaken from sleep. A study of auditory arousal thresholds in enuretic boys, using a graduated pure tone terminating at 120 dB, resulted in complete behavioral arousal in only 40% of trials in normal, healthy control boys age 7 to 12 years (29). Arousal was more difficult in the first third of the night, occurring only after 12% of trials. Arousal became more frequent as the night progressed, reaching 60% of trials in the latter third of the night. Enuretic boys were more difficult to arouse than the control group, awakening after only 25% of trials, suggesting that an arousal deficit may play a role in nocturnal enuresis (29). A similar study of arousal thresholds in normal and hyperkinetic prepubertal boys found comparable results, with only about one-half of acoustic challenges resulting in arousal and only one-third in complete awakening despite sound levels of 123 dB (30).

Badr and coworkers studied normal adults in NREM sleep with auditory stimuli ranging from 45 to 85 dB (31). Arousal was defined by the ASDA scoring rules and occurred in about 60% of trials. In addition to EEG arousals, the authors also examined the effect of the stimuli on ventilation. They found that hyperpnea resulted from auditory stimuli, but only in the presence of an arousal response (31). Blood pressure and heart rate increased with auditory stimulation during sleep, even in the absence of cortical arousal, and these physiological responses were further augmented by cortical arousal (31). Somewhat different findings were described by Carley and coworkers from a group of healthy young adults exposed to 85-dB tones during NREM sleep (32). Arousal occurred in response to this stimulus in 42% of trials in stages 1 and 2 sleep, and in 31% of trials in stages 3 to 4 sleep. They also documented hyperpnea in response to auditory stimuli but noted that the increase in ventilation was seen even in the absence of cortical arousal (32).

Two studies are available comparing auditory arousal in different age groups, and both demonstrate a fall in arousal thresholds with increasing age (easier to arouse). McDonald and coworkers studied adult men and women in three age groups, 18 to 25, 40 to 48, and 52 to 71 years (33). Arousal thresholds fell in both NREM and REM sleep with advancing age in men and in NREM sleep in women. More recently, Busby and coworkers studied male children, preadolescents, adolescents, and young adults and found that awakenings occurred more frequently in response to lower stimulus intensities with advancing age (34). Children did not exhibit differences in arousal thresholds between sleep stages, whereas adults were more difficult to awaken in NREM sleep than REM sleep.

Thus, arousal in response to sensory stimuli requires less intense stimuli in older subjects. Infants and children are generally more difficult to arouse with auditory stimuli than adults.

VI. Spontaneous Arousals

In addition to induced arousal responses to external stimuli, examination of spontaneous arousals can provide information about the maturation of the arousal response. Spontaneous arousals define the characteristics of undisturbed sleep. Naturally occurring arousals were studied in normal infants at a mean age of 9.6 weeks and in normal children at a mean age of 4.6 years by McNamara and associates (35). Spontaneous arousals occurred about once every 3 to 6 min in infants and every 6 to 10 min in the children in both quiet and active sleep, suggesting more sleep fragmentation in the infants (35). Boselli and coworkers studied EEG arousals using the ASDA rules in healthy people in four age groups: 1) teenagers age 10 to 19 years; 2) young adults age 20 to 39 years; 3) middle-aged adults age 40 to 59 years; and 4) the elderly, older than 60 years (36). Ten subjects were included in each group. Overnight polysomnograms were scored for arousals, with arousal indices calculated for total sleep and for each sleep stage. Extensive precautions in the testing procedure and in preparation for the study night were used to ensure that the data collected represented normal sleep. Arousal indices increased linearly with age for total sleep, NREM sleep, and stages 1 to 2 sleep (36). Arousal indices did not change with age in stages 3 to 4 and in REM sleep (36). The length of each arousal was stable across age groups (about 15 sec), and there were no differences in arousal lengths in NREM compared to REM sleep. The authors concluded that aging is physiologically associated with a progressive increase in sleep fragmentation (36). Their study provides normative data; however, the upper limit of normal spontaneous arousal indices remains to be described.

Thus, it appears that both induced and spontaneous arousals are more common with advancing age and that school-age children are particularly difficult to arouse from sleep. Parallel to the changes in arousal responsiveness, there is also a decrease in NREM sleep, which first becomes apparent in adolescents and is most obvious when the elderly are examined (37). The explanations for these changes vary widely. Some view spontaneous EEG arousals as a normal feature rather than an indication of sleep disturbance. The fall in NREM sleep has been seen as a reflection of the normal decline in cortical metabolism, increased dendritic pruning, and decreased cortical synaptic activity. Others simply view this as a marker of aging. The young age of onset is explained by the evolutionary context of human life expectancy of 20 to 30 years in the premodern era (38). If arousal responses are considered to be an important protective mechanism from danger-signaling stimuli during sleep, then perhaps the elderly could be seen as more vulnerable and in greater need of protective vigilance. Shore and colleagues addressed this question by studying spontaneous and apnea-related arousals in healthy elderly subjects and compared them to patterns obtained from young adults (39). The elderly subjects had more sleep apnea and significantly more arousals than the younger subjects. Apneic episodes were frequently terminated by arousals, but there were many spontaneous arousals in the elderly subjects unrelated to apnea. In fact, arousals occurred with equal frequency in apneic and nonapneic elderly subjects (39).

Thus, spontaneous arousals become more common during sleep with advancing age. They are less common in infants and increase in childhood, adulthood, and elderly life.

VII. Respiratory-Related Arousals and Apnea-Induced Arousals

The consequences of frequent arousals in adults, caused by OSAS or induced experimentally, have been well documented. Excessive daytime sleepiness and neurobehavioral abnormalities of vigilance and reaction time are the sequelae of frequent arousals in adults. The arousal response in a patient with sleep-disordered breathing is a two-edged sword. Arousal from sleep can be a lifesaving event, rescuing the patient from asphyxia. However, if frequent arousals result in sleep disruption, then sleep is not restorative and daytime function is impaired (2). Experimental sleep fragmentation, induced by nonrespiratory stimuli, results in severe daytime sleepiness in the absence of exposure to airway obstruction or hypoxemia. Even stimuli that only cause transient elevations in blood pressure, or "autonomic arousals," have been shown to result in increased daytime sleepiness (40). Evidence suggests that sleep fragmentation or deprivation may contribute to impaired arousal responsiveness and that this may play a role in adults with OSAS. Adults with OSAS have impaired arousal responses to airway occlusion compared to normal individuals (41). Even when the same subject is studied over one night, an increase in apnea length and increased inspiratory effort at apnea termination can be seen as the night progresses (42). The relative contributions of sleep fragmentation, habituation to repetitive stimuli, or genetic predisposition to impaired arousal responsiveness in OSAS are not known. In support of an inherent predisposition are studies showing persistently high arousal thresholds in OSAS patients receiving long-term therapy with continuous positive airway pressure (CPAP) (43–45). Impaired arousal responses in adults with OSAS may actually result in the beneficial effect of allowing some sleep to occur despite the presence of multiple afferent stimuli. Overall, the situation for adults with OSAS can be viewed as a tug of war between the need for sleep and the need to arouse and respond to dangerous stimuli.

Like that in the adult population, pediatric obstructive sleep apnea has been reported to have neurobehavioral sequelae, but excessive daytime sleepiness is less common in pediatric OSAS than in adults (46). This may be due to the fact that obstructive apneas, even when accompanied by hypoxemia, frequently do not result in cortical arousal in children. McNamara and coworkers studied apnea-related arousals in infants and children with OSAS and found that only 39% and 38% of apneas in NREM and REM sleep, respectively, were terminated by an arousal response (35). Obstructive apneas were more likely to result in arousal than central apneas. The number of respiratory-related arousals increased as age increased (35). Infants and children with OSAS had less active or REM sleep than their normal counterparts. However, the overall frequency of arousal did not differ from that of normal children.

Therefore, disruptions of sleep architecture are not as severe in OSAS children as those in OSAS adults, so there is less sleep fragmentation and deprivation in pediatric OSAS (35). Marcus and coworkers evaluated arousal responses to hypercapnia and hypoxia in children with OSAS (47). They found no difference in arousal to hypoxia between OSAS and normal children. However, children with OSAS did have slightly elevated arousal thresholds to hypercapnia, although all subjects did arouse (47). A few children with OSAS were studied again following adenotonsillectomy, and they had lower arousal thresholds to hypercapnia after treatment (increased arousal) (47). Therefore, abnormalities of arousal responsiveness appear to exist in both adults and children with OSAS, but the clinical manifestations and sequelae are different. It is not known if the differences seen in children with OSAS, as compared to adults, are due to decreased arousability, an increased drive to maintain sleep, or a lower intensity of the stimuli for arousal. Decreased chemoreceptor function is unlikely because children have higher ventilatory responses to hypoxia and hypercapnia than adults (48). It may be that the need for sleep in children and adolescents overrides the protective advantage of frequent arousal responses, either spontaneous or induced.

Thus, children have decreased arousal in response to respiratory stimuli than adults. Children with OSAS have less arousal, sleep fragmentation, and excessive daytime sleepiness than adults with OSAS.

VIII. Hypoxic and Hypercapnic Arousal Responses

Hypoxic and hypercapnic arousal responses are mediated by the central and peripheral chemoreceptors with transmission to the reticular activating system. Ventilatory responses to hypoxia and hypercapnia depend on the transmission of afferent information from the peripheral and central chemoreceptors to the brainstem respiratory centers. Although the arousal and ventilatory responses are distinct (49–52), the arousal response plays a facilitatory role in the ventilatory response to respiratory stimuli (5).

Hypercapnia during NREM sleep is a potent stimulus to arousal. In normal human adults and infants, the Pa_{CO_2} arousal threshold is about 50 to 60 torr, with arousal occurring in essentially 100% of trials (3,50,53). The arousal threshold in adults during REM sleep is somewhat higher (54,55). Fewell and coworkers have demonstrated a decreased frequency of arousal responses to hypercapnia, in both quiet and REM sleep, in lambs with carotid denervation, suggesting that peripheral chemoreceptors play a role in the generation of arousal responses to hypercapnia (56).

Hypoxia is a less effective stimulus to arousal. Most normal infants less than 6 months of age fail to arouse from quiet sleep in response to a fractional inspired oxygen concentration of 11% to 12% (57,58). The earliest study of hypoxic arousal responses in infants was performed in 1955 by Miller and Smull (57), who described arousal from sleep in 5 of 9 (56%) 1-day old full-term infants challenged with an FI_{O_2} of 12% via mask for 5 min. Sleep and arousal were determined by behavioral criteria. No attempt to stage sleep was made (57). These results suggested that a slight majority of infants are born with an arousal response to hypoxia, which presumably has some protective function (57). In adults, progressive arterial oxygen desaturation to as low as 70% fails to elicit an arousal response in over 50% of trials in both REM and NREM sleep (59–61).

Gingras and colleagues (62) evaluated hypoxic arousal responses in 10 healthy term infants during the first week of life according to the method of Davidson Ward et al. (58) and of van der Hal et al. (3). Complete behavioral arousal from quiet sleep was elicited in 89% of hypoxic challenge tests (62). Garg and associates found that the infants with bronchopulmonary dysplasia, studied at term-corrected age, had intact hypoxic arousal responses (52). Therefore, the newborn hypoxic arousal response is intact and appears to differ from that of older infants, children, and adults, in whom arousal to hypoxia is less likely (58–62). This is an interesting contrast to the unique hypoxic ventilatory response in newborn infants, which is characterized by respiratory depression.

Davidson Ward and colleagues studied hypoxic arousal responses using an F_{IO_2} of 0.11 in normal infants 6 months of age and less (58). They found that only approximately 40% of normal infants aroused from quiet sleep in response to a 3-min hypoxic challenge. Further, when those infants who aroused were compared to those who failed to arouse, there was a trend for the younger infants to arouse (58). It was also found that periodic breathing or apnea was unusual during hypoxia but occurred in the majority of infants who failed to arouse following hypoxia (58). These results suggest a maturational pattern in the hypoxic arousal response. Infants appear to be born with a hypoxic arousal response, which is presumably brainstem-mediated. As they enter the age when the incidence of SIDS increases (approximately 2 months of age), a majority of infants lose this hypoxic arousal response. The mechanism for this loss is unclear, but it may relate to maturation of cortical areas of the brain, which may suppress more "primitive" brainstem function (58). It is tempting to postulate that infants may be at increased risk for SIDS beginning at about 2 months of age, in part because they lose a potentially protective hypoxic arousal response at about this age (58,62).

Ariagno and coworkers described arousal from quiet sleep in 4 of 5 (80%) healthy infants between the ages of 1 and 4 months using an F_{IO_2} of 15% via mask (63). Hunt demonstrated arousal in 15 of 21 (71%) control infants at about 2 months of age challenged with an F_{IO_2} of 15% using a nasal mask (64). Therefore, in studies using a face mask to deliver the hypoxic mixture, arousal occurred in 56% to 80% of challenges. However, the presence of the mask itself may have contributed to arousal in some cases, resulting in the apparent increased frequency of arousal in these infants compared to those in other studies (58,63,64).

McCulloch and coworkers reported arousal from quiet sleep in 14 of 20 (70%) control infants at about 2 months of age using an F_{IO_2} of 15% via head hood (65). Brady described arousal responses from quiet sleep in response to an F_{IO_2} of 17% via head hood in 30% of trials performed on 7 control infants at 2 to 3 months of age (66).

Milerad and associates documented arousal from quiet sleep in 6 of 18 (32%) control infants 4 to 14 weeks of age employing an FI_{O_2} of 15% for up to 10 min delivered via head hood (67). Arousal occurred predominantly in infants younger than 10 weeks of age and was uncommon in older infants. These studies agree with those of Davidson Ward et al. (58), suggesting that hypoxic arousal occurs in less than half of normal infants and that younger infants show greater hypoxic arousal responsiveness.

Utilizing a protocol with stepwise reduction in oxygen concentration over a 15-min period, Lewis and Bosque elicited complete behavioral arousal during a daytime nap from quiet sleep in 85% of control infants at a mean age of 2 months (19). In a study of siblings of SIDS victims and infants with apnea, Dunne and associates exposed three groups of normal infants during quiet sleep to an FI_{O_2} of 0.15 for 20 min and elicited complete behavioral arousal in about two-thirds of infants at 4 days, 6 weeks, and 13 weeks of age (68). Arousal responses did not vary between the different ages, suggesting no effect of maturation. In comparing these two studies with other investigations, it must be noted that false positives may occur secondary to spontaneous arousals from sleep when lengthy challenge protocols are used. van der Hal and coworkers reported no failures to arouse from quiet sleep in nine control infants at a mean age of 7 months challenged with an FI_{O_2} of 11% via head hood (3). Failure to arouse was defined as no arousal on two consecutive challenges. There were two infants in this study less than 7 months of age who failed to arouse on one of two challenges (3).

In a study of arousal responses in prepubertal children with obstructive apnea, Marcus and colleagues included a group of normal healthy children, yielding important information on the normal arousal response to respiratory stimuli in the school-age child (47). They found hypoxia to be a relatively poor stimulus to arousal, with arousal occurring in one-fourth of trials, a slightly lower percentage than has been reported in both infants (58) and adults (59–61). They used a 3-min hypoxic challenge with a minimum arterial oxygen saturation of 75% and noted considerable variability in the responses within individuals (47)—a finding also reported in adults (59). As has been reported in other age groups, hypercapnia was a potent stimulus to arousal, and all children aroused during hypercapnic challenges (47). However, they did find an elevated hypercapnic arousal threshold (PET_{CO_2} of 59 ± 5 mmHg), compared to that reported in infants (52 mmHg), adolescents (46 mmHg), and adults (49 mmHg) (3,70,71).

Studies of hypoxic arousal responses from NREM sleep in normal adults suggest that isolated acute hypoxia is a poor stimulus to arousal (59–61). All but one study reported failure to arouse in the majority of trials (69). Berthon-Jones and Sullivan studied arousal to hypoxia from both NREM and REM sleep in normal adults using a face mask delivery system and allowed saturation to fall as low as 70% (59). They elicited arousal in about 50% of challenges in both REM and NREM sleep. Marcus and coworkers reported similar findings in older children (47). Gleeson reported failure to arouse in only 25% of trials, but the subjects had an esophageal balloon in place, which may have affected arousal thresholds (69). In those studies that included both female and male subjects, there were no differences in hypoxic arousal responsiveness between the sexes (59,61).

The arousal threshold is affected by sleep state. In adult animals, an arousal response to hypoxia occurs at a lower oxygen saturation during REM compared to NREM sleep. That is, it is more difficult to arouse from REM sleep (or active sleep) than it is from NREM (or quiet sleep). Newborn animals also awaken at a lower oxygen saturation during REM sleep compared to NREM (10,11). NREM sleep arousal occurs at similar arterial oxygen saturations in both newborns and adults. However, REM sleep arousal thresholds may occur at lower oxygen saturations in the newborn than in adults (57). A maturational change in arousal threshold through gestation and postnatally is suggested by studies in human infants. Although not controlled for sleep state, term infants tended to awaken sooner than preterm infants when placed in a 12% oxygen environment (57). When retested several weeks later, most infants awoke more promptly in response to a hypoxic challenge (57).

Fewell and coworkers have extensively studied hypoxic arousal responses in lambs (72–75). They have delineated a number of characteristics of the response. The hypoxic arousal response is subject to habituation, with repetitive exposure to hypoxia resulting in a progressively lower Sa_{O_2} required to achieve arousal (72). The hypoxic arousal response is dependent on the carotid body, with carotid denervation significantly reducing arousal responsiveness (73). Simultaneous hypercapnia facilitates arousal to hypoxia, especially when some degree of habituation to hypoxia has occurred (74). Hypoxic arousal may play a role in arousal from active sleep but not quiet sleep in response to upper airway obstruction (75). How the responses of the lamb might differ from those of human infants is not known.

The mechanisms for arousal in response to hypoxia are not clear. Several possibilities exist. One pathway would be via afferents from peripheral chemoreceptors to the reticular activating system, with subsequent cortical activation. Support for this comes from studies demonstrating decreased hypoxic arousal responses in carotid body–denervated animals (73,76). However, peripheral chemoreceptors are also responsible for the hypoxic ventilatory response, and it has been postulated that it is the increased ventilatory effort sensed via mechanoreceptors of the chest that stimulates the reticular activating system and results in arousal. In support of this, Gleeson and colleagues demonstrated that arousal occurred in adult males in response to hypoxia, hypercapnia, and increased resistive load at similar levels of ventilatory effort as measured by peak esophageal pressures (69). Phillipson and coworkers also speculated that an increase in minute ventilation is responsible for arousal, as arousal occurred in response to various hypoxic and hypercapnic mixtures at similar levels of ventilation (77). However, a subsequent study by Bowes and coworkers reported no significant change in hypoxic arousal thresholds despite vagal blockade (76). Clouding the issue is the possible existence of phrenic nerve afferents carrying mechanical information centrally (78). Further, Marcus and associates showed that hypoxic and hypercapnic arousal responses occurred in children with congenital central hypoventilation syndrome receiving assisted ventilation (50). These patients did not mount a ventilatory response to hypoxia or hypercapnia (49). Further, they were supported by mechanical assisted ventilation during the arousal response testing, so ventilatory effort did not change (50). The fact that these children did arouse in response to hypoxia and hypercapnia indicates that a respiratory arousal response can occur in the absence of increased ventilatory effort (50). Garg and associates also showed that infants with bronchopulmonary dysplasia, studied at term-corrected age, had intact hypoxic arousal responses, but had inadequate ventilatory responses (52). Many of the infants studied had prolonged apneas despite arousal, and some required stimulation to restore normal breathing (52). It is also possible that the reticular activating system receives collateral information from both the peripheral chemoreceptors and mechanoreceptors and that both systems play a role in the generation of the arousal response. A direct effect of hypoxia on the central nervous system, causing arousal, has also been postulated (79).

Because the majority of infants, children, and adolescents fail to arouse to hypoxia, mechanisms for failure to arouse are perhaps more germane than the pathways leading to arousal. Habituation could play a role. However, it is doubtful that normal infants have spent a significant amount of their postnatal lifetime exposed to the degree of hypoxia utilized in the laboratory setting. Carotid body failure is unlikely. A generalized decrease in arousal responsiveness is unlikely, as the majority of infants who did not respond to hypoxia had prompt arousal responses to auditory stimuli (29,80). Sleep disruption and fragmentation have been shown in animal models to decrease arousal responsiveness (15,81). However, the infants in most reported studies were not sleep-deprived. Inhibitory inputs from the cortex have been postulated. Decortication markedly potentiates the ventilatory response to hypoxia and produces intense arousal in cats (82). Tenney and Ou hypothesized that arousal depends on facilitatory inputs from the hypothalamus. Because hypoxia may have a depressant effect on the hypothalamus, the inhibitory effect of the cortex predominates (82).

The presence of a ventilatory response to hypoxia does not ensure that arousal will occur. Fewell and coworkers demonstrated habituation of the arousal response to hypoxia with apparent preservation of the hypoxic ventilatory responses in lambs (72). Conversely, Marcus et al. demonstrated arousal to hypoxic and hypercapnic challenges in patients with congenital central hypoventilation syndrome without a ventilatory responses to these stimuli (50). Similarly, Garg and coworkers demonstrated hypoxic arousal in infants with bronchopulmonary dysplasia without a ventilatory response (52). Thus, arousal and ventilatory responses may occur independently. However, characterization of the relationship between these two important defense mechanisms of the respiratory system in human infants is needed.

In the clinical setting, acute hypoxia is frequently accompanied by other respiratory stimuli, such as hypercapnia or airway occlusion, both of which are potent stimuli to arousal (3,4,23,35,50,54,64,70,71,75,83–85). There are also gasping reflexes that may cause autoresuscitation during severe hypoxia (86). Therefore, in many instances, there are other protective responses that will be operable during respiratory events. In addition, it is also possible that more severe hypoxia would result in arousal responses in a higher percentage of infants. Although arousal to hypoxia may play a role in the clinical setting, hypoxic challenges do not appear to have any value as a screening test for SIDS risk.

It should be noted that all of the studies reporting hypoxic arousal responses in normal infants have been performed during daytime naps, and most have studied responses during quiet sleep (3,10,16,57,58,62–65,67–68). Responses to hypoxia during nighttime sleep or during active sleep may differ from those studied during quiet sleep in the daytime.

Thus, arousal is less likely to occur in response to hypoxia in infants between 1 and 6 months of age than in older or younger subjects. Hypoxia is not a potent stimulus for arousal in subjects outside the newborn period. Hypoxic arousal is affected by sleep state, and is less likely during REM sleep than NREM sleep. Hypoxic arousal is inhibited by sleep fragmentation, though this effect seems less significant in infants and children than in adults. Hypercapnia is a potent stimulus for arousal in infants, children, and adults.

IX. Hypoxic and Hypercapnic Arousal Response Testing

It has been suggested that arousal responses to hypoxia or hypercapnia may be useful clinical tools for the diagnosis of respiratory control dysfunction (51). However, the majority of normal infants, children, and adults fail to arouse from sleep in response to hypoxia (58–61). Further, children with absent ventilatory responses to hypoxia and hypercapnia can arouse in response to hypercapnia (49,50,52). Thus, the interpretation of these test results is complicated. Arousal responses might be useful in assessing central and peripheral chemoreceptor function in infants or children who are totally apneic, thus eliminating the need to use ventilatory responses (4,50). Gases with any desired concentration of oxygen or CO_2 can be introduced through the ventilator circuit of an apneic child and a nonventilatory response (arousal) used to assess chemoreceptor function (4,50,51). Details of testing procedures have been described elsewhere (3,50,51).

Since normal infants, children, and adults often fail to arouse in response to hypoxia, this does not in and of itself indicate any abnormality in respiratory control. However, if a patient does arouse to hypoxia, one can reasonably assume that peripheral chemoreceptors detect hypoxia. Special care should be taken to be sure that arousal is in response to hypoxia rather than a coincidental spontaneous arousal. If a patient fails to arouse to hypoxia, this may be a normal response and does not make the diagnosis of peripheral chemoreceptor dysfunction or a respiratory control disorder.

Hypercapnia is a potent stimulus for arousal in normal infants, children, and adults (3,20,50,64,65,70,71). Infants with unexplained apnea arouse to hypercapnia (3,64,65), as do the majority of children with congenital central hypoventilation syndrome (50). Infants with myelomeningocele and Arnold-Chiari type II malformation have brainstem dysfunction, which may affect central chemoreceptors (4,87). A significant percentage of this group of infants fail to arouse in response to hypercapnia

(4). Failure to arouse to hypercapnia is generally seen only in infants and children with evidence of significant brainstem and/or respiratory control dysfunction.

X. Summary

Arousal from sleep is an important defense mechanism against danger-signaling stimuli during sleep. Spontaneous arousals occur throughout the night in normal individuals. There is a tendency for spontaneous arousals to increase as an individual ages. Humans also respond to sensory stimuli, such as auditory stimuli, by arousal from sleep. Arousal to sensory stimuli appears to occur less during infancy and childhood, whereas adults arouse more readily. Arousal may also occur in response to respiratory stimuli, including hypoxia, hypercapnia, and airway occlusion. Hypoxia is a relatively poor stimulus for arousal in all but newborn infants. Hypercapnia is a potent arousal stimulus in normal infants, children, and adults. However, patients with brainstem disorders have failed to arouse in response to hypercapnic stimuli. Arousal responses are not necessarily linked to ventilatory responses, as patients have been able to arouse to hypoxia or hypercapnia without mounting a ventilatory response. The environment and sleep history also affect arousal responses. Sleep fragmentation and habituation to the arousal stimulus may inhibit arousal. In general, it appears that arousal thresholds decrease with increasing age, although proper longitudinal studies in the same subjects have not been performed to confirm this.

References

1. Phillipson EA, Bowes G. Control of breathing during sleep. In: The Handbook of Physiology: Sec. 3. The Respiratory System. Vol. II. Part 2. Baltimore, MD: American Physiological Society, 1986:649–690.
2. Bedard MA, Montplaiser J, Richer F, Rouleau I, Malo J. Obstructive sleep apnea syndrome: pathogenesis of neurophysiological deficits. J Clin Exp Neuropsychol 1991; 13:950–964.
3. van der Hal AL, Rodriguez AM, Sargent CW, Platzker ACG, Keens TG. Hypoxic and hypercapnic arousal responses and prediction of subsequent apnea in apnea of infancy. Pediatrics 1985; 75:848–854.
4. Davidson Ward SL, Nickerson BG, van der Hal AL, Rodriguez AM, Jacobs RA, Keens TG. Absent hypoxic and hypercarbic arousal responses in children with myelomeningocele and apnea. Pediatrics 1986; 78:44–50.
5. Phillipson EA, Sullivan CE. Arousal: the forgotten response to respiratory stimuli. Am Rev Respir Dis 1978; 118:807–808.
6. Badia P, Harsh J, Balkin T, O'Rourke D, Burton S. Behavioral control of respiration in sleep and sleepiness due to signal-induced sleep fragmentation. Psychophysiology 1985; 22:517–524.
7. Horner RL. Autonomic consequences of arousal from sleep: mechanisms and implications. Sleep 1996; 19:S193–S195.
8. Jones BE. Basic mechanisms of sleep-wake states. In: Kryger MH, Roth T, Dement WC, eds. Principles and Practice of Sleep Medicine. Philadelphia: Saunders, 1989:121–138.

9. American Sleep Disorders Association. EEG arousals: scoring rules and examples: a preliminary report from the Sleep Disorders Atlas Task Force of the American Sleep Disorders Association. Sleep 1992; 15:174–184.
10. Henderson-Smart DJ, Read DJC. Ventilatory responses to hypoxaemia during sleep in the newborn. J Dev Physiol 1979; 1:195–208.
11. Jeffrey HE, Read DJC. Ventilatory responses of newborn calves to progressive hypoxia in quiet and active sleep. J Appl Physiol 1980; 48:892–895.
12. Chugh DK, Weaver TE, Dinges DF. Neurobehavioral consequences of arousals. Sleep 1996; 19:S198–S201.
13. Douglas NJ, Martin SE. Arousals and the sleep apnea/hypopnea syndrome. Sleep 1996; 19:S196–S197.
14. White DP, Douglas NJ, Pickett CK, Zwillich CW, Weil JV. Sleep deprivation and the control of ventilation. Am Rev Respir Dis 1983; 128:984–986.
15. Phillipson EA, Bowes G, Sullivan CE, Woolf GM. The influence of sleep fragmentation on arousal and ventilatory responses to respiratory stimuli. Sleep 1980; 3:281–288.
16. Thomas DA, Poole K, McArdle EK, Goodenough PC, Thompson J, Beardsmore CS, Simpson H. The effect of sleep deprivation on sleep states, breathing events, peripheral chemoresponsiveness and arousal propensity in healthy 3 month old infants. Eur Respir J 1996; 9:932–938.
17. Tirosh E, Libon D, Bader D. The effect of maternal smoking during pregnancy on sleep respiratory and arousal patterns in neonates. J Perinatol 1996: 16:435–348.
18. Franco P, Hainaut M, Pardou A, Groswasser J, Kahn A. Prenatal exposure to cigarette smoke increases auditory arousal thresholds in infants. Pediatr Pulmonol 1996; 22:426.
19. Lewis KW, Bosque EM. Deficient hypoxia awakening response in infants of smoking mothers: possible relationship to sudden infant death syndrome. J Pediatr 1995; 127:691–699.
20. Davidson Ward SL, Bautista DB, Woo MS, Chang M, Scheutz S, Wachsman L, Sehgal S, Bean X. Responses to hypoxia and hypercapnia in infants of substance-abusing mothers. J Pediatr 1992; 121:704–709.
21. Mosko S, Richard C, McKenna J. Infant arousals during mother-infant bed sharing: implications for infant sleep and sudden infant death syndrome research. Pediatrics 1997; 100:841–849.
22. Newman NM, Trinder JA, Phillips KA, Jordon K, Cruickshank J. Arousal deficit: mechanism of the sudden infant death syndrome? Aust Paediatr J 1989; 25:196–201.
23. Newman NM, Frost JK, Bury L, Jordon K, Phillips K. Responses to partial nasal obstruction in sleeping infants. Aust Paediatr J 1986; 22:111–116.
24. Fleming PJ, Blair PS, Bacon C, Bensley D, Smith I, Taylor E, Berry J, Golding J, Tripp J. Environment of infants during sleep and risk for sudden infant death syndrome: results of 1993-5 case-control study for confidential inquiry into stillbirths and deaths in infancy. BMJ 1996; 313:191–195.
25. Skadberg BT, Markestad T. Infant behavior in response to a change in body position from side to prone during sleep. Eur J Pediatr 1996; 155:1052–1056.
26. Lijowska AS, Reed NW, Mertins Chiodini BA, Thach BT. Sequential arousal and airway-defensive behavior in asphyxial sleep environments. J Appl Physiol 1997; 83:219–228.
27. Clark S, Sabey P, Jolley K. Nonstress testing with acoustic stimulation and amniotic fluid volume assessment: 5973 tests without unexpected fetal death. Am J Obstet Gynecol 1989; 160:694–697.

28. Kahn A, Picard E, Blum D. Auditory arousal thresholds of normal and near-miss SIDS infants. Dev Med Child Neurol 1986; 28:299–302.
29. Wolfish NM, Pivik RT, Busby KA. Elevated sleep arousal thresholds in enuretic boys: clinical implications. Acta Paediatr 1997; 86:381–384.
30. Busby K, Pivik RT, Auditory arousal thresholds during sleep in hyperkinetic children. Sleep 1985; 8:332–341.
31. Badr MS, Morgan BJ, Finn L, Toiber FS, Crabtree DC, Puleo DS, Skatrud JB. Ventilatory response to induced auditory arousals during NREM sleep. Sleep 1997; 20: 707–714.
32. Carley DW, Applebaum R, Basner RC, Onal E, Lopata M. Respiratory and arousal responses to acoustic stimulation. Chest 1997; 112:1567–1571.
33. McDonald CS, Zepelin H, Zammit GK. Age and sex patterns in auditory awakening thresholds. Sleep Res 1985; 14:115.
34. Busby KA, Mercier L, Pivik RT. Ontogenetic variations in auditory arousal threshold during sleep. Psychophysiology 1994; 31:182–188.
35. McNamara F, Issa FG, Sullivan CE. Arousal pattern following central and obstructive breathing abnormalities in infants and children. J Appl Physiol 1996; 81:2651–2657.
36. Boselli M, Parrino L, Smerieri A, Terzano MD. Effect of age on EEG arousals in normal sleep. Sleep 1998; 21:351–357.
37. Carskadon MA, Dement WC. Normal human sleep: An overview. In: Kryger MH, Roth T, Dement WC, eds. Principles and Practice of Sleep Medicine. Philadelphia: Saunders, 1994:16–25.
38. Bliwise DL. Normal aging. In: Kryger MH, Roth T, Dement WC, eds. Principles and Practice of Sleep Medicine. Philadelphia: Saunders, 1994:26–39.
39. Shore ET, Millman RP, Silage DA, Chung D-CC, Pack PI. Ventilatory an arousal patterns during sleep in normal young and elderly subjects. J Appl Physiol 1985; 59:1607–1615.
40. Martin SE, Wraith PK, Deary IJ, Douglas NJ. The effect of nonvisible sleep fragmentation of daytime function. Am J Resp Crit Care Med 1997; 155:1596–1601.
41. Kimoff RJ, Olha AE, Charbonneau M, Cheong TH, Cosio MG, Gottfried SB. Mechanisms of apnea termination in obstructive sleep apnea: role of mechanoreceptor and chemoreceptor stimuli. Am Rev Respir Dis 1994; 149:707–714.
42. Charbonneau M, Marin JM, Olha AE, Kimoff RJ, Levy RD, Cosio MG. Changes in obstructive sleep apnea characteristics across the night. Chest 1994; 106:1695–1701.
43. Berry RB, Gleeson K. Respiratory arousal from sleep: mechanisms and significance. Sleep 1997; 20:654–675.
44. Berry RE, Kouchi K, Der DE, Dickel MJ, Light RW. Sleep apnea impairs the arousal response to airway occlusion. Chest 1996; 109:1490–1496.
45. Boudewyns A, Sforza E, Zamagni M, Krieger J. Respiratory effort during sleep apneas after interruption of long-term CPAP treatment in patients with obstructive sleep apnea. Chest 1996; 110:120–127.
46. Davidson Ward SL, Marcus CL. Obstructive sleep apnea in infants and young children. J Clin Neurophysiol 1996; 13:198–207.
47. Marcus CL, Lutz J, Carroll JL, Bamford O. Arousal and ventilatory responses during sleep in children with obstructive sleep apnea. J Appl Physiol 1998; 84:1926–1936.
48. Marcus CL, Glomb WB, Basinski DJ, Davidson Ward SL, Keens TG. Developmental pattern of hypercapnic and hypoxic ventilatory responses from childhood to adulthood. J Appl Physiol 1994; 76:314–320.

49. Paton JY, Swaminathan S, Sargent CW, Keens TG. Hypoxic and hypercapnic ventilatory responses in awake children with congenital central hypoventilation syndrome. Am Rev Respir Dis 1989; 140:368–372.
50. Marcus CL, Bautista DB, Amihyia A, Davidson Ward SL, Keens TG. Hypercapneic arousal responses in children with congenital central hypoventilation syndrome. Pediatrics 1991; 88:993–998.
51. Davidson Ward SL, Keens TG. Ventilatory and arousal responses. In: Beckerman RC, Brouillette RT, Hunt CE, eds. Respiratory Control Disorders in Infants and Children. Baltimore, MD: Williams & Wilkins, 1992:112–124.
52. Garg M, Kurzner SI, Bautista DB, Keens TG. Hypoxic arousal responses in infants with bronchopulmonary dysplasia. Pediatrics 1988; 82:59–63.
53. Belville JW, Howland WS, Seed JC, Loude RW. The effect of sleep on the respiratory response to carbon dioxide. Anesthesiology 1959; 20:628–634.
54. Phillipson EA, Kozar LF, Rebuck AS, Murphy E. Ventilatory and waking responses to CO_2 and lung inflation in sleeping dogs. Am Rev Respir Dis 1977; 115:251–259.
55. Sullivan CE, Murphy E, Kozar LF, Phillipson EA. Ventilatory responses to CO_2 and lung inflation in tonic vs. phasic REM sleep. J Appl Physiol Respir Environ Exerc Physiol 1979; 47:1304–1310.
56. Fewell JE, Kondo CS, Dascalu V, Filyk SC. Influence of carotid denervation on the arousal and cardiopulmonary responses to alveolar hypercapnia in lambs. J Develop Physiol 1989; 12:193–199.
57. Miller HC, Smull NW. Further studies on the effects of hypoxia on the respiration of newborn infants. Pediatrics 1955; 16:93–102.
58. Davidson Ward SL, Bautista DB, Keens TG. Hypoxic arousal responses in normal infants. Pediatrics 1992; 89:860–864.
59. Berthon-Jones M, Sullivan CE. Ventilatory and arousal responses to hypoxia in sleeping humans. Am Rev Respir Dis 1982; 125:623–629.
60. Douglas NJ, White DP, Weil JV, Pickett CK, Martin RI, Hudgel DW, Zwillich CW. Hypoxic ventilatory response decreases during sleep in normal men. Am Rev Respir Dis 1982; 125:286–289.
61. Gothe B, Goldman MD, Cherniack NS, Mantey P. Effect of progressive hypoxia on breathing during sleep. Am Rev Respir Dis 1982; 126:97–102.
62. Gingras JL, Muelenaer A, Dalley LB, O'Donnell KJ. Prenatal cocaine exposure alters postnatal hypoxic arousal responses and hypercarbic ventilatory responses but not pneumocardiograms in prenatally cocaine-exposed term infants. Pediatr Pulmonol 1994; 18: 13–20.
63. Ariagno R, Nagel L, Guilleminault C. Waking and ventilatory responses during sleep in infants near-miss for sudden infant death syndrome. Sleep 1980; 3:351–359.
64. Hunt CE. Abnormal hypercarbic and hypoxic sleep arousal responses in near-miss SIDS infants. Pediatr Res 1981; 15:1462–1464.
65. McCulloch K, Brouillette RT, Guzzetta AJ, Hunt CE. Arousal responses in near-miss sudden infant death and in normal infants. J Pediatr 1982; 101:911–917.
66. Brady JP, McCann EM. Control of ventilation in subsequent siblings of victims of sudden infant death syndrome. J Pediatr 1985; 106:212–217.
67. Milerad J, Hertzberg T, Wennergren G, Lagercrantz H. Respiratory and arousal responses to hypoxia in apnoeic infants reinvestigated. Eur J Pediatr 1989; 148:565–570.
68. Dunne KP, Fox GPP, O'Regan M, Matthews TG. Arousal responses in babies at risk of sudden infant death syndrome at different postnatal ages. Irish Med J 1992; 85:19–22.

69. Gleeson K, Zwillich CW, White DP. The influence of increasing ventilatory effort on arousal from sleep. Am Rev Resp Dis 1990; 142:295–300.
70. Livingston FR, Arens R, Bailey SL, Keens TG, Davidson Ward SL. Hypercapnic arousal responses in Prader-Willi syndrome. Chest, 1995; 108:1627–1631.
71. Hedemark LL, Kronenberg RS. Ventilatory and heart rate responses to hypoxia and hypercapnia during sleep in adults. J Appl Physiol 1982; 53:307–312.
72. Fewell JE, Konduri GG. Influence of repeated exposure to rapidly developing hypoxaemia on the arousal and cardiopulmonary response to developing hypoxaemia in lambs. J Dev Physiol 1989; 11:77–82.
73. Fewell JE, Kondo CS, Dascalu V, Filyk SC. Influence of carotid denervation on the arousal and cardiopulmonary response to rapidly developing hypoxemia in lambs. Pediatr Res 1989; 25:473–477.
74. Fewell JE, Konduri GG. Repeated exposure to rapidly developing hypoxemia influences the interaction between oxygen and carbon dioxide in initiating arousal from sleep in lambs. Pediatr Res 1988; 24:28–33.
75. Fewell JE, Williams BJ, Szabo JS, Taylor BJ. Influence of repeated upper airway obstruction on the arousal and cardiopulmonary response to upper airway obstruction in lambs. Pediatr Res 1988; 23:191–195.
76. Bowes G, Townsend ER, Kozar LF, Bromley SM, Phillipson EA. Effects of carotid body denervation on arousal response to hypoxia in sleeping dogs. J Appl Physiol 1981; 51: 40–45.
77. Phillipson EA, Sullivan CE, Read DJC, Murphy E, Kozar LF. Ventilatory and waking responses to hypoxia in sleeping dogs. J Appl Physiol 1978; 44:512–520.
78. Frazier DT, Revelette WR. Role of phrenic nerve afferents in the control of breathing. J Appl Physiol 1991; 70:491–496.
79. Neubauer JA, Santiago TV, Edelman NH. Hypoxic arousal in intact and carotid chemodenervated sleeping cats. J Appl Physiol 1981; 51:1294–1299.
80. Davidson Ward SL, Bautista DB, Sargent CW, Keens TG. Arousal responses to sensory stimuli in infants at increased risk for sudden infant death syndrome. Am Rev Respir Dis 1990; 141:809A.
81. Bows G, Woolf GM, Sullivan CE, Phillipson EA. Effect of sleep fragmentation on ventilatory and arousal responses of sleep dogs to respiratory stimuli. Am Rev Respir Dis 1980; 122:899–908.
82. Tenny SM, Ou LC. Ventilatory responses of decorticate and decerebrate cats to hypoxia and CO_2. Respir Physiol 1977; 29:81–92.
83. Fewell JE, Baker SB. Arousal and cardiopulmonary responses to hyperoxic hypercapnia in lambs. J Dev Physiol 1989; 12:21–26.
84. Phillipson EA, Kozar LF, Rebuck AS, Murphy E. Ventilatory and waking responses to CO_2 in sleeping dogs. Am Rev Respir Dis 1977; 115:251–259.
85. Issa FG, Sullivan CE. Arousal and breathing responses to airway occlusion in healthy sleeping adults. J Appl Physiol 1983; 55:1113–1119.
86. Lawson EE, Thach BT. Respiratory patterns during progressive asphyxia in newborn rabbits. J Appl Physiol 1977; 43:468–474.
87. Swaminathan S, Paton JY, Davidson Ward SL, Sargent CW, Jacobs RA, Keens TG. Abnormal control of ventilation in adolescents with myelomeningocele. J Pediatr 1989; 115: 898–903.

5

Cultural Influences on Infant and Childhood Sleep Biology and the Science That Studies It

Toward a More Inclusive Paradigm

JAMES J. McKENNA

University of Notre Dame
Notre Dame, Indiana

I. Introduction

... we try to keep in mind cultural influences on the advice we give. We remind ourselves that much of what comes to the pediatrician's attention, as problematic sleep behavior—children who have difficulty falling asleep alone at bedtime, who wake at night and ask for parental attention, or who continue to nurse at night—is problematic only in relation to our society's expectations, rather than to some more general standard of what constitutes difficult behavior in the young child. Our pediatric advice on transitional objects, breast feeding, cosleeping may be unknowingly biased toward traditional Euroamerican views of childrearing, especially those about bedtime and nighttime behavior. Thus, in giving advice about sleep, pediatric health professionals might do well to be aware of their own cultural values, to examine closely their patients' cultural and family contexts, and to assess parental reactions to children's sleep behaviors. (1)

Who sleeps by whom is not merely a personal or private activity. Instead, it is social practice, like burying the dead or expressing gratitude for gifts or eating meals with your family, or honoring the practice of a monogamous marriage, which (for those engaged in the practice) is invested with moral and social meaning for a person's reputation and good standing in the community. (2)

In clinical pediatrics, cosleeping is the political third rail. If you touch it, you die. (3)

This chapter provides a cultural background to our thinking about what constitutes "normal, healthy, and desirable" infant sleep and show the interconnectedness between scientific research, cultural values, concerns for morality, and sleeping arrangements characteristic of Western society. Specific biological and psychological evidence is put forth supporting Sadeh and Anders (4,5) and Anders' (6) views on the importance of understanding what is "appropriate" infant sleep *based on the overall social and physical context within which it occurs*.

To illustrate this viewpoint, I selected data on a variety of topics demonstrating how culturally guided parental child-care choices, including those involved in sleeping arrangements, set in motion a cascade of interconnected changes that affect the biology and behavior of the participants *appropriate to those choices*. I suggest that clinicians generally fail to convey to parents the legitimacy of different choices and that the widely accepted research paradigm fails scientifically to include alternatives to the model of the solitary-sleeping, bottle-, or minimally breast-fed infant. The diversity of sleep-related arrangements and practices alter infant sleep development significantly in the first years of life, and this argues against a simple cultural definition of infant sleep progression implied by the widely accepted (traditional) model.

Relatedly, perhaps no other issue has been so often misrepresented and grossly oversimplified as parent–infant cosleeping. New data on the subject highlight the extent to which cultural ideologies, cultural judgments, and concerns for morality are often mistaken for science in this area. For example, data collected exclusively on the solitary-sleeping, bottle-fed infant continue to provide the basis for definitions of clinically "normal" infant sleep-wake patterns and research into them. These data continue to serve as the "gold standard" against which, eventually, parents and professionals evaluate infant sleep development, despite significant contextual differences that may invalidate the comparisons. Almost no consideration is given to other sleeping arrangements, however healthy they may be.

New data from psychology are presented, raising the possibility that clinicians have overestimated the need for infants to sleep separately in order to assure "independence" from their parents. Recent biological data described here suggest that sleep researchers underestimate the importance of maternal proximity and breast-feeding in regulating infant sleep physiology and thus to understanding "normal" infant sleep. By using data from only one type of sleeping arrangement and implying that there is only one context within which healthy infant sleep emerges—i.e., the solitary one—pediatric sleep research is held captive by Western ethnocentrism.

I conclude that to forge effective partnerships between parents and health professionals in our ever more multicultural society, pediatric sleep medicine must come to terms with cultural biases embedded in sleep research medicine in general and clinical interpretations and advice in particular. At this point in the history of Western societies, where an unprecedented convergence of cultural practices is under way—not the least of which involves sleeping arrangements—it is critical that clinicians and researchers broaden their thinking about what constitute appropriate and desirable childhood sleep practices. Failure do so will continue to limit both the accuracy of pediatric sleep science and the effectiveness of care.

II. Culture and Childhood Sleep

The importance of local cultural influences, including health professional and family values on infant and childhood sleep, was anticipated more than a decade ago by Lozoff and colleagues (1). In the first of the three passages quoted above, they acknowledge, as eloquently as any group of anthropologists or psychologists have done, the critical if not pivotal role that personal beliefs, experiences, and societal values can play in pediatric research. The same applies to the advice given to parents regarding a range of nighttime sleep–related issues, problems, and possible solutions. Across different cultures, ideas vary about how, where, and why infants and children *should* sleep as well as what constitutes "normal" sleep and "sleep problems" (2,7,8). Ethnographic studies of this variability worldwide are important because the data help to establish the extent to which specieswide sleep biology and development are subject to environmental manipulation and regulation. Local customs and traditions, irrespective of whether the society is industrialized or is structured around a hunting-and-gathering economy, all play roles (9–14).

Even within a single society, infant and childhood sleeping patterns and the social values and relationships that influence them are diverse, and significant differences cut across subgroups in unexpected but important ways (15–17). For example, Anders and Taylor (8) point out that infants and children who are not able to sleep alone and "through the night" are not uniformly regarded in our own culture as having a "sleep problem." Most conceptualizations of sleep problems are based on culturally and parentally constructed definitions and expectations, not biology. In reality, infant sleep development plays out extraordinarily differently in diverse family settings, wherein infant feeding and nighttime nurturing behaviors as well as parental needs and goals vary. These, in turn, affect both long and short term developmental processes. Yet the legitimacy of these variations continues to be largely ignored in both professional as well as popular discourse and a "one size should fit all" approach to sleeping arrangements continues to be advocated (18).

A. How Do Social Values and Cultural Goals Influence Infant Sleep Practices?

That a critical relationship exists between the cultural ideologies underlying sleep practices and desired developmental outcomes (even when they are not achieved) is made dramatically clear when one compares Asian, Guatemalan, and American values, conceptualizations of infants at birth, and desired developmental outcomes. For example, interdependence and group harmony are positively valued in Japan, where parent–child cosleeping is practiced. As Christopher describes it, "One monkey that does perch on the back of nearly all Japanese is a deeply engrained feeling that individual gratification is possible only in a group context—a feeling which, like the taste for dependence, clearly stems from childhood experiences (19).

American children are presumed to be trained to be self-reliant and to display their individuality by sleeping alone, and Japanese children are taught to "harmonize with the group" and hence "cosleep" with their parents. These observations relate to the different attitudes that Japanese and American parents have concerning the "nature" of the infant at birth, what developmental outcomes are desired, and what sleeping arrangement are presumed necessary to achieve them. For example, Caudill and Weinstein (20), cited in Shand (21), state that: "In Japan, the infant is seen more as a separate biological organism who from the beginning, in order to develop, needs to be drawn into increasingly interdependent relations with others. In America, the infant is seen more as a dependent biological organism who in order to develop, needs to be made increasingly independent of others."

Indeed, according to Brazleton (22), "the Japanese think the U.S. culture rather merciless in pushing small children toward such independence at night." Kawakami (23, as cited in 24) describes American and Japanese differences this way: "An American mother-infant relationship consists of two individuals.... On the other hand, a Japanese mother-infant relationship consists of only one individual, i.e., mother and infants are not divided." Japanese infants and children usually sleep next to their mothers on futons, with space availability playing a minor role in this arrangement; in general, children sleep with someone (fathers or extended family members) through the age of 15 (24,25).

Like the Japanese, Mayan mothers from Guatemala *do not believe in* separate sleeping quarters for infants, children, and parents. In fact, sleeping alone is considered so difficult for adult Guatemalans that, in the absence of family members, it is not uncommon for adults to seek out friends with whom they can share sleep (24). Upon hearing that American babies are made to sleep alone, Mayan women respond with "shock, disapproval and pity" and think of the practice as "tantamount to child neglect" (24). This evaluation contrasts dramatically with one offered by Ferber of the United States, who advocates that all infants should be taught to sleep alone. In his popular book, *How To Solve Your Child's Sleep Problems*, Ferber provides mothers who may be emotionally predisposed to sleep with their infants with a reason to ponder the status of their own mental health. He advises: "If you find that you actually prefer to have your child in bed, you should examine your feelings very carefully" (26).

The study of Guatemalan (Mayan) women is one of the best cross-cultural (comparative) studies of childhood sleep to date. Morelli et al. examined a group of middle-class American (Caucasian) and contemporary Mayan (Guatemalan) mothers and found that all the 14 Mayan mothers slept in the same bed with their infants and 8 older toddlers slept with their fathers. In the middle-class American sample, none of the newborn infants regularly slept with their mothers. Mayan parents believe that cosleeping is the only "reasonable way" for a parents and infants to sleep, while the Americans in the sample of Morelli et al. felt comfortable keeping newborns and neonates next to their beds "to make sure that they were still breathing" (24) but were not comfortable having them in the same bed. After their children's third to sixth months of life, the Americans parents felt that their infants were no longer so vulnerable. Fearful of interfering with the infant's progress toward independence and autonomy, most American parents in the sample moved their infants to a separate room.

In another study, conducted in Australia, an immigrant Vietnamese mother was told about the sudden infant death syndrome (SIDS), with which she was unfamiliar. She surmised that "the custom of being with the baby must prevent this disease. If you are sleeping with your baby, you always sleep lightly. You notice if his breathing changes.... Babies should not be left alone." Further to the point, another of the Vietnamese mothers added: "Babies are too important to be left alone with nobody watching them" (27).

Of 40 Chinese women interviewed (in Chinese) at Guagzho University Hospital by Wilson (28), over 66% of new mothers were intending to have their infants sleep with them in the marital bed, and all of her sample were planning to have their infants sleep alongside their beds. One informant represented many when she stated that the baby is "too little to sleep alone" and that cosleeping "make babies happy." Another Chinese informant tells Wilson: that "the parents' breathing affects the baby, so cosleeping is good" and, later, that cosleeping permits mothers to know "if the baby [was] too hot or too cold" and "to hear the baby's sounds" (28).

B. Is Moral Character a Function of the Sleep Environment?

What might come as a surprise to some researchers is the work of cultural psychologist Shweder and his colleagues at the University of Chicago (e.g., the second passage quoted at the opening of this chapter). They show explicitly that concerns for "moral goods" (taken here to mean concerns or preferences for particular personal qualities or behavior and personality or character outcomes) are deeply embedded in and reflective of notions about proper sleeping arrangements, regardless of whether these notions are scientifically based or simply folk assumptions (2). Their cross-cultural comparisons reveal that in choosing sleeping arrangements, parents feel a powerful concern for what looks morally acceptable and for practices they have come to believe lead to certain moral traits. At least initially, it is believed not only that certain types of sleeping arrangements produce certain types of children but that these arrangements reflect certain types of parents (i.e., good or moral parents) who are themselves judged by family, friends, and community on where they place their infants or children for nighttime sleep (2,29).

Schweder and colleagues showed specifically that where and with whom some American children are allowed to sleep is guided by concerns for three specific moral issues: the sacredness-separateness (from children) of the husband-wife relationship; the appearance of incest avoidance; and the importance of teaching the child self-reliance and independence by enforcing the practice of sleeping alone.

Perhaps the overriding importance of these moral goods in certain segments of American society helps to explain why culture-based "folk" and scientific understandings of infant and childhood sleep often intermingle and mutually reinforce one another. In pediatric sleep medicine, for example, it is often difficult to distinguish between what is passed on to parents as proven scientific findings—in relation to how sleeping arrangements affect marriages, personality development, self-confidence, independence, and/or overall satisfaction with life—and what is simply personal judgment on the part of the advice giver (18,22).

Interestingly, the "moral" outcomes parents desire to instill in their children through choices for particular sleeping arrangements contrast and often conflict with the sleep-management strategies parents think they need to employ to obtain those outcomes. For example, Western parents generally seek to instill sensitivity, kindness, trust, and empathy in their children (30). At the same time, they want to create separateness, self-reliance, and/or autonomy through enforced solitary sleep, which can be facilitated through first withdrawing and then eliminating nighttime feedings and parental contact (26). Such emotionally conflicted parents will often display inconsistent (on-again, off-again) enforcement of solitary sleep, alternating between some form of cosleeping and separate sleeping arrangements. This pattern of cosleeping, first introduced by Madansky and Edelrock (31), is referred to as "reactive cosleeping" and has proven to be distinct in form and function from situations where parents elect or prefer to cosleep. Reactive cosleeping only exacerbates parent-child sleep struggles, and certainly does not eliminate them, as these investigators' study illustrates (31).

C. Do Solitary or Social Infant Sleeping Arrangements Produce Independent, Satisfied (Moral) Children and Adults? Is This the Right Question?

The absence of systematic studies on the relationship between acquired infant/child personality characteristics and routine sleeping arrangements probably explains why Western conventional understandings about the relationship between solitary infant sleeping arrangements and early independence are imprecise and misleading at best. Recent systematic studies are beginning to provide evidence that contradicts conventional wisdom on solitary sleep in early childhood. Consider:

Heron's (17) recent cross-sectional study of middle-class English children shows that among the children who "never" slept in their parents' bed, there was a trend to be harder to control, less happy, and to exhibit a greater number of tantrums. Moreover, he found that those children who were never permitted to bedshare were actually *more* fearful than children who always slept in their parents' bed for all of the night (17).

In a survey of adult college-age subjects, Lewis and Janda (32) report that males who coslept with their parents between birth and 5 years of age had significantly higher self-esteem, experienced less guilt and anxiety, and reported greater frequency of sex. Boys who coslept between 6 and 11 years of age also had higher self-esteem. For women, cosleeping during childhood was associated with less discomfort about physical contact and affection as adults.

(While these traits may be confounded by parental attitudes, such findings are clearly inconsistent with the folk belief that cosleeping has detrimental long-term effects on psychosocial development.)

Crawford (33) found that women who coslept as children had higher self-esteem than those who did not. Indeed, cosleeping appears to promote confidence, self-esteem, and intimacy, possibly by reflecting an attitude of parental acceptance (32).

A study of parents of 86 children in clinics of pediatrics and child psychiatry (ages 2 to 13 years) on military bases (offspring of military personnel) revealed that cosleeping children received higher evaluations of their comportment from their teachers than did solitary-sleeping children, and they were *underrepresented* in psychiatric populations compared with children who did not cosleep. The authors state:

> Contrary to expectations, those children who had not had previous professional attention for emotional or behavioral problems coslept more frequently than did children who were known to have had psychiatric intervention, and lower parental ratings of adaptive functioning. The same finding occurred in a sample of boys one might consider Oedipal victors (e.g., 3-year-old and older boys who sleep with their mothers in the absence of their fathers)—a finding which directly opposes traditional analytic thought. [16]

Again, in England, Heron (17) found that it was the solitary-sleeping children who were harder to handle (as reported by their parents), who dealt less well with stress, and who were rated as being *more* (not less) dependent on their parents than were the cosleepers!

And in the largest and possibly most systematic study to date, conducted on five different ethnic groups from both Chicago and New York involving 1411 subjects, Mosenkis (34) found far more positive adult outcomes for individuals who coslept as a children among almost all ethnic groups (African Americans and Puerto Ricans in New York and Puerto Ricans, Dominicans, and Mexicans in Chicago) than there were negative findings. An especially robust finding, which cut across all the ethnic groups included in the study, was that cosleepers exhibited a feeling of satisfaction with life.

But Mosenkis's main finding went beyond trying to determine causal links between sleeping arrangements and adult characteristics or experiences. Perhaps his most important finding was that the interpretation of "outcome" of cosleeping had to be understood within the context specific to each cultural milieu and within the relational matrix in which it occurs. For the most part, cosleeping as a child did not correlate with *anything* in any simple or direct way. He concluded that there is no one "function" of cosleeping, but that cosleeping as a child interacts with a variety of cultural, social, and unique developmental characteristics of the relational setting (34)—also that the sleeping arrangement is but a small part of a larger system affecting adult characteristics (34).

D. Beliefs About the Consequences of Nontraditional Sleeping Arrangements: Science or Religion?

Judging from public discourse at least, the validity of predicted outcomes associated with particular sleeping arrangements need not be demonstrated or proven scientifically as long as people *believe* that they are valid or that the outcomes promised reflect, complement, or in some way support the prevailing values and goals that justified the recommended practice in the first place. For example, in contrast with situations where parents and children sleep together (cosleep), solitary childhood sleeping arrangements are *believed* to foster more independent infants and children. The problem is that no study has ever defined what exactly is meant by independence, how it should be measured, or—assuming that it can be measured or achieved at a young age—whether this quality or character is causally linked to childhood satisfaction, competence, or happiness. Furthermore, no study has ever determined if the ability to sleep alone through the night at an early age relates to the emergence of other skills or personality characteristics unavailable to infants and children sleeping under different conditions.

When discussions turn to nontraditional sleeping arrangements, much is presumed but little or nothing is proven. For example, it is often implied or stated outright that cosleeping exacerbates or creates a parent–child sleep problems, but this appears to be true where parents do not value cosleeping, as when parents permit a child to sleep in their bed as a response to ongoing sleep difficulties. Furthermore, Hayes et al. (35) studied cosleeping among 51 children 3 to 5 years old and found, in the subgroup considered difficult sleepers, that all but one had developed sleep problems in the context of sleeping alone; that is, originally all the children who developed into "problem sleepers" as defined by their parents had been placed in a separate bed from infancy. Even where cosleeping parents report problems, this does not mean that solitary sleeping is not the preferred sleeping arrangement.

Whether a child is sleeping alone or socially, the functions of the sleep environment change in relation to age (36,37), and/or changing circumstances. For example, the physiological consequences of a mother sleeping beside her 1-month-old infant are enormously different from the physiological consequences associated with her sleeping with this same child 13 months later, when its cognitive and psychological systems are much more mature. At 1 month, and owing to the human infant's extreme neurological immaturity at birth and continuing slow development, the mother's body acts as a cue or trigger in regulating the baby's body temperature, breathing, arousal patterns, cortisol levels, and sleep architecture (38–41). But at 2 and/or 5 or 13 years of age, children will actively interpret the relational meaning and affects of cosleeping with their parents while the initial important physiological effects will diminish. Indeed, whether the consequences of the sleeping arrangement is beneficial, benign, or deleterious (at any given age) will depend not simply on the location—where the sleep occurs—but also on the social meaning and psychological content of the relationship of the participants as expressed within the family, *of which the sleep-*

ing arrangements per se are but a small reflection and part. Such critical analytic distinctions are mostly absent when the potential value of nontraditional sleeping arrangements (especially cosleeping) are addressed (42).

III. Conventional Western Understandings of "Healthy, Normal" Infant and Childhood Sleep: Where Did They Come From? Is One Form of Sleep as Good as Any Other?

It is tempting to use the concept of cultural relativism to argue that regardless of differences in the *ways* infants or children's sleep worldwide, each culturally based strategy is equally valid and appropriate. Such a simplistic perspective is fallacious, however, in a number of ways. First, it presumes that parents in all societies are equally satisfied with the way their infants and children sleep, or that parents (and children) are equally well rested despite differences in how or where they sleep. Though it is hard to make comparisons across all cultures, the impression of many anthropologists is that, in general, parents living in Western industrialized societies are much less satisfied with how their children sleep than are parents in non-Western societies, and that in industrialized societies, nightly infant and childhood sleep comes about under more stressful conditions (43,44).

A second fallacy is the erroneous assumption that any society (including our own) necessarily produces a sleep management strategy that is appropriate for all, and that it is optimal (promotes maximum health) for all, or is always compatible with the short- or long-term biological needs of the infant. Parental caregiving choices that satisfy parental best interests are not, for example, necessarily the same as those which best serve the infant's (40). Although modern lifestyles and/or technology offer some effective substitutes for parental nurturing (contact, protection, and support), it is worthwhile to recall Bruner's warning that "it would be a mistake to leap to the conclusion that because human immaturity makes possible high flexibility in later adjustment, anything is possible for the species.... we would err if we assumed a priori that man's inheritance places no constraint on his power to adapt" (45).

A third problem with the relativist perspective is that it erroneously implies that within any given society each family's values and goals are the same, and that publicly preferred or "ideal" sleeping arrangements are those which are actually practiced. We now have evidence that there is much more variability regarding sleep practices, especially in the United States and the United Kingdom, than has ever been acknowledged (16,46–48).

Obviously, each culture is unique, and there must be some compatibility between family behaviors and the society within which they live. My criticism is that the pediatric sleep community continues to make it uncomfortable for many parents to practice sleeping and nighttime feeding arrangements that differ from their own. More importantly, I regret that the "science" of infant sleep continues, for the most part, to disregard the biological significance of the mother's presence as a regulator of infant sleep, as it unfolds and develops within the cosleeping/breast-feeding adaptive complex. I argue that this disregard precludes a full understanding of infant sleep physiology and development; therefore, it also precludes a full understanding of the likely etiology of so many sleep-related problems that infants, children, and parents experience in Western societies.

In my own work, no particular sleeping arrangement is advocated for any particular family. Rather, data from ethnographic studies and human infant evolutionary studies are used to provide a perspective from which other kinds of analysis and concerns can proceed. An evolutionary perspective provides a more objective context, I believe, for understanding infant responses to the diverse sleep environments different cultures provide (49–51). As a conceptual tool, evolution offers a beginning point to consider how social factors come to predominate over and influence infant and childhood sleep biology and development (42). For example, anthropological studies that incorporate an evolutionary framework reveal that infant sleep physiology evolved in the context of continuous maternal contact, including baby-controlled nighttime breast feeding (52,53). This fact permits us to argue that in order to understand specieswide infant sleep-wake patterns and/or sleep architecture, infant sleep must first be studied under conditions that mimic this "environment of adaptedness" (54).

In Western cultures (as described above), clinicians generally continue to advocate only one form of sleep for infants and children (i.e., solitary sleep) and sleep *management* strategies aimed at sharply reducing, as early in life as possible, parental handling and feeding of infants at bedtime. Parents are encouraged not to permit infants to associate falling asleep with food (including breast-feeding) or parental touch (18,26,55,56), the very context within which the infant's "falling asleep" evolved. Breast-feeding rates in the United States have increased to reach a historic high (57). If the infant falling asleep at the breast is as common and as biologically appropriate as cross-cultural data suggest (43), then the recommendation by Western clinicians to prevent it will not only fail but will continue to prove problematic for many mothers and infants.

Given the historical context within which infant sleep studies were begun, these contemporary recommendations are better understood. Both clinicians and pediatricians encounter parents who need practical, immediate solutions to ongoing problems associated with solitary infant/child sleeping arrangements. Thus, a clinician's impressions is colored by families in crisis and mostly limited to them. Clinicians hear little testimony from parents who have found alternative sleeping arrangements (to the solitary model) and who enjoy alternative choices. Recall that infant sleep studies were first conducted by researchers in the fifties and sixties, a time period in which breast-feeding rates were at an all-time low. Mother-infant cosleeping was regarded as being aberrant, a sleeping arrangement definitely to be avoided. Since the significance of mother-infant cosleeping with nighttime breast-feeding was considered neither biologically nor culturally appropriate, it is not surprising that patterns of childhood sleep development considered clinically "healthy" and "normal" were those patterns expressed by bottle-fed infants sleeping alone in sleep laboratories.

A. The Traditional Sleep Research Paradigm Is Inadequate for the Diversity of Family Sleep Practices It Must and Should Accommodate

> It is hypothesized that the progressive organization of sleep and wakefulness at night in infancy reflects the integration of constitutional propensities of the infant [temperament] in interaction with the infant's multiple contexts.... Contextual relationships are mediated by the infant's primary relationships, which are different from, but have their origins in, the infant's social dyadic interactions. (6)

Anders suggests, in the quote above, that patterns of "normal" and "appropriate" infant sleep development are extremely variable and responsive to a variety of environmental—i.e., contextual—processes. Some of these processes involve family interactional factors that characterize the nature and affectional structure of the social relationships each parent experiences with his or her infant or child during the day (58). If fully realized by researchers and clinicians alike, the "transactional" model that Anders (6) and Sadeh and Anders (4) envision offers a revolutionary approach to studying and understanding infant sleep development and for creating the inclusive paradigm for which this chapter argues.

Indeed, a transactional approach takes Lozoff and her colleagues one step further. The approach acknowledges at the outset that "normal" infant sleep development can vary not only within different cultural subgroups but also from one infant to the next, depending upon the interplay of intrinsic and extrinsic variables significant to each developing child. Intrinsic factors can include but are not limited to infant temperament, growth rate, and neurological status (constitutional needs) at birth. Extrinsic factors, with which intrinsic variables interact, can involve such things as whether infants are breast- or bottle-fed (59); whether or not the infant feeds on its own or on its parent's schedule (60); whether the infant sleeps in the same bed, in the same room, or in a different room (alone) (61,62); whether the infant sleeps on its back, side, or belly (63); whether the family generally favors nighttime contact or discourages or resists it (17); and whether the infant has siblings or is an only child. All of these factors (and others) can alter the trajectory of infant sleep development in important ways.

Unfortunately for parents, popular discourse about how babies should sleep does not ordinarily make reference to these factors, and neither do clinicians. Harkness et al. (64) point out that the traditional theoretical models, explanations, and clinical treatments of infants with dysomnias and parasomnias continue to be predicated on the notion that the ontogeny or maturation of infant sleep is, in the vernacular, fairly clean, neat, and predictable. Changes in infant sleep architecture, particularly the reversal of the predominance of active to quiet sleep, is reported to follow an orderly, unfolding pattern *dominated by endogenous mechanisms*. For example, during the first year of life, a more stable "adult-like" pattern of sleep emerges. The infant sleeps for longer and longer (relatively uninterrupted) periods in increasingly deeper (delta-wave) sleep, which is thought to reflect an increase in the level of "integrity and maturity" of the central nervous system (64). Indeed, the ability of infants to return to sleep unassisted after awakening (to self-soothe)—to "sleep through the night" as early in life as possible with minimal parental contact—continues to be a developmental benchmark against which infants and their caregivers are evaluated, even when sleeping through the night is not an important issue for the parents. Such a criterion used to evaluate "developmental progress" may do more harm than good, if the sleeping arrangements actually practiced are not the same as the one for which the method of evaluation was intended.

B. Examples of How Culturally Guided "Choices" Concerning Sleeping Arrangements and Related Sleep Practices Matter Biologically to the Infant and Change "Normative" Sleep Development

Infant Sleep Position and Susceptibility to Sudden Infant Death Syndrome

It is worthwhile to consider how sensitive the infant's sleep behavior, physiology, and health is to culturally guided decisions about how, where, and with whom (if anyone) infants should sleep. Indeed, while Lozoff and her colleagues hinted at it, they never could have anticipated the degree to which culturally based decisions regarding infant and childhood sleep affect development and nightly sleep physiology, including the chances of an infant dying from the sudden infant death syndrome (SIDS). In fact, the sleeping position of the infant has proven to be the single most important factor for reducing the chances of an infant dying of SIDS (65), although the reasons for increased risk remain unknown. The discovery that, merely by placing infants in the supine rather than in the prone sleep position, SIDS rates could decline as much as 90% in some countries continues to astonish many SIDS researchers worldwide (66). The decision to recommend the prone sleeping position emerged from the widely accepted belief that if prone sleeping helped premature infants to breathe and sleep better, it could probably do the same for older, term infants. The possibility that supine infant sleep could make the infant vulnerable to choking (esophageal reflux) only added to the resolve of physicians to place infants prone for sleep (67).

Do infantile arousal mechanisms needed to protect infants during respiratory crises follow the same time course of development as the neurological mechanisms that promote longer periods of deeper sleep (delta wave, stages 3 and 4)? This is an important question as pertains to susceptibility to SIDS (68). Over 20 years ago, Douthitt and Brackbill (69) found that prone-sleeping newborns slept longer and deeper (aroused less and slept longer) than did supine-sleeping infants. They showed that infants sleeping on their backs experienced twice as many motor activities during sleep and more awakenings than did prone-sleeping newborns, findings recently confirmed by Kahn et al. (70). Since the goal of both parents and health professionals in Western societies was and continues to be to promote sleep and not awakenings, it is easy to understand why these earlier data provided support for the argument that infants should be placed in the prone position to sleep. Yet, it has been suggested that some infants who die of SIDS perhaps cannot arouse or awaken easily or fast enough to terminate a cardiorespiratory crisis during sleep, especially while in deep sleep, where arousal thresholds are higher (68). These findings raise the possibility that supine sleep might well be safer *precisely because of the increased arousal and motor activity accompanying it*, even though the implications of this possibility conflict with cultural strategies to promote early "deep" sleep in infants as early in life as possible.

There are other parent-controlled "social" precautions that lower the risks of SIDS. Mitchell (71) found that the presence of a responsible adult sleeping in the same room as an infant reduced the chances of the infant's dying from SIDS by fourfold. This protective effect did not generalize to cosleeping among siblings, indicating that a responsible role played by the caregiver is likely critical in reducing the chances of the infant dying. Moreover, the largest epidemiological study to date, conducted in Great Britain, also shows increased risks for infants sleeping in rooms alone as well as for babies sleeping in their mother's beds, *if the mother smokes*. Other dangerous conditions include the use of a duvet pulled up over the infant's head as well as the use of a soft mattress. Overheating by overwrapping an infant also significantly increased the SIDS risk. All of these new data illustrate the extent to which infant sleep physiology is directly mediated by parental intervention (see Chap. 21).

Feeding Practices

Bottle-fed infants exhibit significantly different nightly sleep profiles than do breast-fed infants. Infants who are breast-fed for a year or more develop different sleep patterns than do infants breast-fed for only the first 3 months (15). Oberlander et al. (72) found that among newborns, a complete milk formula feed increased postfeed sleep by 46% and 118% compared respectively to water and carbohydrate-only feedings. Furthermore, the most recent Ross survey of breast-feeding in the United States indicates that 62% of contemporary mothers are breast-feeding when they leave the hospital (57). New evidence suggests that at least for the first 3 or 4 months of life, mothers continue to provide their infants with at least two breast-feedings or more from midnight through to the morning (59).

That so many more mothers are now breast-feeding their infants for increasingly longer periods makes sleep models based entirely on data from infants fed artificial or cow's milk (from bottles) highly problematic for at least half of the population of contemporary American infants. And while breast-feeding drops to 26% at 6 months, the number of mothers who breast-feed in the United States continue to rise (57). This is particularly significant since, as described below, in addition to sleep differences induced by breast versus cow's milk, sleep proximity to mother also influences the frequency and duration of feedings (59). Maternal proximity in the form of bed sharing, in addition to breast feeding, especially changes the infant's nightly sleep architecture, including arousals and sleep period time. Developmental models of infant sleep in the first year of life that do not take into account feeding method and frequency in relationship to sleeping arrangements are therefore not appropriate for many infants.

That feeding affects sleep physiology, including infant cardiac patterns, was demonstrated over 25 years ago. In fact, Harper and colleagues (73) argued that feeding behavior plays an underestimated role in regulating infant sleep physiology and sleep architecture. He and his colleagues found that among bottle-fed, solitary-sleeping infants, the waking periods associated with feeding increased the probability of a subsequent rapid-eye-movement (REM) period, a finding consistent with previous work on small mammals. They suggested that because REM sleep and quiet sleep followed each other in sequential fashion, a change in the relative distribution of REM sleep altered the likely sequence of state. Their laboratory research on bottle-fed infants showed that feeding tended to entrain the subsequent REM-QS cycle in that the percentage of REM increased after feeding and then dropped sharply approximately 20 min later, with a corresponding increase in quiet sleep. They concluded that "the interpretation of behavior resulting from maternal-infant interaction should be viewed within the framework of incorporation of food, in that satiety play a large role in regulation of state integration and cardiac response" (73). Despite this finding, infant sleep research papers rarely include information on feeding method and frequency.

"Choice" of sleeping arrangement was found to greatly increase not only the number of breast-feedings but the total nightly duration of breast-feeding and the average intervals between the feeding sessions. For example, among 70 nearly exclusively breast-feeding mothers of Latin-American descent and their 2- to 4-month-old infants, we found that when mother and child were bed sharing, the average interval between the breast feedings was approximately 1½ hr. When they were sleeping apart in separate bedrooms (but still within earshot), however, the interval was at least twice as long (about 3 hr). Moreover, on their bed-sharing nights, we found that babies breast-fed twice as often for three times the total nightly duration than they did when they slept alone (59).

These differences in feeding were part of a broader complex of differences, a cascade of interconnected changes induced by the presence of the mother. Mother-infant cosleeping altered not only feeding behavior within what was supposed to be a homogenous breast-feeding group but also infant and maternal arousal patterns (74–76), sleep architecture (61), mother-baby body orientations in bed (77), infant respiratory behavior (78)—in short, almost every major parameter important in understanding infant and maternal sleep physiology (see Figs. 1 and 2 and discussion below).

Infant and Maternal Arousals, Temporal Correspondences, and Sleep Architecture Among Solitary and Bed-sharing Mother-Baby Pairs

> Separate normative values for infant sleep need to be developed for infants who bed-share, and existing norms should be reinterpreted within the cultural context in which they were established. (61)

In three in-house laboratory studies of one form of mother-infant cosleeping—bed sharing—we used standardized polysomnography and infrared photography to quantify differences in the behavior and physiology of mother-infant pairs as they shared a bed or slept apart. These data show that during bed sharing, a significant amount of

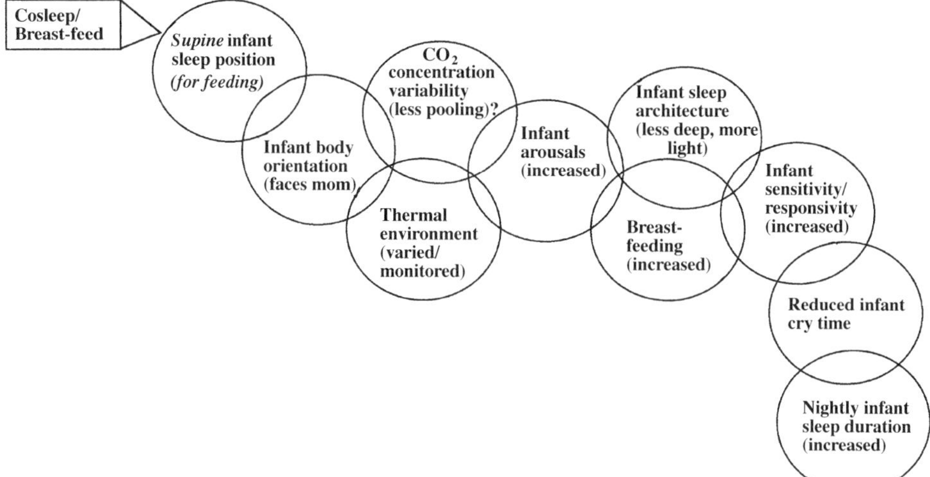

Figure 1 For the breast-fed infant, "Choice" of sleeping arrangement sets in motion a cascade of potentially beneficial biobehavioral effects for the mother-infant dyad (from the infant's perspective).

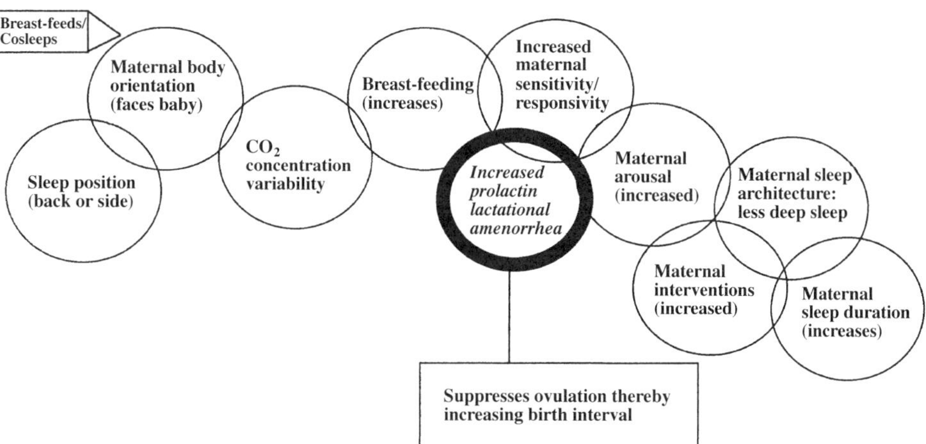

Figure 2 Cosleeping sets in motion a cascade of biobehavioral effects and events relevant to mothers (from the mother's perspective).

temporal correspondence occurred between the sleeping pair's transient (brief) arousals and between their larger epochal awakenings (75). We also found that bed-sharing mother-infant pairs exhibited a trend toward greater simultaneous overlap in all sleep stages (i.e., stages 1 and 2, 3 and 4, and REM). This synchronization of sleep states was not explained by chance and is not found when the sleep/wake activity of infants is compared to randomly selected mothers with whom they did not cosleep (50,79).

In our most extensive 3-year study, we reported that in general, small, electroencephalographically defined transient infant arousals were facilitated in the bed-sharing environment, albeit selectively; even when routinely bed-sharing infants slept alone, they continued to exhibit more transient arousals than did routinely solitary-sleeping infants sleeping alone (75). Furthermore, bed sharing significantly shortened the amount of time per episode infants remained in deeper stages of sleep (stages 3 and 4) compared with when they slept alone but increased amounts of time spent in stages 1 and 2. Bed-sharing infants also experienced more total time asleep (61), in part because they cried significantly less while sleeping with their mothers than they did when sleeping alone (51).

We also documented an acute sensitivity on the part of the routinely bed-sharing mothers to their infants' presence in the bed. That is, compared to the number of overlapping arousals (in which the infant aroused first), routinely solitary-sleeping mothers on their bed-sharing night in the laboratory exhibited significantly less overlapping arousals than the routinely bed-sharing mothers did, indicating that bed-sharing mothers do not habituate to the presence of their babies but become more sensitized to their behavior (75).

Although routinely bed-sharing mothers aroused and fed their infants more frequently while sleeping next to them, they received as much sleep on average as solitary-sleeping breast-feeding mothers did. Moreover, bed-sharing mothers evaluated their bed-sharing sleep experiences (in the laboratory) at least as positively as did routinely solitary-sleeping mothers following the night they slept alone (76).

All together, these documented differences between the bed-sharing and solitary-sleep environments elucidate some of the processes accounting for how and why the presence of the mother routinely in bed with the infant leads to significant changes in sleep development over the infant's first year of life—patterns confirmed by the ethnographic data discussed below. *This kind of "normative" trajectory of first-year sleep development, while appropriate for situations in which parents choose to routinely bed share, is not presently accommodated by the traditional paradigm.*

Culture (Versus Sleeping Arrangements) Regulates Infant Breathing?

Richard and colleagues (78) showed that characteristics of the sleep environment also affect the infant's nightly breathing patterns. For example, the bed-sharing environment is associated with more central apneas, fewer obstructive apneas, and more periodic breathing in infants than is the solitary sleep environment. During bed sharing, irrespective of the routine sleeping arrangement at home, the infant experiences a higher frequency of central apneas during stages 1 to 2 and REM sleep (and overall). Among routinely solitary-sleeping infants who then slept with their mothers in the same bed in the laboratory, this increase largely reflected an increase in the shortest apneas (3 to 5.9 sec) in stages 1 and 2; in routinely bed-sharing infants, it reflected increases in apneas in the 6 to 8.9-sec range during REM and in the apnea range of 9 to 11.9 sec during stages 1 to 2. In contrast to central apneas, however, obstructive apneas were decreased by bed sharing, but only among routinely solitary-sleeping infants (while bed sharing) who had a lower frequency overall and specifically in stages 1 and 2 and REM (78).

The amount of periodic breathing was also significantly increased in the bed-sharing environment. Routinely bed-sharing infants had a higher frequency of periodic breathing and a longer mean duration over the entire night (overall) while bed sharing and specifically during REM sleep. Routinely solitary-sleeping infants exhibited more frequent periodic breathing only during stages 3 and 4 while bed sharing in the laboratory with their mothers (78).

Social Determinants of Total Infant Sleep Time and Length of Average Sleep Period

The ethnographic studies of infant sleep in diverse settings confirm just how extensively the infant's endogenous mechanisms *transact* with parental behavior. Outside of the laboratory, it is clear that the total amount of daily sleep an infant experiences is regulated by the environment and cannot (strictly speaking) be considered dependent on endogenous factors. For example, in a recent in-home longitudinal study, Harkness et al. (64) studied 36 American families from Cambridge, Massachusetts. The children ranged in age from birth to 36 months and were studied for over a year. The sleep behavior of these children was compared to that of a sample from 66 Dutch families (living near Leiden and Amsterdam) with children of different ages, ranging from 6 months to 8 years. Analysis was based on diaries kept by parents in both settings. The researchers found that, on average, Dutch babies slept 2 hr longer (15 versus 13 hr) than American infants did, and the parent-infant sleep "struggles," ubiquitous among the Americans, were not as familiar to the Dutch (64).

The authors explained these differences between the American and Dutch infants' sleep behavior in terms of the importance of the three "R's" of Dutch child rearing: *rust* (rest), *regelmaat* (regulation), and *rein held* (cleanliness). The three "R's" reflect Dutch social values that justify and provide the rationale for the preferred infant sleep context and other aspects of daytime child care. For example, Harkness et al. (64) describe how Dutch parents bring to their child rearing an "ethnohistory," or set of beliefs, which explains why infants need a great deal of sleep and must not, therefore, be overstimulated either during the day or night. Not only are babies put down to sleep earlier in the evenings but—rather than worrying about whether their infants are receiving enough intellectual stimulation during the day, as American parents do—Dutch parents are concerned that they may be receiving too much stimulation, potentially threatening the infants' ability to sleep at night (64).

In another study, Elias et al. (15) compared the development of sleep in infants of "standard-care" mothers (those following Dr. Spock's recommendations to minimize contact and feeding during the night) with the sleep of infants whose mothers practice care recommended by the La Leche League, a worldwide voluntary health organization committed to promoting prolonged breast-feeding, physical contact, and cosleeping. Among infants receiving standard, minimal nighttime contact care, the maximum period of unbroken sleep increased from an average of 6.5 hr at 2 months of age to 8 hr at 4 months and to more than 8 hr during the second year. Infants of La Leche League mothers at 2 months of age slept an average of 5 hr during their longest sleep period. Not until they were 20 months old did these infants sleep significantly longer than 5 hr during their longest sleep period. In contrast to the consolidated sleep of the standard-care infants, their sleep was characterized by shorter sleep periods and frequent awakenings at night.

In addition to the length of sleep periods, total sleep time developed differently for cosleepers. La Leche League infants slept a total of 15 hr at 2 months, 12.5 hr at 4 months, and just over 11 hr by 2 years. Standard-care infants continued to sleep 13 to 14 hr per day throughout the 2-year monitoring period (15). As such, Elias et al. concluded that weaning status and bed sharing have major effects on the development of sleep patterns. Indeed, in their sample, these two factors explained 67% of the variance in the length of sleep periods (80,81).

These data are consistent with those from babies born to mothers from a very different society but whose patterns of nighttime sleep and feeding were approximately the same as those from infants whose mothers practiced baby care as recommended by the La Leche League. For example, for the first year of life and longer, Super and Harkness (43) documented significant differences in nighttime infant sleep behavior between the Kipsigis people of rural Kenya and infants living in Los Angeles. The ten Kipsigis infants were observed over a 24-hr cycle on a series of days during the first 8 months of life, with records kept on their sleep-wake states and feeding patterns. Comparison data for the Los Angeles sample were provided by work conducted by Parmelee and colleagues (82). Kipsigis babies breast-fed throughout the night in close contact with their mothers in one-room dwellings, while American babies slept either in their own rooms or own beds. Whereas the American babies averaged 8 hr of nighttime sleep by 16 weeks of age, the Kipsigis babies continued to wake at intervals of 3 to 4 hr up to 8 months of age, the oldest age for which the researchers kept data. Super and Harkness also found that over the 24-hr cycle by the third and fourth months of age, American babies were sleeping about 2 hr longer (43).

Thumb Sucking and Transitional Objects

Winnicott (83) first described the use of "sleep aids" by young children as part of the process by which they learn to sleep alone. In the absence of a parent or attachment figure, a young child might adopt a "special object" (blanket, favored toy, or stuffed animal) to which he or she attributes special qualities. These objects serve to comfort a young child during awakenings or while falling asleep (4). In Western cultures, these *transitional objects* are so ubiquitous that current psychological models of development imply that their use is a natural stage through which all children pass. Use of such objects, however, is not universal but dependent upon the social context within which a child's nightly sleep experience begins and ends. As discussed in their review, Wolf and Lozoff (84) report that American toddlers (mean age 21.7 months) who had an adult present when they fell asleep were significantly less likely to use an attachment object (such as a blanket or doll) or to suck their thumbs, practices that appear to provide a sense of security in the absence of parental contact.

In Japan and Korea, where cosleeping is the norm, children as a general rule do not suck their thumbs at night or use transitional objects. One of the most convincing studies showing that thumb sucking may be correlated with infants falling asleep alone comes from a study conducted among Turkish children. In one group, children between the ages of 1 and 7 years of age sucked their thumbs; 96% of them had been left alone (as infants) to fall asleep. In contrast, all of the children in the non-thumb-sucking group (the majority of the total sample) had some type of adult contact or body contact, such as either being held or breast-fed while falling asleep. Even in American samples, children whose parents stayed with them at bedtime were less likely to suck their thumbs than were children who fell asleep alone (as cited in 84; 85,86).

Among contemporary Mayan children, on only a rare occasion were objects used to ease the transition to sleep, and there were no preparations for bedtime or bedtime rituals, including special nighttime clothes. Babies mostly fell asleep in their mothers' arms or were breast-fed to sleep, and only one child observed by Morelli et al. (24) used a security (transitional) object while falling asleep. As they explain, among the Mayans infant sleep occurred in the same company with which the babies spend their days and "no coaxing of any type is needed to get the infant to sleep" (24).

In sum, culture (including medical views) guides parental decisions regarding infant sleep position, feeding method and distribution, whether the baby sleeps alone or with its mother. In turn, parental decisions influence infant sleep behavior and physiology, including infant sleep architecture, maternal and infant arousals, sensitivity to the presence of the other, breathing, amount of feeding, amount of sleep, nightly infant crying time, as well as thumb sucking and the use of transitional objects. These documented, interrelated effects support Anders' (6) "transactional model," which sees the emergence of infant sleep patterns in terms of a dynamic "transaction" between extrinsic and intrinsic factors. He phrases it this way: "the progressive organization of sleep and wakefulness at night in infancy reflects the integration of constitutional propensities of the infant (temperament) *in interaction with the infant's multiple contexts....* Contextual influences are mediated by the infant's primary relationships, which are different from, but have their origins in, the infant's social dyadic interactions."

Do Solitary Infant Sleep and Rigid Parental Expectations Foster Infant-Parent Sleep Difficulties?

That infant sleep biology changes much more slowly than do the cultural values that underlie and regulate it raises the possibility that the most biologically optimal sleep environments for infants may not be the ones promoted by the larger society within which an infant's family lives. And, of course, it is highly probable that widely accepted infant sleep-management strategies are sufficient for some infants and children but unsuitable for others, who vary emotionally or psychologically. Moreover, some families may apply widely accepted developmental sleep norms established for one kind of sleep environment to their own when it is inappropriate to do so. This can lead to parental disappointment or to parents concluding wrongly that their own parenting skills are deficient or that their infant or child is uncooperative or poorly developed. Ironically, this situation might best describe what occurs in developed countries such as the United States, Great Britain, and Australia, where approximately 35% of otherwise healthy children, have "problems" falling or staying asleep after having first been conditioned to sleep alone (17,35,87). Such high percentages likely do not reflect infant or caregiver deficiencies but perhaps unrealistic or inappropriate definitions and expectations about how infants *should* sleep, including the rigidity by which parents hear, interpret, and apply popular and scientific information about infant sleep.

Indeed, the degree of rigidity by which parents are socialized to hold onto these expectations can, in some instances, be used to predict the relative likelihood that infant-child sleep problems will manifest themselves. Parents with more rigid expectations are more likely to report dissatisfaction with their child's sleep behavior than parents less committed to any particular expectation (17,80). As Anders and Taylor (8) astutely point out, night awakenings constitute a problem only for those parents who expect their children to sleep through the night at very definite ages (4,5).

Only in the last 100 years or so, in a relatively small number of world cultures, have parents and health professionals become concerned with how infants *should* be conditioned to sleep—and concerned with accelerating sleep development. And only in Western cultures are infants thought to need to "learn" to sleep, in this case alone and without parental contact. Most cultures simply take infant sleep for granted. Consider this remarkable insight offered by Harkness et al.:

> ... in the sense that normal children everywhere will eventually sleep throughout the night, will need less sleep as they get older and will go to bed and get up at approximately the same hours as other members of the family, and they will eventually fall asleep (and wake up) without immediate support from their mothers or fathers, all four of the major behavioral stages or components of infant sleep are "developmentally based." [64]

IV. Infant–Parent or Child Cosleeping: The "Political Third Rail"? Why So Controversial?

> ... Although taking your child into bed with you for a night or two may be reasonable if he is ill or very upset about something, for the most part this is not a good idea. (26)

> ... The parents have to be firm and committed to returning the child to bed ... parents have to learn to ignore crying until the child falls asleep. Sometimes children can cry for

> a couple of hours. Children may vomit with crying and so parents need to be prepared to go in to clean up the child and change the bedclothes quickly and, with the minimum of fuss, put the child back to bed, and walk out. (56)
>
> ... sleeping in your bed can make your child feel confused and anxious rather than relaxed and reassured. Even a young toddler may find this repeated experience overly stimulating [26].
>
> ... advice against cosleeping may be overly simplistic. (88)

Infant–parent cosleeping is a *generic* concept referring to the diverse ways in which a primary (responsible) caregiver, usually the mother, sleeps within close proximity (arm's reach) of the infant or child. This permits each to detect and respond to a variety of each other's sensory stimuli (sound, movement, smells, sights, touch). Cosleeping represents the universal (species-specific) evolved context of human infant sleep development. It is not, therefore, surprising that the breast-feeding/mother-infant cosleeping arrangement is for the majority of contemporary people inevitable and inseparable and not a choice. This fact suggests that any universal biological understanding of infant sleep physiology (and sleep-related difficulties) that neglects the evolved connections between nighttime mother-infant proximity, breast-feeding, and infant sleep must be regarded as inaccurate, incomplete, and/or fundamentally flawed.

Bedsharing is but one form of cosleeping. Another is futon cosleeping or letting the infant sleep alongside but not on the same surface as the mother. This occurs, for instance, when infants sleep in a basket or hammock above or on the side of the mother or when mothers and infants lie beside each other on a mat on the floor. There can be no one outcome associated with cosleeping—benign, beneficial, or deleterious—just as there can be no one outcome associated with solitary infant sleeping arrangements. Physiological or psychological outcomes depend on the infant's or child's age as well as on the nature of the relational setting, social conditions, and physical circumstances within which cosleeping occurs.

A. How Cultural/Scientific Bias Manifests Itself Against the Choice to "Cosleep": A Social Critique

The idea of parent–infant cosleeping as a legitimate and appropriate choice for parents remains controversial in Western societies. The controversy exists because so many negative consequences are speculated to be associated with it, although they are rarely contextualized or systematically documented. In popular parenting books, childcare bulletins and child-care magazines, cosleeping can be 1) mostly described as if it were a unitary concept; 2) ignored completely; or 3) presented to parents in terms of the likely or inevitable "problems" that will, might, or could, arise if it were practiced. Sometimes, it is explicitly discouraged (26); other times, the message is a bit more subtle (18). It is usually implied that by avoiding cosleeping, marriages might best be nurtured and preserved, infant/child individualism and autonomy promoted, incest and suffocation avoided, social (childhood) competence maximized, gender and sexual identities strengthened, and the chances of short- and long-term life satisfaction (for all family members) potentially realized (29,47).

Indeed, where a "problem" or potential problem with cosleeping can be identified—rather than being considered simply a "problem to be solved"—the putative problem becomes the argument against the practice, as if all families who cosleep will experience the same "problem." Furthermore, possible problems associated with cosleeping are presented as if they could not be solved in the same manner as, for example, problems associated with conditioning infants to sleep alone can be solved. Throughout the literature, cosleeping is described as the cause of marital discord (58), though recent data from Sweden refutes this notion (89), or the cause of sibling jealousies—which, while possible, may be only one of hundreds of causes of sibling jealousy! Moreover, without considering whether the particular parents involved consider cosleeping a "bad" or a "good" habit, parents are warned that cosleeping creates a "bad habit," one "difficult to break." Furthermore, cosleeping is said to "confuse" the infant or child emotionally or sexually or to induce "overstimulation." But no evidence is offered that specifies how, when, and under what circumstances these negative consequences arise (26). As the work of Shweder and colleagues suggests, a child *needs* to sleep alone; it is also said that this is necessary (26) in order to create a sense of self, or comfort with aloneness, or skills that presumably foster self-reliance—all of which constitute "moral goods" and not biological gains. Again, no specifics are given as to how only this arrangement produces these outcomes, leaving the reader to assume that solitary sleep is the only way.

Certainly, concerns for infant safety top the list of reasons why some health professionals suggest that all cosleeping should be avoided. It is true that many modern beds were not designed for infant safety. Suffocation and SIDS, which are mostly indistinguishable from each other, are argued to be two potential consequences of parents-infant cosleeping (71). Indeed, where mattresses are soft, the mother smokes, and/or any adult cosleeper is desensitized by drugs, bed sharing should definitely be avoided—and there are many other conditions that would make bed sharing less than an ideal choice, including parental discomfort with the idea. But recognizing when and where cosleeping in the form of bed sharing should be avoided is different from assuming that all bed sharing is dangerous—as laboratory (49,59,61,75,76,90,91), home (46), and epidemiological studies of unexpected deaths in infants are making clear (see Chapt. 23).

Cosleeping/bedsharing is not synonymous with dangerous sleep environments, although dangerous conditions are used inappropriately as a proxy for the act itself (i.e., mothers and infants lying side by side), as current debates about cosleeping are beginning to reveal (92,93). The exaggerated fear of suffocating an infant while cosleeping may stem partly from Western cultural history. During the last 500 years, many economically destitute women living in Paris, Brussels, Munich, and London (to name but a few locales) confessed to Catholic priests to having murdered their infants by lying on top of them in order to control family size (94–96). Under the priests' leadership and the threat of ex-communication, fines or imprisonment (for actual deaths), infants were banned from parental beds. The legacy of this particular historical condition in Western history probably converged with other changing social mores and customs (values favoring privacy, self-reliance, and individualism) in providing a philosophical foundation for contemporary cultural beliefs. This foundation makes it far easier to find dangers associated with cosleeping than to find (or assume) hidden benefits.

The proliferation and expansion of the idea of "romantic love" throughout Europe, coupled with the belief in the importance of the "conjugal" (husband–wife) relationship, probably also promoted separate sleeping quarters. It has been proposed that this physical separation, especially of the father from his children, maximized his ability to dispense religious training and to display moral authority (96,97).

As with many relational issues, parent–child cosleeping may require unique solutions to assure, in this case, safety and "private" adult time. However, the fact that problems can be associated with cosleeping is no more an argument against its legitimacy than is the fact that thousands of parents purchase books to solve the problems associated with solitary infant sleep.

As Kuhn (98) has noted, scientific paradigms change neither quickly nor easily. The controversy surrounding cosleeping and the value of mother–infant cosleeping studies might partially be explained by the fact that these topics are part of a new paradigm that is not readily or necessarily easily assimilated by those who have worked all of their scientific lives to document the normality of solitary infant sleep and who have accepted uncritically the alleged deleterious consequences of infant-parent cosleeping. Researchers, clinicians, and parents alike share many common cultural experiences. This common background probably means that most or very few routinely coslept with their own parents—a factor that strongly influences one's comfort with the practice (99). Perhaps an appreciation of diverse child-care practices including cosleeping will come only when non-European immigrants come to dominate Western countries. As demographics on that score suggest, the question is not whether the paradigm will change, but when.

B. Cosleeping/Bed Sharing in Western Societies: How Often? How Much of the Night? Who Really Knows?

Infant–parent cosleeping represents the universal, specieswide pattern of sleep for children worldwide. Barry and Paxson (10) surveyed the sleeping practices of 186 independent societies in a sample representative of all known major cultural types in the world. Of the 119 cultures with reliable ethnographic data on parental nighttime sleeping proximity to infants, mothers slept in the same bed with their infants in 76 cultures (64%). In 20% of these cases, the father slept in the same bed as well. *In none of the cultures was the infant actually isolated at bedtime.* Always, the baby was placed in sensory proximity of another person, but did not necessarily sleep on the same surface.

Few studies have addressed the prevalence of parent–infant cosleeping in the United States, and most surveys are now dated. It is a difficult subject on which to collect accurate information. Some American subgroups are comfortable reporting that they cosleep while others are not. Fear of censure and/or parental perceptions that bed sharing is outside of the cultural norm probably leads to underreporting (58,99, 100). Until recently, popular parenting books and magazines warned parents about the psychological consequences of cosleeping. That parents might fear disapproval and be reluctant to admit to cosleeping is justified. One survey in 1984 found that 94% of pediatricians disapproved of cosleeping. Although that number is likely considerably lower today, negative opinions about cosleeping probably remain high (88).

That said, even within Western industrialized cultures, it appears that diverse forms of cosleeping are not uncommon. For example, Abbott (29) found that in eastern Kentucky (Appalachia), infant-parent cosleeping is prevalent among white Americans who seem not "to care what doctors say," believing rather that "it is best for the mother and child to be together." Says another informant, "These new mothers are losing two of the greatest blessings that God gave mothers: the pleasure of sleeping with your child and letting it nurse" (29). Abbot argues that the eastern Kentucky practice of parents sleeping with or near their infants throughout the first 2 years of life is a strategy used by parents in this subgroup to induce interdependence, which is preferred to independence. As one eastern Kentucky woman phrased it, "How can you expect to hold on to them later in life, if you begin their lives by pushing them away?" (29).

In the well-cited study of parent–infant cosleeping conducted among urban Americans in Cleveland, Lozoff et al. (88) found that 35% of poor urban whites and 79% of poor urban blacks routinely slept with their children, who ranged in age from 6 months to 4 years. In contrast, Anders and Keener (36) recorded the nighttime sleep of 40 newborns and found that between the time the infant was initially laid in the crib and the time it was removed in the morning, at 2 and 4 weeks of life, the infant spent less than 20% of the night outside the crib. After the age of 20 weeks (5 months) through to the first birthday, infants spent less than 3% of the night outside their cribs.

Of the 150 mothers in the Cleveland area, 71% indicated that they did not practice cosleeping during the month before the interview, and 65% disclosed that they did not provide any body contact to their child at bedtime (88). However, what parents say and what they actually do are often two different things. For example, in this same survey, fewer than 35% of these mothers indicated that they were "firm" in adhering to these stated practices when their child continued to awaken during the night, was ill, or was frightened.

In the Boston metropolitan area (Worcester), Madansky and Edelbrock (31) found similar differences between black and white families. The majority of parents in the sample, (55%) reported that their 2- to 3-year-olds had slept in their beds at least once in the last 2 months, and 14% reported cosleeping several times a week. Of the African-American families, 76% coslept, while 53% of the white families did. African-American families were more than twice as likely as whites to cosleep more than twice a week (50% to 21% respectively). A relatively recent study of cosleeping in Harlem by Schacter-Fuchs et al. (48) reveals that 20% of Hispanic Americans slept with their children all night at least three nights a week, compared with only 6% of the white families sampled there.

The La Leche League—a worldwide organization committed to promoting frequent nursing, late weaning, and close parent–infant physical contact–reports that U.S. mothers frequently share a bed with their infants and children. Elias et al. (15) showed that between 2 to 13 months of age, 60% to 90% of La Leche League infants slept with their mothers. Especially for upper-middle-class families, nighttime nurturing in the form of cosleeping is one way that mothers and fathers feel they can compensate for time spent apart from their children during the day. Says one career woman interviewed in southern California: "Sleeping with my baby lets me make up some time I couldn't spend with her during the day, since my husband and I do not return to the house until early evening. Cosleeping gives me more time to feel and nurture my baby."

Among middle- to upper-class (Caucasian) families, cosleeping no longer appears to be taboo, as it was just a decade ago (46). The fact that over half of all American mothers are breast-feeding for between 3 and 6 months or longer (57) makes it even more likely that increasing numbers of mothers are sleeping with or near their infants or children to facilitate nighttime feedings. Breast-feeding is known to promote bed sharing (100). Still, fear of censure by pediatricians, family, and friends prevent many parents from discussing their nighttime caregiving practices if they happen to vary from the expected "norms" (88,99,101).

C. Closet Cosleepers, Changing Demographics of Cosleeping Families, and "Dear Abby"

That many more parents sleep with their infants or children in Western societies than is ever reported is further indicated by recent anthropological field studies in Great Britain. Ball and Hooker (46) studied a white working-class community in northeast England. They found that parents often respond to questions regarding the place where the infant sleeps at night by identifying the place where the infant *starts* the night or where the infant "is *supposed* to sleep" but not necessarily with where the infant spends most of the night. Ball and Hooker filmed nighttime parenting behavior using infrared cameras placed in the parents' bedroom. In addition, they conducted two sets of interviews—one before the infant was born and the other when the infant was 2 months old. Their study revealed that unless researchers specifically asked parents if the babies were moved during the night, possibly as many as half the infants who actually were cosleepers would not have been identified as such (46).

Attitudes regarding the validity of the choice to cosleep are changing in Western countries. Perhaps advice columnist Abigail van Buren (alias "Dear Abby") reflects where popular culture is headed on this issue. Recently a letter written to her, from a husband who signed: "Crowded Bed," was published in the *Chicago Tribune*. He complained about his wife's insistence that their 16-month-old daughter, Alicia, be permitted to sleep in their bed, and asked for Abby's opinion. She responded: "Dear Crowded Bed: In some cultures, it is normal for a baby to share the parents' bed until mid-childhood. An infant will adjust to the style parents choose.... but Alicia can learn to sleep comfortably in her own bed if that is what you choose to teach her" (102).

V. Conclusions, Recommendations, Afterthoughts

> People order their universe through social bias. By bringing these biases out in the open, we will understand better which policy issues can be reconciled and which cannot. [103]

Lozoff and her colleagues were correct. Culture and medical practice affect each other in powerful ways. I like to keep in mind that cultural biases in science do not invalidate or make any less important the methods or insights that science provides (to change Lozoff's phrasing just a bit). Biases do, however, require scientists to constantly rethink what questions are asked, which are ignored, and why. This reconsideration must include examining what cultural assumptions underlie, direct, and ultimately limit the interpretation of data. That scientists strive to be objective cannot, of course, ameliorate intellectual prejudice.

This essay revisits insights offered over a decade ago. Lozoff and her colleagues (1) suggested that it is important to be conscious of Euro-American biases regarding "proper" childhood sleep habits that find expression in the pediatrician's office. This chapter builds on their work. I call attention to the way specific ideologies continue to affect and constrain pediatric and clinical sleep practice and pediatric research. I believe that by broadening working models of the childhood sleep and by encouraging the use of a more diverse range of concepts to be used by parents, researchers, and clinicians, the chances of finding a better fit between family characteristics, sleeping arrangements, and the needs of particular infants, children, and parents is greatly enhanced. It is time to dispense with the "one size should fit all" approach to infant and childhood sleeping arrangements.

This critique is not meant to malign any of my colleagues—whose work makes my own possible. I am aware that my own training and research experiences (in anthropology) lead to yet another type of bias. But this is precisely why the intersection of different perspectives and disciplines is so critical. Unstated assumptions in each area of inquiry are made explicit. Furthermore, we are made aware that each discipline's biases shape and limit research. All of this means simply that no one discipline can do it all.

Along these lines many different ideas and issues are proposed in this chapter. Perhaps the most important are the following:

In pediatric practice, physicians should be prepared to give advice relevant to culturally diverse parental child-care goals, attitudes, desires, and approaches, and attempts should be made to inform parents about a broad range of sleeping and feeding patterns. This means discussing choices that might differ from those personally favored by the physician. The potential advantages and disadvantages of all sleeping arrangements should be raised, and mention of safety precautions for all choices should be included in discussions.

Problems associated with nontraditional sleeping arrangements, such as cosleeping, do not by themselves constitute arguments against the validity of the choice. Nor does the existence of "problems" suggest that they cannot be solved or that particular problems are intrinsic to the practice and inevitable.

The human infant's extreme neurological immaturity at birth makes social care (including the sleeping arrangements of young infants) practically synonymous with physiological regulation. This is an extraordinarily important and unique aspect of the importance of the sleep environment for the human infant—a significance that is not acknowledged by the traditional paradigm or, in general, by pediatricians and sleep clinicians.

Unless it is determined that mothers want to reduce nighttime breast-feeding, it should not automatically be assumed by sleep clinicians or pediatricians that the best approach is always "the fewer the nighttime feeds the better." The potential benefits of breast milk, including nighttime breast-feedings, are far too significant to the infant, as recent scientific studies have revealed. The choice belongs to fully informed parents, not to advice givers.

Regardless of where parents want their children to sleep, parents should be reminded that as a beginning point for understanding, infants, children and their parents are biologically and psychologically designed to sleep close. It is perfectly appropriate that some parents, perhaps many, may choose not to do so. However, it should be explained to parents that some infants' inability to "sleep through the night" or to sleep alone easily, should not be interpreted as a deficiency or as manipulation on the part of the infant. Such an knowledge may help prevent parents from evaluating their own caregiving skills negatively and/or their infants' or children's behavior as abnormal, bizarre, or deficient.

A more scientifically accurate and "user friendly" approach to infant-child sleep problems and potential solutions requires sensitivity to the legitimacy of diverse familial choices. The transactional model described by Anders (6) and Sadeh and Anders (4,5) can and, in my opinion should, guide both research and clinical practice into the new millennium. They describe a model that can accommodate biological, sociocultural, and family-based psychological influences on sleep development. Indeed, it is a model that regards these factors as inseparable. This *way of thinking* about infant and childhood sleep, I argue, can assist researchers in formulating new questions, further demonstrating how culturally guided choices influence infant sleep and potentially induce significant physiological regulatory effects—some of which, among infants, might be lifesaving.

References

1. Lozoff B, Wolf A, Davis NS. Sleep problems seen in pediatric practice. Pediatrics 1985; 75:477–483.
2. Shweder R, Jensen LA, Goldstein WM. Who sleeps by whom revisited: a method for extracting moral goods implicit in practice. In: Goodnow JJ, Miler PJ, Kessel F, eds.

Cultural Practices as Contexts for Development. San Francisco: Jossey-Bass, 1995: 21–40.

3. Shifrin D. A nod to family togetherness. In: Feeney S. New York Daily News, August 1997, p. 32.
4. Sadeh A, Anders TF. Infant sleep problems: origins, assessment, interventions. Infant Ment Health J 1993; 14(1):17–34.
5. Sadeh A, Anders TF. Sleep disorders. In: Zeanah CH, ed. Handbook of Infant Mental Health. New York: Guilford Press, 1993:305–316.
6. Anders TF. Infant sleep, nighttime relationships, and attachment. Psychiatry 1994; 57: 11–21.
7. Anders TF, Eiben LA. Pediatric sleep disorders: a review of the past 10 years. J Am Acad Child Adolesc Psychiatry 1997; 36:9–20.
8. Anders TF, Taylor TR. Babies and their sleep environment. Child Environ 1994; 11: 123–134.
9. Balararian R, Raleigh VS, Botting B. Sudden infant death syndrome and post-neonatal mortality in immigrants in England and Wales. BMJ 1989; 298:716–720.
10. Barry H III, Paxson LM. Infancy and early childhood: cross-cultural codes. Ethology 1971; 10:466–508.
11. Chisholm JS. Navajo Infancy. Hawthorne, NY: Aldine, 1983.
12. LeVine R, Dixon S, LeVine S. Child Care and Culture: Lessons from Africa. Cambridge, UK: Cambridge University Press, 1994.
13. LeVine R. A cross-cultural perspective on parenting. In: Fantini MD, Cardenas R, eds. Parenting in a Multicultural Society. San Diego: Academic Press, 1980.
14. Whiting JWM. Environmental constraints on infant care practices. In: Munroe RH, Munroe RL, Whiting JM, eds. Handbook of Cross-Cultural Human Development. New York: Garland STPM Press, 1981:155–164.
15. Elias MF, Nicholson N, Bora C, Johnston J. Sleep-wake patterns of breast-fed infants in the first two years of life. Pediatrics 1986; 77:322–329.
16. Forbes JF, Weiss DS, Folen RA. The co-sleeping habits of military children. Mil Med 1992; 157:196–200.
17. Heron P. Nonreactive Co-sleeping and Child Behavior: Getting a Good Night's Sleep All Night, Every Night. Masters Thesis. Bristol, UK: University of Bristol, 1994.
18. Godfrey AB, Kilgore A. An approach to help young infants sleep through the night. Zero to Three 1998; 19(2):15–21.
19. Christopher RC. The Japanese Mind: The Goliath Explained. New York: Linden Press/Simon and Schuster, 1983.
20. Caudill W, Weinstein H. Maternal care and infant behavior in Japan and America. Psychiatry 1969; 32:12–43.
21. Shand N. Culture's influence in Japanese and American maternal role perception and confidence. Psychiatry 1985; 48:52–67.
22. Brazelton T. Parent-infant co-sleeping revisited. Ab Initio 1990; 2:1.
23. Kawakami K. Comparison of mother-infant relationships in Japanese and American Families. Paper presented at the meetings of the International Society for the Study of Behavioral Development, Tokyo, Japan, 1987.
24. Morelli GA, Rogoff B, Oppenheim D, Goldsmith D. Cultural variation in infants' sleeping arrangements: questions of independence. Dev Psychol 1992; 28:604–613.
25. Caudill W, Plath DW. Who sleeps by whom? Parent-child involvement in urban Japanese families. Psychiatry 1966; 29:344–366.

26. Ferber R. Solve Your Child's Sleep Problems. New York: Simon and Schuster, 1985.
27. Yelland J, Gifford S, MacIntyre M. Explanatory models about maternal and infant health and sudden infant death syndrome among Asian born mothers. Asian mothers, Australian birth, pregnancy, childbirth and child rearing: the Asian experience in an English speaking country. Rice, PL, ed. Melbourne: Ausmed Publication, 1994:175–190.
28. Wilson E. Sudden Infant Death Syndrome (SIDS) and Environmental Perturbations in Cross-Cultural Context. Master's thesis. University of Calgary, Calgary, Alberta, Canada: 1990.
29. Abbott S. Holding on and pushing away: comparative perspectives on an eastern Kentucky child-rearing practice. Ethos 1992; 20(1):33–65.
30. Lewis M, Havilland J. The Handbook of Emotion. New York: Guilford Press, 1993.
31. Mandansky D, Edelbrock C. Co-sleeping in a community of 2- and 3-year-old children. Pediatrics 1990; 86:1987–2003.
32. Lewis RJ, Janda LH. The relationship between adult sexual adjustment and childhood experience regarding exposure to nudity, sleeping in the parental bed, and parental attitudes toward sexuality. Arch Sex Behav 1988; 17:349–363.
33. Crawford M. Parenting practices in the Basque country: Implications of infant and childhood sleeping location for personality development. Ethos 1994; 22(1):42–82.
34. Mosenkis J. The Effects of Childhood Cosleeping on Later Life Development. Master's Thesis. Chicago: University of Chicago, 1998.
35. Hayes MJ, Roberts SM, Stowe R. Early childhood cosleeping: parent-child and parent-infant interactions. Infant Mental Health J 1996; 17:348–357.
36. Anders TF, Keener MA. Developmental course of nighttime sleep-wake patterns in full-term and premature infants during the first year of life: I. Sleep 1985; 8:173–192.
37. Weissbluth M. Naps in children: 6 months–7 years. Sleep 1995; 18:82.
38. Hofer M. Parental contributions to the development of offspring. In: Gubernick D, Klopfer P, eds. Parental Care in Mammals. New York: Academic Press, 1981:77–115.
39. Hofer M. The Roots of Human Behavior. San Francisco: Freeman, 1981.
40. McKenna JJ. An anthropological perspective on the sudden infant death syndrome (SIDS): the role of parental breathing cues and speech breathing adaptations. Med Anthropol 1986; 10:9–53.
41. McKenna JJ. The potential benefits of infant-parent co-sleeping in relation to SIDS prevention: overview and critique of epidemiological bed sharing studies. In: Rognum TO, ed. Sudden Infant Death Syndrome: New Trends in the Nineties. Oslo: Scandinavian University Press, 1995:256–265.
42. McKenna JJ. SIDS in cross-cultural perspective: is infant-parent cosleeping protective? Annu Rev Anthropol 1996; 25:201–216.
43. Super CM, Harkness S. The infant's niche in rural Kenya and metropolitan America. In: Adler LL, ed. Cross Cultural Research at Issue. New York: Academic Press, 1987: 47–56.
44. Konner M, Super C. Sudden infant death syndrome: an anthropological hypothesis. In: Harkness S, Super C, eds. The Role of Culture in Developmental Disorder. New York: Academic Press, 1987:95–108.
45. Bruner J. Nature and uses of immaturity. Am Psychol 1972; 27:687–708.
46. Ball H, Hooker E. The North Tees cosleeping project: the first three years. Am Anthropol. In press.
47. Medoff D, Schaefer CE. Children sharing the parental bed: a review of the advantages and disadvantages of co-sleeping. Psychol J Hum Behav 1993; 30(1):1–9.

48. Schachter FF, Fuchs ML, Bijur PE, Stone RK. Co-sleeping and sleep problems in Hispanic-American urban young children. Pediatrics 1989; 84:522–530.
49. McKenna JJ, Thoman E, Anders T, Sadeh A, Schechtman V, Glotzbach S. Infant-parent co-sleeping in evolutionary perspective: implications for understanding infant sleep development and the sudden infant death syndrome (SIDS). Sleep 1993; 16:263–282.
50. Mosko S, McKenna JJ, Dickel M, Hunt L. Parent-infant co-sleeping: the appropriate context for the study of infant sleep and implications for SIDS research. J Behav Med 1993; 16:589–610.
51. McKenna JJ, Mosko S, Richard C, Drummond S, Hunt L, Cetal M, Arpaia J. Mutual behavioral and physiological influences among solitary and co-sleeping mother-infant pairs: implications for SIDS. Early Hum Dev 1994; 38:182–201.
52. Konner MJ. Evolution of human behavior development. In: Munroe RH, Munroe RL, Whiting JM, eds. Handbook of Cross-Cultural Human Development. New York: Garland STPM Press, 1981:3–52.
53. Konner MJ, Worthman C. Nursing frequency, gonadal function and birth spacing among Kung hunter-gatherers. Science 1979; 207:788–791.
54. Bowlby J. Attachment and Loss, Vol. I. London: Pergamon Press, 1959.
55. Cuthbertson J, Schevill S. Helping Your Child Sleep Through the Night. New York: Doubleday, 1985.
56. Douglas J. Behaviour Problems in Young Children. London: Tavistock/Routledge, 1989.
57. Ross Mothers Survey (1997). Published and available through Ross Laboratories. Ross Products Division of Abbot Laboratories.
58. Kaplan SL, Poznanski E. Child psychiatric patients who share a bed with a parent. J Am Acad Child Psychiatry 1974; 13:344–356.
59. McKenna J, Mosko S, Richard C. Bedsharing promotes breast feeding. Pediatrics 1997; 100:214–219.
60. Pinilla T, Birch LL. Help me make it through the night: behavioral entrainment of breast-fed infants' sleep patterns. Pediatrics 1993; 91:436–444.
61. Mosko S, Richard C, McKenna J, Drummond S. Infant sleep architecture during bedsharing and possible implications for SIDS. Sleep 1996; 19:677–684.
62. Fleming P, Blair P, Bacon C, Bensley D, Smith I, Taylor E, Berry J, Golding J, Tripp J. Environments of infants during sleep and the risk of the sudden infant death syndrome: results of 1993–1995 case control study for confidential inquiry into stillbirths and deaths in infancy. BMJ 1996; 313:191–195.
63. Kahn A, Picard E, Blum D. Auditory arousal thresholds of normal and near-miss SIDS infants. Dev Med Child Neurol 1986; 28:299–302.
64. Harkness S, Super C, Keefer CH, van Tijen N, van der Vlugt E. Cultural influences on sleep patterns in infancy and early childhood. Meeting of the American Association for the Advancement of Science, Atlanta, February 1995.
65. Guntheroth WG, Spiers P. Sleeping prone and the risks of the sudden infant death syndrome. JAMA 1992; 2:359–363.
66. Rognum TO, ed. SIDS in the 90s. Oslo: Scandinavian University Press, 1995.
67. Fleming P, Blair P. Safe environments for infant sleep: community and laboratory investigations or folk wisdom? Symposium on Breast Feeding, Parental Proximity and Contact in Promoting Infant Health. Notre Dame, IN: University of Notre Dame, 1998.
68. Sterman MB, Hodgman J. The role of sleep and arousal in SIDS. In: PJ Swartz, The Sudden Infant Death Syndrome. New York: New York Academy of Sciences, 1988: 48–61.

69. Douthitt TC, Brackbill Y. Differences in sleep, waking and motor activity as a function of prone or supine resting position in the human neonate. Psychophysiology 1972; 9:99–100.
70. Kahn A, Grosswater J, Scottiaux M, Rebuffat E, Franco P, Dramaix M. Prone or supine position and sleep characteristics in infants. Pediatrics 1993; 91:1112–1115.
71. Mitchell EA, Thompson JMD. Cosleeping increases the risks of the sudden infant death syndrome, but sleeping in the parent's bedroom lowers it. In: Rognum TO. Sudden Infant Death Syndrome in the Nineties. Oslo: Scandinavian University Press, 1995: 266–269.
72. Oberlander TF, Barr R, Young S, Brian JA, Short TR. Effects of feed composition on sleeping and crying in newborn infants. Pediatrics 1992; 90:733–740.
73. Harper R, Hoppenbrouwers T, Bannett D, Hodgman J, Sterman MB, McGinty DJ. Effects of feeding on state and cardiac regulation in the infant. Dev Psychobiol 1976; 10:507–517.
74. Mosko SS, Richards C, McKenna JJ, Drummond D, Mukai D. Infant sleeping position and the CO_2 environment during co-sleeping: the parents' contribution. Amer J Phys Anthropol 1997; 103:315–328.
75. Mosko S, Richard C, McKenna J. Infant arousals during mother-infant bedsharing: implications for infant sleep and SIDS research. Pediatrics 1997; 100:841–849.
76. Mosko S, Richard C, McKenna J. Maternal sleep and arousals during bedsharing with infants. Sleep 1996; 20(2):142–150.
77. Richard C, Mosko S, McKenna J. Sleeping position, orientation, and proximity in bedsharing infants and mothers. Sleep 1996; 19:667–684.
78. Richard C, Mosko S, McKenna J. Apnea and periodic breathing in the bedsharing infant. Am J Appl Physiol 1998; 84:1374–1380.
79. McKenna JJ, Mosko S, Dungy C, McAninch P. Sleep and arousal patterns of co-sleeping human mothers/infant pairs: a preliminary physiological study with implications for the study of sudden infant death syndrome (SIDS). Am J Phys Anthropol 1990; 83: 331–347.
80. Spock B. Baby and Child Care. New York: Pocket Books, 1968.
81. Minturn L, Lambert WW. Mothers of Sleep Cultures: Antecedents of Child Rearing. New York: Wiley, 1964.
82. Parmalee AH, Wenner AN, Schultz HR. Infant sleep patterns: from birth to sixteen weeks of life. J Pediatr 1964; 65:576–582.
83. Winnicott DH. Transitional objects and transitional phenomena. In: Collected Papers of D.W. Winnicott. New York: Basic Books, 1958:23–45.
84. Wolf AW, Lozoff B. Object attachment, thumbsucking, and the passage to sleep. J Am Acad Child Adolesc Psychiatry 1989; 28:287–292.
85. Ozturk M, Ozturk OM. Thumbsucking and falling asleep. Br J Med Psychol 1977; 50:95–103.
86. Litt CJ. Children's attachment to transitional objects. Am J Orthopsychiatry 1979; 51: 131–139.
87. Wolfson A, Lacks P, Futterman A. Effects of parent training on infant sleeping patterns, parents' stress, and perceived parental competence. J Counsel Clin Psychol 1992; 60(1):41–48.
88. Lozoff B, Wolf AW, Davis NS. Co-sleeping in urban families with young children in the United States. Pediatrics 1984; 74:171–182.
89. Klackenberg G. Sleep behaviour studied longitudinally. Acta Paediatr Scand 1982; 71:501–506.

90. Young J, Pollard KS, Blair P, Fleming PJ, Sawczenko A. Sleep position, proximity, orientation and physical contact between mother-infant pairs: a longitudinal study of room-sharing and bed-sharing. Early Hum Dev. In press.
91. Fleming PJ. Infant sleep physiology: does mum make a difference? Ambul Child Health 1998; 4(suppl 1):153–154.
92. McKenna J. Bedsharing promotes breast feeding and the AAP task force on infant positioning and SIDS. Pediatrics 1998; 102:663–664.
93. Hauck F, Kemp J. Bedsharing promotes breast feeding and the AAP task force on infant positioning and SIDS. Pediatrics 1998; 102:662–663.
94. Flandrin JL. Families in Former Times: Kinship, Household and Sexuality. New York: Cambridge University Press, 1979.
95. Kellum BA. Infanticide in England in the later Middle Ages. Hist Child J Psychohist 1974; 1:367–388.
96. Stone L. The Family, Sex and Marriage in England, 1500–1800. New York: Harper & Row, 1977.
97. Aries P. Centuries of Childhood. New York: Vintage Press, 1962.
98. Kuhn TS. The Structure of Scientific Revolutions. Chicago: University of Chicago Press: 1962.
99. Hanks CC, Rebelsky FG. Mommy and the nighttime visitor: a study of occasional cosleeping. Psychiatry 1977; 40:277–280.
100. Mitchell EA, Scragg L, Clements M. Factors related to infant bedsharing. NZ Med J 1994; 107:466–467.
101. Oleinick MS, Bahn AK, Eisenberg L, Lilienfeld AM. Early socialization experiences and intrafamilial environment: a study of psychiatric outpatient and control group children. Psychiatry 1966; 15:344–353.
102. "Dear Abby." Chicago Tribune, January 27, 1998.
103. Douglas M, Wildarsky A. Risk and Culture. Berkeley, CA: University of California Press, 1982.

6

Hormonal and Metabolic Changes During Sleep in Children

RONALD R. GRUNSTEIN

University of Sydney
Sydney, Australia

I. Introduction

Endocrine and metabolic physiology in humans is strongly influenced by state—in particular, sleep and wakefulness. There has been an expanding knowledge base in this area as the development of more exact measurements of endocrine function have paralleled the advances in sleep research. Although a significant proportion of data has been collected in adults, in some cases there are equivalent data in infants or children.

One example of state-dependent change is the fluctuation in plasma levels of pituitary and other hormones across the 24-hr period. These endocrine rhythms have often been labeled either *sleep-related* (when the predominant change in fluctuation is nocturnal) or *circadian* (when the rhythm appears to be regulated by an internal clock rather than periodic changes in the external environment). The predominant influences are intrinsic circadian rhythmicity and sleep, which interact to varying degrees to produce the characteristic 24-hr rhythm of each hormone. Other factors such as meals and exercise may also cause some changes in hormone level (1). In children, two important endocrine and metabolic "outcomes" are normal growth and sexual development. In both these areas, there are physiologically important changes involving sleep-related hormone secretion. Alteration of sleep-related hormone secretion may result in delay or other abnormalities in growth or puberty.

The recognition of breathing disorders in sleep has paralleled the advances in understanding of neuroendocrine and metabolic biology. However, despite the existence of sleep apnea as a unique mix of sleep fragmentation and hypoxic exposure, little is known about the interrelationships between endocrine and metabolic pathophysiology and sleep apnea. There are numerous areas of common interest. Epidemiological features of sleep apnea in adults include marked male preponderance (2,3). The most common human metabolic disorder, obesity, is closely linked to sleep apnea (4). Sleep apnea has also been linked to impaired life quality, sexual dysfunction in adults, poor growth and delayed puberty in children, and endocrine conditions such as acromegaly, hypothyroidism and Cushing's disease. Hormonal treatments such as progesterone have been used therapeutically in sleep apnea, while other treatments such as growth hormone or testosterone may worsen sleep disordered breathing. One can speculate whether there are links between altered hypothalamic function due to sleep fragmentation and/or hypoxia and positive energy balance in obese children with sleep apnea.

Sleep apnea may interact with endocrine rhythms via a number of mechanisms. First, repetitive apneas will cause sleep fragmentation and disorganization of sleep stages and cycles. Second, hypoxia may have direct central effects on neurotransmitters (5), which, in turn, would affect hypothalamic pituitary hormone production. Third, sudden arousal from sleep may produce a central "stress" response leading to hormonal changes (6). Fourth, daytime sleep episodes may interact with daytime hormone rhythms. Finally, all the above factors may interact and lead to changes in the central control of sleep and endocrine rhythms.

The purpose of this chapter is *not* to provide an exhaustive review of hormonal and metabolic physiology as it relates to sleep and wakefulness. Given that the focus of this book is sleep and breathing in children, deliberate emphasis is given to those aspects most pertaining to sleep breathing disorders. It must be stated at this point that little information is available on the effect of childhood sleep breathing disorders on hormonal and metabolic function. Therefore, some use is made of adult data and its relevance to the pediatric population discussed. Given the dearth of knowledge, there is also speculation on future avenues of research.

II. Potential Factors Influencing Endocrine and Metabolic Function in Pediatric Sleep Breathing Disorders

A. Hypoxia and Hormones

Hypoxia has long been known to influence certain endocrine parameters, but these studies have been performed in fetal or adult animal models, altitude simulations, or hypocapnic hypoxia exposure in exercise studies (7). Most have been performed without measurement of arterial O_2 saturation, and typically the CO_2 level has not been controlled. Studies simulating the type of repetitive hypoxia seen in sleep apnea are unknown. The effects of hypercapnic hypoxic exposure has also not been researched.

In animal models, reduction of maternal inspired gas concentrations have been used to assess the hormonal responses of the fetus in animals. Short hypoxic exposure leads to rapid increases in plasma adrenocorticotropic hormone (ACTH) and cortisol (8). Longer exposure (24 hr) leads to sustained elevation in these hormones (9). After weeks to months of hypoxic exposure, there is adaptation and ACTH and cortisol levels return to normal and cortisol responses to exogenous ACTH are attenuated (9,10).

There are few data from studies of children with chronic hypoxic exposure. Two groups have reported elevated fasting growth hormone (GH) in children with cyanotic congenital heart disease (11,12). This does not necessarily mean increased growth in these groups as tissue receptors for GH or insulin-like growth factor 1 (IGF-1) may be downregulated. A number of studies have indicated that chronic fetal hypoxia may modulate IGF-1 regulation and contribute to growth retardation. Interestingly, hypoxic exposure in postnatal rats will lead to reduction in somatic growth but increase in cardiac mass relative to body weight. Therefore, hypoxia may lead to different patterns of growth depending on the organ system (13,14).

B. Obesity

Obesity, particularly central adiposity, may influence endocrine function (15). Some of these hormonal changes are reversible with weight reduction, suggesting that a common underlying disorder—for example, in the hypothalamus—may lead to both endocrine dysfunction and obesity. Confounding can be controlled for with multivariate analysis or by treatments that eliminate the disease process—e.g., weight reduction for obesity or continuous positive airway pressure (CPAP) for sleep apnea. However, in analyzing the confounding effect of obesity in sleep apnea, weight reduction may not answer the question, as both sleep apnea and obesity could resolve in parallel.

C. Stress

The influence of stressors on endocrine function are controversial. The classic "fear and flight" hormones, cortisol and catecholamines, typically rise in response to stress, as do growth hormone and prolactin (16). Testosterone tends to fall following exposure to stressful stimuli (17). The "sick euthyroid" syndrome with a decrease in triiodothyronine (T3) levels is said to be an example of a chronic stress response. Many different endocrine responses to a variety of stressful stimuli have been recorded (6,16,17). There are many disparate views on what constitutes a stressful stimulus as well as significant individual variation in these responses. Most human chronic stress studies have demonstrated gradual adaptation to stimuli. Intermittent stress exposure has rarely been investigated in humans and virtually all studies occur in the awake patient. In one study, we examined the response of patients with sleep apnea who had been on long-term CPAP treatment, to sudden withdrawal of this therapy (6). We postulated that sudden re-exposure to asphyxia in patients who had lost adaptation to such a stimulus would have produced an increase in catecholamines and ACTH. However, no such response occurred, suggesting either that the stimulus was not enough to produce an increase in stress hormones or that years of untreated sleep apnea had led to permanent adaptation to the stress. In the pediatric population, chronic psychosocial stress has been observed to result in reduced growth hormone secretion, possibly in genetically susceptible individuals (18).

III. Growth Hormone, Sleep, and Sleep Apnea

A. Introduction

Growth hormone (GH) is a polypeptide released by the anterior pituitary whose major known function is to stimulate growth. Growth is a slow, continuous process that takes place over more than a decade. It might be expected, therefore, that concentrations of GH in blood would be fairly static. However, frequent measurements of GH concentrations in blood plasma throughout the day reveal wide fluctuations, indicative of multiple episodes of secretion (15). Because the metabolism of GH is generally thought to be reasonably constant, changes in its plasma concentration imply changes in secretion. In rats, GH is secreted in regular pulses every 3.0 to 3.5 hr in what has been called an ultradian rhythm. In humans, GH secretion is also pulsatile, but the pattern of changes in blood concentrations is less obvious than in rats. Frequent bursts of secretion occur throughout the day, with the largest being associated with the early hours of sleep (19–21).

In addition, stressful changes in the internal and external environment can produce brief episodes of hormone secretion (22). Little diagnostic insight can therefore be obtained from a single random measurement of the concentration of GH in blood. Secretory episodes are only brief; therefore multiple, frequent measurements are needed to evaluate the functional status of GH secretion relative to physiological events. Alternatively, it is possible to withdraw small amounts of blood continuously over the course of a day and, by measuring GH in the pooled sample, obtain a 24-hr integrated concentration of GH in blood.

B. GH Secretion

GH may act directly on tissues, but in most body organs GH acts through an intermediate mediator somatomedin C, now known as insulin-like growth factor 1 (IGF-1) which is synthesized in the liver and other organs in response to GH (23). GH secretion from the pituitary is regulated by two hypothalamic hormones released into the pituitary portal circulation: growth hormone releasing hormone (GH-RH), which stimulates GH output, and somatostatin, which is inhibitory. Inhibitory modulation of GH secretion by somatostatin is dominant across the 24-hr period, but reduction in inhibitory inputs and unopposed GHRH secetion leads to GH secretory "bursts." The control of GH release is mediated through several long and short predominantly negative feedback loops involving GH itself and IGF-1 (23). As GH is secreted in a pulsatile fashion and has a relatively short serum half-life (22 min), a single random GH level provides little information on the 24-hr GH production of an individual (23). In adults, a single IGF-1 level has a reasonable level of correlation with 24-hr mean plasma GH and can be used clinically as an index of GH status (23). In children, the value of IGF-1 is less clear. There is also considerable overlap in 24-hr GH secretory profiles in children with short stature, where there may be a complex interplay of genetics, GH responses to provocative testing, as well as 24-hr GH profiles (24).

GHRH has been used pharmacologically as a test of the ability of the pituitary to produce GH in response to stimuli (24). Analogues of somatostatin have been used to inhibit GH production in acromegaly, a state of GH excess (23). These hypothalamic hormones themselves are under the excitatory and inhibitory control of several neurotransmitters, including dopamine, serotonin, and norepinephrine (alpha-adrenergic receptors).

C. Function of GH and Consequences of GH Deficiency

Attainment of adult size is absolutely dependent on GH; deficiency of GH results in growth limitation (25). GH is crucial to skeletal development, with effects at the cellular level promoting endochondral ossification, elongation of chondrocyte columns, and widening of epiphyseal plates. Many of these growth processes are dependent on local tissue and remote production of IGF-1. GH also increases muscle protein stores and has anabolic effects on body composition. GH is also a metabolic hormone. Initially, GH produces a brief insulin-like response that includes a decrease in blood glucose concentration accompanied by increased uptake and utilization of glucose by muscle and fat. After about 2 hr, glucose metabolism is inhibited in both muscle and adipose tissue. There is not only a decrease in the rate of glucose uptake but glycogen stores in muscle are preserved. In adipose tissue, GH promotes the breakdown of stored triglyceride, which increases the concentration of free fatty acids (FFA) in blood. This effect , coupled with inhibition of glucose metabolism and hence synthesis of fatty acids, accounts for relative loss of body fat (26).

Lack of GH in childhood leads to pituitary dwarfism. This disorder becomes obvious from the end of the first year of life. The pituitary dwarf, left untreated, may only reach heights of 3 to 4 ft. "Baby fat" retention and small facial bones result in a juvenile appearance. GH deficiency may be isolated or combined with lack of other pituitary hormones (26).

Available studies show an exponential decline in the calculated daily GH secretion rate as a function of age in healthy men ("somatopause") (15,24–26). Every 7 years of advancing age beyond ages 18 to 21 results in an approximately 50% decline in the amount of GH secreted per day. At puberty and in fact at all adult ages, gonadal steroid hormone concentrations positively influence GH release. Serum estradiol and testosterone concentrations are proportionate to GH secretory mass burst and mean serum GH concentrations. Central obesity is a powerful negative determinant of GH secretion.

D. GH and Sleep

Growth hormone secretion is pulsatile and episodic but, unlike many other hormones, it does not have a dominant independent circadian rhythm. The first studies measuring GH during polygraphically monitored sleep indicated that there was a consistent relationship between GH secretion and slow-wave sleep (SWS) (27,28). Though subsequent investigators have challenged this observation (29,30), recent studies, using more frequent sampling to better characterize GH secretory bursts, have found a close association between GH and SWS (19–21). Although the presence of SWS is not obligatory for GH secretion, Van Cauter and coworkers observed that 70% of GH pulses occurring during sleep were associated with SWS (20,21). Another group, using 30-sec sampling, observed maximal GH concentrations within minutes of SWS onset (19). Other work has shown that drugs that enhance SWS, such as ritanserin (31) or gammahydroxybuytrate (32), increase GH secretion. GH pulses are closely related to delta-wave electroencephalographic activity (33). Experimental arousals during SWS will reduce the magnitude of GH-RH–induced GH secretory pulses (21).

The temporal relationship between the first few hours of sleep and the secretion of GH is present in both sexes from early childhood (34). The highest levels of GH are present in the adolescent growth spurt. However, there does not appear to be a relationship between idiopathic or genetic short stature and GH secretory pattern in sleep (35). Certain stressful conditions interfering with sleep, such as depression (36) and other psychosocial problems (37), are believed to affect GH secretion during sleep. For example, children with psychosocial dwarfism exhibit a decrease in SWS (38). Sleep deprivation supresses GH secretion (39). In animals, exposure to certain stressors rapidly reduces GH gene expression in the brain (40). Even some of the earliest GH studies in children showed little variation in nocturnal GH with varying stature, but reduced GH levels are seen in childhood obesity (41).

Studies of the GH-sleep association are hampered by the lack of an animal model, as GH secretion in sleep is a consistent finding only in humans. Interestingly, only rhesus monkeys with well developed non–rapid-eye-movement/rapid-eye-movement (NREM/REM) sleep cycles had GH secretory peaks in sleep, while animals with fragmented sleep tended to have less secretion at night (42). Humans with fragmented sleep also tend to have less GH secretion. One example of this is aging, when sleep becomes more fragmented, SWS less, and GH secretion in sleep diminished (43). Twenty-four-hour growth hormone production and IGF-1 levels are lower in healthy elderly men than in younger male subjects. Patients with narcolepsy, although characterized by excessive daytime sleepiness, often have fragmented sleep, and GH secretion occurs irregularly without any relation to sleep cycles (44). In obesity, GH production is decreased in both 24-hr mean levels and in response to stimuli (15,25). This reduction in GH output is related to increased fat mass rather than weight. Most studies suggest that the reduced GH output in obesity is reversed with weight loss (15,25). IGF-1 levels are reduced in obesity (45).

Somatotropic peptides, including GH-RH and GH have sleep-promoting effects (33). In patients with GH deficiency, reduced SWS has been reported (33).

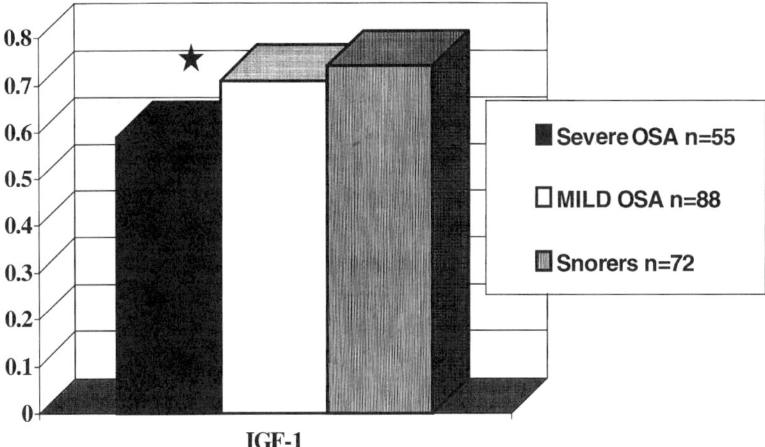

Figure 1 Insulin-like growth factor -1 (IGF-1) µm/L levels in patients with severe obstructive sleep apnea (severe OSA), mild obstructive sleep apnea (mild OSA) and snorers. Severe OSA patients have significantly reduced IGF-1 levels ($p < .008$).

E. Growth Hormone and Sleep-Disordered Breathing

In adults, there is evidence that sleep apnea leads to a reduction in GH concentrations. In a cross-sectional study of 225 men undergoing sleep studies (45), IGF-1 levels were reduced in men with sleep apnea and this was related to the severity of the apnea (both desaturations per hour and minimum oxygen saturation in sleep) (Fig. 1). The decreased IGF-1 levels were also related to aging and coexisting obesity, but also independently to sleep apnea. The role of sleep apnea in these cross-sectional results was confirmed by the reversal of these reduced IGF-1 levels with 3 months of nasal CPAP treatment without any significant accompanying weight change (45) (Fig. 2). As circulating IGF-1 levels are dependent on GH secretion, these data suggest that the lower plasma IGF-1 levels reflect reduced GH secretion. The best evidence supporting a role for sleep apnea in reducing GH secretion in sleep is provided by studies measuring GH concentrations before and after elimination of sleep apnea without change in confounding variables. Data are also available suggesting nocturnal GH secretion increases following reversal of apnea and sleep fragmentation with the use of CPAP (46–49). After CPAP treatment, GH pulses were 11 times more likely to be preceded by an epoch of SWS compared with the baseline (49) (Fig. 3).

In the pediatric age group, GH data on sleep apnea are more limited. In a case report (50), a 9-year-old male with achondroplasia, growth failure (3 cm/year), and severe obstructive sleep apnea had repeated sampling for sleep-entrained GH before and after therapeutic tracheostomy. GH concentrations during sleep were normalized after tracheostomy and led to a sustained increase in growth rate. Detailed studies of GH secretion in otherwise healthy children with sleep apnea are lacking. Waters and coworkers (51) examined GH secretion in sleep in 19 subjects with achondroplasia

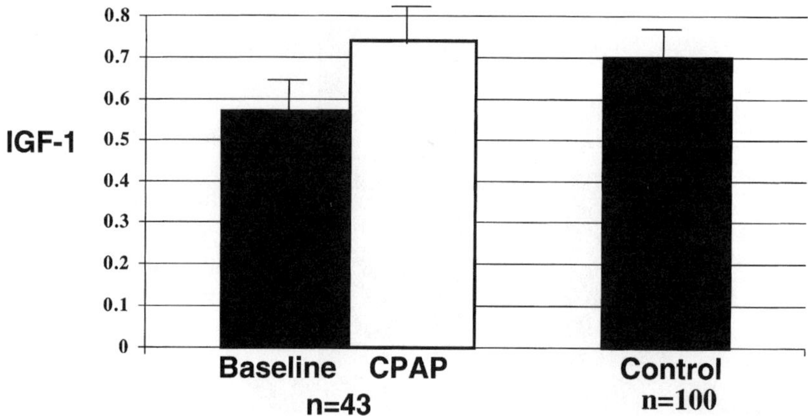

Figure 2 Insulin-like growth factor 1 (IGF-1) µm/L levels in 43 men with sleep apnea before (black bar) and after (white bar) 3 months of nasal continuous positive airway pressure CPAP. These results are contrasted with 100 men of similar age used to establish normative values for IGF-1.

with a mean age of 11 years. There was no relationship between OSA severity and GH secretion. Five subjects were restudied after treatment for OSA. In this group, improved respiratory distress index and reduced sleep-state transitions were not associated with significant changes in GH secretion by sleep stage. However, a GH secretion peak during the first 2 hr of SWS was initially absent, appearing only after treatment of OSA. In a recent report, Bar and colleagues (52) investigated 13 prepu-

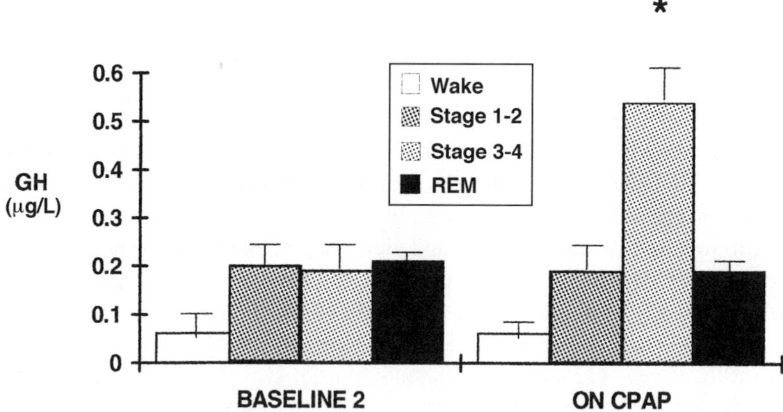

Figure 3 Increased GH concentrations in stages 3 and 4 sleep compared with other sleep stages in nine men on nasal CPAP. There is no difference in GH concentrations in different sleep stages during two baseline sleep studies.

bertal children before and 3 to 12 months after adenotonsillectomy. They observed a reduction in apneic events and increased IGF-1 and growth in most of the children posttonsillectomy.

There are a number of possible reasons why GH secretion may be reduced in sleep apnea. Sleep is fragmented and SWS is markedly reduced or absent in sleep apnea (53), and this may cause a reduction in sleep-entrained GH secretion. Fragmentation of SWS by apnea-induced arousals may reduce both the frequency and magnitude of the pulse of GH associated with SWS. Support for this hypothesis is provided by experimental data in healthy volunteers. GH secretion in response to GH-RH infusion is enhanced at night, particularly in SWS, as opposed to REM when the response to GH-RH is similar to wakefulness (21). Arousals following GH-RH infusion interrupt the normal GH response, which is restored following resumption of sleep (21). As the pulsatile secretion of GH results from the interaction of GH-RH and somatostatin at the level of the somatotrope, it is certainly possible that repetitive arousal in sleep apnea may impair the GH response to endogenous bursts of GH-RH into the pituitary portal circulation. Interestingly, patients with fibromyalgia are characterized by intrusions of alpha electroencephalographic (EEG) (awake) activity; fragmenting SWS and low GH concentrations have been reported in this condition (54).

It is also possible that GH secretion may be attenuated by hypoxia (7). A direct effect of intermittent hypoxia on hypothalamic or other central regulation of endocrine rhythms is possible, although we have found no independent effect of awake P_{O_2} or P_{CO_2} on endocrine function (45). Cornil and coworkers (55) also failed to find an effect of acute and chronic respiratory failure in patients with chronic lung disease on GH secretion. Nevertheless, intermittent severe hypoxemia may well have a different effect centrally than milder sustained hypoxia.

Finally, most patients with sleep apnea exhibit daytime sleepiness and decreased activity during the day. Exercise is a stimulus to GH secretion (22). It is possible that reduced exercise and activity in sleep apnea may lead to reduced daytime pulses of GH and decreased IGF-1. With restoration of normal alertness with nasal CPAP, IGF-1 levels could increase. Nevertheless the precise neurotransmitter changes caused by sleep apnea and their relationship to GH regulation by somatostatin and GH-RH secretion remain to be elucidated. The location of the defect in GH secretion is either hypothalamic or pituitary. Tests of pituitary GH reserve, such as the GH-RH stimulation test, have not been performed in patients with sleep apnea. However, a hypothalamic origin for reduced secretion is more likely in view of preserved gonadotrophin reserve in sleep apnea (56). Moreover, the potential effects of sleep apnea, such as sleep fragmentation, are more likely to have effects at the hypothalamic rather than the pituitary level.

One note of caution needs to be introduced. Although it is possible that sleep apnea leads to relative GH deficiency, some cases of GH-induced sleep apnea have been reported in GH-deficient children receiving GH replacement (57). This may be plausible, as GH excess is associated with sleep apnea (see below).

F. Possible Implications of Reduced GH Levels in Sleep Apnea in Children: Does Sleep Apnea Cause Failure to Thrive?

Severe sleep apnea in the pediatric population is often characterized by failure to thrive, short stature, and other growth disturbances that can be corrected by elimination of the upper airway obstruction. There are many studies, particularly in the ear, nose, and throat (ENT) literature, documenting improved growth following surgical correction of upper airway obstruction (58,59).

It is possible that impaired GH secretion may play a role in these observations, but based on current data, this is entirely speculative. Apart from reduced GH secretion, other mechanisms have been postulated to explain failure to thrive. For example, tonsillitis may produce swallowing difficulty and reduced energy intake. Alternatively, other workers have proposed increased energy expenditure during sleep due to increased work of breathing (60). This study employed a canopy-hood technique to document this altered energy expenditure. Similar increases in energy expenditure, measured by whole-room indirect calorimetry during obstructed breathing in sleep, have been reported in adults (61). Interestingly, in the pediatric population, sleep apnea is associated with impaired growth, yet it is often linked to progressive weight gain in adults. This may reflect differences in daytime energy expenditure. In contrast to the sleepy or sedentary response to chronic sleep fragmentation/apnea in the adult, infants and children may exhibit greater daytime activity levels.

G. Sleep Apnea, Acromegaly, and Gigantism

Acromegaly is a condition of GH excess in adults, characterized by the insidious development of coarsening of facial features, bony proliferation, and soft tissue swelling (23). It is usually secondary to a GH-producing pituitary adenoma, which may be either a micro-or macroadenoma. Rarely, the GH excess commences prior to puberty and closure of the epiphyses; then the condition is termed *gigantism*. Arguably, the most famous giant was Robert Wadlow, the "Alton giant," who was the tallest human ever measured (62). His death at a young age highlights the morbidity associated with this rare condition.

The mortality of untreated or partially treated acromegaly is about double the expected rate in healthy subjects matched for age (63). Acromegaly was first described as a clinical entity by Marie in 1886. Ten years later, Roxburgh and Collis (64) described daytime sleepiness and Chappell and Booth (65) observed upper airway obstruction as features of acromegaly, but the association between sleep apnea and acromegaly was only described 80 years later (66).

Sleep-disordered breathing is extremely common in acromegaly, with a prevalence of at least 60% irrespective of treatment status (67). In a recent Finnish case-control study, Pelttari and coworkers (68) compared the prevalence of sleep apnea in treated acromegaly with a community sample using the static charged bed respiratory screening device. They found that 10 of their 11 patients had sleep apnea (91%) compared with 29.4% of the general population.

There are no reported data specifically on gigantism. In our accumulated database of over 90 patients with acromegaly, we have studied only 1 patient with gigantism. He had repetitive central apnea (see below). There is a much higher than expected prevalence of central apnea in acromegaly (67), and possible reasons for this are discussed in detail elsewhere (67,69,70). In brief, although macroglossia and upper airway soft tissue narrowing is common in acromegaly, endoscopy during apnea in these patients does not necessarily show collapse of the tongue blocking the airway (68,71). The high prevalence of central apnea in acromegaly suggests that abnormalities of central respiratory control are involved. This has been supported by the finding that patients with central sleep apnea have significantly lower awake arterial carbon dioxide levels than those with obstructive apnea (67–70) and increased ventilatory responsiveness to chemical stimuli (69). Central apnea occurs in association with a wide range of disorders, and many potential mechanisms have been described, including disordered central respiratory control (72). We have speculated that, as acromegaly is possibly caused by altered function in somatostatin neurons (67,69,70), similar defects in somatostatin neural pathways may exist in the brainstem, where somatostatin is inhibitory to respiratory neurons (73,74). Hypofunction in these inhibitory neurons could explain the heightened chemosensitivity and central apnea pattern in these patients. Another possible mechanism is that elevated GH or IGF-1 affects central respiratory control, either directly or by altering metabolic rate, thus inducing central apnea. This is supported by the correlation between GH hypersecretion and the prevalence of central apnea (67,69). Interestingly, apparent central apneas have been observed in beagles exposed to medroxyprogesterone, which, in turn, causes GH increases and an acromegaly-like condition (75). Treatment with somatostatin analogue reduces sleep apnea, particularly central apnea (70).

Our patient with gigantism had severe central apnea with extremely high GH secretion. Initial treatment with somatostatin analogue had a marked effect on reducing sleep apnea, but out-of-hospital noncompliance with injections of somatostatin analogue occurred. We have also observed one case of severe sleep apnea in a 14-year-old girl with cerebral gigantism (Sotos syndrome). In this syndrome, no GH abnormalities are observed and sleep apnea is presumed to be secondary to craniofacial abnormalities.

It is important to recognize the adverse health consequences of GH excess, including cardiorespiratory morbidity and mortality and increased risk of anesthetic death (76).

IV. Sex Hormones

A. The Hypothalamic Pituitary Gonadal Axis

Human sexual and reproductive function involves a complex interaction between neural and endocrine events. In humans, pituitary gonadal function is regulated by the feedback effects of gonadal steroid hormones (progestogens, estrogens, and androgens) and by the hypothalamus (77). The hypothalamus releases luteinizing hormone-releasing hormone (LH-RH) under the influence of central neurotransmitters and the feedback of pituitary and gonadal hormones. In response to LH-RH, the pituitary releases luteinizing hormone (LH) and follicle-stimulating hormone (FSH). These peptides, in turn, influence the gonads to secrete testosterone (testes) and estrogen and progesterone (ovaries). This very simplistic outline deliberately ignores the role of organs such as the adrenals in sex hormone regulation.

In patients with hypogonadism due to gonadal damage, LH and FSH levels are elevated with decreased gonadal hormone levels. In central lesions, LH and FSH levels do not increase despite reduced gonadal hormone levels. An example of this is the castrated male. LH and FSH levels are high, with testosterone levels greatly reduced. In a man with a large pituitary tumor destroying gonadotropin-producing cells, LH and FSH levels are low, as is the testosterone level. Hypothalamic and pituitary lesions can be differentiated by measuring the pituitary response to administered LH-RH.

Higher estrogen, decreased total testosterone, and sex hormone–binding globulin (SHBG) levels occur in obesity (78). The concentration of the free testosterone is normal. In massively obese men more than 250% above their ideal body weight, there can be a decrease in the free testosterone level in spite of the decrease in SHBG (78). Sleep also influences sex hormone levels. LH and testosterone secretion are augmented by sleep (79,80). Testosterone levels fall with prolonged physical stress and sleep deprivation in military exercises (81).

B. Puberty

Initiation and maintenance of the reproductive axis in the human is contingent upon the pulsatile secretion of gonadotropin-releasing hormone (Gn-RH) from the hypothalamus (82–84). The pattern of Gn-RH secretion is constantly changing across development, from high levels during the neonatal period through a period of quiescence in midchildhood, followed by sleep entrained reactivation of the reproductive axis at the onset of puberty, ultimately culminating in the adult pattern of pulsatile secretion, which in the male is approximately every 2 hr and in the female varies with the stage of the menstrual cycle.

Recent availability of sensitive assays has shown that the first increase in sleep-entrained Gn-RH/LH secretion occurs some 2 years before the clinical onset of puberty. From midchildhood to sexual maturity, the LH production rate increases 39-fold, though Gn-RH/LH pulse frequency shows only a relatively small (1.8-fold) increment from midchildhood to the clinical onset of puberty, with no subsequent changes to continuing development toward adulthood (83). Thus most of the increment in LH plasma concentration from childhood to sexual maturity is due to amplification of a preexisting ultradian rhythm of secretion with a steadily and markedly increasing mass of LH secreted per burst. The duration of secretory burst and apparent half-life of plasma LH disappearance remains constant from mid-childhood through puberty to adulthood. However, sleep-associated LH/Gn-RH secretion is eventually lost in young adulthood.

In effect, the onset of puberty in humans is heralded by the reawakening of a partially quiescent Gn-RH pulse generator. This predominantly involves an amplification of a preexisting pattern of hypothalamic Gn-RH secretion, leading to a major augmentation of the total quantity of LH molecules released per burst. The almost twofold increment in Gn-RH pulse frequency contributes to the pubertal process before the clinical onset of puberty, possibly by enhancing gonadotropic sensitivity to increase the mass of LH produced per burst. The relative constancy of Gn-RH pulse frequency in the gonad-intact hypothalamic pituitary testicular axis from pubertal onset to adulthood implies that testicular steroidal feedback plays a role in restraining the burst frequency of the GnRH pulse generator during pubertal development and adulthood (84).

The onset of puberty is a centrally driven process, the detailed mechanisms of which are not known. It is translated into an increased activity of the hypothalamic Gn-RH pulse generator. This, in turn, is seen as increased pituitary pulsatile secretion of LH and FSH. LH pulses are observed even in mid-childhood, particularly after the onset of sleep. Onset of puberty is associated with a greater increase in LH pulse amplitude than frequency and a much greater increase in LH and FSH. A progressive increase in daytime pulsatility occurs, with a gradual reduction of sleep-entrained amplification. Prepubertal FSH concentrations are relatively high in girls, and continuous ovarian follicular growth and atresia take place, with estradiol concentrations being higher than in boys. Only after the steep early pubertal increase in LH, ovarian steroidogenesis is activated, with increases in androgen and estrogen secretion. Under further FSH stimulation, follicular growth and maturation proceed. The first menstrual cycles are mostly anovulatory for 1 to 2 years. Luteal-phase insufficiency is common the first 5 years after menarche.

C. Androgens and Sleep Apnea

It is possible that repetitive sleep disruption in prepuberty or even during puberty would cause a delay in sexual maturation. Mosko and colleagues (85) have described a case where a 20-year-old hypogonadal man was discovered to have had obstructive sleep apnea syndrome, spanning the years of puberty, secondary to hypertrophied tonsils, adenoids, and uvula. LH concentrations (sampling at 20-min intervals) were performed before and after surgery. At baseline, the patient was hypogonadotropic. Daytime LH concentrations were in the low normal range for an adult male, and concentrations fell dramatically during nocturnal sleep, in contrast to normal secretory patterns. LH concentrations rose dramatically long term, with relief of sleep apnea postoperatively. However, no evidence of continued sexual development beyond that achieved preoperatively was observed. This case suggests that sleep apnea during puberty may impair sexual development by preventing the sleep-related elevation in LH secretion normally observed during a critical period spanning puberty. More cases are obviously needed to support this hypothesis.

Some support for an effect of sleep apnea on sex-hormone physiology in childhood and during puberty are provided by data from adults with sleep apnea. Low testosterone levels have been reported in men with sleep apnea independent of age, degree of obesity, and presence of awake hypoxemia and hypercapnia. Testosterone levels increase with treatment of sleep apnea using nasal CPAP or even successful uvulopalatopharyngoplasty (45,86). Androgen abnormalities reported in adult sleep apnea (decreased SHBG and free and total testosterone) are qualitatively as well as quantitatively distinct from those reported in aging (increased SHBG, decreased free and total testosterone) and obesity (decreased SHBG and total testosterone, normal free testosterone). Importantly, despite the fall in plasma free and total testosterone levels, there was no increase in basal plasma gonadotrophin (LH, FSH) levels. It is possible that the sexual dysfunction reported in patients with sleep apnea may be mediated by the sex hormone changes seen in sleep-disordered breathing. The low testosterone levels may also interact with low IGF-1 levels and impair anabolism.

These findings, together with the retention of pituitary sensitivity to exogenous GN-RH in sleep apnea (56), point to a hypothalamic abnormality as the cause of the fall in testosterone levels in adult sleep apnea. This explanation would be similar to the postulated level of the dysfunction of the GH IGF-1 axis in sleep apnea. There are no data on LH and FSH pulsatility in sleep apnea. These adult data certainly indicate the potential importance of treating sleep apnea in the child to avoid any potential delay in puberty. However, again, data are lacking in the pediatric population to support this.

V. Effect of Sex Hormone Therapy on Sleep Apnea

A. Testosterone

Several case reports in the early 1980s described development of sleep apnea following testosterone therapy (87,89). Johnson et al. (90) reported the development of sleep apnea in a 54-year-old woman with renal failure following androgen administration. The sleep apnea resolved upon withdrawal of the medication and recurred when the drug was reintroduced. They also observed an increase in supraglottic resistance following androgen administration. These cases suggest that testosterone may be important in the regulation of breathing during sleep and the pathogenesis of sleep apnea. Two studies have systematically examined the sleep breathing effects of exogenous testosterone on hypogonadal patients. Matsumoto et al. (91) studied five patients and observed development of sleep apnea in one patient and worsening of preexisting sleep apnea in another. There was no effect in the other three patients. Schneider and coworkers (92) investigated 11 hypogonadal men before and after testosterone replacement. There was a significant increase in apneas in the group as a whole, but clinically significant increases occurred in only three patients. These two studies suggest that testosterone-induced or exacerbated sleep apnea is not a consistent finding in hypogonadal patients.

We have also observed a case (93) where testosterone exacerbated sleep apnea in a 13-year-old male. Testosterone was being used to reduce growth and was associated with an increase in upper airway collapsibility during sleep (reduced closing pressure). Cessation of testosterone led to reduction in apnea severity (Fig. 4).

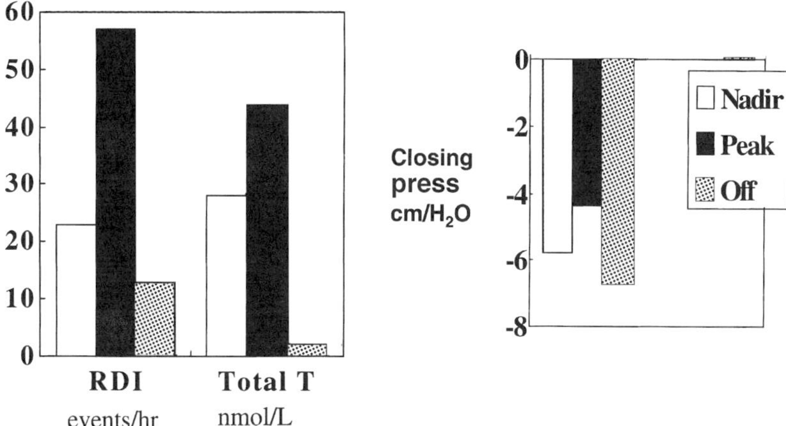

Figure 4 Change in respiratory disturbance index (RDI), total testosterone (Total T) and closing pressure in a 13-year-old male with Marfan's syndrome commenced on high-dose testosterone to attenuate his growth. RDI increases and closing pressure decreases with peak testosterone levels (black bar) compared with nadir level (white bar) and untreated conditions (gray bar). (Adapted from Ref. 93.)

B. Progesterone and Estrogen

Progesterone levels fall after menopause and progestigins have been shown to stimulate ventilation during the luteal phase of the menstrual cycle, in pregnancy, in normal male subjects, and in conditions of alveolar hypoventilation (94). Progesterone has little effect in men with sleep apnea (94,95). Block et al. (96) were unable to demonstrate a protective effect of progesterone upon postmenopausal females with sleep apnea syndrome. The apparent "protection" of premenopausal status against sleep apnea has provoked some interest in hormone replacement as a therapy for sleep apnea in women. Pickett and coworkers (97) used combined therapy with both progestogen and estrogen in women who had a surgical menopause. They demonstrated improvement, but the pretreatment apnea was very mild. In sleep disordered-breathing, estrogen alone or in combination with progesterone had no effect on sleep apnea in 15 postmenopausal women with moderate obstructive sleep apnea despite a doubling of serum estrogen (98). It is still possible that longer-term or higher-dose treatment may provide more positive results.

C. Antiandrogens

If testosterone has an apnea-promoting effect, one might postulate that androgen antagonists could improve sleep apnea. The nonsteroidal androgen antagonist flutamide was used for 1 week in seven males with sleep apnea. Despite endocrine evidence of androgen antagonism, short-term flutamide did not alter sleep-disordered breathing or awake ventilatory drive (99).

VI. Hypothyroidism

Apneic breathing in myxedema was noted by Massumi and Winnacker (100) and the presence of sleep apnea was later confirmed by others (101–107). Though myxedema coma is now rare, in retrospect, many cases were probably due to severe sleepiness and obtundation secondary to severe sleep apnea coupled with the hypercapnic respiratory failure of sleep apnea.

The exact nature of the association between sleep apnea and hypothyroidism is unclear. Although small groups of hypothyroid patients appear to have a high prevalence of sleep apnea, screening for hypothyroidism in sleep clinic cohorts is controversial. Pelttari and coworkers (108) compared 26 patients with hypothyroidism with 188 euthyroid controls. Some 50% of the hypothyroid patients and 29.3% of the control subjects had at least some episodes of partial or complete upper airway obstruction. Severe obstruction with episodes of repetitive apnea was present in 7.7% of the patients and in 1.5% of the controls. However, this association was largely explained by coexisting obesity and male gender. There is no large body of prospectively collected data on the prevalence of sleep apnea in patients with hypothyroidism. It has been asserted that the prevalence of sleep apnea in this group is high based on small cohorts (106).

The effect of adequate thyroid hormone replacement on sleep apnea in hypothyroidism has been variable. Some cures have been described (103–107), but in other studies the experience has been different (106,107). The failure of sleep apnea to resolve after thyroxine treatment supports the view of a chance rather than causal association, although an alternative explanation may be that hypothyroidism induces long-term changes in upper airway mechanics or breathing control that do not resolve immediately after a euthyroid state is achieved. In one study, Petrof and coworkers (109) investigated the effects of hypothyroidism on myosin heavy chain (MHC) expression in the sternohyoid, geniohyoid, and genioglossus muscles of adult rats. Hypothyroid muscles showed a reduction of fast twitch fibers relative to control muscles.

One would expect sleep apnea to be prevalent in infant or childhood hypothyroidism, but no specific data are available. In hypothyroidism, mucoproteins can be deposited in the tongue (causing macroglossia) and pharyngeal tissues (103,104), narrowing the airway. Airway narrowing is exacerbated by an increase in muscle volume, including the genioglossus (107). In addition, upper airway muscle function may be impaired by hypothyroid myopathy.

VII. Adrenocorticotrophic Hormone, Cortisol, and Cushing's Syndrome

In a preliminary report, Rapaport et al. (110) found that nocturnal adrenocorticotrophic hormone (ACTH) levels in patients with sleep apnea fell on the first night of CPAP treatment compared to a night with untreated sleep apnea. They interpreted these findings as demonstrating the "stress" effect of sleep apnea. In contrast, no effect on plasma cortisol, ACTH, or catecholamines was observed with CPAP withdrawal in long-term users (6). Morning cortisol levels appear unaffected by sleep apnea (45). Patients with corticosteroid excess secondary to Cushing's disease are characterized by truncal obesity, hypertension, and depression. In the only published data, about one-third of patients appear to have sleep apnea (111). There are no reported data on sleep apnea in children with steroid excess.

VIII. Diabetes

In adult sleep apnea, there is an association between diabetes and sleep apnea. Hyperinsulinemia is linked to sleep apnea independent of body mass (112) (Fig. 5). However, in community cohorts, insulin resistance does not appear to be increased in mild to moderate asymptomatic sleep apnea compared with controls (113). In contrast, we have shown that insulin sensitivity improves with CPAP treatment of sleep apnea (114).

Recent data on diabetes, sleep, and circadian physiology suggest that sleep disruption can influence diabetes or even insulin sensitivity (115). Studies in subjects receiving continuous intravenous glucose infusion have shown that major alterations of glucose tolerance occur during sleep and that sleep quality markedly influences glucose utilization. Short-term laboratory-supervised sleep-debt studies indicate that sleep loss results in decreased insulin sensitivity (116). Other work has shown decreased epinephrine and norepinephrine responses to hypoglycemia during sleep, in-

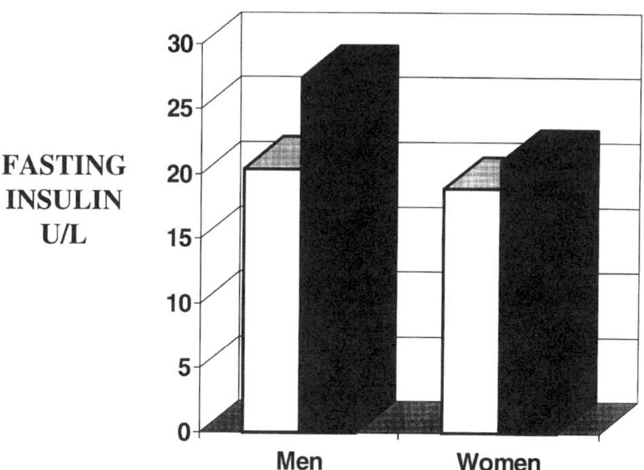

Figure 5 Fasting insulin levels are higher in severely obese men and women with a high likelihood of sleep apnea (black bars, $n = 338$ men and 155 women) versus those with low likelihood sleep apnea (white bars, $n = 216$ men and 481 women). (Adapted from Ref. 112.)

dicating that sleep also interferes with the counterregulatory responses to hypoglycemia (117).

These studies suggest that more work is needed to elucidate the influence of sleep apnea on insulin and glucose regulation. For example, sleep disruption by apnea (at least acutely) may improve counterregulatory responses to hypoglycemia with sympathetic activation due to apnea-induced arousal and hypoxemia. In contrast, chronic sleep fragmentation and sleep "loss" may lead to insulin resistance in the long term.

IX. Neuroendocrine Changes, Obesity, and Sleep Apnea: Speculations and Future Research

A. Central Obesity and Sleep Apnea

The health risks of obesity are well known (118). Recent work has shown that body fat distribution (i.e., predominantly upper-body obesity) is often a more crucial determinant of morbidity and mortality than total adiposity (118,119). In terms of measurement, this means that morbidity and mortality are more closely related to waist-hip ratio (an elevated ratio is a measure of upper body obesity) than body-mass index (BMI). This concept has clarified much of the confusing, contradictory research on the health risks of obesity. Upper-body-obese individuals have an increased risk of cardiovascular and cerebrovascular disease, diabetes, hypertension, hyperlipidemia, hyperuricemia, and insulin resistance relative to lower-body-obese individuals. The clustering of diseases associated with upper-body obesity is really a rediscovery of the concept of "android" obesity (excess fat in the upper body) versus "gynoid" obesity (excess fat in the gluteofemoral region). Similar data show the development of central fat distribution in young males and the role of central fat as a potential health risk factor in adolescents (120).

Obesity is the commonest metabolic abnormality in sleep apnea, where the predominant pattern of obesity is central (121). There is a plethora of data linking central obesity to poor health outcomes (122,123). Clearly, the health risks of obesity and sleep apnea are similar and data are complicated by mutual confounding variables (121). Attempts at separating out the two disorders have suggested that both are additive in the pathogenesis of obesity related morbidity.

B. Does Sleep Apnea Promote Central Obesity? Future Research Issues

Obesity is a powerful epidemiological predictor of sleep apnea (2–4), and weight reduction may lead to marked improvement in the severity of sleep apnea (124). However, there are certainly less data addressing the reverse possibility—that sleep apnea may promote the development of obesity (125). Unfortunately, no long-term longitudinal studies of sleep apnea development exist. Over 50% of the first 100 patients commenced on home CPAP had a measured weight loss of greater than 5 kg at the time of long-term follow up (126). In addition, we have frequently observed dramatic weight loss following commencement of nasal CPAP in patients who have previously been resistant to active weight-loss programs. It is tempting to think that chronic intermittent hypoxia and sleep fragmentation over years in patients with sleep apnea can lead to changes in central control of energy regulation, appetite control, feeding, and metabolism, which would promote weight gain and thus worsen sleep apnea further. Moreover, if this is the case, could this vicious cycle be broken by successful CPAP therapy? Or are there clear interindividual differences in underlying hypothalamic function, leading to divergent responses in energy balance in patients with sleep apnea?

During sleep, energy expenditure (EE) typically falls relative to the awake basal state (127). In severe sleep apnea, sleep EE appears to increase during apneic sleep and falls with CPAP therapy (61). This would seem to be paradoxical, since such EE changes would favor weight loss prior to CPAP and weight gain after CPAP. However, the 24-hr EE may be different in untreated sleep apnea with reduced spontaneous physical activity (fidgeting, routine physical activities) due to fatigue and sleepiness producing a net decrease in EE, despite increased EE in sleep due to respiratory effort and sleep fragmentation. Other intriguing data suggest that patients with sleep apnea may have altered serotinergic sensitivity in the hypothalamus. Hudgel and coworkers observed that the cortisol response to L 5 HTP, a serotonin precursor, was elevated relative to control nonapneic subjects and was not readily explained by changes in weight (128). Subsequent data have shown that treatment with nasal CPAP reverses the elevated cortisol response to serotoninergic stimulation (129). These investigators have speculated that the exaggerated cortisol responses in sleep apnea indicate supersensitivity of postsynaptic serotinergic receptors in the hypothalamus caused by a serotonergic-"deficient" state induced by sleep apnea. Certainly short periods of sleep deprivation in humans and animals produce evidence of increased serotonin turnover (130). Whether chronic sleep fragmentation and hypoxemia in sleep apnea produce serotonin depletion in the hypothalamus and other regions, is entirely speculative.

Interestingly, there are parallel findings of a serotonin- deficient state in central obesity (123). Bjorntorp has described a cluster of disorders associated with central obesity, including abnormalities of the hypothalamic pituitary end-organ axes (low GH and testosterone, high cortisol), a "defeat" reaction to stress, with psychosocial disability and carbohydrate craving promoted by a low serotoninergic state (123). Specific serotoninergic agonists have been used as treatments in central obesity. The observed low testosterone and GH in sleep apnea also occur in central obesity, where recombinant GH appears to reduce central body fat (131). Perhaps restoration of GH secretion during sleep with nasal CPAP in sleep apnea may have similar effects. A recent report suggests that nasal CPAP will reduce visceral fat deposits without change in BMI in patients with sleep apnea (132).

Another area of common ground is insulin sensitivity. Central obesity is associated with hyperinsulinemia and insulin resistance (123). Certainly some data also point to increased insulin levels in sleep apnea independent of weight and central obesity (112). Nasal CPAP also improves insulin sensitivity in non-insulin-dependent di-

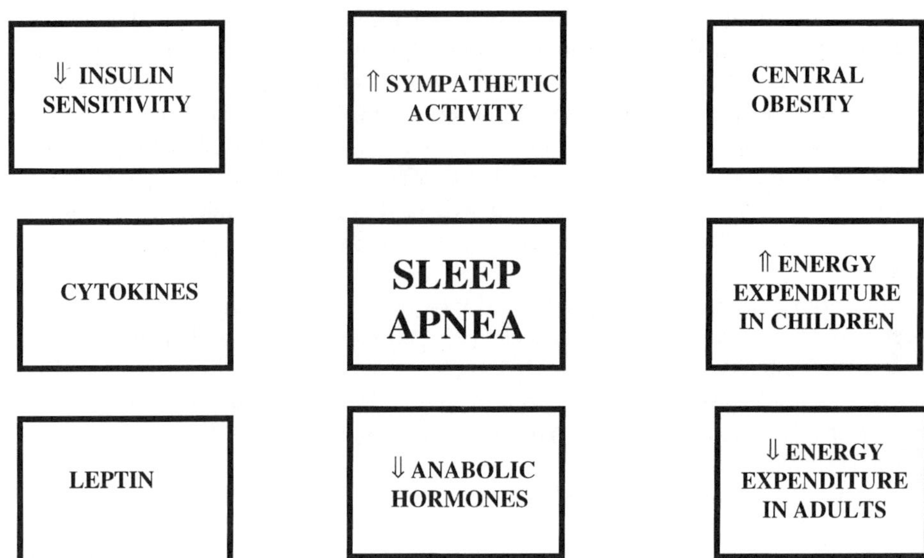

Figure 6 Some of the metabolic and hormonal factors interacting in sleep apnea, potentially leading to weight gain. See text for details.

abetes mellitus (114). Sleep "loss" appears to reduce insulin sensitivity. However, in community cohorts, any relationship between sleep apnea and insulin resistance appears to be mediated by obesity (113). Normal sleep disturbs the counterregulatory responses to hypoglycemia. Other areas of speculative interest include products of fat mass, which include the hypothalamic weight regulator leptin and certain cytokines, such as tumor necrosis factor alpha (TNF-α) (133). TNF-α is involved in promoting sleep (134) and also, via separate actions, insulin resistance. Recent data indicate that the circadian rhythm of TNF-α, measured by a bioassay, is altered in patients with sleep apnea versus controls (135). The rhythm is not normalized by nasal CPAP. TNF-α levels, measured by direct assay, are elevated in sleep apnea and related to severity of disease. It is possible that TNF- α may be involved in exacerbating somnolence, low activity levels, and even promoting insulin resistance in sleep apnea. Interestingly, it has been claimed that even obese individuals without sleep apnea have more somnolence than controls (136). How all these data would be confounded by more accurate measures of central obesity is unknown. Moreover, the exact role of the sympathetic nervous system in the relationship between obesity and sleep apnea is unclear. Sympathetic activity appears to be increased in men with sleep apnea (137), but low sympathoadrenal activity seems to be a risk factor for weight gain among certain genetically obese groups (138).

Leptin has only recently been discovered to promote motor activity, energy expenditure, and weight loss (139). One brief report suggests that a plasma leptin (one sample only) is increased in sleep apnea and reduced with nasal CPAP (140). Leptin levels are high in obesity due to increased production and leptin "resistance" at the hypothalamic level (139). Moreover leptin production appears to be pulsatile with nocturnal components (141). Could control of sleep apnea with nasal CPAP improve leptin sensitivity (suggested by lower leptin levels) and promote weight loss by this mechanism? At this stage of knowledge, there is no direct evidence of a coherent unifying mechanism or series of mechanisms to suggest that sleep apnea will promote weight gain. Inactivity, sleepiness, low levels of anabolic hormones, altered central serotinergic "tone," TNF-α and other cytokines all may promote central fat accumulation (Fig. 6). Future research into the links between central obesity, neuroendocrine function, and sleep apnea may provide not only insights into the pathophysiology of sleep breathing disorders, but also clues to novel pharmacological therapies.

References

1. Van Cauter E, Refetoff S. Multifactorial control of the 24 hour secretory profiles of pituitary hormones. J Endocrinol Invest 1985; 8:381–391.
2. Young T, Palta M, Dempsey J, Skatrud J, Weber S, Badr S. Occurrence of sleep disordered breathing among middle aged adults. N Engl J Med 1993; 328:1230–1235.
3. Bearpark H, Elliott L, Grunstein R, Cullen S, Schneider H, Althaus W, Sullivan C. Snoring and sleep apnea: a population study in Australian men. Am J Respir Crit Care Med 1995; 151:1459–1465.
4. Grunstein RR, Wilcox I, Yang TS, Gould Y, Hedner JA. Snoring and sleep apnoea in men: association with central obesity and hypertension. Int J Obesity 1993; 17:533–540.
5. Pastuszko A, Wilson DF, Ericinsk M. Neurotransmitter metabolism in rat brain synaptosomes: effect of anoxia and pH. J Neurochem 1982; 38:1657–1667.
6. Grunstein RR, Stewart DA, Lloyd H, Akinci M, Cheng N, Sullivan CE. Acute withdrawal of nasal CPAP in obstructive sleep apnea does not cause a rise in stress hormones. Sleep 1996; 19:774–782.
7. Cargill RI, McFarlane LC, Coutie WJ, Lipworth BJ. Acute neurohormonal responses to hypoxemia in man. Eur J Appl Physiol 1996; 72:256–260.
8. Jackson BT, Morrison SH, Cohn HE, Piasecki GJ. Adrenal secretion of glucocorticoids during hypoxemia in fetal sheep. Endocrinology 1989; 125:2751–2757.
9. Hooper SB, Coulter CL, Dayton J, Harding R. Fetal endocrine responses to prolonged hypoxemia in sheep. Am J Physiol 1989; 256:R1348–R1354.
10. Harvey LM, Gilbert RD, Longo LD, Ducsay CA. Changes in ovine fetal adrenocortical responses after long term hypoxemia. Am J Physiol 1993; 264:E741–E747.
11. Fahrer M, Gruneiro L, Rivarolo M, Bergada C. Levels of plasma growth hormone in children with congenital heart disease. Acta Endocrinol 1974; 77:451–459.
12. Ikkos DD, Thanopoulos V, Ikkos DG. 24 h plasma levels of growth hormone in growth retardation of children with congenital heart disease. Helv Pediatr Acta 1974; 29: 583–588.
13. McClellan KC, Hooper SB, Bocking AD. Prolonged hypoxia induced by a reduction of maternal uterine blood flow alters insulin like growth factor binding protein (IGFBP 1) and IGFBP 2 gene expression in the ovine fetus. Endocrinology 1992; 131: 1619–1628.

14. Russel Jones DL, Leach RM, Ward JP, Thomas CR. Insulin like growth factor 1 gene expression is increased in the right ventricular hypertrophy induced by chronic hypoxia in the rat. J Mol Endocrinol 1993; 10:99–102.
15. Veldhuis JD, Iranmanesh A. Physiological regulation of the human growth hormone (GH) insulin like growth factor type I (IGF I) axis: predominant impact of age, obesity, gonadal function, and sleep. Sleep 1996; 19:S221–S224.
16. Chrousos GP. Ultradian, circadian, and stress related hypothalamic pituitary adrenal axis activity: a dynamic digital to analog modulation. Endocrinology 1998; 139:437–440.
17. Gonzalez Santos MR, Gaja Rodriguez OV, Alonso Uriarte R, Sojo Aranda I, Cortes Gallegos V. Sleep deprivation and adaptive hormonal responses of healthy men. Arch Androl 1989; 22:203–207.
18. Skuse D, Albanese A, Stanhope R, Gilmour J, Voss L. A new stress related syndrome of growth failure and hyperphagia in children, associated with reversibility of growth hormone insufficiency. Lancet 1996; 348:353–358.
19. Holl RW, Hartman ML, Veldhuis JD, Taylor WM Thorner MO. Thirty second sampling of plasma growth hormone in man: correlation with sleep stages. J Clin Endocrinol Metab 1991; 72:854–861.
20. Van Cauter E, Kerkofs M, Caufriez A, van Onderbergen A, Thorner MO, Copinschi G. A qualitative estimation of growth hormone secretion in normal man: reproducibility and relation to sleep and time of day. J Clin Endocrinol Metab 1992; 74:1441–1450.
21. Van Cauter E, Caufriez A, Kerkofs M, van Onderbergen A, Thorner MO, Copinschi G. Sleep, awakenings, and insulin like growth factor 1 modulate the growth hormone (GH) secretory response to GH releasing hormone. J Clin Endocrinol Metab 1992; 74: 1451–1459.
22. Kanaley JA, Weltman JY, Veldhuis JD, Rogol AD, Hartman ML, Weltman A. Human growth hormone response to repeated bouts of aerobic exercise. J Appl Physiol 1997; 83:1756–1761.
23. Melmed S. Acromegaly. N Engl J Med 1990; 322:966–977.
24. Merriam GR, Buchner DM, Prinz PN, Schwartz RS, Vitiello MV. Potential applications of GH secretagogs in the evaluation and treatment of the age related decline in growth hormone secretion. Endocrine 1997; 1:49–52.
25. Veldhuis JD, Iranmanesh A, Weltman A. Elements in the pathophysiology of diminished growth hormone (GH) secretion in aging humans. Endocrine 1997; Aug,7(1):41–48.
26. Carroll PV, Christ ER, Bengtsson BA, Carlsson L, Christiansen JS, Clemmons D, Hintz R, Ho K, Laron Z, Sizonenko P, Sonksen PH, Tanaka T, Thorner M. Growth hormone deficiency in adulthood and the effects of growth hormone replacement: a review. Growth Hormone Research Society Scientific Committee. J Clin Endocrinol Metab 1998; 83:382–395.
27. Takahashi Y, Kipnis DM, Daughaday WH. Growth hormone secretion in sleep. J Clin Invest 1968; 47:2079–2090.
28. Sassin JF, Parker DC, Mace JW, Gotlin RW, Johnson LC, Rossman LG. Human growth hormone release: relation to slow wave sleep and sleep waking cycles. Science 1969; 165:513–515.
29. Steiger A, Herth T, Holsber F. Sleep electroencephalography and the secretion of cortisol and growth hormone in normal controls. Acta Endocrinol (Copenh) 1987; 116:36.
30. Jarrett DB, Greenhouse JB, Miewald JM, Fedorka IB, Kupfer DJ. A reexamination of the relationship between growth hormone secretion and slow wave sleep using delta wave analysis. Biol Psych 1990; 27:497–509.

31. Gronfier C, Luthringer R, Follenius M, Schaltenbrand N, Macher JP, Muzet A, Brandenberger G. A quantitative evaluation of the relationships between growth hormone secretion and delta wave electroencephalographic activity during normal sleep and after enrichment in delta waves. Sleep 1996; 19:817–824.
32. Van Cauter E, Plat L, Scharf MB, Lepoult R, Cespedes S. L'Hermite Baleriaux M, Copinschi G. Simultaneous stimulation of slow wave sleep and growth hormone secretion by gamma hydroxybutyrate in normal young men. J Clin Invest 1997; 100:745–753.
33. Steiger A, Holsboer F. Neuropeptides and human sleep. Sleep 1997; 20:1038–1052.
34. Van Cauter E, Plat L. Growth of hormone secretion during sleep. J Pediatr 1996; 128: S32–S37.
35. Buzi F, Zanotti P, Tiberti A, Monteleone M, Lombardi A, Ugazio AG. Overnight growth hormone secretion in short children: independence of the sleep pattern. J Clin Endocrinol Metab 1993; 77:1495–1499.
36. Dahl RE, Ryan ND, Williamson DE, Ambrosini PJ, Rabinovich H, Novacenko H, Nelson B, Puig Antich J. Regulation of sleep and growth hormone in adolescent depression. J Am Acad Child Adolesc Psychiatry 1992; 31:615–621.
37. Uhde TW, Tancer ME, Rubinow DR, Roscow DB, Boulenger JP, Vittone B, Gurguis G, Geraci M, Black B. Post RM Evidence for hypothalamic growth hormone dysfunction in panic disorder: profile of growth hormone (GH) responses to clonidine, yohimbine, caffeine, glucose, GRF and TRH in panic disorder patients versus healthy volunteers. Neuropsychopharmacology 1992; 6:101–118.
38. Taylor BJ, Brook CGD. Sleep EEG in growth disorders. Arch Dis Child 1986; 61: 754–760.
39. Radomski MW, Hart LE, Goodman JM, Plyley MJ. Aerobic fitness and hormonal responses to prolonged sleep deprivation and sustained mental work. Aviat Space Environ Med 1992; 63:101–106.
40. Fujikawa T, Yoshizato H, Soya H, Nakashima K. Dynamic alterations in growth hormone receptor mRNA levels in rat brain during stress tolerance. Endocrinol J 1996; 43:S119–S122.
41. Quabbe HJ, Helge H, Kubicki S. Nocturnal growth hormone secretion: correlation with sleeping EEG in adults and pattern in children and adolescents with non-pituitary dwarfism, overgrowth and with obesity. Acta Endocrinol (Copenh) 1971; 67: 767–783.
42. Quabbe H, Gregor M, Bumke Vogt C, Eckhof A, Witt I. Twenty four hour pattern of growth hormone secretetion in the rhesus monkey: studies including alterations of the sleep/wake and sleep stage cycles. Endocrinology 1981; 109:513–518.
43. Vermeulen A. Nyctohemeral growth hormone profiles in young and aged men: Correlation with somatomedin C levels. J Clin Endocrinol Metab 1987; 64:884–888.
44. Higuchi T, Takahashi Y, Takahashi K, Niimi Y, Miyasita A. Twenty four hour secretory patterns of growth hormone, prolactin, and cortisol in narcolepsy. J Clin Endocrinol Metab 1979; 49:197–204.
45. Grunstein RR, Handelsman DJ, Lawrence S, Blackwell C, Caterson ID, Sullivan CE. Neuroendocrine dysfunction in sleep apnea: reversal by nasal continuous positive airway pressure. J Clin Endocrinol Metab 1989; 8:352–358.
46. Grunstein R, McNamara SG, Caterson I, Turtle JR, Sullivan CE. Nocturnal growth hormone secretion in sleep apnea: changes with CPAP therapy. Aust NZ J Med 1986; (suppl 3):16:629.
47. Saini J, Krieger J, Brandenberger G, Wittersheim G, Simon C, Follenius M. Continous

positive airway pressure treatment: effects on growth hormone, insulin and glucose profiles in obstructive sleep apnea patients. Horm Metab Res 1993; 25:375–381.

48. Cooper BG, White JES, Ashworth L, Alberti KGMM, Gibson GJ. Hormonal and metabolic profiles in subjects with obstructive sleep apnoea syndrome and the acute effects of nasal continuous positive airway pressure treatment. Sleep 1995; 18:172–179.
49. Grunstein RR. Metabolic aspects of sleep apnea. Sleep 1996; 19(10 suppl):S218–S220.
50. Goldstein SJ, Wu RHK, Thorpy MF, Shprintzen RJ, Marion RE, Senger P. Reversibility of deficient sleep entrained growth hormone secretion in a boy with achondroplasia and obstructive sleep apnoea. Acta Endocrinol (Copenh) 1987; 16:95–97.
51. Waters KA, Kirjavainen T, Jimenez M, Cowell CT, Sillence DO, Sullivan CE. Overnight growth hormone secretion in achondroplasia: deconvolution analysis, correlation with sleep state, and changes after treatment of obstructive sleep apnea. Pediatr Res 1996; 39:547–553.
52. Bar A, Tarasiuk A, Segev Y, Phillip M, Tal A. The effect of adenotonsillectomy in children with obstructive sleep apnea syndrome on serum insulin like growth factor 1 and growth. Am Rev Respir Crit Care Med 1998; 157:A534.
53. Issa FG, Sullivan CE. The immediate effects of nasal continuous positive airway pressure treatment on sleep pattern in patients with obstructive sleep apnea syndrome. Electroencephalogr Clin Neurophysiol 1986; 136:755–761.
54. Bennett RM, Clark SR, Campbell SM, Burckhardt CS. Low levels of somatomedin C in patients with the fibromyalgia syndrome. Arthritis Rheum 1992; 35:1113–1116.
55. Cornil A, Glinoer D, Leclerq R, Copinschi G. Adrenocortical and somatotrophic secretions in acute and chronic respiratory insufficiency. Am Rev Respir Dis 1975; 112:77–81.
56. Stewart DA, Grunstein RR, Sullivan CE, Handelsman DJ. Neuroendocrine changes in sleep apnea are not related to a pituitary defect. Sleep Res 1989; 18:308.
57. Gerard JM, Garibaldi L, Myers SE, Aceto T Jr, Kotagal S, Gibbons VP, Stith J, Weber C. Sleep apnea in patients receiving growth hormone. Clin Pediatr (Phila) 1997; 36: 321–326.
58. Stradling JR, Thomas G, Williams P, Warley AH, Freeland A. Effect of adenotonsillectomy on nocturnal hypoxemia, sleep disturbance and symptoms in snoring children. Lancet 1990; 335:249–253.
59. Freezer NJ, Bucens IK, Robertson CF. Obstructive sleep apnea presenting as failure to thrive in infancy. J Pediatr Child Health 1995; 31:172–175.
60. Marcus CL, Carroll JL, Koerner CB, Hamer A, Lutz J, Loughlin GM. Determinants of growth in children with OSA syndrome. J Pediatr 1994; 125:556–562.
61. Stenlof K, Grunstein RR, Hedner J, Sjostrom L. Energy expenditure in obstructive sleep apnea: effects of treatment with continuous positive airway pressure. Am J Physiol 1996; 271:E1036–E1043.
62. Behrens LH, Barr DP. Hyperpituitarism beginning in infancy: the Alton giant. Endocrinology 1932; 16:120–122.
63. Wright AD, Hill DM, Lowy C, Fraser TR. Mortality in acromegaly. Q J Med 1970; 39:116–128.
64. Roxburgh F, Collis AJ. Notes on a case of acromegaly. BMJ 1886; 2:63–65.
65. Chappell WF, Booth JA. A case of acromegaly with laryngeal symptoms and pharyngeal symptoms. J Laryngol Otol. 1886; 10:142–150.
66. Laroche C, Festal G, Poenaru S, Caquet R, Lemaigre D, Auperin A. Une observation de respiration periodique chez une acromegalie. Ann Med Intern 1976; 127:381–385.

67. Grunstein RR, Ho KY, Sullivan CE. Acromegaly and sleep apnea. Ann Intern Med 1991; 115:527–532.
68. Pelttari L, Polo O, Rauhala E, Vuoriluoto J, Aitasalo K, Hyyppa MT, Kronholm E, Irjala K, Viikari I. Nocturnal breathing abnormalities in acromegaly after adenomectomy. J Clin Endocrinol (Oxf) 1995; 43:175–182.
69. Grunstein RR, Ho KY, Berthon Jones M, Stewart D, Sullivan CE. Central sleep apnea is associated with increased ventilatory response to carbon dioxide and hypersecretion of growth hormone in patients with acromegaly. Am J Respir Crit Care Med 1994; 150: 496–502.
70. Grunstein RR, Ho KK, Sullivan CE. Effect of octreotide, a somatostatin analog, on sleep apnea in patients with acromegaly. Ann Intern Med 1994; 121:478–483.
71. Cadieux RJ, Kales A, Santen RJ, Bixler EO, Gordon R. Endoscopic findings in sleep apnea associated with acromegaly. J Clin Endocrinol Metab 1982; 55:18–22.
72. Neubauer JA. Mechanisms of apnea. Curr Opin Pulmon Med 1995; 1:491–497.
73. Kalia M, Fuxe K, Agnati LF, Hokfelt T, Harfstrand A. Somatostatin produces apnea and is localised in medullary respiratory nuclei: a possible role in apneic syndromes. Brain Res 1984; 296:339–344.
74. Chen Z, Hedner T, Hedner J. Local application of somatostatin in the rat ventrolateral brain medulla induces apnea. 1990; 69:2233–2238.
75. Concannon P, Altszuler N, Hampshire J, Butler WR, Hansel W. Growth hormone, prolactin, and cortisol in dogs developing mammary nodules and an acromegaly like appearance during treatment with medroxyprogesterone acetate. Endocrinology 1980; 106:1173–1177.
76. Southwick JP, Katz J. Unusual airway difficulty in the acromegalic patient, indications for tracheostomy. Anesthesiology 1979; 51:72–73.
77. Veldhuis JV, Evans WS, Johnson ML, Rogol AD. Physiological properties of the luteinizing hormone pulse signal: impact of intensive and extended venous sampling paradigms on their characterization in healthy men and women. J Clin Endocrinol Metab 1986; 62:881–888.
78. Glass AR. Endocrine aspects of obesity. Med Clin North Am 1989; 73:139–160.
79. Pietrowsky R, Meyrer R, Kern W, Born J, Fehm HL. Effects of diurnal sleep on secretion of cortisol, luteinizing hormone, and growth hormone in man. J Clin Endocrinol Metab 1994; 78:683–687.
80. Pincus SM, Mulligan T, Iranmanesh A, Gheorghiu S, Godschalk M, Veldhuis JD. Older males secrete luteinizing hormone and testosterone more irregularly, and jointly more asynchronously, than younger males. Proc Natl Acad Sci USA 1996; 93:14100–14105.
81. Elman I, Breier A. Effects of acute metabolic stress on plasma progesterone and testosterone in male subjects: relationship to pituitary adrenocortical axis activation. Life Sci 1997; 61:1705–1712.
82. Hayes FJ, Crowley WF Jr. Gonadotropin pulsations across development. Ann NY Acad Sci 1997; 816:9–21.
83. Wu FC, Butler GE, Kelnar CJ, Huhtaniemi I, Veldhuis JD. Ontogeny of pulsatile gonadotropin releasing hormone secretion from mid-childhood, through puberty, to adulthood in the human male: a study using deconvolution analysis and an ultrasensitive immunofluorometric assay. J Clin Endocrinol Metab 1996; 81:1798–1805.
84. Yen SS, Apter D, Butzow T, Laughlin GA. Gonadotrophin releasing hormone pulse generator activity before and during sexual maturation in girls: new insights. Hum Reprod 1993; 8(suppl 2):66–71.

85. Mosko SS, Lewis E, Sassin JF. Impaired sexual maturation associated with sleep apnea syndrome during puberty: a case study. Sleep 1980; 3:13–22.
86. Santamaria JD, Prior JC, Fleetham JA. Reversible reproductive dysfunction in men with obstructive sleep apnea. Clin Endocrinol 1988; 28:461–470.
87. Sandblom RE, Matsumoto AM, Schoene RB, Lee KA, Giblin EC, Bremner WJ, Pierson DJ. Obstructive sleep apnea induced by testosterone administration. N Eng J Med 1983; 308:506–510.
88. Strumpf IJ, Reynolds SF, Vash P, Tashkin DP. A possible relationship between testosterone, central control of ventilation, and the Pickwickian syndrome. Am Rev Respir Dis 1978; 117:A183.
89. Harman E, Wynne JW, Block AJ. The effect of weight loss on sleep disordered breathing and oxygen desaturation in morbidly obese men. Chest 1982; 82:291–293.
90. Johnson MW, Arch AM, Remmers JE. Induction of the obstructive sleep apnea syndrome in a woman by exogenous androgen administration. Am Rev Respir Dis 1984; 129:1023.
91. Matsumoto AM, Sandblom RE, Schoene RB, Lee KA, Giblin EC, Pierson DJ, Bremner WJ. Testosterone replacement in hypogonadal males: effects on obstructive sleep apnea, respiratory drives and sleep. Clin Endocrinol 1985; 22:713–717.
92. Schneider BK, Pickett CK, Zwillich CW, Weil JV, McDermott MT, Santen RJ, Varano LA, White DP. Influence of testosterone on breathing during sleep. J Appl Physiol 1986; 61:618–624.
93. Cistulli PA, Grunstein RR, Sullivan CE: Effect of testosterone administration on upper airway collapsibility during sleep. Am J Respir Crit Care Med 1994; 149:530–532.
94. Robinson RW, Zwillich CW. The effects of drugs on breathing during sleep. Clin Chest Med 1985; 6:603–614.
95. Cook WR, Benich JJ, Wooten SA. Indices of severity of obstructive sleep apnea syndrome do not change during medroxyprogesterone acetate therapy. Chest 1989; 96:262–266.
96. Block AJ, Wynne JW, Boysen PG, Lindsey S, Martin C, Cantor B. Menopause, medroxyprogesterone and breathing during sleep. Am J Med 1980; 70:506–510.
97. Pickett CK, Regensteiner JG, Woodard WD, Hagerman DG, Weil JV, Moore LG. Progestogen and estrogen reduce sleep disordered breathing in post menopausal women. J Appl Physiol 1989; 66:1656–1661.
98. Cistulli PA, Barnes DJ, Grunstein RR, Sullivan CE. Effect of short term hormone replacement in the treatment of obstructive sleep apnea in postmenopausal women. Thorax 1994; 49:699–702.
99. Stewart DA, Grunstein RR, Berthon Jones M, Handelsman DJ, Sullivan CE. Androgen blockade does not affect sleep disordered breathing or chemosensitivity in men with obstructive sleep apnea. Am Rev Respir Dis 1992; 146:1389–1393.
100. Massumi RA, Winnaker JL. Severe depression of the respiratory center in myxedema. Am J Med 1964; 36:876–882.
101. Duron B, Quinchard J, Fullana N. Nouvelles recherches sur le mechanisme des apnecs du syndrome de pickwick. Bull Physiopathol Respir 1972; 8:1277–1288.
102. Yamamoto T, Hirose N, Miyoshi K. Polygraphic study of periodic breathing and hypersomnolence in a patient with severe hypothyroidism. Eur Neurol 1977; 15:188–193.
103. Orr WC, Males JL, Imes NK. Myxedema and obstructive sleep apnoea. Am J Med 1981; 70:1061–1066.

104. Skatrud J, Iber C, Ewart R, Thomas G, Rasmussen H, Schultze B. Disordered breathing during sleep in hypothyroidism. Am Rev Respir Dis 1981; 124:325–329.
105. Millman RP, Bevilacqua J, Peterson DD, Pack AL. Central sleep apnea in hypothyroidism. Am Rev Respir Dis 1983; 127:504–507.
106. Rajagopal KR, Abbrecht PH, Derderian SS, Pickett C, Hofeldt F, Tellis CJ, Zwillich CW. Obstructive sleep apnea in hypothyroidism. Ann Intern Med 1984; 101:471–474.
107. Grunstein RR, Sullivan CE. Hypothyroidism and sleep apnea: mechanisms and management. Am J Med 1988; 85:775–779.
108. Pelttari L, Rauhala E, Polo O, Hyyppa MT, Kronholm E, Viikari J, Kantola I. Upper airway obstruction in hypothyroidism. J Intern Med 1994; 236:177–181.
109. Petrof BJ, Kelly AM, Rubinstein NA, Pack AI. Effect of hypothyroidism on myosin heavy chain expression in rat pharyngeal dilator muscles. J Appl Physiol 1992; 73:179–187.
110. Rapaport D, Rothenberg SA, Hollander CS, Goldring RM. Obstructive sleep apnea (OSA) alters ultradian rhythm of ACTH secretion. Am Rev Respir Dis 1989; 139:A80.
111. Shipley JE, Schteingart DE, Tandon R, Starkman MN. Sleep architecture and sleep apnea in patients with Cushing's disease. Sleep. 1992; 15:514–518.
112. Grunstein RR, Stenlof K, Hedner J, Sjostrom L. Impact of obstructive sleep apnea and sleepiness on metabolic and cardiovascular risk factors in the Swedish Obese Subjects (SOS) study. Int J Obesity 1995; 151:410–418.
113. Stoohs RA, Facchini F, Guilleminault C. Insulin resistance and sleep disordered breathing in healthy humans. Am J Respir Crit Care Med 1996; 154:170–174.
114. Brooks B, Cistulli PA, Borkman M, McGee S, Ross G, Grunstein RR, Sullivan CE, Yue D. Effect of nasal continuous positive airway pressure treatment on insulin sensitivity in patients with type II diabetes and obstructive sleep apnea. J Clin Endocrinol Metab 1994; 79:16t81–1685.
115. Scheen AJ, Van Cauter E. The roles of time of day and sleep quality in modulating glucose regulation: clinical implications. Horm Res 1998; 49:191–201.
116. Scheen AJ, Byrne MM, Plat L, Leproult R, Van Cauter E. Relationships between sleep quality and glucose regulation in normal humans. Am J Physiol 1996; 271(2 Pt 1):E261–E270.
117. Jones TW, Porter P, Sherwin RS, Davis EA, O'Leary P, Frazer F, Byrne G, Stick S, Tamborlane WV. Decreased epinephrine responses to hypoglycemia during sleep. N Engl J Med 1998; 338:1657–1662.
118. Kissebah AH, Freedman DS, Peiris AN. Health Risks of Obesity. Med Clin North Am 1989; 73:111–138.
119. Bjorntorp P. Obesity. Lancet 1997; 350:423–426.
120. Caprio S, Hyman LD, Limb C, McCarthy S, Lange R, Sherwin RS, Shulman G, Tamborlane WV. Central adiposity and its metabolic correlates in obese adolescent girls. Am J Physiol. 1995; 269(1 pt 1):E118–E126.
121. Grunstein RR, Stenlof K, Hedner J, Sjostrom L. Impact of self reported sleep apnea symptoms on psychosocial performance in the Swedish Obese Subjects (SOS) study. Sleep 1995; 18:635–643.
122. Vanhala MJ, Pitkajarvi TK, Kumpusalo EA, Takala JK. Obesity type and clustering of insulin resistance associated cardiovascular risk factors in middle aged men and women. Int J Obesity 1998; 22:369–374.
123. Bjorntorp P. Neuroendocrine abnormalities in human obesity. Metabolism 1995; 44(2 suppl 2):38–41.

124. Strobel RJ, Rosen RC. Obesity and weight loss in obstructive sleep apnea: a critical review. Sleep 1996; 19:104–115.
125. Grunstein RR. Endocrine and metabolic disturbances in obstructive sleep apnea. In: Saunders NA, Sullivan CE, eds. Sleep and Breathing, 2d ed. New York: Marcel Dekker, 1993.
126. Grunstein RR, Dodd MJ, Costas L, Sullivan CE. Home nasal CPAP for sleep apnea acceptance of home therapy and its usefulness. Aust NZ J Med 1986; 16:635.
127. Bonnet MH, Berry RB, Arand DL. Metabolism during normal, fragmented and recovery sleep. J Appl Physiol 1991; 71:1112–1118.
128. Hudgel DW, Gordon EA, Meltzer HY. Abnormal serotenergic stimulation of cortisol production in obstructive sleep apnea. Am J Respir Crit Care Med 1995; 152:186–192.
129. Hudgel DW, Gordon EA. Serotonin induced cortisol release in CPAP treated obstructive sleep apnea patients. Chest 1997; 111:632–638.
130. Heiser P, Dickhaus B, Opper C, Schreiber W, Clement HW, Hasse C, Hennig J, Krieg JC, Wesemann W. Platelet serotonin and interleukin 1 beta after sleep deprivation and recovery sleep in humans. J Neural Transm 1997; 104:1049–1058.
131. Johannsson G, Marin P, Lonn L, Ottosson M, Stenlof K, Bjorntorp P, Sjostrom L, Bengtsson BA. Growth hormone treatment of abdominally obese men reduces abdominal fat mass, improves glucose and lipoprotein metabolism, and reduces diastolic blood pressure. J Clin Endocrinol Metab 1997; 82:727–734.
132. Chin K, Nakamura T, Narai N, Shimziu K, Kita Y, Oku M, Mishima M, Ohi M. Changes in intrabdominal visceral fat in patients with obstructive sleep apnea syndrome following long term nasal CPAP therapy. Am J Respir Crit Care Med 1998; 157:A58.
133. Katsuki A, Sumida Y, Murashima S, Murata K, Takarada Y, Ito K, Fujii M, Tsuchihashi K, Goto H, Nakatani K, Yano Y. Serum levels of tumor necrosis factor alpha are increased in obese patients with noninsulin dependent diabetes mellitus. J Clin Endocrinol Metab 1998; 83:859–862.
134. Vgontzas AN, Papanicolaou DA, Bixler EO, Kales A, Tyson K, Chrousos GP. Elevation of plasma cytokines in disorders of excessive daytime sleepiness: role of sleep disturbance and obesity. J Clin Endocrinol Metab 1997; 82:1313–1316.
135. Entzian P, Linnemann K, Schlaak M, Zabel P. Obstructive sleep apnea syndrome and circadian rhythms of hormones and cytokines. Am J Respir Crit Care Med 1996; 153:1080–1086.
136. Vgontzas AN, Bixler EO, Tan TL, Kantner D, Martin LF, Kales A. Obesity without sleep apnea is associated with daytime sleepiness. Arch Intern Med 1998; 158:1333–1337.
137. Waradekar NV, Sinoway LI, Zwillich CW, Leuenberger UA. Influence of treatment on muscle sympathetic nerve activity in sleep apnea. Am J Respir Crit Care Med 1996; 153:1333–1338.
138. Tataranni PA, Young JB, Bogardus C, Ravussin E. A low sympathoadrenal activity is associated with body weight gain and development of central adiposity in Pima Indian men. Obesity Res 1997; 5:341–347.
139. Tataranni PA. From physiology to neuroendocrinology: a reappraisal of risk factors of body weight gain in humans. Diabetes Metab 1998; 24:108–115.
140. Saarelainen S, Lahtela J, Kallonen E. Effect of nasal CPAP treatment on insulin sensitivity and plasma leptin. J Sleep Res 1997; 6:146–147.
141. Licinio J, Mantzoros C, Negrao AB, Cizza G, Wong ML, Bongiorno PB, Chrousos GP, Karp B, Allen C, Flier JS, Gold PW. Human leptin levels are pulsatile and inversely related to pituitary adrenal function. Nature Med 1997; 3:575–579.

Part Two

BREATHING

7

Breathing and "Sleep States" in the Fetus and at Birth

CARLOS E. BLANCO

University Hospital Maastricht
Maastricht, The Netherlands

MARK A. HANSON

University College London
London, England

PREM KUMAR

University of Birmingham
School of Medicine
Birmingham, England

I. Introduction

At birth breathing must change from a periodic non-air intrauterine breathing pattern to a continuous air-breathing pattern. This clear, obligatory, and irreversible change happens after the exclusion of the umbilical circulation and simultaneously with several other adaptations, such as full perfusion of the lungs, thermoregulation, changes in behavioral state, a large increase in metabolism, increase in afferent input to the central nervous system, and many other changes associated with the transition from the intrauterine to the extrauterine environment. The understanding of the process and the identification of the crucial mechanisms involved in starting continuous breathing at birth may help to find new insight into the pathological conditions such as apnea or sudden infant death syndrome (SIDS). Therefore, the study of the physiological mechanisms involved in the process of birth is of interest not only to the physiologist but also very important to the neonatologist and pediatrician.

II. Fetal Breathing Movements

Breathing activity in utero is the consequence of rhythmic activation of respiratory neurons in the brainstem (1,2). Breathing movements are present in utero from very early in gestation, but it is not known why. Barcroft and Barron (3) described a spasm of the diaphragm at the 38th day of gestation (term, 147 days) in the fetal lamb followed by the first rhythmic movements of the diaphragm at the 40th day of gestation. The earliest chronic recordings from fetal lambs in utero were performed at approximately 50 days of gestation. Two types of diaphragmatic activity could be seen: 1) unpatterned discharge and 2) patterned, bursting discharge (4). In the human fetus, thoracic movements were observed from the 10 to 12th week of gestation (5).

Later in gestation (75 to 110 days), movements of the fetal lamb diaphragm start to become periodic (Fig. 1). At this age they are often but not always associated with nuchal and lateral rectus muscle activity (6,7). From 108 to 120 days of gestation, breathing movements begin to be organized into a more complex state, now associated with the presence of rapid eye movements and nuchal muscle activity (Fig. 2) (6–9). At this time in gestation the electrocorticogram (ECoG) is still undifferentiated. By 120 to 125 days of gestation, electrocortical activity shows a clear differentiation into low-voltage high-frequency activity [13 to 30 Hz; low-voltage electrocorticogram (LVECoG)] and high-voltage low-frequency activity [3 to 9 Hz; high-voltage electrocorticogram (HVECoG)] (6,10–12). At this time in gestation, breathing movements are rapid and irregular, with a frequency of 0.1 to 4 Hz and an amplitude of 3 to 5 mmHg; they produce small movements of tracheal fluid (< 1 mL) (13). This activity is exclusively associated with a fetal behavioral state that consists of LVECoG, inhibition of nuchal muscle activity, rapid eye movements, and inhibition of polysynaptic spinal reflexes (14) (Fig. 3). During HVECoG, fetal breathing activity is absent (15).

It is clear that the periodicity of breathing in utero is determined by the electrocortical state, being present during low-voltage activity [equivalent to rapid-eye-movement (REM)-like sleep] and absent during high-voltage activity (equivalent to quiet sleep). This implies either that breathing activity is facilitated or even stimulated during LVECoG and/or that it is inhibited during HVECoG. During LVECoG, there is more neural activity in cortical and subcortical structures, including the brainstem reticular formation. This facilitatory state could increase the sensitivity for basal stimuli, such as the level of arterial CO_2, and generate respiratory output. This hypothesis is supported by the observation that during hypocapnia, breathing activity is not present even in the LVECoG state (16). In the high-voltage ECoG state, absence of breathing could be due to a disfacilitation, as reported during quiet sleep, when slow waves appear in the electroencephalogram (EEG) (17). Other evidence leads us to believe that during HVECoG, there is an active inhibition of breathing activity. This evidence comes from experiments where fetal breathing activity and ECoG were dissociated after the brainstem was transected at the level of the colliculi (15). Furthermore, fetal breathing response to hypercapnia is limited to LVECoG activity in the intact fetus, but hypercapnia can produce continuous breathing in both LV and HVECoG after small bilateral lesions in the lateral pons (18). The mechanisms, origin, and location for this inhibition are not clear, but it is known that it is of central origin, that it can be overridden in utero by different mechanisms and that it is overridden at the time of birth, when breathing activity becomes continuous.

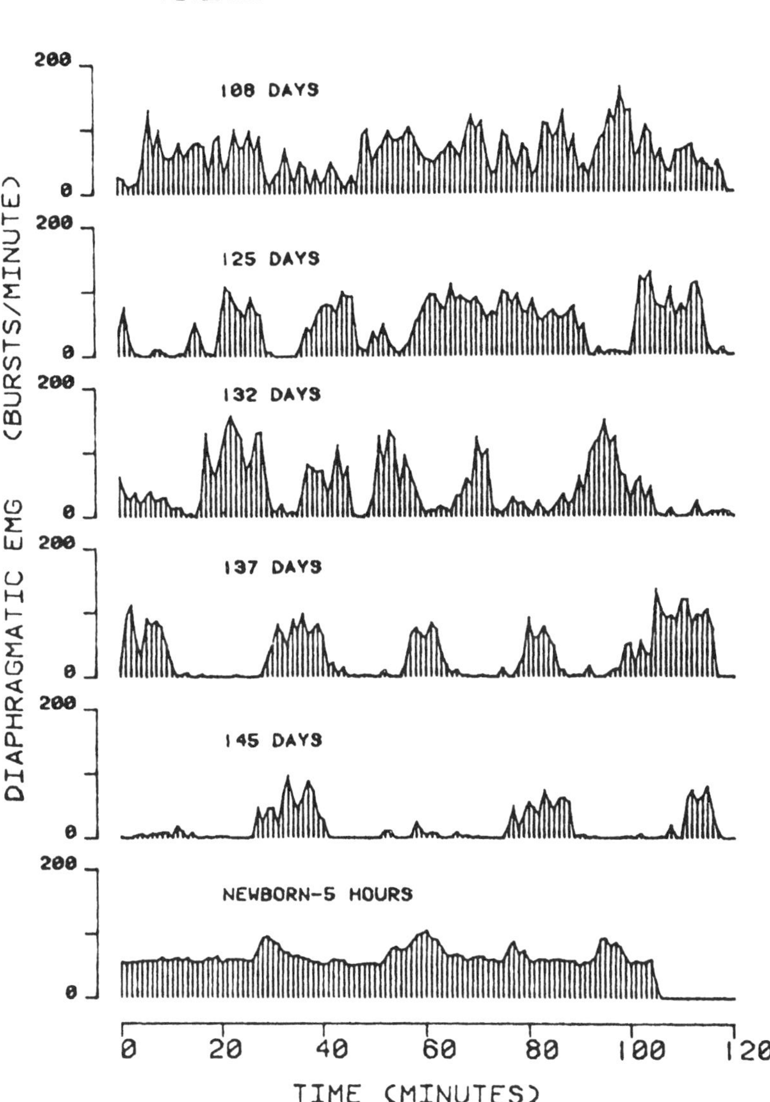

Figure 1 Analysis of a diaphragmatic EMG of one fetus at five differing gestational ages and as a newborn. Each graph displays time, in minutes, on abscissa, and diaphragmatic EMG activity, in bursts per minute, on ordinate. Gestational age, in days, is displayed on each graph, as is postdelivery time, in hours, for newborn. Note: the newborn recording is only 105 min long. (From Ref. 8.)

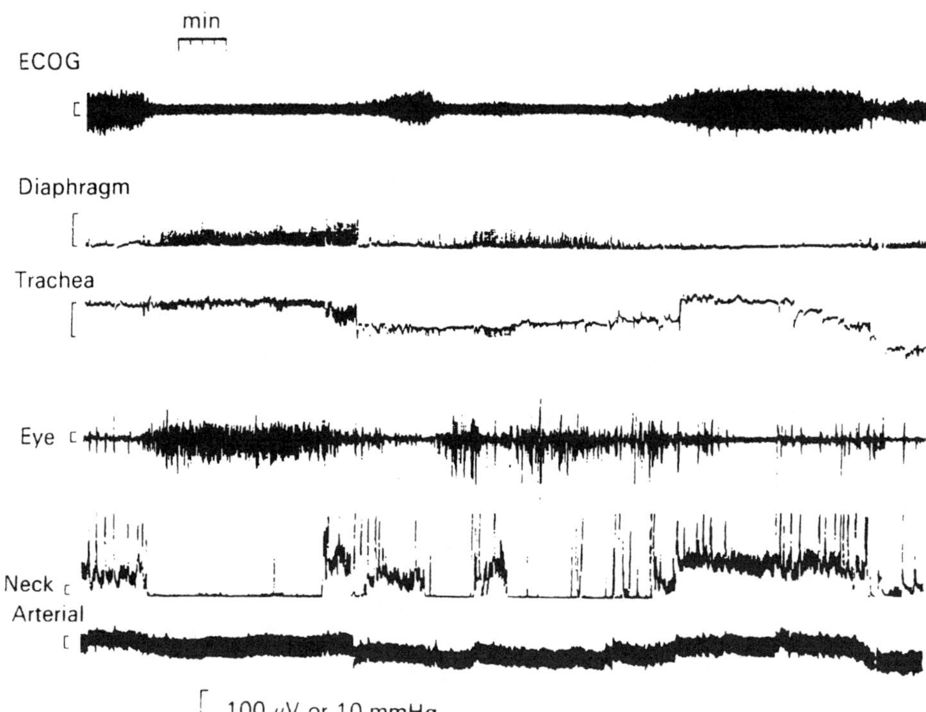

Figure 2 One-hour polygraph recording from unanesthetized sheep fetus in utero at 141 days gestation showing electro-oculo-(eye) and electrocorticograms (ECoG), fetal breathing movements (diaphragm EMG and tracheal pressure) neck EMG, and carotid arterial pressure. (From Ref. 101.)

A. Chemoreceptor Function In Utero

The concept that peripheral chemoreceptors could produce effects on breathing can be traced to experiments conducted over 50 years ago (19), in which breathing was shown to be stimulated in exteriorized midgestation animal fetuses by hypoxia or cyanide (20). In late gestation, the descending inhibitory effects on breathing arising from the fetal brainstem in hypoxia and with HVECoG (see above) dominate. It was perhaps the increasing interest in these processes that caused the scientific community to lose sight of the implications of the earlier observations, and the idea became prevalent that the carotid chemoreceptors were quiescent in utero and were activated at birth, perhaps by the increase in sympathetic nervous activity that occurs then. In addition, when it became clear that normal fetal arterial P_{O_2} in late gestation, both in the sheep and the human fetus, was about 25 mmHg, it was thought that if the chemoreceptors were functional, they would be so intensely stimulated that powerful reflex

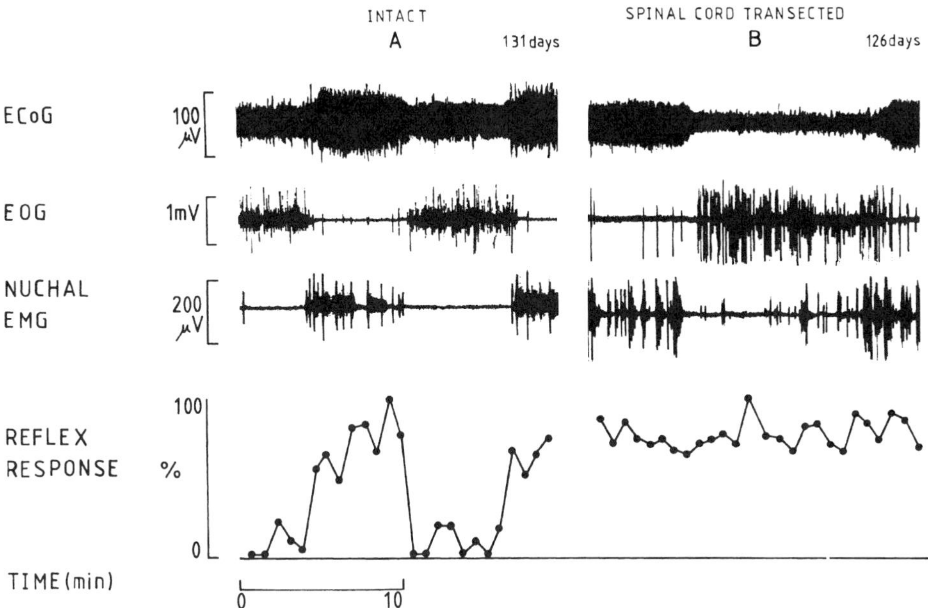

Figure 3 Changes in the sensitivity of the lumbar polysynaptic reflex (lowest record) in different phases of electrocortical or electro-ocular and nuchal EMG activity in an intact fetal lamb at 131 days gestation (A) and in a lamb at 126 days after transection of the spinal cord several days previously (B). Note that gain of reflex is reduced in LVECoG in the intact but not in the transected fetus. (From Ref. 14.)

effects would be induced continuously. This was clearly not the case, although it had been shown that brainstem transection removed inhibitory effects on breathing (19,21) and permitted a stimulation in hypoxia. It was therefore essential to readdress the question of arterial chemoreceptor function in utero; when this was done in the sheep, it was found that both carotid (22) and aortic (23) chemoreceptors were spontaneously active at the normal fetal arterial P_{O_2} and that they responded with an increase in discharge if P_{O_2} fell or P_{CO_2} rose. There were several very important implications of these findings. First, it was clear that the peripheral chemoreceptors would be able to stimulate fetal breathing under some circumstances, but that it was the balance between this stimulatory input and the normally dominant, inhibitory input from higher centers that determined the characteristics of fetal breathing (see above). Second, it redirected attention to the role that particularly the carotid chemoreceptors play in initiating *cardiovascular* reflex responses to hypoxia (24,25). As such reflexes are the first-line defense of the fetus against reduced oxygen supply from the placenta, understanding them is of clinical as well as scientific importance. Last, the observation that the fetal peripheral chemoreceptors discharge spontaneously (at about 5 Hz) at the normal fetal arterial P_{O_2} made it clear that the rise in P_{O_2} at birth would silence them. Their sensitivity to P_{O_2} would then have to reset to the adult range postnatally. The mechanisms and consequences of this have now been studied extensively (see elsewhere in this volume).

B. Neural Mechanisms Involved in Control of Fetal Breathing Movements and "Behavioral States"

The work of Barcroft and Karnoven (19) gave rise to the concept that inhibitory mechanisms that descend from higher centers are involved in producing apneic periods in the fetus. This inhibitory control develops in the second half of gestation. These workers also showed that the inhibition of fetal breathing movements (FBM) in hypoxemia is not seen early in gestation and, once again, it appears that the descending inhibitory processes develop later. While the inhibition of FBM in HVECoG and in hypoxia both involve descending inhibitory processes, they do not necessarily utilize the same neural mechanisms. Barcroft employed similar brainstem transection techniques to those of Lumsden (26) to show that neural structures above approximately the level of the pons do not exert significant control over FBM. These studies were extended by Dawes and coworkers (21), who had employed the technique of transection in the chronically instrumented late-gestation fetal sheep. They showed that transection at the level of upper midbrain/caudal hypothalamus resulted in FBM that were episodic but not related to the ECoG. These FBM were still inhibited by hypoxia. This makes it clear that the processes that mediate the inhibition of FBM in HVECoG are different from those that produce the inhibition in hypoxia. Transection through the rostral pons/caudal midbrain produced FBM that occurred almost continuously and were not inhibition by hypoxia. This focused attention on the upper pons in the inhibition of fetal breathing movements in hypoxia. Gluckman and Johnston (27) pursued this by making lesions in the rostral lateral pons and compiled a diagram showing areas not needed for the inhibition to be manifest and the location of an area in the lateral pons which, if lesioned bilaterally, prevented the inhibition (Fig. 4).

One of the key questions to emerge from these brainstem studies was whether the descending inhibitory mechanism must be capable of inhibiting the input from peripheral chemoreceptors: once it had been established that the peripheral chemoreceptors are active in utero and respond to natural stimuli such as hypoxia or hypercapnia (see above), it was no longer necessary to view the effect of modest hypoxia in inhibiting FBM as a direct *depression* of the medulla. It was also clear that the descending processes must directly inhibit the respiratory neurons and/or prevent the peripheral chemoreceptors from exerting a stimulatory effect on them in hypoxia. The results of transection and lesion studies suggested that a stimulation of FBM occurred in hypoxia after the damage to the brainstem, as if a stimulatory effect of the peripheral chemoreceptors had been unmasked. Direct confirmation of this idea came from the study of Johnston and Gluckman (28), who conducted a two-stage procedure: first lesions were placed as before to prevent the inhibition of FBM in hypoxia or to give an overt stimulation; this was then prevented by chemodenervation at a second operation.

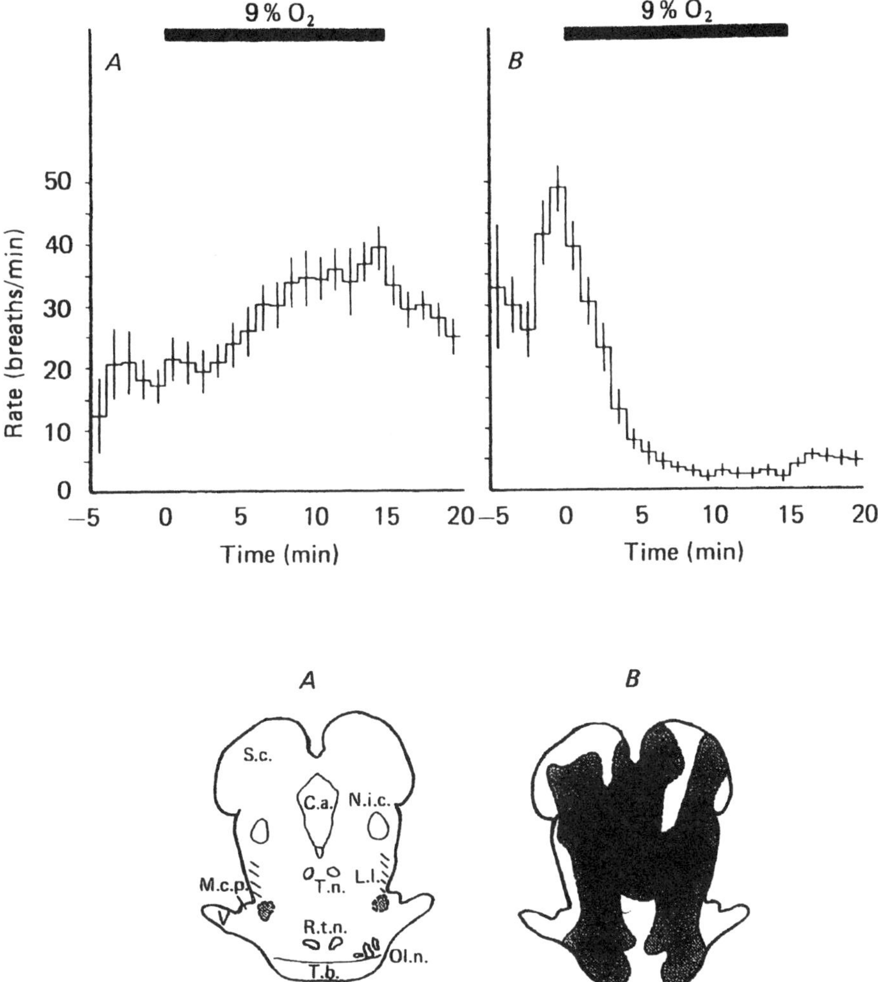

Figure 4 Effect of lesioning bilaterally in the pons on the frequency of fetal breathing movements in hypoxia (9% O_2 given to ewe) in late-gestation fetal sheep. In panels on left (A), small bilateral lesions in the pons permit breathing to continue or be stimulated in hypoxia. In panels on right (B), a composite of lesions destroying a large area of the pons still permits the inhibition of breathing in hypoxia that would be seen in intact fetuses. (From Ref. 27.)

The nature (and indeed the location) of the inhibitory processes is not known. Because the inhibition occurs even in chemodenervated fetuses (29), it is clear that the neurons involved do not receive an excitatory input from the chemoreceptors. They may therefore be chemoreceptors themselves or receive an input from other cells thought to be sensitive to hypoxia—e.g., in the rostral ventrolateral medulla (RVLM) (30). The neural activity as a whole behaves as a chemoreceptor, because the chemoreceptor stimulant drug almitrine mimics the effects of hypoxia in inhibiting FBM irrespective of the integrity of the peripheral chemoreceptors (31). As expected from the discussion above, the stimulatory effect of the drug on the peripheral chemoreceptors becomes manifest only when lesions were placed in the lateral pons (32), unmasking its peripheral actions.

C. Insights from the Neonate

Studies to identify the brainstem mechanism have been conducted in the neonate, in which hypoxia also inhibits breathing, but after a transient chemoreceptor-mediated stimulation. The reasoning is therefore that the secondary fall in ventilation is produced by similar inhibitory processes to those operating in the fetus. Transection of the brainstem through the rostral pons does indeed remove the secondary fall in ventilation (33), as does placement of lesions in the lateral pons (34). However, these studies did not identify any clear group of neurons involved in mediating the effect. Attention has recently focused on the red nucleus, located above the pons in the mesencephalon. The transection studies implicate structures in either the rostral pons or caudal mesencephalon, so it is likely that the red nucleus would have been affected. In neonatal rabbits, electrical stimulation of the red nucleus produces a profound inhibition of respiratory output, and bilateral lesions in the red nucleus prevent the inhibition of respiratory output in hypoxia while not affecting the cardiovascular responses. Evidence that neurons in the red nucleus are involved in this effect comes from the observation that chemical stimulation with glutamate also produces an inhibition of respiratory output (35). Interestingly, the efferent pathway for these cells, the rubrospinal tract, runs in precisely the ventrolateral region of the pons lesioned by Gluckman and Johnston in their fetal studies (27).

The observations on the red nucleus are interesting because, in postnatal life, it has been implicated in producing the hypotonia of postural muscles that occurs in REM sleep. Such hypotonia also occurs in the fetus (21), but at that time it is associated with presence and not absence of FBM. Once again, behaviorally related and hypoxia-induced inhibition of FBM appears to be distinct. In addition, the brainstem reticular formation and related nuclei associated with sleep and arousal have not been greatly studied in the postnatal period. In one study, Moore et al. (36) reported that cooling the locus ceruleus by a few degrees, sufficient to reduce neuronal activity but not conducted action potentials, prevented the secondary fall in ventilation in hypoxia in neonatal lambs. The locus ceruleus has been implicated in producing arousal at birth (37). There are also reports that structures as high in the brain as the thalamus are implicated in the descending inhibition of breathing during hypoxia (38).

While the effects of acute hypoxia on FBM have been widely studied, the effects of prolonged hypoxemia are quite different. Over a period of 6 to 12 hr, FBM return to their control incidence, as does cycling of the ECoG (39). Recent studies reveal that the peripheral chemoreceptors are necessary for the return of fetal breathing movements during sustained hypoxia produced by reduced uterine blood flow, but the mechanisms involved are not known (Stein et al., unpublished observations).

D. Pharmacology of Fetal Breathing Movements and Behavioral States

A range of agents that would be expected to lower tissue P_{O_2} in the central nervous system (CNS) mimic hypoxia, thus inhibiting fetal breathing movements—e.g., CO poisoning (40), oligomycin B (41), and anemia (42). Adenosine is also released in neural tissue in hypoxia and exerts a range of actions: it stimulates the peripheral chemoreceptors but reduces respiratory output in the fetus and neonate. The stimulation of FBM by adenosine after caudal brainstem transection (43) is explicable in terms of the removal of descending inhibitory processes referred to above.

In addition, the role of glutamate receptors in these processes has recently been addressed in the fetus and the neonate (44,45).

Adrenergic agonists and antagonists have also been used to investigate catecholamines in the control of FBM. Murata et al. (46), working on the rhesus monkey, showed that noradrenaline inhibits FBM, while isopreterenol, α-adrenergic agonist, had a stimulatory effect on FBM. However, Bamford et al. (47) showed that the α_2-agonist clonidine increased FBM and the α_2-antagonist idazoxan inhibits it. As α_2-adrenoreceptors exert a presynaptic inhibition on noradrenaline release, this suggests that noradrenaline stimulates FBM rather than inhibiting it, as indicated by Murata et al. (46). In a subsequent study, Bamford and Hawkins (48) showed that the α_2-adrenergic antagonist MSDL 657743 also stimulated FBM in normoxia and also allowed FBM to continue in hypoxia, an effect that Giussani et al. (49) have reported of phentolamine, an α_1-and α_2-antagonist. Furthermore, Joseph and Walker (50) blocked the reuptake of noradrenaline from the synaptic cleft and showed that FBM were initially increased and then decreased, presumably owing to a depletion of presynaptic stores of noradrenaline. The conclusion is that noradrenaline stimulates FBM, but that the predominant action of drugs is on the presynaptic α_2-adrenergic receptor, which, when stimulated, inhibits endogenous release of noradrenaline.

Prostaglandins exert a powerful influence on FBM and postnatal breathing. Prostaglandin E_2 (PGE_2) decreases the incidence of FBM (51) and meclofenamate and indomethacin, inhibitors of its synthesis increase FBM (52–54). The effect of prostaglandins appears to be central, as it is independent of the peripheral chemoreceptors (55) and because central administration of meclaphenamates stimulates FBM (56,57). The same effects can be produced postnatally, with PGE_2 decreasing (58) and meclofenamate and indomethacin increasing ventilation in lambs (58,59). However, the change in the concentration of PGE_2 that occurs around birth cannot be solely responsible for either the decrease in FBM seen immediately before birth (60,61) or the onset of continuous breathing postnatally (62). The well-established effects of ethyl alcohol to reduce the incidence of FBM (63) are mediated by adenosine rather than by prostaglandin (64) and/or adenosine (65).

Bennet et al. (66) showed that large doses of thyrotropin-releasing hormone (TRH) can induce stimulation of FBM. This effect may be at the level of the respiratory neurons, where TRH can be localized, but its physiological significance is not known. This may also be true of the effects of the cholinergic agonist pilocarpine and the 5-HT precursor L-5-HTP (67,68). Both these agents stimulate FBM, but pilocarpine induces LVECoG and L-5-HTP HVECoG. This stresses again that the coincidental rather than causal unknown link between FBM and LVECoG to 5-HT has been implicated in neural mechanisms controlling sleep but that the site of action in the fetus is not known. A range of opiates have effects on FBM (69), but the physiological localization of this effect has not been established.

Last, one of the striking aspects of FBM is that they cease 24 to 48 hr before parturition. The mechanism involved is not known. Kitterman et al. (52) excluded a rise in plasma PGE_2 and Parkes et al. (70) showed that it did not occur if the fall in plasma progesterone was prevented.

E. Changes in Breathing and Behavior at Birth

At birth, breathing activity must become continuous in order to fulfill the gas exchange function despite the fact that HVECoG is still generated. After cord occlusion, the neonatal ECoG still cycles between low-and high-voltage states, and they seem to have identical characteristics to the fetal states, LVECoG activity is associated with absence of nuchal muscle activity, REM, inhibition of polysynaptic reflexes and HVECoG is associated with presence of nuchal muscle activity, lack of rapid eye movements, presence of polysynaptic reflexes (71). Despite the fact that after birth, the HVECoG state seems to be similar to the fetal state, breathing activity is present. We do not know why breathing is present during HVECoG after birth. It may be that answering this question will require detailed power spectral analysis of the ECoG from different areas of the brain before and during the first hours of birth. But it is worth noting that some mammals—such as the rat, cat and rabbit—develop organized behavioral states 2 to 3 weeks after birth; in utero, however, they do not breathe continuously. So clearly it is not simply the development of the HVECoG state that makes breathing episodic in the late-gestation fetus.

Studies of the mechanisms involved in the establishment of continuous breathing at birth have followed two lines: (1) attempts to induce continuous breathing in utero or (2) observation of establishment of continuous breathing during situations aimed at mimicking birth.

Induction of Continuous Breathing In Utero

It is well established that the inhibition of fetal breathing activity during HVECoG can be overridden, as demonstrated by the presence of continuous breathing during metabolic acidosis (72,73), administration of prostaglandin synthetase inhibitors (52,53,57), or by 5-hydroxytryptophan (74,68), catecholamines (75), pilocarpine (67), TRH (76), corticotrophin-releasing factor (66), central or peripheral fetal cooling (77,78) and by lesions in certain centers or pathways within the CNS—for instance in the lateral pons (18). These experiments show that fetal breathing can become continuous through the operation of various mechanisms, including disinhibition during HVECVoG, direct stimulation of breathing, changes in the balance between stimulatory and inhibitory neuromodulators, increased arousability, and changes in chemoreceptor sensitivity (79). Some of these mechanisms (but not necessarily all) are surely active at the moment of birth.

Observation of Establishment of Continuous Breathing During Simulated Birth

Experiments designed to observe changes in breathing activity after cord occlusion have led to two main hypotheses: 1) The exclusion of fetal-placental circulation leads to the disappearance of hormones or neuromodulators which exert continuous tonic inhibition (through the CNS) during fetal life and this allows breathing activity (80–83). There are reports indicating that an unidentified substance originating from placental tissue can inhibit fetal breathing activity (84). Although this is a possible explanation, it is not yet demonstrated that such a substance is responsible for the modulation by ECoG of breathing activity in utero; 2) Breathing activity is dependent on the level of Pa_{CO_2} in utero and at birth (16). It is known that during hypocapnia fetal and neonatal breathing are reduced (80). Hence lowering Pa_{CO_2} reduces breathing even after it has been experimentally produced by cord occlusion in the sheep fetus (Fig. 5). Hypercapnia stimulates breathing activity, but in utero this is inhibited during quiet sleep (81) (Fig. 6). However, this inhibition can be overridden after lesions in the lateral pons (18) or when hypercapnia is combined with cooling (78). This might be explained by changes in the CO_2 sensitivity of central and/or peripheral chemoreceptors or due to changes in the balance between central inhibitory and excitatory (arousability) mechanisms caused by an increase in afferent input at birth.

We conclude that changes in afferent input from chemo- and thermoreceptors to the CNS are important in the transition from fetal to neonatal breathing. Changes in the plasma level of a placental neuromodulator at birth may then serve to maintain breathing after its initiation (Fig. 6). More insight into these mechanisms will offer explanations for apnea periods after birth.

F. Postnatal Adaptation of Chemoreflexes

The influence of CO_2 and of ambient and core temperatures upon respiratory chemoreflexes in postnatal life has been ascertained in a series of studies on unanesthetized kittens. In these, peripheral chemosensitivity was quantified as the reflex respiratory response to an alternating inspiratory O_2 or CO_2 stimulus. All experiments were performed in quiet sleep, as judged behaviorally, as electrocortical states are relatively undifferentiated in kittens below 1 month of age (85). In accordance with similar studies performed in unanesthetized rats (86), kittens (87), lambs (88), and newborn babies (89), the reflex sensitivity to hypoxia was either low or absent in kittens aged 3 to 7 days and only increased after this age. These results were predicted from the postnatal increase in the hypoxic sensitivity (resetting) of both carotid (22) and aortic (90) chemoreceptors. In contrast, sensitivity to CO_2 was present at all ages from birth and remained elevated throughout the longitudinal study, such that the responses to both

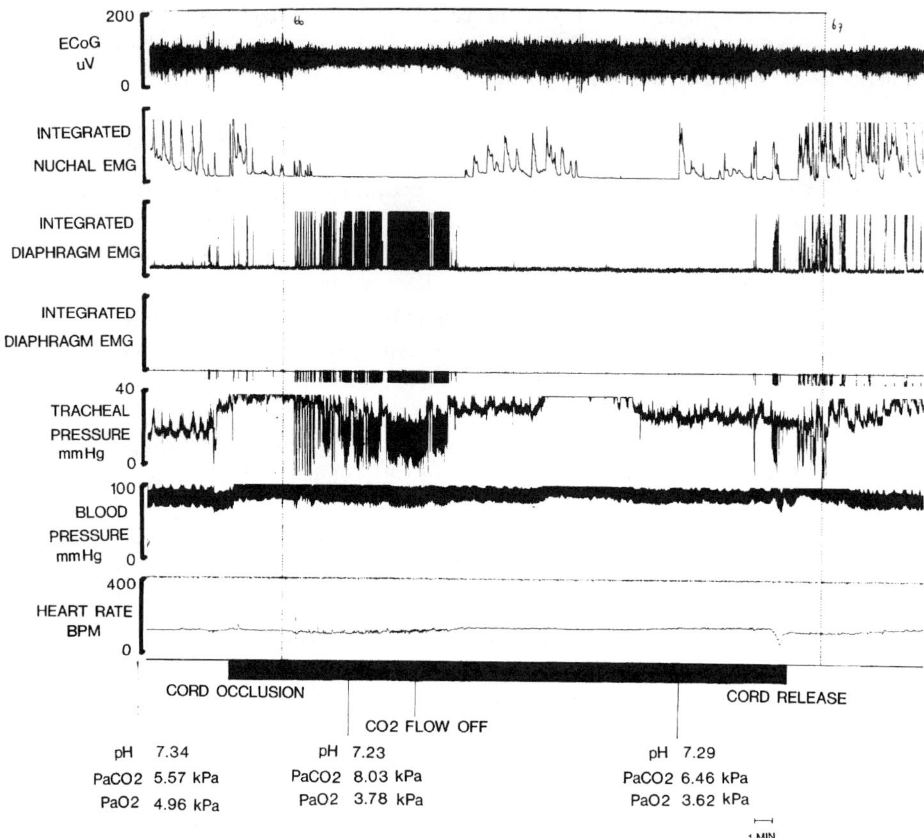

Figure 5 Late-gestation fetal sheep maintained in utero as extracorporeal circuit. Traces for the top are ECoG, nuchal EMG, integrated diaphragm EMG (two traces), tracheal pressure, blood pressure, heart rate, and event marker. Arterial blood gas values (kPa) and pHa are given at bottom. A period of cord occlusion does not initiate fetal breathing until the Pa_{CO2} has risen substantially and Pa_{O2} has also fallen. Lowering Pa_{CO2} by removing the CO_2 flowing to the membrane (CO_2 flow off) then stops breathing. Normal fetal breathing occurs only when the ECoG switches from HV to LV. (From Ref. 16.)

hypoxia and CO_2 were similar in terms of the pattern of breathing only by 35 to 39 days. These findings were confirmed by direct recording of sinus nerve chemoafferents in the lamb in response to a similar, alternating stimulus profile (91), where a steady-state response to CO_2 was present at all ages from birth and increased with increasing postnatal age. This maturation of steady-state responses to CO_2 might reflect an increase in the degree of interaction between CO_2 and hypoxia at the peripheral

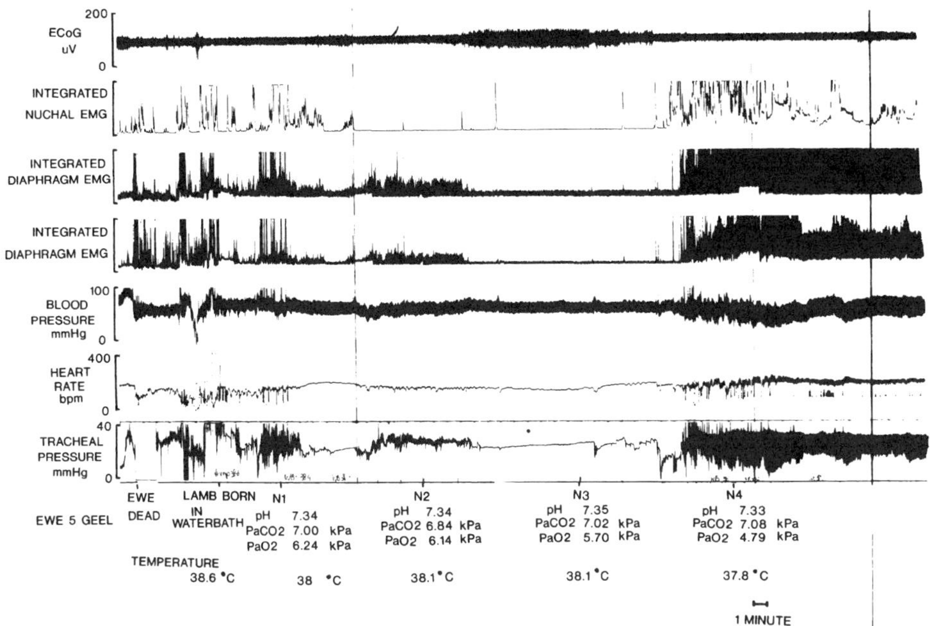

Figure 6 Recording of a neonatal lamb in the warm saline bath at 133 days of gestation, 6 days after surgery, and connected to the extracorporeal membrane oxygenation (ECMO) system. Tracings are, from the top: electrocortical activity, integrated nuchal EMG, integrated diaphragm EMG (two traces), blood pressure, heart rate, and tracheal pressure. Blood gas and pH samples were taken at the times indicated. Note that breathing movements were still present periodically for 36 min after delivering the neonate into the saline bath. Continuous breathing activity became present after 36 min. Nuchal muscle activity was still modulated by electrocortical activity. This figure demonstrates that breathing with neonatal characteristics does not start immediately after cord occlusion if the neonate is kept warm and the gases near fetal values. However, a slower switch to continuous breathing occurs later. (From Ref. 78.)

chemoreceptor (22,92–95). However, the dynamic sensitivity to CO_2, as measured by the amplitude of the oscillating chemoreceptor response to the alternating CO_2 blood gas stimulus (91), while present at birth, was unaffected both by increasing levels of hypoxia and by increasing postnatal age, suggesting that this component of the response was independent of arterial P_{O_2}, as had been previously proposed (96).

Using the same technique for assessing chemoreflex sensitivity in unanesthetized kittens, Watanabe et al. (97) demonstrated that peripheral chemosensitivity could be attenuated by increasing environmental temperature from 25° to 30°C. At all ages from 3 to 39 days, this increase in environmental temperature significantly increased rectal temperature and decreased O_2 consumption. Similar increases in rectal temperature with an increased oxygen consumption were obtained (98) in kittens aged 27 to 35 days and at about 25°C by the intravenous administration of the pyrogen interleukin-1. In contrast to the reflex respiratory responses observed when similar increases in rectal temperature were obtained by external heating, however (99), in these animals there was no difference in the chemoreflex response to hypoxia or CO_2, in terms of either the pattern or of the amplitude of alternation. This suggests that the increase in gain of chemoreflex observed during external cooling is not due to an increase in metabolism. It is possible, therefore, that cutaneous thermoreceptor input to the CNS could bias the gain of the chemoreflexes. Such a change could also be accompanied by a change in the incidence of sleep/wakefulness states which may, in turn, be associated with a change in chemoreflex gain as—at least in the lamb—the O_2 saturation at which arousal from sleep occurs is lower in active than in quiet sleep (100). Additionally, it may be that endocrine changes produced by the fall in environmental temperature are responsible for altering the chemoreflex gain.

III. Conclusion

Birth clearly involves some irreversible processes, the transition to continuous breathing being one. However, breathing remains linked to behavioral and sleep states in the neonate as in the fetus, and clearly there is continuity of some control processes from late gestation to early postnatal life. Some of these processes mature relatively slowly after birth: in this review, we have highlighted resetting of chemoreceptor hypoxia sensitivity and the diminishing influence of descending inhibitory effects on breathing in hypoxia. Research has demonstrated how inhibitory effects on breathing that appear to be more fetal in character can be involved postnatally under certain conditions—e.g., chronic hypoxia or hyperthermia. An understanding of these effects will be of vital importance to the prevention of SIDS and the care of newborn, especially preterm babies.

References

1. Bystrzycka E, Nail B, Purves MJ. Central and peripheral neural respiratory activity in the mature sheep foetus and newborn lamb. Resp Physiol 1975; 25:199–215.
2. Bahoric A, Chernick V. Electrical activity of phrenic nerve and diaphragm in utero. J Appl Physiol 1975; 39:513–518.
3. Barcroft J, Barron DH. The genesis of respiratory movements in the fetus of the sheep. 1937; 88:56–61.
4. Cooke IRC, Berger PH. Precursor of respiratory pattern in the early gestation mammalian fetus. Brain Res 1990; 522:333–336.
5. Vries de JIP, Visser GHA, Prechtl HFR. The emergence of fetal behaviour: 1. Qualitative aspects. Early Hum Dev 1982; 7:301–322.
6. Clewlow R, Dawes GS, Johnston BM, Walker DW. Changes in breathing, electrocortical and muscle activity in unanaesthetized fetal lambs with age. J Physiol 1983; 341:463–476.

7. Ioffe S, Jansen AH, Chernick V. Maturation of spontaneous fetal diaphragmatic activity and fetal response to hypercapnia and hypoxemia. J Appl Physiol 1987; 62:609–622.
8. Bowes G, Adamson TM, Ritchie BC, Dowling MH, Wilkinson MH, Maloney JE. Development of patterns of respiratory activity in unanaesthetized fetal sheep in utero. J Appl Physiol 1981; 50:693–700.
9. Szeto HH, Cheng PY, Decena JA, Wu D-L, Dwyer G. Developmental changes in continuity and stability of breathing in the fetal lamb. Am J Physiol 1992; 262:R452–R458.
10. Dawes GS, Fox HE, Leduc BM, Liggins GC, Richards RT. Respiratory movements and rapid eye movements sleep in the fetal lamb. J Physiol Lond 1972; 404:587–589.
11. Szeto HH, Vo TDH, Dwyer G, Dogromajian ME, Cox MJ, Senger G. The ontogeny of fetal lamb electrocortical activity: a power spectral analysis. Am J Obstet Gynecol 1985; 153:462–466.
12. Szeto HH. Spectral edge frequency as a simple quantitative measure of maturation of electrocortical activity. Pediatr Res 1990; 27:289–292.
13. Harding R, Bocking AD, Sigger JN. Influence of upper respiratory tract on liquid flow to and from fetal lungs. J Physiol 1986; 61:68–71.
14. Blanco CE, Dawes GS, Walker DW. Effects of hypoxia on polysynaptic hind-limb reflexes of unanaesthetized fetal and new-born lambs. J Physiol 1983; 339:453–454.
15. Dawes GS, Gardner WN, Johnston BM, Walker DW. Breathing in fetal lambs: the effects of brain stem section. J Physiol 1983; 335:535–553.
16. Kuipers IM, Maertzdorf WM, De Jong DS, Hanson MA, Blanco CE. Effects of mild hypocapnia on fetal breathing and behavior in unanesthetized normoxic fetal lambs. J Appl Physiol 1994; 76:1476–1480.
17. Steriade M, Contreras D, Amzica F. Synchronised sleep oscillations and their paroxysmal developments. Trends in Neurosciences 1994; 17:199–208.
18. Johnston BM, Gluckman PD. Lateral pontine lesion affects central chemosensitivity in unanesthetized fetal lambs. J Physiol 1989; 67:1113–1118.
19. Barcroft J. Researches on Pre-natal Life. Oxford: Blackwell, 1946.
20. Hanson MA. Peripheral chemoreceptor function before and after birth. In: Johnson BM, Gluckman P, eds. Respiratory Control and Lung Development in the Fetus and Newborn. Ithaca, NY: Perinatology Press, 1986: 311–330.
21. Dawes GS. The central control of fetal breathing and skeletal muscle movements. J Physiol 1984; 346:1–18.
22. Blanco CE, Dawes GS, Hanson MA, McCooke, HB. The response to hypoxia of arterial chemoreceptors in fetal sheep and newborn lambs. J Physiol 1984; 351:25–37.
23. Blanco CE, Dawes GS, Hanson MA, McCooke HB. The arterial chemoreceptors in fetal sheep and newborn lambs. J Physiol 1982; 330:38P.
24. Bartelds B, Van Bel F, Teitel DF, Rudolph AM. Carotid, not aortic, chemoreceptors mediate the fetal cardiovascular response to acute hypoxemia in lambs. Pediatr Res 1993; 34(1):51–55.
25. Giussani DA, Spencer JAD, Moore PJ, Bennet L, Hanson MA. Afferent and efferent components of the cardiovascular reflex responses to acute hypoxia in term fetal sheep. J Physiol 1993; 461:431–449.
26. Lumsden T. Observations on the respiratory centres. J Physiol 1923; 57:354–367.
27. Gluckman PD, Johnston BM. Lesions in the upper lateral pons abolish the hypoxic depression of breathing in unanaesthetized fetal lambs in utero. J Physiol 1987; 382: 373–383.

28. Johnston BM, Gluckman PD. Peripheral chemoreceptors respond to hypoxia in pontine-lesioned fetal lambs in utero. J Appl Physiol 1993; 75:1027–1034.
29. Moore PJ1, Moore PJ, Parkes MJ, Nijhuis JG, Hanson MA. The incidence of breathing movements in fetal sheep in normoxia and hypoxia after peripheral chemodenervation and brain stem transection. J Dev Physiol 1989; 11:147–151.
30. Nolan PC, Dillon GH, Waldrop, TG. Central hypoxic chemoreceptors in the ventro-lateral medulla and caudal hypothalamus. Adv Exp Med Biol 1995; 393:261–266.
31. Moore PJ, Hanson MA, Parkes MJ. Almitrine inhibits breathing movements in fetal sheep. J Dev Physiol 1989; 11:277–281.
32. Johnston BM, Moore PJ, Bennet L, Hanson MA, Gluckman PD. Almitrine mimics hypoxia in fetal sheep with lateral pontine lesions. J Appl Physiol 1990; 69:1330–1335.
33. Martin-Body RL. Brain transections demonstrate the central origin of hypoxic ventilatory depression in carotid body-denervated rats. J Physiol 1988; 407:41–52.
34. Martin-Body, RL, Johnston BM. Central origin of the hypoxic depression of breathing in the young rabbit. Respir Physiol 1988; 71:25–32.
35. Ackland GL, Noble R, Hanson MA. Red nucleus inhibits breathing during hypoxia in neonates. Respir Physiol 1997; 110:251–260.
36. Moore PJ, Ackland GL, Hanson MA. Unilateral cooling in the region of locus coeruleus blocks the fall in respiratory output during hypoxia in anaesthetised neonatal sheep. Exp Physiol 1996; 81:983–994.
37. Lagercrantz H. Stress, arousal and gene activation at birth. Pediatr Res 1996; 11:214–218.
38. Chau AF, Matsurura M, Koos B. Glutamate receptors in the thalamus stimulate breathing and modulate sleep state in fetal sheep. J Soc Gynecol Invest 1996; 3:252A/388.
39. Bocking AD, Harding R. Effects of reduced uterine blood flow on electrocortical activity, breathing and skeletal muscle activity in fetal sheep. Am J Obstet Gynecol 1986; 154:655–662.
40. Koos BJ, Matsuda K, Power GG. Fetal breathing and sleep state responses to graded carboxyhemoglobinemia in sheep. J Appl Physiol 1988; 65:2118–2123.
41. Koos BJ, Sameshima H, Power GG. Fetal breathing movement, sleep state and cardiovascular responses to an inhibitor of mitochondrial ATPase in sheep. J Dev Physiol 1986; 8:67–75.
42. Matsuda K, Ducsay C, Koos BJ. Fetal breathing, sleep state and cardiovascular adaptations to anaemia in sheep. J Physiol 1992; 445:713–723.
43. Koos BJ, Chao A, Doany W. Adenosine stimulates breathing in fetal sheep with brain stem section. J Appl Physiol 1992; 72:94–99
44. Bissonnette JM, Hohimer AR, Knopp SJ. Non-NMDA receptors modulate respiratory drive in fetal sheep. J Physiol 1997; 501:415–424.
45. Navarro H, Suguihara C, Soliz A, Hehre D, Huang J, Bancalari E. Effect of L-aspartate on the ventilatory response to hypoxia in sedated newborn piglets. Biol Neonate 1998; 73:387–394.
46. Murata Y, Martin CB, Miyake K, Socol M, Druzin M. Effects of catecholamines on fetal breathing activity in rhesus monkeys. Am J Obstet Gynecol 1981; 139:942–947.
47. Bamford OS, Dawes GS, Ward RA. Effects of α_2-adrenergic agonist clonidine and its antagonist idazoxan on the fetal lamb. J Physiol 1986; 381:29–37.
48. Bamford OS, Hawkins LH. Central effects of an α_2-adrenergic antagonist on the fetal lamb: a possible mechanism for hypoxic apnea. J Dev Physiol 1990; 13:353–358.
49. Giussani DA, Moore PJ, Spencer JAD, Hanson MA. a1 and a2-adrenoreceptor actions

of phentolamine and prazosin on breathing movements in fetal sheep in utero. J Physiol 1995; 486:249–255.

50. Joseph SA, Walker DW. Catecholamine neurons in fetal brain: effects on breathing movements and electrocorticogram J Appl Physiol 1990; 69:1903–1911.
51. Kitterman JA, Liggins GC, Fewell JE, Tooley WH. Inhibition of breathing movements in fetal sheep of sodium meclofenamate. J Physiol 1983; 54:687–692.
52. Kitterman JA, Liggins GC, Clements JA, Tooley WH. Stimulation of breathing movements in fetal sheep by inhibitors of prostaglandin synthesis. J Dev Physiol 1979; 1: 453–466.
53. Wallen LD, Murai DT, Clyman RI, Lee CH, Mauray FE, Kitterman JA. Regulation of breathing movements in fetal sheep by prostaglandin E_2. J Appl Physiol 1986; 60:526–531.
54. Patrick J, Challis JRG, Cross J. Effects of maternal indomethacin administration on fetal breathing movements in sheep. J Dev Physiol 1987; 9:295–300.
55. Murai DT, Wallen LD, Lee CC, Clyman RI, Mauray F, Kitterman JA. Effects of prostaglandins in fetal breathing do not involve peripheral chemoreceptors. J Appl Physiol 1987; 62:271–277.
56. Koos BJ. Central effects on breathing in fetal sheep of sodium meclofenamate. J Physiol 1982; 330:50-1P.
57. Koos BJ. Central stimulation of breathing movements in fetal lambs by prostaglandin synthetase inhibitors. J Physiol 1985; 362:455–466.
58. Guerra FA, Savich RD, Clyman RI, Kitterman JA. Meclofenamate increases ventilation in lambs. J Dev Physiol 1988; 11:1–6.
59. Long WA. Prostaglandins and control of breathing in newborn piglets. J Appl Physiol 1988; 64:409–418.
60. Patrick J, Challis JRG, Cross J. Effects of maternal indomethacin administration on fetal breathing movements in sheep. J Dev Physiol 1987; 9:295–300.
61. Wallen LD, Murai DT, Clyman RI, Lee CH, Mauray FE, Kitterman JA. Effects of meclofenamate on breathing movements in fetal sheep before delivery. J Appl Physiol 1988; 64:759–766.
62. Lee DS, Choy P, Davi M, Caces R, Gibson D, Hasan SU, Cates D, Rigatto H. Decrease in plasma prostaglandin E_2 is not essential for the establishment of continuous breathing at birth in sheep. J Dev Physiol 1989; 12:145–151.
63. Smith GN, Brien JF, Homan J, Carmichael L, Treissman D, Patrick J. Effect of ethanol on ovine fetal and maternal plasma prostaglandin E_2 concentrations and fetal breathing movements. J Dev Physiol 1990; 14:23–28.
64. Smith GN, Brien JF, Homan J, Carmichael L, Patrick J. Indomethacin reversal of ethanol-induced suppression of ovine fetal breathing movements and relationship to prostaglandin E_2. J Dev Physiol 1990; 14:29–35.
65. Watson CS, Challis JRG, Bocking, AD. Ethanol-induced inhibition of fetal breathing movements is associated with a decrease in fetal cerebral extracellular prostaglandin E_2. J Soc Gynecol Invest 1998; 5:154A/T476.
66. Bennet L, Johnston BM, Vale WW, Gluckman PD. The central effects of thyrotropin-releasing factor and two antagonists on breathing movements in fetal sheep. J Physiol 1990; 421:1–11.
67. Hanson MA, Moore PJ, Nijhuis JG, Parkes MJ. Effects of pilocarpine on breathing movements in normal, chemodenervated and brain stem-transected fetal sheep. J Physiol 1988; 400:415–424.

68. Fletcher DJ, Hanson MA, Moore PJ, Nijhuis JG, Parkes MJ. Stimulation of breathing movements by L-5-hydroxytryptophan in fetal sheep during normoxia and hypoxia. J Physiol 1988; 404:7575–7589.
69. Hasan SU, Lee DS, Gibson DA, Nowaczyk BJ, Cates DB, Sitar DS, Pinsky C, Rigatto H. Effect of morphine on breathing and behavior in fetal sheep. J Appl Physiol 1988; 64:2058–2065.
70. Parkes MJ, Moore PJ, Hanson MA. The effects of inhibition of 3-B hydroxysteroid dehydrogenase activity in sheep fetuses in utero. Cairn, Australia: Proceedings of The Society for the Study of Fetal Physiology, 1988.
71. Blanco CE, Dawes GS, Walker DW. Effects of hypoxia on polysynaptic hind-limb reflexes in new-born lambs before and after carotid denervation. J Physiol 1983; 339:467–474.
72. Molteni RA, Melmed MH, Sheldon RE, Jones MD, Meschia G. Induction of fetal breathing by metabolic acidemia and its effects on blood flow to the respiratory muscles. Am J Obstet Gynecol 1980; 136:609–620.
73. Hohimer AR, Bissonnette JM. Effects of metabolic acidosis on fetal breathing movements in utero. Respir Physiol 1981; 43:99–106.
74. Quilligan EJ, Clewlow F, Johnston BM, Walker DW. Effects of 5-hydroxytryptophan on electrocortical activity and breathing movements of fetal sheep. Am J Obstet Gynecol 1994; 141:271–275.
75. Jansen AH, Loffe S, Chernick V. Stimulation of fetal breathing activity by beta-adrenergic mechanisms. J Appl Physiol 1986; 60:1938–1945.
76. Bennet L, Gluckman PD, Johnston BM. The effects of corticotrophin-releasing hormone on breathing movements and electrocortical activity of the fetal sheep. J Physiol 1988; 23:72–75.
77. Gluckman PD, Gunn TR, Johnston BM. The effect of cooling on breathing and shivering in unanaesthetized fetal lambs in utero. J Physiol 1983; 343:495–506.
78. Kuipers IM, Masertzdorf EJ, De Jong DS, Hanson MA, Blanco CE. Initiation and maintenance of continuous breathing at birth. Pediatr Res 1997; 42:163–168.
79. Lagercrantz H, Pequignot JM, Hertzberg T, Holgert H, Ringstedt T. Birth-related changes of expression and turnover of some neuroactive agents and respiratory control. Biol Neonate 1994; 65:145–148.
80. Adamson SL, Richardson BS, Homan J. Initiation of pulmonary gas exchange by fetal sheep in utero. J Appl Physiol 1987; 62:989–998.
81. Boddy K, Dawes GD, Fisher R, Pinter S, Robinson JS. Fetal respiratory movements, electrocortical activity and cardiovascular responses to hypoxaemia and hypercapnia in sheep. J Physiol 1974; 243:599–618.
82. Adamson SL, Kuipers IM, Olson DM. Umbilical cord occlusion stimulates breathing independent of blood gases and pH. J Appl Physiol 1991; 70:1796–1809.
83. Sawa R, Asakura H, Power G. Changes in plasma adenosine during simulated birth of fetal sheep. J Appl Physiol 1991; 70:1524–1528.
84. Alvaro RE, Rehan V, de Almeida Z, Robertson M, Jansen A, Cates DB, Rigatto H. Specificity of a placental factor inhibiting breathing in fetal sheep. Reprod Fertil Dev 1996; 8:423–429.
85. Jouvet-Mounier D, Astic I, Lacote D. Ontogenesis of the states of sleep in the rat, cats and guinea pig during the first postnatal month. Dev Psychobiol 1969; 2:216–239.

86. Eden GJ, Hanson MA. Maturation of the respiratory response to acute hypoxia in the newborn rat. J Physiol 1987; 392:1–9.
87. Blanco CE, Martin CB Jr, Hanson MA, McCooke HB. Determinants of the onset of continuous air breathing at birth. Eur J Obstet Gynecol Reprod Biol 1987; 26:183–192.
88. Hanson MA, Kumar P, Williams BA. The effect of chronic hypoxia on the development of respiratory chemoreflexes in newborn kittens. J Physiol 1989; 411:563–574.
89. Williams BA, Hanson MA. Role of carotid chemoreceptors in the respiratory response of newborn lambs to alternate breaths of air and a hypoxic gas. J Dev Physiol 1990; 13:157–164.
90. Williams BA, Smyth J, Boon AW, Hanson MA, Kumar P, Blanco CE. Development of respiratory chemoreflexes in response to alterations of fractional inspired oxygen in the newborn infant. J Physiol 1991; 442:81–90.
91. Kumar P, Hanson MA. Re-setting of the hypoxic sensitivity of aortic chemoreceptors in the new-born lamb. J Dev Physiol 1989; 11:199–206.
92. Calder NA, Kumar P, Hanson MA. Development of carotid chemoreceptor dynamic and steady-state sensitivity to CO_2 in the newborn lamb. J Physiol 1997; 503:187–194.
93. Mulligan E. Single fiber carotid-body chemoreceptor responses in the piglet. FASEB 1988; Journal 2.
94. Marchal F, Bairam A, Haouzi P, Crance JP, Digiulio C, Vert P, Lahiri S. Carotid chemoreceptor response to natural stimuli in the newborn kitten. Respir Physiol 1992; 87:183–192.
95. Carroll JL, Bamford OS, Fitzgerald RS. Postnatal maturation of carotid chemoreceptor responses to O_2 and CO_2 in the cat. J Appl Physiol 1993; 75:2383–2391.
96. Pepper DR, Landauer RC, Kumar P. Postnatal development of CO_2–O_2 interaction in the rat carotid body in vitro. J Physiol 1995; 485:531–541.
97. Torrance RW, Bartels EM, McLaren A. Update of the bicarbonate hypothesis. In: Data PG, Acker H, Lahiri S, eds. Neurobiology and Cell Biology of Chemoreception: Advances in Experimental Medicine and Biology. New York: Plenum Press 1993: 243–250.
98. Watanabe T, Kumar P, Hanson MA. Development of respiratory chemoreflexes to hypoxia and CO_2 in unanaesthetized kittens. Respir Physiol 1996; 106:247–254.
99. Watanabe T, Kumar P, Hanson MA. Elevation of metabolic rate by pyrogen administration does not affect the gain of respiratory peripheral chemoreflexes in unanaesthetised kittens. Pediatr Res 1998; 44:357–362.
100. Watanabe T, Kumar P, Hanson MA. Effect of ambient temperature on respiratory chemoreflex in unanaesthetized kittens. Respir Physiol 1996; 106:239–246.
101. Fewell JE, Kondo CS, Dascalu V, Filyk SC. Influence of carotid denervation on the arousal and cardiopulmonary response to rapidly developing hypoxaemia in lambs. Pediatr Res 1989; 25:473–477.
102. Parkes MJ. Sleep and wakefulness: do they occur in utero? In: Hanson MA, ed. The Fetal and Neonatal Brainstem. New York: Cambridge University Press, 1991.

8

Maturation of Breathing During Sleep
Infants Through Adolescents

CAROL LYNN ROSEN

Case Western Reserve University and
Rainbow Babies and Children's Hospital
University Hospitals of Cleveland
Cleveland, Ohio

I. Introduction

The objective of this chapter is to describe the maturational changes of breathing during sleep that contribute to the unique features of sleep-disordered breathing in children. Understanding these developmental changes is important for clinicians dealing with common childhood problems such as apnea of prematurity, apparent life-threatening events, sudden infant death syndrome (SIDS), and obstructive sleep apnea/hypoventilation syndrome. This knowledge is also relevant to children with conditions such as trisomy 21, cerebral palsy, craniofacial anomalies, achondroplasia, muscular dystrophy, and myelodysplasia. Such children are at high risk for severe sleep-dissordered breathing that can further compromise developmental potential.

This chapter is not meant to duplicate previous encyclopedic reviews of respiratory adaptation to sleep (1,2) but to provide an updated summary of maturation of breathing during sleep. Specific topics include ventilatory mechanics of the upper airways and chest, respiratory patterns and apnea, ventilation and gas exchange, ventilatory and arousal responses, and the interactions between apnea, bradycardia, and desaturations. References focus on human data. Maturational changes in sleep and more details about arousal responses are discussed in Chapters 3 and 4, respectively.

Developmental changes in heart rate, heart rate variability, and autonomic function are reviewed in Chap. 9.

II. Normal Respiration During Sleep: An Overview

Ventilation during sleep is decreased compared to the awake state and varies with the state of sleep. During non–rapid-eye-movement (NREM) sleep, the behavioral influence on ventilation is absent and ventilation is governed by metabolic factors. Breathing is regular, but tidal volume and respiratory rate are lower, which results in a decline in minute ventilation. In adolescents and adults, the minute ventilation during sleep decreases by 8 to 15% compared to wakefulness (3,4). This decline, in combination with the supine position and decrease in intercostal muscle tone, results in a decrease in functional residual capacity (FRC) (5). Furthermore, a sleep-related decrease in upper-airway tone and lung volume results in a marked increase in upper-airway resistance (6,7). During rapid-eye-movement (REM) sleep, breathing is irregular, with variable respiratory rate and tidal volume and frequent central apneas. Inhibition of tonic activity of the intercostal muscles during REM results in a further decline in FRC. Hypotonia of the upper airway muscles occurs in the presence of unchanged diaphragmatic contractions, predisposing the subject to obstructive apnea. Finally, hypoxic and hypercapnic ventilatory drives decrease during sleep. During sleep, normal children experience an increase in the partial pressure of carbon dioxide and a decrease in arterial oxyhemoglobin saturation. These effects are exaggerated in children with underlying pulmonary or upper airway problems.

III. Ventilatory Mechanics During Sleep

In early life, the ventilatory response to loaded breathing is limited. Differences between the newborn and adult respiratory systems that make the infant more vulnerable to ventilatory failure are summarized in Table 1.

A. Upper Airways

Route of Breathing

The claim that infants are obligate nose breathers because of the presence of a veloepiglottic sphincter formed by the apposition of the soft palate and epiglottis (8) has been rejected. Although resting infants and adults preferentially breathe through their noses, newer studies have shown that infants can switch to mouth breathing in a manner similar to that of adults—that is, by detaching the soft palate from the tongue and opening the oropharyngeal isthmus (9–11). However, the ability to establish mouth breathing varies with age and behavioral state. Younger, sleeping infants respond more slowly than older, awake infants (9,12,13). In preterm infants, the prevalence of oral breathing is low and almost exclusively associated with body movement

Table 1 Differences Between the Newborn and Adult Respiratory Systems

Upper airway
Greater difficulty switching from nasal to oral route of breathing
Laryngeal reflexes with prominent cardiorespiratory depressant syndrome
Chest wall properties impairing load compensation
Increased chest wall compliance
Circular "barrel-shaped" chest wall with horizontal position of the ribs
Smaller diaphragmatic zone of apposition
Softer, cartilaginous ribs
Greater percentage of sleep time in REM when stabilizing intercostal muscles are inhibited
Lower resting functional residual capacity
Low specific lung compliance
Higher metabolic rate
Immature respiratory control

(14). When nasal passages are obstructed, mouth breathing is established more slowly and less effectively during REM than during NREM sleep (15,16).

Upper Airway Reflexes

In human infants, reflexes originating in the upper airway can induce profound apnea and bradycardia (17–20). The best studied reflex, the laryngeal chemoreflex, has been elicited in humans by water or saline instillation into the pharynx. Components of the laryngeal chemoreflex include central apnea, airway closure, cardiac deceleration, peripheral vasoconstriction with increased blood pressure and blood flow redistribution, swallowing, arousal, and possibly cough (21). The severity of the apnea and bradycardia elicited by this reflex is increased by respiratory syncytial virus infection (22) and hypoxemia (23). Hypoxia intensifies the cardioinhibitory effect on peripheral chemoreceptors during apnea because pulmonary stretch receptor input is suppressed (24). The respiratory depressant component of the laryngeal chemoreflex decreases with maturation. Prolonged apnea is more prominent in preterm than in full-term infants (25). Although most studies on laryngeal chemoreflexes were performed during sleep, the influence of sleep state on the magnitude of the response is not known. The clinical importance of this reflex outside the newborn period is also unknown.

During the neonatal period, stimulation of other upper airway receptors can alter respiratory patterns. In human infants, trigeminal airway stimulation can elicit a cardiorespiratory response characterized by heart rate slowing in preterm infants, cardiac acceleration in term and older infants, and respiratory rate slowing in both ages (26,27). The ventilatory component of trigeminal stimulation is blunted with maturation (27). The importance of this reflex in sleep-disordered breathing in children is unknown.

Upper Airway Collapsibility

Upper airway stability and response to inspiratory loading are limited in the infant, but improve with maturation from preterm to full-term (28,29). In fact, upper-airway stability in prepubertal children is greater than in the adult (30).

B. Lung and Chest Wall Mechanics

Maturational changes in the mechanical properties of the chest wall influence the evolution of respiratory adaptation during sleep. In the preterm, the chest wall is so compliant that in conditions of mild load, the diaphragm dissipates a substantial fraction of its power pulling in the ribs rather than fresh air (31). Furthermore, mechanisms capable of stabilizing the thorax appear to be switched off in REM sleep, the predominant state of the preterm (32).

Growth results in major changes in rib cage geometry and composition. At birth, the ribs are composed mainly of cartilage and extend almost at right angles from the vertebral column. Consequently, the rib cage is more barrel-shaped than in adults and lacks mechanical efficiency (33). In adults, rib cage volume can be increased by elevating the ribs. In infants, the ribs are already elevated, so that rib cage motion contributes little to tidal volume in unstressed conditions. At 1 month of age, the contribution of the rib cage to tidal breathing is estimated at 34% during REM sleep (34). By 1 year of age, the rib cage contribution to tidal breathing is similar to that seen in adolescents during NREM sleep: 60% (4). Other maturational changes in chest wall mechanics include 1) progressive mineralization of the ribs and 2) a change from a flattened, horizontal diaphragm with a small zone of apposition to a more curved position with a larger area of apposition (35). These maturational changes in shape and structure play a central role in stiffening the rib cage and increasing mechanical efficiency.

Chest wall compliance relative to lung compliance is high in newborn mammals (36) but decreases with advancing postnatal age (37,38). Tonic contraction of the chest wall muscles augments the rigidity of the relatively compliant infant rib cage, which would otherwise be pulled inward by the contraction of the diaphragm. However, the compliant rib cage of the newborn is easily deformed when the diaphragm is vigorously contracted or when the stabilizing effect of the intercostal muscles is inhibited (32). During REM sleep, the intercostal muscles are inhibited and phasic inspiratory diaphragm contractions cause the rib cage to move inward rather than outward (32). In full-term newborns, rib cage distortion occurs during nearly 100% of REM sleep periods (39). With this distortion, other derangements occur in healthy preterm and/or full-term newborns, including 1) a decrease in transcutaneous partial pressure of O_2 (40) 2) an increase in the diaphragmatic work of breathing (41) and 3) a decrease in the functional residual capacity (FRC) (42,43). However, there is no consensus on the decrease in FRC during REM sleep in healthy newborns (32).

Chest wall compliance also has a major influence on maintenance of lung volume. In the newborn, chest wall compliance is relatively high relative to lung compliance and outward recoil of the chest wall is very small (36). Since FRC is defined as the static passive balance of forces between lung and chest wall, one might expect that the FRC in infants would be very small. Fortunately, the dynamic end-expiratory lung volume in newborns and infants is maintained substantially above the passively determined FRC (44). In contrast to the adult, expiration in the newborn is terminated at substantial flow rates suggesting active interruption of a passive expiration (44). Newborns use two mechanisms to actively slow expiration: 1) postinspiratory activity of the diaphragm and 2) laryngeal narrowing during expiration (45). However, it is well documented that expiratory airflow braking mechanisms are disabled during REM sleep in premature infants (46). Changes in end-expiratory lung volume associated with sleep state may be more marked in newborns than in older infants. The age at which the end-expiratory lung volume is no longer dynamically elevated above the passive FRC has been estimated to be 12 months (47).

REM sleep is the predominant state during early life. Full-term neonates spend more than 50% of their total sleep time in REM sleep, and REM sleep is even more prominent in premature infants. This places the newborn at increased risk for hypoxemia and airway collapse due to the mechanical disadvantage of a highly compliant chest wall. Chest wall muscle contraction helps stabilize the compliant infant rib cage; minimizing inward displacement of the rib cage diaphragmatic contraction. When the stabilizing effect of intercostal muscles is inhibited during REM sleep, paradoxical inward motion of the motion of the rib cage occurs during inspiration. After 6 months of age, the duration of inspiratory paradoxical rib cage motion during REM sleep decreases as postnatal age increases (48). Paradoxical motion is rare or absent after 3 years of age. In healthy adolescents, paradoxical movement of the rib cage was absent in REM sleep (4).

These maturation differences in the mechanical properties of the chest wall have clinical implications for children with underlying respiratory disorders associated with increased resistive loads. For example, young infants with croup or bronchopulmonary dysplasia experience thoracoabdominal asynchrony even during NREM sleep (49–51). As growth proceeds and the thoracic cage becomes less compliant, increases in resistive loads lead to increased activation of the inspiratory thoracic muscles, which maintains inspiratory rib cage movement (52). However, when inhibition of inspiratory intercostal muscles occurs during REM sleep or a greater negative pressure is needed during inspiration, the destabilized rib cage may move paradoxically (52). In chronic lung diseases such as cystic fibrosis, worsening of hypoxemia with thoracoabdominal asynchrony can occur during REM sleep (53).

The respiratory muscle recruitment strategies to increased mechanical respiratory loads depend on thoracoabdominal wall mechanics and state of wakefulness (54). With growth, there is a progressive change in bulk, fiber composition, fiber size, and oxidative capacity. Maximum pressures exerted by infants are surprisingly high compared to those of adults. Inspiratory and expiratory pressures of about 120 cmH_2O have been recorded during crying in normal infants (55). However, despite the relatively high maximal static inspiratory pressure, the inspiratory force reserve of respiratory muscles is reduced in infants with respect to adults because inspiratory pressure demand at rest is greater (54).

IV. Ventilation, Respiratory Pattern, and Apneas

In children, studies of respiration during sleep have focused mainly on respiratory frequency and apnea, whereas data on tidal volume and minute ventilation are scarce. Although there are extensive data about preterm and full-term infants in the first year of life, data on children and adolescents are limited. Furthermore, it is difficult to compare studies because measurement conditions and methods vary widely between studies.

Respiratory Frequency

The respiratory rate is high in the neonatal period and decreases during infancy and early childhood, until it reaches that of the adult (57). This observation is consistent with the well-known inverse relationship between resting respiratory rate and body size across mammalian species. Smaller, younger infants and children have higher respiratory rates per unit body weight than larger, older children. Respiratory rate decreases exponentially with increasing body weight (58). The changes in respiratory frequency with maturation are shown in Fig. 1. In general, respiratory frequency is higher during REM sleep than during NREM sleep in newborns and infants (1). In children, the respiratory frequency was lowest during stage 2 NREM sleep and during the second half of the night (59). In adolescents, respiratory frequency was highest and most variable during REM sleep and lowest during stages 3 and 4 NREM sleep (4). These sleep state differences are most prominent in infants, but clinically trivial in children and adolescents.

Tidal Volume and Minute Ventilation

Respiration is measured by minute ventilation, which is defined as the product of respiratory frequency and tidal volume. To increase minute ventilation, a child can increase the volume of each breath, the breathing frequency or both. In the newborn and young child, increasing respiratory rate (rather than tidal volume) is the most energy efficient strategy to cope with higher ventilation needs (60). This strategy of changing respiratory frequency rather than tidal volume agrees with data in resting humans showing that both tidal volume and dead space per body weight remains essentially unchanged from birth to adulthood (about 6 mL/kg for tidal volume and 2.2 mL/kg for dead space) (61).

The scant data on tidal volume and minute ventilation during sleep come only from newborn and adolescent age groups (1,4). In general, minute ventilation is slightly higher in REM than in NREM sleep, consistent with the higher respiratory rates in REM. As expected, minute ventilation decreases with age (from 250 mL/kg

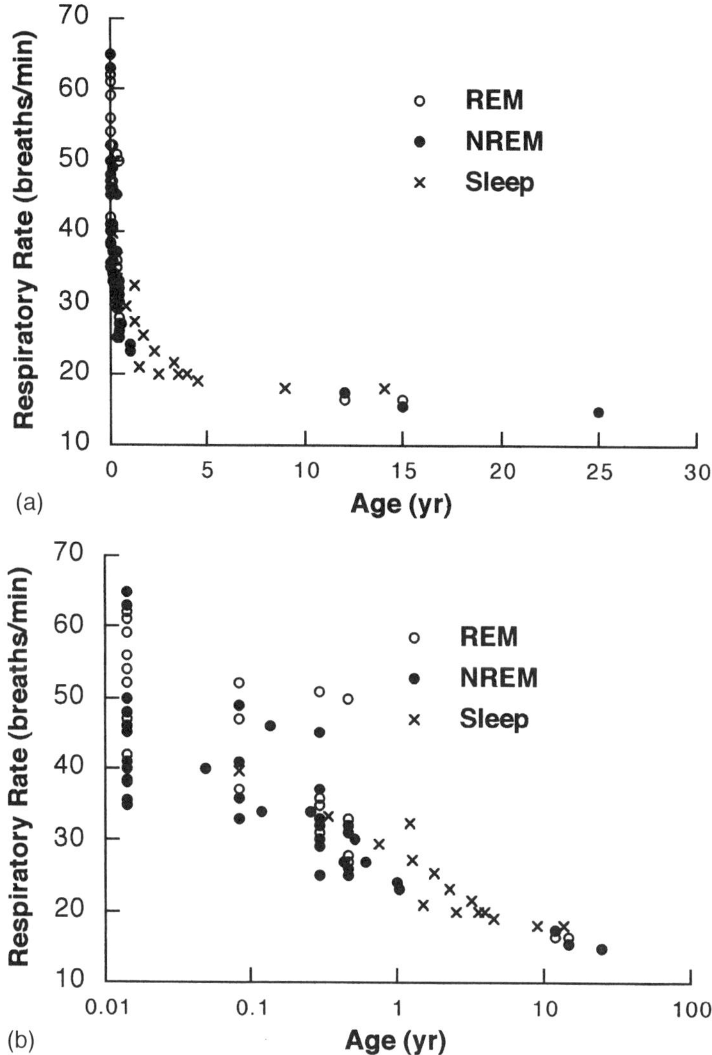

Figure 1 Respiratory rate changes with age. Data are mean, median, or 50th centile values extrapolated from references (4,59,63,64,94,98,139,157–172). If results in the original reference were summarized for a specific age range, then the midpoint of that age range was used to define data points for this graph. Specific sleep state is noted when available. Data from this graph are *not* meant to represent normative ranges. Data with a linear age axis (a). Data with a log age axis (b).

per minute in newborns to 100 mL/kg per minute in adolescents) and parallels the maturational changes in respiration frequency and metabolic needs.

Apnea Type, Duration, and Frequency

Numerous studies have investigated the occurrence and duration of apnea in newborns and infants in the first year of life. However, the varying methods and measurement condition make it difficult to compare data from different studies. Furthermore, not all studies attempted to characterize sleep states by neurophysiological criteria. In general, central apneas of short duration (less than 10 sec) are common in neonates and occur more often during REM than NREM sleep (62). A potential mechanism underlying the greater respiratory instability in infants during REM sleep compared to NREM sleep include the association of overall brainstem center immaturity with phasic inhibitory-excitatory mechanisms inherent to REM sleep (63).

A. Apnea in Preterm Infants

Preterm infants have significantly more apneic pauses and periodic breathing when they reach term than infants who are born at term (64,65), particularly if they have a previous history of apnea of prematurity (66). Apneas in preterm infants appear to be related to underlying oscillatory breathing patterns (67,68). The frequency of apneic pauses in preterm infants decreases by more than 80% between 40 and 52 weeks gestational age, by which time preterm infants have fewer apneic pauses than do term infants of similar gestational age (65). However, extremely preterm infants (gestational ages 24 to 28 weeks) experience persistent apneic and bradycardic episodes for longer time periods, frequently beyond term postconceptional age (69,70).

Obstructive and mixed apneas are more frequently seen in preterm than in full-term infants (65), but there is no consensus regarding the incidence of such events. In two studies, the incidence of obstructive apnea was found to be very low (64,71). In other studies, the incidence of obstructive apnea ranged from 6.5% to 14% of the total number of apneas and the percentage of mixed apnea ranged from 31% to 49.5% (68,72,73). The difficulty in distinguishing central apneas (no effort, no airflow) from obstructive apneas (effort, but no airflow) was highlighted in a study by Upton and colleagues (72). They found that airway closure (as detected by the absence of cardiogenic pulsations in the airflow signal) was present in 47% of "central apneas" and in 72% of mixed apnea in preterm infants at a mean gestational age of 29 weeks (72).

Upper-airway obstruction may be an important risk factor for apnea in preterm infants. Continuous positive airway pressure has been shown to selectively reduce obstructive apnea occurrence in preterm infants (74). Obstructive apnea decreases with increasing postconceptional age (75). This may be related to the improvement of extrathoracic airway stability with maturation (76). In addition, apneic pauses may be triggered by chronic hypoxemia or may themselves cause episodic hypoxemia. In healthy preterm infants, desaturation triggers for apnea decrease over time because of developmental improvements in chest wall stability (77) and in ventilation-perfusion matching (78).

B. Apnea in Full-Term Infants

In full-term infants, most apneas are central (79). Several studies have shown that obstructive and mixed apneas are rare in healthy infants (79–81). In full-term infants aged 3 weeks to 6 months, no obstructive apnea longer than 10 sec were recorded after 4.5 months (79). Obstructive apnea occurs mainly during REM sleep (82). The sleeping position (prone or supine) does not alter the incidence, duration, or type of apnea in healthy infants and infants with a history of apnea (83). The incidence of both central and obstructive apneas decreases with increasing postgestational age (75,79).

C. Periodic Breathing and Sighs

Periodic breathing is a common respiratory pattern in preterm infants that is usually not of clinical significance (84). It is defined as three episodes of apnea lasting longer than 3 sec, separated by continued respiration of 20 sec or less (85). This oscillatory breathing pattern is closely related to peripheral chemoreflex gain (86), temperature regulation (87), and other factors such as central chemosensitivity, circulation time, and sleep. Periodic breathing is more frequent in preterm infants, varies across studies in full-term infants, and decreases during the first year of life (1,85,88,89). Many factors can increase periodic breathing in neonates and infants, including hypoxia (90), hyperthermia (91), and sleep deprivation (92). Older studies suggesting that increased periodic breathing was a marker for increased risk of SIDS have been challenged (84,93,94).

Sighs are large (more than twice baseline tidal volume), augmented breaths that are necessary to reopen airways and recruit underventilated zones. Sighs are initiated by an inspiration-augmenting reflex arising in vagal afferents, probably from rapidly adapting pulmonary mechanoreceptors. This vagally mediated stimulus triggers an end-inspiratory reinforcement gasp that is superimposed near the peak of an apparently normal breath. Sighs are more frequent on the first days of life in preterm compared to term infants and in REM compared to quiet sleep (95,96). There is no strong association between sighs and apnea, with apnea being equally distributed either before or after a sigh. Hypoxia augments the frequency of sighs induced by airway occlusions (96). Sigh-related heart rate changes are dependent on maturation and behavioral state. In full-term and near-term infant, sighs during quiet sleep are accompanied by heart rate acceleration and then deceleration. During active (REM) sleep, only heart rate acceleration is observed. In 35- to 36-week preterm infants, only heart rate acceleration is observed in quiet or active sleep. In 31- to 34-week preterm infants, these heart rate changes are absent (97).

D. Apnea Beyond the First Year of Life

Respiratory pauses are a part of the normal pattern of breathing during sleep in children and adolescents. The frequency of respiratory pauses (as measured by impedance plethysmography) remains constant from ages 2 to 16 years (98) and is similar to that observed in healthy infants in the first year of life (99). However, the duration of the pauses increases with increasing age. Obstructive apneas of any length are rare in both normal full-term infants and children (1,79,100–103). Obstructive apneas occur mainly in REM and lighter NREM sleep. They can be associated with short total sleep time and frequent arousal (104–107).

Normative data for apneas in children beyond the first year of life and in which sleep state was monitored are summarized in Table 2 (4,59,103,104,108). The main findings of these studies are 1) obstructive apnea of any length is extremely rare and 2) central pauses are occasionally seen, including pauses up to 25 sec. Pauses are most commonly found in stage 1 NREM sleep followed by REM sleep (59,104). Further investigations are clearly needed to define normal respiratory behavior during sleep in children and to develop better criteria for the recognition of abnormal breathing patterns.

V. Gas Exchange and Metabolism

Most of our current information about gas exchange in sleeping children comes from noninvasive techniques such as pulse oximetry monitoring of oxygen saturation (Sp_{O_2}), transcutaneous monitoring of partial pressures of oxygen and carbon dioxide (Ptc_{O_2} and Ptc_{CO_2}, respectively), and end-tidal carbon dioxide monitoring of expired gases (Et_{CO_2}). There are considerable normative data on Sp_{O_2} values from infancy through adolescence but relatively little normative data on Et_{CO_2} values. Reliable Ptc_{O_2} and Ptc_{CO_2} values in older children and adolescents as estimates of arterial P_{O_2} and P_{CO_2} are limited by technical difficulties, although trend data may be useful in some clinical settings. Available data suggest that gas exchange during sleep improves with advancing postconceptional age.

During sleep in normal adults, there is an increase in P_{CO_2} of 3 to 7 mmHg, a decrease in P_{O_2} of 3 to 9 mmHg, and a decrease in Sp_{O_2} of 2%, as compared to wakefulness (3). Similar changes occur in normal children and adolescents, with a mean increase in Et_{CO_2} of 7 mmHg (103) and a decrease in Sa_{O_2} of 1% to 4% (3,4,103,109). These normal phenomena will be exaggerated in children with lung disease or upper-airway obstruction.

Sp_{O_2}

Over the past decade, considerable normative data for arterial oxygen saturation as measured by pulse oximetry (Sp_{O_2}) were obtained in healthy preterm and full-term infants. Preterm infants (29 to 34 weeks gestation) without cardiorespiratory disease have a mean sleeping Sp_{O_2} of 92% ± 3% (range, 86% to 96%) (110). Oxygenation improves with increasing postconceptional age rather than postnatal age (110). The baseline sleeping Sp_{O_2} of preterm infants measured at term is usually the same as that of normal full-term infants (110). Oxygenation is lowest during the first week of life (111) and increases over the next 1 to 3 months (112). Some 95% of older preterm

Table 2 Normative Respiratory Data During Nocturnal Sleep in Children

Source	Carskadon (173)	Guilleminault (174)	Tabachnick (175)	Marcus (176)	Acebo (177)
No. of children	22	27	9	50	45
Ages (years)	9–13	2–16	12–17	1–17	9–16
Apnea definition by length (sec)	>5	>10	>10	Central, >10 Mixed, >4 Obstructive, all	>10
Apnea types seen	Central only	Central only	Central only	Central Obstructive	Defined by absent airflow
No. of apneas	3–40 per study	<5 per study	5.5 per study	Obstructive 0.1 ± 0.5 per hr Range: 0–3.1 per hr	1–5.4 per hr
Apnea duration (sec)	7–10 (mean range)	—	—	Range: Central, 10–18 Obstructive, <10	14.1 ± 2.5 (mean ± SD)
Longest apnea (sec)	Central, 25	—	Central, 24	Central, 26 Obstructive, 10	≤30
Sleep stages with apnea	Stage 1 NREM REM	Stage 1 NREM REM	Stage 2 REM	Staging by EOG and behavior	NREM REM

infants had baseline Sp_{O_2} values between 95% and 100%, and 95% of term infants studied during the first 4 weeks of life had values between 92% and 100%; all term infants studied at 2 to 12 months of age had values between 97% and 100% (99, 113–117). Brief desaturations frequently occur in association with central apnea or periodic breathing in normal infants (111,116). Hourly transient desaturations to <80% occurring in conjunction with short central apneas, were seen in 80% of the 1- to 2-month-old infants studied (116).

Gestational age influences the development of stability in arterial oxygenation. Although healthy preterm infants have baseline Sp_{O_2} values in the same range as full-term infants, the variability about that baseline is greater in preterm infants. During the regular breathing of quiet (NREM) sleep, most infants do not have episodes of desaturation or when episodes do occur, they are brief. In contrast, during active (REM) sleep, the brief apneic pauses are more likely to be associated with a desaturation. The frequency of transient desaturation episodes to ≤80% varies considerably with age and between individual patients, with rates being highest in preterm infants and lowest in term infants studied at around 1 year of age (113,114,116,117). Although infrequent, desaturation episodes occurred in 68% of preterm infants ready for discharge. Similarly, 60% of full-term infants had desaturation episodes in the first 2 to 4 weeks of life, but this decreased to 16% of term infants by 6 weeks of life. The majority of these episodes were associated with pauses in respiratory efforts, often during periods of irregular breathing. Sleeping position does not influence baseline oxygen saturation or frequency of intermittent episodes of desaturation in non-preterm infants (83,118–120), although infants sleep more when placed in the prone position (83).

In healthy children 2 to 16 years of age, the frequency of transient desaturations is much lower than in infants and decreases with advancing age (98). Desaturation episodes to ≤ 80% disappear. Using a desaturation criteria of ≤ 90%, the majority of children (63%) did not show any episodes of desaturation. During sleep, normal children and adolescents rarely show more than an 8% drop in Sp_{O_2} (4,103,109), more than four desaturations episodes per hour (103,121), or an Sp_{O_2} nadir below 90% (103,108).

This increased stability in oxygenation may be explained by developmental changes in the relationship between lung volume and oxygen consumption. Infants have a highly compliant chest wall, resulting in a functional residual capacity that is significantly lower than that of adults when compared on the basis of metabolism (122). Lung volume in infants decreases even further during apneic pauses (123) and during REM sleep (42). Since lung volume at the onset of breath-holding is a major determinant of the severity of resulting hypoxemia, the increase in the stability of oxygenation with age is likely due to increased and more stable lung volumes relative to oxygen consumption in the older child.

Carbon Dioxide

There is little information about partial pressure of carbon dioxide during sleep in children. Both transcutaneous CO_2 (Ptc_{CO_2}) and end-tidal CO_2 (Et_{CO_2}) measurements have been used to estimate arterial P_{CO_2}, and each method has advantages and disadvantages (124). Transcutaneous P_{CO_2} values during sleep changed little with postnatal age during the first 18 months of life (94,112). Basal P_{CO_2} values during sleep are generally between 36 to 42 mmHg in newborns and infants (1), but few data exist for older children and adolescents. Normal children have shown an increase in Et_{CO_2} values of 4 to 10 mmHg during sleep (103). In 50 normal children ranging in age from 1.1 to 17.4 years, the mean maximal Et_{CO_2} value during sleep was 46 ± 4 mmHg (range, 38 to 53) (103). Statistically, the P_{CO_2} values are lower in REM than NREM sleep, but clinically this 1 to 2 mmHg difference is trivial.

VI. Ventilatory and Arousal Responses

Ventilatory and arousal responses are modified during sleep, but most of these data come from studies in adults. Compared to the awake state, hypoxic and hypercapnic ventilatory drives decrease during NREM sleep, and decrease even further during REM sleep (125). Hypercapnia and airway occlusion are potent stimuli to arousal in humans of all ages (125,126). In contrast, hypoxia is a poor stimulus to arousal (125,127).

Ventilatory Responses

In the newborn, steady state hypoxia produces a transient increase in ventilation followed by a decrease back to or below the baseline level. This biphasic response to hypoxia changes to a sustained ventilatory response with maturation. In contrast, the newborn has a sustained ventilatory response to hypercapnia (2). Hypercapnic and hypoxic ventilatory responses during wakefulness are highest in childhood and then decrease through adolescence into adulthood (128–130). With increasing age, peripheral chemoreceptors undergo progressive decrements in their relative sensitivity to hypoxia through childhood until maturation is complete during early adulthood (131,132). Furthermore, there are developmental changes in ventilatory responses depending on how the stimulus is presented (133).

Studies of ventilatory differences between sleep states have been examined only in newborns. In preterm infants, hypoxic ventilatory responses are smaller in REM compared to NREM sleep (134). For hypercapnic ventilatory responses, the data have been conflicting (2), but studies using the rebreathing technique consistently show significantly reduced ventilatory responses to CO_2 during REM compared to NREM sleep (135–138).

Arousal Responses

Arousal from sleep is the most important protective response to dangerous conditions during sleep. Arousal responses to hypoxia, hypercapnia, airway occlusion, gastroesophageal reflux, airway irritants, and noise as well as spontaneous arousals have been studied in infants. Some stimuli, for example, hypoxia and hypercapnia, can interact to amplify the response. It is unclear whether arousal responses change with maturation because of the different criteria used to define arousals and the variety of stimuli used to trigger arousals. For a more detailed evaluation of arousal, see Chap. 4.

Behavioral arousal to hypercapnic stimuli has been studied in healthy infants and young children during NREM sleep (126,139,140). Hypercapnia is a potent stimulus causing arousal from NREM sleep. All tested infants and young children had behavioral arousal from sleep when the end-tidal P_{CO_2} was raised to between 48 and 52 mmHg. In one study examining ventilatory responses to CO_2 in preterm infants, behavioral arousal occurred in only one-third of tests during REM sleep versus 93% during NREM sleep (137).

Compared to hypercapnia, hypoxia is less effective in causing arousal from sleep. Several studies have reported the incidence of behavioral arousal during NREM sleep in response to hypoxic stimuli (127,139–141). These findings are quite variable. One study on healthy infants (mean age, 8.4 months) found that arousal consistently occurred to a hypoxic challenge (140). However, the proportion of infants who aroused was much lower in the other studies, ranging from 32% to 70%.

Arousal from sleep is thought to be a principal determinant in the termination of apnea, although the mechanism is incompletely understood. Mechanoreceptor feedback is thought to play an important role in adults (142,143), but there are no data on the role of these receptors in children. Arousal can be accompanied by cortical electroencephalographic (EEG) changes, autonomic phenomena (heart rate or blood pressure changes) or body movements. The occurrence of behavioral arousals was studied in term infants and preterm infants with and without apnea. Fewer than 10% of apnea episodes ended with an arousal (144). Furthermore, behavioral arousals were more commonly associated with long versus short, mixed versus central, and severe versus mild apnea (144). In prepubertal children with obstructive sleep apnea syndrome, only 12% of obstructive sleep apneas in NREM sleep were terminated with EEG arousal and the remainder with a movement arousal (105). In REM sleep, all obstructive apneas ended with a movement arousal (105). Using only EEG criteria for arousal, McNamara and colleagues examined the arousal pattern following central and obstructive breathing abnormalities in infants and children (107). They found that the majority of respiratory events were not terminated with arousal. In children (mean age, 5 years), arousal terminated slightly more than one-third of respiratory events in either REM or NREM sleep. In infants (mean age 9 weeks), the percentage was even lower—around 8%. In both age groups, respiratory related arousals occurred more frequently after obstructive compared to central events. In contrast, other investigators using both EEG and movement criteria concluded that most obstructive events in children were terminated by arousal (106).

Other stimuli can lead to arousal from sleep in infants. The importance of arousal from sleep in facilitating acid clearance from the esophagus has been demonstrated in adults (145). In a sleeping infant with a history of an apparent life-threatening event, behavioral arousals did not occur after a reflux episode, but 50% of the reflux episodes were preceded by an arousal (146). In near-term infants, the esophageal acid infusion test induced increases in the frequency and duration of EEG arousals during REM sleep (147). Auditory arousal thresholds decrease with maturation between 44 and 52 weeks postconceptional age (148). Finally, other factors may decrease arousability such as prone position (83) and phenothiazines (149).

VII. Relationships Between Apnea, Bradycardia, and Desaturation

Bradycardia, apnea, and hypoxemia are closely related in preterm infants. However, the precise mechanisms underlying these relationships remain controversial (150). In preterm infants, 83% of bradycardic episodes were associated with apnea and 86% with desaturation (151). There is a rapid onset of bradycardia after the start of the apnea, consistent with a reflex mechanism similar to that seen after breath-holding. This deceleration is likely due to the absence of lung inflation, a stimulus usually responsible for heart rate acceleration in the face of a vagally mediated reflex (24). Sleep state exerts a measurable influence on the heart rate changes during apneas in healthy full-term infants studied from 1 to 4 months of age (152). Apneas were more likely to be associated with a fall in heart rate during NREM sleep than during REM sleep.

Hypoxia also enhances reflex bradycardia during apnea (23). The direct, inhibitory effects of peripheral chemoreceptors on heart rate are normally counteracted by influences from the pulmonary stretch receptors (153). The Sa_{O_2} level before an apneic event also has a profound effect on the degree of bradycardia. Thus, maintaining the baseline Sa_{O_2} at an optimum value may be effective in preventing or limiting severe bradycardia that can accompany an apneic event.

Other reflex bradycardia episodes can occur in response to vagal stimuli in preterm infants. In studying a variety of reflexes, Ramet and colleagues found that these responses are usually more pronounced during REM than NREM sleep because sympathetic activity is enhanced in REM (27,154,155). Sympathetic activity amplifies the cardiodepressant effect of direct vagal stimulation. Furthermore, the cardiac deceleration in response to vagal stimulation becomes increasing blunted with advancing postconceptional age in healthy infants during REM sleep.

The regulation of breathing during sleep is predominantly influenced by chemical control, and oxygen levels change far more rapidly than carbon dioxide levels (156). The proportion of apneic pauses leading to desaturation is extremely variable and depends not only on the duration of the pause but also on the breathing pattern in which it occurs (116). Furthermore, desaturation can also occur without complete cessation of breathing movements, airflow, or both. This observation has important implications for monitoring vulnerable infants. In a study of well preterm infants (mean gestational age, 35 weeks) in the first days of life, only 2% of the prolonged desaturation episodes ($\leq$ 80% Sp_{O_2} lasting > 20 sec) were associated with an apneic pause of 20 sec or longer and only 16% with a bradycardia event that would have triggered an alarm from a cardiorespiratory monitor (115).

VIII. Summary

Respiratory adaptation during sleep changes with growth and development as a result of maturation of the mechanics of the respiratory pump and the respiratory control center. The last three decades have expanded our knowledge of normal development of cardiorespiratory adaptation to sleep. However, the paucity of data beyond infancy continues to hinder our understanding in this field. Furthermore, the numerous techniques developed to characterize sleep and quantitate breathing at different ages make it difficult to compare data from different studies and to identify developmental changes. Multicenter investigations using standardized methods are needed to gather additional normative data beyond the infant age group. One major reason for the lack of data on young children is that the tools for physiological measurements of sleep and respiration are often poorly tolerated. For example, even a simple nasal cannula for end-tidal carbon dioxide measurement may be unacceptable to a young child. Development of improved noninvasive techniques will facilitate studies in children. Standards for normal pediatric respiratory parameters during sleep have not been established. Continued research in this area is important to better define normal respiratory behavior and to better identify abnormal conditions.

References

1. Gaultier C. Respiratory adaptation during sleep from the neonatal period to adolescence. In: Guilleminault C, ed. Sleep and Its Disorders in Children. New York: Raven Press, 1987: 67–97.
2. Gaultier C. Cardiorespiratory adaptation during sleep in infants and children. Pediatr Pulmonol 1995; 19(2):105–117.
3. Krieger J. Breathing during sleep in normal subjects. In: Kryger M, Roth T, Dement W, eds. Principles and Practice of Sleep Medicine. 2d ed. Philadelphia: Saunders, 1994: 212–223.
4. Tabachnik E, Muller NL, Bryan AC, Levison H. Changes in ventilation and chest wall mechanics during sleep in normal adolescents. J Appl Physiol 1981; 51(3):557–564.
5. Hudgel DW, Devadatta P. Decrease in functional residual capacity during sleep in normal humans. J Appl Physiol 1984; 57(5):1319–1322.
6. Hudgel DW, Martin RJ, Johnson B, Hill P. Mechanics of the respiratory system and breathing pattern during sleep in normal humans. J Appl Physiol 1984; 56(1):133–137.
7. Lopes JM, Tabachnik E, Muller NL, Levison H, Bryan AC. Total airway resistance and respiratory muscle activity during sleep. J Appl Physiol 1983; 54(3):773–777.
8. Moss M. The veloepiglottic sphincter and obligate nose breathing in the neonate. J Pediatr 1965; 67:330–331.
9. Rodenstein DO, Perlmutter N, Stanescu DC. Infants are not obligatory nasal breathers. Am Rev Respir Dis 1985; 131(3):343–347.
10. Miller MJ, Martin RJ, Carlo WA, Fouke JM, Strohl KP, Fanaroff AA. Oral breathing in newborn infants. J Pediatr 1985; 107(3):465–469.
11. Rodenstein DO, Stanescu DC. The soft palate and breathing. Am Rev Respir Dis 1986; 134(2):311–325.

12. Shaw EB. Sudden unexpected death in infancy syndrome. Am J Dis Child 1970; 119(5):416–418.
13. Miller MJ, Carlo WA, Strohl KP, Fanaroff AA, Martin RJ. Effect of maturation on oral breathing in sleeping premature infants. J Pediatr 1986; 109(3):515–519.
14. de Almeida V, Alvaro R, al-Alaiyan S, Haider Z, Rehan V, Cates D, Nowaczyk B, Kwiatkowski K, Rigatto H. Prevalence and characterization of spontaneous oral breathing in preterm infants. Am J Perinatol 1995; 12(3):185–188.
15. Swift PG, Emery JL. Clinical observations on response to nasal occlusion in infancy. Arch Dis Child 1973; 48(12):947–951.
16. Purcell M. Response in the newborn to raised upper airway resistance. Arch Dis Child 1976; 51(8):602–607.
17. Haddad GG, Mellins RB. The role of airway receptors in the control of respiration in infants: a review. J Pediatr 1977; 91(2):281–286.
18. Fisher JT, Sant'Ambrogio G. Airway and lung receptors and their reflex effects in the newborn. Pediatr Pulmonol 1985; 1(2):112–126.
19. Davies AM, Koenig JS, Thach BT. Upper airway chemoreflex responses to saline and water in preterm infants. J Appl Physiol 1988; 64(4):1412–1420.
20. Pickens DL, Schefft G, Thach BT. Prolonged apnea associated with upper airway protective reflexes in apnea of prematurity. Am Rev Respir Dis 1988; 137(1):113–118.
21. Wennergren G, Bjure J, Hertzberg T, Lagercrantz H, Milerad J. Laryngeal reflex. Acta Paediatr Suppl 1993; 82(suppl 389):53–56.
22. Pickens DL, Schefft GL, Storch GA, Thach BT. Characterization of prolonged apneic episodes associated with respiratory syncytial virus infection. Pediatr Pulmonol 1989; 6(3):195–201.
23. Wennergren G, Hertzberg T, Milerad J, Bjure J, Lagercrantz H. Hypoxia reinforces laryngeal reflex bradycardia in infants. Acta Paediatr Scand 1989; 78(1):11–17.
24. Daly MD, Angell-James JE, Elsner R. Role of carotid-body chemoreceptors and their reflex interactions in bradycardia and cardiac arrest. Lancet 1979; 1(8119):764–767.
25. Pickens DL, Schefft GL, Thach BT. Pharyngeal fluid clearance and aspiration preventive mechanisms in sleeping infants. J Appl Physiol 1989; 66(3):1164–1171.
26. Allen LG, Howard G, Smith JB, McCubbin JA, Weaver RL. Infant heart rate response to trigeminal airstream stimulation: determination of normal and deviant values. Pediatr Res 1979; 13(3):184–187.
27. Ramet J, Praud JP, D'Allest AM, Dehan M, Gaultier C. Trigeminal airstream stimulation: Maturation-related cardiac and respiratory responses during REM sleep in human infants. Chest 1990; 98(1):92–96.
28. Duara S, Silva Neto G, Claure N. Role of respiratory muscles in upper airway narrowing induced by inspiratory loading in preterm infants. J Appl Physiol 1994; 77(1):30–36.
29. Duara S, Rojas M, Claure N. Upper airway stability and respiratory muscle activity during inspiratory loading in full-term neonates. J Appl Physiol 1994; 77(1):37–42.
30. Marcus CL, McColley SA, Carroll JL, Loughlin GM, Smith PL, Schwartz AR. Upper airway collapsibility in children with obstructive sleep apnea syndrome. J Appl Physiol 1994; 77(2):918–924.
31. Davis GM, Coates Al, Papageorgiou A, Bureau MA. Direct measurement of static chest wall compliance in animal and human neonates. J Appl Physiol 1988; 65(3):1093–1098.
32. England S, Gaultier C, Bryan A. Chest wall mechanics in the newborn. In: Roussos C, ed. The Thorax, Lung Biology in Health and Disease. 2d ed. New York: Marcel Dekker, 1995:1541–1556.

33. Openshaw P, Edwards S, Helms P. Changes in rib cage geometry during childhood. Thorax 1984; 39(8):624–627.
34. Hershenson MB, Colin AA, Wohl ME, Stark AR. Changes in the contribution of the rib cage to tidal breathing during infancy. Am Rev Respir Dis 1990; 141(4 pt 1):922–925.
35. Devlieger H, Daniels H, Marchal G, Moerman P, Casaer P, Eggermont E. The diaphragm of the newborn infant: anatomical and ultrasonographic studies. J Dev Physiol 1991; 16(6):321–329.
36. Agostini E. Volume-pressure relationship to the thorax and lung in the newborn. J Appl Physiol 1959; 14:909–913.
37. Gerhardt T, Bancalari E. Chest wall compliance in full-term and premature infants. Acta Paediatr Scand 1980; 69(3):359–364.
38. Sharp JT, Druz WS, Balagot RC, Bandelin VR, Danon J. Total respiratory compliance in infants and children. J Appl Physiol 1970; 29(6):775–779.
39. Curzi-Dascalova L. Thoraco-abdominal respiratory correlations in infants: constancy and variability in different sleep states. Early Hum Dev 1978; 2(1):25–38.
40. Martin RJ, Okken A, Rubin D. Arterial oxygen tension during active and quiet sleep in the normal neonate. J Pediatr 1979; 94(2):271–274.
41. Guslits BG, Gaston SE, Bryan MH, England SJ, Bryan AC. Diaphragmatic work of breathing in premature human infants. J Appl Physiol 1987; 62(4):1410–1415.
42. Henderson-Smart DJ, Read DJ. Reduced lung volume during behavioral active sleep in the newborn. J Appl Physiol 1979; 46(6):1081–1085.
43. Walti H, Moriette G, Radvanyi-Bouvet MF, Chaussain M, Morel-Kahn F, Pajot N, Relier JP. Influence of breathing pattern on functional residual capacity in sleeping newborn infants. J Dev Physiol 1986; 8(3):167–172.
44. Kosch PC, Stark AR. Dynamic maintenance of end-expiratory lung volume in full-term infants. J Appl Physiol 1984; 57(4):1126–1233.
45. Kosch PC, Hutchinson AA, Wozniak JCWA, Stark AR. Posterior cricoarytenoid and diaphragm activities during tidal breathing in neonates. J Appl Physiol 1988; 64(5):1968–1978.
46. Stark AR, Cohlan BA, Waggener TB, Frantz ID III, Kosch PC. Regulation of end-expiratory lung volume during sleep in premature infants. J Appl Physiol 1987; 62(3):1117–1123.
47. Colin AA, Wohl ME, Mead J, Ratjen FA, Glass G, Stark AR. Transition from dynamically maintained to relaxed end-expiratory volume in human infants. J Appl Physiol 1989; 67(5):2107–2111.
48. Gaultier C, Praud JP, Canet E, Delaperche MF, D'Allest AM. Paradoxical inward rib cage motion during rapid eye movement sleep in infants and young children. J Dev Physiol 1987; 9(5):391–397.
49. Sivan Y, Deakers TW, Newth CJ. Thoracoabdominal asynchrony in acute upper airway obstruction in small children. Am Rev Respir Dis 1990; 142(3):540–544.
50. Allen JL, Wolfson MR, McDowell K, Shaffer TH. Thoracoabdominal asynchrony in infants with airflow obstruction. Am Rev Respir Dis 1990; 141(2):337–342.
51. Allen JL, Greenspan JS, Deoras KS, Keklikian E, Wolfson MR, Shaffer TH. Interaction between chest wall motion and lung mechanics in normal infants and infants with bronchopulmonary dysplasia. Pediatr Pulmonol 1991; 11(1):37–43.
52. Goldman MD, Pagani M, Trang HT, Praud JP, Sartene R, Gaultier C. Asynchronous chest wall movements during non-rapid eye movement and rapid eye movement sleep

in children with bronchopulmonary dysplasia. Am Rev Respir Dis 1993; 147(5): 1175–1184.

53. Muller NL, Francis PW, Gurwits D, Levison H, Bryan AC. Mechanism of hemoglobin desaturation during rapid-eye-movement sleep in normal subjects and in patients with cystic fibrosis. Am Rev Respir Dis 1980; 121(3):463–469.
54. Gaultier C. Respiratory muscle function in infants. Eur Respir J 1995; 8(1):150–153.
55. Shardonofsky FR, Perez-Chada D, Carmuega E, Milic-Emili J. Airway pressures during crying in healthy infants. Pediatr Pulmonol 1989; 6(1):14–18.
57. Iliff A, Lee V. Pulse rate, respiratory rate and coding temperature of children between two months and eighteen years of age. Child Dev 1952; 23:237–252.
58. Gagliardi L, Rusconi F. Respiratory rate and body mass in the first three years of life: the working party on respiratory rate. Arch Dis Child 1997; 76(2):151–154.
59. Carskadon MA, Harvey K, Dement WC, Guilleminault C, Simmons B, Anders TF. Respiration during sleep in children. West J Med 1978; 128:477–481.
60. Mortola JP. Some functional mechanical implications of the structural design of the respiratory system in newborn mammals. Am Rev Respir Dis 1983; 128(2 pt 2): S69–S72.
61. Polgar G, Weng TR. The functional development of the respiratory system from the period of gestation to adulthood. Am Rev Respir Dis 1979; 120(3):625–695.
62. Gaultier C. Apnea and sleep state in newborns and infants. Biol Neonate 1994; 65(3–4): 231–234.
63. Haddad GG, Epstein RA, Epstein MA, Leistner HL, Marino PA, Mellins RB. Maturation of ventilation and ventilatory pattern in normal sleeping infants. J Appl Physiol 1979; 46(5):998–1002.
64. Curzi-Dascalova L, Christova-Gueorguieva E. Respiratory pauses in normal prematurely born infants: a comparison with full-term newborns. Biol Neonate 1983; 44(6): 325–332.
65. Albani M, Bentele KH, Budde C, Schulte FJ. Infant sleep apnea profile: preterm vs. term infants. Eur J Pediatr 1985; 143(4):261–268.
66. Hageman JR, Holmes D, Suchy S, Hunt CE. Respiratory patterns at hospital discharge in asymptomatic preterm infants. Pediatr Pulmonol 1988; 4(2):78–83.
67. Waggener TB, Stark AR, Cohlan BA, Frantz ID III. Apnea duration is related to ventilatory oscillation characteristics in newborn infants. J Appl Physiol 1984; 57(2): 536–544.
68. Waggener TB, Frantz ID III, Cohlan BA, Stark AR. Mixed and obstructive apneas are related to ventilatory oscillations in premature infants. J Appl Physiol 1989; 66(6): 2818–2826.
69. Barrington KJ, Finer N, Li D. Predischarge respiratory recordings in very low birth weight newborn infants. J Pediatr 1996; 129(6):934–940.
70. Eichenwald EC, Aina A, Stark AR. Apnea frequently persists beyond term gestation in infants delivered at 24 to 28 weeks. Pediatrics 1997; 100(3 pt 1):354–359.
71. Thach BT, Stark AR. Spontaneous neck flexion and airway obstruction during apneic spells in preterm infants. J Pediatr 1979; 94(2):275–281.
72. Upton CJ, Milner AD, Stokes GM. Upper airway patency during apnoea of prematurity. Arch Dis Child 1992; 67(4 spec no):419–424.
73. Finer NN, Barrington KJ, Hayes BJ, Hugh A. Obstructive, mixed, and central apnea in the neonate: physiologic correlates. J Pediatr 1992; 121(6):943–950.

74. Miller MJ, Carlo WA, Martin RJ. Continuous positive airway pressure selectively reduces obstructive apnea in preterm infants. J Pediatr 1985; 106(1):91–94.
75. Hoppenbrouwers T, Hodgman JE, Cabal L. Obstructive apnea, associated patterns of movement, heart rate, and oxygenation in infants at low and increased risk for SIDS. Pediatr Pulmonol 1993; 15(1):1–12.
76. Duara S, Silva Neto G, Claure N, Gerhardt T, Bancalari E. Effect of maturation on the extrathoracic airway stability of infants. J Appl Physiol 1992; 73(6):2368–2372.
77. Heldt GP. Development of stability of the respiratory system in preterm infants. J Appl Physiol 1988; 65(1):441–444.
78. Woodrum DE, Oliver TK Jr, Hodson WA. The effect of prematurity and hyaline membrane disease on oxygen exchange in the lung. Pediatrics 1972; 50(3):380–386.
79. Guilleminault C, Ariagno R, Korobkin R, Nagel L, Baldwin R, Coons S, Owen M. Mixed and obstructive sleep apnea and near miss for sudden infant death syndrome: 2. Comparison of near miss and normal control infants by age. Pediatrics 1979; 64(6):882–891.
80. Flores-Guevara R, Plouin P, Curzi-Dascalova L, Radvanyi MF, Guidasci S, Pajot N, Monod N. Sleep apneas in normal neonates and infants during the first 3 months of life. Neuropediatrics 1982; 13(suppl):21–28.
81. Kahn A, Groswasser J, Sottiaux M, Rebuffat E, Sunseri M, Franco P, Dramaix M, Bochner A, Belhadi B, Foerster M. Clinical symptoms associated with brief obstructive sleep apnea in normal infants. Sleep 1993; 16(5):409–413.
82. Kahn A, Groswasser J, Rebuffat E, Sottiaux M, Blum D, Foerster M, Franco P, Bochner A, Alexander M, Bachy A, Richard P, Verghote M, Le Polain D, Wayenberg JL. Sleep and cardiorespiratory characteristics of infant victims of sudden death: a prospective case-control study. Sleep 1992; 15(4):287–292.
83. Kahn A, Groswasser J, Sottiaux M, Rebuffat E, Franco P, Dramaix M. Prone or supine body position and sleep characteristics in infants. Pediatrics 1993; 91(6):1112–1115.
84. Glotzbach SF, Baldwin RB, Lederer NE, Tansey PA, Ariagno RL. Periodic breathing in preterm infants: incidence and characteristics. Pediatrics 1989; 84(5):785–792.
85. Kelly DH, Stellwagen LM, Kaitz E, Shannon DC. Apnea and periodic breathing in normal full-term infants during the first twelve months. Pediatr Pulmonol 1985; 1(4): 215–219.
86. Cherniack NS, von Euler C, Homma I, Kao FF. Experimentally induced Cheyne-Stokes breathing. Respir Physiol 1979; 37(2):185–200.
87. Fleming PJ, Levine MR, Long AM, Cleave JP. Postneonatal development of respiratory oscillations. Ann NY Acad Sci 1988; 533:305–313.
88. Richards JM, Alexander JR, Shinebourne EA, de Swiet M, Wilson AJ, Southall DP. Sequential 22-hour profiles of breathing patterns and heart rate in 110 full-term infants during their first 6 months of life. Pediatrics 1984; 74(5):763–777.
89. Kelly DH, Riordan L, Smith MJ. Apnea and periodic breathing in healthy full-term infants, 12–18 months of age. Pediatr Pulmonol 1992; 13(3):169–171.
90. Manning DJ, Stothers JK. Sleep state, hypoxia and periodic breathing in the neonate. Acta Paediatr Scand 1991; 80(8–9):763–769.
91. Berterottiere D, D'Allest AM, Dehan M, Gaultier C. Effects of increase in body temperature on the breathing pattern in premature infants. J Dev Physiol 1990; 13(6): 303–308.
92. Canet E, Gaultier C, D'Allest AM, Dehan M. Effects of sleep deprivation on respiratory events during sleep in healthy infants. J Appl Physiol 1989; 66(3):1158–1163.

93. Glotzbach S, Ariagno R. Periodic breathing. In: Beckerman R, Brouillette R, Hunt C, eds. Respiratory Control Disorders in Infants and Children. Baltimore: Williams & Wilkins, 1992: 142–160.
94. Schäfer T, Schäfer D, Schlafke ME. Breathing, transcutaneous blood gases, and CO_2 response in SIDS siblings and control infants during sleep. J Appl Physiol 1993; 74(1): 88–102.
95. Thach BT, Taeusch HW Jr. Sighing in newborn human infants: role of inflation-augmenting reflex. J Appl Physiol 1976; 41(4):502–507.
96. Alvarez JE, Bodani J, Fajardo CA, Kwiatkowski K, Cates DB, Rigatto H. Sighs and their relationship to apnea in the newborn infant. Biol Neonate 1993; 63(3):139–146.
97. Eiselt M, Curzi-Dascalova L, Leffler C, Christova E. Sigh-related heart rate changes during sleep in premature and full-term newborns. Neuropediatrics 1992; 23(6):286–291.
98. Poets CF, Stebbens VA, Samuels MP, Southall DP. Oxygen saturation and breathing patterns in children. Pediatrics 1993; 92(5):686–690.
99. Poets CF, Stebbens VA, Southall DP. Arterial oxygen saturation and breathing movements during the first year of life. J Dev Physiol 1991; 15(6):341–345.
100. Guilleminault C. Obstructive sleep apnea and its treatment in children: areas of agreement and controversy. Pediatr Pulmonol 1987; 3:429–436.
101. Kahn A, Blum D, Rebuffat E, Sottiaux M, Levitt J, Bochner A, Alexander M, Grosswasser J, Muller MF. Polysomnographic studies of infants who subsequently died of sudden infant death syndrome. Pediatrics 1988; 82(5):721–727.
102. Kahn A, Mozin MJ, Burniat W, Shepherd S, Muller MF. Sleep pattern alterations and brief airway obstructions in overweight infants. Sleep 1989; 12(5):430–438.
103. Marcus CL, Omlin KJ, Basinki DJ, Bailey SL, Rachal AB, Von Pechmann WS, Keens TG, Ward SL. Normal polysomnographic values for children and adolescents. Am Rev Respir Dis 1992; 146(5 pt 1):1235–1239.
104. Guilleminault C, Korobkin R, Winkle R. A review of 50 children with obstructive sleep apnea syndrome. Lung 1981; 159:275–287.
105. Praud JP, D'Allest AM, Nedelcoux H, Curzi-Dascalova L, Guilleminault C, Gaultier C. Sleep-related abdominal muscle behavior during partial or complete obstructed breathing in prepubertal children. Pediatr Res 1989; 26(4):347–350.
106. Mograss MA, Ducharme FM, Brouillette RT. Movement/arousals: description, classification, and relationship to sleep apnea in children. Am J Respir Crit Care Med 1994; 150(6 pt 1):1690–1696.
107. McNamara F, Issa FG, Sullivan CE. Arousal pattern following central and obstructive breathing abnormalities in infants and children. J Appl Physiol 1996; 81(6):2651–2657.
108. Acebo C, Millman RP, Rosenberg C, Cavallo A, Carskadon MA. Sleep, breathing, and cephalometrics in older children and young adults: Part I. Normative values. Chest 1996; 109(3):664–672.
109. Chipps BE, Mak H, Schuberth KC, Talamo JH, Menkes HA, Scherr MS. Nocturnal oxygen saturation in normal and asthmatic children. Pediatrics 1980; 65:1157–1160.
110. Mok JY, Hak H, McLaughlin FJ, Pintar M, Canny GJ, Levison H. Effect of age and state of wakefulness on transcutaneous oxygen values in preterm infants: a longitudinal study. J Pediatr 1988; 113(4):706–709.
111. Mok JY, McLaughlin FJ, Pintar M, Hak H, Amaro-Galvez R, Levison H. Transcutaneous monitoring of oxygenation: what is normal? J Pediatr 1986; 108(3):365–371.
112. Hoppenbrouwers T, Hodgman JE, Arakawa K, Durand M, Cabal LA. Transcutaneous

oxygen and carbon dioxide during the first half year of life in premature and normal term infants. Pediatr Res 1992; 31(1):73–79.

113. Poets CF, Stebbens VAJR, Arrowsmith WA, Salfield SA, Southall DP. Oxygen saturation and breathing patterns in infancy. 2: Preterm infants at discharge from special care. Arch Dis Child 1991; 66(5):574–578.
114. Poets CF, Stebbens VA, Alexander JR, Arrowsmith WA, Salfield SA, Southall DP. Arterial oxygen saturation in preterm infants at discharge from the hospital and six weeks later. J Pediatr 1992; 120(3):447–454.
115. Richard D, Poets CF, Neale S, Stebbens VA, Alexander JR, Southall DP. Arterial oxygen saturation in preterm neonates without respiratory failure. J Pediatr 1993; 123(6):963–968.
116. Stebbens VA, Poets CF, Alexander JR, Arrowsmith WA, Southall DP. Oxygen saturation and breathing patterns in infancy: 1. Full term infants in the second month of life. Arch Dis Child 1991; 66(5):569–573.
117. Poets CF, Stebbens VA, Lang JA, O'Brien LM, Boon AW, Southall DP. Arterial oxygen saturation in healthy term neonates. Eur J Pediatr 1996; 155(3):219–223.
118. Peirano P, Guidasci S, Monod N. Effect of sleep position on transcutaneous oxygen tension in SIDS siblings. Early Hum Dev 1986; 13(3):303–312.
119. Levene S, McKenzie SA. Transcutaneous oxygen saturation in sleeping infants: prone and supine. Arch Dis Child 1990; 65(5):524–526.
120. Poets CF, Rudolph A, Neuber K, Buch U, von der Hardt H. Arterial oxygen saturation in infants at risk of sudden death: influence of sleeping position. Acta Paediatr 1995; 84(4):379–382.
121. Stradling JR, Thomas G, Warley AR, Williams P, Freeland A. Effect of adenotonsillectomy on nocturnal hypoxaemia, sleep disturbance, and symptoms in snoring children. Lancet 1990; 335(8684):249–253.
122. Cook C, Cherry R, O'Brien D, Karlberg P, Smith C. Studies of the respiratory physiology in the newborn infant: 1. Observation on normal premature and full-term infants. J Clin Invest 1955; 34:975–982.
123. Olinsky A, Bryan MH, Bryan AC. Influence of lung inflation on respiratory control in neonates. J Appl Physiol 1974; 36(4):426–429.
124. Morielli A, Desjardins D, Brouill Hospital QC. Transcutaneous and end-tidal carbon dioxide pressures should be measured during pediatric polysomnography. Am Rev Respir Dis 1993; 148(6 pt 1):1599–1604.
125. Douglas N. Control of ventilation during sleep. In: Kryger M, Roth T, Dement W, eds. Principles and Practice of Sleep Medicine, 2d ed. Philadelphia: Saunders, 1994:204–211.
126. Marcus CL, Bautista DB, Amihyia A, Ward SL, Keens TG. Hypercapneic arousal responses in children with congenital central hypoventilation syndrome. Pediatrics 1991; 88(5):993–998.
127. Ward SL, Bautista DB, Keens TG. Hypoxic arousal responses in normal infants. Pediatrics 1992; 89(5 pt 1):860–864.
128. Honda Y, Ohyabu Y, Sato M, Masuyama H, Nishibayashi Y, Maruyama R, Tanaka Y, Nakajo I, Shirase H, Hayashida K. Hypercapnic and hypoxic ventilatory responses during growth. Jpn J Physiol 1986; 36(1):177–187.
129. Gratas-Delamarche A, Mercier J, Ramonatxo M, Dassonville J, Prefaut C. Ventilatory response of prepubertal boys and adults to carbon dioxide at rest and during exercise. Eur J Appl Physiol 1993; 66(1):25–30.

130. Marcus CL, Glomb WB, Basinski DJ, Davidson SL, Keens TG. Developmental pattern of hypercapnic and hypoxic ventilatory responses from childhood to adulthood (see comments). J Appl Physiol 1994; 76(1):314–320.
131. Cooper DM, Kaplan MR, Baumgarten L, Weiler-Ravell D, Whipp BJ, Wasserman K. Coupling of ventilation and CO_2 production during exercise in children. Pediatr Res 1987; 21(6):568–572.
132. Springer C, Cooper DM, Wasserman K. Evidence that maturation of the peripheral chemoreceptors is not complete in childhood. Respir Physiol 1988; 74(1): 55–64.
133. Gozal D, Arens R, Omlin KJ, Marcus CL, Keens TG. Maturational differences in step vs. ramp hypoxic and hypercapnic ventilatory responses. J Appl Physiol 1994; 76(5):1968–1975.
134. Rigatto H, Kalapesi Z, Leahy FN, Durand M, MacCallum M, Cates D. Ventilatory response to 100% and 15% O_2 during wakefulness and sleep in preterm infants. Early Hum Dev 1982; 7(1):1–10.
135. Homma Y, Wilkes D, Bryan MH, Bryan AC. Rib cage and abdominal contributions to ventilatory response to CO_2 in infants. J Appl Physiol 1984; 56(5):1211–1216.
136. Moriette G, Van Reempts P, Moore M, Cates D, Rigatto H. The effect of rebreathing CO_2 on ventilation and diaphragmatic electromyography in newborn infants. Respir Physiol 1985; 62(3):387–397.
137. Praud JP, Egreteau L, Benlabed M, Curzi-Dascalova L, Nedelcoux H, Gaultier C. Abdominal muscle activity during CO_2 rebreathing in sleeping neonates. J Appl Physiol 1991; 70(3):1344–1350.
138. Cohen G, Xu C, Henderson-Smart D. Ventilatory response of the sleeping newborn to CO_2 during normoxic rebreathing (see comments). J Appl Physiol 1991; 71(1):168–174.
139. McCulloch K, Brouillette RT, Guzzetta AJ, Hunt CE. Arousal responses in near-miss sudden infant death syndrome and in normal infants. J Pediatr 1982; 101(6):911–917.
140. van der Hal AL, Rodriguez AM, Sargent CW, Platzker AC, Keens TG. Hypoxic and hypercapneic arousal responses and prediction of subsequent apnea in apnea of infancy. Pediatrics 1985; 75(5):848–854.
141. Milerad J, Hertzberg T, Wennergren G, Lagercrantz H. Respiratory and arousal responses to hypoxia in apnoeic infants reinvestigated. Eur J Pediatr 1989; 148(6): 565–570.
142. Gleeson K, Zwillich CW, White DP. The influence of increasing ventilatory effort on arousal from sleep. Am Rev Respir Dis 1990; 142(2):295–300.
143. Kimoff RJ, Cheong TH, Olha AE, Charbonneau M, Levy RD, Cosio MG, Gottfried SB. Mechanisms of apnea termination in obstructive sleep apnea: role of chemoreceptor and mechanoreceptor stimuli. Am J Respir Crit Care Med 1994; 149(3 pt 1):707–714.
144. Thoppil CK, Belan MA, Cowen CP, Mathew OP. Behavioral arousal in newborn infants and its association with termination of apnea. J Appl Physiol 1991; 70(6):2479–2484.
145. Orr WC, Robinson MG, Johnson LF. Acid clearance during sleep in the pathogenesis of reflux esophagitis. Dig Dis Sci 1981; 26(5):423–427.
146. Kahn A, Rebuffat E, Sottiaux M, Blum D, Yasik EA. Sleep apneas and acid esophageal reflux in control infants and in infants with an apparent life-threatening event. Biol Neonate 1990; 57(3–4):144–149.
147. Ramet J, Egreteau L, Curzi-Dascalova L, Escourrou P, Dehan M, Gaultier C. Cardiac, respiratory, and arousal responses to an esophageal acid infusion test in near-term infants during active sleep. J Pediatr Gastroenterol Nutr 1992; 15(2):135–140.

148. Kahn A, Picard E, Blum D. Auditory arousal thresholds of normal and near-miss SIDS infants. Dev Med Child Neurol 1986; 28(3):299–302.
149. Kahn A, Hasaerts D, Blum D. Phenothiazine-induced sleep apneas in normal infants. Pediatrics 1985; 75(5):844–847.
150. Poets CF, Stebbens VA, Samuels MP, Southall DP. The relationship between bradycardia, apnea, and hypoxemia in preterm infants. Pediatr Res 1993; 34(2):144–147.
151. Upton CJ, Milner AD, Stokes GM. Apnoea, bradycardia, and oxygen saturation in preterm infants. Arch Dis Child 1991; 66(4 spec no):381–385.
152. Haddad GG, Bazzy AR, Chang SL, Mellins RB. Heart rate pattern during respiratory pauses in normal infants during sleep. J Dev Physiol 1984; 6(4):329–337.
153. Henderson-Smart DJ, Butcher-Puech MC, Edwards DA. Incidence and mechanism of bradycardia during apnoea in preterm infants. Arch Dis Child 1986; 61(3):227–232.
154. Ramet J, Praud JP, D'Allest AM, Carofilis A, Dehan M. Effect of maturation on heart rate response to ocular compression test during rapid eye movement sleep in human infants. Pediatr Res 1988; 24:477–480.
155. Ramet J, Praud JP, d'Allest AM, Dehan M, Guilleminault C, Gaultier C. Cardiac and respiratory responses to esophageal dilatation during REM sleep in human infants. Biol Neonate 1990; 58(4):181–187.
156. Sullivan CE, Kozar LF, Murphy E, Phillipson EA. Primary role of respiratory afferents in sustaining breathing rhythm. J Appl Physiol 1978; 45(1):11–17.
157. Adamson TM, Cranage S, Maloney JE, Wilkinson MH, Wilson FE, Yu VY. The maturation of respiratory patterns in normal full term infants during the first six postnatal months: 1. Sleep states and respiratory variability. Aust Paediatr J 1981; 17(4):250–256.
158. Andersson D, Gennser G, Johnson P. Phase characteristics of breathing movements in healthy newborns. J Dev Physiol 1983; 5(5):289–298.
159. Bolton DP, Herman S. Ventilation and sleep state in the new-born. J Physiol (Lond) 1974; 240(1):67–77.
160. Carse EA, Wilkinson AR, Whyte PL, Henderson-Smart DJ, Johnson P. Oxygen and carbon dioxide tensions, breathing and heart rate in normal infants during the first six months of life. J Dev Physiol 1981; 3(2):85–100.
161. Coup A, Coup D, Weathall S, Withy S. The development and abnormalities of breathing patterns. In: Tildon J, Roeder L, Steinscheider A, eds. Sudden Infant Death Syndrome. New York: Academic Press, 1983; 423–449.
162. Davi M, Sankaran K, MacCallum M, Cates D, Rigatto H. Effect of sleep state on chest distortion and on the ventilatory response to CO_2 in neonates. Pediatr Res 1979; 13(9):982–986.
163. Finer NN, Abroms IF, Taeusch HW Jr. Ventilation and sleep states in newborn infants. J Pediatr 1976; 89(1):100–108.
164. Haddad GG, Leistner HL, Epstein RA, Epstein MA, Grodin WK, Mellins RB. CO_2-induced changes in ventilation and ventilatory pattern in normal sleeping infants. J Appl Physiol 1980; 48(4):684–688.
165. Hathorn MK. The rate and depth of breathing in new-born infants in different sleep states. J Physiol (Lond) 1974; 243(1):101–113.
166. Hoppenbrouwers T, Harper RM, Hodgman JE, Sterman MB, McGinty DJ. Polygraphic studies on normal infants during the first six months of life: II. Respiratory rate and variability as a function of state. Pediatr Res 1978; 12(2):120–125.
167. Hoppenbrouwers T, Hodgman JE, Harper RM, Sterman MB. Respiration during the first

six months of life in normal infants: IV. Gender differences. Early Hum Dev 1980; 4(2):167–177.

168. Katona PG, Egbert JR. Heart rate and respiratory rate differences between preterm and full-term infants during quiet sleep: possible implications for sudden infant death syndrome. Pediatrics 1978; 62(1):91–95.
169. Litscher G, Pfurtscheller G, Bes F, Poiseau E. Respiration and heart rate variation in normal infants during quiet sleep in the first year of life. Klin Paediatr 1993; 205(3):170–175.
170. Marks MK, South M, Carlin JB. Reference ranges for respiratory rate measured by thermistry (12–84 months). Arch Dis Child 1993; 69(5):569–572.
171. Rusconi F, Castagneto M, Gagliardi L, Leo G, Pelliegatta A, Porta N, Razon S, Braga M. Reference values for respiratory rate in the first 3 years of life. Pediatrics 1994; 94(3):350–355.
172. Steinschneider A, Weinstein S. Sleep respiratory instability in term neonates under hyperthermic conditions: age, sex, type of feeding, and rapid eye movements. Pediatr Res 1983; 17(1):35–41.
173. Carskadon MA, Harvey K, Dement WC, Guilleminault C, Simmons B, Anders TF. Respiration during sleep in children. West J Med 1978; 128:477–481.
174. Guilleminault C, Korobkin R, Winkle R. A review of 50 children with obstructive sleep apnea syndrome. Lung 1981; 159:275–287.
175. Tabachnik E, Muller NL, Bryan AC, Levison H. Changes in ventilation and chest wall mechanics during sleep in normal adolescents. J Appl Physiol 1981; 51(3):557–564.
176. Marcus CL, Omlin KJ, Basinki DJ, Bailey SL, Rachal AB, Von Pechmann WS, Keens TG, Ward SL. Normal polysomnographic values for children and adolescents. Am Rev Respir Dis 1992; 146(5 pt 1):1235–1239.
177. Acebo C, Millman RP, Rosenberg C, Cavallo A, Carskadon MA. Sleep, breathing, and cephalometrics in older children and young adults. Part I—Normative values. Chest 1996; 109(3):664–672.

9

New Insights into Maturation of Central Components in Cardiovascular and Respiratory Control

DAVID GOZAL

Kosair Children's Hospital Research Institute
University of Louisville School of Medicine
Louisville, Kentucky

RONALD M. HARPER

University of California at Los Angeles
Los Angeles, California

I. Introduction

The ability to rapidly adjust to changes in environmental, state, and/or metabolic conditions while maintaining tightly controlled homeostasis is one of the major adaptive mechanisms underlying survival. In mammalian species, sophisticated systems have evolved to allow for preservation of homeostasis. However, these systems may not be fully integrated or operational during the initial stages of postnatal life, thereby leading to the emergence of vulnerable states under certain circumstances. Examples of such situations include the onset of apnea and/or bradycardia during sleep, common problems in the neonate and infant, which often result in the need for prolonged hospitalization and home cardiorespiratory monitoring.

It is now quite clear that major differences in respiratory activity exist between wakefulness and sleep. Such differences include a fall in ventilation, decreased metabolic rate, an increase in alveolar P_{CO_2}, a decrease in responsiveness to ventilatory stimuli, and an increase in airflow resistance (1). Such changes appear to reflect conflicting state-dependent drives (2). However, within sleep states, there is considerable variability in respiratory patterns, such that during non–rapid-eye-movement (NREM) or slow-wave sleep (SWS), respiratory rate decreases and tidal volume may either increase or remain unchanged, while during phasic rapid-eye-movement (REM) sleep, breathing becomes irregular, rapid, and shallow (3,4). Thus, sleep states exert major effects on moment-to-moment expression of breathing and autonomic control as well as on evoked responses to specific challenges. The momentary changes are typically far out of proportion to demands dictated by metabolic needs; thus, a portion of the variation associated with state reflects neural processes other than mechanisms essential for homeostasis, and, in some instances, may compromise vital needs.

A detailed review of each of the central systems underlying homeostatic defense and adaptation during wakefulness and sleep is clearly beyond the scope of this review. Thus, we focus on three selected and illustrative aspects of maturation in this context: 1) the hypoxic ventilatory response; 2) central chemosensitivity; and 3) autonomic nervous system tone.

II. Hypoxic Ventilatory Response

The adult mammalian ventilatory response to acute hypoxia is biphasic. There is an initial rise in ventilation, followed by a later ventilatory reduction to a level above prehypoxic values, the latter being termed *roll-off* (5). This phenomenon is particularly pronounced in developing mammals, such that, dependent on the severity of the hypoxic environment and the postnatal age of the animal, the early ventilatory enhancement is comparatively reduced, and the sustained ventilatory response in developing mammals may decrease to stable values markedly below those measured in normoxia (6,7). The fall in minute ventilation ($\dot{V}_E$) cannot be accounted for by changes in pulmonary mechanics, altered peripheral chemoreceptor activity, or respiratory muscle fatigue; thus, a central inhibitory process that gradually abates with increasing maturation has been postulated (5,7). The mechanism(s) of this centrally mediated biphasic response remain unclear. While glutamatergic processes have been implicated in the early component of the $\dot{V}_E$-enhanced response (8–10), the mechanisms by which hypoxic ventilatory depression (HVD) occurs remain obscure. Adenosine (11) and γ-aminobutyric acid (GABA) concentrations in the brain are increased during roll-off and specific antagonists attenuate but do not completely abolish HVD (12,13). Sustained hypoxia has been associated with increasing formation of GABA, which is inhibitory to respiration (12). Increased GABA is probably related to the availability of α-ketoglutarate, since the latter is important in the degradation of GABA and synthesis of glutamate. During sustained or severe hypoxia, the level of α-ketoglutarate declines rapidly, since the Krebs cycle intermediates depend on aerobic metabolism. With a reduction in α-ketoglutarate, GABA cannot be degraded, but it can still be formed from glutamate because glutamic acid decarboxylase, the enzyme necessary for conversion of glutamate to GABA, is an anaerobic enzyme and allows GABA formation to proceed during hypoxia (14). Thus, Kazemi and colleagues have proposed an elegant model whereby the balance between excitatory (glutamate) and inhibitory (GABA) inputs during hypoxic challenge determine overall ventilatory output during hypoxic conditions (12,15). However, this early model does not fully account for potential changes occurring during the hypoxic response, namely 1) release and/or formation of other factors that may exert a modulatory effect on *N*-methyl-D-aspartate (NMDA) glutamate receptor channel function and 2) temporal changes in intracellular second-messenger systems following NMDA glutamate receptor activation.

Previous work from our and other laboratories has identified nitric oxide (NO) as a putative neurotransmitter with a dual role in the hypoxic chemotransduction pathway. Indeed, while NO derived from endothelial nitric oxide synthase (eNOS) exerts an inhibitory effect at the carotid body (16–20), NO derived from the neuronal NOS isoform (nNOS) plays a significant excitatory role on ventilation (21,22). Indeed, we have previously shown that both selective and nonselective blockers of constitutive nitric oxide synthase (NOS) induce marked ventilatory reductions during sustained hypoxia in the adult rat, thereby enhancing ventilatory roll-off (21). Since HVD is greater in developing mammals during the late phases of hypoxic exposure, we hypothesized that limited NOS activity may play a role in the late arm of the ventilatory response. To test our hypothesis, 5-, 10-, and 15-day-old rat pups underwent a 30-min hypoxic challenge (10% O_2) before and following administration of 100 mg/kg *N*-nitro-L-arginine methyl ester (L-NAME), a competitive NOS inhibitor. Ventilation ($\dot{V}_E$) was measured using whole-body plethysmography in awake animals. In 5-day pups, early $\dot{V}_E$ hypoxic responses were enhanced and late $\dot{V}_E$ responses were similar following L-NAME. In contrast, in 15-day hypoxic pups, L-NAME administration was associated with smaller early $\dot{V}_E$ increments and significantly larger $\dot{V}_E$ reductions when compared to pretreatment conditions. The role of central nervous system NO in the development of these ventilatory changes was further assessed by Western blots of protein equivalents from the nucleus tractus solitarius (NTS), the first central relay for peripheral chemoreceptor afferent input, which revealed increasing neuronal NOS expression with age. Furthermore, immunohistochemical straining of neurons in the NTS for NADPH diaphorase, a marker of nNOS, revealed increased positively labeled neuronal populations within subnuclei of this structure with advancing postnatal age. Thus, nNOS increasing expression with advancing postnatal age parallels the ability to sustain $\dot{V}_E$ during the late phase of an hypoxic challenge (23).

As mentioned above, a substantial body of evidence indicates that the early response to hypoxia is predominantly glutamatergic and, more recently, that this response is primarily mediated via NMDA glutamate receptors (8–10,15,24,25). The cytoplasmic domain of the NMDA receptor displays multiple serine/threonine phosphorylation sites (26), and there is substantial experimental evidence to suggest an important modulatory role for protein kinase C (PKC) in NMDA receptor activity (27–29). Furthermore, changes in PKC activity may also exert significant regulatory effects in presynaptic neurons, such that changes in neurotransmitter release ensue (30). Thus, alterations in PKC activity could modify synaptic transmission both presynaptically and postsynaptically within the NTS. However, the second-messenger systems recruited by NMDA receptor activation and the temporal changes in second-messenger system activity occurring during the course of the hypoxic ventilatory response have not been thoroughly investigated.

Protein kinase C (PKC) is a ubiquitous histone protein kinase, highly expressed in neural tissue, which can be activated by Ca^{2+}, phospholipids, and/or diacylglycerol (DAG; 31), and has been implicated in the transduction of multiple extracellular signals into the neuronal cell (32). The PKC family consists of 12 major isoenzymes divided into three subgroups, namely the classic or Ca^{2+}-dependent PKC (α, $\beta 1$, $\beta 2$, and γ), the novel or Ca^{2+}-independent PKC isoforms (δ, ε, υ, η, and μ), and the atypical PKC isoforms (ζ, ι, and λ) (33,34). The functional relevance of PKC to respiratory control has only started to emerge in recent years. For example, Champagnat and Richter have reported that PKC activation with phorbol ester, a nonphysiological PKC activator, leads to increased respiratory drive potentials (35). Similarly, the excitability of expiratory bulbar neurons is dependent on endogenous PKC (36). To further determine the role of PKC in respiratory control, we initially conducted experiments in which adult rats received a systemic PKC inhibitor, the bisindolylmaleimide Ro 32-0432 (37). In addition to significant prolongation of expiratory duration, marked attenuation of the hypoxic but not the hypercapnic ventilatory response emerged (37). Since the NTS is the first central relay of afferent inputs originating from the peripheral chemo-and baroreceptors, the membrane-permeable phorbol ester phorbol 12-myristate 13-acetate (PMA) was microinjected into the commissural NTS of chronically instrumented unrestrained rats. Animals developed significant cardiorespiratory enhancements that lasted for at least 4 hr and resulted from similar tidal volume and respiratory frequency contributions. Furthermore, administration of vehicle or of the inactive phorbol ester 4 α–phorbol, 12,13-didecanoate failed to elicit $\dot{V}_E$ changes. Hypoxic $\dot{V}_E$ responses (10% O_2) were measured in 19 additional animals following NTS microinjection of bisindolylmaleimide (BIM) I, a PKC inhibitor, BIM V (inactive analogue), or control vehicle. In the latter, $\dot{V}_E$ increased from 139 ± 9 mL/min in room air (RA) to 285 ± 26 mL/min in hypoxia. Following BIM V administration, both RA and hypoxic $\dot{V}_E$ responses were not affected (p = NS vs. control). BIM I did not affect RA $\dot{V}_E$, but markedly attenuated hypoxia-induced $\dot{V}_E$ increases (128 ± 12 to 167 ± 19 mL/min; $p < .02$ vs. control and BIM V). When BIM I was microinjected to the cerebellum ($n = 4$), cortex ($n = 4$), or spinal cord ($n = 4$), $\dot{V}_E$ responses were similar to control. Western blots of subcellular fractions of NTS lysates revealed translocation of PKC α, β, γ, δ, ε, and ι isoenzymes during acute hypoxia (15 min 10% O_2). Enhanced overall PKC activity was further confirmed in the particulate fraction of NTS lysates harvested after 15-min hypoxic challenges. Thus, these studies suggest that, in the adult rat, PKC activation in the NTS mediates essential components of the acute hypoxic ventilatory response (38–40). The developmental characteristics of a putative NMDA-PKC pathway model (Fig. 1) are now under intense investigation. Preliminary results demonstrate that the ability of the neonatal rat to mount a hypoxic response is not as critically dependent on the presence of NMDA glutamate receptors as is the case for the adult rat (25). Similarly, systemic PKC inhibition does not modify the hypoxic response characteristics in the young animals, although it exerts sub-

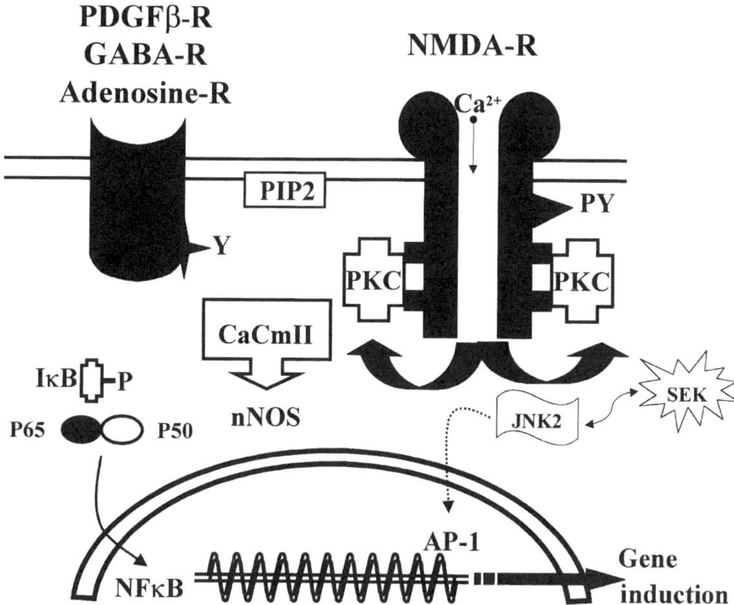

Figure 1 Representative diagram of a postsynaptic neuron in the NTS. Hypoxia elicits glutamate release (10,15), NMDA receptors are activated in the dorsocaudal brainstem, and initiate a signal transduction cascade which results in transient phosphorylation of NR1 tyrosine residues (PY) (51), activation of various PKC isoforms (39), as well as calcium calmodulin kinase II (CaCm II) with nNOS induction and NO release (20–23). In addition, activation of the SEK-JNK2-AP-1 (52) and NF-κB pathways occurs (53). AP-1 and NF-κB activation could in turn induce or inhibit the expression of particular genes.

With ongoing hypoxia, PDGF-β, GABA, and/or adenosine receptors are activated, phosphorylate intracellular receptor domain tyrosine residues, and may catalyze via activation of kinases such as PLC-γ the breakdown of phosphatidylinositol-4,5-biphosphate (PIP2), and produce inositol-1,3,4-triphosphate (IP3) which will bind its receptor and induce release of calcium (Ca^{2+}) from endoplasmic reticulum (ER). As proposed by Valenzuela et al. (54), activation of protein phosphatases (PP) type 1 and/or 2A ensues, leading to inactivation of PKC isoforms involved in NMDA receptor activation, and attenuation of NMDA receptor currents and synaptic transmission.

stantial modifications on respiratory patterning during normoxia (41,42). Thus, marked postnatal changes in the overall role of NMDA glutamate receptors and in the second-messenger systems mediating the ventilatory response to hypoxia occur and may ultimately lead to either inefficient or otherwise less robust neural network recruitment, particularly during situations such as sleep, a condition in which other respiratory drives are either removed or diminished.

III. Effect of Sleep on Hypoxic Responses

Developmental changes in ventilatory response patterns to acute hypoxia immediately after birth have been extensively studied. Dynamic changes in the peripheral chemoreceptor sensitivity "set point" to hypoxia during the early postnatal period have been demonstrated in human infants (43,44). Furthermore, it has become evident that the evolution of the hypoxic response over time varies dependent on the state of vigilance and the level of maturation at which such challenge is conducted. For example, the preterm infant responds to a mild hypoxic challenge (15% O_2) by sustained ventilatory increments during NREM sleep, progressive ventilatory depression during REM sleep, and the typical biphasic response when awake (45). Similar findings were found in calves, whereby the ventilatory increase associated with application of the hypoxic stimulus lasted longer during quiet sleep compared to active sleep (46). In contrast, studies in other mammalian species, such as the dog and rat, have found conflicting results compared to the newborn human. Indeed, decreased or unchanged hypoxic responses in dogs (47), and even increased responses in rats were reported (48).

The mechanisms underlying the resetting of chemoreceptors during postnatal development and the brain regions involved in the transition from transient to sustained increases in ventilation during hypoxia in humans are currently unknown. In addition, sleep states and sleep deprivation, as well as environmental conditions such as ambient P_{O_2}, may independently affect the maturation pattern of one or more of the structures involved in the hypoxic response and therefore alter the balance between peripheral and central contributions in response to acute hypoxia (49,50).

IV. Central Chemosensitivity

Since the early 1960s, areas of the ventrolateral medulla oblongata (VLM) have become accepted as the sites of central chemoreception of CO_2 and/or H^+, after Mitchell and colleagues reported that localized application of acid or of CO_2-saturated solutions to the VLM elicited significant cardioventilatory enhancements (55–57). Since these fundamental studies, several laboratories have expanded on the concept that central chemoreceptors are not restricted to the VLM regions originally described as the sites for central chemoreception, and that neurons exhibiting CO_2 chemosensitivity can be found in many other brain regions (58–61). In addition, although the possibility exists that multiple neurotransmitters may be involved in the process of chemosensitivity, the presence of cholinergic muscarinic receptors in those brainstem areas traditionally associated with CO_2 chemosensitivity suggests that acetyl choline exerts important modulatory roles on the ventilatory response to hypercapnia (62). It remains unclear, however, whether all widely distributed chemosensitive neurons participate in a functionally meaningful fashion on the generation of the ventilatory response to hypercapnia. Furthermore, maturational changes occurring in muscarinic receptor expression and in the functional implications of such chemosensitive sites remain undefined. Indeed, it has been suggested that central CO_2 chemosensory mechanisms may not be fully functional or mature at birth (63); for example, topical application of H^+ to the ventral brainstem is associated with smaller increases in neuronal activity in neonatal cats compared to adult animals (64). However, very few studies have systematically addressed these issues.

It should also be stressed that separation of central and peripheral contributions to the ventilatory response to hypercapnia and/or hypoxia is arduous when one is testing human subjects. Although the ventilatory response to hypercapnia is generally believed to indicate the activity of brainstem chemoreceptors, abrupt elevation of inspired CO_2 concentrations will also elicit a significant contribution from peripheral chemoreceptors (65). Such peripheral contributions to the hypercapnic response are also present in young children, as evidenced from a recent study in preterm infants which demonstrated larger ventilatory slopes in the response to either endogenous or bolus CO_2 when compared to rebreathing or steady-state methods (66). Independent of such technical considerations, the ventilatory response to hypercapnia in premature infants was lower than that found in term infants, and CO_2 responses increased with postnatal age (67,68). It was further proposed that decreased CO_2 responsivity may underlie determinants of periodic breathing in newborn animals (69), sleep apnea in preterm infants (70), or even be involved in the pathophysiological mechanisms underlying sudden infant death syndrome (SIDS) (71).

Beyond the infancy period, little is known about the development of central chemoreceptor function. In awake prepubertal children, using rebreathing techniques, Marcus and colleagues found increased CO_2 ventilatory responses to hypercapnia in prepubertal children compared to adults provided that correction of the slopes for body size was performed (72). Similarly, significant developmental differences in CO_2 responses emerged when the CO_2 stimulus was presented in a step or a ramp fashion (73). These findings in older children suggest that some time during the transition from childhood to adulthood, significant changes in the relative contributions of peripheral and central chemoreceptor activity occur. It remains unclear which mechanisms mediate these maturation changes and whether they are operative at the carotid body, neural transmission, or brainstem level.

V. Effect of Sleep on CO_2 Responses

It is now clear that when hypercapnic ventilatory responses are conducted in the adult sleeping subject, CO_2 sensitivity is reduced, especially during REM sleep epochs (74,75). Although studies in infants are not always in close agreement (76,77), it appears that, as in adult subjects, a decrease in central chemosensitivity occurs during REM sleep in the young infant when the rebreathing technique is employed (78–80). Thus, the transition from wakefulness to the sleep state will elicit significant reductions in hypercapnic drive, and such changes are further accentuated during REM sleep.

VI. Autonomic Development: Interactions with Breathing and Sleep

Maintenance of homeostasis requires close interaction of autonomic and somatic motor systems, as even gross examination of cardiovascular and respiratory control mechanisms indicates. Transient blood pressure elevation suppresses respiratory activity (preferentially in the upper airway musculature, and thus a particular danger for airway obstruction), slows breath-to-breath timing, and induces arousal (81,82), while lowering of blood pressure stimulates ventilation (83). Conversely, respiratory efforts vary cardiac rate, with cardiac acceleration accompanying inspiration and deceleration associated with expiration, resulting from stretch and aortic receptor activity responding to venous return. Both the pressor effects on breathing and respiratory modulation of cardiac rate are accentuated by sleep (82). A large number of motor or vocalization events, central or obstructive apnea during sleep, or increased inspiratory or expiratory loading can initiate large blood pressure changes, which can then reflexively modify subsequent motor events. Hypoxia developing from inadequate ventilation initiates a substantial reorganization of metabolic rate and sympathetic outflow, with consequences to heart rate, blood pressure, and body temperature (84). Acute hypoxia apparently reduces metabolism in the very young, eliciting an appropriate decline in minute ventilation (85). Thus, any examination of autonomic nervous system development must consider the interactions between brain areas mediating temperature, sympathetic outflow to the cardiovascular system, and somatomotor (e.g., respiratory) systems. Overriding all of these interactions are the effects of sleep state, which often result in substantial reorganization of influences of one brain area on another, or in nearly-complete inactivation of systems—e.g., the diminution of hypothalamic influences on temperature regulating systems and the paralysis of the somatic motor system in REM sleep.

VII. Developmental Trends in Cardiovascular and Respiratory Measures

The manner in which infants respond to ventilatory or cardiovascular challenges during sleep bears on a number of critical clinical issues, including SIDS, since SIDS apparently occurs in close temporal relationship to sleep (86). Reaction to provocative challenges are superimposed on levels of background rate and variability, which vary remarkably with age and state. Basal heart rate rises over the first month of life before declining over the next 6 months of life (87); overall variability declines during quiet sleep over the first month before rising. The most substantial portion of that variation—i.e., that arising from respiratory sources—follows a similar time course as overall variability (88). The respiratory influences on heart rate variation arise principally from blood pressure and stretch afferent activity exerted by thoracic sources and are mediated primarily by vagal contributions to the heart. Determination of the proportion of vagal influences relative to sympathetic outflow on heart rate variation has been frequently used to evaluate development of cardiovascular activity in the infant and has been suggested as a useful index of risk in certain cardiac failure syndromes (89). Infants who later succumb to SIDS as well as infants who are at risk for SIDS and those afflicted with congenital central hypoventilation syndrome show diminished respiratory-related variation during particular sleep states (88,90). Conversely, infants who later succumb to SIDS also show a diminished incidence of short apnea (91). Since such apnea may arise from blood pressure perturbations resulting from minor movement, the loss of breathing variation might result from a loss of blood pressure influences on cyclic respiratory patterning.

Heart rate responses to head tilt, which induces blood pressure increases and decreases, suggest a substantial effect of age, with younger infants (1 to 2 days) showing markedly increased heart rate compensatory changes to head-up tilt, and with older (2 to 4 months) infants showing either a reduced or no response; respiratory responses are present at both young and older ages (Fifer, personal communication). The findings from head-tilt challenge demonstrate a significant role for vestibular and cerebellar input to blood pressure regulation that varies with age. The age dependency of baroreflex responses is an important issue, since at least some SIDS victims succumb to a loss of blood pressure and bradycardia, rather than a respiratory failure (92). Thus, the functional development of neural structures underlying control of blood pressure and slowing of the heart, especially in conditions which could trigger a shock-like reaction, are of interest.

VIII. Neural Structures Involved in Autonomic and Respiratory Regulation: Cerebellum and Vestibular Regions

Among the structures mediating the extent of heart rate response to a hypotensive or hypertensive challenge, such as head tilt, are structures within the cerebellum, especially areas within the fastigial nucleus. Bilateral lesions of fastigial nucleus sites abolish the compensatory heart rate responses to blood pressure loss to the point that the subject may succumb (93). Similarly, the bradycardia accompanying hypertensive challenges is lost with comparable lesions (94). The function of the fastigial nuclei may be that of “dampening” an evoked autonomic response in a fashion comparable to the manner in which the range of certain somatic motor actions are modulated by regions within the cerebellum. Fastigial cerebellar sites as well as other regions within the cerebellum also show functional magnetic resonance image (MRI) signal changes to a cold pressor or Valsalva challenge, which elevate blood pressure (95). Although the cerebellum is traditionally associated with aspects of motor rather than autonomic control, its role in cardiovascular function has been known for over 50 years (96), and those functions are now under active investigation (97,98).

Fastigial nuclei also apparently mediate aspects of respiratory control; electrical stimulation induces apnea or tachypnea, depending on frequency of the stimulus (99). Other evidence indicates a role for the cerebellum in respiratory loading

(100–102). Both inspiratory and expiratory loading as well as hypercapnia activate sites within the cerebellum, as indicated by functional MRI (103–105). The cerebellar regions activated by loaded breathing may be responsive to both blood pressure and respiratory modulation; contributions of cerebellar influences on breathing and cardiovascular control during development, however, are relatively unexplored.

The potential for cerebellar regions to play a role in limiting the extent of blood pressure responses to a hypotensive challenge is of particular interest in considering the mechanism of failure in the fatal event of SIDS; some infants succumb with bradycardia and hypotension (92). A ventral medullary surface site, the arcuate nucleus, has been implicated as being deficient in muscarinic and kainate receptors in a proportion of infants who later succumb to SIDS (71,106). The arcuate nucleus has classically been described to project to the cerebellum and could well mediate a vestibulocerebellar fastigial nucleus–mediated compensatory response to a marked loss of blood pressure. Kinney and colleagues also report that the arcuate nucleus projects to the caudal midline medullary raphe in humans (107). Excitation of the caudal midline medullary raphe evokes hypotension and bradycardia, although the area contributes little to routine maintenance of blood pressure (108). Thus, reduced muscarinic and kainate receptor binding in the arcuate nucleus may well result in an ineffective ability to compensate for challenges that provoke a profound and sudden loss of blood pressure.

The rapid adjustments in vasomotor activity to body position changes, such as rising from the supine position or even more modest body movements, indicate that central circulatory compensatory mechanisms other than baroreflexes must be operating. Vestibular systems play an essential role in regulation of blood pressure to head tilt (109), an entirely expected finding considering the liaisons between vestibular and cerebellar structures. Vestibular nuclei have prominent projections to midline caudal raphe nuclei as well as to the rostral ventrolateral medulla; both regions, in turn, project to the intermediolateral column of the spinal cord, the motor column for sympathetic outflow (for review, see Ref. 110). The conditions under which vestibular nuclei mediate vasomotor tone through the midline caudal raphe, a structure implicated in the sympathoinhibition associated with shock, are not clear. However, the vestibular/caudal raphe relationships are of interest to investigators examining the cardiovascular collapse that accompanies some cases of SIDS (92). The vestibular system projections to the ventrolateral medulla may also play a critical role in the SIDS event. Any of the potential relationships between structures could be greatly affected by sleep states, a thus far untested assumption. Sympathetic control, however, is profoundly changed during REM sleep.

IX. Sleep-State Effects

Sleep states exert substantial effects on instantaneous cardiac rate variability and vasomotor activity, particularly in REM sleep (111,112). In infants, during quiet sleep, most variation arises from respiratory-related sources, while in REM sleep, variation derives from both respiratory-related sources and marked, longer-term accelerations and decelerations (113). Phasic increases in heart rate and coronary blood flow accompanied by momentary decreased coronary vasculature resistance occur during phasic episodes of the REM state in adult animals (114,115), while pauses in heart rate also occur associated with coronary vasodilation; these pauses appear to be baroreflex-mediated (116). However, bursts of vagally mediated bradycardia *not* preceded by tachycardia or blood pressure changes and not accompanied by expected respiratory rate changes occur in tonic periods of that state (117). The latter finding is significant, because the centrally mediated bradycardia points to the existence of state-related mechanisms that can potentially adversely affect perfusion in the absence of reflex control. The fatal event in some SIDS victims appears to be one circumstance in which bradycardia and hypotension occur, but normal reflexes between heart rate, blood pressure, and breathing apparently are not operative (92).

The vasomotor phenomena that occur during REM sleep present a number of other circumstances which generate concern. In lambs, a substantial increase in systemic vascular resistance occurs during the REM state, preventing a severe loss in blood pressure during that state, and coronary vascular resistance increases during phasic events, preventing substantial increases in coronary flow (118); these circumstances compromise coronary perfusion at a time when an increasing work load is placed on the heart. Further compromises that could occur in infants, such as hypoxia, might place the individual at risk.

X. Ventral Medullary Surface Activity

The central mechanisms underlying the substantial phasic variation in heart rate, coronary flow, and systemic vascular resistance during the REM state are still unclear, as are the sources for the momentary increases and pauses in breathing. Areas within the rostral ventral medullary surface (VMS) which, when cooled, induce a loss of blood pressure show very large "spontaneous" variation in activity during REM sleep compared to quiet sleep states (199). Intermediate areas of the VMS of the cat show similar phasic changes (120). Correlations between rostral VMS optical activity and momentary arterial pressure suggest that increased activity precedes blood pressure changes and that those correlations preferably occur during REM sleep (121). These findings indicate a more prominent role for regions within the VMS during REM over other states in mediating blood pressure changes, but the nature of that mediation is unknown. In addition to "spontaneous" changes, VMS responses to pressor and ventilatory challenges are also state-dependent. The VMS responses to pressor and ventilatory challenges differ markedly in the waking state from anesthetic and sleep states. Elevating blood pressure elicits a widespread, profound decline in VMS activity during both halothane and barbiturate anesthesia, as indicated by optical studies in cats and goats; microelectrode recording from nearby structures in the cat also show marked cell discharge slowing during a similar challenge (122). During waking, however, the response to pressor challenge is only a minor increase in activity (123). Hypoxia increases VMS activity in the anesthetized goat; during waking, the response is dramatically accentuated (124). The response to hypercapnia under anesthesia is a decline in VMS activity; in waking, activity in the rostral VMS increases transiently before declining (125). Cooling a portion of the rostral VMS elicits marked apnea during anesthesia and sleep but not during waking (126). Changes in state-induced baseline VMS activity may underlie the state-dependent responses to challenges.

A region on the goat VMS ventral to the retrotrapezoid nucleus activates under both anesthesia and waking to a rapid lowering of blood pressure, a challenge that elicits enhanced drive to breathing (83). Cooling this area during anesthesia or sleep elicits apnea (126). Although the rostral VMS areas may not be analogous in both the cat and goat, the response of increased activity to the depressor challenge occurs in both species (123,126). Conversely, the decline in VMS activity to blood pressure elevation is associated with a marked loss of respiratory muscle activity and slowing of breathing. Part of the interaction between blood pressure lowering and stimulation of breathing may occur at rostral VMS sites.

Appropriate functioning of the VMS depends on the integrity of vagal and carotid sinus nerve afferents, since carotid nerve transection abolishes VMS responses (a decline in intermediate area activity) to chemoreceptor stimulation by intravenous cyanide (128). Sinus nerve transection also enhances the VMS responses (the response is an activity decline, but the decline is enhanced) to pressor challenge, while vagotomy nearly abolishes the response (129). These findings suggest that carotid sinus chemoreceptor input to the nucleus of the solitary tract (NTS) (which then projects to the VMS) causes the NTS to exert a disfacilitatory or inhibitory influence on intermediate area VMS neurons and that transection releases that influence. Afferent activity from vagal fibers, however, appears to exert an excitatory influence on VMS neurons. Similarly, transient hypoxia challenge (two breaths of N_2 to preferentially stimulate peripheral chemoreceptors) increases intermediate area VMS activity, an effect enhanced by sinus nerve section and abolished by vagotomy (129,130). Thus, these data suggest a functionally more excitatory role on the VMS for vagal afferents.

XI. Rostral Brain Influences

Rostral brain structures have the potential to modify respiratory and autonomic patterns in a major fashion and play a particularly large role in mediating sleep-related patterns, alterations induced by affect, or the considerable effects of core temperature manipulation. We define "rostral structures" as hypothalamic, limbic, and cortical areas, although a number of other motor regions, (e.g., the basal ganglia), and midbrain areas (e.g., the periaqueductal gray), could also be included and almost certainly contribute to both cardiovascular and breathing control during development. The influence of sleep states on descending neural influences on breathing and autonomic control is substantial, with REM sleep normally eliciting nearly total suppression of upper airway and thoracic wall respiratory muscle activity as well as sympathetic output; in some syndromes, the paralysis of respiratory muscles extends to the diaphragm (131–134). Basal forebrain sites initiate and maintain quiet sleep, whereas pontine mechanisms underlie the major characteristics of REM sleep (135). Although medullary regions maintain respiratory rhythmogenesis and cerebellar/vestibular regions appear to exert dampening effects to minimize variations from homeostasis, descending forebrain influences appear to elicit transient respiratory or cardiovascular changes to particular stimuli or alter background "tone" to provocative challenges.

The descending influences include more than traditional voluntary pathways, since affective "drive" can elicit diaphragmatic movement, bypassing classic pyramidal respiratory control mechanisms—e.g., capsular lesions prevent voluntary diaphragmatic movements which still can be elicited with laughter (136). The latter finding emphasizes the potential for descending affective influences to modify breathing.

The major descending projection systems to structures mediating brainstem respiratory and autonomic control include limbic descending projections from the central amygdala nucleus, red nucleus of the stria terminalis, and the paraventricular nucleus of the hypothalamus (137–139). The paraventricular hypothalamus projects to the VMS in a wide area just lateral to the pyramids (140) and sends reciprocal projections to the bed nucleus of the stria terminalis and central nucleus of the amygdala. The latter two structures contain respiratory-related neurons (141–143); moreover, the central amygdala nucleus paces breathing by single-pulse stimulation, an effect obliterated by sleep (144), and cooling of the central amygdala abolishes conditioned blood pressure responses (145). The paraventricular hypothalamus (as well as the red nucleus) shows substantial *c-fos* expression on blood pressure manipulation (146); the hypothalamus activates to transient respiratory pauses (147) and, on stimulation, regionally activates the VMS. Since the pathways from rostral sites to midbrain and medullary areas may take a period of time to develop, descending influences may follow a time course of expression; those time courses have yet to be described for most influences.

Functional MRI shows activation of hypothalamic sites in addition to VMS areas to loaded breathing (104,105). Since increased airway resistance often accompanies sleep (and is substantial, or nearly infinite, in obstructive sleep apnea), the responses of these regions to such loading during sleep are of particular interest in determining mechanisms of arousal from obstruction. The hypothalamic activation may result from that structure, generating sympathetic influences associated with the blood pressure changes accompanying enhanced airway resistance, or to recruitment of cells that project to dorsal pontine areas mediating adrenergic activation.

Descending forebrain systems may be recruited under certain behavioral conditions, such as those conditions associated with stress, vocalization, or affective influences to respiratory control areas. The paraventricular hypothalamus is a major component in pituitary-adrenocortical activation and exhibits cellular activity changes after exposure to stress (148,149). The paraventricular hypothalamus projects to the rostral NTS; to the rat (150) and cat (140) dorsal vagal nucleus; to A1, A2, and A5 noradrenergic brainstem nuclei, and nucleus raphe magnus (151). It also sends projections directly to the intermediolateral column of the spinal cord (152); the structure can thus modify both parasympathetic and sympathetic efferent activity.

Respiratory rate and effort are profoundly influenced by core or anterior hypothalamic temperature, an effect that is greatly reduced in REM sleep in both the cat and developing kitten (153,154). Appropriate rapid breathing responses to hypothalamic warming require a period of time to develop in the kitten; very young animals cannot maintain adequate ventilation with such warming and switch intermittently to slower breathing, risking hyperthermic damage (154). Hypothalamic warming effects on breathing are most likely mediated through descending projections to the parabrachial pons, nucleus of the solitary tract, and periaqueductal gray (140). Thermal influences are important for maintaining breathing early in life, at least for some species; lambs kept apart from maternal warmth show increased apnea (155). REM sleep also abolishes at least some descending rostral influences on autonomic control, including transient hypertension induced by stimulation of the central amygdala nucleus (141). The near abolition of descending hypothalamic temperature-related influences on breathing and cardiovascular control by REM sleep poses certain clinical implications; excessively high core temperatures have been found postmortem in SIDS victims (156), and infants with life-threatening events are sometimes found drenched in sweat (157), indicative of intense sympathetic activation. Heat dissipation in the human relies heavily on sympathetic mechanisms by means of sweating and vasodilation; such actions are at least partially mediated through ventral medullary structures (158). Withdrawal of influences from hypothalamic sites during sleep may modulate some of the state-related physiological changes mediated by the VMS.

XII. Summary

The multiplicity of central systems whose function is to preserve homeostasis and the elevated number of interdependencies occurring between functionally related structures in the central network usually ensure proper activation of backup defense systems and overall system stability during state transitions. However, perturbations can coincide with normally functioning transitional states and can lead to disrupted responses or to generation of vulnerable states—e.g., sleep-associated periodic breathing and hypoxemia, bradycardia, or hypotension. Similarly, dynamic changes within individual components in the network and their connectivity to other network elements occur during and even after maturation. The characteristics of such developmental changes are dictated at least in part by environmental, metabolic, and state conditions as well as the overall neuronal activity of each network compartment, thereby creating infinite permutation possibilities in the overall network—i.e., individual and temporal variabilities. Thus, careful consideration of behavioral states and developmental stage must be incorporated in experimental or clinical settings to allow for improved understanding and interpretation of central cardiovascular and respiratory control mechanisms and their responses to particular stimuli.

Acknowledgments

DG is supported by grants from the National Institutes of Health (HD-01072 and HL-65270), and the American Lung Association (CI-002-N). RMH is supported by National Institutes of Health grants HD-22506, HD-22695, HL-22418, and HL-60296.

References

1. Phillipson EA, Bowes G. Control of breathing during sleep. In: Handbook of Physiology: Sec. 3, Vol. II, Pt2. The Respiratory System—Control of Breathing. Bethesda, MD: American Physiological Society, 1986: 649–690.
2. Trinder J, Whitworth F, Kay A, Wilkin P. Respiratory instability during sleep onset. J Appl Physiol 1992; 73:2462–2469.
3. Douglas NJ, White DP, Pickett CK, Weil JV, Zwillich CW. Respiration during sleep in normal man. Thorax 1982; 37:840–844.
4. Orem J. The wakefulness stimulus for breathing. In: Saunders NA, Sullivan CE, eds. Sleep and Breathing, 2d ed. New York: Marcel Dekker, 1995: 113–155.
5. Vizek M, Pickett CK, Weil JV. Biphasic ventilatory response of adult cats to sustained hypoxia has central origin. J Appl Physiol 1987; 63:1658–1664.
6. Bureau MA, Zinman R, Foulon P, Begin R. Diphasic ventilatory response to hypoxia in the newborn lamb. J Appl Physiol 1984; 56:84–90.
7. Eden GJ, Hanson MA. Maturation of the respiratory response to acute hypoxia in the newborn rat. J Physiol (Lond) 1987; 392:1–9.
8. Soto-Arape I, Burton MD, Kazemi H. Central amino acid neurotransmitters and the hypoxic ventilatory response. Am J Respir Crit Care Med 1995; 151:1113–1120.
9. Lin J, Suguihara C, Huang J, Hehre D, Devia C, Bancalari E. Effect of *N*-methyl-D-aspartate receptor blockade on hypoxic ventilatory response in unanesthetized piglets. J Appl Physiol 1996; 80:1759–1763.
10. Mizusawa A, Ogawa H, Kikuchi Y, Hida W, Kurosawa H, Okabe S, Takishima T, Shirato K. In vivo release of glutamate in nucleus tractus solitarii of the rat during hypoxia. J Physiol (Lond) 1994; 478:55–65.
11. Neylon M, Marshall JM. The role of adenosine in the respiratory and cardiovascular response to systemic hypoxia in the rat. J Physiol (Lond) 1991; 440:529–545.
12. Kneussl MP, Pappagianopolous P, Hoop B, Kazemi H. Reversible depression of ventilation and cardiovascular function by ventriculo-cisternal perfusion with gamma-aminobutyric acid in dogs. Am Rev Respir Dis 1986; 133:1024–1028.
13. Easton PA, Anthonisen NR. Ventilatory response to sustained hypoxia after pretreatment with aminophylline. J Appl Physiol 1988; 64:1445–1450.
14. McGeer PL, McGeer EG. Amino acid neurotransmitters. In: Siegel CJ, Albers RW, Katzman R, Agranoff BW, eds. Basic Neurochemistry. Boston: Little, Brown, 1981:233–252.
15. Kazemi H, Hoop B. Glutamic acid and gamma-aminobutyric acid neurotransmitters in central control of breathing. J Appl Physiol 1991; 70:1–7.
16. Prabhakar NR, Cherniack NS, Haxhiu MA. Inhibitory and excitatory effects of nitric oxide on respiratory responses to hypoxia. In: Trouth OC, Millis RM, Kiwull-Schöne HF, Schläfke ME, eds. Ventral Brainstem Mechanisms and Control of Respiration and

Blood Pressure: Lung Biology in Health and Disease. New York: Marcel Dekker, 1995: 393–404.

17. Prabhakar NR, Kumar GK, Chang CH, Agani FH, Haxhiu MA. Nitric oxide in the sensory function of the carotid body. Brain Res 1993; 625:16–22.
18. Chugh DK, Katayama M, Mokashi A, Dehout DE, Ray DK, Lahiri S. Nitric oxide-related inhibition of carotid chemosensory nerve activity in the cat. Respir Physiol 1994; 97:147–156.
19. Wang ZZ, Stensaas LJ, Dinger BG, Fidone SJ. Nitric oxide mediates chemoreceptor inhibition in the cat carotid body. Neuroscience 1995; 65:217–229.
20. Gozal D, Gozal E, Gozal YM, Torres JE. Nitric oxide synthase isoforms and peripheral chemoreceptor stimulation in conscious rats. Neuroreport 1996; 7:1145–1148.
21. Gozal D, Torres JE, Gozal YM, Littwin SM. Effect of nitric oxide synthase inhibition on cardiorespiratory responses in the conscious rat. J Appl Physiol 1996; 81:2068–2077.
22. Torres JE, Kreisman NR, Gozal D. Nitric oxide modulates in vitro intrinsic optical signal and neural activity in the nucleus tractus solitarius of the rat. Neurosci Lett 1997; 232:175–178.
23. Gozal D, Gozal E, Torres JE, Gozal YM, Nuckton TJ, Hornby PJ. Nitric oxide modulates ventilatory responses to hypoxia in conscious developing rats. Am J Respir Crit Care Med 1997; 155:1755–1762.
24. Ang RC, Hoop B, Kazemi H. Role of glutamate as the central neurotransmitter in the hypoxic ventilatory response. J Appl Physiol 1992; 72:1480–1487.
25. Ohtake PJ, Torres JE, Gozal YM, Graff GR, Gozal D. NMDA receptors mediate cardiorespiratory responses to afferent peripheral chemoreceptor input in the conscious rat. J Appl Physiol 1998; 84:853–861.
26. Moriyoshi K, Masu M, Ishii T, Shigemoto R, Mizuno N, Nakanishi S. Molecular cloning and characterization of the rat NMDA receptor. Nature 1991; 354:31–37.
27. Chen L, Huang LYM. Protein kinase C reduces Mg^{2+} block of NMDA-receptor channels as a mechanism of modulation. Nature 1992; 356:521–523.
28. Tingley WG, Roche KW, Thompson AK, Huganir RL. Regulation of NMDA receptor phosphorylation by alternative splicing of the C-terminal domain. Nature 1993; 364: 70–73.
29. Urushihara H, Tohda M, Nomura Y. Selective potentiation of N-methyl-D-aspartate-induced current by protein kinase C in *Xenopus* oocytes injected with rat brain mRNA. J Biol Chem 1992; 267:11697–11700.
30. Dekker LV, De Graan PNE, Gispen WH. Transmitter release: target of regulation by protein kinase C? Prog Brain Res 1991; 89:209–233.
31. Inoue M, Kishimoto A, Takai Y, Nishizuka Y. Studies on a cyclic nucleotide-independent protein kinase and its proenzyme in mammalian tissue: II. Proenzyme and its activation by calcium dependent protease from the rat brain. J Biol Chem 1977; 252:7610–7616.
32. Tanaka C, Nishizuka Y. The protein kinase C family for neuronal signaling. Annu Rev Neurosci 1994; 17:551–567.
33. Nishizuka Y. The molecular heterogeneity of protein kinase C and its implications for cellular regulation. Nature 1988; 334:661–665.
34. Nishizuka Y. Intracellular signalling by hydrolysis of phospholipids and activation of protein kinase C. Science 1992; 258:607–614.
35. Champagnat J, Richter DW. Second messenger-induced modulation of the excitability of respiratory neurones. Neuroreport 1993; 4:861–863.

36. Haji A, Pierrefiche O, Lalley PM, Richter DW. Protein kinase C pathways modulate respiratory pattern generation in the cat. J Physiol (Lond) 1996; 494:297–306.
37. Gozal D, Graff GR, Torres JE, Khicha SG, Nayak GS, Simakajornboon N, Gozal E. Cardiorespiratory responses to systemic administration of a protein kinase C inhibitor in the conscious rat. J Appl Physiol 1998; 84:641–648.
38. Gozal D, Gozal E. Hypoxic ventilatory roll-off is associated with decreases in protein kinase C activation within the nucleus tractus solitarius of the rat. Brain Res 1997; 774:246–249.
39. Gozal E, Roussel AL, Holt GA, Gozal L, Gozal YM, Torres JE, Gozal D. Protein kinase C modulation of the ventilatory response to hypoxia in the nucleus tractus solitarius of the conscious rat. J Appl Physiol 1998; 84:1982–1990.
40. Gozal D, Graff GR, Gozal E, Torres JE. Modulation of the hypoxic ventilatory response by Ca^{2+}-dependent and Ca^{2+}-independent protein kinase C in the nucleus tractus solitarii of conscious rats. Respir Physiol 1998; 112:283–290.
41. Bandla HPR, Graff GR, Gozal D. Post-natal changes in the ventilatory response to systemic protein kinase C (PKC) inhibition in the rat. Am J Respir Crit Care Med 1998; 157:A341.
42. Bandla HPR, Simakajornboon N, Graff GR, Gozal D. Developmental changes in the hypoxic ventilatory response after systemic protein kinase C (PKC) inhibition in the rat. Pediatr Res 1998; 43:330A.
43. Hertzberg T, Lagercrantz H. Postnatal sensitivity of the peripheral chemoreceptors in newborn infants. Arch Dis Child 1987; 62:1238–1241.
44. Walker DW. Peripheral and central chemoreceptors in the fetus and newborn. Annu Rev Physiol 1984; 46:687–703.
45. Rigatto H. Control of ventilation in the newborn. Ann Rev Physiol 1984; 46:661–674.
46. Jeffrey HE, Read DJC. Reduced lung volume during behavioral active sleep in the newborn. J Appl Physiol 1979; 46:1081–1085.
47. Phillipson EA, Sullivan CE, Read DJC, Murphy E, Kozar LF. Ventilatory and waking responses to hypoxia in sleeping dogs. J Appl Physiol 1978; 44:512–520.
48. Pappenheimer J. Sleep and respiration of rats during hypoxia. J Physiol (Lond) 1977; 266:191–207.
49. Eden GJ, Hanson MA. The effect of chronic hypoxia from birth on the ventilatory response to acute hypoxia in the newborn rat. J Physiol (Lond) 1987; 392:11–19.
50. Hanson MA, Kumar P, Williams BA. The effect of chronic hypoxia upon the development of respiratory chemoreflexes in the newborn kitten. J Physiol (Lond) 1989; 411:563–574.
51. Czapla MA, Holt GA, Gozal D. Putative role of tyrosine kinase activation within the nucleus tractus solitarii (nTS) in the hypoxic ventilatory response of the conscious rat. Am J Respir Crit Care Med 1998; 157:A249.
52. Gozal E, Simakajornboon N, El-Dahr S, Gozal D. Hypoxia induces selective in vivo SAPK/JNK-AP-1 pathway activation in the nucleus tractus solitarius (NTS) of the rat. Am J Respir Crit Care Med 1998; 157:A249.
53. Gozal E, Simakajornboon N, Gozal D. NF-κB induction during in vivo hypoxia in the dorsocaudal brainstem of the rat: effect of MK801 and L-NAME. J Appl Physiol 1998; 85:372–376.
54. Valenzuela CF, Xiong Z, MacDonald JF, Weiner JL, Frazier CJ, Dunwiddie TV, Kazlauskas A, Whiting PJ, Harris RA. Platelet-derived growth factor induces a long-term

inhibition of *N*-methyl-D-aspartate receptor function. J Biol Chem 1996; 271: 16151–16159.

55. Loeschcke HH, Koepchen HP. Versuch fur Lokatisation des Angriffsortes de, Atmungs- und Kreislaufwirkung von Novocain im Liquor cerebrospinalis. Pflugers Arch 1958; 266:623–641.
56. Mitchell RA, Loeschcke HH, Massion WH, Severinghaus JW. Respiratory responses mediated through superficial chemosensitive areas on the medulla. J Appl Physiol 1963; 18:523–533.
57. Schlaefke ME. Central chemosensitivity: A respiratory drive. Rev Physiol Biochem Pharmacol 1981; 90:172–244.
58. Bruce EN, Cherniack NS. Central chemoreceptors. J Appl Physiol 1987; 62:389–402.
59. Dean JB, Lawing WL, Millhorn DE. CO_2 decreases membrane conductance and depolarizes neurons in the nucleus tractus solitarii. Exp Brain Res 1989; 76:656–661.
60. Sato M, Severinghaus JW, Basbaum A. Medullary CO_2 chemoreceptor identification by c-fos immunocytochemistry. J Appl Physiol 1992; 73:96–100.
61. Coates EL, Li A, Nattie EE. Widespread sites of brainstem ventilatory chemoreceptors. J Appl Physiol 1993; 75:5–14.
62. Nattie EE, Wood J, Mega A, Goritski W. Rostral ventrolateral medulla muscarinic receptor involvement in central ventilatory chemosensitivity. J Appl Physiol 1989; 66: 1462–1470.
63. Moss IR, Scarpelli EM. Generation and regulation of breathing in utero: Fetal CO_2 response test. J Appl Physiol 1979; 47:527–531.
64. Whittaker JAC, Trouth CO, Pan Y, et al. Age differences in responsiveness of brainstem chemosensitive neurons to extracellular pH changes. Life Sci 1990; 46:1699–1705.
65. Gabel RA, Kronenborg RS, Severinghaus JW. Vital capacity breaths of 5% or 15% CO_2 in N_2 or O_2 to test carotid chemosensitivity. Respir Physiol 1973; 17:195–208.
66. Rigatto H, Kwiatowski KA, Hasan SU, Cates DB. The ventilatory response to endogenous CO_2 in preterm infants. Am Rev Respir Dis 1991; 143:101–104.
67. Frantz ID III, Alder SM, Thach BT, Taeusch WH Jr. Maturational effects on respiratory response to carbon dioxide in premature infants. J Appl Physiol 1976; 41:41–45.
68. Rigatto H, Brady JP, de la Torre Verduzco R. Chemoreceptor reflexes in preterm infants: II. The effect of gestational and postnatal age on the ventilatory response to inhaled carbon dioxide. Pediatrics 1975; 55:614–621.
69. Wennergren G, Wennergren M. Respiratory effects elicited in newborn animals via the central chemoreceptors. Acta Physiol Scand 1980; 108:309–311.
70. Gerhardt T, Bancalari E. Ventilatory response to CO_2 in premature infants with apnea. Pediatr Res 1979; 13:534.
71. Kinney HC, Filiano JJ, Sleeper LA, Mandell F, Valdes Dapena M, White WF. Decreased muscarinic receptor binding in the arcuate nucleus in sudden infant death syndrome. Science 1995; 269:1446–1450.
72. Marcus CL, Glomb WB, Basinski DJ, Davidson Ward SL, Keens TG. Developmental pattern of hypercapnic and hypoxic ventilatory responses from childhood to adulthood. J Appl Physiol 1994; 76:314–320.
73. Gozal D, Arens R, Omlin KJ, Marcus CL, Keens TG. Maturational differences in step vs. ramp hypoxic and hypercapnic ventilatory responses. J Appl Physiol 1994; 76: 1968–1975.
74. Berthon Jones M, Sullivan CE. Ventilation and arousal responses to hypercapnia in normal sleeping humans. J Appl Physiol 1984; 57:59–67.

75. Douglas NJ, White DP, Weil JV. Hypercapnic ventilatory responses in sleeping adults. Am Rev Respir Dis 1982; 126:758–762.
76. Davi M, Sankaran K, McCallum M, Cates D, Rigatto H. Effect of sleep state on chest distortion and on the ventilatory response to CO_2 in neonates. Pediatr Res 1979; 13: 982–986.
77. Haddad GG, Leistner HL, Epstein RA, Epstein MAF, Grodin WK, Mellins RB. CO_2-induced changes in ventilation and ventilatory pattern in normal sleeping infants. J Appl Physiol 1980; 48:684–688.
78. Honma Y, Wilkes D, Bryan MH, Bryan AC. Ribcage and abdominal contributions to the ventilatory response to CO_2 in infants. J Appl Physiol 1984; 56:1211–1216.
79. Moriette G, Van Reempts P, Moore M, Cates D, Rigatto H. The effect of rebreathing CO_2 on ventilation and diaphragmatic electromyography in newborn infants. Respir Physiol 1985; 62:387–397.
80. Cohen G, Xu C, Henderson-Smart D. Ventilatory response of the sleeping newborn to CO_2 during normoxic rebreathing. J Appl Physiol 1991; 71:168–174.
81. Marks JD, Harper RM. Differential inhibition of the diaphragm and posterior cricoarytenoid muscles induced by transient hypertension across sleep states in intact cats. Exp Neurol 1987; 95:730–742.
82. Trelease RB, Sieck GC, Marks JD, Harper RM. Respiratory inhibition induced by transient hypertension during sleep. Exp Neurol 1985; 90:173–186.
83. Ohtake PJ, Jennings DB. Ventilation is stimulated by small reductions in arterial pressure in the awake dog. J Appl Physiol 1992; 73:1549–1557.
84. Clark DJ, Fewell JE. Decreased body-core temperature during acute hypoxemia in guinea pigs during postnatal maturation: a regulated thermoregulatory response. Can J Physiol Pharmacol 1996; 74:331–336.
85. Mortola JP, Rezzonico R. Metabolic and ventilatory rates in newborn kittens during acute hypoxia. Respir Physiol 1988; 73:55–63.
86. Beckwith JB. Pathology discussion. In: Bergman AB, Beckwith FB, Ray CG, eds. Sudden Infant Death Syndrome: Proceedings of the Second International Conference on Causes of Sudden Death in Infants. Seattle, WA: University of Washington Press, 1970: 120–122.
87. Harper RM, Leake B, Hodgman JE, Hoppenbrowers T. Developmental patterns of heart rate and heart rate variability during sleep and waking in normal infants and infants at risk for the sudden infant death syndrome. Sleep 1982; 5:28–38.
88. Kluge KA, Harper RM, Schechtman VL, Wilson AJ, Hoffman HJ, Southall DP. Spectral analysis assessment of respiratory sinus arrhythmia in normal infants and infants who subsequently died of sudden infant death syndrome. Pediatr Res 1988; 24:677–682.
89. Woo MA, Stevenson WG, Moser DK, Trelease RB, Harper RM. Patterns of beat-to-beat heart rate variability in advanced heart failure. Am Heart J 1992; 123:704–710.
90. Woo MS, Woo MA, Gozal D, Jansen MT, Keens TG, Harper RM. Heart rate variability in congenital central hypoventilation syndrome. Pediatr Res 1992; 31:291–296.
91. Schechtman VL, Harper RM, Wilson AJ, Southall DP. Sleep apnea in infants who succumb to the sudden infant death syndrome. Pediatrics 1991; 87:841–846.
92. Harper RM, Bandler R. Finding the failure mechanism in the sudden infant death syndrome. Nature Med 1998; 4:157–158.
93. Lutherer LO, Lutherer BC, Dormer KJ, Janssen HF, Barnes CD. Bilateral lesions of the fastigial nucleus prevent the recovery of blood pressure following hypotension induced by hemorrhage or administration of endotoxin. Brain Res 1983; 269:251–257.

94. Chen CH, Williams JL, Lutherer LO. Cerebellar lesions alter autonomic responses to transient isovolaemic changes in arterial pressure in anaesthetized cats. Clin Auton Res 1994; 4:263–272.
95. Harper RM, Bandler R, Alger J, Bockhorst KHJ, Mintorovitch J, Spriggs D. Functional magnetic resonance imaging of hippocampal and cerebellar activation to pressor challenges. Soc Neurosci Abstr 1997; 23:425.
96. Moruzzi G. Paleocerebellar inhibition of vasomotor and respiratory carotid sinus reflexes. J Neurophysiol 1940; 3:20–32.
97. Paton JFR, Spyer KM. Brain stem regions mediating the cardiovascular responses elicited from the posterior cerebellar cortex in the rabbit. J Physiol 1990; 427:533–552.
98. Reis DJ, Golanov EV. Autonomic and vascular regulation. Int Rev Neurobiol 1997; 41:121–149.
99. Williams JL, Everse SJ, Lutherer LO. Stimulating fastigial nucleus alters central mechanisms regulating phrenic activity. Respir Physiol 1989; 76:215–227.
100. Xu F, Frazier DT. Cerebellar role in the load-compensating response of expiratory muscle. J Appl Physiol 1994; 77:1232–1238.
101. Xu F, Owen J, Frazier DT. Cerebellar modulation of ventilatory response to progressive hypercapnia. J Appl Physiol 1994; 77:1073–1080.
102. Huang Q, Zhou D, St John WM. Cerebellar control of expiratory activities of medullary neurons and spinal nerves. J Appl Physiol 1993; 74:1934–1940.
103. Gozal D, Hathout GM, Kirlew KAT, Tang H, Woo MS, Zhang J, Lufkin RB, Harper RM. Localization of putative neural respiratory regions in the human by functional magnetic resonance imaging. J Appl Physiol 1994; 76:2076–2083.
104. Gozal D, Omidvar O, Kirlew KAT, Hathout GM, Hamilton R, Lufkin RB, Harper RM. Identification of human brain regions underlying responses to inspiratory loading with functional magnetic resonance imaging. Proc Nat Acad Sci USA 1995; 92:6607–6611.
105. Gozal D, Omidvar O, Kirlew KAT, Hathout GM, Lufkin RB, Harper RM. Functional magnetic resonance imaging reveals brain regions mediating the response to resistive expiratory loads in humans. J Clin Invest 1996; 97:47–53.
106. Panigrahy A, Filiano JJ, Sleeper LA, Mandell F, Valdes-Dapena M, Krous HF, Rava LA, White WF, Kinney HC. Decreased kainate receptor binding in the arcuate nucleus of the sudden infant death syndrome. J Neuropath Exper Neurol 1997; 56:1253–1261.
107. Zec N, Filiano JJ, Kinney HC. Anatomic relationships of the human arcuate nucleus of the medulla: a DiI labeling study. J Neuropath Exper Neurol 1997; 56:509–522.
108. Henderson LA, Keay KA, Bandler R. The ventrolateral periaqueductal gray projects to caudal brainstem depressor regions: a functional-anatomical and physiological study. Neuroscience 1998; 82:201–221.
109. Doba A, Reis DJ. Role of the cerebellum and vestibular apparatus in regulation of orthostatic reflexes in the cat. Circ Res 1974; 34:9–18.
110. Yates BJ. Vestibular influences on the autonomic nervous system. In: Highstein SM, Cohen B, Buttner-Ennever JA, eds. New Directions in Vestibular Research. Ann NY Acad Sci 1996; XX:458–470.
111. Mancia G, Baccelli G, Adams DB, Zanchetti A. Vasomotor regulation during sleep in the cat. Am J Physiol 1971; 220:1086–1093.
112. Gassel M, Ghelarducci B, Marchiafava PL, Pompeiano O. Phasic changes in blood pressure and heart rate during the rapid eye movement episodes of desynchronized sleep in unrestrained cats. Arch Ital Biol 1964; 102:530–544.

113. Harper RM, Schechtman VL. Physiological measurements as predictive tests for SIDS. Rognum TO, ed. Sudden Infant Death Syndrome: New Trends in the Nineties. Oslo: Scandinavian University Press, 1995: 314–319.
114. Kirby DA, Verrier RL. Differential effects of sleep stage on coronary hemodynamic function. Am J Physiol 1989; 256:H1378–H1383.
115. Dickerson LW, Huang AH, Thurnher MM, Nearing BD, Verrier RL. Relationship between coronary hemodynamic changes and the phasic events of rapid eye movement sleep. Sleep 1993; 16:550–557.
116. Dickerson LW, Huang AH, Nearing BD, Verrier RL. Primary coronary vasodilation associated with pauses in heart rhythm during sleep. Am J Physiol 1993; 264:R186–R196.
117. Verrier R, Lau TR, Wallooppillai U, Quattrochi J, Nearing BD, Moreno R, Hobson JA. Primary vagally mediated decelerations in heart rate during tonic rapid eye movement sleep in cats. Am J Physiol 1998; 274:R1136–R1141.
118. Fewell JE. Influence of sleep on systemic and coronary hemodynamics in lambs. J Dev Physiol 1993; 19:71–76.
119. Rector DM, Gozal D, Forster HV, Ohtake PJ, Pan LG, Lowry TF, Harper RM. Imaging of goat ventral medullary surface activity during sleep-waking states. Am J Physiol 1994, 267:R1154–R1160.
120. Rector DM, Oguri M, Harper RM. Imaging of ventral medullary surface changes in the freely behaving cat. Soc Neurosci Abstr 1996; 22:852.
121. Harper RM, Rector DM, Poe G, Forster HV, Ohtake PJ, Pan LG, Lowry TF, Gozal D. Ventral medullary surface activity changes during momentary blood pressure variation within sleep states. Soc Neurosci Abstr 1995; 21:1015.
122. McAllen RM. Identification and properties of sub-retrofacial bulbospinal neurones: a descending cardiovascular pathway in the cat. J Auton Nerv Syst 1986; 17:151–164.
123. Harper RM, Gozal D, Forster HV, Ohtake PJ, Pan LG, Lowry TF, Rector DM. Imaging of ventral medullary surface activity during blood pressure challenges in awake and anesthetized goats. Am J Physiol 1996; 39:R182–R191.
124. Forster HV, Gozal D, Harper RM, Lowry TF, Ohtake PJ, Pan LG, Rector DM. Ventral medullary surface activity during hypoxia in awake and anesthetized goats. Respir Physiol 1996; 103:45–56.
125. Gozal D, Ohtake PJ, Rector DM, Lowry TF, Pan LG, Forster HV, Harper RM. Rostral ventral medullary surface activity during hypercapnic challenges in awake and anesthetized goats. Neurosci Lett 1995; 192:89–92.
126. Forster HV, Ohtake PJ, Pan LG, Lowry TF, Korducki MJ, Aarons EA. Effects on breathing of cooling the ventrolateral medulla (VLM) in anesthetized and awake goats. Proceedings of the International Union of Physiological Science, 33d Congress, Vol. 4 (abstr). Glasgow, 1993: 194.
127. Harper RM, Gozal D, Aljadeff G, Carroll JL, Dong XW, Rector DM. Optical imaging of pressor-induced neural activation of the cat ventral medullary surface. Am J Physiol 1995; 268:R324–R333.
128. Carroll JL, Gozal D, Rector DM, Aljadeff G, Harper RM. Peripheral chemoreceptor afferent contributions to the intermediate area of the ventral medullary surface of the cat. Neuroscience 1996; 73:989–998.
129. Gozal D, Aljadeff G, Carroll JL, Rector DM, Harper RM. Afferent contributions to intermediate area of the cat ventral medullary surface during mild hypoxia. Neurosci Lett 1994; 178:73–78.

130. Aljadeff G, Gozal D, Carroll JL, Rector DM, Harper RM. Ventral medullary response to hypoxic and hyperoxic transient ventilatory challenges in the cat. Life Sci 1995; 57:319–324.
131. Severinghaus JW, Mitchell RA. Ondine's curse: failure of respiratory automaticity while asleep. Clin Res 1962; 10:122.
132. Harper RM, Sauerland EK. The role of the tongue in sleep apnea. In: Guilleminault C, Dement WC, eds. Sleep Apnea Syndromes. New York: Liss, 1978: 219–234.
133. Remmers JE, Degroot WJ, Sauerland EK, Auch AM. Pathogenesis of upper airway occlusion during sleep. J Appl Physiol 1978, 44:931–938.
134. Baust W, Weidinger H, Kirchner F. Sympathetic activity during natural sleep and arousal. Arch Ital Biol 1968; 106:379–390.
135. Jouvet M. Recherches sur les structures nerveuses et les mecanismes responsables des differentes phases du sommeil physiologique. Arch Ital Biol 1962; 100:125–206.
136. Munschauser FE, Mader MJ, Ahuja A, Jacobs L. Selective paralysis of voluntary but not limbically influenced automatic respiration. Arch Neurol 1991; 48:1190–1192.
137. Holstege G. Anatomical study of the final common pathway for vocalization in the cat. J Comp Neurol 1989; 284:242–252.
138. Holstege G, Meiners L, Tan K. Projections of the bed nucleus of the stria terminalis in the mesencephalon, pons, and medulla oblongata in the cat. Exp Brain Res 1985; 58: 379–391.
139. Hopkins DA, Holstege G. Amygdaloid projections to the mesencephalon, pons and medulla oblongata in the cat. Exp Brain Res 1978; 32:529–547.
140. Holstege G. Some anatomical observations on the projections from the hypothalamus to brainstem and spinal cord: an HRP and autoradiographic tracing study in the cat. J Comp Neurol 1987; 260:98–126.
141. Frysinger RC, Zhang J, Harper RM. Cardiovascular and respiratory relationships with neuronal discharge in the central nucleus of the amygdala during sleep-waking states. Sleep 1988; 11:317–332.
142. Terreberry RR, Oguri M, Harper RM. State-dependent respiratory and cardiac relationships with neuronal discharge in the bed nucleus of the stria terminalis. Sleep 1995; 18:139–144.
143. Zhang JX, Harper RM, Frysinger RC. Respiratory modulation of neuronal discharge in the central nucleus of the amygdala during sleep and waking states. Exp Neurol 1986; 91:193–207.
144. Harper RM, Frysinger RC, Trelease RB, Marks JD. State-dependent alteration of respiratory cycle timing by stimulation of the central nucleus of the amygdala. Brain Res 1984; 306:1–8.
145. Zhang JX, Harper RM, Ni H. Cryogenic blockade of the central nucleus of the amygdala attenuates aversively conditioned blood pressure and respiratory responses. Brain Res 1986; 386:136–145.
146. Li Y-W, Dampney RAL. Expression of Fos-like protein in brain following sustained hypertension and hypotension in conscious rabbits. Neuroscience 1994; 61:613–634.
147. Kristensen MP, Poe GR, Rector DM, Harper RM. Activity changes of the cat paraventricular hypothalamus during phasic respiratory events. Neuroscience 1997; 80: 811–819.
148. Coveñas R, de León M, Cintra A, Bjelke B, Gustafsson J-Å, Fuxe K. Coexistence of *c-Fos* and glucocorticoid receptor immunoreactivities in the CRF immunoreactive neu-

rons of the paraventricular hypothalamic nucleus of the rat after acute immobilization stress. Neurosci Lett 1993; 149:149–152.

149. Kristensen MP, Rector DM, Poe GR, Harper RM. Reflectance imaging of the hypothalamic paraventricular region demonstrates biphasic cellular activation patterns in freely behaving cats during noise exposure. First World Congress on Stress, Bethesda, Maryland, 1994, p. 56.
150. Swanson LW, Kuypers HGJM. The paraventricular nucleus of the hypothalamus: cytoarchitectonic subdivisions and organization of projections to the pituitary, dorsal vagal complex, and spinal cord as demonstrated by retrograde fluorescence double labelling methods. J Comp Neurol 1980; 194:555–570.
151. Luiten PGM, ter Horst GJ, Karst H, Steffens AB. The course of paraventricular hypothalamic efferents to autonomic structures in medulla and spinal cord. Brain Res 1995; 329:374–378.
152. Saper CB, Loewy AD, Swanson LW, Cowan WM. Direct hypothalamo-autonomic connections. Brain Res 1976; 117:305–312.
153. Parmeggiani PL, Azzaroni A, Cevolani D, Ferrari G. Responses of anterior hypothalamic-preoptic neurons to direct thermal stimulation during wakefulness and sleep. Brain Res 1983; 269:382–385.
154. Ni H, Schechtman VL, Zhang J, Glotzbach SF, Harper RM. Respiratory responses to preoptic/anterior hypothalamic warming during sleep in kittens. Reprod Fertil Dev 1996; 8:79–86.
155. Johnson P. Airway reflexes and the control of breathing in postnatal life. Ann NY Acad Sci 1988; 533:262–275.
156. Stanton AN. Overheating and cot deaths. Lancet 1984; 24:1199–1201.
157. Kahn A, Blum D. Sudden infant death syndrome and phenothiazines. Pediatrics 1983; 71:986–988.
158. Lovick TA, Hilton SM. Vasodilator and vasoconstrictor neurones of the ventrolateral medulla in the cat. Brain Res 1985; 331:353–357.

10

Postnatal Development of Carotid Chemoreceptor Function

JOHN L. CARROLL

Johns Hopkins University School of Medicine
New Haven, Connecticut

DAVID F. DONNELLY

Yale University School of Medicine
Baltimore, Maryland

I. Overview

Regulation of arterial oxygen levels is critically important in mammals, particularly during early life. Peri- and postnatal hypoxia may lead to death, impaired cognitive development, and abnormalities in cardiovascular function, breathing control maturation, and lung function (1–3).

The main sensors of arterial O_2 tension are the carotid body chemoreceptors, which are located bilaterally at the bifurcations of the common carotid arteries. Carotid chemoreceptor sensory afferents, via the carotid sinus nerves (CSN), project to the nucleus tractus solitarius and other brainstem nuclei, providing the major source of O_2-mediated ventilatory drive. Neural signals from the carotid chemoreceptors to brainstem cardiorespiratory control nuclei also mediate critically important respiratory reflexes such as arousal from sleep during hypoxia and cardiovascular reflexes that modulate heart rate and blood pressure (4).

Perhaps surprisingly, given their importance, the carotid chemoreceptors have a low sensitivity to hypoxia at the time of birth and become more sensitive to hypoxia over the first few days of life. In some species, a slower phase of carotid chemoreceptor maturation has been described, with O_2 sensitivity increasing slowly over weeks or months (5). This enhanced hypoxia sensitivity of arterial chemoreceptors (rightward shifting of the O_2 response curve) after birth is termed *resetting*, and it occurs in both carotid and aortic chemoreceptors (6). Although it is clear that the increase in oxygen tension at birth is a major factor initiating carotid chemoreceptor resetting (7), the exact mechanism and sites of maturation are unknown.

The critical importance of carotid chemoreceptor function during infancy has been demonstrated by experiments in which the carotid sinus nerves are severed just after birth. Adults survive bilateral carotid denervation (CD) (8). In sharp contrast, bilateral CD in newborns leads to hypoventilation, increased frequency of central apnea, prolonged duration of apnea, abnormal breathing pattern development, and mortality rates as high as 66% during the neonatal period (9–12).

Taken together, available data suggest that a "vulnerable period" exists in mammalian postnatal development during which functioning carotid chemoreceptors are crucial for maintaining normal respiration. Abnormalities in respiration or respiratory pattern may be especially critical in neonates because of their low pulmonary O_2 stores and higher ratio of O_2 consumption to body surface area. This leads to rapid oxyhemoglobin desaturation (rapidly developing hypoxemia) during periods of hypoventilation due to apnea, upper airway obstruction, rebreathing (e.g., bedding material covering the face) or illness.

In addition to hypoxia, the carotid chemoreceptors also respond to changes in CO_2, pH, temperature, osmolarity, elevated K^+, and several pharmacological stimuli. Lowering of the P_{O_2} increases carotid chemoreceptor sensitivity to CO_2, and raising CO_2 increases sensitivity to hypoxia, a phenomenon known as O_2–CO_2 interaction. A detailed description of the response to all of these stimuli as well maturational changes in the responses is beyond the scope of this chapter. Instead, we focus on 1) the role of the carotid chemoreceptors in normal breathing control during development, 2) maturation of the response to hypoxia, 3) developmental changes in carotid chemoreceptor neural responses to natural stimuli, 4) mechanisms of carotid body development, and 5) the carotid chemoreceptors in selected states of abnormal cardiorespiratory control.

II. The Carotid Chemoreceptors in Normal Breathing Control in Childhood

As noted above, the function of carotid chemoreceptors may be grossly assessed by comparing subjects whose chemoreceptors have been resected with normal subjects. This is more readily undertaken in animal studies; therefore, much of the information on the carotid chemoreceptors in maturation of breathing control derives from studies in rats, rabbits, cats, goats, ponies, dogs, and pigs. In the past, a population of human patients underwent carotid body resection for the treatment of intractable asthma and thus became a useful study population (13). Today, studies of human subjects necessarily employ indirect techniques, such as the Dejours transient O_2 test, which measure complex integrated responses. Although a great deal has been learned from the denervation approach, it is worth noting that the extent to which these studies can be extrapolated to human respiratory control maturation remains unclear.

A. Onset of Breathing at Birth

Studies in lambs show that the carotid chemoreceptors are not necessary for the onset of normal breathing at birth (14,15). However, they play important roles in a variety of other respiratory responses during development and in the mature mammal. Several studies using the carotid denervation approach have revealed striking effects on cardiorespiratory control during postnatal development. It should be noted that the neural output from carotid sinus baroreceptors also runs in the CSN, therefore cutting the CSN also results in denervation of carotid sinus baroreceptors in addition to chemoreceptors. Clearly, this complicates interpretation of studies using this approach.

B. Breathing Control Development

Denervation of carotid chemoreceptors in the newborn period has been shown to cause severe respiratory abnormalities in piglets, rats, and sheep. For instance, Donnelly and Haddad compared piglets undergoing CD and, in some cases, carotid and aortic denervation (CAD) at < 9 days of age to piglets undergoing denervation at ~ 30 days of age (10). Studies on the days following denervation showed abnormalities in breathing control in the young pig, characterized by prolonged apneas and desaturation. Of particular note, about 60% of the young denervated piglets died 3 to 7 days following surgery, while none in the older denervated or SHAM operated groups died (10). Coté et al. subsequently performed a more extensive study of denervated piglets with surgery performed at ~ 5, 10, 15, and 21 days of age. CD again resulted in prolonged apnea, severe hypoxemia, and flattening of the electroencephalogram (EEG), but the effect was confined to the 15-day group and only during quiet sleep. Prolonged apnea and hypoxemia were not observed at other ages or during active sleep at any age. Although the reasons for the difference in mortality rates between the studies is unclear, it is clear that the effect of denervation around the first weeks of life can have major effects on the generation of respiratory rhythm (16).

As in piglets, denervation in other species results in breathing abnormalities and increased mortality. Newborn lambs CD at 1 to 2 days of age died suddenly and unexpectedly in 43% of the cases between 4 and 5 weeks of age, suggesting that the carotid chemoreceptors become important for survival within a particular age range during development (9). These investigators also reported that minute ventilation (VE) in intact lambs, adjusted for body weight, decreased with age between 7 and 70 days, accompanied by characteristic changes in breathing pattern. In contrast, lambs CD just after birth exhibited hypoventilation and little change in $\dot{V}_E$ or breathing pattern during the same time frame (9). Similarly, CD in immature rats resulted in hypoventilation, especially during rapid-eye-movement (REM) sleep, and mortality rates of ~ 50% (11,12). Sectioning of the aortic depressor nerves alone did not have this effect.

Thus, it is clear that CD is associated with cardiorespiratory control abnormalities and an increased probability of mortality in immature mammals across species. However, caution must be exercised in the interpretation of survival data. The reasons for increased mortality in these studies is unknown. In addition, the extent to which the increased mortality was related to chemo- versus barodenervation or to other factors is unclear. Nevertheless, it seems clear that neural input from the carotid chemoreceptors, baroreceptors, or both is critically important for ensuring survival during a vulnerable period of postnatal development.

C. Central Apnea Termination

Central apnea is common in infants but is usually not prolonged beyond ~ 20 to 25 sec, is not associated with bradycardia, and is generally not accompanied by severe or prolonged hypoxemia (17). In general these apneas terminate spontaneously; however, considering the vulnerability of the newborn to rapid desaturation, termination of spontaneous apnea must be considered of vital importance. Therefore, the mechanisms responsible for the termination of central apnea and resumption of normal breathing are of particular interest, and here the carotid body appears to play a vital role.

Studies on the unanesthetized, awake lamb have indicated that carotid chemoreceptors have a major influence on the blood-gas threshold for the resumption of breathing following apnea (18). Apnea was induced by passive hyperventilation in lambs aged 1 day and 15 days under normoxic, hyperoxic, and hypoxic conditions. The apnea termination threshold (ATT) was determined by measuring the Pa_{O_2} and Pa_{CO_2} at which breathing resumed. The effect of carotid denervation was also examined in lambs < 2 days old. The results were striking. Figure 1 shows the apnea threshold for Pa_{O_2} ($PATT_{O_2}$) plotted against the apnea threshold for Pa_{CO_2} ($PATT_{CO_2}$). In 14-day-

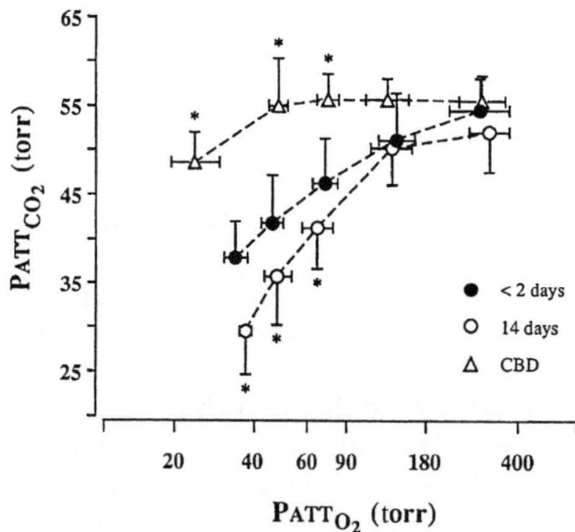

Figure 1 Mean $PATT_{CO_2}$ values calculated for each $PATT_{O_2}$ range (severe hypoxia, moderate hypoxia, normoxia, moderate hyperoxia, hyperoxia) in each group of lambs [groups were (●) < 2 days carotid body (CB) intact, (○) 14 days CB intact, (△) < 2 days carotid body denervated]. $PATT_{O_2}$ is plotted on a logarithmic scale. Values are mean ± SD. *Significant difference from 1-day-old lamb group, $p < .05$. (From Ref. 18.)

old lambs, as Pa_{O_2} was lowered from ~ 150 to ~ 40 mmHg, the CO_2 threshold for resumption of breathing became progressively lower, from ~ 50 to ~ 30 mmHg (Fig. 1, open circles). A similar relationship, although not as steep, was observed for the < 2-day-old lambs (Fig. 1, filled circles). In sharp contrast, in the CD group (open triangles), across the full range of Pa_{O_2} from ~ 400 to 30 mmHg, $PATT_{CO_2}$ remained elevated at ~ 50 to 55 mmHg (Fig. 1, triangles). Thus, in the absence of functioning carotid chemoreceptors, the Pa_{CO_2} threshold for resumption of breathing during central apnea is abnormally high and independent of Pa_{O_2}. In other words, input from the carotid chemoreceptors appears to modulate the level of Pa_{CO_2} at which breathing resumes after central apnea. Another important finding of this study was that hypoxia consistently failed to suppress the reinitiation of breathing after apnea, even in CD lambs. Therefore, although it appears the input from carotid chemoreceptors modulates the Pa_{CO_2} apnea threshold, the carotid chemoreceptors are not required for reinitiation of breathing.

D. Bradycardia

In mammals, stimulation of the carotid chemoreceptors may lead to profound vagally mediated bradycardia and negative inotropic effects (4,19). However, the situation is complex, as input from the carotid chemoreceptors to brainstem cardiovascular control areas is gated by respiratory phase, modulated by the level of Pa_{CO_2}, and modulated by the level of input from pulmonary stretch receptors (19). Nevertheless, prolonged expiratory apnea is a particularly dangerous condition for developing infants, because rapidly developing hypoxemia is likely and the resulting, powerful hypoxia-driven cardioinhibitory reflexes are unopposed by cardiostimulatory input from pulmonary stretch receptors (20). Although in the term fetal sheep hypoxia induces profound bradycardia via reflex mechanisms driven by the carotid chemoreceptors (21), little is known about the same reflex during postnatal life.

Carotid chemoreceptors may also significantly modulate reflex effects induced by other respiratory afferents. For instance, laryngeal stimulation (LCR) by water or foreign substances in the larynx causes a reflex effect consisting of apnea, bradycardia, arousal from sleep, swallowing, hypertension, and blood flow redistribution (22). Part of this pattern is due to the consequences of carotid body stimulation, particularly the bradycardia and hypertension components of this reflex (22,23). In addition, the same investigators found that CD markedly attenuated the arousal response to laryngeal stimulation during sleep, indicating yet another role for the carotid chemoreceptors in defensive responses of the developing infant (22). Wennergren et al., studying the LCR in human infants, found that mild hypoxia caused powerful enhancements of the bradycardic and apneic components of the response (24). More recent studies examining the effects of hypoxia on the LCR in piglets (25) and lambs (26) report that peripheral chemoreceptor stimulation enhances the bradycardia component. Taken together, these studies indicate an important role for the carotid chemoreceptors in the modulation of heart rate during hypoxia as well as significant interactions with other reflexes such as the LCR.

E. Respiratory Control Stability

The breathing pattern of the newborn and developing neonate is characterized by instability and exaggerated responses to perturbations such as sigh, movement, or apnea (27). Studies in adult mammals indicate a significant role for the carotid chemoreceptors in maintaining respiratory stability (28). Indirect evidence and theoretical modeling suggest that the carotid chemoreceptors play a role in newborn respiratory pattern instability, such as post-sigh apnea or oscillation (27,29,30). Although it is plausible that postnatal maturation of carotid chemoreceptor sensitivity plays a role in the development of respiratory system stability, and modeling approaches support this, direct evidence is lacking.

F. Arousal from Sleep

Arousal from sleep in response to hypoxic or hypercapnic challenge is a critically important defense mechanism. Fewell and Baker studied arousal from sleep in response to rapidly developing hypoxemia by challenging lambs with mild, moderate, or severe hypoxia during sleep (31). More severe levels of hypoxia resulted in a markedly faster rate of arterial desaturation. Arousal from sleep in response to hypoxia occurred in ~ 94% of the challenges and, during quiet sleep, the lambs aroused at an Sa_{O_2} of about 80%, no matter how rapidly Sa_{O_2} fell. However, during active sleep, more rapidly developing hypoxemia correlated with arousal occurring at progressively lower Sa_{O_2} levels. Interestingly, repeated exposure to rapidly developing hypoxemia further impaired the arousal response (32). The same authors later showed that carotid denervation markedly blunted arousal from sleep in response to rapidly developing hypoxemia, with only 28% of challenges resulting in arousal before Sa_{O_2} reached 30% (33). Because CD also denervates the carotid sinus baroreceptors, these authors could not determine the relative contribution of the chemo- vs. baroreceptors to their findings. However, it was clear that the carotid chemo- and/or baroreceptors play a major role in arousal from sleep in response to rapidly developing hypoxemia.

Arousal from sleep in response to upper airway obstruction or hypercapnia are other crucial defense mechanisms in the developing infant. Igras and Fewell showed, in 3- to 4-week-old lambs, that nasal or tracheal airway occlusion usually results in arousal from sleep, although the arousal response is significantly delayed in active compared to quiet sleep (34). Repeated airway obstruction further delayed the arousal response in active sleep (35). Carotid denervation markedly impaired the arousal response to airway obstruction. Following CD, although airway obstruction still produced arousal from sleep, the response was markedly delayed and occurred at lower Sa_{O_2} levels (36). In addition to mediating arousal responses to hypoxia and airway obstruction, Fewell et al. also reported that the carotid chemoreceptors play a major role in the arousal response to alveolar hypercapnia (37). Taken together, these studies indicate that the carotid chemoreceptors play a significant role in modulating arousal responses to hypoxemia, hypercapnia, and airway obstruction and that active sleep is a condition during which infants are likely to be particularly vulnerable to these stressors.

G. Ventilatory Response to Hypoxia: Selected Aspects

The neonatal ventilatory response to hypoxia is complex, reflecting a balance between increased neural input from the carotid chemoreceptors, central nervous system (CNS) inhibition (38,39), and hypoxic hypometabolism (40,41). The carotid chemoreceptors provide nearly all of the stimulatory input driving the ventilatory response to hypoxia (see Ref. 42 for review). Over three decades ago, Schwieler reported that carotid denervation in kittens eliminates the ventilatory response to hypoxia (43), and numerous studies have confirmed the key role of the carotid chemoreceptors in driving the $\dot{V}_E$ response to hypoxia in developing mammals.

In all mammalian species studied to date, the increase in $\dot{V}_E$ during hypoxia is relatively small in the newborn and increases with age (44–48). Furthermore, at all ages, the increased minute ventilation in response to a constant level of hypoxia is not sustained. Initially, upon exposure to hypoxia, minute ventilation rises, reaching maximum within several minutes; thereafter, $\dot{V}_E$ slowly declines (termed the *late decline in ventilation*, *biphasic response*, or *VE roll-off*) (Fig. 2). The major differences between mature and immature responses to hypoxia are that in mature mammals, the $\dot{V}_E$ response declines more slowly and is ultimately sustained at a higher level compared to that in neonates. The late decline in $\dot{V}_E$ during hypoxia is particularly pronounced in neonates, especially premature infants and nonhuman species that are relatively immature at birth.

There is strong evidence that the late $\dot{V}_E$ decline during hypoxia is mediated by inhibitory mechanisms operating at the level of the CNS. Possible mechanisms underlying the late $\dot{V}_E$ decline are discussed further in Chapter 23 and are not repeated here. However, intriguing results from recent studies raise interesting questions about a possible role for the carotid chemoreceptors in the late-phase $\dot{V}_E$ decline during hypoxia.

Figure 3 shows the effect on a 17-day-old anesthetized kitten of breathing 6% O_2. After an initial rise in breathing frequency and tidal volume, both fell progressively during the 4.5-min challenge. Blood pressure declined as well. However, throughout this classic example of the biphasic $\dot{V}_E$ response, neural output from the carotid chemoreceptors was sustained. This would appear to be consistent with the mechanism outlined above; stimulation from the carotid chemoreceptors is counteracted or "gated out" by depression at the CNS level. However, several lines of evidence suggest that it is not that simple and, to the contrary, suggest that the carotid chemoreceptors may mediate *both* the excitatory and significant proportions of the inhibitory components.

Schramm and Grunstein in 1987 reported that ventilatory depression occurred during hypoxia in 1- to 33-day-old rabbits, but that it required intact carotid chemoreceptors (49). Carotid denervation abolished both the excitatory and inhibitory components of the $\dot{V}_E$ response (Fig. 2). Similarly, Long et al. as well as Miller and Tenney reported that mild to moderate hypoxia failed to induce hypoventilation in CD awake adult cats (50,51). A similar lack of $\dot{V}_E$ depression during hypoxia was reported in awake, unanesthetized CD neonatal lambs (52). In contrast to results obtained with-

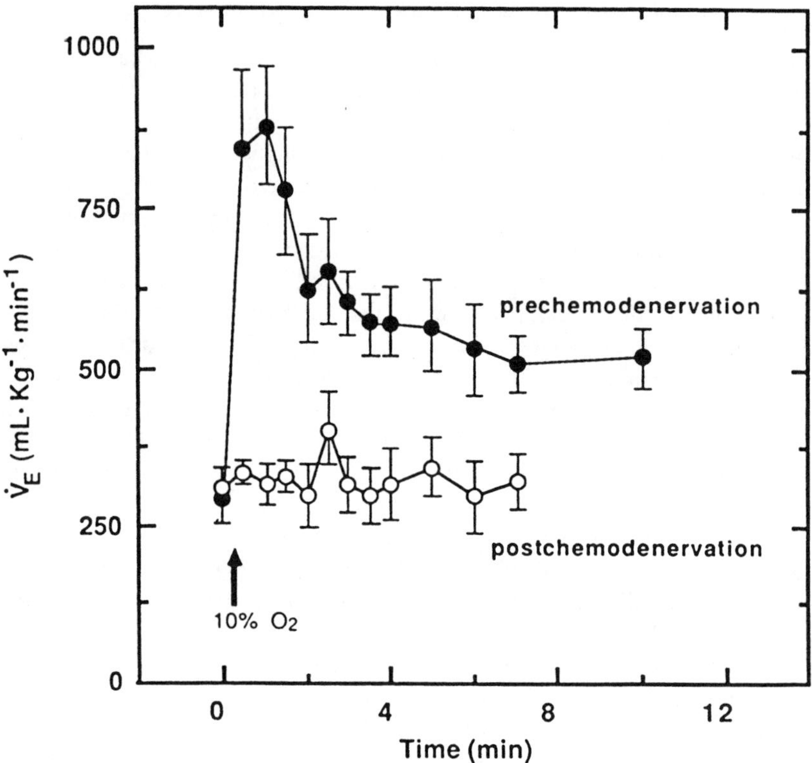

Figure 2 Time course of ventilatory responses to acute hypoxia in five rabbits before (filled circles) and after (open circles) peripheral chemodenervation. Data represent mean ± SE of minute ventilation adjusted for body weight. Note that after CD, there is no VE response to hypoxia but also no ventilatory depression. (From Ref. 49.)

out anesthesia, studies in anesthetized subjects have reported $\dot{V}_E$ depression during hypoxia following CD, but this is probably caused by the effects of anesthesia (50). While controversial, these findings suggest that central hypoxia cannot account for the ventilatory depression in the newborn. This suggests that input from the peripheral chemoreceptors plays a role in both the ventilatory excitation as well as the subsequent depression.

Several recent studies, taking a completely different approach, support the hypothesis that peripheral chemoreceptors stimulate central nuclei, which cause ventilatory depression. In vagotomized, paralyzed, decerebrate ~ 26-day-old rabbits, Waites et al. demonstrated that bilateral small lesions in the red nucleus abolished the late $\dot{V}_E$ (phrenic nerve output) decline, resulting in a sustained $\dot{V}_E$ response to hypoxia (53). Moore et al., studying anesthetized 3- to 8-day-old lambs, demonstrated that focal cooling in the dorsal pons, at the locus ceruleus, also eliminated (reversibly) the

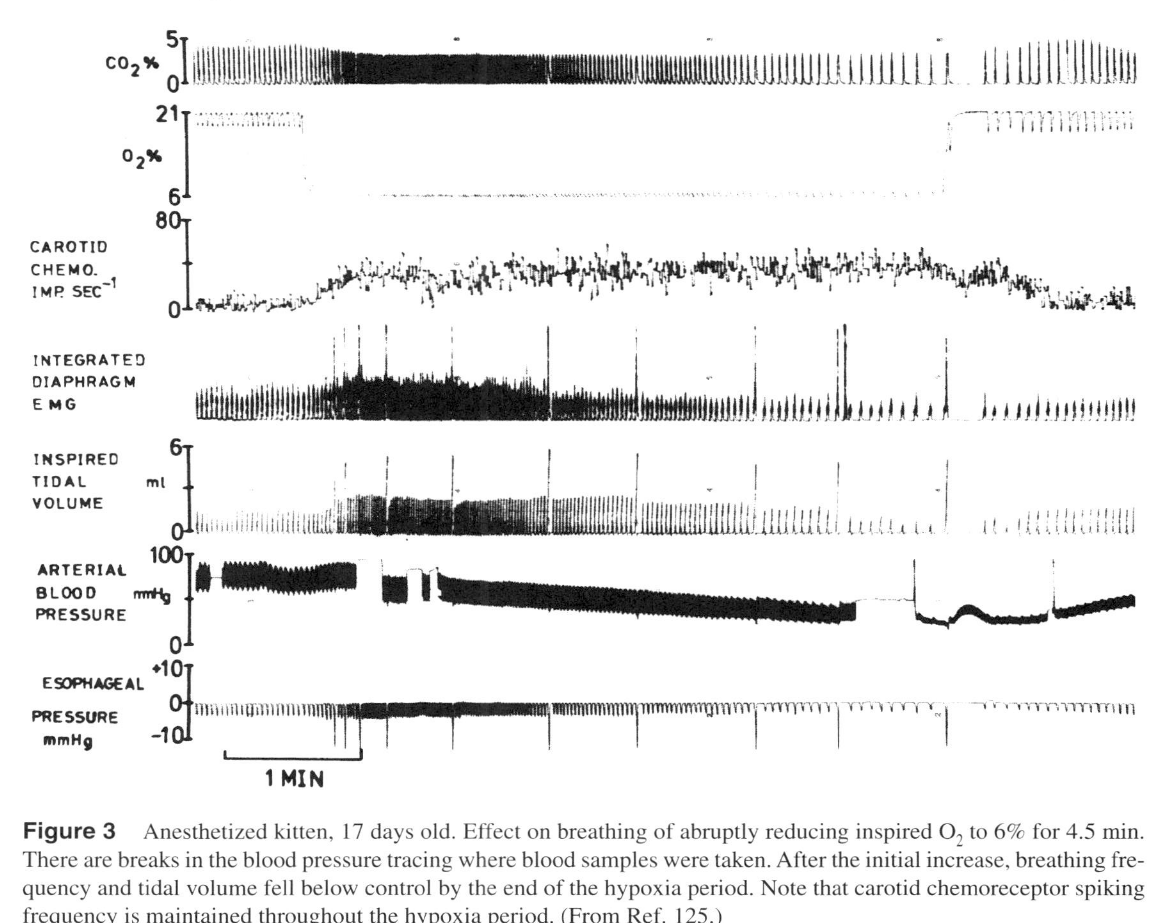

Figure 3 Anesthetized kitten, 17 days old. Effect on breathing of abruptly reducing inspired O_2 to 6% for 4.5 min. There are breaks in the blood pressure tracing where blood samples were taken. After the initial increase, breathing frequency and tidal volume fell below control by the end of the hypoxia period. Note that carotid chemoreceptor spiking frequency is maintained throughout the hypoxia period. (From Ref. 125.)

late decline in respiratory output during hypoxia (54). Thus, lesioning or cooling specific brainstem areas abolished the late $\dot{V}_E$ decline in spite of continued brain hypoxia. These results are consistent with the hypothesis that the late $\dot{V}_E$ decline during hypoxia is mediated by stimulation of brainstem neurons that are inhibitory to respiratory output (54). Combined with the observation that the late $\dot{V}_E$ decline in hypoxia (at least in unanesthetized subjects) depends on having intact carotid chemoreceptors, these data suggest that the neurons inhibiting the $\dot{V}_E$ response to hypoxia are stimulated by neural input from the carotid chemoreceptors.

The studies described above raise some intriguing possibilities. If the degree of cardiorespiratory depression during hypoxia depends on a complex balance between chemoreceptor-driven excitatory versus inhibitory neuron pools, then differences in rates of maturation of neurons involved in the $\dot{V}_E$ response to hypoxia could result in imbalances and vulnerability during particular periods of development. Little is known about potential sources of developmental vulnerability to hypoxic stress and more work is needed in this critically important area.

III. Developmental Changes in O_2 Chemoreflexes

Numerous studies have attempted to assess the role of the carotid chemoreceptors in the maturation of breathing control using the transient O_2 test developed by Dejours (55). In this test, the inspired gas is suddenly switched from room air to 100% O_2 for a few breaths, causing Pa_{O_2} to rise suddenly and peripheral chemoreceptors abruptly to reduce their spiking rates. As a result, minute ventilation falls, and the drop in $\dot{V}_E$ is proportional to the amount of $\dot{V}_E$ drive arising from the carotid chemoreceptors at the moment of the test (55). Using this approach, it was shown that in human infants transient exposure to 100% O_2 had no effect in 2- to 6-hr-old newborns but caused an ~ 10% fall in $\dot{V}_E$ in 2- to 6-day-old infants (56). Comparable results were obtained in other species (46,56,57). Because hyperoxia is applied systemically, the response includes contributions by the entire peripheral and CSN neural pathway; it does not assess peripheral chemoreceptor output per se. Maturational changes in the relative contribution of the peripheral chemoreceptors to overall $\dot{V}_E$ drive may be entirely due to changes in central gating or processing of chemoreceptor inputs. In addition, the magnitude and time profile of the stimulus may be affected by lung function.

There are several alternative methods of assessing peripheral chemoreceptor function in developing intact animals. In the opposite sense to the Dejours test, peripheral chemoreceptors may be selectively stimulated by switching to a few breaths of N_2 or brief injection of a low dose of cyanide. When a subject is suddenly exposed to two or three breaths of pure N_2, there is a sudden large drop in Pa_{O_2} and a corresponding transient increase in minute ventilation. Theoretically, this should allow measurement of the immediate, dynamic $\dot{V}_E$ response to hypoxia without the confounding effects of hypocapnia, blood pH shifts, and brain hypoxia that occur with more prolonged challenges. Using this test in lambs, Canet et al. reported that the $\dot{V}_E$ response to three breaths of N_2 nearly doubled between ~ 24 hr of age versus 12 days

(58). As with the transient O_2 test, this one also uses $\dot{V}_E$ as an output measure and is therefore not a direct test of peripheral chemoreceptor output. A variation on this approach involves administration of intravenous NaCN to stimulate the peripheral chemoreceptors in developing animals. With this method, it was demonstrated in lambs that the $\dot{V}_E$ response to 0.1 mg/kg of intravenous NaCN increased nearly fourfold between 2 and 10 days of age, with no further increase at 21 days (46). However, this test also uses $\dot{V}_E$ as the outcome measure and suffers from the limitations described above.

Still another method of assessing O_2 chemoreflex maturation is the alternating breath technique, which alternates Fi_{O_2} between normoxia and hypoxia every other breath. This oscillating input function, sensed by the peripheral chemoreceptors, generates an alternating output function in the form of breath-to-breath alternation of instantaneous $\dot{V}_E$. The degree of $\dot{V}_E$ alternation produced by the alternating of Fi_{O_2} is taken as a measure of peripheral chemoreceptor sensitivity. With this method it was demonstrated, in unanesthetized kittens, that the alternation response was absent on day 1 and increased after day 4 of age, again indicating a developmental increase in the O_2 chemoreflex response (59). This test, which shares the limitations discussed in the preceding paragraphs, has also been used in human infants. Calder et al. used this method on human infants, reporting that the alternation response was present by ~ 43 hr and was not increased further at 47 days (60). They concluded that, in humans, the "resetting" of peripheral chemoreceptor responses to hypoxia was almost complete by 24 to 48 hr of age. However, they did not study older infants or intermediate ages, leaving open the possibility for a missed peak (at an intermediate age between 2 and 47 days) or a slower rate of maturation over many months. In any case, by any method of testing, it is clear that developmental changes in O_2 chemoreflex strength occur in all species studied to date.

IV. Developmental Changes in Afferent Chemoreceptor Nerve Activity

As discussed above, the carotid chemoreceptors modulate resting respiratory control as well as driving ventilatory, arousal, and other critically important defensive responses to stressors such as hypoxia. Therefore, it is noteworthy that important developmental changes also occur at the level of the peripheral chemoreceptors (61). In the newborn, the sensitivity of the neural response to hypoxia and hypercapnia is less than in the adult, and the neural response is more poorly sustained than in the adult.

The concept of hypoxia sensitivity may be viewed from two perspectives. First, from the viewpoint of a relative change in nerve activity, and this is usually assessed by recording from many nerve fibers simultaneously and normalizing all measurements to baseline activity or peak activity. Alternatively, chemoreceptor activity may be considered as an absolute—that is, in terms of spiking activity of individual axons. This type of recording represents the minimal unit of chemoreceptor activity, since no further subdivision of a functioning chemoreceptor unit is possible. When viewed from both perspectives, significant developmental changes occur in peripheral chemoreceptor function.

V. Hypoxia Sensitivity and Response

On both absolute and relative scales, the level of spiking activity for a given level of hypoxia is less in the newborn than in the adult, and maturation appears to occur in the first 2 weeks after birth. This was first unequivocally demonstrated by Mulligan in piglets, in which she employed single-axon recordings in vivo from cell bodies of chemoreceptor neurons in the petrosal ganglion (Fig. 4) (62). Based on recordings from a population of single axons, the increase in spiking activity in response to graded hypoxia was approximately twofold greater in 12- to 20-day-old piglets than in 1- to 5-day-old piglets (Fig. 4).

Not only was the peak frequency of discharge greater in the older piglets, but the response curve was shifted to the right (sensitivity increased). Similar rightward shifts in the response curves were also found in kittens (5,63) and lambs (61). This developmental increase in hypoxia sensitivity is not limited to the carotid chemoreceptors, since a 50% increase in the response to hypoxia was also observed in recordings from aortic chemoreceptors in vivo (6). This increased responsiveness is of some import, because the chemoreceptor response curve is not linear but approximates the hyperbolic dissociation curve of hemoglobin (64). The right shift of the chemoreceptor response curve with development would thus provide a greater safety margin in avoiding significant oxygen desaturation.

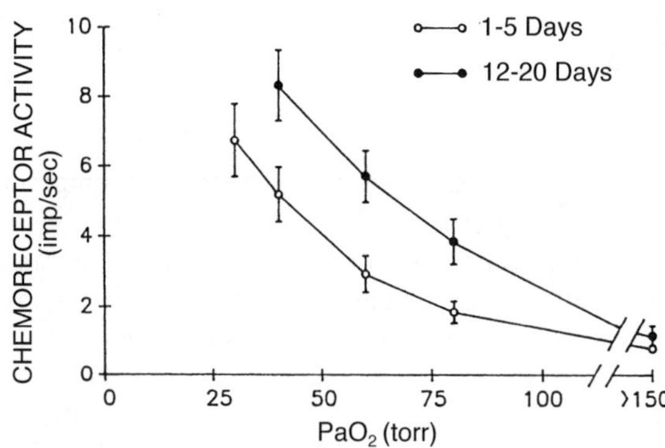

Figure 4 Single-cell carotid chemoreceptor afferent responses to isocapnic hypoxia in young (1- to 5-day-old) and older (12- to 20-day-old) piglets. (Mean ± SEM, n = 10 for each age group). Chemoreceptor activity was significantly greater in the older age group at all P_{O_2} levels except hyperoxia. (From Ref. 68.)

Before birth, chemoreceptor activity is even more reduced as compared to the newborn. Some studies indicate that fetal chemoreceptor activity is low or absent and, when present, fails to respond to hypoxia, at least in the presence of normal sympathetic activity (65,66). Results of other studies indicate that fetal chemoreceptor activity is present but the response curve is far left-shifted compared to the newborn and adult response curves. For instance, it was necessary to reduce fetal Pa_{O_2} to below 20 mmHg in order to increase chemoreceptor nerve activity by two- to fourfold (61). In comparison, a Pa_{O_2} of 60 to 70 mmHg would be expected to increase chemoreceptor activity threefold in the adult (67).

In addition to a reduced sensitivity to hypoxia, the newborn may also be less able to sustain a neural carotid chemoreceptor response to hypoxia. Mulligan noted this in her piglets, in which a strong hypoxic stimulus (below 30 mmHg) resulted in a decrease rather than an increase in spiking activity (68). Several of her axons, in fact, ceased to continue spiking and required reoxygenation in order to resume spiking. This observation was confirmed and extended by Marchal et al. and Carroll et al., who observed significant accommodation to a hypoxic stimulus. Using single-fiber recording of kitten chemoreceptors, Marchal observed that 46% of 1- to 3-day-old kitten chemoreceptor fibers accommodated to a hypoxic stimulus, but this was not observed in fibers recorded from 15-day-old kittens (63). Similar results were obtained using whole-nerve recordings in kittens (5).

A. CO_2 Sensitivity and Response

As compared to experiments addressing hypoxia sensitivity, less data are available on the developmental changes in CO_2 sensitivity, and some of these data have been inconsistent. Recordings of single-fiber chemoreceptor nerve activity from kittens indicate some developmental increase in hypercapnia sensitivity over the first 2 weeks of life (63), and a similar developmental increase in single-fiber nerve activity was reported by Calder and colleagues in lambs (69). Other data suggest that the developmental increase continues over a much longer period. In studies of kitten chemoreceptors, there was no significant change in the whole-nerve response to hypercapnia between 1 week and 8 weeks of age, but there was a significant increase to adulthood, suggesting that maturation of the CO_2 response is quite slow in this species (5). On the other hand, some studies indicate that the response to hypercapnia is unchanged after birth (70) or that, while the steady-state response to CO_2 may increase after birth, the dynamic response to CO_2 is unchanged (69). Finally, Bamford et al., using multifiber CSN recording in excised superfused carotid bodies from rats aged term-fetal to 21 days, found no significant maturational increase in the response to 15% CO_2 (71).

Confounding a clear interpretation to these (sometimes) conflicting data are uncertainties introduced by normalization parameters. For instance, one study calculated the percent increase in nerve RMS voltage during application of a 6% inspired CO_2 stimulus and determined that this increased with age (5). However, normalization to whole-nerve baseline spiking activity may have introduced an age bias if the newborn had a greater level of nonchemoreceptor activity or higher baseline spiking rates than the adult. In another study, nerve activities were normalized to that obtained during superfusion of a chemoreceptor in vitro, with saline equilibrated to 70 mmHg P_{O_2}. In this case, it was claimed that hypercapnia sensitivity did not change with age (70). However, since spiking rates during hypoxia are higher in older animals (62,72) normalization to the higher spiking rates may have obscured a developmental increase in hypercapnic responsiveness. A recent study of Bamford et al., also using an in vitro superfusion approach, also found no developmental increase in the CO_2 response during the first 3 weeks of life in rats (71). This study did not employ normalization. It is clearly difficult or even impossible to fully appreciate the biases introduced by normalization procedures applied to multifiber nerve activities, but it is worthwhile keeping in mind that they may introduce a variable that may have a significant effect on the conclusions.

Despite some evidence that the carotid sinus nerve response to CO_2 increases with age, the increased responsiveness does not appear to be reflected in the ventilatory output. Analysis of the ventilatory response to a transient hypercapnia stimulus (which is assumed to specifically stimulate the peripheral chemoreceptors) showed no developmental change in lambs over the course of 1 to 12 days of age in the response to 13% CO_2 in air (58). Similar results were obtained in maturing piglets using a sophisticated systems analysis to isolate the fast (peripheral) chemoreceptor part of the ventilatory response to CO_2 (73). Taken together, these observations suggest that there may be a developmental increase in CO_2 sensitivity in some species, but the magnitude is smaller and time course is slower than maturation of the hypoxia response.

B. Interactions in CO_2 and Oxygen

Hypoxia and acidity not only stimulate chemoreceptor activity but also interact together, enhancing activity beyond that expected for a simple summation of stimuli. This is perhaps best observed in the family of CO_2 response curves as developed against several different P_{O_2} backgrounds. The slope of the CO_2 response line is steeper as the level of oxygen is decreased (5). In contrast, the same experiment in the newborn yields CO_2 response curves that show little interaction between CO_2 and hypoxia (5).

This observation was placed on a more quantitative basis by Kumar and colleagues, who deconvolved the response of rat chemoreceptors recorded in vitro into three components: 1) a response to hypoxia alone, 2) response to CO_2 alone, and 3) a term CO_2 multiplied by hypoxia. In this case, all chemoreceptor activities were normalized to 100% (defined as the spiking activity observed during superfusion with 70 mmHg oxygen). Using this normalization scheme, there was no change with age in the sensitivity to CO_2 alone or to hypoxia alone, but age significantly enhanced the stimulus interaction between CO_2 and hypoxia. The effect of the combined stimuli was superadditive in the adult but not in the newborn. These findings are consistent with a recent study from Bamford et al., which used multifiber CSN recording in excised superfused carotid bodies from rats aged term- fetal to 21 days (71). Although they found no developmental increase in the carotid body response to CO_2, O_2-CO_2 interaction was absent in carotid bodies from rats term-fetal to 11 days, but increased fivefold by 16 to 21 days of age (71). Thus, it appears that development specifically targets O_2–CO_2 interaction and not the response to hypercapnia per se.

VI. Mechanisms of Developmental Changes

An overview of the carotid chemoreceptor is shown in Fig. 5. The chemoreceptor complex consists of the afferent nerve fibers whose cell bodies are in the petrosal ganglia. The axons enter the carotid body, bifurcate, and terminate on O_2-sensitive secretory cells (glomus cells). The terminations may be quite extensive. A cat carotid body contains approximately 10,000 glomus cells, each of which averages a single nerve terminal. The sinus nerve contains about 500 axons, resulting in an estimated 20 glomus cells per single chemoreceptor axon (74). Because of the synaptic arrangement, it is universally speculated that hypoxia and acidity are transduced by glomus cells resulting in the release of an excitatory transmitter(s). The purported excitatory transmitter causes nerve depolarization and enhanced spiking activity on the afferent nerve.

Although this transduction path is reasonable based on some biophysical responses of glomus cells (described below), it is hardly established. Most lacking is the identification of an excitatory transmitter, since pharmacologic blockade of many candidate neurotransmitters yields no change in afferent nerve activity or increased, not decreased, afferent nerve activity. For instance, application of an antagonist to

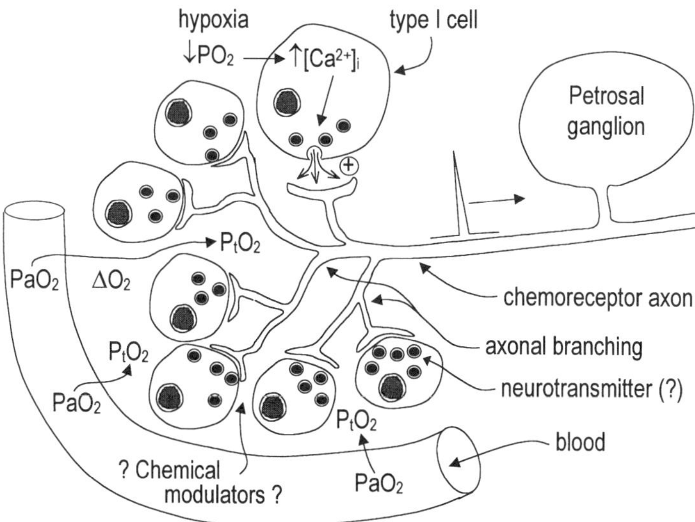

Figure 5 Schematic drawing of mammalian carotid body. See text for explanation.

dopamine D_2 receptors, which should block the effects of released catecholamine (a major candidate transmitter of the glomus cell) causes an enhancement of the nerve response to hypoxia, especially in rats exposed to chronic hypoxia (75). In addition, there is a body of evidence suggesting that the afferent nerve terminals may possess an endogenous sensitivity to hypoxia, thus obviating the necessity to postulate the existence of an excitatory neurotransmitter (76). Data are currently lacking to reach a definite conclusion regarding the mechanism of afferent nerve excitation, but for the purposes of this chapter we will stay with the conventional model in which the glomus cell is the transducing element and releases a neurotransmitter that excites the afferent nerve endings. On occasion we will speculate on alternate models.

A. Changes in Organ Anatomy

Despite the high level of blood flow to the carotid body, the tissue oxygen tension is considerably lower than arterial blood, and it is the level of tissue oxygen pressure which undergoes developmental change. Measurements of carotid body tissue P_{O_2} indicate that tissue oxygenation decreases over the first week of life and that the alveolar $\dot{V}_{O_2}$ difference increases following the increase an arterial oxygen tension (such as occurs after birth) (77). This likely reflects changes in blood vessel control, since no anatomical vascular changes occur over this time period (78,79), thus strengthening the case for the importance of local neural control of the circulation. This is further supported by the observations that sympathetic stimulation causes afferent activity to increase (80) and that parasympathetic stimulation causes nerve activity to decrease (81), apparently related to local blood flow changes (77). This modulation may be particularly potent around the time of birth, because chemoreceptor activity may be switched from absent to present by sympathetic stimulation in the fetus (66).

B. Changes in Humoral Factors

In addition to local flow changes, factors in the blood may modulate chemoreceptor activity, such as changes in serum K^+, Na^+, or osmolarity. For instance, the slight increase in K^+ that occurs with exercise causes a 20% to 30% increase in the sensitivity to hypoxia (82). In addition, an isotonic decrease in sodium by 20% may reduce chemoreceptor spiking rates by over 50% (126), and a small increase in serum osmolarity also decreases afferent nerve activity (83). Whether these circulatory factors contribute to the postnatal changes in chemosensitivity in the newborn period remains unexplored.

Circulatory neurochemicals may also potentially modulate carotid chemoreceptor activity in the newborn period. Endorphins levels decrease in the newborn period, and application of exogenous endorphins causes an inhibition of hypoxia sensitivity (84). Thus, the postnatal enhancement of chemoreceptor activity may be partly due to a reduction in endorphin-based inhibition. An additional but unidentified neurochemical is also implicated based on the work of Joels and Neil in 1968. These investigators noted that chemoreceptors perfused with artificial plasma became unresponsive over time but could be functionally restored by the addition of as little as 5% blood to the perfusate, suggesting the presence of a vital factor in blood which is not present in artificial plasma (85). On the other hand, fetal blood may contain an inhibitory modulator based on the observation that chemoreceptor nerve activity is difficult to record in situ but may be readily recorded from the same chemoreceptor after removal and perfusion with saline (66).

C. Morphological Changes in Synapses and Nerve Terminals

In addition to developmental changes in vascular control or hormonal factors, there is strong evidence that developmental changes occur within the chemoreceptor complex itself. Removal and superfusion of the organ with oxygenated saline would be expected to eliminate all circulatory factors. Under these conditions, the level of spiking activity recorded on individual axons during severe hypoxia clearly increases with age (72). This correlates well with results of an anatomical study demonstrating that the number of synapses between afferent nerve endings and glomus cells increase four to five times between birth and 20 days of age (86).

What is less clear is whether there is an actual increase in hypoxia sensitivity as compared to an increase in spike generation sites. While it is well established that the nerve activity at a given P_{O_2} is less in the newborn (Fig. 4), there are two ways to interpret this difference. The newborn response may be "left- shifted" from the adult, such that one may overlay the response lines by shifting the adult curve to the left by approximately 30 mmHg, suggesting a change in the sensitivity of the oxygen sensor. On the other hand, the lines may be superimposed by multiplying the newborn response by a constant without changing the apparent sensitivity to hypoxia, suggesting no change in sensitivity but an increase in spike-generating sites. There are insufficient data to discriminate between these possibilities based on published studies from recordings in vivo. However, from rat chemoreceptors in vitro, the apparent sensitivity to hypoxia (here expressed as a rate constant for a decrease in activity with an increase in superfusate P_{O_2}) was unchanged with development, suggesting no change in the sensor's sensitivity for hypoxia.

D. Glomus Cell Anatomy and Physiologic Responses

A general schema for the release of an excitatory transmitter from glomus cells may involve three steps: 1) glomus cell depolarization and activation of voltage-dependent calcium currents, 2) a rise in intracellular calcium, and 3) enhanced neurotransmitter secretion due to the rise in intracellular calcium. None of these steps are unequivocally established, but they nevertheless provide a framework for addressing some developmental changes in glomus cell properties.

Glomus Cell Membrane Depolarization with Hypoxia

Depolarization of the glomus cell by hypoxia is likely the first critical step in the transduction cascade, but the mechanism for the depolarization is far from resolved. Several investigators have proposed that hypoxia inhibits a K^+ current, which leads to cell depolarization. Several different types K^+ currents that are inhibited by hypoxia have been described in glomus cells and can be broadly categorized as 1) transient (87), 2) calcium- dependent (88), and 3) background or "leak" (89). Of all these O_2-sensitive K^+ currents, the P_{O_2} current inhibition relatinship of the background K^+ current (89) most closely matches the P_{O_2}–$[Ca^{2+}]_i$ relationship of dissociated glomus cells (90–92) and the tissue P_{O_2}–nerve activity relationship of the carotid body (93). In the case of the transient K^+ current, the sensitivity to hypoxia appears to be abnormally high, with complete inhibition at P_{O_2} levels considerably higher than that for the $[Ca^{2+}]_i$ response or organ response to hypoxia (94). The O_2-response curve for the calcium-dependent current has not been elucidated, to date. Whether or not an hypoxia-sensitive background K^+ conductance is responsible for depolarizing glomus cells in response to hypoxia remains to be demonstrated.

To date, formal developmental studies have been undertaken only for the calcium-dependent current, and preliminary studies have been undertaken on the background K^+ current. Both currents are found to mature in the newborn period. The magnitude of the calcium-dependent current increases with age over the first 1 to 2 weeks of life (Fig. 6) (95), and this current is reduced by raising the animals in chronically hypoxic conditions (96). This experimental maneuver appears to eliminate the physiological signal for chemoreceptor maturation, and it is established that animals so treated maintain an immature response to hypoxia (59). Similarly, recent preliminary data from one of our laboratories (Carroll) demonstrated that the O_2 sensitivity of the background or "leak" K^+ conductance (89) is small in glomus cells from newborn rats and increases over the first 2 weeks of life (MJ Wasicko and JL Carroll, unpublished observations). Although the maturational time course for both currents matches the known time course of glomus cell $[Ca^{2+}]_i$ response maturation (91) and nerve activity hypoxia response maturation (72), a causal nature to the relationship has not been established for either oxygen-sensitive current.

Calcium Responses of Glomus Cells

Depolarization of the glomus cell leads to activation of voltage-dependent calcium currents and a rise in intracellular calcium. Based on recording from a large number of glomus cells, the magnitude of the calcium response is significantly greater in glomus cells harvested from older animals compared to younger animals (91,97). Wasicko et al. recently characterized the $[Ca^{2+}]_i$ response to graded hypoxia in glomus cells isolated from term-fetal, 1-, 3-, 7-, 11-, 14-, and 21-day-old rats (91). The response was hyperbolic at all ages. Two major developmental changes were noted, an increase in the maximal $[Ca^{2+}]_i$ response to anoxia and an apparent rightward shift in the response curve with age (Fig. 7). The developmental increase in the $[Ca^{2+}]_i$ response to graded hypoxia occurred between 3 and 11 to 14 days of age, which agrees well with the reported time course for maturation of carotid body nerve responses to anoxia (72).

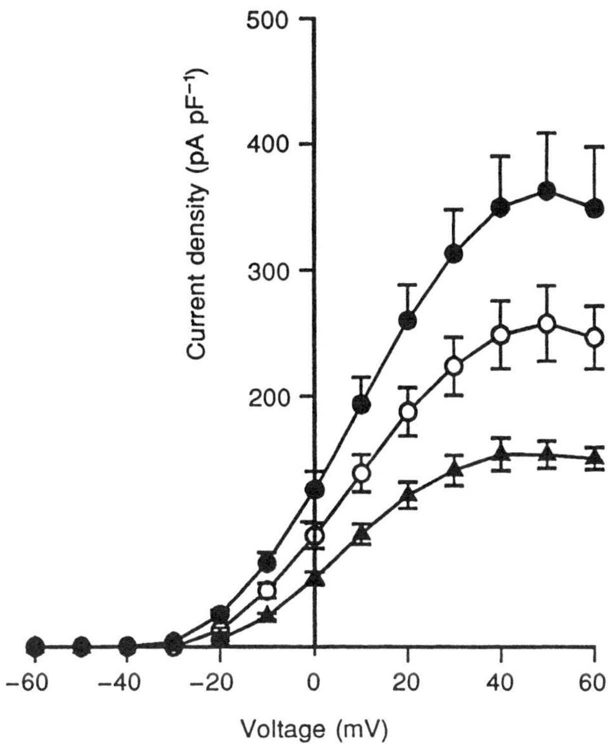

Figure 6 Current density-voltage plots of glomus cell K^+ currents from 4-day-old (▲, *n* = 40 cells), 10-day-old (○, *n* = 47 cells), and adult rats (●, *n* = 46 cells). Currents were evoked by step depolarizations from −70 mV to between − 30 and +50 mV in 20 mV increments. (From Ref. 95.)

The smaller calcium response of the immature cell does not appear to be due to a lack of voltage-gated calcium channels, since the calcium channel density is similar between 4- and 10-day-old rats (95). In addition, Wasicko et al. found no change in the glomus cell $[Ca^{2+}]_i$ response to elevated extracellular K^+ between 3 and 14 days of age, the same time frame during which all of the developmental increase in the $[Ca^{2+}]_i$ response to hypoxia occurred (91). If elevated K^+ is taken to be a nonspecific depolarization stimulus, these results indicate that the immature glomus cell is capable of mobilizing large amounts of $[Ca^{2+}]_i$ with depolarization, suggesting that maturation of the $[Ca^{2+}]_i$ response is not due to changes in voltage-gated calcium channels. Furthermore, chronic hypoxia after birth increases, not decreases, the magnitude of the whole-cell calcium current in response to a depolarization (98), although this may largely be caused by the hypertrophy associated with chronic hypoxia (99). In addition, a recent study reported that glomus cells harvested from 11-day-old rats reared in chronic hypoxia had minimal or no $[Ca^{2+}]_i$ response to hypoxia, while $[Ca^{2+}]_i$ re-

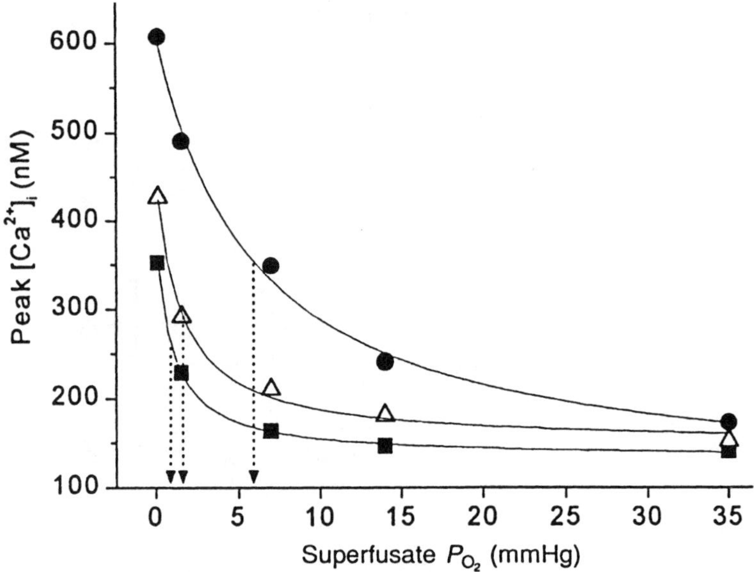

Figure 7 Rightward/upward shift in glomus cell $[Ca^{2+}]_i$ response to hypoxia with age. Mean peak $[Ca^{2+}]_i$ responses of dissociated carotid chemoreceptor cells from three age groups plotted versus superfusate P_{O_2}. Age groups were as follows: ■ = fetal–1 day (*n* = 28 glomus cell clusters), △ = 3–7 days (*n* = 15 clusters), ● = 11–21 days (*n* = 34 clusters). Arrows indicate superfusate P_{O_2} at half-maximal $[Ca^{2+}]_i$ response. (From Ref. 91.)

sponses to elevated extracellular K^+ and CO_2 were unaffected (100). Taken together, these results suggest that the postnatal development of glomus cell $[Ca^{2+}]_i$ response to hypoxia depends on maturation of an O_2 sensor or its ability to depolarize the cell.

A second possible area of maturation is in the number of responding cells. Several studies conclude that a significant number of glomus cells fail to deporalize with hypoxia (101) and many glomus cells fail to increase their intracellular calcium levels with hypoxia (97,102–104). Why many cells fail to respond is presently unclear, although methods of cell preparation and stimulus strength may be important. For example, Bright et al. used 35 mmHg superfusate P_{O_2} as the "hypoxia" challenge and found that only 20% of isolated glomus cells responded with an increase in $[Ca^{2+}]_i$ (102). However, 35 mmHg $P_{O_2}$is in the normoxic range of carotid body microvascular (tissue) P_{O_2} (93), which may explain the low proportion of glomus cell $[Ca^{2+}]_i$ responses reported by these authors. In a recent study using superfusate P_{O_2}'s of 0, 2, 7, and 14 mmHg, the great majority of glomus cells significantly raised $[Ca^{2+}]_i$ in response to hypoxia (91). Nevertheless, patch-clamp recordings of intact glomus cells demonstrate a suppression of calcium-dependent K^+ current in many cells under normoxic conditions (105), suggesting that calcium currents may be inhibited in situ. If so, then the number of responding cells may (potentially) increase postnatally, providing an enhanced response with development.

E. Secretory Responses

As in adrenal chromaffin cells, an increase in intracellular calcium influx leads to enhanced secretion by the glomus cells. Since a major constituent of the dense cored vesicles in glomus cell cells is catecholamine, catecholamine release is often used as an index of glomus cell secretion. Consistent with a role of catecholamine release in afferent nerve excitation are the observations that catecholamine release occurs in close temporal association with nerve excitation and treatments that eliminate catecholamine release—for instance, perfusion with calcium- free saline also eliminates hypoxia-induced changes in nerve activity (106).

The magnitude of the catecholamine secretory response for a given stimulus increases in the postnatal period, as does the magnitude of the response to hypoxia. This was first demonstrated by observing the response to an anoxic stimulus, which rapidly increases both nerve activity and free tissue catecholamine (Fig. 8) (107,108). A similar increase in the total release of catecholamine following a 1-hr incubation in solution equilibrated with 8% oxygen was recently described for isolated rabbit carotid bodies in which release as a proportion of total dopamine was larger in 25-day and adult rabbit than in rabbit pups (109).

The increased secretion of catecholamine is paralleled by an increased expression of D_2 receptors in the petrosal ganglia (location of the cells bodies whose axons innervate the carotid body) and in the carotid body itself. D_2-receptor mRNA in both the ganglia and carotid body increases by fivefold in rabbits between 1 and 25 days of age (110). However, in the opposite sense, pharmacological antagonism of D_2 receptors with domperidone has a greater effect on the hypoxia sensitivity in the newborn compared to the older cat (111). Although the role of dopamine receptors in organ function is presently unresolved, it is clear that catecholamine secretion as well as catecholamine receptors undergo changes in the postnatal period.

In addition to the proposed excitatory role for catecholamines, there is evidence that some catecholamine receptors are inhibitory. Application of dopamine antagonists generally excite rather than inhibit chemoreceptor activity in both the newborn and adult (64,111). This demonstrated inhibitory effect gave rise to an alternate theory of the lower sensitivity in the newborn period. Instead of a lack of excitation, it was proposed that excessive secretion of catecholamines may lead to an active inhibition in the newborn period (57,112). This is supported by data showing a higher turnover rate for catecholamine in rat carotid body immediately after birth and decreasing over the first 12 to 18 hr after birth (57). Furthermore, postnatal hypoxia, which appears to impair maturation of the normal adult pattern, perpetuates the high turnover of catecholamine (112). While this alternative model offers some explanation for the postnatal maturation, it appears that the maturation of the turnover rate occurs too rapidly. The period of high catecholamine turnover occurs only within the

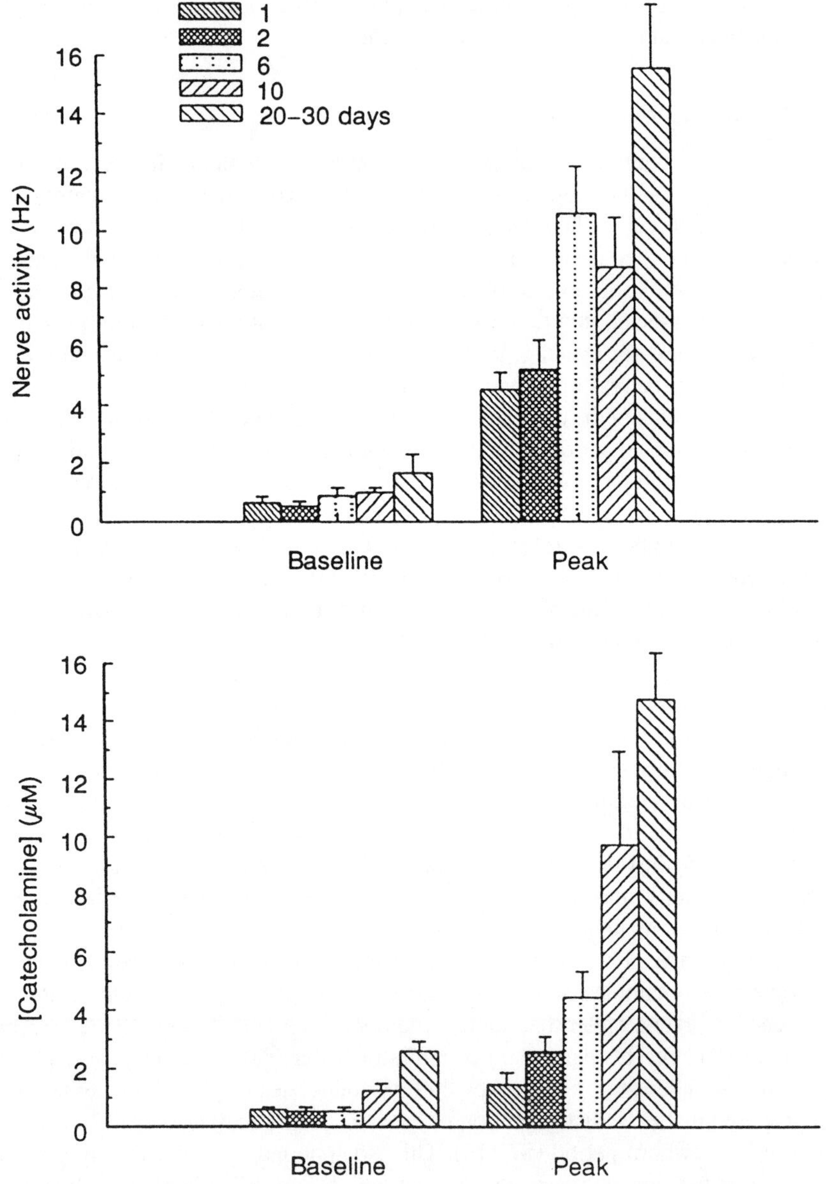

Figure 8 Baseline and peak values for rat carotid sinus nerve activity and carotid body catecholamines. Mean ± SEM for carotid bodies harvested from rats aged 1 ($n = 6$), 2 ($n = 6$), 6 ($n = 5$), 10 ($n = 7$), and 20 to 30 days ($n = 11$). Note age-dependent increase in both tissue catecholamines and CSN response to anoxia. (From Ref. 107.)

first 6 hr after birth, while the developmental changes in nerve and calcium responses appear to occur over the first 1 to 2 weeks (71,72,91,97).

VII. The Carotid Chemoreceptors and Abnormal Breathing Control in Children

Much has been written elsewhere about the possible roles of the carotid chemoreceptors in disease states affecting human infants and children. However, most of this literature consists of inferences from indirect evidence and direct evidence is sometimes conflicting. Although there is no question that disorders such as bronchopulmonary dysplasia (58,113–115) or prematurity (58,116) are associated with marked abnormalities in ventilatory or arousal responses to hypoxia, it is less clear how much this involves abnormal carotid chemoreceptor function per se versus abnormal CNS processing of chemoreceptor inputs. Breathing control in premature infants is discussed elsewhere (Chap. 23).

Pathological conditions such as sudden infant death syndrome, bronchopulmonary dysplasia and apparent life threatening events (ALTE) may be associated with chronic or recurrent hypoxia. Therefore, it is noteworthy that chronic hypoxia, from birth markedly blunts carotid chemoreceptor maturation. Using the alternating breath technique to assess peripheral chemoreflex strength, Hanson et al. reported that kittens born into and reared in Fi_{O_2} 0.13 to 0.15 exhibited marked impairment of arterial chemoreflex maturation during the first 2 weeks of life (117). Similarly, chronic hypoxia from birth in rats has been shown to attenuate the maturation of CO_2–O_2 interaction at the carotid body (118). These results are consistent with reports that glomus cells from rats reared in hypoxia do not depolarize in response to acute hypoxia (96) and do not exhibit $[Ca^{2+}]_i$ responses to acute hypoxic challenge (100). Although the mechanisms remain to be worked out, it is clear that chronic hypoxia may profoundly affect maturation of carotid chemoreceptor sensitivity. Further work is needed to determine the precise role(s) played by carotid chemoreceptor abnormalities in disorders such as SIDS, ALTE, BPD, and prematurity.

Chronic or recurrent hypoxia has been implicated in SIDS, although the cause or causes of SIDS remain unknown (20). Involvement of the carotid bodies in the pathogenesis of SIDS is controversial; several investigators have reported specific carotid body abnormalities in SIDS victims (119–121), while others have not found abnormalities (122,123). Reported abnormalities—such as reduction of dense cytoplasmic granules of the carotid chemoreceptor cells, reduction of glomus cell number and size (120), and 10-fold higher concentrations of dopamine compared to carotid bodies from age-matched control infants (121)—may result from chronic hypoxia or from postmortem artifact and do not necessarily implicate the carotid bodies in the pathogenesis. Other studies looking for similar abnormalities in structure and catecholamine levels did not find differences between SIDS victims and controls (122,123). In any case, impairment of carotid chemoreceptor O_2 sensitivity and neural output may not be detectable on postmortem examination. It should also be noted that carotid chemoreceptors need not be abnormal to play a role in SIDS. Normal maturation of carotid body O_2 sensitivity may underlie, in part, developmental vulnerability to stressors such as airway obstruction or asphyxia due to sleeping position or bedding materials covering the infant's face (20,124). Finally, carotid chemoreceptor function may start out normal and become blunted by recurrent or chronic hypoxia, which may then further increase vulnerability to hypoxic stress (20). Much more work is necessary before conclusions can be reached concerning the role of the carotid chemoreceptors in SIDS.

VIII. Summary

The carotid chemoreceptors play a critically important role in numerous aspects of respiratory and cardiovascular control, particularly in defensive responses that are important during sleep. In addition, the effects of carotid chemoreceptor stimulation are complex, with inputs to key brainstem cardiorespiratory cell groups being inhibitory in some cases and stimulatory in others. Complex integrated responses to hypoxia depend on a balance between multiple effects of carotid chemoreceptor stimulation as well as other effects of hypoxia on cardiorespiratory control centers. Although the carotid chemoreceptors drive vitally important responses—such as arousal from sleep in response to hypoxia, the ventilatory response to hypoxia, hypoxia-induced bradycardia and apnea termination—their chemosensory function is immature at birth and increases with age. As maturation may be impaired or delayed by common clinical conditions such as chronic hypoxia, it is important to understand the numerous key roles played by the carotid chemoreceptors and the changes that occur during postnatal development.

References

1. Nyakas C, Buwalda B, Luiten PG. Hypoxia and brain development. Prog Neurobiol 1996; 49:1–51.
2. Hudlicka O, Brown MD. Postnasal growth of the heart and its blood vessels. J Vasc Res 1996; 33:266–287.
3. Okubo S, Mortola JP. Long-term respiratory effects of neonatal hypoxia in the rat. J Appl Physiol 1988; 64:952–958.
4. Marshall JM. Peripheral chemoreceptors and cardiovascular regulation. Physiol Rev 1994; 74:543–594.
5. Carroll JL, Bamford OS, Fitzgerald RS. Postnatal maturation of carotid chemoreceptor responses to O_2 and CO_2 in the cat. J Appl Physiol 1993; 75:2383–2391.
6. Kumar P, Hanson MA. Re-setting of the hypoxic sensitivity of aortic chemoreceptors in the new-born lamb. J Dev Physiol 1989; 11:199–206.
7. Blanco CE, Hanson MA, McCooke HB. Effects on carotid chemoreceptor resetting of pulmonary ventilation in the fetal lamb in utero. J Dev Physiol 1988; 10:167–174.
8. Whipp BJ, Ward SA. Physiologic changes following bilateral carotid-body resection in patients with chronic obstructive pulmonary disease. Chest 1992; 101:656–661.

9. Bureau MA, Lamarche J, Foulon P, Dalle D. Postnatal maturation of respiration in intact and carotid body–chemodenervated lambs. J Appl Physiol 1985; 59:869–874.
10. Donnelly DF, Haddad GG. Prolonged apnea and impaired survival in piglets after sinus and aortic nerve section. J Appl Physiol 1990; 68:1048–1052.
11. Hofer MA. Lethal respiratory disturbance in neonatal rats after arterial chemoreceptor denervation. Life Sci 1984; 34:489–496.
12. Hofer MA. Role of carotid sinus and aortic nerves in respiratory control of infant rats. Am J Physiol 1986; 251:R811–R817.
13. Nakayama K. Surgical removal of the carotid body for bronchial asthma. Dis Chest 1961; 40:595–604.
14. Jansen AH, Ioffe S, Russell BJ, Chernick V. Effect of carotid chemoreceptor denervation on breathing in utero and after birth. J Appl Physiol 1981; 51:630–633.
15. Herrington RT, Harned HSJ, Ferreiro JI, Griffin CA. The role of the central nervous system in perinatal respiration: studies of chemoregulatory mechanisms in the term lamb. Pediatrics 1971; 47:857–864.
16. Cote A, Porras H, Meehan B. Age-dependent vulnerability to carotid chemodenervation in piglets. J Appl Physiol 1996; 80:323–331.
17. Hunt CE, Hufford DR, Bourguignon C, Oess MA. Home documented monitoring of cardiorespiratory pattern and oxygen saturation in healthy infants. Pediatr Res 1996; 39:216–222.
18. Delacourt C, Canet E, Bureau MA. Predominant role of peripheral chemoreceptors in the termination of apnea in maturing newborn lambs. J Appl Physiol 1996; 80:892–898.
19. Daly MD. Carotid chemoreceptor reflex cardioinhibitory responses: comparison of their modulation by central inspiratory neuronal activity and activity of pulmonary stretch afferents. Adv Exp Med Biol 1993; 337:333–343.
20. Marshall JM. Chemoreceptors and cardiovascular control in acute and chronic systemic hypoxia. Braz J Med Biol Res 1998; 31:863–888.
21. Giussani DA, Spencer JA, Moore PJ, Bennet L, Hanson MA. Afferent and efferent components of the cardiovascular reflex responses to acute hypoxia in term fetal sheep. J Physiol (Lond) 1993; 461:431–449.
22. Grogaard J, Kreuger E, Lindstrom D, Sundell H. Effects of carotid body maturation and terbutaline on the laryngeal chemoreflex in newborn lambs. Pediatr Res 1986; 20:724–729.
23. Grogaard J, Lindstrom DP, Stahlman MT, Marchal F, Sundell H. The cardiovascular response to laryngeal water administration in young lambs. J Dev Physiol 1982; 4:353–370.
24. Wennergren G, Hertzberg T, Milerad J, Bjure J, Lagercrantz H. Hypoxia reinforces laryngeal reflex bradycardia in infants. Acta Paediatr Scand 1989; 78:11–17.
25. Woodson GE, Brauel G. Arterial chemoreceptor influences on the laryngeal chemoreflex. Otolaryngol Head Neck Surg 1992; 107:775–782.
26. Sladek M, Grogaard JB, Parker RA, Sundell HW. Prolonged hypoxemia enhances and acute hypoxemia attenuates laryngeal reflex apnea in young lambs. Pediatr Res 1993; 34:813–820.
27. Fleming PJ, Goncalves AL, Levine MR, Woollard S. The development of stability of respiration in human infants: changes in ventilatory responses to spontaneous sighs. J Physiol (Lond) 1984; 347:1–16.
28. Daristotle L, Berssenbrugge AD, Engwall MJ, Bisgard GE. The effects of carotid body hypocapnia on ventilation in goats. Respir Physiol 1990; 79:123–135.

29. Tehrani FT. A model study of periodic breathing, stability of the neonatal respiratory system, and causes of sudden infant death syndrome. Med Eng Phys 1997; 19:547–555.
30. Cleave JP, Levine MR, Fleming PJ. The control of ventilation: a theoretical analysis of the response to transient disturbances. J Theor Biol 1984; 108:261–283.
31. Fewell JE, Baker SB. Arousal from sleep during rapidly developing hypoxemia in lambs. Pediatr Res 1987; 22:471–477.
32. Fewell JE, Konduri GG. Repeated exposure to rapidly developing hypoxemia influences the interaction between oxygen and carbon dioxide in initiating arousal from sleep in lambs. Pediatr Res 1988; 24:28–33.
33. Fewell JE, Kondo CS, Dascalu V, Filyk SC. Influence of carotid denervation on the arousal and cardiopulmonary response to rapidly developing hypoxemia in lambs. Pediatr Res 1989; 25:473–477.
34. Igras D, Fewell JE. Arousal response to upper airway obstruction in young lambs: comparison of nasal and tracheal occlusion. J Dev Physiol 1991; 15:215–220.
35. Fewell JE, Williams BJ, Szabo JS, Taylor BJ. Influence of repeated upper airway obstruction on the arousal and cardiopulmonary response to upper airway obstruction in lambs. Pediatr Res 1988; 23:191–195.
36. Fewell JE, Taylor BJ, Kondo CS, Dascalu V, Filyk SC. Influence of carotid denervation on the arousal and cardiopulmonary responses to upper airway obstruction in lambs. Pediatr Res 1990; 28:374–378.
37. Fewell JE, Kondo CS, Dascalu V, Filyk SC. Influence of carotid-denervation on the arousal and cardiopulmonary responses to alveolar hypercapnia in lambs. J Dev Physiol 1989; 12:193–199.
38. Lawson EE, Long WA. Central origin of biphasic breathing pattern during hypoxia in new borns. J Appl Physiol 1983; 55:483–488.
39. Martin-Body RL. Brain transections demonstrate the central origin of hypoxic ventilatory depression in carotid body- denervated rats. J Physiol (Lond) 1988; 407:41–52.
40. Frappell P, Saiki C, Mortola JP. Metabolism during normoxia, hypoxia and recovery in the newborn kitten. Respir Physiol 1991; 86:115–124.
41. Mortola JP, Rezzonico R, Lanthier C. Ventilation and oxygen consumption during acute hypoxia in newborn mammals: a comparative analysis. Respir Physiol 1989; 78:31–43.
42. Gonzalez C, Almaraz L, Obeso A, Rigual R. Carotid body chemoreceptors: from natural stimuli to sensory discharges. Physiol Rev 1994; 74:829–898.
43. Schwieler GH. Respiratory regulation during postnatal development in cats and rabbits and some of its morphological substrate. Acta Physiol Scand Suppl 1968; 304:1–123.
44. Belenky DA, Standaert TA, Woodrum DE. Maturation of hypoxic ventilatory response of the newborn lamb. J Appl Physiol 1979; 47:927–930.
45. Bonora M, Marlot D, Gautier H, Duron B. Effects of hypoxia on ventilation during postnatal development in conscious kittens. J Appl Physiol 1984; 56:1464–1471.
46. Bureau MA, Begin R. Postnatal maturation of the respiratory response to O_2 in awake newborn lambs. J Appl Physiol 1982; 52:428–433.
47. Eden GJ, Hanson MA. Maturation of the respiratory response to acute hypoxia in the newborn rat. J Physiol (Lond) 1987; 392:1–9.
48. Haddad GG, Gandhi MR, Mellins RB. Maturation of ventilatory response to hypoxia in puppies during sleep. J Appl Physiol 1982; 52:309–314.
49. Schramm CM, Grunstein MM. Respiratory influence of peripheral chemoreceptor stimulation in maturing rabbits. J Appl Physiol 1987; 63:1671–1680.

50. Long WQ, Giesbrecht GG, Anthonisen NR. Ventilatory response to moderate hypoxia in awake chemodenervated cats. J Appl Physiol 1993; 74:805–810.
51. Miller MJ, Tenney SM. Hypoxia-induced tachypnea in carotid-deafferented cats. Respir Physiol 1975; 23:31–39.
52. Bureau MA, Lamarche J, Foulon P, Dalle D. The ventilatory response to hypoxia in the newborn lamb after carotid body denervation. Respir Physiol 1985; 60:109–119.
53. Waites BA, Ackland GL, Noble R, Hanson MA. Red nucleus lesions abolish the biphasic respiratory response to isocapnic hypoxia in decerebrate young rabbits. J Physiol (Lond) 1996; 495:217–225.
54. Moore PJ, Ackland GL, Hanson MA. Unilateral cooling in the region of locus coeruleus blocks the fall in respiratory output during hypoxia in anaesthetized neonatal sheep. Exp Physiol 1996; 81:983–994.
55. Dejours P. Chemoreflexes in breathing. Physiol Rev 1962; 42:335–357.
56. Hertzberg T, Lagercrantz H. Postnatal sensitivity of the peripheral chemoreceptors in newborn infants. Arch Dis Child 1987; 62:1238–1241.
57. Hertzberg T, Hellstrom S, Lagercrantz H, Pequignot JM. Development of the arterial chemoreflex and turnover of carotid body catecholamines in the newborn rat. J Physiol (Lond) 1990; 425:211–225.
58. Canet E, Kianicka I, Praud JP. Postnatal maturation of peripheral chemoreceptor ventilatory response to O_2 and CO_2 in newborn lambs [published errata appear in J Appl Physiol 1996; 81:1861 and 2766]. J Appl Physiol 1996; 80:1928–1933.
59. Eden GJ, Hanson MA. Effects of chronic hypoxia from birth on the ventilatory response to acute hypoxia in the newborn rat. J Physiol (Lond) 1987; 392:11–19.
60. Calder NA, Williams BA, Kumar P, Hanson MA. The respiratory response of healthy term infants to breath-by-breath alternations in inspired oxygen at two postnatal ages. Pediatr Res 1994; 35:321–324.
61. Blanco CE, Dawes GS, Hanson MA, McCooke HB. The response to hypoxia of arterial chemoreceptors in fetal sheep and new-born lambs. J Physiol (Lond) 1984; 351:25–37.
62. Mulligan E, Alsberge M, Bhide S. Carotid chemoreceptor recording in the newborn piglet. In: Eyzaguirre C, Fidone S, Fitzgerald RS, Lahiri S, McDonald D, eds. Arterial Chemoreception. New York: Springer-Verlag, 1990:285–289.
63. Marchal F, Bairam A, Haouzi P, Crance JP, Di Giulio C, Vert P, Lahiri S. Carotid chemoreceptor response to natural stimuli in the newborn kitten. Respir Physiol 1992; 87:183–193.
64. Donnelly DF, Smith EJ, Dutton RE. Neural response of carotid chemoreceptors following dopamine blockade. J Appl Physiol 1981; 50:172–177.
65. Biscoe TJ, Purves MJ, Sampson SR. Types of nervous activity which may be recorded from the carotid sinus nerve in the sheep foetus. J Physiol (Lond) 1969; 202:1–23.
66. Jansen AH, Purves MJ, Tan ED. The role of sympathetic nerves in the activation of the carotid body chemoreceptors at birth in the sheep. J Dev Physiol 1980; 2:305–321.
67. Mulligan E, Lahiri S, Storey BT. Carotid body O_2 chemoreception and mitochondrial oxidative phosphorylation. J Appl Physiol 1981; 51:438–446.
68. Mulligan EM. Discharge properties of carotid bodies: developmental aspects. In: Haddad GG, Farber JP, eds. Developmental Neurobiology of Breathing. New York: Marcel Dekker, 1991: 321–340.
69. Calder NA, Kumar P, Hanson MA. Development of carotid chemoreceptor dynamic and steady-state sensitivity to CO_2 in the newborn lamb. J Physiol (Lond) 1997; 503:187–194.

70. Pepper DR, Landauer RC, Kumar P. Postnatal development of CO_2–O_2 interaction in the rat carotid body in vitro. J Physiol (Lond) 1995; 485:531–541.
71. Bamford OS, Sterni LM, Wasicko MJ, Montrose MH, Carroll JL. Postnatal maturation of carotid body and type I cell chemoreception in the rat. Am J Physiol 1999; 276:L875–884.
72. Kholwadwala D, Donnelly DF. Maturation of carotid chemoreceptor sensitivity to hypoxia: in vitro studies in the newborn rat. J Physiol (Lond) 1992; 453:461–473.
73. Wolsink JG, Berkenbosch A, DeGoede J, Olievier CN. Maturation of the ventilatory response to CO_2 in the newborn piglet. Pediatr Res 1993; 34:485–489.
74. McDonald DM, Mitchell RA. The innervation of glomus cells, ganglion cells and blood vessels in the rat carotid body: a quantitative ultrastructural analysis. J Neurocytol 1975; 4:177–230.
75. Tatsumi K, Pickett CK, Weil JV. Decreased carotid body hypoxic sensitivity in chronic hypoxia: role of dopamine. Respir Physiol 1995; 101:47–57.
76. Kienecker EW, Knoche H, Bingmann D. Functional properties of regenerating sinus nerve fibres in the rabbit. Neuroscience 1978; 3:977–988.
77. Acker H, Lubbers DW, Purves MJ, Tan ED. Measurements of the partial pressure of oxygen in the carotid body of fetal sheep and newborn lambs. J Dev Physiol 1980; 2:323–328.
78. Clarke JA, de Burgh D, Ead HW. Comparison of the size of the vascular compartment of the carotid body of the fetal, neonatal and adult cat. Acta Anat (Basel) 1990; 138:166–174.
79. Moore PJ, Clarke JA, Hanson MA, Daly MD, Ead HW. Quantitative studies of the vasculature of the carotid body in fetal and newborn sheep. J Dev Physiol 1991; 15:211–214.
80. Biscoe TJ, Purves MJ. Carotid body chemoreceptor activity in the new-born lamb. J Physiol (Lond) 1967; 190:443–454.
81. Neil E, O'Regan RG. The effects of electrical stimulation of the distal end of the cut sinus and aortic nerves on peripheral arterial chemoreceptor activity in the cat. J Physiol (Lond) 1971; 215:15–32.
82. Band DM, Linton RA. The effect of potassium on carotid body chemoreceptor discharge in the anaesthetized cat. J Physiol (Lond) 1986; 381:39–47.
83. Gallego R, Eyzaguirre C, Monti-Bloch L. Thermal and osmotic responses of arterial receptors. J Neurophysiol 1979; 42:665–680.
84. Pokorski M, Lahiri S. Effects of naloxone on carotid body chemoreception and ventilation in the cat. J Appl Physiol 1981; 51:1533–1538.
85. Joels N, Neil E. The idea of a sensory transmitter. In: Torrance RW, ed. Arterial Chemoreceptors. Oxford, UK: 1968: 153–178.
86. Kondo H. An electron microscopic study on the development of synapses in the rat carotid body. Neurosci Lett 1976; 3:197–200.
87. Lopez-Lopez JR, De Luis DA, Gonzalez C. Properties of a transient K+ current in chemoreceptor cells of rabbit carotid body. J Physiol (Lond) 1993; 460:15–32.
88. Peers C. Hypoxic suppression of K+ currents in type I carotid body cells: selective effect on the Ca2(+)-activated K+ current. Neurosci Lett 1990; 119:253–256.
89. Buckler KJ. A novel oxygen-sensitive potassium current in rat carotid body type I cells. J Physiol (Lond) 1997; 498:649–662.
90. Buckler KJ, Vaughan-Jones RD. Effects of hypoxia on membrane potential and intracellular calcium in rat neonatal carotid body type I cells. J Physiol (Lond) 1994; 476:423–428.

91. Wasicko MJ, Sterni LM, Bamford OS, Montrose MH, Carroll JL. Resetting and postnatal maturation of oxygen chemosensitivity in rat carotid chemoreceptor cells. J Physiol (Lond) 1999; 514:493–503.
92. Montoro RJ, Urena J, Fernandez-Chacon R, Alvarez DT, Lopez-Barneo J. Oxygen sensing by ion channels and chemotransduction in single glomus cells. J Gen Physiol 1996; 107:133–143.
93. Rumsey WL, Iturriaga R, Spergel D, Lahiri S, Wilson DF. Optical measurements of the dependence of chemoreception on oxygen pressure in the cat carotid body. Am J Physiol 1991; 261:C614–C622.
94. Ganfornina MD, Lopez-Barneo J. Single K+ channels in membrane patches of arterial chemoreceptor cells are modulated by O_2 tension. Proc Natl Acad Sci USA 1991; 88: 2927–2930.
95. Hatton CJ, Carpenter E, Papper DR, Kumar P, Peers C. Developmental changes in isolated rat type I carotid body cell K+ currents and their modulation by hypoxia. J Physiol (Lond) 1997; 501:49–58.
96. Wyatt CN, Wright C, Bee D, Peers C. O_2- sensitive K+ currents in carotid body chemoreceptor cells from normoxic and chronically hypoxic rats and their roles in hypoxic chemotransduction. Proc Natl Acad Sci USA 1995; 92:295–299.
97. Sterni LM, Bamford OS, Tomares SM, Montrose MH, Carroll JL. Developmental changes in intracellular Ca^{2+} response of carotid chemoreceptor cells to hypoxia. Am J Physiol 1995; 268:L801–L808.
98. Hempleman SC. Increased calcium current in carotid body glomus cells following in vivo acclimatization to chronic hypoxia. J Neurophysiol 1996; 76:1880–1886.
99. Peers C, Carpenter E, Hatton CJ, Wyatt CN, Bee D. Ca^{2+} channel currents in type I carotid body cells of normoxic and chronically hypoxic neonatal rats. Brain Res 1996; 739: 251–257.
100. Sterni LM, Bamford OS, Wasicko MJ, Carroll JL. Chronic hypoxia abolished the postnatal increase in carotid body type I cell sensitivity to hypoxia. Am J Physiol 1999; 277: L645–652.
101. Pang L, Eyzaguirre C. Different effects of hypoxia on the membrane potential and input resistance of isolated and clustered carotid body glomus cells. Brain Res 1992; 575: 167–173.
102. Bright GR, Agani FH, Haque U, Overholt JL, Prabhakar NR. Heterogeneity in cytosolic calcium responses to hypoxia in carotid body cells. Brain Res 1996; 706:297–302.
103. Donnelly DF, Kholwadwala D. Hypoxia decreases intracellular calcium in adult rat carotid body glomus cells. J Neurophysiol 1992; 67:1543–1551.
104. Roumy M. Cytosolic calcium in isolated type I cells of the adult rabbit carotid body: effects of hypoxia, cyanide and changes in intracellular pH. Adv Exp Med Biol 1994; 360:175–177.
105. Donnelly DF. Modulation of glomus cell membrane currents of intact rat carotid body. J Physiol (Lond) 1995; 489:677–688.
106. Donnelly DF. Electrochemical detection of catecholamine release from rat carotid body in vitro. J Appl Physiol 1993; 74:2330–2337.
107. Donnelly DF, Doyle TP. Developmental changes in hypoxia-induced catecholamine release from rat carotid body, in vitro. J Physiol (Lond) 1994; 475:267–275.
108. Fidone S, Gonzalez C, Yoshizaki K. Effects of low oxygen on the release of dopamine from the rabbit carotid body in vitro. J Physiol (Lond) 1982; 333:93–110.

109. Bairam A, Basson H, Marchal F, Cottet-Emard JM, Pequignot JM, Hascoet JM, Lahiri S. Effects of hypoxia on carotid body dopamine content and release in developing rabbits. J Appl Physiol 1996; 80:20–24.
110. Bairam A, Dauphin C, Rousseau F, Khandjian EW. Expression of dopamine D2-receptor mRNA isoforms at the peripheral chemoreflex afferent pathway in developing rabbits. Am J Respir Cell Mol Biol 1996; 15:374–381.
111. Tomares SM, Bamford OS, Sterni LM, Fitzgerald RS, Carroll JL. Effects of domperidone on neonatal and adult carotid chemoreceptors in the cat. J Appl Physiol 1994; 77:1274–1280.
112. Hertzberg T, Hellstrom S, Holgert H, Lagercrantz H, Piquignot JM. Ventilatory response to hyperoxia in newborn rats born in hypoxia—possible relationship to carotid body dopamine. J Physiol (Lond) 1992; 456:645–654.
113. Garg M, Kurzner SI, Bautista D, Keens TG. Hypoxic arousal responses in infants with bronchopulmonary dysplasia. Pediatrics 1988; 82:59–63.
114. Katz-Salamon M, Jonsson B, Lagercrantz H. Blunted peripheral chemoreceptor response to hyperoxia in a group of infants with bronchopulmonary dysplasia. Pediatr Pulmonol 1995; 20:101–106.
115. Katz-Salamon M, Eriksson M, Jonsson B. Development of peripheral chemoreceptor function in infants with chronic lung disease and initially lacking hyperoxic response. Arch Dis Child Fetal Neonatal Ed 1996; 75:F4–F9.
116. Katz-Salamon M, Lagercrantz H. Hypoxic ventilatory defence in very preterm infants: attenuation after long term oxygen treatment. Arch Dis Child Fetal Neonatal Ed 1994; 70:F90–F95.
117. Hanson MA, Kumar P, Williams BA. The effect of chronic hypoxia upon the development of respiratory chemoreflexes in the newborn kitten. J Physiol (Lond) 1989; 411:563–574.
118. Landauer RC, Pepper DR, Kumar P. Effect of chronic hypoxaemia from birth upon chemosensitivity in the adult rat carotid body in vitro. J Physiol (Lond) 1995; 485:543–550.
119. Naeye RL, Fisher R, Ryser M, Whalen P. Carotid body in the sudden infant death syndrome. Science 1976; 191:567–569.
120. Cole S, Lindenberg LB, Galioto FM Jr, Howe PE, DeGraff AC Jr, Davis JM, Lubka R, Gross EM. Ultrastructural abnormalities of the carotid body in sudden infant death syndrome. Pediatrics 1979; 63:13–17.
121. Perrin DG, Cutz E, Becker LE, Bryan AC, Madapallimatum A, Sole MJ. Sudden infant death syndrome: increased carotid-body dopamine and noradrenaline content. Lancet 1984; 2:535–537.
122. Lack EE, Perez-Atayde AR, Young JB. Carotid bodies in sudden infant death syndrome: a combined light microscopic, ultrastructural, and biochemical study. Pediatr Pathol 1986; 6:335–350.
123. Perrin DG, Cutz E, Becker LE, Bryan AC. Ultrastructure of carotid bodies in sudden infant death syndrome. Pediatrics 1984; 73:646–651.
124. Henderson-Smart DJ, Ponsonby AL, Murphy E. Reducing the risk of sudden infant death syndrome: a review of the scientific literature. J Paediatr Child Health 1998; 34:213–219.
125. Blanco CE, Hanson MA, Johnson P, Rigatto H. Breathing pattern of kittens during hypoxia. J Appl Physiol 1984; 56:12–17.
126. Donnelly DF, Panisello JM, Boggs D. Effect of sodium perturbations on rat chemoreceptor spike generation: implications for a Poisson model. J Physiol (Lond.) 1998; 511: 301–311.

11

Upper Airway Muscle Function During Sleep

SHIROH ISONO

Chiba University School of Medicine
Chiba, Japan

I. Introduction

The upper airway is composed of the nose, pharynx, larynx, and extrathoracic trachea. The upper airway system is a complex but well-designed organ for multiple purposes such as vocalization, ingestion, airway protection, and respiration. Although coordination and interdependence between the segments are key for the performance of the upper airway, the function of each segment is considered separately in this chapter. The segments of greatest interest are the pharynx and larynx, where partial and/or complete airway obstruction occurs during sleep in patients with obstructive sleep apnea (OSA). Under supervision of neural and chemical controls, contraction of the pharyngeal muscles surrounding the collapsible conduit of the pharynx modulates its size and stiffness according to the purpose. For instance, the pharyngeal airway constricts to efficiently propel food into the esophagus during swallowing. Pharyngeal size and stiffness change dynamically during speech, partly—in addition to fine tuning by the larynx—determining the tone of the voice. By contrast, maintenance of a rigid and patent upper airway is mandatory for achieving adequate respiration. Thus, the inherent collapsibility of the pharynx predisposes to impaired respiration when the regulation of the pharyngeal muscles is impaired, and falling asleep appears to induce derangement of this regulation to some extent. The larynx plays a significant role in vocalization and airway protective responses. Dynamic laryngeal closure and opening occurs during laryngeal reflex responses such as coughing, expiration reflex, and laryngospasm, which prevent aspiration of foreign materials into the respiratory tract. Exaggeration of these reflexes interrupts stable respiration, leading to hypercapnia and hypoxemia, and may possibly be responsible for apnea during sleep in infants or even for the sudden infant death syndrome. Among the upper-airway functions, maintenance of a patent upper airway and airway protective reflex responses are two major tasks for the upper airway during sleep. Accordingly, this chapter focuses on describing normal upper airway muscle function during sleep and shaping new information that possibly relates to the pathophysiology of sleep-disordered breathing. Unfortunately, current knowledge of upper airway function in infants and children is limited, whereas it has been examined extensively in adults. The readers must take special care in reviewing the experiments to take note of the experimental population, whether it was made up of infants, children, or adults.

II. Anatomy and Development of the Upper Airway

As demonstrated in Figure 1, the configuration of the upper airway changes with maturation (1). The infant has a relatively large epiglottis that is at the level of the first vertebra, and the tip of the epiglottis reaches the caudal margin of the soft palate, as in many mammals. The swallowed bolus passes through the lateral channels of the epiglottis and the inhaled air passes behind the epiglottis through the nasal passage, thus, during feeding, there is minimal interference with ventilation. Presumably, for the development of vocalization, the epiglottis descends to the level of the fourth ver-

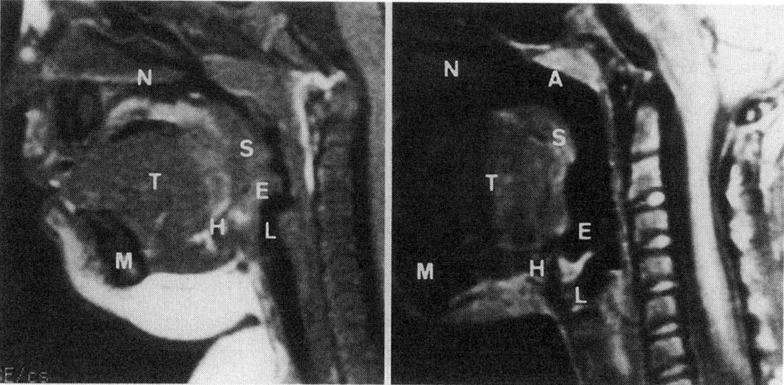

Figure 1 Longitudinal MRI images of the upper airway showing developmental changes in the structures. T, tongue; S, soft palate; N, nose; M, mandible; H, hyoid bone; E, epiglottis; L, larynx; A, adenoid. Note that the position of the larynx in a 10-month-old boy (left panel) is higher than that in an 8-year-old girl (right panel), resulting in approximation of the soft palate and the epiglottis. Although the pharyngeal airway appears to be narrower in the younger child, the image was taken under sedation in this child, whereas the older girl was awake.

tebra and is separate from the soft palate by the first or second year of life. The larynx and the hyoid bone also descend and locate posteriorly, while the pharynx elongates and becomes tortuous with growth. As discussed in this chapter, these changes in the upper airway configuration appear to link the ability to maintain upper airway patency and to prevent aspiration of foreign materials into the lower respiratory tract.

III. Pharynx

A. Limitations of Investigating Upper Airway Muscle Function

Approximately 30 pairs of muscle are responsible for the complicated behavior of the upper airway. Although contraction of each muscle usually results in unidirectional movement of the structure, the actual movement is determined by the sum of vector forces produced by the group of upper airway muscles participating in the specific function. Accordingly, evaluation of a single muscle contraction does not necessarily represent actual behavior of the upper airway. Furthermore, one should also recognize electromechanical uncoupling in interpretation of changes in electromyographic (EMG) activities. For instance, an increase in EMG activity of the genioglossus muscle, which is a major pharyngeal dilator muscle, does not always imply an increase in the cross-sectional area of the pharyngeal airway. Another limitation in interpreting EMG data is the difficulty in comparing between subjects. In the genioglossus, some researchers normalize EMG activity using 100% of the maximum activity obtained by a reproducible procedure, such as swallowing or maximum protrusion of the tongue, although this is controversial (2–4). Keeping in mind these limitations, in numerous previous studies, EMG activities of several "representative" muscles were simultaneously measured during the evaluation of actual mechanical changes of the upper airway, including resistance and airway size, in order to correlate observed changes of EMG activities with mechanical changes.

B. Pharyngeal Muscle Function for Stable Respiration

A simple classification of the pharyngeal muscles greatly aids in understanding the principal role of each muscle for stable respiration. Table 1 lists the representative pharyngeal muscles investigated by various researchers in the past two decades. At the level of the pharynx, the surrounding muscles are divided into pharyngeal dilators and constrictors. Major constrictor muscles of the pharynx consist of the superior, middle, and inferior pharyngeal constrictors; however, dilators are numerous. At the oropharyngeal airway (between the tip of the epiglottis and the edge of the soft palate), the genioglossus muscle dilates the airway for respiration, while its fan-like projection of muscle fibers produces complicated movements of the tongue. The genioglossus is the most extensively explored muscle, since reduction of its activity is known to be associated with an increase in upper airway resistance (5). At the hypopharyngeal airway (between the vocal cords and the tip of the epiglottis), net vector forces of the suprahyoid muscles, which attach superiorly to the hyoid bone (i.e.,

Table 1 Pharyngeal Muscles

UA segment	Muscle	Function	Nerve
Pharynx	Pharyngeal constrictors		
	Superior	Constrictor	9,10
	Middle	Constrictor	9,10
	Inferior	Constrictor	9,10
Nasopharynx	Palatoglossus	Nasal breathing	10
	Palatopharyngeal	Nasal breathing	10
	Tensor veli palatini	Oral breathing	5
	Levator veli palatini	Oral breathing	9,10
Oropharynx	Genioglossus	Anterior movement of the tongue	12
Hypopharynx	Suprahyoid muscles	Anterior-cranial movement of the hyoid bone	
	Geniohyoid		C1,C4
	Mylohyoid		C1,C4
	Infrahyoid muscles	Caudal movement of the hyoid bone	
	Sternohyoid		C1,C4
	Thyrohyoid		C1,C4
	Omohyoid		C1,C4

geniohyoid and myohyoid), and the infrahyoid muscles, which attach inferiorly to the hyoid bone (i.e., sternohyoid, thyrohyoid, omohyoid), determine the position of the hyoid bone, play a role in dilatation of this segment. The position of the hyoid bone and the direction of the muscle fibers significantly influence the net vector forces of these muscles (6–9). At the nasopharyngeal airway (between the edge of the soft palate and the end of the nasal septum), the role of each muscle depends on the preferred breathing route. Contraction of the palatoglossus and the palatopharyngeal muscle opens the retropalatal airway, allowing for nasal breathing. These muscles are therefore considered to be the dilators during nasal breathing (2,3). The tensor veli palatini and the levator veli palatini, which elevate the soft palate, are considered to be the dilators during oral breathing.

Net vector forces of the two antagonistic muscle groups, the dilators and constrictors, determine the airway size in the static condition, i.e., absence of airflow through the airway. Feroah et al. demonstrated that balance between the stylopharyngeus (dilator) and inferior pharyngeal constrictor modulated the isolated pharyngeal airway size in awake goats (10). In addition to the regulation of the pharyngeal airway size, recent evidence obtained by EMG recording of the pharyngeal constrictor suggests another important function of the pharyngeal muscles. Kuna et al. observed that inspiratory phasic activation of the superior pharyngeal constrictor was frequently associated with airway reopening on arousal in patients with OSA (Fig. 2) (11). The behavior of the constrictor was similar to that of pharyngeal dilators during spontaneous and induced apnea. Although their findings appear to disagree with the

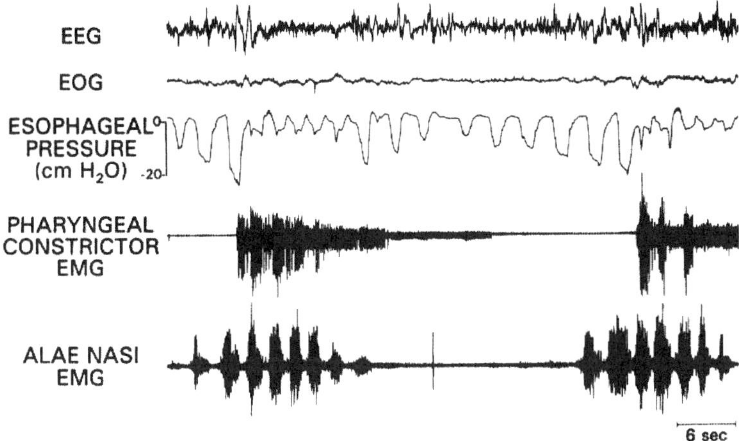

Figure 2 Superior pharyngeal constrictor and alae nasi activity during an obstructive apnea in an adult patient with OSA. Note that sudden pharyngeal constrictor activation during inspiration at the end of apnea is associated with a less negative esophageal pressure. (From Ref. 11.)

simple dilator-constrictor model, construction of an extended model of the pharyngeal airway may possibly solve this seeming contradiction. As many dilator muscles exhibit phasic inspiratory activity, especially during mechanical loading (12–16) or chemical stimuli (17,18), inspiration is the most critical phase for airway maintenance, since development of negative intraluminal pressure opposes the dilator forces during this period (5,19). Therefore, reciprocal inhibition of the constrictors may be preferable in facilitating dilator muscle function in the simple dilator-constrictor model. However, Kuna's data do not support this idea. One possible interpretation of these data is the resultant stiffening of the pharyngeal airway wall by contraction of the constrictor muscle, which assists in maintenance of a patent airway reestablished by a burst of the genioglossus upon arousal. Increases in tonic EMG activity often observed in dilator muscles during mechanical loading and chemical stimuli may also contribute to stiffening of the pharyngeal airway wall. Pharyngeal muscles not only act as dilators or constrictors in controlling the pharyngeal airway size but also as stiffeners in regulating compliance of the pharyngeal airway wall. In order to accomplish their primary role of ensuring stable respiration, the pharyngeal muscles' dilation of the airway is insufficient, since an airway with a larger cross section and higher compliance tends to collapse easily during inspiration, resulting in limitation of airflow. In contrast, an airway with a smaller cross section and lower compliance tends to allow sufficient airflow, in accordance with increased respiratory drive. Recent evidence from electric stimulation of the pharyngeal muscles strongly supports the function of the pharyngeal muscles as stiffeners. In anesthetized dogs with an isolated upper airway, Hida et al. measured the static pressure/volume relationship of the upper airway

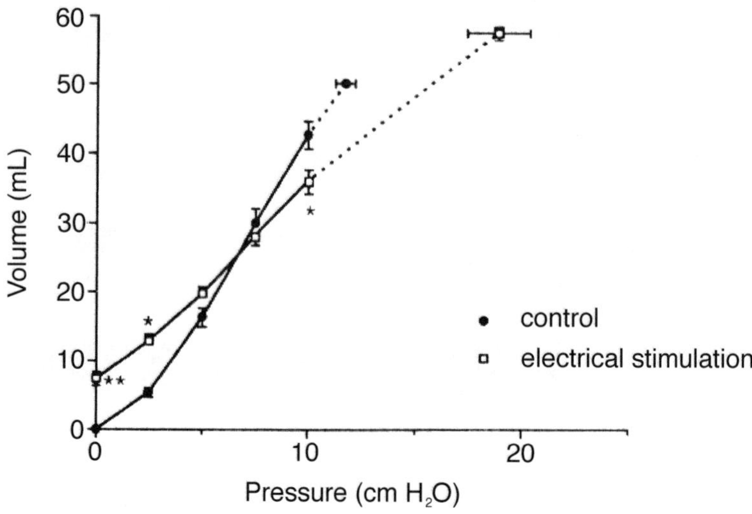

Figure 3 Effect of electrical stimulation of bilateral hypoglossal nerves on static pressure/volume relationship in dogs with an isolated upper airway. Note that the slope of the relationship, i.e., the compliance of the upper airway, decreased following stimulation. (From Ref. 20.)

with and without electrical stimulation of the branches of the hypoglossal nerve (20). As clearly demonstrated in Figure 3, compliance of the upper airway, which is the slope of the pressure/volume relationship, decreased by contraction of pharyngeal dilators. It should also be noted that electrical stimulation at a lower airway pressure increased upper airway volume, which indicates that the pharyngeal muscles act as dilators when upper airway volume is small. In contrast, electrical stimulation at higher airway pressure resulted in reduction of upper airway volume, indicating that the pharyngeal dilators act as constrictors when upper airway volume is large. Accordingly, the pharyngeal muscles have two significant functions for respiratory stabilization: controlling airway size and regulating airway compliance.

The activating pattern of pharyngeal muscles differs from that of primary inspiratory muscles. Strohl et al. demonstrated that activation of the alae nasi occurred before the onset of inspiratory airflow, which was more clearly evident during sleep (21). This sequence is considered to act as a stiffener for the collapsible pharynx against the collapsing forces of inspiratory efforts developed by the primary inspiratory muscles. EMG activity of the diaphragm gradually increases during inspiration and peaks during the late inspiratory phase. In contrast, pharyngeal muscle activity peaks during the early inspiratory phase, and higher activity is maintained throughout inspiration. Some researchers believe that the differences in the configuration of the EMG activities contributes to stabilization of respiration.

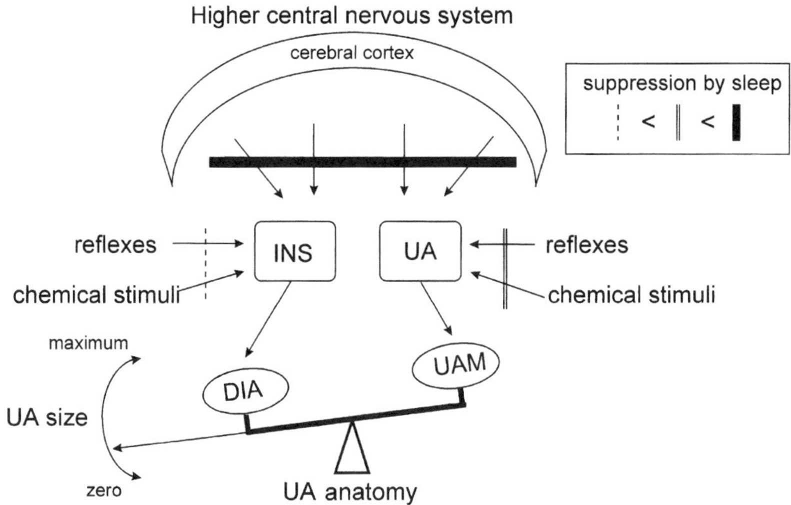

Figure 4 Various factors influencing the upper airway (UA) size. INS, the center of diaphragm motor neurons in the medulla; UA, the center of upper airway respiratory motor neurons in the medulla; DIA, diaphragmatic activity; UAM, upper airway muscle activity. Differences of suppression by sleep between the UAM and DIA result in a reduction of UA size during sleep.

C. State-Dependent Pharyngeal Muscle Activities

Pharyngeal patency during wakefulness is ensured by the continuous supervision of the higher central nervous system, including the cerebral cortex, which regulates and coordinates the action of more than 30 pairs of pharyngeal muscles in conjunction with neural and chemical inputs (Fig. 4). Negative pharyngeal pressure (22–24), increased nasal airflow (25), and nasal obstruction (12,26) are known to immediately augment pharyngeal muscle activity. Chemical responses of the pharyngeal muscles also contribute to pharyngeal patency during wakefulness. The pharyngeal muscle activity, which ensures pharyngeal patency, counterbalances the primary inspiratory muscle activity, which promotes pharyngeal narrowing (5,27). Mezzanotte et al. demonstrated that patients with OSA have significantly greater genioglossus muscle activity than normal subjects during wakefulness, presumably owing to compensation for their structurally narrowed pharynx (4).

Sleep depresses the higher central nervous system and influences the chemical and neural regulation of the pharyngeal muscle activity, leading to suppression of pharyngeal muscle activity (28–31). The extent of pharyngeal muscle suppression is much greater during rapid-eye-movement (REM) sleep than during non–rapid eye movement (NREM) sleep, as with many other skeletal muscles. Atonia of the upper airway muscle activity is one criterion for staging REM sleep. Parisi et al. reported that the genioglossal responses to hypoxia and hypercapnia decreased during sleep as opposed to wakefulness in goats (awake > NREM > REM) (17,18). The pattern of genioglossal responses to hypoxia was observed to differ significantly from that of the diaphragm, in that the genioglossus was activated only below an Sa_{O_2} threshold, whereas diaphragmatic activity increased monotonously in response to progressive hypoxia. Therefore, the imbalance between the pharyngeal dilating forces and inspiratory collapsing forces favors pharyngeal narrowing during sleep, as demonstrated by Remmers et al. (5). Although abnormally depressed pharyngeal muscle activity may lead to severe pharyngeal narrowing, no study has successfully tested this important hypothesis for the pathogenesis of upper airway obstruction. An alternative factor that determines pharyngeal patency during sleep is the intrinsic mechanical properties of the pharynx, shown by a fulcrum in Figure 4. Isono et al. suggested that the fulcrum of normal subjects is located to the left of patients with sleep-disordered breathing, indicating that the anatomy of the pharynx favors pharyngeal narrowing in sleep apneics (32). This mechanism was evident in both children (33) and adults (32). Henke pondered the necessity of pharyngeal muscle activity for stable respiration during sleep in normal subjects and performed the following study (34). Nasal CPAP was applied to significantly reduce the genioglossal activity (35). This was followed by an abrupt reduction of mask pressure to atmospheric pressure for a single breath, during which the suppressed muscle activity was maintained. Despite the marked reduction of genioglossal activity, upper airway resistance did not increase in normal young men during NREM sleep. In complete contrast, as Remmers et al. consistently report, OSA patients with anatomical abnormalities of the pharynx require pharyngeal muscle activity to maintain a patent airway, thereby producing stable respiration (36–38).

D. The Pharyngeal Airway as a Collapsible Tube

The pharynx behaves like a collapsible tube. Collapsible tubes have long been used as a mechanical model for pulmonary circulation (39) and expiratory flow limitation in the lung (40,41). Thach et al. first characterized the pharyngeal airway as a collapsible tube in infants and children (42–44). Schwartz et al. successfully applied a Starling resistor model to the pharyngeal airway and elegantly accounted for mechanisms of inspiratory flow limitation by the pharynx in sleeping adult humans (45–48). Marcus et al. extended these findings to sleeping children (49). Remmers and colleagues further supported their approach by describing static mechanics of the hypotonic pharynx and pharyngeal behavior during inspiratory flow limitation (36–38,50).

Behavior of a Collapsible Tube

Most pharyngeal behavior is demonstrable by a collapsible tube in a rigid chamber, as illustrated in Fig. 5 (27,51). In this model, the cross-sectional area of the tube is determined by transmural pressure (P_{tm}), the difference between intraluminal and tissue pressure ($P_{tm} = P_l - P_{ti}$), according to a "tube law" representing intrinsic mechanical properties of the tube (Fig. 6). P_l is defined as the lateral wall pressure acting on

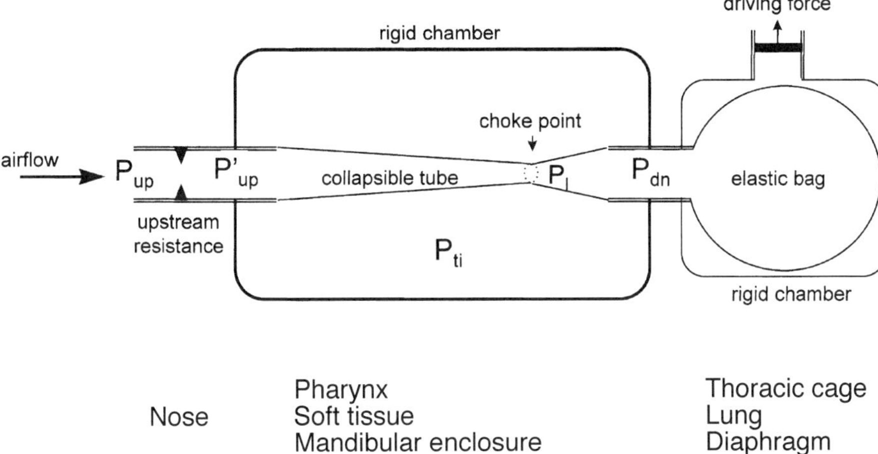

Figure 5 Schematic presentation of the experimental setting of a collapsible tube (latex Penrose tube, ID = 12 mm, length = 8 cm), as a mechanical model of the upper airway. Airflow through the collapsible tube is produced by applying a negative driving pressure around an elastic bag in a chamber which is analogous to the thorax. P_{up}, upstream pressure; P'_{up}, pressure upstream to the tube and downstream to a rigid upstream resistance; P_{ti}, pressure in the chamber; P_l, intraluminal pressure at choke point; P_{dn}, downstream pressure.

the luminal surface of the tube, while P_{ti} is defined as the tissue pressure acting on the outside surface of the tube. The behavior of the tube depends upon the experimental conditions, which are prescribed by the upstream pressure (P_{up}), chamber pressure (P_{ti}), and the tube law. A constant driving force is periodically created inside of another chamber in order to mimic a subject breathing through a collapsible pharynx. Inflation of an elastic bag produces airflow through the collapsible tube. In a variety

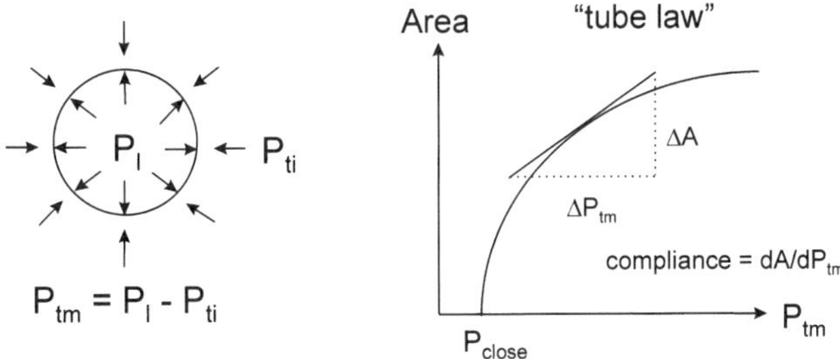

Figure 6 Definition of transmural pressure (P_{tm}) and "tube law." P_l, intraluminal pressure; P_{ti}, tissue pressure; P_{close}, closing pressure. A decrease in P_{tm} results in a decrease in cross-sectional area of the tube, in accordance with the tube law. The slope of the tube law represents the compliance of the tube, which varies with P_{tm}.

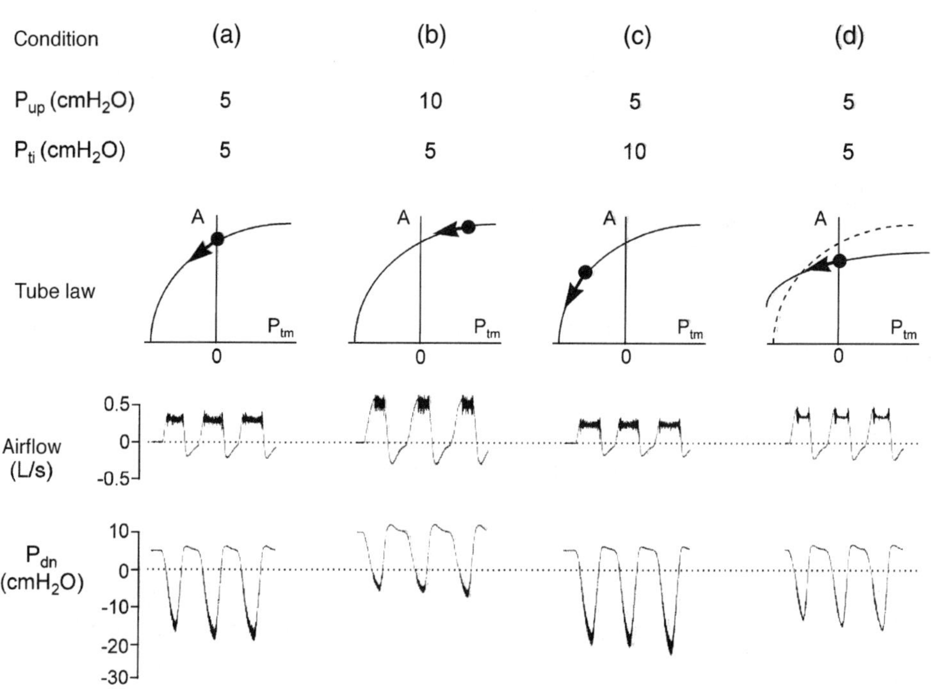

Figure 7 Airflow limitation by a collapsible tube in a variety of conditions. The experimental setting is shown in Figure 5. (a) $P_{up} = P_{ti}$; (b) $P_{up} > P_{ti}$; (c) $P_{up} < P_{ti}$; (d) stretching of the tube. See text for detailed explanation.

of conditions, we evaluated maximum airflow and downstream pressure (P_{dn}), as demonstrated in Figure 7 a through d.

In the following study, a simple condition was produced in which P_{up} and P_{ti} were held constant (P_{up} and $P_{ti} = 5$) (Fig. 7a). Whereas no pressure gradient exists in P_l along the tube in the static condition, introduction of airflow by a driving force produces progressive reduction of P_l along the tube due to two mechanisms: acceleration of airflow through the tube and energy dissipation at upstream resistance. The former is due to a conversion of energy from static to kinetic, caused by an increase in airflow velocity accompanied by reduction of the luminal size (Bernoulli's theory). P_l reduction causes narrowing of the cross-sectional area according to the tube law. At the downstream site, the pressure gradient along the tube produces P_l reduction, creating constriction, which, in turn, stimulates a further increase in the kinetic energy of air flowing through the constriction, leading to further P_l reduction. In this manner, the collapsible tube progressively narrows with increases in the driving force. Ultimately, "a choke point," which limits airflow, may develop. Airflow reaches a maximum value ($\dot{V}_{Imax}$) following an initial increase; thereafter, the airflow does not increase further but often shows a decrease (negative effort dependence) despite a progressive increase in the driving force. This situation is referred to as flow limitation. Further increases in the driving force produce high frequency vibrations of the tube with audible sound, as is evident in the airflow tracing. During flow limitation, a point of minimum lateral pressure locates downstream of the constriction (40), and the area between these two points is called the *region of elastic jump*, as described by Dawson and Elliott (41). This phenomenon relates to flow separation due to abrupt area expansion, leading to marked reduction of P_{dn} (Fig. 8). A notable point here is that the flow profile upstream of the constriction is more likely to be laminar without evidence of wall vibration, whereas the flow downstream of the constriction becomes turbulent, causing deformation of the wall (52).

Although in the previous condition we assumed that P_{up} and P_{ti} are constant and that the tube law does not change, these variables significantly influence the dynamic behavior of the collapsible tube, as demonstrated in Figures 7b and c. It is a well-known important characteristic of this model that the level of $\dot{V}_{Imax}$ depends upon the level of P_{up} (39). When P_{up} is maintained above P_{ti}, as illustrated in Figure 7b, P_l at the constriction site of the tube increases, which results in increased P_{tm}. This shifts the starting point of the progressive reduction of P_l on the tube law to that with a larger cross-sectional area and lower compliance. Accordingly, reduction of the cross-sectional area during progressive reduction of P_l is less severe compared to condition of Figure 7a, leading to a marked increase in $\dot{V}_{Imax}$ with a lesser extent of progressive reduction of P_{dn}. A linear relationship between P_{up} and $\dot{V}_{Imax}$ exists, allowing for the calculation of critical closing pressure at zero flow, where presumably the tube completely collapses (45–47).

When P_{ti} is higher than P_{up} (Fig. 7c), P_{tm} decreases. The starting point of progressive P_l reduction on the tube law shifts to the point with a smaller cross-sectional

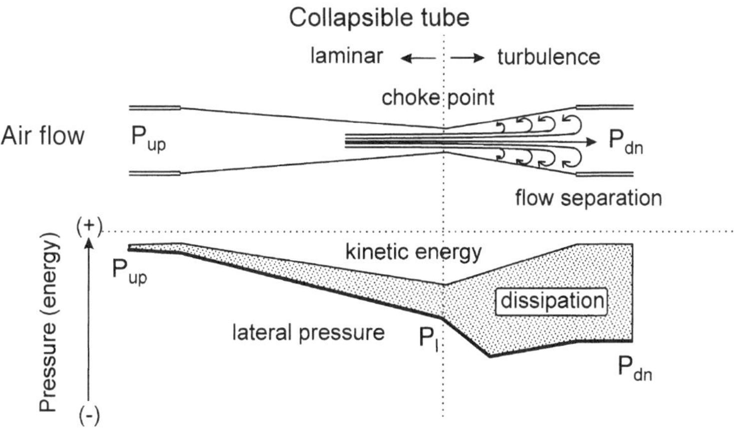

Figure 8 Aerodynamics in a collapsible tube. See text for detailed explanation.

area and with higher compliance. During progressive reduction of P_l, severe pharyngeal narrowing occurs, which results in severe flow limitation (reduction of $\dot{V}_{Imax}$) with greater reduction of P_{dn}.

Changes in the tube law significantly influence the dynamic behavior of the pharynx (Fig. 7d). In the collapsible tube model, the tube law can easily be altered by changing the longitudinal forces—i.e., stretching forces of the tube. When the longitudinal forces are increased, the tube stiffens, thereby decreasing the slope of the tube law. Assuming that P_{up} and P_{ti} are constant (P_{up} and $P_{ti} = 5$), narrowing of the tube for a given reduction of P_{tm} during progressive reduction of P_l becomes less severe, leading to increases in $\dot{V}_{Imax}$ with smaller decrease in P_{dn}.

Numerous theories—such as the waterfall model (39), wave-speed theory (41,27,53) and more complicated mathematical models—have been developed to account for the behavior of the collapsible tube in the last three decades. These have yet to be applied to flow limitation by the pharynx during sleep.

Behavior of the Pharynx During Breathing

The pharynx behaves just like a collapsible tube, as described above. Isono et al. reported that static pressure/area relationships of the passive pharynx in adult patients with OSA are exponential, being flat at higher airway pressures and steep at lower airway pressures, as shown in Figure 9 (36). The pressure/area relationship predicts behavior of the pharynx during inspiration, although the relationship is not a tube law. During inspiration, starting at a higher airway pressure, the cross-sectional area nar-

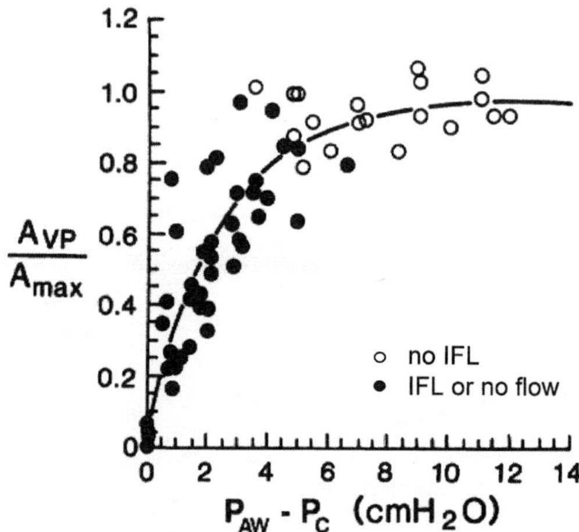

Figure 9 Static pressure/area relationship of the passive pharynx in adult patients with OSA. IFL, inspiratory flow limitation; A_{VP}, cross-sectional area of the velopharynx; A_{max}, maximal velopharyngeal area; P_{AW}, airway pressure; P_C, closing pressure. (From Ref. 36.)

rows slightly for a given reduction of airway pressure as the curve is flat, resulting in absence of airflow limitation. In contrast, during inspiration, starting at a lower airway pressure, the pharynx supposedly narrows substantially, since the slope of the curve is steep, resulting in inspiratory flow limitation. In fact, no inspiratory flow limitation occurred when mask pressure exceeded a closing pressure of greater than 5 cmH_2O. Inspiratory flow limitation, however, was consistently observed when mask pressure did not exceed the closing pressure of more than 5 cmH_2O. Isono et al. further described the dynamic behavior of the passive pharynx during inspiration in detail (50). As clearly demonstrated in Figure 10, the observed dynamic behavior of the pharynx during inspiration completely agrees with the behavior of the collapsible tube described above, confirming an analogy of the collapsible tube to the pharyngeal airway. The pharyngeal airway progressively narrowed during inspiration, leading to progressive increases in pharyngeal resistance and the kinetic energy of air at constriction. Dependence of $\dot{V}_{Imax}$ on mask pressure (upstream pressure) was evident, in

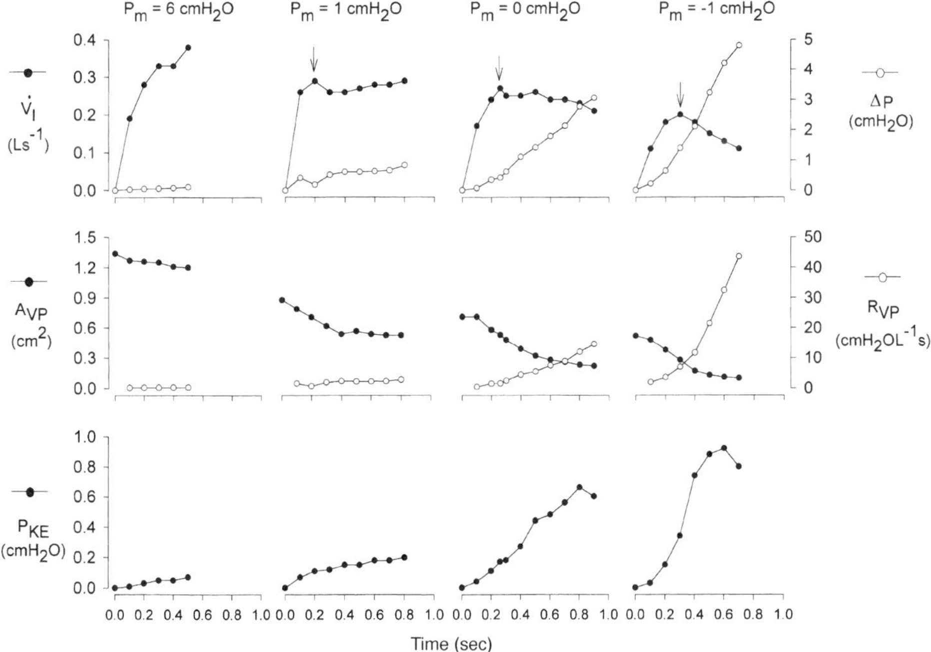

Figure 10 Dynamic behavior of the passive pharynx at a variety of mask pressures (P_m) in a sleeping patient with OSA and a primary site of narrowing at the velopharynx. Data were obtained from the beginning of inspiration to the peak of inspiratory effort. V_I, airflow; A_{VP}, cross-sectional area of the velopharynx; P_{KE}, kinetic energy at the velopharynx; P, pressure difference across the velopharynx; R_{VP}, velopharyngeal resistance. Note the similarity of the behavior of the pharynx to that of a collapsible tube. (From Ref. 32.)

accordance with the results of Schwartz et al. (45–49). The pharyngeal area at the beginning of inspiration also depended on mask pressure. Isono et al. presented a mathematical expression describing the mutual interdependence among the cross-sectional area of the pharynx (A), pressure difference across the pharynx (ΔP), and inspiratory airflow (V_I) for flow-limited and non-flow-limited inspirations by $V_I = K(A/A_{max})\Delta P^{1/3}$, where K is a constant and A_{max} is maximal A. Although ΔP is a driving force for air movement, ΔP produces a simultaneous impedance of airflow by also narrowing the collapsible pharynx. The balance between the driving force and the impedance determines airflow. Airflow increases up to the onset of flow limitation since the driving force is predominant; however, after the onset of flow limitation, impedance dominates the driving force causing flow limitation. Pharyngeal narrowing during inspiration is key to the understanding of the mechanisms of inspiratory flow limitation at the pharynx.

Current understanding of P_{ti} of the pharynx for airway maintenance is limited because of difficulty in the measurement of P_{ti}. P_{ti} may differ among subjects, and varies depending on airway size. The pharyngeal airway is surrounded by soft tissues such as the pharyngeal muscles, lymphoid tissue, connective tissue and fat tissue, and is enclosed by bony structures such as the cervical spine and the mandible. P_{ti} is a tissue pressure acting on the outer surface of the pharyngeal wall, and is determined by a number of factors, some of which operate at a considerable distance from the pharyngeal wall. For instance, mass loading on the submandibular area may increase P_{ti} leading to narrowing of the pharynx (54), and neck flexion may compress the submandibular area similarly to mass loading (42), causing an increase in P_{ti}. Increased volume of the pharyngeal fat pads (55), often seen in MRI images of obese patients with OSA (56,57), and a thickened lateral pharyngeal wall (58) may also increase P_{ti}. A smaller mandibular enclosure, reported in OSA patients (59), as well as micrognathia and retrognathia, may also increase P_{ti}, while mandibular advancement may decrease P_{ti} (60). Enlarged volume of the tongue (61) and the soft palate (62) is considered to increase P_{ti}. This gravitational impact can be offset by the lateral or seated position (63). In children, hypertrophied tonsils and adenoids can significantly increase P_{ti} (33,49).

The longitudinal tension of the pharynx appears to be an important determinant of airflow, although data are limited due to difficulty in measuring tension. Van de Graaff demonstrated that caudal traction of the trachea improved airflow in dogs (64). Thut et al. confirmed his finding in using a paralyzed cat preparation, and further indicated that improvement of airflow is primarily due to alterations in upper airway length, presumably by an increase in the longitudinal tension of the upper airway (65). They also examined the effects of neck position on airflow dynamics and concluded that these effects are also related to changes in upper airway length. Since lung inflation causes caudal movement of the larynx, thereby increasing longitudinal tension of the pharynx, the lung volume dependence of pharyngeal cross-sectional area and upper airway resistance reported previously may possibly be explained by this mechanism (66–68). Pharyngeal muscle contraction may be another cause of increased longitudinal tension of the pharynx, as discussed below.

E. Developmental Changes in Anatomical and Neural Factors

Since $P_{tm} = P_l - P_{ti}$, the P_l-area relationship shifts according to the degree of P_{ti} and the P_{tm}-area relationship (tube law). Accordingly, a reduction of P_{ti} may shift the P_l-area relationship to the left, leading to a decrease in closing pressure of the collapsible tube. Dilating muscular forces of the pharynx can be considered to decrease P_{ti}, shifting the P_l-area relationship of the pharynx to the left, which results in reduction of the critical closing pressure, while a stiffening muscular effect on the pharynx reduces the slope of the P_l-area relationship. Accordingly, evaluation of the P_l-area relationship allows us to estimate relative contributions of anatomical and neural factors to pharyngeal patency. Figure 11 summarizes developmental changes in the closing pressures of the passive and active pharynx, both in normal subjects and patients with sleep-disordered breathing, reported in the literature, although the methods and background theories differ among studies. Wilson et al. obtained the passive closing pressure in infants after death (42), while Roberts et al. measured the active closing pressure in normal and micrognathic infants by the nasal occlusion technique (44). Isono et al. measured the closing pressure of the passive pharynx endoscopically in adults and children (32,33), whereas Marcus et al. obtained the critical pressure of the active pharynx in children by applying the Starling resistor model to the upper airway (49). Gleadhill et al. measured critical pressure in adults (48).

Anatomical differences between generations may be assessed by comparison of the closing pressure of the passive pharynx. The mean highest closing pressure of the passive pharynx in normal infants (-0.7 ± 2.0 cmH_2O) significantly decreases in

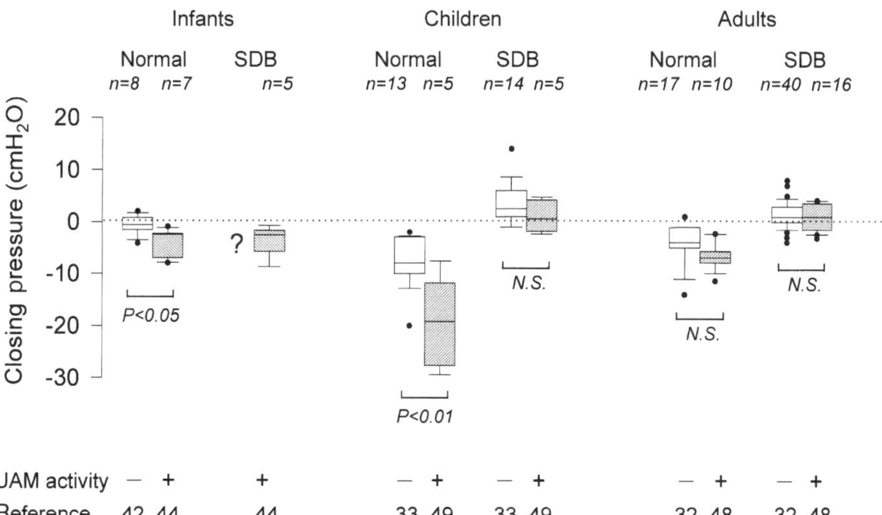

Figure 11 Closing pressures of the passive and active pharynx both in normals and patients with sleep-disordered breathing (SDB) are presented for each generation. Previously published data were used for comparison, as indicated by the reference numbers.

normal children (-7.4 ± 4.9 cmH$_2$O), and increases in normal adults (-3.8 ± 3.4 cmH$_2$O). This indicates that the pharynx is structurally most collapsible in infancy, becomes less collapsible during childhood, and increases in collapsibility thereafter. It should be noted also that the closing pressure of the passive pharynx in patients (both children and adults) with sleep-disordered breathing is greater than atmospheric pressure, while that of normal subjects is less than atmospheric pressure, indicating that the disease process relates to anatomical abnormalities of the pharynx.

The difference between the closing pressures of the passive and active pharynx is presumably due to neuromuscular mechanisms maintaining pharyngeal patency. As evident in Figure 11, the difference is significant in normal children and infants, but insignificant in normal adults. This does not necessarily suggest that pharyngeal muscles are active during sleep in infants and children in maintaining airway patency. Since the passive closing pressure is significantly less than atmospheric pressure in children, muscle activity does not need to be present at atmospheric pressure to maintain airway patency. This agrees with the finding of Jeffries et al., who reported that phasic inspiratory activity of the upper airway muscles was absent in normal children (69). It is important to be aware of the experimental methods used in obtaining active closing pressures. Roberts recruited muscle activity using nasal airway occlusion (44), while Marcus and Gleadhill applied negative airway pressure, activating the pharyngeal muscles (48,49). The differences between passive and active closing pressures suggest that neuromuscular compensatory mechanisms are capable of stabilizing the pharynx in normal infants and children during sleep, although they contribute little in adults. EMG evidence suggests that the immediate augmenting responses of the pharyngeal muscles in response to nasal occlusion or added load appears to be more prominent in infants and children (14–16,26) than in adults (12,13), which also supports this speculation. The relatively smaller contribution of the arousal response in reestablishing the airway patency in infants and children compared to adults may be explained by this difference (70). Notably, the difference is absent in children and adults with sleep disordered breathing, suggesting that the disease process also relates to neuromuscular abnormalities.

In summary, both anatomical and neural factors determining the collapsibility of the pharynx change with maturation. The pharyngeal airway of children appears to be less collapsible than that of adults, whereas information on pharyngeal collapsibility in infants is insufficient. This coincides with the well-known evidence that the prevalence of disordered breathing during sleep increases with aging and that the normal values for apnea frequency are lower in children than in adults (71).

F. Role of Nasal Resistance in Pharyngeal Behavior During Breathing

The nose is responsible for approximately half of the total respiratory resistance in normal humans at rest (72). The extent of vascular engorgement of the mucous membranes lining the nasal cavity mainly determines the nasal resistance. It is highly variable among subjects, and even within the subject. Although the external nares and the nasal cavity could possibly limit airflow during augmented inspiratory efforts (73), the nose is believed not to be a responsible site for inspiratory flow limitation during sleep. It may be assumed that the nose is a relatively rigid resistance upstream to the pharynx, where the flow-limiting segment usually exists during sleep. In the collapsible tube model described in Figure 5, placement of a rigid upstream resistance decreases the pressure immediately upstream to the collapsible tube (P'_{up}); therefore, P_l at the choke point decreases more when air flows through it (Fig. 12). More severe narrowing of the tube during progressive increments of the driving pressure occurs according to the tube law, leading to more severe flow limitation with marked reduction of P_{dn}. The observations of the model suggest that increased nasal resistance may be a significant factor worsening the inspiratory flow limitation. In fact, acute increases in nasal resistance are reported to induce sleep-disordered breathing (74), and a recent epidemiological survey indicates an association between a history of high nasal resistance and the presence of sleep-disordered breathing (75). The efficacy of nasal surgery in the treatment of OSA, however, is controversial, probably because the primary site of narrowing is not the nose (76,77). Accordingly, high nasal resistance may be a risk factor for development of sleep disordered breathing.

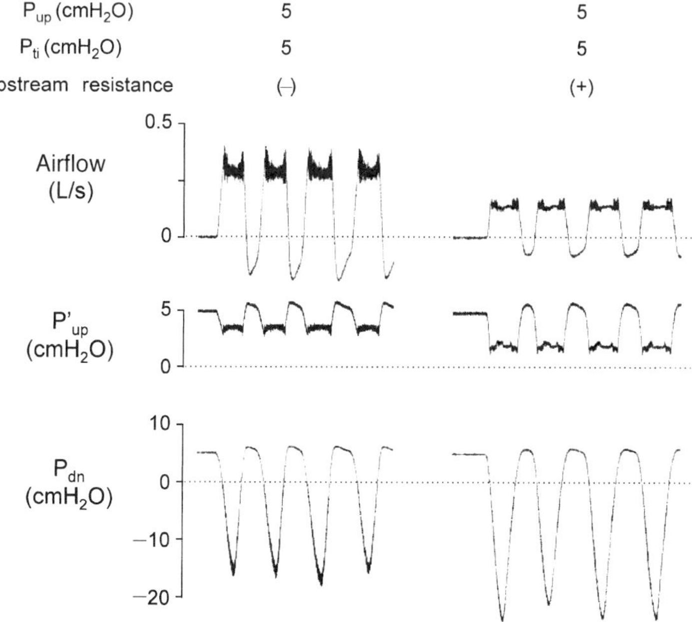

Figure 12 Influence of a rigid upstream resistance (a rigid tube with 8-mm ID and 30-cm length) on the airflow dynamic of a collapsible tube. See Figure 5 illustrating the experimental setting.

G. Role of Surface Adhesive Forces of the Pharynx

Surface adhesive forces between the opposed luminal surfaces contribute to airway patency. In human infant cadavers, Wilson et al. reported that P_{open}, defined as a pressure required to reopen the closed airway, is greater by 6 cmH_2O than P_{close}, defined as the pressure at which the airway completely closes (42). Roberts et al. demonstrated this fact in living human infants (44). This partly explains why upper airway muscle activity at the termination of apnea is much greater than that of quiet breathing during wakefulness. If surface adhesive forces on the pharyngeal mucosa cause the pressure difference between P_{open} and P_{close}, alteration of surface adhesive forces can be expected to change the pressure difference. All previous studies examining the influence of surface adhesive forces on pharyngeal patency in rabbits (78), dogs (79) and awake humans (80) agree that reduction of surface adhesive forces leads to decreases in P_{open} indicating that reopening of the pharynx is easier with reduction of surface tension, although the behavior of P_{close} is controversial. Van der Touw et al. reported a reduction of P_{close} after application of surfactant to the pharynx (80) whereas Olson et al. showed a reduction of P_{close} after an increase in pharyngeal secretions (78). Our preliminary report indicates that P_{open} decreased without changing P_{close} in anesthetized and completely paralyzed humans after application of surfactant (81).

The role of surface adhesive forces in the partially collapsed airway has not been examined, although the evidence mentioned above indicates the significance of surface tension in the completely closed upper airway. Figure 13 exhibits the velopharyngeal behavior during flow-limited inspiration and expiration. Cross-sectional area progressively decreases up to the maximum inspiratory effort, and increases at late inspiration and expiration. Notably, the second inspiration starts with a smaller cross-sectional area than the first inspiration, and the maximum inspiratory airflow of the second inspiration is smaller than the first inspiration, although P_{up} is maintained constant. One possible explanation for this is that the narrowed airway during inspiration

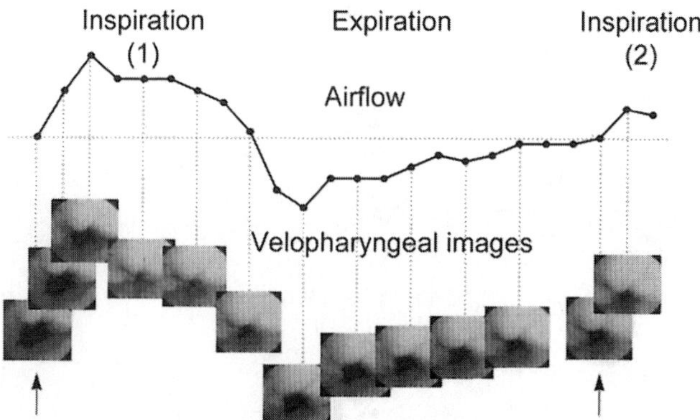

Figure 13 Dynamic behavior of the velopharynx following an abrupt reduction of mask pressure (P_m) from 16 cmH_2O to 3 cmH_2O in a spontaneously breathing, anesthetized patient with OSA.

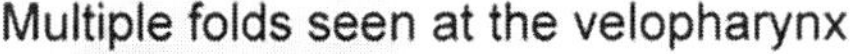

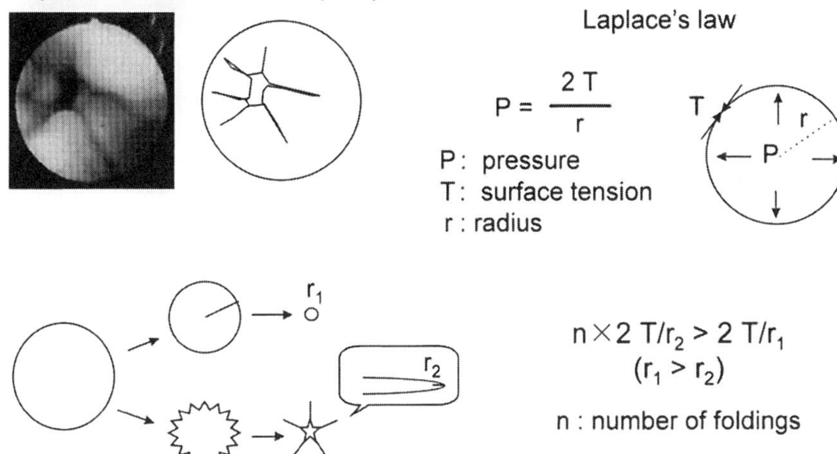

Figure 14 Theoretical prediction of the role of surface adhesive forces in a partially collapsed airway. Multiple folds often seen at the partially collapsed velopharynx possibly increase surface adhesive forces on the pharyngeal mucosa.

does not recover due to the effect of surface adhesive forces on the pharyngeal mucosa. Surface tension is calculated by Laplace's law, as shown in Figure 14. The calculated pressure needed to balance the surface tension appears to depend upon the radius and the number of folds of the pharynx. Endoscopic images of the pharynx often show multiple folds, particularly in a narrowed pharynx as in Figure 14. Since the surface tension at each fold is believed to resist reopening of the airway, surface tension possibly modulates the pharyngeal behavior even in the partially collapsed airway.

H. Sites of Pharyngeal Narrowing

Endoscopic evaluation of anesthetized and totally paralyzed subjects allowed us to determine the most collapsible segment in the passive pharynx, which had the highest closing pressure along the pharyngeal segments (32,33). Figure 15 illustrates the distribution of the most collapsible segment in children and adults with and without sleep-disordered breathing. In half of the normal children, the most collapsible segment was located at the oropharynx, whereas it was located at the nasopharynx in more than 80% of normal adults. Reed et al. reported that the oropharynx was the most compliant segment in the passive pharynx of infant cadavers (43). This evidence suggests that the most collapsible segment shifts from the caudal to the cranial segment with maturation. It should also be noted that the developmental changes in the site of the most collapsible segment were accompanied by increases in the closing pressure, as demonstrated in Figure 11. Although further studies are necessary to elucidate the underlying mechanisms, developmental changes in upper airway configuration may account for these interesting findings. Despite the presence of sleep dis-

Most collapsible site		Children Normal	Children SDB	Adults Normal	Adults SDB
Nasopharynx	Adenoids	0	57	0	0
Nasopharynx	Soft palate	54	29	82	88
Oropharynx	Tonsils	15	14	0	0
Oropharynx	Tongue	31	0	18	12

(%)

Figure 15 Distribution of the pharyngeal segment with the highest closing pressure in children and adults with and without sleep-disordered breathing (SDB). (Adapted from Refs. 32 and 33.)

ordered breathing, adults had the most collapsible segment at the nasopharynx. In contrast, increased collapsibility at the nasopharynx, due mainly to hypertrophied adenoids, was responsible for the development of the disease in children.

I. Switching from Nasal to Oral Breathing

In both adults and children, nasal air passages are most likely to be initially blocked during sleep. In response to nasal occlusion, switching from nasal to oral breathing is necessary to maintain ventilation. Although infants were previously believed to be obligatory nasal breathers, Rodenstein et al. demonstrated the presence of a shift to oral breathing during wakefulness (82). Like many other reflex responses, the reflex switching is accomplished by the combined actions of the peripheral receptors at the nose and pharynx, central nervous system regulation, and pharyngeal muscles, as illustrated in Figure 16. Any depression or derangement at any site involved in this reflex leads to failure or impairment of the switching from nasal to oral breathing. Konno et al. induced hypoventilation by nasal packing in infants and children during sleep (74), and Nishino et al. demonstrated prolongation of the latent period of the switching under sedation (83). This evidence demonstrates the importance of the level of consciousness in modulating the reflex. Sleep stages also influence responsiveness: the response is greatly depressed during REM sleep (84,85). Since receptors in the nose and the pharynx also play a significant role in controlling the shift of breathing route, as shown by Nishino et al. (86), pharyngeal edema or damage of the receptors may result in impairment of the reflex, especially in patients with sleep-disordered breathing in whom the augmenting reflex response to negative airway pressure was

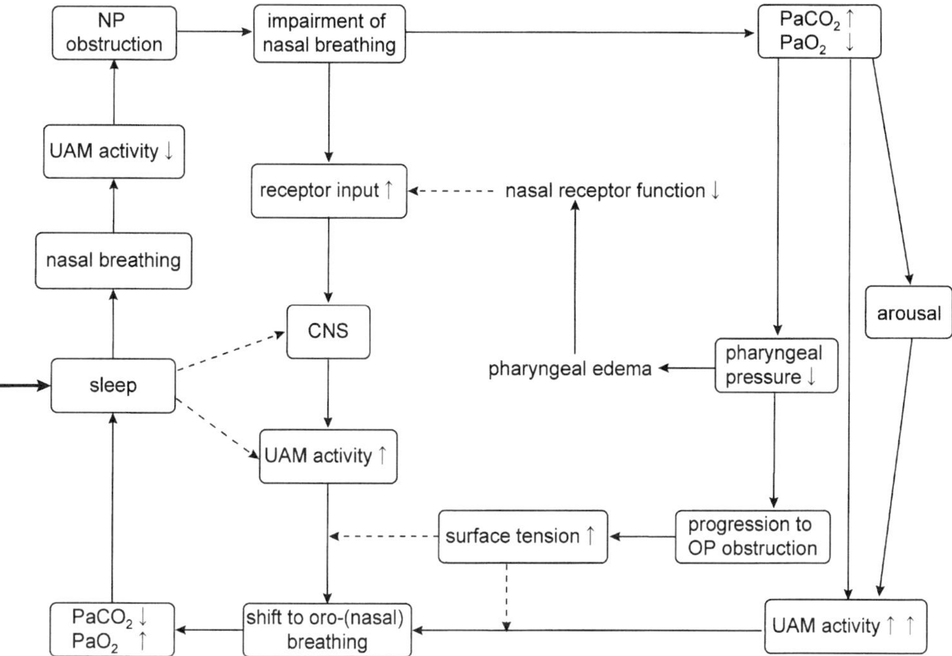

Figure 16 A schematic diagram explaining the sequential causal events leading to periodic ventilatory apnea/hypopnea cycles focusing on the mechanisms involved in switching from nasal to oral breathing. Dashed lines indicate suppression. CNS, central nervous system; UAM, upper airway muscle; NP, nasopharynx; OP, oropharynx.

reported to be depressed (24). Increased surface adhesive tension with progressive oropharyngeal narrowing would also impede the switching mechanism. Figure 16 schematically illustrates a diagram of sequential events involved in the switching from nasal to oral breathing during sleep. According to detailed analysis of polysomnographic records of infants and children, arousal is likely to be unimportant in the termination of respiratory events, in contrast to adults (12,70). This is probably due to difference in the responsiveness of pharyngeal muscles or differences in the switching mechanisms between generations.

IV. Larynx

A. Actions of Intrinsic Laryngeal Muscles

Intrinsic laryngeal muscles control the behavior of the laryngeal aperture. Functionally, they can be classified into two antagonistic muscle groups: the adductors, which close the vocal cords, and the abductors, which open the vocal cords. The former includes the transverse arytenoids, the lateral cricoarytenoids (LCA), the interarytenoids, and the thyroarytenoids (TA), all of which are innervated by the recurrent laryngeal nerve. Abduction of the vocal cords is performed solely by the posterior cricoarytenoids (PCA), which are also innervated by the recurrent laryngeal nerve branches. The muscle actions can be understood by their attachments and rotation of the arytenoid cartilages produced by the contraction of the muscles, as illustrated in Figure 17 (1). The PCA abducts the vocal cords, as contraction of the PCA, which is attached to the muscular process located at the lateral side of the arytenoid cartilage, approximates the muscular processes while rotating the cartilage. The LCA adducts the vocal cords as the LCA pulls the muscular process anteriorly, rotating the arytenoids in the opposite direction. The contraction of the cricothyroids (CT) alone narrows the vocal cords by tilting the anterior part of the cricoid cartilage cranially with dorsal movement of the arytenoids, as well as stretching the vocal cords. Contraction of the CT muscle together with the PCA muscle, however, makes the glottic airway larger than during sole PCA contraction (1,87). The CT muscle is innervated by a branch of the superior laryngeal nerve. The size of the glottic airway is determined mainly by the balance between the adductors and the abductors of the larynx, although the extrinsic laryngeal muscles also modulate the vocal cord position (1).

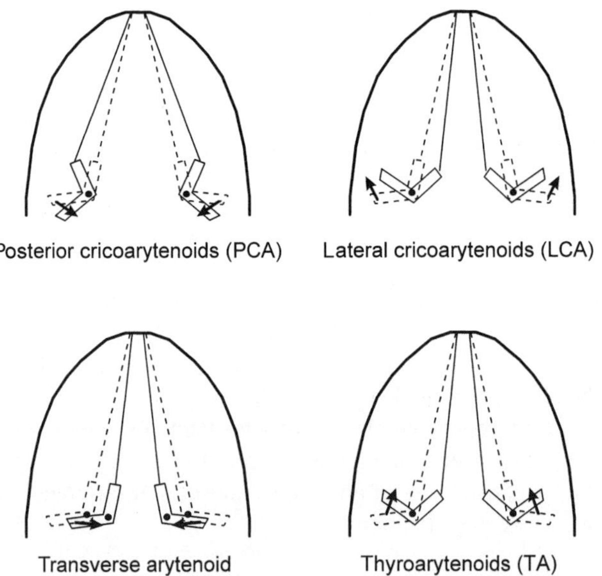

Figure 17 Schematic explanation of the action of each intrinsic laryngeal muscle leading to laryngeal closure or opening. The neutral positions of the arytenoid cartilages and the vocal cords are shown by dashed lines. The direction of contraction of each muscle is indicated by the arrows. Note the importance of the site of muscle attachment and resultant rotation of the L-shaped arytenoid cartilages.

B. Regulation of Respiratory Airflow by the Larynx

The laryngeal muscles exhibit respiratory-related activity, indicating that these muscles play a role in regulating airflow through the larynx by adjusting the laryngeal resistance during breathing. During quiet breathing, the glottic aperture is greater during inspiration than during expiration (88–90). Phasic activity of the abductors, such as the PCA muscle, which usually starts just prior to contraction of the inspiratory pump muscles such as the pharyngeal dilators, is believed to contribute to the widening of the glottic aperture during inspiration in both the awake and sleeping states (88,91,92). Phasic expiratory activity recorded in the adductors, such as the TA and arytenoideus muscles, is likely to counterbalance the tonic expiratory activity of the PCA muscle, leading to active return of the vocal cords towards the midline during wakefulness (93,94). During sleep, the tonic activity of the PCA as well as the phasic activity of the adductors during expiration disappears, while the PCA preserves its phasic inspiratory activity (93). Accordingly, Kuna et al. suggested that inspiratory dilation and expiratory narrowing of the laryngeal aperture is actively controlled by the antagonistic laryngeal muscles during wakefulness, whereas the return of the vocal cords toward the midline during expiration appears to be a passive phenomenon during sleep (95). When ventilation is stimulated by hypoxia or hypercapnia, the size of the laryngeal aperture increases and the laryngeal resistance decreases, whereas hypocapnia leads to narrowing of the laryngeal aperture and increased laryngeal resistance (96,97). The laryngeal caliber appears to be controlled in relation to the magnitude of respiratory activity.

The inspiratory dilation is believed to be beneficial for efficient breathing, and expiratory narrowing may play a role in braking expiratory airflow while controlling lung volume (89,98). Inspiratory airflow limitation by the vocal cords does not usually occur in normal subjects, even during sleep, when PCA activity decreases. However, airflow limitation is evident when the bilateral recurrent laryngeal nerves are damaged or when laryngospasm is induced. Vocal cord dysfunction in Shy-Drager syndrome is known to produce a distinctive stridor during inspiratory flow limitation. Laryngomalacia in newborn infants is another condition that causes inspiratory airflow limitation at increased ventilation. Although complete paralysis of the vocal cords does not lead to complete laryngeal closure, the narrowed laryngeal aperture narrows progressively because of increases in kinetic energy during constriction (Bernoulli effect) at inspiration.

C. Laryngeal Muscle Functions for Airway Protection

Stimulation of receptors on the upper airway mucosa is known to elicit various reflex responses, such as swallowing, coughing, the expiration reflex, apnea, and laryngeal closure, all of which contribute to a powerful airway clearance mechanism (99). The larynx plays a significant role in these reflexes while coordinating with other muscles groups, such as those of the pharynx and chest wall. Complete closure of the larynx just before exhalation and full opening of the larynx during exhalation increases the efficiency of coughing in order to blow foreign material out of the airway. Complete laryngeal closure during apnea serves to prevent aspiration of the material into the respiratory tract, passively but with certainty.

The types of upper airway reflex responses depend upon the site of receptor stimulation (100), the level of consciousness (101), sleep state (102), depth of anesthesia and the anesthetic agents used (103,104), chemical stimuli (105,106), and maturation (107–109). To cover all these in detail is beyond the scope of this chapter. Therefore, a general flowchart is presented in Figure 18. This is not based entirely on reported observations and hence is speculative. The reflex responses can be classified into two types: active and passive. The former includes swallowing, coughing, and the expiration reflex, which accompanies the dynamic elimination of foreign material from the respiratory tract. Apnea and laryngeal closure may be included in the latter, since they do not actively result in the removal of foreign material. Sullivan et al. reported that typical responses to laryngeal stimulation during wakefulness and slow-wave sleep were active, whereas prolonged apnea was typical during REM sleep in tracheotomized dogs (102). No study has examined the effects of sleep stage on human responses. Nishino et al. examined the influence of anesthetic depth on adult human responses to laryngeal stimulation with a small amount of distilled water and found that increasing depths of anesthesia with either enflurane or propofol plus fentanyl changed the responses from active to passive (103,104). Interestingly, the duration of

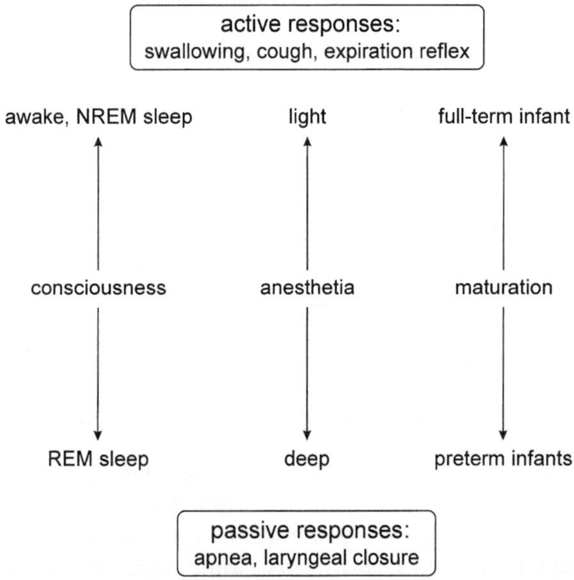

Figure 18 Modification of upper airway reflex responses by the level of consciousness, maturation, and depth of anesthesia.

responses was much shorter in awake adult subjects than in anesthetized subjects, although the predominant responses were the cough and the expiration reflex in both states (101). Pickens et al. compared the reflex response patterns elicited by saline injection into the pharynx between full-term and preterm infants during sleep and found that the prolonged apnea response was much more common in preterm than in full-term infants, although the amount of saline eliciting the response was significantly less in preterm infants (107). This agrees with the findings of lamb and dog studies, in which the prolonged apnea observed immediately after birth disappeared in a few weeks (108,109). The predominant responses in newborn animals and infants are swallowing and apnea and differ from those of adult animals and humans, which are cough and the expiration reflex.

V. Summary

Descent of the larynx and elongation of the pharynx with development may be key to explaining changing collapsibility of the pharynx.

Pharyngeal constrictors as well as dilators act as stiffeners of the pharyngeal tube.

Sleep suppresses pharyngeal muscle activity.

The pharyngeal airway behaves like a collapsible tube.

The concept of the "tube law" of the pharynx is helpful for better understanding the pathophysiology of pharyngeal obstruction during sleep.

Pharyngeal muscles appear to contribute little to maintenance of a patent airway during sleep in normal subjects.

Patients with obstructive sleep apnea have anatomical abnormalities of the pharynx.

The capability of neuromuscular compensation in response to pharyngeal airway narrowing declines with maturation.

The pharyngeal structure of normal children appears to be less collapsible than that of normal adults.

High nasal resistance is a risk factor for the development of sleep-disordered breathing.

Surface adhesive forces on the pharyngeal mucosa are likely to play a role in partial pharyngeal narrowing as well as complete closure.

Sites of pharyngeal narrowing shift from caudal to cranial segment with maturation.

Switching from nasal to oral breathing is depressed by sleep.

The position of the vocal cords is determined mainly by the balance between the adductors and abductors of the larynx.

Sleep abolishes adductor muscle activity and greatly reduces abductor activity.

The patterns of upper airway reflex responses are modulated by sleep stages and maturation.

Acknowledgments

The author is grateful to Professor Takashi Nishino of the Department of Anesthesiology, Chiba University School of Medicine, for his constructive comments. The MRI images of Figure 1 were kindly offered by Dr. Naokatsu Saeki of the Department of Neurosurgery, Chiba University School of Medicine. Dr. Atsuko Tanaka, my colleague, assisted me in performing an experiment of the collapsible tube. Dr. Sara Shimizu helped me greatly to improve this manuscript.

References

1. Bartlett D Jr. Upper airway motor system. In Cherniack NS, Widdicombe JG, eds. Handbook of Physiology: The Respiratory System. Control of Breathing, Part 1. Bethesda, MD: American Physiological Society, 1986: 223–245.
2. Mortimore IL, Mathur R, Douglas NJ. Effects of posture, route of respiration, and negative pressure on palatal muscle activity in humans. J Appl Physiol 1995; 79:448–454.
3. Tangel DJ, Mezzanotte WS, White DP. Respiratory related control of palatoglossus and levator palatini muscle activity. J Appl Physiol 1995; 78:680–688.
4. Mezzanotte WS, Tanjel DJ, White DP. Waking genioglossal electromyogram in sleep apnea patients versus normal controls: a neuromuscular compensatory mechanism. J Clin Invest 1992; 89:1571–1579.
5. Remmers JE, deGroot WJ, Sauerland EK, Anch AM. Pathogenesis of upper airway occlusion during sleep. J Appl Physiol 1978; 44:931–938.
6. van de Graaff WB, Gottfried SB, Mitra J, van Lunteren E, Cherniack NS, Strohl KP. Respiratory function of hyoid muscles and hyoid arch. J Appl Physiol 1984; 57:197–204.
7. Roberts JL, Reed WR, Thach BT. Pharyngeal airway-stabilizing function of sternohyoid and sternothyroid muscles in the rabbit. J Appl Physiol 1984; 57:1790–1795.
8. van Lunteren E, Haxhiu MA, Cherniack NS. Relation between upper airway volume and hyoid muscle length. J Appl Physiol 1987; 63:1443–1449.
9. van Lunteren E, Haxhiu MA, Cherniack NS. Mechanical function of hyoid muscles during spontaneous breathing in cats. J Appl Physiol 1987; 62:582–590.
10. Feroah TR, Forster HV, Rice T, Pan L, Lowry T. Reciprocal activity of inferior pharyngeal constrictor and stylopharyngeus correlate with changes in retroglossal area. Am J Respir Crit Care Med 1997; 155:A413.
11. Kuna ST, Smickley JS. Superior pharyngeal constrictor activation in obstructive sleep apnea. Am J Respir Crit Care Med 1997; 156:874–880.
12. Kuna ST, Smickley J. Response of genioglossus muscle activity to nasal airway occlusion in normal sleeping adults. J Appl Physiol 1988; 64:347–353.
13. Hudgel DW, Mulholland M, Hendricks C. Neuromuscular and mechanical responses to inspiratory resistive loading during sleep. J Appl Physiol 1987; 63:603–608.
14. Cohen G, Henderson-Smart DJ. Upper airway muscle activity during nasal occlusion in newborn babies. J Appl Physiol 1989; 66:1328–1335.
15. Duara S, Rojas M, Claure N. Upper airway stability and respiratory muscle activity during inspiratory loading in full-term neonates. J Appl Physiol 1994; 77:37–42.

16. Roberts JL, Reed WR, Mathew OP, Thach BT. Control of respiratory activity of the genioglossus muscle in micrognathic infants. J Appl Physiol 1986; 61:1523–1533.
17. Parisi RA, Santiago TV, Edelman NH. Genioglossal and diaphragmatic EMG responses to hypoxia during sleep. Am Rev Respir Dis 1988; 138:610–616.
18. Parisi RA, Neubauer JA, Frank MM, Edelman NH, Santiago TV. Correlation between genioglossal and diaphragmatic responses to hypercapnia during sleep. Am Rev Respir Dis 1987; 135:378–382.
19. Brouillette RT, Thach BT. A neuromuscular mechanism maintaining extrathoracic airway patency. J Appl Physiol 1979; 46:772–779.
20. Hida W, Kurosawa H, Okabe S, Kikuchi Y, Midorikawa J, Chung Y, Takishima T, Shirato K. Hypoglossal nerve stimulation affects the pressure-volume behavior of the upper airway. Am J Respir Crit Care Med 1995; 151:455–460.
21. Strohl KP, Hensley MJ, Hallett M, Saunders NA, Ingram RH Jr. Activation of upper airway muscles before onset of inspiration in normal humans. J Appl Physiol 1980; 49:638–642.
22. Horner RL, Innes JA, Holden HB, Guz A. Afferent pathway(s) for pharyngeal dilator reflex to negative pressure in man: a study using upper airway anaesthesia. J Physiol Lond 1991; 436:31–44.
23. van der Touw T, O'Neill N, Brancatisano A, Amis T, Wheatley J, Engel LA. Respiratory-related activity of soft palate muscles: augmentation by negative upper airway pressure. J Appl Physiol 1994; 76:424–432.
24. Mortimore IL, Douglas NJ. Palatal muscle EMG response to negative pressure in awake sleep apneic and control subjects. Am J Respir Crit Care Med 1997; 156:867–873.
25. McNicholas WT, Coffey M, Boyle T. Effects of nasal airflow on breathing during sleep in normal humans. Am Rev Respir Dis 1993; 147:620–623.
26. Carlo WA, Miller MJ, Martin RJ. Differential response of respiratory muscles to airway occlusion in infants. J Appl Physiol 1985; 59:847–852.
27. Isono S, Remmers JE. Anatomy and physiology of upper airway obstruction. In: Kryger MH, Roth T, Dement WC, eds. Principles and Practice of Sleep Medicine. Philadelphia: Saunders, 1994: 642–656.
28. Sauerland EK, Harper RM. The human tongue during sleep: electromyographic activity of the genioglossus muscle. Exp Neurol 1976; 51:160–170.
29. Anch AM, Remmers JE, Sauerland EK, deGroot WJ. Oropharyngeal patency during waking and sleep in the Pickwickian syndrome: electromyographic activity of the tensor veli palatini. Electromyogr Clin Neurophysiol 1981; 21:317–330.
30. Tangel DJ, Mezzanotte WS, White DP. Influence of sleep on tensor palatini EMG and upper airway resistance in normal men. J Appl Physiol 1991; 70:2574–2581.
31. Mezzanotte WS, Tanjel DJ, White DP. Influence of sleep onset on upper airway muscle activity in apnea patients versus normal controls. Am J Respir Crit Care Med 1996; 153:1880–1887.
32. Isono S, Remmers JE, Tanaka A, Sho Y, Sato J, Nichino T. Anatomy of pharynx in patients with obstructive sleep apnea and in normal subjects. J Appl Physiol 1997; 82:1319–1326.
33. Isono S, Shimada A, Utsugi M, Konno A, Nishino T. Comparison of static mechanical properties of the passive pharynx between normal children and children with sleep disordered breathing. Am J Respir Crit Car Med 1998; 157:1204–1212.

34. Henke KG. Upper airway muscle activity and upper airway resistance in young adults during sleep. J Appl Physiol 1998; 84:486–491.
35. Alex CG, Aronson RM, Onal E, Lopata M. Effects of continuous positive airway pressure on upper airway and respiratory muscle activity. J Appl Physiol 1987; 62:2026–2030.
36. Isono S, Morrison DL, Launois SH, Feroah TR, Whitelaw WA, Remmers JE. Static mechanics of the velopharynx of patients with obstructive sleep apnea. J Appl Physiol 1993; 75:148–154.
37. Launois SH, Feroah TR, Campbell WN, Issa FG, Morrison DL, Whitelaw WA, Isono S, Remmers JE. Site of pharyngeal narrowing predicts outcome of surgery for obstructive sleep apnea. Am Rev Respir Dis 1993; 147:182–189.
38. Morrison DL, Launois SH, Isono S, Feroah TR, Whitelaw WA, Remmers JE. Pharyngeal narrowing and closing pressure in patients with obstructive sleep apnea. Am Rev Respir Dis 1993; 148:606–611.
39. Permutt S, Riley RL. Hemodynamics of collapsible vessels with tone: the vascular waterfall. J Appl Physiol 1963; 18:924–932.
40. Webster PM, Sawatzky RP, Hoffstein V, Leblanc R, Hinchey MJ, Sullivan PA. Wall motion in expiratory flow limitation: choke and flutter. J Appl Physiol 1985; 59:1304–1312.
41. Dawson SV, Elliott EA. Wave-speed limitation on expiratory flow: a unifying concept. J Appl Physiol 1977; 43:498–515.
42. Wilson SL, Thach BT, Brouillette RT, Abuosba YK. Upper airway patency in human infant: influence of airway pressure and posture. J Appl Physiol 1980; 48:500–504.
43. Reed WR, Roberts JL, Thach BT. Factors influencing regional patency and configuration of the human infant upper airway. J Appl Physiol 1985; 58:635–644.
44. Roberts JL, Reed WR, Mathew OP, Menon AA, Thach BT. Assessment of pharyngeal stability in normal and micrognathic infants. J Appl Physiol 1985; 58:290–299.
45. Schwartz AR, Smith PL, Wise RA, Gold AR, Permutt S. Induction of upper airway occlusion in sleeping individuals with subatmospheric nasal pressure. J Appl Physiol 1988; 64:535–542.
46. Schwartz AR, Smith PL, Wise RA, Bankman I, Permutt S. Effects of positive nasal pressure on upper airway pressure-flow relationships. J Appl Physiol 1989; 66:1626–1634.
47. Smith PL, Wise RA, Gold AR, Schwartz AR, Permutt S. Upper airway pressure-flow relationships in obstructive sleep apnea. J Appl Physiol 1988; 64:789–795.
48. Gleadhill IC, Schwartz AR, Schubert N, Wise RA, Permutt S, Smith PL. Upper airway collapsibility in snorers and in patients with obstructive hypopnea and apnea. Am Rev Respir Dis 1991; 143:1300–1303.
49. Marcus CL, McColley SA, Carroll JL, Loughlin GM, Smith PL, Schwartz AR. Upper airway collapsibility in children with obstructive sleep apnea syndrome. J Appl Physiol 1994; 77:918–924.
50. Isono S, Feroah TR, Hajduk EA, Brabt R, Whitelaw WA, Remmers JE. Interaction of cross-sectional area, driving pressure and airflow of passive velopharynx. J Appl Physiol 1997; 83:851–859.
51. Kamm RD, Pedley TJ. Flow in collapsible tubes: a brief review. J Biomech Eng 1989; 111:177–179.
52. Pedley TJ, Drazen JM. Aerodynamic theory. In: Macklem P, Mead J, eds. Handbook of Physiology: The Respiratory System. Mechanics of Breathing, Part 1. Bethesda, MD: American Physiological Society, 1986: 41–54.

53. Mead J. Expiratory flow limitation: a physiologist's point of view. Federation 1980; 39:2771–2775.
54. Koenig JS, Thach. Effects of mass loading on the upper airway. J Appl Physiol 1988; 64:2294–2299.
55. Winter WC, Gampper T, Gay SB, Suratt PM. Enlargement of the lateral pharyngeal fat pad space in pigs increases upper airway resistance. J Appl Physiol 1995; 79:726–731.
56. Shelton KE, Woodson H, Gay S, Suratt PM. Pharyngeal fat in obstructive sleep apnea. Am Rev Respir Dis 1993; 148:462–466.
57. Horner RL, Mohiaddin RH, Lowell DG, Shea SA, Burman ED, Longmore DB, Guz A. Sites and sizes of fat deposits around the pharynx in obese patients with obstructive sleep apnoea and weight matched controls. Eur Respir J 1989; 2:613–622.
58. Schwab RJ, Gupta KB, Gefter WB, Metzger LJ, Hoffman EA, Pack AI. Upper airway soft tissue anatomy in normals and patients with sleep disordered breathing: significance of the lateral pharyngeal walls. Am J Respir Crit Care Med 1995; 152:1673–1689.
59. Shelton KE, Gay SB, Hollowell DE, Woodson H, Suratt PM. Mandible enclosure of upper airway and weight in obstructive sleep apnea. Am Rev Respir Dis 1993; 148:195–200.
60. Isono S, Tanaka A, Sho Y, Konno A, Nishino T. Advancement of the mandible improves velopharyngeal airway patency. J Appl Physiol 1995; 79:2132–2138.
61. Lowe AA, Gionhaku N, Takeuchi K, Fleetham JA. Three- dimensional reconstructions of tongue and airway in adults subjects with obstructive sleep apnea. Am J Orthod Dentofacial Orthop 1986; 90:364–374.
62. Jamieson A, Guilleminault C, Partinen M, Quera-Salva MA. Obstructive sleep apnea patients have craniomandibular abnormalities. Sleep 1986; 9:469–477.
63. Neill AM, Angus SM, Sajkov D, McEvoy RD. Effects of sleep posture on upper airway stability in patients with obstructive sleep apnea. Am J Respir Crit Care Med 1997; 155:199–204.
64. van de Graaff WB. Thoracic influence on upper airway patency. J Appl Physiol 1988; 65:2124–2131.
65. Thut DC, Schwartz AR, Roach D, Wise RA, Permutt S, Smith PL. Tracheal and neck position influence upper airway airflow dynamics by altering airway length. J Appl Physiol 1993; 75:2084–2090.
66. Series F, Marc I. Influence of lung volume dependence of upper airway resistance during continuous negative airway pressure. J Appl Physiol 1994; 77:840–844.
67. Begle RL, Badr S, Skatrud JB, Dempsey JA. Effect of lung inflation on pulmonary resistance during NREM sleep. Am Rev Respir Dis 1990; 141:854–860.
68. Hoffstein V, Zamel N, Phillipson EA. Lung volume dependence of pharyngeal cross-sectional area in patients with obstructive sleep apnea. Am Rev Respir Dis 1984; 130:175–178.
69. Jeffries B, Brouillette RT, Hunt CE. Electromyographic study of some accessory muscles of respiration in children with obstructive sleep apnea. Am Rev Respir Dis 1984; 129:696–702.
70. McNamara F, Issa FG, Sullivan CE. Arousal pattern following central and obstructive breathing abnormalities in infants and children. J Appl Physiol 1996; 81:2651–2657.
71. Marcus CL, Omlin KJ, Basinki DJ, Bailey SL, Rachal AB, Von Pechmann WS, Keens TG, Ward SLD. Normal polysomnographic values for children and adolescents. Am Rev Respir Dis 1992; 146:1235–1239.

72. Ferris BG Jr, Mead J, Opie LH. Partitioning of respiratory flow resistance in man. J Appl Physiol 1964; 19:653–658.
73. Bridger GP, Proctor DF. Maximum nasal inspiratory flow and nasal resistance. Ann Otol Rhinol Laryngol 1970; 79:481–488.
74. Konno A, Togawa K, Hoshino T. The effect of nasal obstruction in infancy and early childhood upon ventilation. Laryngoscope 1980; 90:699–707.
75. Young T, Finn L, Kim H. Nasal obstruction as a risk factor for sleep-disordered breathing: The University of Wisconsin Sleep Respiratory Research Group. J Allergy Clin Immunol 1997; 99:S757–S762.
76. Series F, Pierre SS, Carrier G. Effects of surgical correction of nasal obstruction in the treatment of obstructive sleep apnea. Am Rev Respir Dis 1992; 146:1261–1265.
77. Heimer D, Scharf SM, Lieberman A, Lavie P. Sleep apnea syndrome treated by repair of deviated nasal septum. Chest 1983; 84:184–185.
78. Olson LG, Strohl KP. Airway secretions influence upper airway patency in the rabbit. Am Rev Respir Dis 1988; 137:1379–1381.
79. Miki H, Hida W, Kikuchi Y, Chonan T, Satoh M, Iwase N, Takishima T. Effects of pharyngeal lubrication on the opening of obstructed upper airway. J Appl Physiol 1992; 72:2311–2316.
80. van der Touw T, Crawford ABH, Wheatley JR. Effects of a synthetic lung surfactant on pharyngeal patency in awake human subjects. J Appl Physiol 1997; 82:78–85.
81. Tanaka A, Isono S, Nishino T. Modulation of reopening of the passive pharynx in humans: a role of surface adhesive forces. Am J Respir Crit Care Med 1997; 155:A412.
82. Rodenstein DO, Perlmutter N, Stanescu DC. Infants are not obligatory nasal breathers. Am Rev Respir Dis 1985; 131:343–347.
83. Nishino T, Kochi T. Effects of sedation produced by thiopentone on responses to nasal occlusion in female adults. Br J Anaesth 1993; 71:388–392.
84. Issa FG, Edwards P, Szeto E, Lauff D, Sullivan CE. J Appl Physiol 1988; 64:543–549.
85. Purcell M. Response in the newborn to raised upper airway resistance. Arch Dis Child 1976; 51:602–607.
86. Nishino T, Sugiyama A, Tanaka A, Ishikawa T. Effects of topical nasal anaesthesia on shift of breathing route in adults. Lancet 1992; 339:1497–1500.
87. Konrad HR, Rattenborg CC. Combined action of laryngeal muscles. Acta Otolaryngol 1969; 67:646–649.
88. England SJ, Barlett D Jr, Daubenspeck JA. Influence of human vocal cord movements on airflow and resistance during eupnea. J Appl Physiol 1982; 52:773–779.
89. Bartlett D Jr, Remmers JE, Gautier H. Laryngeal regulation of respiratory airflow. Respir Physiol 1973; 18:194–204.
90. Campbell CJ, Murtagh JA, Raber CF. Laryngeal resistance to airflow. Ann Otol Rhinol Laryngol 1963; 72:5–30.
91. Brancatisano TP, Dodd DS, Engel LA. Respiratory activity of posterior cricoarytenoid muscle and vocal cords in humans. J Appl Physiol 1984; 57:1143–1149.
92. Carlo WA, Kosch PC, Bruce EN, Strohl KP, Martin RJ. Control of laryngeal muscle activity in preterm infants. Pediatr Res 1987; 22:87–91.
93. Kuna ST, Insalaco G, Woodson GE. Thyroarytenoid muscle activity during wakefulness and sleep in normal adults. J Appl Physiol 1988; 65:1332–1339.
94. Tully A, Brancatisano A, Loring SH, Engel LA. Relationship between thyroarytenoid activity and laryngeal resistance. J Appl Physiol 1990; 68:1988–1996.

95. Kuna ST, Smickley JS, Insalaco G. Posterior cricoarytenoid muscle activity during wakefulness and sleep in normal adults. J Appl Physiol 1990; 68:1746–1754.
96. Campbell CJ, Murtagh JA, Raber CF. Chemical agents and laryngeal reflex control of laryngeal glottis. Ann Otol Rhinol Laryngol 1963; 72:589–604.
97. Bartlett D Jr. Effects of hypercapnia and hypoxia on laryngeal resistance to airflow. Respir Physiol 1979; 37:293–302.
98. Remmers JE, Bartlett D Jr. Reflex control of expiratory airflow and duration. J Appl Physiol 1977; 42:80–87.
99. Widdicombe JG. Reflexes from the upper respiratory tract. In: Cherniack NS, Widdicombe JG, eds. Handbook of Physiology: The Respiratory System. Control of Breathing. Part 1. Bethesda, MD: American Physiological Society, 1986: 363–394.
100. Nishino T, Kochi T, Ishii M. Differences in respiratory reflex responses from the larynx, trachea, and bronchi in anesthetized female subjects. Anesthesiology 1996; 84:70–74.
101. Nishino T, Tagaito Y, Isono S. Cough and other reflexes on irritation of airway mucosa in man. Pulm Pharmacol 1996; 9:285–292.
102. Sullivan CE, Murphy E, Kozar LF, Phillipson EA. Waking and ventilatory responses to laryngeal stimulation in sleeping dogs. J Appl Physiol 1978; 45:681–689.
103. Nashino T, Honda Y. Respiratory reflex responses to stimulation of tracheal mucosa in enflurane-anesthetized humans. J Appl Physiol 1988; 65:1069–1074.
104. Tagaito Y, Isono S, Nishino T. Upper airway reflexes during a combination of propofol and fentanyl anesthesia. Anesthesiology 1998; 88:1459–1466.
105. Nishino T, Yonezawa T, Honda Y. Modification of laryngospasm in response to changes in Pa_{CO_2} and Pa_{O_2} in the cat. Anesthesiology 1981; 55:286–291.
106. Nishino T, Hiraga K, Honda Y. Inhibitory effects of CO_2 on airway defensive reflexes in enflurane-anesthetized humans. J Appl Physiol 1989; 66:2642–2646.
107. Pickens DL, Schefft GL, Thach BT. Pharyngeal fluid clearance and aspiration preventive mechanisms in sleeping infants. J Appl Physiol 1989; 66:1164–1171.
108. Marchal F, Corke BC, Sundell H. Reflex apnea from laryngeal chemostimulation in the sleeping premature newborn lamb. Pediatr Res 1982; 16:621–627.
109. Boggs DF, Bartlett D Jr. Chemical specificity of a laryngeal apneic reflex in puppies. J Appl Physiol 1982; 53:455–462.

12

Craniofacial Development and the Airway During Sleep

NALTON F. FERRARO

Children's Hospital
Boston, Massachusetts

I. Introduction

Patency of the upper airway during sleep is integrally related to craniofacial morphology, but craniofacial structure is only one element in the equation that defines airway patency. If a tube is narrow enough, its walls collapsible enough, and the transluminal pressure differential great enough, the tube will fail as a conduit. This happens in the obstructive sleep apnea (OSA) syndrome; but this tube, the upper airway, has daunting structural complexity and variability. There are two main intake ports in this tube; internally it has recesses, multiple valves, movable baffles, and glands that can swell or fill parts of the tube with mucus. The rigidity of the tube can change very quickly secondary to both internal and external control factors; parts of this tube can grow into the lumen (e.g., tonsils), the tube carries multiple fluids, and it works better in certain positions than others. This is the normal human upper airway and it functions beautifully most of the time.

To fully understand the upper airway, it will be useful to examine the normal airway, the congenitally abnormal airway (nature's experiments), and therapeutic interventions that attempt to change the airway. In this way, one can gain insight into the impact that structure has on the function of this complex system. Much of what goes on in the upper airway is controlled centrally (1). Neuromuscular control, tone, and central feedback loops are ultimately what determine airway patency, but these crucial factors will not be the focus in this discussion of craniofacial development and anatomy. This is, of course, an artifice, because the size and shape of this tortuous tube is under moment-to-moment central nervous system control. This surgery of the craniofacial skeleton is a snapshot—a "still" for the sake of clarity in what is really a moving picture. The airway patency in a retrognathic child, a midface-deficient infant, or even a child with large tonsils is still subject to these central controls, but the structural abnormalities place rather strict limitations on tube patency no matter what the brain tries to do to overcome or compensate.

Conversely, when central and neuromuscular controls are malfunctioning, normal structural anatomy cannot alone maintain airway patency. Such a clinical example is a patient with normal craniofacial structure who develops worsening obstructive sleep apnea because of a progressive myotonia.

The two building blocks for craniofacial development interlock: the bony element and the soft tissue element. Bony growth cannot actually be separated from soft tissue growth and function. For expediency, however, the growth of the bony framework is considered first and the soft tissue elements are added secondarily; much as one first builds the frame for a dwelling.

This bony framework has a complex relationship with its soft tissue envelope that is only partially elucidated. This soft tissue envelope includes muscle, fat, and connective tissue and it is crucial in several functions such as breathing, swallowing, chewing, eating, and speaking. Functional forces have a profound effect on the craniofacial skeleton. According to the functional matrix theory first proposed by Moss in the 1960s, the development of the skeletal framework is controlled at least in part by the soft tissue envelope and the functional forces to which the skeleton is exposed (2). Such a functional force affecting skeletal growth can be seen in the fetus that has an abnormal lie in utero and on whose developing mandible pressure is exerted, with resultant micrognathia and airway difficulties in infancy. After birth, the deformational forces on the mandible are relieved; the mandible then grows and can "catch up," with resultant improvement in the airway. This is a rather straightforward demonstration of functional force affecting skeletal growth (3).

Sometimes the situation is less obvious. A baby with Beckwith-Wiedemann syndrome is a large baby with, among other findings, a large tongue. As the child grows, the mandible tends to be large with relative maxillary deficiency and there may be an anterior open bite. If a significant reduction glossectomy is performed, the open bite will close but the maxillary/mandibular relationship does not change. This indicates that portions of the facial skeletal changes are "reactive" (the open bite)—i.e., secondary to functional forces that are epigenetic, and that other skeletal patterns are genetically programmed into the craniofacial skeletal matrix and not the functional matrix (the relative midface hypoplasia and mandibular prognathism). The Treacher Collins syndrome includes a small mandible and a hypoplastic pharynx; these malformations are genetically determined and not controlled to any great extent by manipulation of the functional matrix (4).

A more common example of the functional matrix dilemma is illustrated by the child with "adenoidal facies." This child has a narrow maxilla, anterior open bite, habitually open mouth, and pinched nares. Evaluation reveals significant degree of nasal obstruction from the adenoids and mucosal swelling secondary to allergies or other nasal/nasopharyngeal abnormalities. This appears to be an obvious example of the functional matrix theory in action. Nasal obstruction shapes the facial skeleton (5). It is legitimate to ask, however, if skeletal development may predispose to nasopharyngeal obstruction. The shape of the facial skeleton results in nasal obstruction. The clinical picture probably develops from multiple contributing factors.

Returning to the example of the newborn with micrognathia secondary to external functional forces, "catch up" to some extent can be expected. In the newborn with a syndromic micrognathia that has a genetic basis, "catch up" cannot be expected. Treatment decisions must account for these distinctions.

Elaboration on airway patency related to specific craniofacial anatomic sites follows. The general principles from this introduction that are of paramount importance in understanding the craniofacial skeleton and its relation to obstructive sleep apnea include:

1. The upper airway is anatomically complex, as is the interplay between craniofacial anatomy and neuromuscular control.
2. Abnormal airways can usually maintain patency because of neural controls despite markedly deranged facial structure.
3. Conversely, seemingly adequate anatomical airways can lose patency because of neural control problems.
4. As the upper airway develops from infancy to adulthood, changes include not just a larger framework but also other dynamic and functional changes. Encroachment on the lumen is not static. Tonsils and adenoids can enlarge and shrink, allergies can cause turbinates to swell, airway rigidity changes, and fat deposition fluctuates. The skeleton must be viewed in light of these dynamic, nonbony changes (5–9).
5. The skeletal framework and the soft tissue envelope have a complex interplay. Bone growth itself is affected by soft tissue and functional forces but genetic control of the skeletal matrix is in evidence in many syndromes that demonstrate abnormal airways (10,11).

II. Principles of Craniofacial Growth

The craniofacial structure has a cephalocaudal gradient of growth. The midface has more postnatal growth potential than the cranium and the mandible has more growth potential than the midface. This growth has both vertical and anteroposterior components. In the newborn, the face is dwarfed by and tucked below the neurocranium. It must grow down and forward (3). In the infant, the tongue is very close to the soft palate and the depth of the pharynx is small; airway patency is generally maintained in babies despite this crowded upper airway.

As the maxilla grows, the bony structure elongates and is displaced forward in the anteroposterior plane and downward in the vertical plane. The mandible follows the same pattern. The net effect is one of a continually enlarging airway as the soft palate is carried away from the posterior pharyngeal wall and as the tongue moves forward and inferiorly. The airway should be continually enlarging. The net result, however, is more complicated. The soft tissues change as the skeleton grows. The soft palate lengthens and thickens, the tongue grows, the nasal cavity elongates but the turbinates enlarge, and, of course, the tonsillar and adenoidal tissue hypertrophies (3,5,12,13). The net effect is, therefore, not as predictable as one might envision.

The bony skeleton itself grows in a complex fashion. There are fields of bone resorption and bone apposition, which processes take place simultaneously with the downward and forward displacement of the whole skeleton in space. This bodily displacement is not well understood but it clearly occurs.

Enlow (3) points out that the nasomaxillary complex relates in a very specific way to the anterior cranial fossa. The anterior margin of the anterior cranial fossa is the anterior margin of the nasomaxillary complex. The posterior boundaries of both structures have the same relationship. The configuration of the palate relates also to the anterior cranial base.

The breadth of the middle cranial fossa determines the lateromedial dimensions of the pharynx. The mandibular rami, which are well within the zygomas in early childhood, grow laterally, so that the adult mandibular rami are equal to the distance from the lateral edge of one middle cranial fossa to the other.

Development of the brain and the neurocranium control to a great degree the depth and width of the nasopharyngeal/oropharyngeal airway. The depth of the pharynx and nasomaxillary complex is a projection of the anterior cranial fossae. The breadth of the pharynx is a projection of the breadth of the middle cranial fossae. This nasomaxillary development is inextricably linked to development of the neurocranium, since the midface is attached to the neurocranium. Enlow notes that there is more variability in mandibular growth than maxillary growth, since the mandibular relationship with the neurocranium is not as intimate as the maxillary relationship. The syndromic midface-deficient growth pattern will highlight this relationship (10,11,14).

Another important concept is basicranial flexure. In other animals, the brain is in line with the spinal column. In humans, the spinal cord comes off the brain at an angle that is somewhat greater than 90 degrees. This allows bipedal activity with the face looking forward; a measurement of this flexure is the angle of the anterior cranial base—the angle formed by lines drawn from nasion point to sella to basion (basion = anterosuperior margin of foramen magnum). As this angle becomes less obtuse and approaches 90 degrees, it correlates with a shortened anterior cranial base and often lack of pharyngeal depth with airway compromise (11,15–17).

The bony resorptive and appositional fields mentioned above are very active in the growing midface. Bone is resorbed along all the inner nasal walls except for the

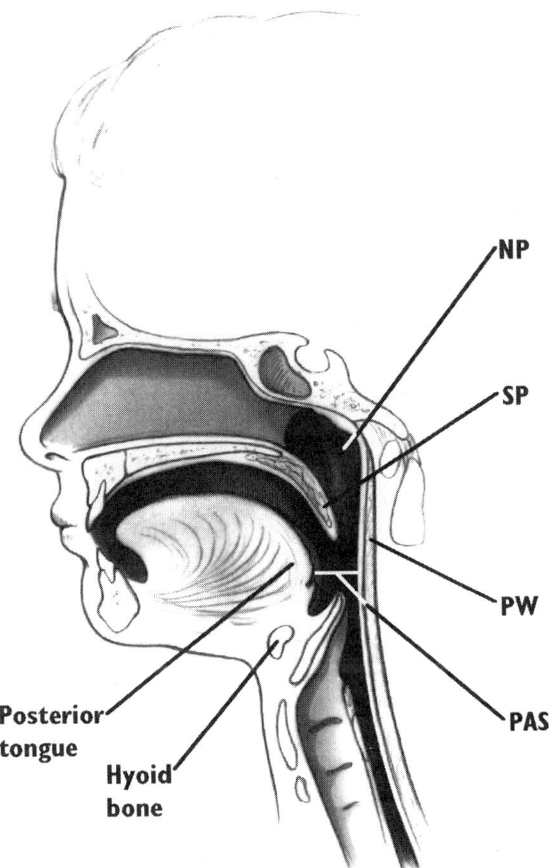

Figure 1 Sagittal view of normal 10-year-old facial skeleton (awake and upright). Note the relationship of the soft palate (SP) to the pharyngeal wall (PW), the depth of the posterior airway space (PAS), the nasopharynx (NP), the relationship of the posterior tongue to the soft palate, and the relationship of the hyoid bone to the mandibular symphysis.

very top of the nasal vault. The net result is an increase in the nasal airway. At the same time, the nasomaxillary complex is displacing anteroinferiorly within the limits of the anterior cranial fossae. This also increases the nasal/nasopharyngeal airway. Maxillary growth "carries" the soft palate also, further enlarging the airway. Nasomaxillary growth transversely under the projection of the middle cranial fossae also increases the airway dimensions (Fig. 1).

It is of particular interest that the resorptive/deposition fields even involve the bony portion of the intranasal septum, which may respond to some minor buckling of the nasal cartilaginous septum. The bone responds to the cartilaginous functional forces, resulting in a bony deviation in the septum. Increased airway resistance is noted because of the deviated bony and cartilaginous septum and because of deficient support of the nasal tip with an abnormal anterior nasal valve (5,18).

Mandibular growth has generally the same vectors as the nasomaxillary complex. However, there are some important differences. The posterior maxilla can accept bone deposition as it enlarges without any significant structural changes. The mandibular body elongates by encroaching on the territory of the mandibular rami. This is dealt with by an active resorptive field at the anterior ramus and bone deposition at the posterior ramus. The ramus in a manner becomes the mandibular body. This lengthening of the body is important to accommodate the tongue. Vertical mandibular growth is also crucial; this carries the tongue base inferiorly away from the soft palate (19). This creates more airway room. The mandible also widens laterally as a projection of the breadth of the middle cranial fossae, and this also improves airway dimension (3).

Recall that the tongue is attached anteriorly to the mandible. A retrognathic mandible is associated with a retropositioned tongue. Within the confines of that mandible, genioglossus and geniohyoid muscle tone control a great deal of the tongue position during sleep (1).

The very small mandible in the infant is often associated with glossoptosis. The tongue is not only retropositioned but is tipped posteriorly. This posterosuperiorly displaced tongue prevents the palatal shelves from achieving their transverse orientation and fusing. As a result, cleft palate is part of the Robin sequence (20,21).

III. Craniofacial Pattern and OSA

Many groups have characterized the craniofacial features that correlate with obstructive sleep apnea in both the pediatric and the adult populations (15,22–26). A straightforward analysis is provided by various measurements on the lateral cephalogram. The lateral cephalogram is a standardized lateral skull radiograph taken with the head in the natural head position (facing straight ahead), and it is used throughout the world to analyze both bony and soft tissue craniofacial relationships. These studies were mainly done with the subject standing and awake, although supine awake lateral cephalogram/OSA studies have been performed.

The craniofacial patterns that have correlated with OSA are provided in the list below and a line tracing of a normal cephalogram is provided as a reference. The craniofacial patterns noted on the lateral cephalogram that correlate with OSA include the following (Fig. 2):

1. SNA (sella-nasion A point) is an angle that measures maxillary retrusion. The more acute the angle, the more retrusion noted. It is in common usage but there are many exceptions to its predictability.
2. SNB (sella-nasion B point) is an angle that measures mandibular retrusion. The statements about SNA apply to SNB.

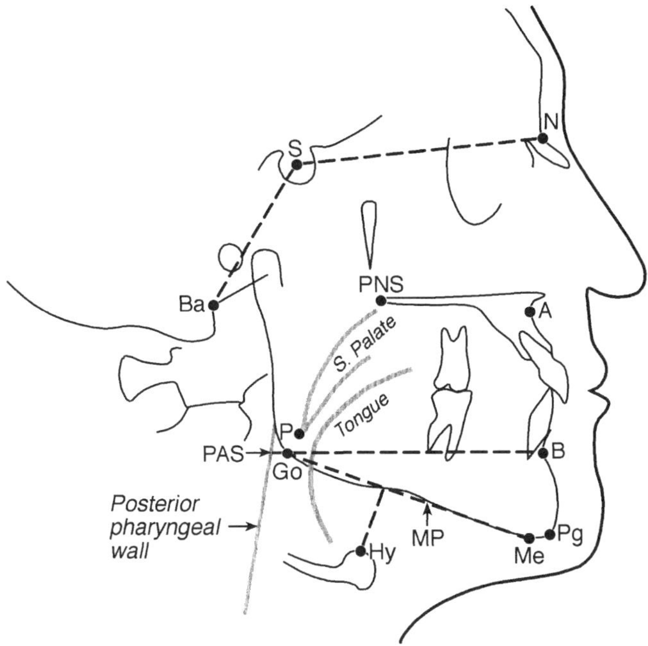

Figure 2 This is a simplified tracing of a lateral cephalogram. The various points have been marked in an obvious fashion for didactic clarity. Various anatomical points may not be as obvious on an actual lateral cephalogram. Straight-line measurements are made from point to point. Angle measurements are constructed by connecting three points. See text for definitions of abbreviations.

3. NSBa (nasion sella basion) is an angle of the anterior cranial base. The less obtuse the angle, the shorter the anterior cranial base. NS (or SN) is a linear measurement of anterior cranial base.
4. The PAS (posterior airway space) is a linear measurement made of the radiolucent airway column made along a line from B point through gonial angle (Go).
5. MP to Hy is a linear measurement of the perpendicular from the mandibular plane (roughly the plane of the mandibular interior border to a tangent at the most superior point of the body of the hyoid).
6. PNS = posterior nasal spine. P = tip of soft palate. PNS - P: linear measurement of the soft palate.
7. Mandibular angle is formed from intersection of MP and SN. The steeper the mandible the less acute is the angle. Steep mandibular angle correlates with OSA.

Maxillary AP deficiency (decreased SNA) (nl = 82°)
Mandibular deficiency (decreased SNB) (nl = 79°)
Short anterior cranial base (decreased SN) (nl = 71 mm)

Less obtuse basicranial flexure angle (decreased NSBa) (nl = 137°)
Short mandibular body (decreased pogonion-gonion; Pg - Go < 88 mm men, 79 mm women)
Steep mandibular plane (less acute SN to MP angle; nl = 37°)
Long soft palate (PNS-P)
Decreased sagittal posterior airway space (decreased PAS; nl ≥ 11 mm)
Increased distance of the hyoid bone from the mandibular inferior border (decreased MP-H) (nl ≤ 15 mm)

Note: Normal measurements are provided as an approximate guide because variability can be great.

Adenoidal tissue may also be seen on the lateral cephalogram. Intranasal structures are not well analyzed on the lateral projection (e.g., turbinates and septal deviations). These are best viewed on coronal projections, as are tongue width and soft palatal and pharyngeal width. Palatine tonsils, if they are very large, can be viewed as a subtle round density overlying the airway space, but this is not an entirely reliable finding. The correlation between the posterior airway space as measured on the lateral cephalogram and calculated posterior airway volume on computed tomography (CT) is very good (28). The lateral cephalogram done awake and standing does not necessarily predict the point or points of obstruction during sleep, but this is also true for the CT scan. However, analysis of the lateral cephalogram reveals the skeletal patterns and some soft tissue patterns that are known to correlate with OSA. In our patients with severe facial deformities, the lateral cephalogram provides a quantitative assessment of the deviation of the skeletal complex from the norm, and it provides a postsurgical treatment gauge of how normalized the structures have become. An obvious abnormality on a cephalogram, however, should be viewed in the totality of the airway. A very small mandible can certainly coexist with narrowed choanae. The former is obvious on lateral cephalogram; the latter is not.

Many groups have systematically evaluated parapharyngeal muscular function in relation to OSA (1,30). During sleep, the airway narrows across the palate, across the oropharynx posterior to the tongue, and in the hypopharyngeal regions. This occurs normally but to a greater extent in OSA subjects. Airway resistance increases. The tensor veli palatini muscle is critical to increased pharyngeal resistance as its tone decreases during sleep. The tensor veli palatini muscle's decrease in activity during sleep is countered by the increased activity of the genioglossus muscle, which is linked to respiration. At times, the genioglossus muscle can be hypoactive, contributing to the posterior tongue position and airway narrowing. Somnofluoroscopy has been used to view the site of airway narrowing and collapse (12). The collapse can begin at the soft palate and spread caudally. It has been suggested that the soft palate can act as a plug in the oropharynx. With increased resistance and increased transpharyngeal pressures, collapse of the airway propagates downstream.

In awake upright and awake supine subjects, these muscles have relative positions that correlate with skeletal anatomy. The tongue and genioglossus muscle are retropositioned in the retrognathic subject. The soft palate, which can act more like a plug, and the decreased postural tone of the tensor veli palatini can together produce a more dramatic effect if the nasomaxillary skeletal complex is posteriorly placed and hypoplastic in relation to the posterior pharyngeal wall. The multifactorial nature of OSA is again underscored (11,16,29,31).

IV. Abnormal Patterns of Craniofacial Growth

Significant maxillary deficiency can predispose to OSA, as found in the syndromic midface deficient craniosynostotic disorders (e.g., Apert, Crouzon, and Pfeiffer syndromes). In this group, the soft palate is against the posterior pharyngeal wall, the anterior cranial base is short, and the nasal cavity is small both in the AP plane and vertically. There is an underbite not because of mandibular prognathism but because of marked nasomaxillary deficiency. In fact, the mandible may be smaller than normal; this underscores how deficient the midface can be. In addition, the posterior choanae can be narrow, mucus can occlude the nose, and the palatal shelves can be thickened (particularly in Apert syndrome). All of this contributes to a very significant encroachment on the upper airway from a strictly structural standpoint before the neuromuscular issues are even considered (10,11,16,32) (Fig. 3).

Despite all of this, the majority of syndromic midface- deficient patients never require tracheostomy, but there are some critical junctures. For example, the midface-deficient newborn may have some airway difficulty when supine or during feeding but is otherwise well compensated. This compensated pattern may continue until physiological adenotonsillar hypertrophy occurs and the balance is upset with the development of frank OSA (often at age 2 or 3 years).

Conversely, an Apert syndrome baby with open cleft palate (30% of Apert infants) may have a compensated airway but then develops OSA after the palate is repaired. The closed palate encroaches on the small midfacial airway and the function of the tensor veli palatini may be poor. In addition, upper respiratory infections frequently tip these children into an obstructive pattern. Awake, these children may look uncomfortable, breathing with the mouth open and the nasal passages invariably filled with mucus. The resistance in the nasal airway can change from night to night because of the variable factors mentioned above.

In our experience, midface advancement via Le Fort III osteotomy does not predictably result in cure of OSA in these children (Ferraro, unpublished data, 1997). According to the lateral cephalogram, the nasomaxillary skeletal complex is placed into a "normal or near normal" position. Why is there this unpredictability with surgery? The recurring theme of soft tissue mass, neuromuscular control, tone, and persistent structural abnormalities (e.g., narrow posterior choanae) can foil the obvious skeletal changes made at operation. Moving the facial skeleton certainly makes the framework larger, but troublesome variables remain.

The child with cleft lip and palate often presents with maxillary hypoplasia; the

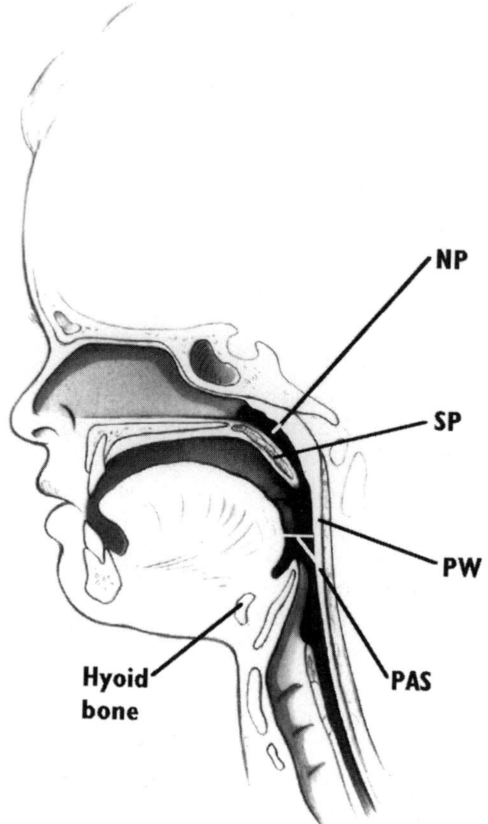

Figure 3 Sagittal view of the 10-year-old Crouzon or Apert facial skeleton (midface deficiency). Note the closeness of the soft palate to the pharyngeal wall, the lack of depth in the nasopharynx (NP), and the shortness of the anterior cranial base from nasion to sella.

anterior cranial base is not short as in the syndromic midface-deficient child. The nasal airway, however, may not be normal because of poor anterior nasal valves due to lack of nasal tip support, deviation of the septum, and compromised soft palatal function. If the repaired palate is short in the sagittal plane, however, this may actually benefit the airway, but at a significant functional cost of hypernasal speech. The mandible may be normal in size or actually retrognathic (it is rarely hyperplastic) despite the presence of an underbite (18,31,33,34).

Mandibular hypoplasia can be syndromic or nonsyndromic; static or progressive. Mild mandibular retrognathia with a class II malocclusion overbite) is the commonest abnormal orthodontic pattern seen in the United States. The spectrum's other end includes nonsyndromic infants with Robin sequence, syndromic micrognathia such as Treacher Collins syndrome, Nager syndrome, and Stickler syndrome. Peri-

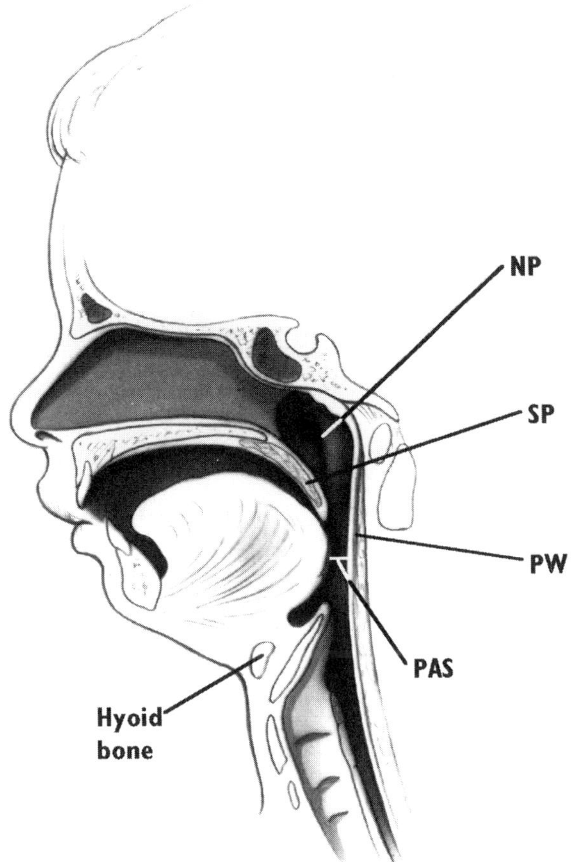

Figure 4 Sagittal view of the 10-year-old facial skeleton with a micrognathic mandible and normal midface. Note the retropositioned tongue, the small PAS, and the inferior displacement of the hyoid bone with a "clockwise" rotation of the tongue. The tongue then acts as an obstruction from the level of the soft palate to the hypopharynx when muscle tone is decreased during sleep.

natal or childhood trauma, infection, and severe juvenile rheumatoid arthritis can also result in micrognathia with OSA (4,19,20,35–38).

Many of these studies confirm the association of the small mandible and OSA. Reports of correction of OSA with mandibular reconstruction or advancement are also numerous. The small mandible results in the posterior and superior displacement of the tongue and its base, including the genioglossus muscle. The soft palate, posterior pharyngeal wall, and tongue meet at a very critical point in the airway (39,40) (Fig. 4). Dental appliances that hold the mandible in a protrusive position are known to treat

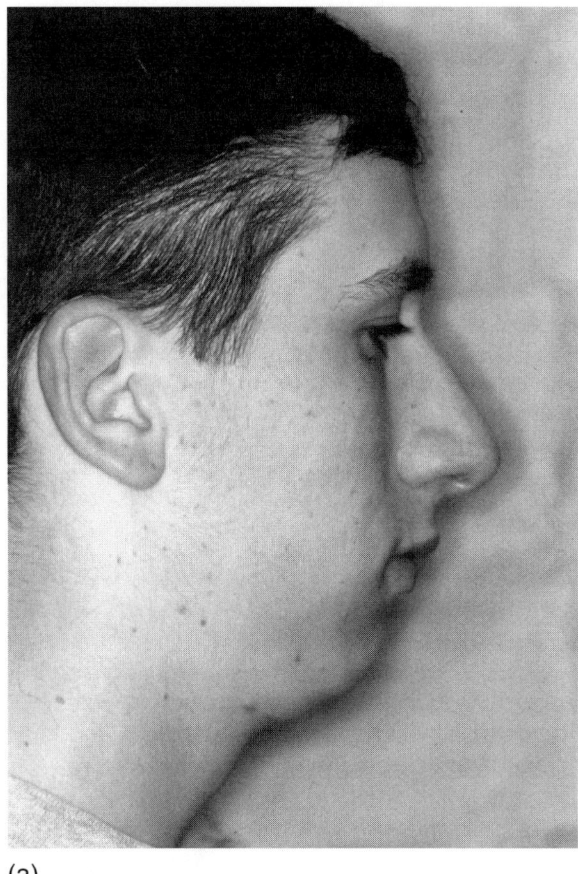

(a)

Figure 5 (a) Retrognathic young man with severe OSA. Note chin position and anterior neck. (b) Same patient's spiral CT sagittal reconstruction. Tongue (T) and soft palate (SP) form a mass of tissue against the pharyngeal wall. This image is taken supine and awake. (c) CT scan axial view demonstrates a pinpoint airway at the level of the tongue.

OSA in certain subjects. It is clear from many different sources that moving the mandible and tongue away from the posterior pharyngeal wall can improve airway patency during sleep (Fig. 5a, b, and c).

A hyoid bone that is at an increased distance from the inferior border of the mandible holds that position because the mandibular rami can be vertically short, the mandibular plane steep, and the tongue posteriorly positioned. Hyoid bone advancement to help open the deep oropharynx/hypopharynx has been proposed. Interestingly, both hyoid advancement toward the mandible and advancement/depression toward the thyroid cartilage are advocated (27,41).

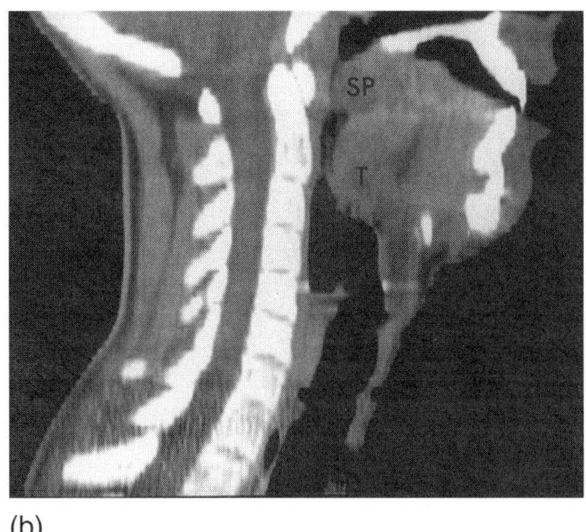

(b)

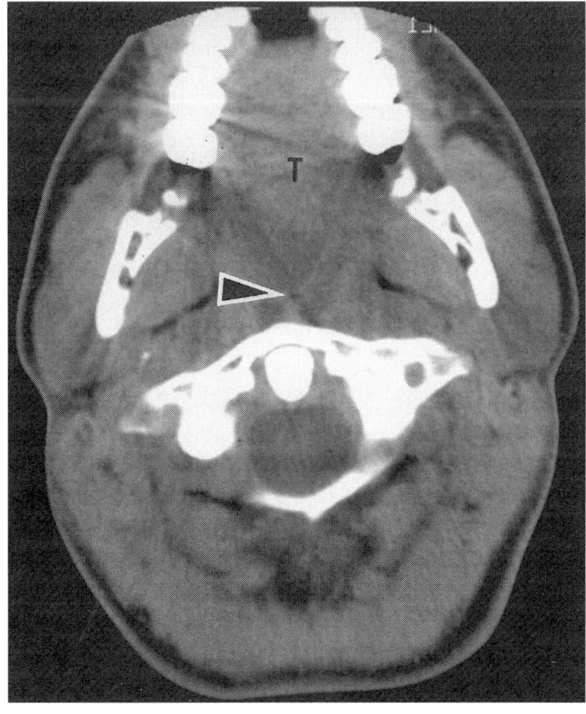

(c)

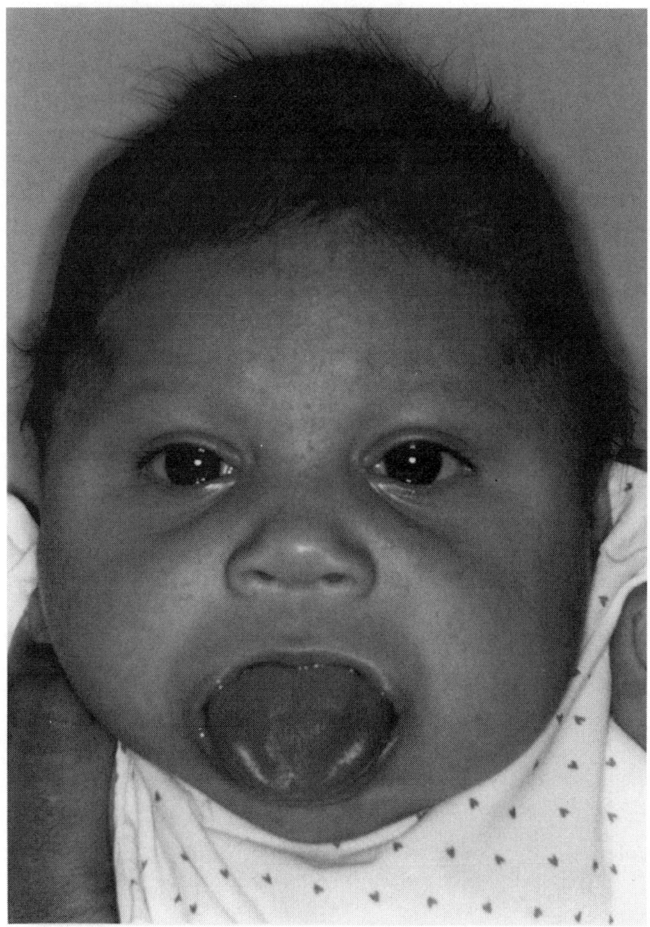

Figure 6 An infant with Beckwith-Wiedemann syndrome. Severe macroglossia and no OSA.

V. Conclusion

Observation of three special clinical groups can help to underscore the complexity of airway function and form.

1. In a Boston Children's Hospital series of 12 babies with Beckwith-Wiedemann syndrome and macroglossia, only one child had a polysomnogram demonstrating OSA. All the children possessed tongues that protruded out of the mouth at rest. Is the lack of OSA in this group secondary to a large airway, an anterior rather than posterior tongue enlargement, or protective neuromuscular tone? This is a group that requires study because of the intriguing lack of OSA (Fig. 6).

2. Mixter et al. reported in a group of syndromic midface-deficient children (including Apert and Pfeiffer syndromes) persistent airway difficulties even after tracheostomy. This group had evidence of tracheomalacia/bronchomalacia. This is a clarion reminder to examine the *whole* airway even in the presence of the obvious structural deformity (42).
3. Pharyngeal flaps are placed for hypernasal speech and other sequelae of velopharyngeal insufficiency. Pharyngeal flaps that partially occlude the nasopharynx are usually very well tolerated; the incidence of OSA is low. However, pharyngeal flaps have occasionally been associated with significant OSA and death. Young children (under the age of 6) are in a higher-risk category for airway complications with pharyngeal flaps (34,43–45). The overwhelming majority of flaps are for cleft lip/palate patients with a short, poorly functioning soft palate. However, flaps that are placed to treat recent-onset velopharyngeal insufficiency (VPI) when there is no obvious palatal shortening can lead to severe OSA. The VPI in these patients is often secondary to unrecognized progressive neuromuscular disease, and partial occlusion of the airway in these hypotonic patients can be disastrous.

These three special situations help highlight themes that have been the core of this discussion. The craniofacial skeleton must be viewed in the context of the soft tissue envelope and the neuromuscular control of the upper airway. At operation, the skeletal framework can be normalized, but soft tissue movement and function have great variability. The airway can be problematic at multiple points. One must "look past" the most obvious structural deformities in conducting the workup.

Muscle tone and neuromuscular control during sleep are critical factors controlling airway patency. The craniofacial skeleton can contribute positively or negatively to this integrated system, and reconstructing the craniofacial skeleton at operation can unquestionably improve an airway. It is neuromuscular and soft tissue function, however, that generally will impose its control on airway patency during sleep. This is the lesson for all who observe and analyze the craniofacial skeleton in patients with obstructive sleep apnea.

References

1. Hudgel DW, Suratt PM. The human airway during sleep. In: Saunders NA, Sullivan CE, eds. Sleep and Breathing, 2d ed. New York: Marcel Dekker, 1994: 191–208.
2. Moss ML. The primary role of functional matrices in facial growth. Am J Orthod 1969; 55:566.
3. Enlow DH. Facial Growth, 3d ed. Philadelphia: Saunders, 1990.
4. Shprintzen RJ, Croft C, Berkman MD. Pharyngeal hypoplasia in Treacher Collins syndrome. Arch Otolaryngol 1979; 105:127–131.
5. Cole P. The Respiratory Role of the Upper Airways. St. Louis: Mosby–Year Book, 1993.
6. Gryczynska D, Powajbo K, Zakrzewaka A. The influence of tonsillectomy on obstructive sleep apnea children with malocclusion. Int J Pediatr Otorhinololaryngol 1995; 32: 225–228.

7. Kahn A, Blum D, Hoffman A, Hamoir M, Moulin D, Spehl M. Obstructive sleep apnea induced by a parapharyngeal cystic hygroma in an infant. Sleep 1985; 8(4):363–366.
8. Fedok FG, Houck JR, Maunders EK. Suction-assisted lipectomy in the management of obstructive sleep apnea. Arch Otolaryngol Head Neck Surg 1990; 116:968–970.
9. Ferguson KA, Ono T, Lowe AA, Ryan CF, Fleetham JA. The relationships between obesity and craniofacial structure in obstructive sleep apnea. Chest 1995; 108(2): 375–381.
10. Ferraro NF. Dental and oral maxillofacial evaluation and treatment in Apert syndrome. In: Upton J, Zuker RM, eds. Clinics in Plastic Surgery. Apert Syndrome. Philadelphia: Saunders, 1991: 291–307.
11. Goldberg JS, Enlow DH, Whitaker LA, Zins JE, Kurihara S. Some anatomical characteristics in several craniofacial syndromes. J Oral Surg 1981; 39:489–498.
12. Gibson SE, Myer CM III, Strife JL, O'Connor DM. Sleep fluoroscopy for localization of upper airway obstruction in children. Ann Otol Rhinol Laryngol 1996; 105(9):678–683.
13. Ward SL, Marcus CL. Obstructive sleep apnea in infants and young children. J Clin Neurophysiol 1996; 13(3):198–207.
14. Cistulli PA, Richard GN, Palmisano RG, Unger G, Berthorn-Jones M, Sullivan CE. Influence of maxillary constriction on nasal resistance and sleep apnea severity in patients with Marfan's syndrome. Chest 1996; 110(5):1184–1188.
15. Jamieson A, Guilleminault C, Partinen M, Quera-Salva MA. Obstructive sleep apnea patients have craniomandibular abnormalities. Sleep 1986; 9:469–477.
16. Peterson-Falzone SJ, Pruzansky S, Parris PJ, Laffer JL. Nasopharyngeal dysmorphology in the syndromes of Apert and Crouzon. Cleft Palate J 1981; 18(4):237–250.
17. Stein berg B, Fraser B. The cranial base in obstructive sleep apnea. J Oral Maxillofac Surg. 1995; 53(10):1150–1154.
18. Josephson GD, Levine J, Cutting CB. Septoplasty for obstructive sleep apnea in infants after cleft lip repair. Cleft Palate Craniofac J 1996; 33(6):473–476.
19. El-Sheikh MM, Medra AM, Warda MH. Bird face deformity secondary to bilateral temporomandibular joint ankylosis. J Craniomaxillofac Surg 1996; 24(3):96–103.
20. Deegan PC, McGlone B, McNicolas WT. Treatment of Robin sequence with nasal CPAP. J Laryngol Otol 1995; 109(4):328–330.
21. Caouette-Laberge L, Bayet B, Larosque Y. The Pierre Rubin sequence: review of 125 cases and evolution of treatment modalities. Plas Reconstr Surg 1993; 93(5):934–942.
22. Frohberg U, Naples RJ, Jones DL. Cephalometric comparison of characteristics in chronically snoring patients with and without sleep apnea syndrome. Oral Surg Oral Med Oral Pathol 1995; 80(1):28–33.
23. Hochban W, Brandenburg U. Morphology of the viscerocranium in obstructive sleep apnea syndrome—cephalometric evaluation of 400 patients. J Craniomaxillofac Surg 1994; 22:205–213.
24. Lowe AA, Santamaria JD, Fleetham JA, Price C. Facial morphology and obstructive sleep apnea. Am J Orthod Dentofac Orthop 1986; 90(6):484–491.
25. Miles PG, Vig PS, Weyant RJ, Forest TD, Rockette HE Jr. Craniofacial structure and obstructive sleep apnea syndrome—a qualitative analysis and meta analysis of the literature. Am J Orthod Dentofac Orthop 1996; 109(2):163–172.
26. Pracharktam N, Nelson S, Hans MG, Broadbent BH, Redline S, Rosenberg C, Strohl KP. Cephalometric assessment in obstructive sleep apnea. Am J Orthod Dentofac Orthop 1996; 109(4):410–419.

27. Riley RW, Powell NB, Guilleminault C. Current surgical concepts for treating obstructive sleep apnea syndrome. J Oral Maxillofac Surg 1987; 45:149–157.
28. Riley, RW, Powell NB, Guilleminault C. Obstructive sleep apnea and the hyoid: a revisesed surgical procedure. Head Neck Surg 1994; 111:717–721.
29. Miyamoto K, Ozbek MM, Lowe AA, Fleetham JA. Effect of body position on tongue posture in awake patients with obstrucive sleep apnoe. Thorax 1997; 52(3):255–259.
30. Cistulli PA, Sullivan CE. Pathophysiology of sleep apnea. In: Saunders NA, Sullivan CE, eds. Sleep and Breathing. 2d ed. New York: Marcel Dekker, 1994; 405–448.
31. Chaisrisookumporn N, Stella JP, Epker BN. Cephalometric profile evaluations in patients with cleft lip and palate. Oral Surg Oral Med Oral Pathol 1995; 80(2):137–144.
32. Lauritzen C, Lilja J, Jarlstedt J. Airway obstruction and sleep apnea in children with craniofacial anomalies. Plast Reconstr Surg 1986; 77(1):1–5.
33. DeLuke DM, Marchand A, Robles EC, Fox P. Facial growth and the need for orthognathic surgery after cleft palate repair: literature review and report of 28 cases. J Oral Maxillofac Surg 1997; 55:694–697.
34. Orr WC, Levine NS, Buchanan RT. Effect of cleft palate repair and pharyngeal flap surgery on upper airway obstruction during sleep. Plast Reconstruct Surg 1987; 80(2): 226–232.
35. Bettega G, Pepin JL, Levy P, Cheikhrouhou R, Raphael B. Surgical treatment of a patient with obstructive sleep apnea syndrome associated with temporomandibular joint destruction by rheumatoid arthritis. Plast Reconstruct Surg 1998; 101(4):1045–1050.
36. James D, Ma L. Mandibular reconstruction in children with obstructive sleep apnea due to micrognathia. Plast Reconstr Surg 1997; 100(5):1131–1138.
37. Perkins JA, Sie KCY, Milczuk H, Richardson MD. Airway management in children with craniofacial anomalies. Cleft Palate Craniofac J 1997; 34(2):135–139.
38. Sugahara T, Mori Y, Kawamoto T, Sakuda M. Obstructive sleep apnea associated with temporomandibular joint destruction by rheumatoid arthritis: report of case. J Oral Maxillofac Surg 52:876–880.
39. Castro Barbosa R, Aloe F, Travares S, Baptista Silva A. Mandibular-lingual repositioning device—MLRD: preliminary results of 8 patients with obstructive sleep apnea syndrome—OSAS. Rev Paul Med 1995; 113(3):888–894.
40. Schmidt-Nowara W, Lowe A, Weigand L, Cartwright R, Perez-Guerra F, Menn S. Oral appliances for the treatment of snoring and obstructive sleep apnea: a review. Sleep 1995; 18(6):501–510.
41. Schmitz JP, Bitonti DA, Lemke RR. Hyoid myotomy and suspension for obstructive sleep apnea syndrome. J Oral Maxillofac Surg 1996; 54:1339–1345.
42. Mixter RC, David DJ, Perloff WH, Green CG, Pauli RM, Popic PM. Obstructive sleep apnea in Apert's and Pfeiffer's syndromes: more than a craniofacial abnormality. Plast Reconstr Surg 1990; 86(3):457–463.
43. Sirois, Michel, Caouette-Laberge L, Spier S, Larocque Y, Egerszegi EP. Sleep apnea following a pharyngeal flap: a feared complication. Plast Reconstruct Surg 1994; 93(5): 943–958.
44. Witt PD, Marsh JL, Muntz HR, Marty-Grames L, Watchmaker GP. Acute obstructive sleep apnea as a complication of sphincter pharyngoplasty. Cleft Palate Craniofac J 1996; 33(3):183–189.
45. Ysunza A, Garcia-Velasco M, Garcia-Garcia M, Haro R, Valencia M. Obstructive sleep apnea secondary to surgery for velopharyngeal insufficiency. Cleft Palate Craniofac J 1993; 30(4):387–390.

Part Three

SLEEP DISORDERS

13

Development of the Human Circadian Cycle

RICHARD P. ALLEN

Johns Hopkins University
Baltimore, Maryland

I. Introduction

Ubiquitous in nature, biological rhythms for plants and animals follow our planet's 24-hr rotation into and out of sunlight. These daily or circadian rhythms extend across phyla far more than does sleep and waking, and they seem almost certain to considerably predate sleep and waking cycles in evolution (1). In this case, for humans, ontogeny initially follows phylogeny and evolution. Circadian rhythms develop early in utero (2,3) apparently before sleep-wake patterns, appear to weaken at birth, but eventually persist as a foundation for the development of sleep patterns. Recognizing this picture is critical to appreciating developmental issues for sleep and the sleep-wake problems of our children.

II. Basic Concepts and Measurements for Development of Circadian Rhythms in Humans

So basic is the circadian or daily biological rhythm that other rhythms are usually defined relative to this one as either ultradian (more than once a day) or infradian (less than once a day—e.g., seasonal rhythms). For mammals, the circadian rhythms are displayed and assessed at several levels, each with somewhat different forms. Core body temperature (CBT), the fundamental and widely accepted physiological measurements in humans and other mammals for circadian rhythms, reflects overall changes in metabolic activity. For humans, this shows abrupt large-magnitude changes on transition from active to inactive periods, with lower-magnitude changes during the active and inactive periods. This circadian temperature rhythm persists for at least several months and apparently indefinitely in humans, even when there are no available external clues for the time of day (temporal isolation) (4). The same is not true for sleep-wake or rest-activity cycles, which, after a few weeks in temporal isolation, may start to vary rapidly, depending on the expectations regarding sleep schedules (5). Thus, in conditions where humans live isolated from time, there must be an internal circadian pacer maintaining a daily temperature cycle that is closely but not completely linked to the sleep-wake cycle.

Since the circadian cycle, particularly for core body temperature, has been found to be both persistent without external cues and stable under a wide variety of external conditions, it seems certain that it is under primary control of a neurological pacemaker. Several studies have provided convincing evidence that this pacemaker is in the bilateral suprachiasmatic nuclei (SCN) in the anterior hypothalamus. These nuclei have been clearly identified and found to be both necessary (6,7) and sufficient (8) for maintaining circadian rhythms in the mammalian brain. Transplanting rat fetal tissue containing SCN cells into a rat with the SCN removed leads to an immediate restoration and resetting of the recipient animal's circadian rhythm to match that of the donor's (9,10). As noted below, the neurological development of the SCN pacemaker parallels the development of circadian rhythms except for the first few postnatal weeks.

The activity of the internal circadian pacer defines three distinct features of the daily cycle: 1) a *period* length, or length of the day for the internal clock, which should not be too different from 24 hr; 2) an *amplitude*, or degree of change over the daily cycle, usually measured by the difference between the high and low points of the cycle; and 3) the *phase* of the cycle in relation to external stimuli, such as the light-dark cycle. The phase is usually measured by the external "time" in the light-dark cycle when the low point or nadir of the internal cycle occurs. The phase must clearly be adjustable in order to permit east-west travel, but it has often been considered that both the amplitude and period length develop early in life and may change slightly with age but remain largely unaffected by external stimuli. This, however, is far too simple a picture. Rats' circadian period length is altered by the period length of prior light-dark training (11). Similarly, the basic length of the human circadian cycle varies with the environmental demands. When measured in temporal isolation conditions encouraging only long sleep episodes, the cycle is greater than 25 hr, but when sleep is encouraged at any time, including short episodes of sleep or "naps," the period length becomes only slightly longer than 24 hr (5). Thus, it seems likely that the developmental patterns for period and amplitude of circadian rhythms are at least somewhat affected by culturally imposed demands on the rest-activity cycle.

Behavioral circadian assessments usually rely upon some measurement of physical activity, such as an ambulatory meter recording the amount of activity at a human's wrist. These measurements in human adults show the rest-activity cycle in an almost square-wave form, with two states: active and rest. Compared to the differences between the states, there is relatively little change within a state, particularly during rest times. As noted below, this rest-activity pattern develops over the first few years of life. Other behavioral assessments, including human performance and cognitive tests, show a far more complicated picture of circadian rhythms with differing optimum performance times for differing types of learning or behavior (12,13). There is also some indication that children show similar differences in circadian patterns depending upon the task; some are better performed in the morning and others the afternoon. It has, therefore, become easy to dismiss gross motor activity assessment as a relatively trivial and inconsequential aspect of circadian rhythms, but the reverse seems more likely. The evolution of circadian rhythms involves the modulation of behavior to match energy conservation, environmental and cultural demands, and, for the child, developmental demands; hence the demand for significant circadian changes in gross activity levels.

Many hormones and other physiological substances show strong circadian variation with varying patterns. Some show pulsatile, rapid increases at certain phases of the circadian cycle (e.g., growth hormone release during early sleep), while others have more modulated variation (e.g., melatonin increases at night). Since sleep and waking generally follow the circadian cycle, it has not always been clear whether normal temporal patterns are controlled by sleep states or the circadian clock. Under conditions of temporal isolation, which is either prolonged or imposed on an abnormal sleep-wake schedule, adult sleep cycles break free from the usual relationship to the phase of the core body temperature (CBT) cycle (14). Growth hormone (15) and prolactin release then tend to primarily follow the sleep cycle (16), cortisol follows the circadian cycle (17), and thyroid-stimulating hormone appears to be significantly affected by both (18).

The expression of sleep itself is only partly under control of the body's circadian rhythm. There are, in effect, two somewhat independent factors determining expression of sleep: a homeostatic sleep drive and the circadian rhythm. In this two-process model, advanced by Borbély among others (19), the homeostatic drive for sleep increases in proportion to the duration of current wakefulness and decreases in proportion to the duration of sleep. The circadian cycle gates the sleep, probably primarily by increasing alertness during certain phases of the cycle and thereby creating times when sleep is difficult. This process in daily life and during development serves to organize the homeostatic expression of sleep into fixed times. Conversely, meeting the homeostatic needs permits waking and activity even during the rest or "down" phase of the circadian cycle, thereby modulating and in this case reducing the time spent inactive.

Finally, since the circadian rhythm adjusts its phase (time of rest or activity) to match changes in the environmental light-dark times, as occurs with east-west travel, there must be inputs from environmental cues indicating the external "time of day." These cues or zeitgebers (givers of time) include the timing of eating, social stimulation, and physical exercise. However, all of these effects are very small compared to the large effect of exposure to the zeitgeber of bright light. For some time, it was thought that humans were entrained to the 24-hr cycle by social cues and were less influenced by light, particularly given their extensive use of artificial lights at night (20). However, this theory failed to consider self-selection of lighting and the effects of bright light. The human circadian phase has been found to be very sensitive to bright light (> 6000 lux), particularly when it is as bright as sunlight about 30 min after sunrise (17,21). Lower levels of illumination have been found to suffice for entrainment of humans to a 24-hr cycle (22). In contrast, nonphotic entrainment, which has been shown to be not uncommon in some mammals, has been very rarely found in humans, even among blind adults, and has not been found at all in a small group of blind children (23). The affect of the light exposure is principally to adjust the phase of the circadian clock, but it may also affect the amplitude or intensity of the circadian rhythm.

The phase-setting effects of light are now fairly well understood. Both dosage and time of exposure alter the amount of change produced. The amount of light is determined by the light intensity on the eye and the duration of exposure. Thus, lower levels of light (bright room lighting level) over long periods may suffice for cycle entrainment, but higher intensities of light for shorter periods of time (≥ 6000 lux for 30 to 60 min) are more effective for acute phase shifts. The dose of light mainly affects the amount of change. The time at which the light exposure occurs has the stronger effect on amount of change and also affects the direction of change, giving a "phase-response curve" for light exposure. Light exposure in the evening and night time delays the circadian rhythm (supporting later bedtime and waking), while exposure in the early to late morning advances the rhythm (supporting earlier bedtime and waking). The amount of change increases in relation to how close the time is to the low point of the cycle (usually measured by the nadir of the CBT), but for brighter lights appears to have some effects at any time of the day, without the apparent "dead zone" of no response shown for nocturnal animals (24). Note that exposure to light in the hour before the nadir produces a large phase delay, while exposure in the hour after produces an equally large advance. This phase-response curve is characteristic of the functioning of the SCN which, as noted below, is probably functioning very early in development. Thus, these same effects of light are expected to operate throughout childhood, after the afferent pathways have developed adequately to provide inputs to the SCN. The exact nature of the needed inputs is, however, not entirely clear. It has long been assumed that the effects of light on the SCN are via visual stimuli using the retinohypothalamic tract, a direct neural pathway from the retina to the SCN. Disruption of this path in moles causes complete loss of SCN entrainment by light (25). This tract develops early in mammals, has been identified in a human newborn infant (26), and could be functional at birth. However, recent studies have shown that exposure of the back of the leg to blue light also produces a phase shifting of the circadian pacer for humans (27). The significance of this source of stimulation and the pathway for its effect on SCN are both unclear at this time.

III. Development of Circadian Sleep–Wake Rhythms

A. Fetal Rhythms

Table 1 presents a summary of the fetal development of the circadian system. The SCN has been shown to start developing in monkeys by at least 3 to 6 weeks of gestation (28). Data from humans have indicated that the SCN are apparent as discrete nuclei starting as early as 18 weeks of gestation, as shown by ^{125}I- melatonin binding to melatonin receptors in the hypothalamus (29). At about this time (20 to 22 weeks gestation), circadian cycles are clearly present in human fetal heart rate, movements and respiration (30), but these rhythms may be driven by the mother's cycles and not directly by the fetal circadian system (31). In the squirrel monkey, fetal SCN rhythms have, however, been shown to be consistent with entrainment to the external environment, indicating that phase could be set by external stimuli if they were available (2). Moreover, fetal circadian rhythms were reported to be absent in one case with anencephaly (32). It therefore seems likely that the fetal SCN directly controls these fetal rhythms. Similarly, for humans, the immature SCN of the fetus is likely to be driving the fetal circadian rhythms. However, without significant external stimuli, it

Table 1 Development of Circadian Sleep–Wake Cycles in Humans: Prenatal to Birth

Gestational age	Cycle characteristics	Significant features
3–6 weeks	Monkey suprachiasmatic nuclei neurogenesis.	Squirrel monkey, also likely for humans.
18 weeks	Human suprachiasmatic nuclei detected.	Melatonin labeling; likely present earlier, but not studied.
	Fetal circadian rhythms develop.	Heart rate, respiration, adrenal function linked to mother's cycle by melatonin, nutrients, etc. (circadian simulation aids development for premature infants).
End of gestation	Suprachiasmatic nuclei show internal circadian metabolic cycle.	Confirmed by studies in monkeys; unknown but assumed for humans.
Birth	Labor onset most likely during early morning.	Linked mostly to maternal cycle; may be influenced by fetal cycles.
	Most infant circadian phases match maternal phases.	Some infants are out of phase with their mothers, uncertain significance of this lack of synchrony.

Table 2 Development of Circadian Sleep–Wake Cycles in Humans: Postnatal to Young Adult

Postnatal age	Cycle characteristic	Significant features
1–2 weeks	Loss of most fetal circadian rhythms. No melatonin rhythm. Some entrainment to low-level lights. Human SCN not fully matured. No clear circadian pattern of activity. Multiultradian sleep-wake cycles.	Fetal heart rate, respiration cycles lost. No clear temperature cycle. Demonstrated for baboons and humans. Vasopressinergic neurons 13% of adult levels. Demonstrated for humans and baboons. Near random alteration of sleep-wake times, mostly sleep.
1–2 months	Circidian activity rhythm develops. Sleep begins to occur more at night.	Temperature nadir in early morning by week 4. Overall decreased activity during the dark/night period.
3–4 months	Sleep mostly at night (70% of children). Ultradian pattern stabilizes. Melatonin production clearly present.	One solid sleep period at night for 70% of children. Midday naps begin to develop—usually 2–3 naps. Melatonin rhythm appears, gradually increases to month 6.
3–6 months	Cortisol circadian pattern develops. Melatonin rhythm develops.	Strongly linked to temperature cycle. Human melatonin light-dark rhythm gradually increases.
6–8 months	Ultradian nap pattern is well developed.	Two to three primary nap times: morning, afternoon, and sometimes a third late-afternoon or early-evening nap.
1 year	SCN more fully developed. 90% of children sleep mostly at night.	Vasopressinergic neurons now close to adult levels. Two to three naps may persist, but midday nap begins to occur.
14–18 months	Ultradian patterns strengthens.	One midday nap develops.
3 years	SCN appears mostly developed. Ultradian pattern of sleep disappears.	VIP neurons reach adult levels. Night sleep becomes well established, with little nap time.
10 years	SCN gender differences develop. Circadian activity cycle well established.	Male vs. female SCN show twice number of VIP neurons. "Square wave" sleep/wake and rest/activity show abrupt changes from one state to the next. Adequate sleep in rest period, alert in active period.

Table 2 Continued

Postnatal age	Cycle characteristic	Significant features
12–16 years	Sleep cycle phase more delayed. Ultradian daytime sleepiness. Day sleepiness starts midpuberty.	Evening alertness, later bedtimes, trouble going to sleep. Difficulty waking; morning and afternoon sleepiness. Chronic insufficient sleep develops.
17–24 years	Sleep cycle phase less delayed. Ultradian sleep pattern developed. Short sleep times are self-selected.	Sleep onset times decrease. Afternoon sleepiness and evening alertness fully developed. Chronic insufficient sleep persists, often gets worse. Extending sleep to 9 to 10 hours restores wakefulness.

Key: SCN, suprachiasmatic nuclei; VIP, vasoactive intestinal peptide.

relies upon maternal signals for setting the circadian phase. If deprived of the maternal signals, it will lose its circadian pattern (33).

The zeitgebers for the fetus could be maternal cycles of melatonin, cortisol, dopamine, nutrients, or possibly maternal activity levels (3). Given the large number of glucocorticoid receptors present in early development of the SCN, maternal rhythms of corticotropin-releasing factor (CRF) and cortisol are likely to be significant for entrainment of the fetal SCN. Blocking maternal cortisol often eliminates some of the fetal circadian rhythms (33). The marked expression of melatonin receptors in the fetal SCN similarly suggests that melatonin also plays a critical role for fetal entrainment, as has been demonstrated for rodents (34,35). It has been further suggested that the circadian rhythm activation by the maternal cycle serves to contribute to fetal development. For preterm infants, an environment simulating aspects of the circadian rhythm, including a light-dark cycle, has been reported to enhance development (36,37).

Birth itself is under circadian control. The timing of births reaches its peak around 4 A.M. for normal, term, live-birth deliveries (38–40) but in the afternoon for stillbirths (41). It is probable that the maternal rhythm provides the circadian signal for timing the start of labor, although the interaction with the fetal rhythm may contribute, at least in other animals (42,43). At birth, the fetal and maternal rhythms are usually well synchronized (44), although this is not always the case for humans (45). There is no clear indication of any clinical significance to lack of synchrony.

B. Neonatal and Early Infant Rhythms

The development of circadian rhythms from birth to adulthood is summarized in Table 2. The development starts out with a striking, virtually complete loss of circadian rhythms immediately after birth for humans (46,47). The infant at birth has a fully functioning although immature SCN, with intact neural connections permitting both circadian rhythms and entrainment by light. Under special conditions, this can sometimes be observed in humans and can clearly be demonstrated experimentally in baboons (48,49). Moreover, prior to birth, the SCN appeared to drive several circadian fetal rhythms. It would now need to rely on an external zeitgeber, but even in the absence of a zeitgeber would be expected to maintain a free-running circadian cycle. Yet almost no circadian rhythm can be observed during the first couple of postnatal weeks. During this time, expressed cycles of sleep and waking have an extremely variable alternation between wake and sleep, sometimes referred to as having mixed ultradian rhythms. This is shown for activity measures for the development of one infant in Figure 1.

This loss of circadian rhythms is somewhat puzzling, especially since the neonate has an immature but intact SCN that sufficed before birth and since other mammals, such as sheep, maintain their rhythms from birth. It has been argued that this demonstrates that the fetal SCN was actually never controlling the fetal rhythms. However, this is not consistent with the experimental data noted above. It is also worth remembering that for a highly altricial (less developed at birth) species such as humans contrasted with precocial (more developed at birth) species such as sheep, rapid-eye-movement (REM) or active sleep strongly dominates the sleep time after birth (50,51). REM sleep may serve the developmental needs of the central nervous system for the very altricial human, which need may be particularly acute immediately after birth. The infant behaves almost as if it needed to wake up to eat and move around a little and then rapidly returns to REM sleep. We may have two competing systems, both supporting developmental demands, namely REM sleep and circadian rhythms, each relatively more important for development at different times. REM sleep is present from birth in a cycle of REM sleep and non–rapid-eye-movement (NREM) sleep of about 50 to 60 min (52). Transition between waking to sleep is often into REM sleep, and this cycling system appears to dominate over circadian rhythms. Immediately after birth, the strong developmental demand for REM sleep may simply overwhelm the expression of the circadian pacer, giving the resulting mixed ultradian pattern of bouts of sleep intermingled with brief awakenings (Fig. 1). However, as the REM sleep demands decrease over the first several weeks of life, the circadian system begins to express itself, with a resulting organization of the sleep patterns. Sleep becomes limited mainly to the nighttime, with a few shorter sleep periods or naps in the day, and there is a gradual development of the slower electroencephalographic (EEG) characteristics of NREM sleep. This gradual development of circadian rhythm of activity is shown in Figure 1 in the usual double-raster plot form (days i and i+1 both shown in line i for i=1 to *n* consecutive days).

Since the circadian patterns are poorly expressed during the first few days of life, it has been suggested that exposure to a 24-hr cycle of light with noise and night with relative quiet would assist the normal development of the circadian cycles, particularly for preterm infants who would normally be receiving temporal cues from

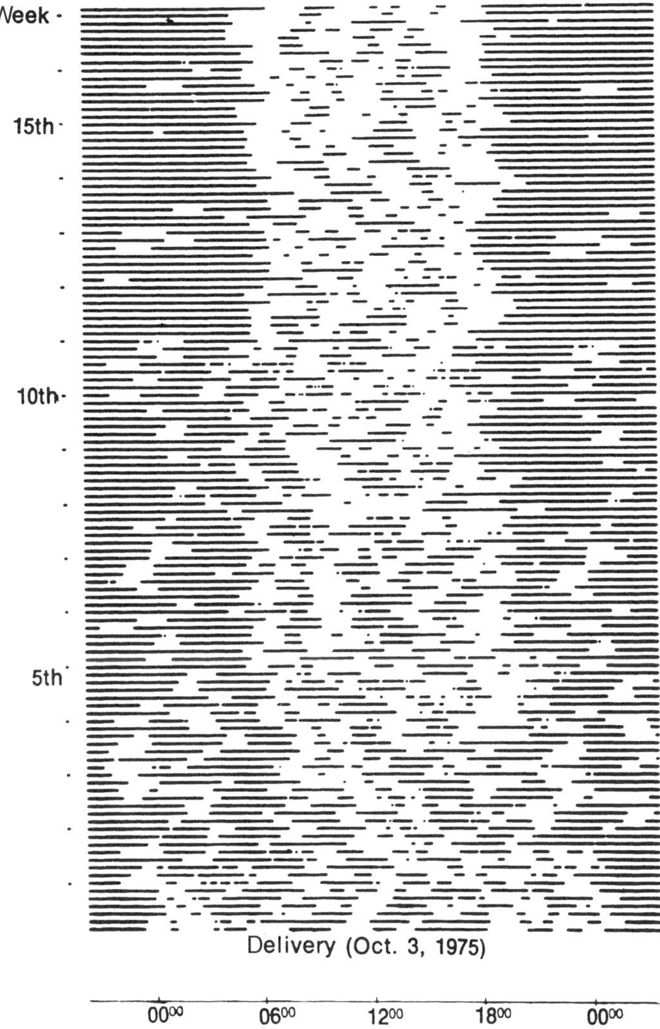

Figure 1 Double raster plot of sleep–wake patterns for one child from age 0 to 110 days, with dark bars indicating sleep. Sleep was judged by the amount of activity. (From Ref. 46.)

their mother. Studies have demonstrated that providing this type of cycle supports this development, at least for the preterm infant (36,37).

C. Infant to Adolescent Rhythms

By postnatal week 4, a body core-temperature cycle has clearly developed, with a nadir in the early morning hours (53). By the end of the second month, most infants will be sleeping more during the night than during the day, and temperature and some other circadian rhythms are likely to be seen. In the third month, most infants show circadian rhythms, with an ultradian pattern of naps reflecting daytime sleepiness. Similarly, by the end of month 3, about 70% of children will have established a 5-hr sleep period at night. Figure 1 shows the development of this pattern for one infant from birth to month 4. The sleep EEG has now developed a somewhat more characteristic slower EEG during NREM sleep. Further brain development is, however, required to provide the neural activity needed to generate the large amplitude, slow EEG characteristic of stage 3 and 4 sleep. During month 3, melatonin production during the night has been documented. It shows a gradual increase in amplitude of the cycle over at least the next 3 months (54). The cortisol circadian rhythm similarly begins to develop at about month 3 and is fully developed by month 6 (55,56).

The ultradian sleep pattern, once developed, is usually first multimodal. By month 3, it shows three main daytime wake periods, with naps in the morning and again in the afternoon. A third nap may also occur in the late afternoon or early evening. This slowly changes over the first 1 ½ years of life to a strong bimodal pattern, with one midday daytime nap. This is usually established by 14 months of age. Even at 12 months of age, there are often some early-evening sleep periods for the child. This development is shown in Figure 2. Generally, when the single midday naptimes develop, they occur earlier than the afternoon sleepiness experienced by adults (57).

The SCN is immature at birth, with only 13 to 20% of the adult levels of vasopressin neurons. These reach nearly adult levels by month 12 (40). Also by month 12, some 90% of infants will have a long (over 5-hr) uninterrupted sleep period at night. The vasoactive intestinal polypeptide (VIP) neurons in the SCN were found in one study to develop even later, usually reaching adult levels by about 3 years of age (58). It is also at about age 3 that the ultradian pattern, with one nap in the day, begins to weaken, slow-wave EEG sleep is fully developed, and the pronounced square-wave circadian pattern of activity begins to dominate. The 3-year-old child begins to be either fully awake or asleep with only, at most, very short periods when the child actually experiences sleepiness without going to sleep. Daytime napping usually disappears before age 6.

The prepubescent child's circadian patterns become well established by age 6 to 9, with marked differences between the somewhat long, deep sleep and the very alert, energetic daytime activities. There appears to be little indication for any ultradian cycle to sleep. If, however, prepubescent children are sleep-deprived, they will show the adult ultradian pattern of afternoon sleepiness with evening alertness. This is not generally experienced by prepubescent children, unlike adults, if they have their normal sleep at night (59). Clinical reports indicate that the phase adjustment of the circadian pattern is readily made by these children, who are apparently very responsive to light stimuli and have less difficulty than adults with adjustment after east-west airplane travel.

After about 10 years of life, the developing SCN shows the adult gender differences with about twice as many VIP neurons for boys than girls (40,58). The role

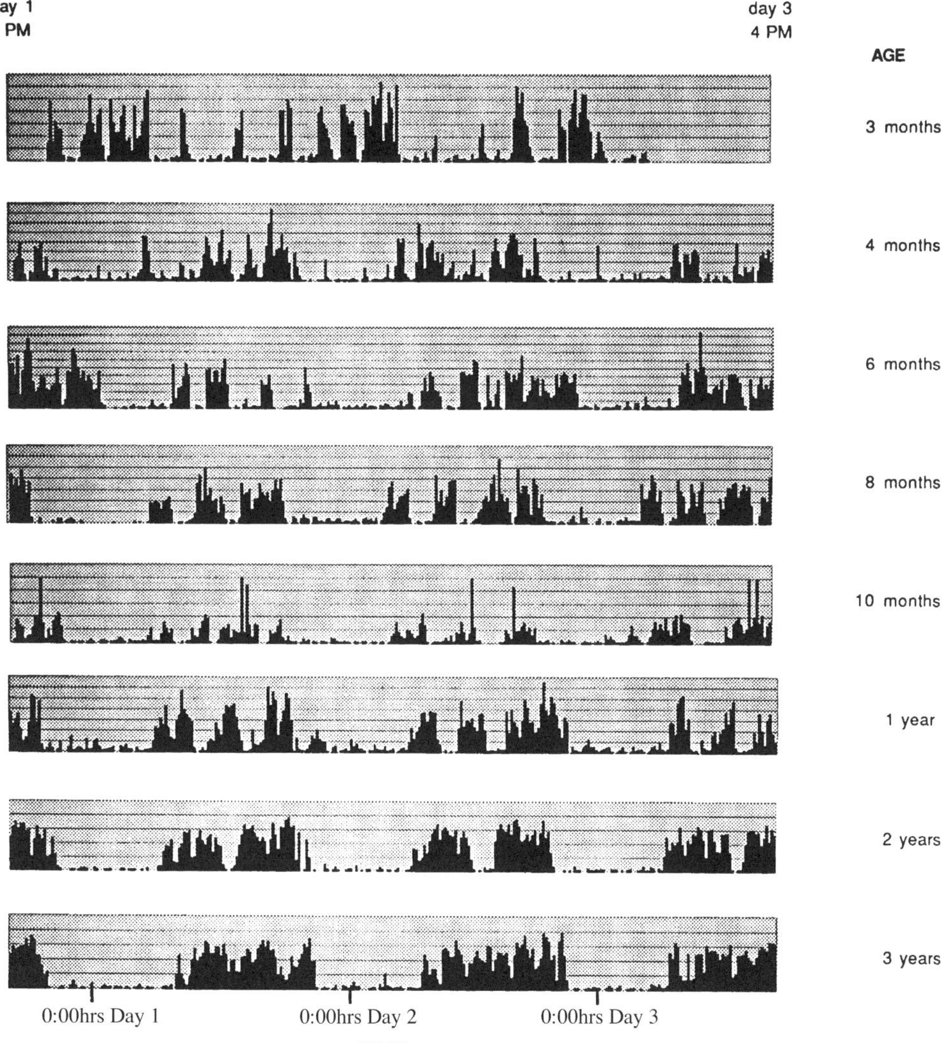

Figure 2 Development of a child's rest-activity cycles for selected ages from age 3 months through 3 years. Average activity is shown for each 15-min period over 3 consecutive days, starting from 4 P.M. Note the gradual development of stability for the nighttime sleep and gradual decrease in number of daytime naps. In particular, note 1) sleeping mostly at night occurs from month 4 but is more stable after month 6; 2) two to three naps each day persist through year 1; 3) one midday nap occurs at year 2; 4) no daytime napping at year 3.

of these neurons in SCN function is unclear. Unlike vasopressinergic neurons, they have not been tightly linked to circadian behaviors. These neurons may relate more to aspects of sex-linked behaviors than to specific circadian behaviors. It has, however, been noted by some that the problems with sleep-phase delay in adolescence discussed below are more pronounced for boys than girls. The adolescent problems with evening sleep onset and morning arousal, particularly when extreme (such as that occurring for adolescent school refusal) (60), have been reported clinically to be worse in boys. In these clinical cases, the obligatory nature of the evening circadian alertness, problems with entrainment, and decreased response to nonphotic entrainment cues may be greater for boys than girls. Other mammals show clear gender differences, with females showing more nonphotic entrainment. Relatively little is known about either the physiology or the gender issues that may be involved with the marked circadian changes the child experiences going through pubescence. Clearly, however, the SCN development of gender differences is occurring during this period of behavioral quiescence preceding the pubescent storm.

D. Adolescent Rhythms: From Pubescence to Young Adult

Several changes in circadian cycles appear to start during puberty. For sleep–wake states, the two most striking are the development of a sleep phase delay and the onset of increased daytime sleepiness, with a marked ultradian pattern of midafternoon sleepiness (61–63). To understand the psychological and psychosocial significance of these changes, it is important to note that they occur against a background of generally good prior sleep. Up to this point in life, the child has essentially not experienced sleepiness or difficulty falling asleep except under exceptional circumstances, e.g., Christmas Eve and jet travel. Now, within as little as 1 school year, as the body rapidly changes, the subjective experience of sleep also profoundly changes. The child experiences, probably for the first time, significant persistent episodes of daytime sleepiness while striving to stay awake. These remarkable but apparently normal developmental changes, and the behavioral adaptation they require, can be difficult for the family and society as well as the child.

The sleep phase delay can be particularly dramatic and cause the most difficulty for behavioral adaptation. The adolescent-preferred sleep phase becomes increasingly later, with preferred sleep times shifting to as late as 1 or 2 A.M. (64–66). There is a complicated debate about the degree to which this is a primary biological change related to the functioning of SCN versus a change secondary to psychosocial factors supporting staying up later at this age. The rapidity of the change was documented in one longitudinal study with Brazilian adolescents, where sleep patterns shifted later by about 30 min within a 6-month period. It is noteworthy that there were no significant social changes or changes in self-reported behavior patterns occurring during this 6-month period to account for this change in sleep phase. The consistency of this change across Western societies and for most adolescents and the rapidity of change in the background of a stable social environment support viewing the change as primarily biological (64–67).

The amount of subjective experience of sleep delay has been correlated with the Tanner scale for pubertal status, at least for females (62). Physiological studies have also demonstrated delayed temperature phase (68) in adolescence. More significantly, using a constant routine, Carskadon et al. (63) demonstrated that a delayed offset phase of melatonin significantly correlated with Tanner stage and age. This provides further support for a developmental delay in SCN phase occurring during pubescence. In an interesting study, 22 adolescent school-refusal patients showed a decreased circadian amplitude and even more marked core-temperature delay than was observed for healthy age-matched adolescents. An extreme degree of the normal delayed sleep phase appears to be a biological feature associated with the school-refusal disorder among adolescents (60).

Neither an obvious evolutionary value nor a relationship to other biological changes serves to provide a reasonable theoretical framework for understanding this change in the developmental context. This could, however, be an adverse consequence of other developmental changes occurring in the context of our social structure. For example, it may relate to the rapid decline in deeper stages of NREM sleep that occurs during this age. Prepubescent children have very deep NREM sleep, with abundant large-amplitude delta EEG and very high arousal thresholds. The sleep pattern shifts during adolescence to the young-adult sleep pattern, with decreased depth of sleep and lowered arousal thresholds during sleep. It could be argued from an evolutionary standpoint that the high arousal threshold during sleep, while advantageous for protected children, would be potentially disastrous for adults. Decreased arousal thresholds could contribute to decreased sleep length and, accordingly, the reappearance of an ultradian sleep cycle with a shorter sleep period in the afternoon complementing the period at night. One of the strong features of such an ultradian pattern is the evening alertness experienced by most adults after a low point in the afternoon. It is, in fact, this evening alertness that causes the most problems for adolescents. They report difficulty falling asleep in the early evening and therefore tend to delay the time for going to bed. It is noteworthy that the human intrinsic circadian rhythm measured in time isolation is lengthened by behavioral demands for one sleep period in a subjective day (5). Failure to take a nap may lengthen the sleep period and thereby contribute to a phase delay. The adolescent phase delay may be in part secondary to difficulty adjusting to the ultradian sleep pattern, particularly at an age where sleep needs appear to be greater than for adults. The problem is compounded by well- established cultural norms against napping and for early rising.

Whatever the basis for the sleep phase delay of adolescents and their experience of daytime sleepiness, it must be seen as a normal, pervasive feature of human development within Western culture. Adolescent behavior and the culture must adapt to respond to this change. It is striking that despite this strong normal developmental trend, our society has chosen to require early morning school attendance for these students. Curiously, as the child's sleep cycle shifts to later times, the school start times in the United States tend to be shifted to earlier times. School start times are often set earlier for adolescents than for the normal adult working day. School starting times for older adolescents between 7 and 7:30 A.M. are not uncommon. It is not clear that adolescents will or can adjust their sleep phase to match this environmental demand. Three surveys (64,67,69) involving schools with late (after 8:30 A.M.) versus early (before 7:30 A.M.) starting times showed that students went to bed on school nights at about the same time in both situations. The adolescents did not go to bed earlier to adjust for the earlier school starting time; they instead went to bed at about the same time and slept less. They reported an evening alertness that makes earlier bedtimes difficult. They did, however, end up sleeping longer on weekends, probably indicating increased sleep deprivation over the school weeks. Yet adolescents will sleep later if the school starts later, and thereby end up getting more sleep each night (Fig. 3). Overall, in a culture discouraging naps, the early-start school schedule effectively imposes significant chronic sleep deprivation on adolescents. There is only partial compensation by longer sleep on weekends.

The adolescent sleep phase should be responsive to the phase-shifting effects of lights, but this has not been well studied. In one study, adolescents with sleep-phase

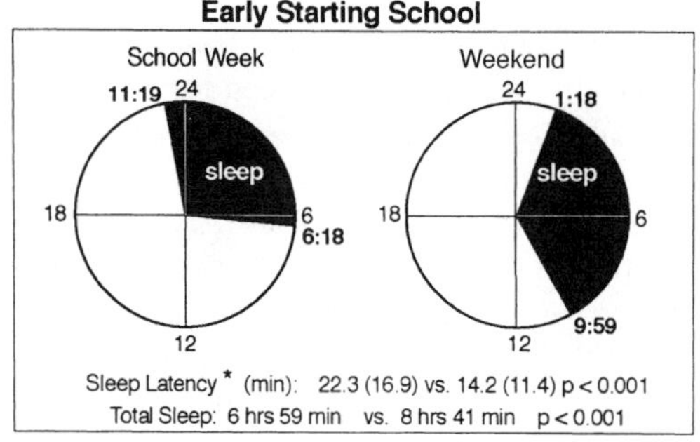

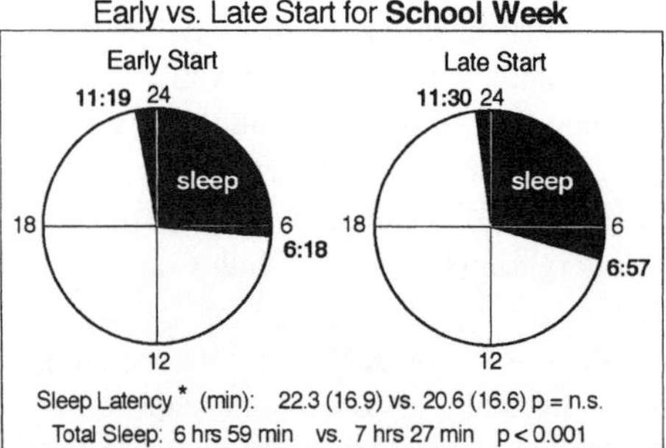

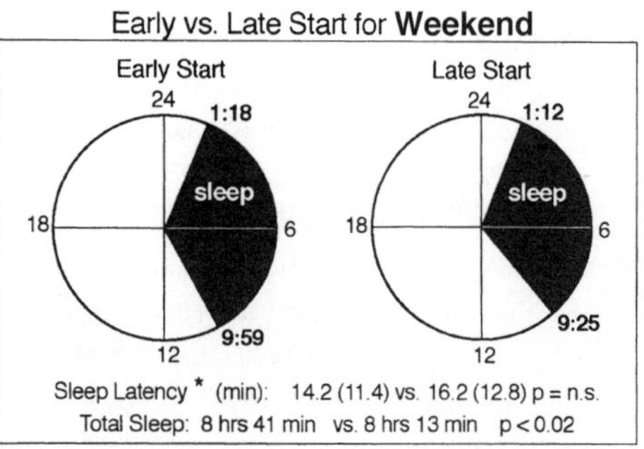

Figure 3 Sleep–wake patterns of adolescents in grades 11–12 during the school year for early-starting (7:20 A.M.) and late-starting (8:40 A.M.) schools. Note the longer sleep during the school week and shorter sleep during the weekend for the late- compared to the early-starting schools. Also note the consistency of the school week and weekend bedtimes. *Shown as: Average (standard deviation)

delay and a non-24-hr rhythm were treated with chronotherapy, a behavioral program of progressively delaying bedtimes until the times correspond to the desired sleep times. While the treatment worked, maintaining the new schedule required extra behavioral treatment and sometimes hypnotic use. Maintaining these patients on the new schedule was reported to be easier for adolescents than for adults with sleep phase delay, but no data were provided to support this clinical impression (70). The benefits of this treatment were maintained for over 1 year for 6 of the 10 adolescents studied (71). Thus, adolescents respond well to at least one of the phase-shifting approaches developed for use with adults. It seems likely that any phase-shifting approach to correct the developmental phase delay will, however, need to be used continually to prevent relapse to the apparent natural rhythm.

The sleepiness commonly reported by adolescents thus appears to have two interdependent developmental bases: first, sleep-phase delay at the time when schools are starting earlier, leading to chronic sleep loss and to morning sleepiness in school, and second, development of the adult ultradian sleep pattern with afternoon sleepiness and evening alertness. These are strong effects altering the life of the adolescent and his or her family.

E. Young Adult Circadian Cycles

Even the young, college-age adult expresses much of the adolescent sleep problem. It is not clear when the natural sleep phase advances to the usual adult pattern of bedtimes at 10 P.M. to 12 A.M., but it seems likely that there is a steady advance over the young adult life. Curiously, in our society, the young adults appear to elect to maintain a chronic, mild sleep deprivation similar to that imposed by the school schedule in adolescence. This seems likely to be a largely cultural issue for many but certainly not all young adults.

IV. Other Circadian Rhythms in Development

The emphasis in this chapter is upon the development of the basic circadian rhythm and its interaction with the sleep–wake cycle. There are, however, multiple other circadian rhythms important for medical care of children and for sleep-related illness. These include blood pressure, airway reactivity, glucose levels, urinary output, and urinary potassium (72). Several studies indicate the importance of these rhythms for management of medical conditions, including asthma and diabetes. There are also circadian rhythms of hormonal expression related to normal pubescent development (73,74). Most of these rhythms develop with their phase tightly linked to that of the SCN, either by direct control from the SCN or by close indirect action of the SCN on other physiological function such as sleep and waking. The more common disturbances of sleep related to problems resulting from these other rhythms include conditions arising with diabetes and asthma. For diabetic adolescents but possibly not normal children (75), there may be a "dawn phenomenon," with a rise in early morning glucose and increased demand for early morning insulin. This is associated with release of growth hormone (76,77) and could interact with sleep maintenance for adolescents who normally prefer to sleep late. There are circadian variations in lung function (78,79) and also significant circadian factors related to administration of drugs and, in particular, plasma levels of theophylline (80,81). Asthma-related disturbances of sleep are not uncommon, and the circadian factors need to be considered in planning treatment.

V. Summary

This chapter emphasizes the parallel development of the neurological circadian system and the behavioral sleep–wake/rest–activity cycle. The developmental patterns noted above for these conditions match at several interesting points and support a reasonable hypothesis about a causal relation between SCN and behavioral development. Loose temporal correlations do not, however, establish causation. The patterns of SCN development, nonetheless, provide a reasonable neurological framework for understanding the developmental changes in sleep–wake circadian cycles. Two developmental features that still do not seem to have an obvious neurophysiological basis are 1) the loss of circadian rhythm in the neonate and 2) the profound sleep phase delay in mid- to late adolescence. The theoretical models advanced above for these features have some rather limited support. They are advanced here as reasonable theoretical positions awaiting further evaluation. Nonetheless, clearly throughout childhood and adolescence, there is a strong developmental interplay between circadian rhythms and sleep. The study of sleep in children essentially always requires recognizing the significant impact of these interacting developmental changes, both for medical care and social planning.

References

1. Pittendrigh CS. Temporal organization: reflections of a Darwinian clock-watcher. Ann Rev Physiol 1993; 55:17–54.
2. Reppert SM, Schwartz WJ. Functional activity of the suprachiasmatic nuclei in the fetal primate. Neuroscience Lett 1984; 46:145–149.
3. Reppert SM. Pre-natal development of a hypothalamic biological clock. Prog Brain Res 1992; 93:119–131; discussion 132.
4. Moore-Ede MC, Czeisler CA, Richardson GS. Circadian timekeeping in health and disease. N Engl J Med 1983; 309:469–476, 530–536.
5. Campbell SS, Dawson D, Zulley J. When the human circadian system is caught napping: evidence for endogenous rhythms close to 24 hours. Sleep 1993; 16:638–640.
6. Moore RY, Eichler VB. Loss of circadian adrenal corticosterone rhythms following suprachiasmatic lesion in the rat. Brain Res 1972; 42:201–206.
7. Stephen FK, Zucker I. Circadian rhythms in drinking behavior and locomotor activity of rats are eliminated by hypothalamic lesions. Proc Natl Acad Sci USA 1972; 69:1583–1586.

8. Inouye ST, Kawamura H. Persistence of circadian rhythmicity in a mammalian hypothalamic "island" containing the suprachiasmatic nucleus. Proc Natl Acad Sci USA 1979; 76:5962–5966.
9. Ralph MR, Foster RG, Davis FC, Menaker M. Transplanted suprachiasmatic nucleus determines circadian period. Science 1990; 247:975–978.
10. DeCoursey PJ, Buggy J. Restoration of circadian locomotor activity in arrhythmic hamsters by fetal SCN transplants. Comp Endocrinol 1988; 7:49–54.
11. Richardson G. Circadian rhythms in mammals: formal properties and environmental influences. In: Kryger MH, Roth T, Dement WC, eds. Principles and Practice of Sleep Medicine. Philadelphia: Saunders, 1994: 277–285.
12. Folkard S, Monk TH. Circadian rhythms in human memory. Br J Psychol 1980 71:295–307.
13. Monk TH. Temporal effects in visual search. In: Clare JN, Sinclair MA, eds. Search and the Human Observer. London: Taylor & Francis, 1979: 30–39.
14. Czeisler CA, Weitzman ED, Moore-Ede MC, Zimmerman JC, Knaurer RS. Human sleep: its duration and organization depend on its circadian phase. Science 1980; 210:1264–1267.
15. Born J, Muth S, Fehm HL. The significance of sleep onset and slow wave sleep for nocturnal release of growth hormone (GH) and cortisol. Psychoneuroendocrinology 1988; 13:233–243.
16. Richardson GS, Lee RM, Sullivan JP. Diurnal variation in human neuroendocrine function. Trends Endocrinol Metab 1998;
17. Czeisler CA, Kronauer RE, Allan JS, Duffy JF, Jewett ME, Brown EN, Ronda JM. Bright light induction of strong (type 0) resetting of the human circadian pacemaker. Science 1989; 244:1328–1333.
18. Parker DC, Pekary AE, Hershman JM. Effect of 64-hour sleep deprivation on the circadian waveform of thyrotropin (TSH): further evidence of sleep-related inhibition of TSH release. J Clin Endocrinol Metab 1987; 64:157–161.
19. Borbély AA, Tobler I. Sleep regulation: relation to photoperiod, sleep duration, waking activity, and torpor. In: Buijs R et al., eds. Progress in Brain Research. Vol. III. Amsterdam: Elsevier, 1996.
20. Wever RA. The Circadian System of Man: Results of Experiments Under Temporal Isolation. New York: Springer-Verlag, 1979.
21. Czeisler CA, Allan JS, Strogatz SH. Bright light resets the human circadian pacemaker independent of the timing of the sleep–wake cycle. Science 1986; 233:667–671.
22. Boivin DB, Duffy JF, Kronauer RE, Czeisler CA. Dose–response relationships for resetting of human circadian clock by light. Nature 1996; 379:540–542.
23. Okawa M, Nanami T, Wada S, Shimizu T, Hishikawa Y, Sasaki H, Nagmine H, Takahashi K. Four congenitally blind children with circadian sleep–wake rhythm disorder. Sleep 1987; 10:101–110.
24. Jewett ME, Rimmer DW, Duffy JE, Klerman EB, Kronauer RE, Czeisler CA. Human circadian pacemaker is sensitive to light throughout subjective day without evidence of transients. Am Physiol Soc 1997; R1800–R1809.
25. Kass JH. Visual system: vision in blind mole rats. Nature 1993; 361:113.
26. Glotzbach SF, Sollars P, Pariagno RL. Development of the human retinohypothalamic tract (abstr). Soc Neurosci Abstr 1992; 18:857.
27. Campbell SS, Murphy PJ. Extraocular circadian phototransduction in humans. Science 1998; 279:396–399.

28. van Eerdenburg FJ, Rakic P. Early neurogenesis in the anterior hypothalamus of the rhesus monkey. Dev Brain Res 1994; 79:290–296.
29. Reppert SM, Weaver DR, Rivkees SA, Stopa EG. Putative melatonin receptors in a human biological clock. Science 1988; 242:78–81.
30. De Vries JIP, Visser GHA, Mulder EJH, Prechtl HFR. Diurnal and other variations in fetal movement and heart rate patterns at 20 to 22 weeks. Early Hum Dev 1987; 15:333–348.
31. Honnebier MBOM, Swaab DF, Mirmiran M. Diurnal rhythmicity during early human development. In: Reppert SM, ed. Development of Circadian Rhythmicity and Photoperiods in Mammals. Ithaca, NY: Perinatology, 1989: 221–244.
32. Mirmiran M, Lunshof S. Perinatal development of human circadian rhythms. Prog Brain Res 1996; 111:217–226.
33. Arduni D, Rizzo G, Parlati E, Dell-Acqua S, Romanini C, Mancuso S. Loss of circadian rhythms of fetal behavior in a totally adrenalectomized pregnant woman. Gynecol Obstet Invest 1987; 23:226–229.
34. Davis FC, Mannion J. Entrainment of hamster pup circadian rhythms by prenatal melatonin injections to the mother. Am J Physiol 1988; 24:R439–R448.
35. Davis FC. Melatonin: role in development (review). J Biol Rhythms 1997; 12(6): 498–508.
36. Fajardo B, Browning M, Fisher D, Paton J. Effect of nursery environment on state regulation in very low birth weight premature infants. Infant Behav Dev 1990; 13:287–303.
37. Mann NP, Haddow R, Stokes L, Goodley S, Rutter N. Effect of night and day on preterm infants in a newborn nursery: randomized trial. Br Med J 1986; 293:1265–1267.
38. Mirmiran M, Kok JH, Boer K, Wolf H. Perinatal development of human circadian rhythms: role of the foetal biological clock (review). Neurosci Biobehav Rev 1992; 16(3): 371–378.
39. Malek J. Der Einfluss des Ichtes und der Dunkelheit auf den klinischen Geburtsbeginn. Gynaecologia 1952; 138:401–405.
40. Swaab DF. Development of the human hypothalamus. Neurochem Res 1995; 20(5): 509–519.
41. DePorte JV. The prevalent hour of stillbirth. Am J Obstet Gynecol 1932; 23:31–37.
42. Umezaki H, Valenzuela GJ, Hess DL, Ducasy CA. Fetectomy alters maternal enocrine and uterine activity rhythms in rhesus macaques during late gestation. Am J Obstet Gynecol 1993; 169:1435–1441.
43. Germain AM, Valenzuela GJ, Ivankovic M, Ducsay CA, Gabella C, Serón-Ferré M. Relationship of circadian rhythms of uterine activity with term and preterm delivery. Am J Obstet Gynecol 1993; 168:1271–1277.
44. Reppert SM. Interaction between the circadian clocks of mother and fetus. Ciba Found Symp 1995; 183:198–207.
45. Parmelee AJ. A study of one infant from birth to eight months of age. Acta Paediatr Scand 1961; 50:160–170.
46. Meier-Koll A, Hall U, Hellwig U, Kott G, Meier-Koll V. A biological oscillator system and the development of sleep-waking behavior during early infancy. Chronobiologia 1978; 5:425–440.
47. Kleitman J, Engleman. Sleep characteristics of infants. J Appl Physiol 1953; 6:269–282.
48. Rivkees SA, Hoffman PL, Fortman J. Newborn primate infants are entrained by low intensity lighting. Proc Natl Acad Sci USA 1997; 94:292–297.
49. Rivkees SA. Developing circadian rhythmicity: basic and clinical aspects (review). Pediatr Clin N Am 1997; 44(2):467–487.

50. Seigel JM, Manger P, Nienhuis R, Fahringer HM, Pettigrew J. Monotremes and the evolution of RLS sleep. Phil Trans R Soc 1998; 353:1147–1157.
51. Zepelin H. Mammalian sleep. In: Kryger M, Roth T, Dement W, eds. Principles and Practice of Sleep Medicine. Philadelphia: Saunders, 1994.
52. Carskadon M, Dement W. Normal human sleep: An overview. In: Kryger M, Roth T, Dement W, eds. Principles and Practice of Sleep Medicine. Philadelphia: Saunders, 1994: 16–25.
53. Weinert D, Sitka U, Minors DS, Waterhouse JM. The development of circadian rhythmicity in neonates. Early Hum Dev 1994; 36:117–126.
54. Attanasio A, Borrelli P, Gupta D. Circadian rhythms in serum melatonin from infancy to adolescence. J Clin Endocrinol Metab 1985; 61:388–390.
55. Kennaway DJ, Stamp GE, Goble FC. Development of melatonin production in infants and the impact of prematurity. J Clin Endocrinol Metab 1992; 75:367–369.
56. Attanasio A, Rager K, Gupta D. Otogeny of circadian rhythmicity for melatonin, serotonin, and N-acetylserotonin in humans. J Pineal Res 1986; 3:251–256.
57. Ma G, Segawa M, Nomura Y, Kondo Y, Yanagitani M, Higurashi M. The development of sleep-wakefulness rhythm in normal. Tokoku J Exp Med 1993; 171(1):29–41.
58. Swaab DF, Zhiu JN, Ehlhart T, Hofman MA. Development of vasoactive intestinal polypeptide (VIP) neurons in the human suprachiasmatic nucleus (SCN) in relation to birth and sex. Dev Brain Res 1994; 79:249–259.
59. Carskadon MA, Dement WC. Multiple sleep latency tests during the constant routine. Sleep 1992; 15:396–399.
60. Tomoda A, Miike T, Yonamine K, Adachi K, Shiraishi S. Disturbed circadian core body temperature rhythm and sleep disturbance in school refusal children and adolescents. Biol Psychiatry 1997; 41(7):810–813.
61. Carskadon MA, Acebo C. Sleep in adolescents—puberty and delayed sleep phase. In: AUS-Sleep '92. Cairns, Australia: 1992.
62. Carskadon MA, Vieira C, Acebo C. Association between puberty and delayed phase preference. Sleep 1993; 16(3):258–262.
63. Carskadon MA, Acebo C, Richardson GS, Tate BA, Seifer R. An approach to studying circadian rhythms of adolescent humans. J Biol Rhythms 1997; 12(3):278–289.
64. Allen RP. School-week sleep lag: sleep problems with earlier starting of senior high schools. Sleep Res 1991; 20:198.
65. Allen R. School sleep lag is less but persists with a very late starting high school. Sleep Res 1995; 24:124.
66. Andrade MM, Benedito-Silva AA, Domenice S, Arnhold IJ, Menna-Barreto L. Sleep characteristics of adolescents: a longitudinal study. J Adolesc Health 1993; 14(5): 401–406.
67. Allen RP. Social factors associated with the amount of school week sleep lag for seniors in an early starting suburban high school. Sleep Res 1992; 21:114.
68. Andrade MM, Benedito-Silva AA, Menna-Barreto L. Correlations between morningness-eveningness character, sleep habits and temperature rhythm in adolescents. Brazil J Med Biol Res 1992; 25(8):835–839.
69. Kowalski NA, Allen RP. School sleep lag is less but persists with a very late starting high school. Sleep Res 1995; 24:124.
70. Ohta T, Iwata T, Kayukawa Y, Okada T. Daily activity and persistent sleep–wake schedule disorders. Prog Neuropsychopharmacol Biol Psychiatry 1992; 16(4):529–537.
71. Ando K, Hayakawa T, Ohta T, Kayukawa Y, Ito A, Iwata T, Okada T. Long-term follow-

up study of 10 adolescent patients with sleep–wake schedule disorders. Jpn J Psychiatry Neurol 1994; 48(1):37–41.

72. Haus R, Halberg E, Haus E, Halberg F, Haus A, Halcomb A, Cornelissen G. Circadian urinary characteristics of adolescents: sensitive dynamic indices complement mean values as new physiologic endpoints. Prog Clin Biol Res 1987; 227B:21–30.
73. Morales AJ, Holden JP, Murphy AA. Pediatric and adolescent gynecologic endocrinology. Curr Opin Obstet Gynecol 1992; 4(6):860–866.
74. Porcu E, Venturoli S, Magrini O, Bolzani R, Gabbi D, Paradisi R, Fabbri R, Flamigni C. Circadian variations of luteinizing hormone can have two different profiles in adolescent anovulation. J Clin Endocrinol Metab 1987; 65(3):488–493.
75. Marin G, Rose SR, Kibarian M, Barnes K, Cassorla F. Absence of dawn phenomenon in normal children and adolescents. Diabetes Care 1988; 11(5):393–396.
76. Edge JA, Matthews DR, Dunger DB. The dawn phenomenon is related to overnight growth hormone release in adolescent diabetics. Clin Endocrinol 1990; 33(6):729–737.
77. Arslanian S, Ohki Y, Becker DJ, Drash AL. Demonstration of a dawn phenomenon in normal adolescents. Horm Res 1990; 34(1):27–32.
78. Casale R, Natali G, Colantonio D, Pasqualetti P. Circadian rhythm of peak expiratory flow. Thorax 1992; 47(10):801–803.
79. Gaultier C, Reinberg A, Girard F. Circadian rhythms in lung resistance and dynamic lung compliance of healthy children: effects of two bronchodilators. Respir Physiol 1977; 31:169–182.
80. Arakawa H, Morikawa A, Shigeta M, Kato M, Kuroume T, Kimura T, Tateno. Plasma theophylline concentrations and airway function in asthmatic. J Asthma 1992; 29(4): 235–242.
81. Godfrey KR. Chronopharmacology and its application to the development of theophylline treatment schedules for asthma (review). Eur J Clin Pharmacol 1989; 36(2):103–109.

14

Disorders of Arousal

GERALD M. ROSEN

University of Minnesota and
Hennepin County Medical Center
Minneapolis, Minnesota

MARK W. MAHOWALD

Hennepin County Medical Center
Minneapolis, Minnesota

Disorders of arousal or partial arousals from sleep comprise a group of common sleep disorders that includes quiet sleepwalking, confusional arousals and sleep terrors that were first characterized as a distinct entity by Broughton in 1968 (1,2). The study of these disorders provides some unique insights into how we understand sleep and wakefulness. These problems are present at some time during the sleep of most children, although they are not always recognized (3–5). All disorders of arousal share a number of important characteristics, including timing in the nighttime sleep cycle, clinical features, genetics, and pathophysiology. Clinical features common to most children experiencing any type of partial arousal from sleep include misperception of and unresponsiveness to the environment, automatic behavior, a high arousal threshold, varying levels of autonomic arousal, and variable retrograde amnesia. Disorders of arousal typically begin abruptly at the transition out of the first period of slow-wave sleep [non–rapid-eye-movement (NREM) stage 4] (Fig. 1) of the night, which accounts for the typical timing 60 to 90 min after sleep onset, and generally terminate with the child's returning to sleep without ever fully awakening. The duration of each event can vary from a few minutes to over 90 min. Although only a single event usually occurs on a given night, some children may have more. When there are multiple events, they often recur at 60- to 90-min intervals during the first half of the night, corresponding to subsequent transitions out of slow-wave sleep (Fig. 1). Successive

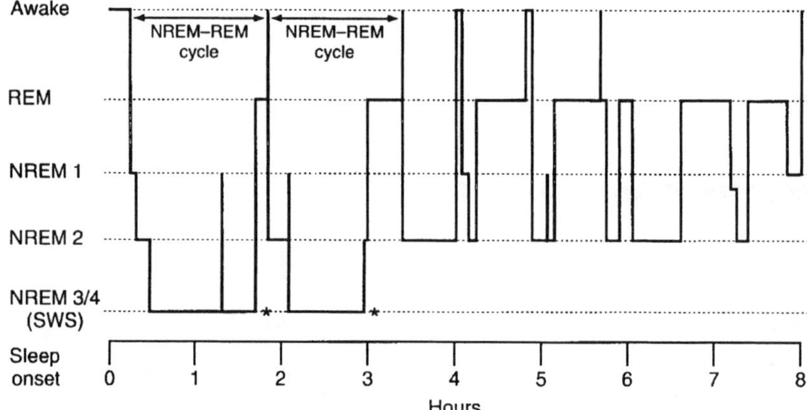

Figure 1 Idealized sleep hypnogram showing ultradian rhythm through the night. NREM-REM cycles are approximately 90 min; the majority of slow-wave sleep (SWS) occurs early in the sleep period; the majority of REM sleep occurs late in the sleep period. Disorders of arousal generally occur at the transition out of SWS (noted by asterisks). (Modified from Ref. 5.)

events on the same night tend to be progressively milder and may also occur in the second half of the night.

The clinical manifestations of disorders of arousal occur along a spectrum, but for ease of description, they have been divided into sleepwalking (calm or agitated), confusional arousals, and sleep terrors (Table 1) (4,5).

I. Clinical Manifestations

A. Sleepwalking

Calm

The stereotypical behavior of calm sleepwalking is fairly similar at all ages. The individual simply gets up and walks about calmly. The young child may walk or crawl about in the crib, but because he or she is quiet, these events often go unnoticed. An older child will usually get up and walk toward the light or parents' room. He or she will often be found simply standing in the living room or quietly next to the parents' bed. Some inappropriate behavior, such as urinating in the corner or next to the toilet, is common. Such a child may easily be led back to bed, perhaps with a stop at the bathroom, with little evidence of complete waking.

The older child may show similar behavior but may be more likely to walk about with his or her own agenda instead of following light, sound, and parents. Occasionally, the child may go to another room and return to sleep. Calm sleepwalking is not dangerous per se, but the child may put himself or herself in harm's way by climbing out a window or leaving the house.

Table 1 Clinical Characteristics of Disorders of Arousal

Clinical characteristics	Quiet sleepwalking	Confusional arousals	Sleep terrors
Usual timing during night	First third	First third	First third
Duration	1–10 min	5–40 min	1–5 min
Agitation	None/mild	Moderate	Marked
Autonomic arousal	None/mild	Moderate	Marked
Incidence	30%	15–30%	1%
Age of peak incidence	Middle childhood/ pre-adolescence	Infant/toddler/pre-school/ middle childhood	Adolescence
Amnesia	Yes	Yes	Yes
Arousal threshold	High	High	High
Family history	Common	Common	Common

Source: Modified from Ref. 5.

Sleepwalking is very common. In Klackenberg's (6) longitudinal study of a group of 212 randomly selected children from Stockholm aged 6 to 16 years, the incidence of quiet sleepwalking was 40%. The yearly prevalence varied from 6% to 17%, although only 2% to 3% had more than one episode per month. The sleepwalking persisted for 5 years in 33% of children and for over 10 years in 12%.

Agitated

Agitated sleepwalking is seen more frequently in older children; the child gets up and walks about in an upset and agitated fashion. There may be more speech, but it is often garbled and unintelligible. The child recoils when touched or held, and the degree of agitation may increase. He or she is more likely to bump into a dresser or otherwise sustain a minor injury than the calm sleepwalker, but even this is unlikely. This type of sleepwalking typically runs a course of a minute to a half-hour or so, after which the child calms and can easily be returned to bed, often without a complete awakening.

B. Confusional Arousals

Confusional arousals are often seen in infants, toddlers, and school-age children (4). These arousals may seem quite bizarre and frightening to observing parents. An arousal usually starts with some movements and moaning, progressing to crying and perhaps calling out, often in association with intense thrashing about in the bed or crib or simply crying inconsolably. Eyes may be open or closed. A look of terror is not described; rather, the child is felt to look very confused, agitated, upset, or "possessed." Like sleepwalking episodes, these can last anywhere from 1 to 2 min up to 30 to 40 min, with 5 to 15 min being typical. Even if the child calls for the parents, he or she often does not recognize them and may appear to "look right through" them. Holding and cuddling do not provide reassurance; instead, the child often resists, arches his or her back, twists, pushes away, and becomes progressively more agitated. Even vigorous attempts to wake the child may be unsuccessful.

C. Sleep Terrors

Sleep terrors are the most dramatic form of disorders of arousal and are uncommon in very young children; instead, they are seen more often in older children and young adults (7,21,22). Such events usually begin precipitously (not gradually, as do confusional events), with the child bolting upright with a "blood-curdling" scream. He or she may continue to cry and scream. The eyes are usually wide open, the heart is racing, and there often is diaphoresis and mydriasis. The facial expression is one of intense fear. In a full-blown episode, a youngster may jump out of bed and run blindly, as if away from some unseen threat. This may be very dangerous, as injury during this frenzied activity is quite possible. Anyone attempting to intervene may also be injured. These events are usually shorter than the confusional arousals, generally terminating within a few minutes. The child may wake before the autonomic storm has died down or may simply return to a quiet sleep without ever having completely awakened. The child may report some memory, but it is most often brief and fragmented, not characteristic of imagery reported from typical dreams or nightmares.

II. Physiology of Sleep

A review of the basic neurophysiology of sleep is helpful in understanding disorders of arousal. First and foremost, sleep must be understood as an active, complex, highly regulated neurological process that involves different neuronal groups at many levels of the neuraxis (8–14). Although the exact purpose of sleep is not fully understood, it is clear that sleep is essential, and that without normal sleep there will not be normal wakefulness. Sleep is composed of two fundamentally different states: rapid eye movement (REM) sleep and non–rapid-eye-movement (NREM) sleep, which share some obvious characteristics—such as posture, unresponsiveness to the environment, reversibility, and lack of consciousness—but have many fundamental differences. During REM sleep as opposed to NREM sleep there are very different patterns of brain blood flow, glucose utilization, predominant neurotransmitter systems, and thalamic functioning. From the perspective of brain function, REM and NREM sleep are as different from each other as each is from wakefulness. Thus, there are really three different states of being that humans can exist in, REM sleep, NREM sleep, and the waking state (10–12). State determination may be made using various criteria. Most commonly, electrographic criteria are used [electroencephalography (EEG), electrooculography (EOG), and chin electromyography (EMG)], as described in the sleep-stage scoring manual of Rechtschaffen and Kales (15). But behavioral criteria may

Table 2 Properties of Three States of Being

	Wake	NREM	REM
Behavioral/cognitive			
Movement	Frequent, voluntary	Infrequent, episodic, involuntary, gross movements	Inhibited; frequent, small brief twitches
Thought	Logical, progressive, remembered	Logical, progressive, not usually remembered	Illogical, bizarre, not remembered (unless awakened)
Sensation and perception	Vividly, externally generated	Dull or absent	Vivid, internally generated
Position	Variable, erect	Recumbent	Recumbent
Level of consciousness	+	−	−
Eyes	Open, moving	Closed, slow or not moving	Closed, moving
Electrographic			
Electroencephalogram	Desynchronized	Synchronized	Desynchronized
Eye movements	+	−	+
Muscle tone	++	+	−

Source: Modified from Ref. 13.

also be used to differentiate the waking state, NREM sleep, and REM sleep, as described in Table 2.

Each sleep state has its own unique neuroanatomical, neurophysiological, neurochemical, and neuropharmacological correlates. Each consists of a number of physiological markers that tend to occur in concert and cycle in a predictable and uniform manner, resulting in the behavioral appearance of a single prevailing state. There is compelling evidence that there is extensive reorganization of the central nervous system as it moves across states of being (11–14). Factors involved in state generation are complex and include a wide variety of neurotransmitters, neuromodulators, neurohormones, and a vast array of "sleep factors," which act upon the multiple neural networks (for review, see Refs. 13 and 14). These facts lead to the conclusion that sleep is a fundamental property of numerous neuronal groups rather than a phenomenon that requires the whole brain.

Consequently, it is possible for different parts of the brain to be in different "states" at the same time. The recognition of this possibility is fundamental to the understanding of a number of sleep disorders, including disorders of arousal, for if different parts of the brain can be in different states simultaneously, then the physical, clinical, and polysomnographic manifestations of these states (waking state, REM sleep, NREM sleep) can also occur simultaneously. When this occurs, the event can be described as a mixed or dissociated state (13,14).

III. Circadian and Ultradian Rhythms

Another fundamental concept important in understanding sleep is the recognition that sleep is not a static phenomenon. There are continuous currents driving and defining the propensity towards NREM sleep, REM sleep, and the waking state. The most apparent biological rhythms are the circadian and ultradian rhythms. The cyclic alternation of waking state, REM sleep, and NREM sleep over the 24-hr light/dark cycle defines the circadian rhythms, while the weaving of these three states over the sleep period defines the ultradian rhythm. Circadian cycling is controlled by a hypothalamic pacemaker located in the suprachiasmatic nucleus (SCN) (16). Virtually every aspect of mammalian life is affected by the circadian rhythm. Sleep/wake cycling is the most obvious manifestations of the circadian rhythm, but equally important are diurnal variations in body temperature, hormone secretion, drug metabolism, pulmonary function, immune response/reactivity, blood pressure, intestinal motility, gastric acid secretion, and the propensity to enter REM sleep.

The ultradian rhythm as shown in the idealized hypnogram in Fig. 1 is defined by the weaving of NREM sleep, REM sleep, and waking over the sleep period. No specific anatomical pacemaker has been identified that controls the ultradian cycling analogous to the SCN, although the brainstem appears to have an important role (12). As the brain cycles between NREM sleep, REM sleep and waking, a dynamic reorganization occurs among multiple neuronal networks and neurotransmitters at many levels of the neuraxis. A complex switching orchestrated in the midbrain and thalamus takes place (11). The transition among states usually occurs smoothly and completely and is behaviorally inapparent, but this is not always the case. The transition may be gradual and variable with the simultaneous appearance or rapid oscillation of multiple state markers, resulting in the behavioral appearance of a mixed state. This is the neurophysiological correlate of the clinical situation that is referred to as *state dissociation* (13,14). Narcolepsy, REM behavior disorder (RBD), and disorders of arousal can all be understood as clinical examples of mixed states of being or dissociated states.

IV. Clinical State Dissociations

State dissociation begins during embryogenesis. Prior to 24 weeks gestation, there are no clear-cut states; rather, there is an admixture of all states occurring simultaneously (17,18). After 24 weeks gestation there is a gradual coalescence of sleep states into active sleep (REM precursor), quiet sleep (NREM precursor), and waking, although a substantial portion of sleep is said to be indeterminate because there is evidence of quiet sleep and active sleep occurring simultaneously. In newborn infants this coalescence of state markers continues, but 25% of sleep is still described as indeterminate by 3 months of age (19).

Narcolepsy is the prototypical example of a clinical syndrome of state dissociation (13). The clinical tetrad of narcolepsy (cataplexy, hypnagogic hallucinations, sleep-onset paralysis, and sleepiness) can be understood as the intrusion of dissociated elements of REM sleep into wakefulness: cataplexy (sudden loss of muscle tone, usually in response to an emotionally laden event) representing REM atonia; hypnagogic hallucinations representing REM (dream) mentation; sleep-onset paralysis representing REM atonia at sleep onset; and excessive daytime sleepiness. REM behavior disorder (RBD) is another clear example of a clinical syndrome that is a direct result of state dissociation (13). RBD is a sleep disorder most commonly seen in older adult males and is the best-studied dissociated state arising from REM sleep. Normally during REM sleep, there is background atonia involving all somatic musculature (except the diaphragm and extraocular muscles). In RBD, the inhibition of muscle tone during REM sleep is lost. This leads to REM sleep dissociated from the muscle atonia, resulting in the literal "acting out" of one's dreams. In narcolepsy, the parent state is wake, and the symptoms can be explained by the dissociated intrusion of some or all of the elements of REM sleep into wakefulness. In RBD, the parent state is REM sleep, and the symptoms can be explained by the loss of one element of REM sleep, muscle atonia.

Disorders of arousal can also be understood as a dissociated state. During disorders of arousal, some facets of wake appear during the transition out of NREM slow-wave sleep. As a consequence, the transition out of NREM sleep that is normally smooth and behaviorally inapparent is dramatic and may be violent. The child appears caught between deep sleep and waking. The child's behavior has elements that we associate with waking (walking, talking, complex motor behaviors) and sleeping (misperception of and unresponsiveness to the environment, high arousal threshold, amnesia, automatic behavior) occurring simultaneously. The electroencephalogram (EEG) during a partial arousal from sleep is typically characterized by a combination of waking and sleeping rhythms with the simultaneous occurrence of alpha, theta, and delta frequencies (as illustrated in Fig. 2).

Many factors may affect the appearance of disorders of arousal; probably the most important of these is a genetic predisposition. A positive family history in a first-degree relative is present in 60% of children with disorders of arousal, compared to 30% in the general population (3). Sleep-state cycling and synchronization is another important factor, probably because disorders of arousal occur at the sleep-state transitions. Sleep-state cycling/synchronization is affected by age, sleep deprivation, circadian factors (shift work, travel across time zones), hormones, drugs, affective disorders, and environmental stress (posttraumatic stress disorder) (13). These factors may also play a role in the clinical appearance of disorders of arousal, particularly in a child who may have a genetic predisposition to such disorders. The association is most likely mediated through the effect these factors have on the duration, timing and intensity of NREM 4 sleep [slow-wave sleep (SWS)]. The intensity of SWS can be quantified using computer analysis of sleep (delta counts). Sleep deprivation, circadian factors, rise in body temperature, and some medications (lithium), which may increase the frequency and/or severity of disorders of arousal, also increase the intensity and/or duration of SWS. Factors that tend to decrease the intensity and duration of SWS—such as increasing age, sleep occurring during successive NREM sleep

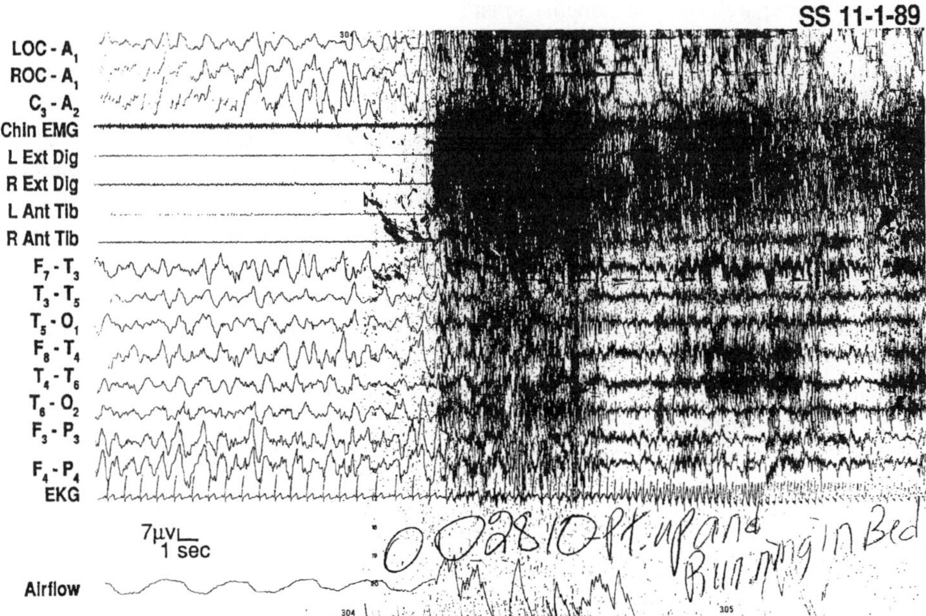

Figure 2 Polysomnogram of partial arousal. Arousal occurred suddenly out of slow-wave sleep. (From Ref. 5.)

periods of the night, and medication (benzodiazepines)—tend to decrease the appearance of disorders of arousal. It is less clear what mediates the effect that environmental stress and affective disorders have on disorders of arousal, although it is clear that in some individuals these factors are important (20).

V. Differential Diagnosis of Nocturnal Arousals

Disorders of arousal are among a number of causes of unusual nocturnal arousals. The differential diagnosis of children with unusual nocturnal awakenings also includes nocturnal seizures, nocturnal dissociative disorders, gastroesophageal reflux, obstructive sleep apnea, nocturnal panic disorder, REM behavior disorder, conditioned arousals, nightmares, posttraumatic stress disorder, and rhythmic movement disorders (5,21,22). The sorting out of these disorders requires a careful clinical sleep history, as described in Table 3, taken by a knowledgeable clinician. The sleep history will delineate the developmental, circadian, behavioral, psychiatric, pharmacologic, cardiorespiratory, neurological, gastrointestinal, and familial factors that affect sleep. The history, together with a physical and neurological examination, is often all that is required to evaluate children with unusual nocturnal arousals. If disorders of arousal are

Table 3 Sleep History

Circadian
- Sleep log for 2 weeks (times in bed, sleep onset, wake time) for weekday/weekend
- 24-hour daily schedule (school, work, meals, play)
- Amount of light in room
- Seasonal variations

Sleep environment
- Describe bedroom (What is in it? Who is there? How much natural light is there? Television? Radio?)

Sleep onset
- How does child fall asleep?
- Who is present at sleep onset and what do they do?
- Are there curtain calls, fears, hypnagogic hallucinations, sleep-onset paralysis, restless legs?
- Headbanging? Bodyrocking?

Arousals

Time of night	Frequency
Triggers	Associated with injury
Description of arousal	How it terminates
Level of agitation/ambulation	How does child return to sleep?
Associated with eating/drinking	Recall the next day
Level of consciousness	Age of onset
Duration	

Other sleep behavior
- Seizures, enuresis, diaphoresis, restlessness, snoring, cough, choking, apnea, periodic movements of sleep, vomiting, nightmares, bruxism

Waking behavior
- Hypnopompic hallucinations, paralysis, headaches

Daytime sleep
- Naps, cataplexy, excessive daytime sleepiness

Medical
- Neurological: Migraine headaches, attention-deficit disorder, seizures, tics, mental retardation, narcolepsy, neuromuscular disease
- Psychiatric: Depression, anxiety, dissociative disorders, conduct disorder, panic disorder, physical/sexual abuse, posttraumatic stress disorder
- Ear, nose, throat: Ear infections, ear effusions, nasal airway obstruction, sinusitis, streptococci infections, swallowing problems
- Cardiorespiratory: Asthma, cough, heart disease, pneumonia
- Gastrointestinal: Vomiting, diarrhea, constipation, swallowing problems
- Growth: Failure to thrive
- Allergies: Milk, seasonal, asthma, eczema
- Drugs: Legal/illegal
- School/behavior: Behavior problems, school/developmental problems
- Acute medical illness

Table 3 Continued

Family history
Sleep apnea/snoring
Arousals (sleepwalking, confusional arousals, night terrors, restless legs/periodic movements)
Psychiatric disease (depression)
Social issues (stress at home, divorce, family violence, drug/alcohol use)
Narcolepsy, hypersomnolence
Restless legs syndrome

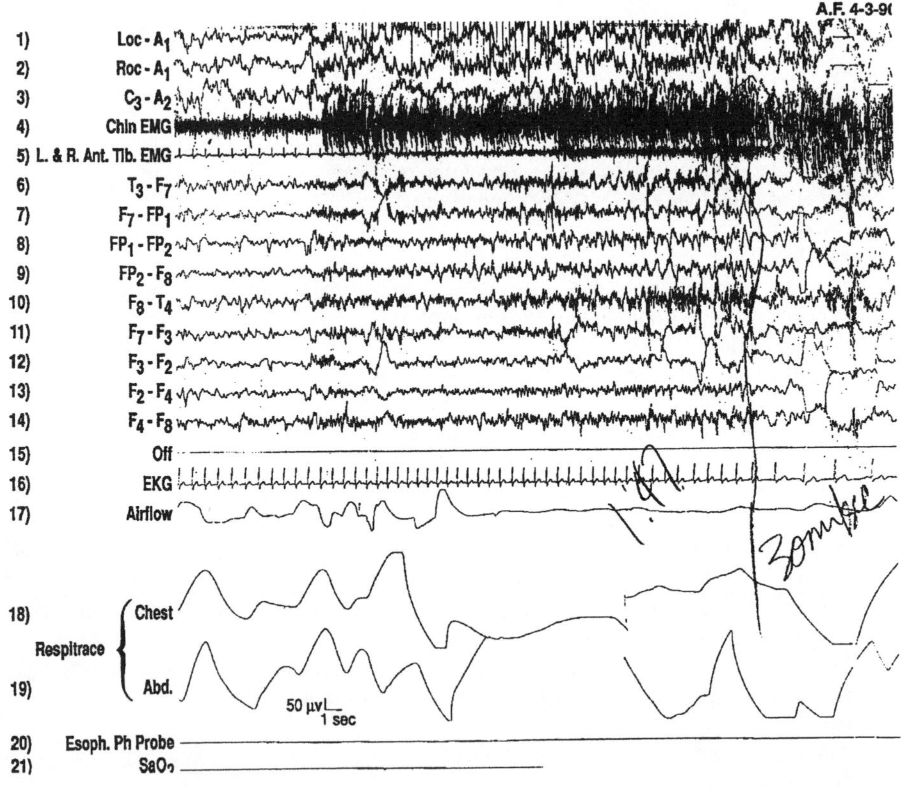

Figure 3 Two consecutive 20-sec epochs on a polysomnogram (A and B) capturing a nocturnal seizure. Note evidence on record of gastroesophageal reflux (drop in esophageal pH) and obstructive sleep apnea (paradoxical chest and abdominal wall movements with absence of airflow and oxyhemoglobin desaturation), both of which are epiphenomena of a nocturnal seizure. (From Ref. 5.)

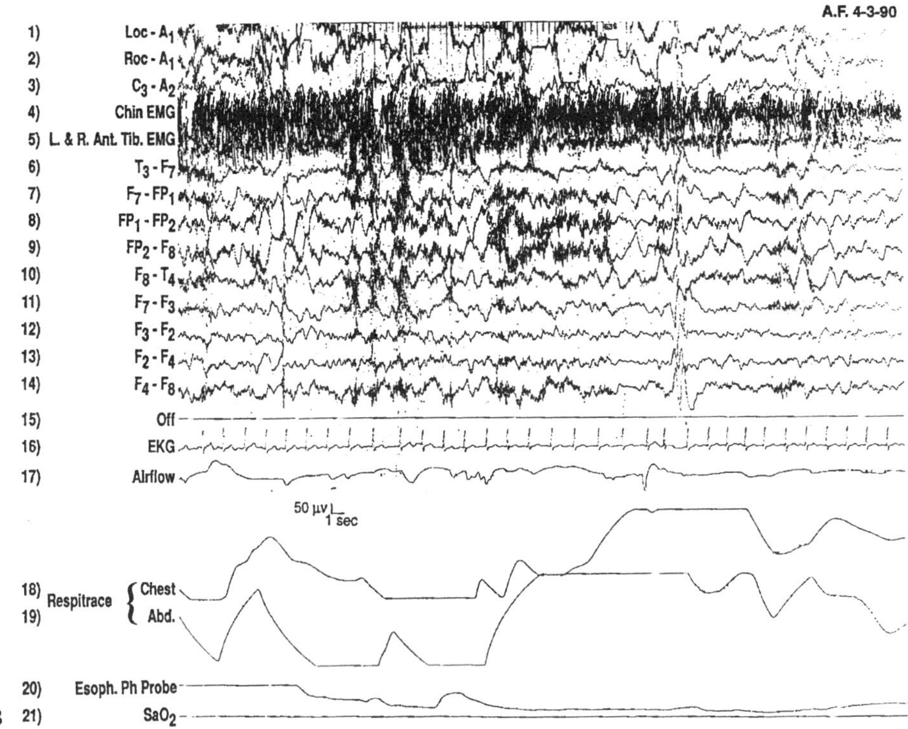

suspected as etiological, then no further diagnostic study is usually indicated unless the behaviors are potentially injurious or violent. Rather, the parent and child should be reassured as to the benign, self-limited nature of these problems; safety measures should be taken to ensure that the child does not put himself or herself in harm's way, and sleep extension should be tried either by getting the child to bed earlier or allowing him or her to sleep later. If significant psychological/psychiatric problems are uncovered, the family should be referred for appropriate evaluation and treatment, with the understanding that these problems may have only a coincidental association with the disorders of arousal.

In some cases further diagnostic studies are important in the evaluation of children with unusual nocturnal arousals. If nocturnal seizures are suspected because the arousals are stereotypical, arise throughout the sleep cycle, or occur upon awakening, a sleep-deprived EEG or video EEG may be diagnostic. A polysomnogram may be an important part of the evaluation of these children if one suspects that sleep-disordered breathing, gastroesophageal reflux, nocturnal dissociative disorder, nocturnal panic, or periodic movements of sleep are playing a role in the arousals. Nocturnal seizures may also be evaluated through polysomnography in centers where the expertise to interpret these complex studies exists. The polysomnogram with an expanded EEG montage at an increased paper speed provides the opportunity to simultaneously evaluate state (wake, REM, NREM) and whatever other physiological parameters are of clinical interest (EEG, esophageal pH, respiratory). This study often provides the necessary information to establish or refute a causal association between an unusual nocturnal arousal and a triggering event (as demonstrated in Figure 3).

To the casual observer, disorders of arousal represent a paradox during which an individual appears to engage in waking behavior while still asleep. With the understanding that sleep and wake are not always mutually exclusive states of being, the paradox disappears. The concept of mixed state or state dissociation provides an explanation for these events that is simple, reasonable, and founded on the current understanding of the neurophysiology of sleep.

References

1. Thorpy MJC, Diagnostic Classification Steering Committee. ICSD—International Classification of Sleep Disorders: Diagnostic and Coding Manual. Rochester, MN: American Sleep Disorders Association, 1990:142–150.
2. Broughton RJ. Sleep disorders: disorders of arousal? Science 1968; 159:1070–1078.
3. Richman N. Surveys of sleep disorders in children in a general population. In: Guilleminault C, ed. Sleep and Its Disorders in Children. New York: Raven Press, 1987: 115–127.
4. Rosen GM, Mahowald MW, Ferber R. Sleepwalking, confusional arousals and sleep terrors in the child. In: Ferber R, Kryger M, eds. The Principles and Practice of Sleep Medicine in the Child. Philadelphia: Saunders, 1995:99–106.
5. Rosen GM, Ferber R, Mahowald MW. Evaluation of parasomnias in children. Child Adolesc Psychiatr Clin North Am 1996; 5:601–616.
6. Klackenberg G. Somnambulism in childhood—prevalence, course and behavior correlates: a prospective longitudinal study (6–16 years). Acta Paediatr Scand 1982; 71: 495–499.
7. Demario FJ, Emergy ES. The natural history of night terrors. Clin Pediatr 1987; 26: 505–511.
8. Jones B. Basic mechanisms of sleep-wake states. In: Kryger MH, Roth R, Dement WC, eds. Principles and Practice of Sleep Medicine. Philadelphia: Saunders, 1994: 145–162.
9. Basics of sleep behavior. In: Chase M, McCarley R, Rechtschaffen A, Roth T, eds. Los Angeles: UCLA Sleep Research Society, 1993:17–78.
10. Hobson JA, Scheibel AB. The brainstem core: sensorimotor integration and behavioral state control. Neurosci Res Prog Bull 1980; 18.
11. Hobson JA, Steriade M. Neuronal basis of behavioral state control. In: Bloom FE, ed. Handbook of Physiology. Vol. 4, Sec. 1. Bethesda, MD: American Physiological Society, 1986:701–823.
12. Hobson JA, Lydic R, Baghdoyan HA. Evolving concepts of sleep cycle generation: from brain centers to neuronal populations. Behav Brain Sci 1986; 9:371–448.
13. Mahowald MW, Schenck CH. Status dissociatus—a perspective on states of being. Sleep 1991; 14:69–79.

14. Mahowald MW, Schenck CH. Dissociated states of wakefulness and sleep. Neurology 1992; 42:44–52.
15. Rechtschaffen A, Kales A. A Manual of Standardized Terminology: Techniques and Scoring System for Sleep Stages of Human Subjects. Los Angeles: UCLA Brain Information Service/Brain Research Institute, 1968.
16. Harrington ME, Rusak B, Mistlberger RE. Anatomy and physiology of the mammalian circadian system. In: Kryger MH, Roth T, Dement WC, eds. Principles and Practice of Sleep Medicine. Philadelphia: Saunders, 1994:286–300.
17. Corner MA. Sleep and the beginnings of behavior in the animal kingdom—studies in ultradian motility cycles in early life. Prog Neurobiol 1977; 8:279–295.
18. Corner MA. Maturation of sleep mechanism in the central nervous system. Exp Brain Res 1984; (suppl 8):50–66.
19. Anders TF, Sadeh A, Appareddy V. Normal sleep in neonates and children. In: Ferber R, Kryger M, eds. Principles and Practice of Sleep Medicine in the Child. Philadelphia: Saunders, 1995: 7–18.
20. Mahowald MW, Ettinger MG. Things that go bump in the night—the parasomnias revisited. J Clin Neurophysiol 1990; 7:119–143.
21. Mahowald MW, Schenck CH. NREM parasomnias. Neurol Clin 1996; 14:675–696.
22. Schenck CH, Mahowald MW. REM parasomnias. Neurol Clin 1996; 14:697–720.

15

A Developmental Perspective on Narcolepsy

SURESH KOTAGAL

Mayo Clinic
Rochester, Minnesota

I. Introduction

In 1880, Gelineau coined the term *narcolepsy* to describe a pathological condition characterized by recurrent brief attacks of sleepiness (1). He recognized that the disorder was accompanied by falls or "astasias" that were subsequently defined as cataplexy. Narcolepsy is a lifelong disorder characterized by the tetrad of sleepiness, cataplexy, hypnagogic hallucinations, and sleep paralysis. Vogel, in 1960, was the first to recognize the presence of sleep-onset rapid eye movement (REM) sleep in narcoleptics (2). The diagnostic criteria were subsequently refined by Rechtschaffen et al. in 1963 (3). This chapter addresses the epidemiology, pathophysiology, clinical features, diagnosis, and management of narcolepsy from a developmental perspective.

II. Epidemiology

The prevalence of narcolepsy has been estimated in Japan at 1 in 600 (4), in the United States between 1 in 1000 to 1 in 10,000 (5), and around 1 in 500,000 in Israel (6). The exact prevalence of childhood narcolepsy is, however, difficult to establish. Between 1957 and 1960, some 400 patients with narcolepsy were seen at the Mayo Clinic by Yoss and Daly (7). Of these, 15 (4%) were 15 years of age or younger. A recent metanalysis (8) of 235 patients derived from three series (9–11) in which the age of onset of symptoms was known reported that 34% of adults with narcolepsy had onset of their symptoms prior to the age of 15 years, 16% prior to age 10 years, and 4.5% prior to age 5 years. Cataplexy, the second major feature of the narcoleptic tetrad, is present only in 50 to 70% of patients (12). Some studies have required that cataplexy be present along with daytime sleepiness for the diagnosis (13), whereas others have not made this stipulation (14). From the epidemiological standpoint, this lack of uniformity in diagnostic criteria has led to disparities in estimating the prevalence (15), both in children as well as adults. It is also frequently difficult to elicit an accurate history of cataplexy in the preadolescent child. There is no specific sex, geographic, or socioeconomic predisposition.

III. Pathogenesis

Certain histocompatibility antigens (HLA), i.e., DRB1*1501 (DR2 subtype under the previous terminology) or DQB1*0602/DQA1*0102 (DQ1 subtype under the previous terminology)—are present in over 95% of subjects with narcolepsy as compared to 20% to 40% prevalence in the general population (16,17). In the black population, assessment for the HLA DQB1*0602/DQA1*0102 is more informative than studies for the DRB1*1501 antigen. The empirical risk for narcolepsy is 40.7 times greater among first-degree relatives than in the general population (18). While these studies affirm a genetic predisposition to narcolepsy and autosomal recessive/dominant as well as X-linked forms of transmission have all been considered, no consistent pattern of vertical transmission has been established. An interplay between genetics and environment seems central to the triggering of narcolepsy; major triggering life events like a personal illness/injury/bereavement have been present in close to 82% of narcoleptics as compared to about 44% of controls ($p < .0001$) (19).

The understanding of the pathogenesis of human narcolepsy has been advanced by the study of canine narcolepsy, which has been described in over 15 breeds of dogs and clearly has a single-gene autosomal recessive transmission (20,21). While no morphological abnormalities have been found in canine narcolepsy, dysfunction in the brainstem noradrenergic and cholinergic systems has been postulated (22). The noradrenergic system not only facilitates cortical arousal, but also inhibits cholinergic mechanisms, the disinhibition of which provokes cataplexy. Microinjection of carbachol into the pontine reticular formation of cats induces cataplectic behavior (23). Specifically, muscarinic type 2 cholinergic receptors have been implicated (22). Decreased activation of the noradrenergic system may lead to decreased cortical arousal as well as to activation of the REM sleep–generating cholinergic mechanisms. Cataplexy, hypnagogic hallucinations, and sleep paralysis are all REM sleep phenomena that begin to intrude onto wakefulness. Patients with narcolepsy do not need to sleep longer than unaffected peers, but do seem to have the need to fall asleep more often at any time of the day (24).

Montplaisir et al. measured the cerebrospinal fluid concentrations of several biogenic amines as well as their breakdown products: serotonin (metabolites 5-hydroxyindoleacteic acid, indoleacetic acid), dopamine (metabolite homovanillic acid), and norepinephrine in patients with narcolepsy, in those with idiopathic hypersomnia, and i normal controls (25). Both groups of sleep subjects (narcoleptics as well as idiopathic hypersomniacs) showed significantly decreased concentrations of dopamine and indoleacetic acid, a metabolite of tryptamine. Dopamine is usually present in high concentrations in the region of the basal ganglia, and its relative deficiency could also be involved in the pathogenesis of hypersomnia. The favorable response of hypersomnia to treatment with dopamine agonists like dextroamphetamine and methylphenidate also supports this hypothesis. Disrupted sleep from periodic leg movements is also fairly common in narcolepsy, and this has been postulated to have a dopaminergic basis, as treatment with levodopa seems to ameliorate symptoms.

IV. Clinical Features in Pre-School-Age Children

It is rare for pre-school-age children to manifest narcolepsy. Yoss and Daly observed (7) that 11.7% of their group of 85 narcolepsy patients were below the age of 5 years. Their series of patients, however, comes from an era in which polysomnographic criteria for the diagnosis of narcolepsy had not yet been established. In a more recent report, Nevsimalova et al. (26) describe a 2 ½-year-old child who developed narcolepsy-cataplexy symptoms at the age of 6 months, with presence of as many as 30 cataplectic attacks per day, that subsided after treatment with monochlorimipramine. A polygraphic recording showed REM sleep several minutes after sleep onset. The electroencephalogram (EEG) showed “discharges of slow waves with a high amplitude” as well as “episodes of spikes and spike-wave complexes.” In another two children, the authors observed a monosymptomatic form of periodic hypersomnia, with onset of symptoms at 6 months and 17 months that responded to treatment with monochlorimipramine. While the polygraphic tracings showed the typical manifestations of REM sleep in all three subjects during these events, there was a positive prenatal history, and the neurological findings suggested “early infantile cerebral palsy.” The validity of the diagnosis of narcolepsy is therefore questionable, as atonic seizures could not be ruled out. Cataplexy secondary to a prenatal/perinatal brainstem lesion may also have been a possibility. Also, daytime napping is a normal developmental feature at this age, and distinguishing physiological from pathological sleepiness is difficult.

The Multiple Sleep Latency Test (MSLT) is a test of degree of daytime sleepiness; it also assesses whether the transition from wakefulness is into REM/NREM sleep (27). Sleep latency is the time from "lights out" to sleep onset. Patients with narcolepsy show the pathognomic features of a shortened mean sleep latency and transition from wakefulness into REM sleep within 15 min of sleep onset during two or more nap opportunities of the MSLT. Based upon the currently available literature, the lower age limit for application of the MSLT norms seems to be 5 or 6 years (28–30). A combination of unequivocal, polysomnographically verified cataplexy and severe hypersomnolence may enable a tentative diagnosis of narcolepsy in this age group, but it should be verified with serial polysomnographic testing over the subsequent months or years.

V. Clinical Features in School-Age Children

The onset of *daytime sleepiness* from proven narcolepsy has been reported as early as 6 years of age by Lenn (29). His patient would fall asleep five to ten times a day. Wittig et al. described a boy 7 years and 5 months old with narcolepsy who tended to fall asleep while watching television for longer than half an hour, at the dinner table, and while seated in his mother's arms at a doctor's office (30). This sleepiness persisted despite sleeping 10 hr every night as well as taking two daily naps of 1 to 1 ½ hr duration. In general, it appears that daytime naps in children with narcolepsy are longer (60 to 90 min) than those of adult patients and are not necessarily followed by a refreshed feeling (31). These attacks of irresistible sleepiness are most likely to occur when the patient is carrying out sedentary activities. Sleep drunkenness may also be seen in the initial, developmental phases of narcolepsy. Automatic behavior, characterized by semipurposive behavior for which the patient is amnestic, occurs in about 80% of all subjects (32). Excessive daytime sleepiness may initially be overlooked by parents and teachers until it starts affecting behavior, attention span, and memory. Daytime sleepiness can also manifest itself as hyperactive behavior. It is not unusual for the child with narcolepsy to present to a pediatrician or pediatric neurologist for the evaluation of a presumed attention-deficit disorder.

Pollack et al. studied the circadian sleep-wake rhythms in subjects with narcolepsy who were isolated from their environmental rhythms (24). They found that the major sleep episode was still about 6 hr long and occurred about once every 24 hr, thus indicating that the circadian clock was functioning normally. Several other body rhythms (e.g., body temperature and cortisol) were also normal. Their work confirms that patients with narcolepsy tend to sleep more often, but not necessarily longer than individuals who do not have narcolepsy.

Cataplexy, the second most important feature of narcolepsy, is characterized by sudden muscular atonia of the extensor musculature triggered by emotions like fright, rage, or laughter. Consciousness is preserved during these attacks, which may last from 1 to 30 min. Extraocular muscles are generally not involved, but transient respiratory muscle weakness may lead to low-volume speech. However, prolonged apnea is not seen. In their metanalysis of 235 children with narcolepsy, Challamel et al. (8)

found that 80.5% of idiopathic narcolepsy patients and 95% of patients with symptomatic narcolepsy manifested cataplexy. While some case reports have noted cataplexy at the very onset in childhood narcolepsy (31), others have noted onset of this symptom to occur 10 or more years after the daytime sleepiness (11).

Sleep paralysis is characterized by a sudden, momentary inability to move the body. It may occur at sleep onset or upon arousal from REM sleep. Consciousness remains intact. The event may be terminated by calling or touching the patient.

Hypnagogic hallucinations are vivid and at times frightening experiences that also occur at the sleep-wake interface. They can be either auditory or visual in nature. The affective response is related to the inappropriateness of the situation in which the hallucinations occur (33). Like cataplexy and sleep paralysis, hypnagogic hallucinations also represent sleep–wake state dissociation and intrusion of fragments of REM sleep onto wakefulness.

Disturbed night sleep is common in childhood narcolepsy. Young and colleagues (34) attributed sleep fragmentation in children with narcolepsy in part to periodic leg movements, which were found in 5 of 8 (63%) of their subjects. They are defined as rhythmic leg muscle contractions of 0.5- to 5.0-sec duration with an interburst interval of 5 to 120 sec, occurring in series of three or more typically in stages I and II of NREM sleep. They may be associated with EEG evidence of arousal and sleep disruption. A sensation of restlessness may or may not accompany the leg jerks. Periodic leg movements could be related to altered dopamine metabolism, as they seem to be ameliorated by the administration of levodopa (35).

Neuropsychological and behavioral impairments are also common in children with narcolepsy, but have not been adequately evaluated. Rogers and Rosenberg carried out a battery of neuropsychological tests on 30 adults with narcolepsy, as well as 30 controls (36). The subjects with narcolepsy experienced more difficulty in maintaining attention than controls, as evidenced by more perseveration errors on Strub and Black's List of Letters. Similar data are unavailable in the pediatric age group. It is not unusual, however, for sleepy children to present with symptoms mimicking an attention-deficit disorder. Adults with narcolepsy have also been found to have selective cognitive deficits in response latency, word recall, and estimation of frequency (37). The investigators propose that a perceptual encoding deficit underlies the problems with memory and complex reaction time.

VI. Symptomatic Narcolepsy

This area has been reviewed in detail by Autret et al. (38). The majority of narcolepsy is idiopathic, but on rare occasions anatomical lesions of the brainstem may precipitate narcolepsy when there is a coexisting biological predisposition. Several forms of brain tumors, including hemangioblastoma (39), third ventricular glioma (40), temporal lobe B-cell lymphoma (41), and craniopharyngoma (42) have been associated with narcolepsy. Aldrich and Naylor (43) reported three patients who fulfilled the clinical and polysomnographic criteria for the diagnosis of narcolepsy. Their brain lesions consisted of a craniopharyngoma, a hypothalamic syndrome of unknown etiology, and obstructive hydrocephalus associated with a sarcoid granuloma in the region of the third ventricle. Only two of the three patients possessed the HLA DR2 antigen, suggesting that the DR2 antigen is not always necessary for the expression of narcolepsy. This author has observed a 10-year-old girl with cerebral palsy secondary to perinatal hypoxic ischemic encephalopathy who manifested daytime sleepiness in association with multiple daily episodes of cataplexy that were provoked by crying and excitement; protryptiline effectively eliminated the cataplexy. Secondary narcolepsy has also been reported following head trauma (44). Kandt et al. reported cataplexy in two patients with Niemann-Pick disease type C (45). These patients cannot be presumed to have narcolepsy, however, as they did not manifest other supportive clinical features. The mechanism(s) underlying the development of secondary narcolepsy are unclear, but may involve decreased activity of the pedunculopontine REM sleep–effector neurons, which might lead to pontine cholinergic supersensitivity and consequent cataplexy (46).

VII. Longitudinal Studies on the Development of Narcolepsy in Children

A key distinction between adults and children with narcolepsy is that adult patients usually present *following* the appearance of all or most of the clinical features, whereas children often present initially only with hypersomnolence and then demonstrate gradual evolution of the entire set of the characteristic clinical and polysomnographic features over months to years. It may also be difficult to elicit a reliable history of cataplexy, hypnagogic hallucinations, or sleep paralysis in a 5- to 6-year-old child. Also, normal values for total sleep time, sleep latency, REM latency, and sleep latency during daytime nap opportunities are constantly changing in the 5- to 15-year age range. Carskadon et al. showed that there was a linear relationship between increases in the Tanner stages of sexual development and increases in degree of daytime sleepiness in normal school-age children (28). In the initial stages, the sleepiness may be mild and the diagnosis can thus easily be overlooked. In a single but well-studied case, Carskadon et al. also reported on longitudinal changes in sleep-wake function during the course of evolution of narcolepsy in a child who had been born to a mother with narcolepsy (47) and who was being evaluated annually at the Stanford University Summer Sleep Camp. There were no sleep-wake complaints when the patient was seen initially at age 12.2 years (Tanner stage I) or at 13.2 years (Tanner stage II). By the age of 14.2 years (Tanner stage IV), however, the patient had begun to take one or two naps per day and to experience about one episode of cataplexy per month. Nighttime sleep measures were abnormal only for a shortened REM latency (time from sleep onset to the first epoch of REM sleep) of 61 min in year 1 (control 114 min), and 40 min in year 3 (control 101 min). The MSLT showed a gradual increase in the level of daytime sleepiness, documented by a corresponding reduction in the mean sleep latency, which fell from 14.1 min in Tanner stage I to 10.3 min in Tanner stage II and finally to 3.8 min in Tanner stage III. Sleep-onset REM periods were not seen during the MSLT in Tanner stages I or II but became apparent during five of six nap opportunities at Tanner stage III, thus becoming diagnostic of narcolepsy.

We recently evaluated the records of 10 children with proven narcolepsy who have been followed prospectively at our institution for pathological daytime sleepiness (48). There were seven boys and three girls. The mean age at onset of daytime sleepiness was 8.4 years (range, 6 to 11.5 years), and the age at the time of the initial sleep laboratory evaluation was 11.7 years (range, 7.8 to 16.8 years). The diagnosis of narcolepsy was based upon the presence of a shortened mean sleep latency of 10 min or less, and the presence of two or more sleep-onset REM periods on the MSLT. These diagnostic features were present on the initial battery of sleep studies only in 3 of 10 subjects. Of the remaining 7 subjects, 6 required a second battery of tests, and 1 a third battery of sleep studies before a definitive diagnosis of narcolepsy could be made. This underscores the need for obtaining serial nocturnal polysomnograms and MSLTs in children who are sleepy with no obvious explanation and in whom narcolepsy is a possibility.

VIII. Nocturnal Sleep in Childhood Narcolepsy

Fragmentation of sleep from an increased number of arousals and periodic leg movements is common in adults with narcolepsy; however, the features of the night sleep of children with narcolepsy have not been adequately evaluated. In a retrospective study (49), we evaluated the nocturnal polysomnographic features of 8 children with proven narcolepsy (Table 1). Their mean age was 11 years (range 6.7 to 16.1; 5 boys and 3 girls), and they were compared to 12 control children with nonnarcoleptic sleep disorders (mean age 8.1 years, range 5 to 12.5 years, 7 boys and 5 girls). The diagnosis of narcolepsy was established on the basis of presence of the characteristic clinical, nocturnal, and multiple sleep latency test findings. Of 8 subjects with narcolepsy, 6 had undergone serial (two or more) batteries of sleep studies in order to establish the diagnosis of narcolepsy. Results are reported only from the final (diagnostically definitive) battery of sleep studies for these 12 subjects. The diagnoses in the controls were epilepsy in 4, idiopathic hypersomnia in 4, idiopathic insomnia in 1, Prader-Willi syndrome in 1, periodic limb movement disorder in 1, and obesity-hypoventilation syndrome in 1. All nighttime polysomnographic data were recorded on a CNS SLEEPLAB system and scored in 30-sec epochs using the standard criteria of Rechtschaffen and Kales (50). There was no significant difference between the two groups with regard to nocturnal sleep latency, mean percentages of stages I, II, III+IV, SREM, sleep efficiency, or the periodic leg movement index. Patients with narcolepsy tended to have a significantly greater number of nocturnal awakenings of 2 min or more duration (mean 14.8, range 2 to 28, SD 11) as compared to controls (mean 7.3,

Table 1 A Study of Nocturnal Sleep in Childhood Narcolepsy Test Subjects

Patient	Sex	Age at symptom onset	Age at diagnosis	Clinical features	HLA profile
1.	Female	6.5	8.8	Daytime sleepiness with 60 to 90 min sleep attacks at school, cataplexy, hypnagogic hallucinations	DR6, DQW1
2.	Male	67	16.7	Daytime sleepiness	Not available
3.	Female	15	15.5	Daytime sleepiness, cataplexy	DR3+, DRw15+
4.	Male	13.8	15.1	Daytime sleepiness, cataplexy	DRw15-ve, DQw6-ve
5.	Female	8.6	9.6	Daytime sleepiness, cataplexy	DRw15+
6.	Male	9	9	Daytime sleepiness, cataplexy	DRw15+
7.	Male	13	13.3	Daytime sleepiness, cataplexy	DRw15+
8.	Male	4	11.5	Daytime sleepiness, cataplexy	DRw15+

range 1 to 15, SD 4.4, $p < .05$ on two-tailed t-test). Nocturnal REM latency in narcoleptic subjects was also significantly reduced (mean 24.5 min, range 0 to 66.5, SD 30) as compared to the controls (mean 143.7 min, range 82.5 to 230.5, SD 50.9, $p < .001$). Another interesting feature about these six narcoleptics with serial studies was that at the time the diagnosis of narcolepsy was equivocal [due to an insufficient number of sleep-onset REM sleep periods (SOREMPs) on the daytime MSLTs], the nocturnal REM latencies were also fairly long (mean 129.6 min, SD 61.1). But by the time they began to show the daytime diagnostic feature of two or more SOREMPs on the MSLT, the nocturnal REM latency had decreased markedly (mean 37.0 min, SD 58.7) (Fig. 1). Nocturnal REM latencies may also be abbreviated in children with depression (51), but are still much longer than those observed in children with narcolepsy. Decreased nocturnal REM latency thus appears to a reliable and fairly robust

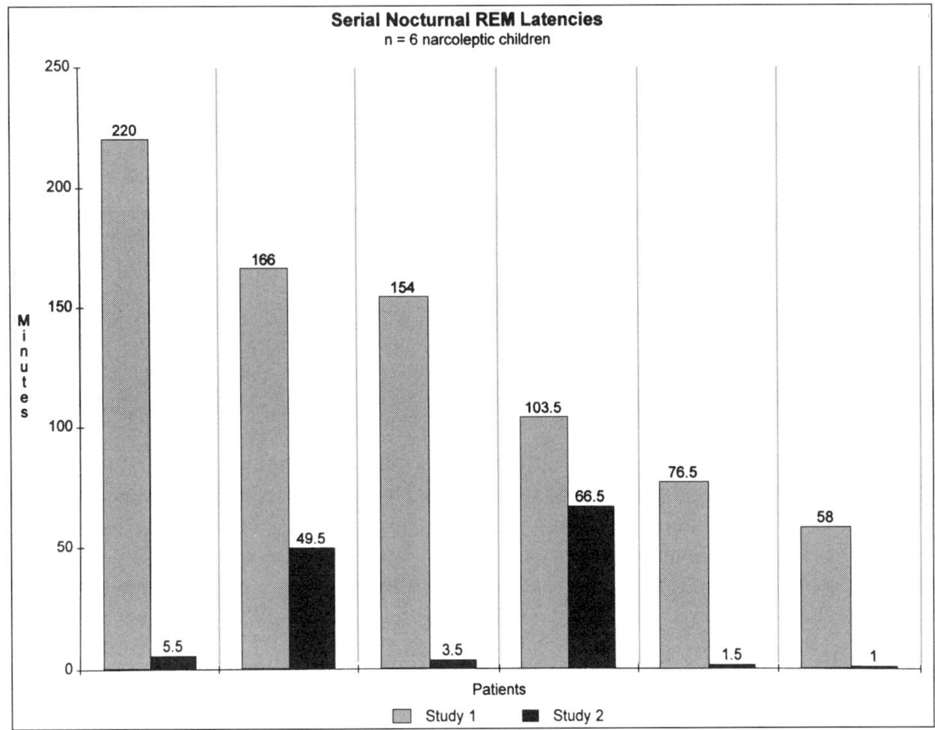

Figure 1 Nocturnal REM latencies in six children with narcolepsy who underwent serial polysomnograms. The light bars indicate nocturnal REM latencies when the diagnosis was uncertain; the solid black bars indicate nocturnal REM latency when the diagnosis of narcolepsy was firmly established.

polygraphic feature of childhood narcolepsy. A similar result was found in the met-analysis of 54 children with idiopathic narcolepsy by Challamel et al. (8). It is also corroborated by the earlier work of Carskadon (47).

IX. The Relationship Between Idiopathic Hypersomnia and Narcolepsy: A Developmental Perspective

The syndrome of idiopathic hypersomnia was initially described by Bedrich Roth and colleagues (52). The International Classification of Sleep Disorders (53) defines it as a disorder associated with nonimperative sleepiness, long unrefreshing naps, difficulty reaching full awakening after sleep, and sleep drunkenness, as well as absence of SOREMPs during the MSLT. Nocturnal polysomnographic recordings are qualitatively and quantitatively normal. The MSLT usually shows shortened mean sleep latencies in the 5- to 10-min range, but two or more SOREMPs suggestive of narcolepsy are not seen.

Six children with narcolepsy from our institution, who underwent serial nocturnal polysomnograms and MSLTs for the assessment of daytime sleepiness had daytime sleepiness as their main presenting symptom (31,49,54). Unrefreshing long naps were common. Even though the initial battery of sleep studies showed moderate daytime sleepiness in the form of shortened mean sleep latencies, they lacked the necessary (two or more) number of SOREMPs to be diagnosed as having narcolepsy. Initially, therefore, they met the diagnostic criteria for idiopathic hypersomnia. Repeat sleep studies several months later, however, showed that two or more SOREMPs, consistent with narcolepsy, had appeared.

Idiopathic hypersomnia was recently reviewed admirably by Bassetti and Aldrich (55). They report 42 subjects who were evaluated at the University of Michigan over a 10-year period. The hypersomnia began at a mean age of 19 ± 8 years (range 6 to 43). Diagnostic criteria were: daytime sleepiness for more than 1 year, mean sleep latency below 10 min, more than 1 SOREMP on the MSLT, apnea plus hypopnea index below 10, no improvement after a trial of increased night sleep time, and no other apparent cause for sleepiness. Almost half the subjects described restless sleep with frequent arousals. Habitual dreaming was present in about 40%. Only 7% were African American, as compared to 27% at their institution with narcolepsy. Habitual snoring was common (45%) but not any more frequent than in narcoleptics. They describe three subforms of idiopathic hypersomnia:

1. The classic form in which sleepiness is not overwhelming and there is a tendency to take long naps, prolonged nighttime sleep, and difficulty awakening.
2. The narcoleptic-like idiopathic hypersomnia, with overwhelming daytime sleepiness, a tendency to take short, refreshing naps, and awakening without difficulty; sleep attacks occur even while standing.
3. The "mixed" idiopathic hypersomnia, in which group the naps are brief but unrefreshing.

Bassetti and Aldrich also remark that there is substantial clinical overlap between idiopathic hypersomnia and narcolepsy. This has also been observed by other clinical investigators (56). Observations on our pediatric subjects fully support these observations and are the first to provide a developmental perspective on the relationship between idiopathic hypersomnia and narcolepsy. *They clearly indicate that in some children, idiopathic hypersomnia represents an initial transitional phase, en route to the development of classic narcolepsy, and that idiopathic hypersomnia and narcolepsy represent the two ends of a spectrum of a single central nervous system disorder of arousal.*

X. Diagnosis

The diagnosis of narcolepsy in childhood rests upon a combination of clinical and polysomnographic findings: the presence of cataplexy, hypnagogic hallucinations, or sleep paralysis along with daytime sleepiness is helpful, but during the early stages these features accompany daytime sleepiness only on an inconsistent basis. In preparation for nocturnal polysomnography, the patient should be withdrawn from all stimulants/psychotropic agents for at least 2 weeks. Long-acting selective serotonin reuptake agents such as fluoxetine can suppress REM sleep for as long as 4 weeks after discontinuation (author's personal experience). During this 2- to 4-week period, the patient is advised to maintain regular sleep-wake schedules. The patient then undergoes nocturnal polysomnography, consisting of monitoring of EEG, eye movements, chin and leg electromyogram, oronasal airflow, respiratory effort, oxygen saturation, and end-tidal carbon dioxide levels. The following day the patient undergoes an MSLT, with provision of four or five nap opportunities at 2-hourly intervals—e.g., at 1000, 1200, 1400, and 1600 hr. A urine drug screen is recommended prior to the MSLT in all adolescents. The patient's level of sexual development should be determined, as normal values for mean sleep latency at various ages are closely linked to the Tanner stages. The diagnosis of narcolepsy rests upon the polysomnographic exclusion of any other significant nocturnal sleep pathology that could lead to daytime sleepiness—e.g., obstructive sleep apnea—as well as upon documenting a short mean sleep latency of less than 5 to 7.5 min on the MSLT, combined with two or more SOREMPs. A repeat nocturnal polysomnogram and MSLT should be considered after some months whenever narcolepsy is suspected, but the polysomnographic features are equivocal. An HLA study for the DRB1*1501, DQA1*0102, and DQB1*0602 antigens provides supportive evidence, but negative studies do not exclude narcolepsy. Nocturnal polysomnography combined with MSLT is therefore still the "gold standard" diagnostic test.

XI. Differential Diagnosis

A detailed sleep-wake history combined with review of a 2- to 3-week-long sleep-wake log goes a long way in identifying the etiology of daytime sleepiness, which frequently presents itself under the guise of inattentiveness, distractibility, and academic/behavioral problems. By far the most common disorder leading to daytime sleepiness in children is *insufficient nocturnal sleep* (57). Teenagers are especially prone to go to bed late for chronobiological as well as environmental reasons and to be relatively sleep-deprived on school nights. Resolution of daytime sleepiness with provision of adequate nighttime sleep is diagnostic. *Delayed sleep-phase syndrome* is a circadian rhythm disorder characterized by a constitutional inability to advance sleep onset time, which can occur only at progressively later and later times at night, once again leading to relative sleep deprivation on most schooldays (58). When unrestricted, sleep is quantitatively and qualitatively normal. Sleep logs 2 to 3 weeks long are invaluable in establishing the diagnosis. The *use of prescription or over-the-counter drugs* (e.g., benzodiazepines, barbiturates, and antihistamines) is frequently overlooked, but is also an easily treatable cause of daytime sleepiness. It is not unusual for children with narcolepsy to present with mild obesity and nocturnal snoring, thus mimicking *obstructive sleep apnea* (OSA), which is most often related to adenotonsillar hypertrophy, craniofacial anomalies such as Down's syndrome, Crouzon syndrome, and neuromuscular disorders such as myotonic dystrophy (59). There is a history of habitual nocturnal snoring that is frequently interrupted by silent pauses (apnea), restless sleep, and bed wetting as well as daytime sleepiness. Nocturnal polysomnography shows frequent obstructive apneas, hypopneas, and oxygen desaturation as well as EEG evidence of sleep fragmentation. *The upper airway resistance syndrome* (UARS) is a form of sleep- disordered breathing that is frequently underrecognized. It can occur at all ages and is characterized by augmentation in the chin EMG activity during sleep in association with snoring and frequent EEG arousals. The clinical symptoms and configuration of the orofacial region are not helpful in distinguishing UARS from OSA; a marked increase in the intraesophageal negative pressure is the key diagnostic feature (60). *Illicit drug use*, especially alcohol, can lead to intermittent sleepiness. Teenagers can be very adept at camouflaging their consumption of alcohol. A high index of suspicion for drug abuse and obtaining a urine drug screen in the sleep laboratory immediately prior to initiating the MSLT is recommended.

The Kleine-Levin syndrome, or periodic hypersomnia, is characterized by recurrent periods of hypersomnia that typically occur weeks to months apart (61). The disorder is common in adolescents, who manifest 18 to 20 hr of sleep during the hypersomnolent periods in association with hyperphagia and hypersexual behavior. There may be a 2- to 5-kg increase in body weight during these periods of apparent binge eating. A monosymptomatic form has also been reported, in which the patient has hypersomnolence without associated hyperphagia and hypersexual behavior. Transient irritability, aggression, hyperactivity, and impulsiveness may be displayed during the sleepy periods. The disorder seems to gradually resolve over time. Nocturnal polysomnography shows a high sleep efficiency, but with decreased time spent in stages 3 and 4 of NREM sleep. The MSLT shows a short mean sleep latency and one or more SOREMPs. *Major depression* is characterized by apathy, mild daytime sleepiness and fatigue, and disturbed night sleep, with a propensity for early morning awakenings and a subsequent inability to fall back to sleep (62). Patients with bipolar disorder may have cycling between periods of depressed mood, normal mood, mania, or hypomania. Nocturnal REM latency is usually shortened (51), but not to the extent observed in narcolepsy. REM sleep may also be inverted, with the longest REM sleep period occurring in the initial third of night sleep rather than in the final third. The density of eye movements during REM sleep as well as the total percentage of time spent in REM sleep may also be increased (63).

XII. Management

Management consists of enhancing daytime alertness, controlling cataplexy, and providing emotional and psychological support. Patients and their families should be informed about the lifelong nature of the disorder. A combination of stimulant medications and planned daytime naps is modestly effective in enhancing alertness. The most common stimulants are pemoline sodium (Cylert) 37.5 to 112.5 mg in one to two divided doses, methylphenidate (Ritalin) 20 to 60 mg/day in two to three divided doses, dextroamphetamine (Dexedrine) 10 to 30 mg/day in one to two divided doses, and a mixture of amphetamine sulfate, amphetamine aspartate, and dextroamphetamine saccharate and sulfate (Adderall) 10 to 30 mg/day in one to two divided doses. These agents enhance catecholamine release from the presynaptic terminals. Mittler evaluated the efficacy of pemoline, methylphenidate, and dextroamphetamine in adults with narcolepsy as well as in age- matched control subjects by using the maintenance of wakefulness test as an objective measure of daytime alertness and the digit-symbol substitution test as a measure of neuropsychological function (64). None of the drugs improved the level of alertness of the narcoleptics above 81% of the controls, and this was seen only with 60 mg/day of methylphenidate. The side effects of stimulant drugs include anorexia and tics as well as difficulty in initiating night sleep. Modafinil, an $alpha_1$-postsynaptic agonist, also appears to be effective in alleviating daytime sleepiness. Billard et al. have studied its effectiveness in adult narcoleptics using a placebo-controlled double blind crossover design (65). Sleep logs indicated that the mean number of daytime naps fell from 1.30 (SD 1.41) on placebo to a mean of 0.95 (SD 0.82) on modafinil ($p = .05$). Data about its effectiveness in children with narcolepsy are thus far unavailable. The provision of one to two planned nap opportunities, each 20 to 30 min in duration (e.g., upon return home from school) also improves daytime alertness and works synergistically with stimulants.

Mild cases of cataplexy might not require any treatment at all. When it becomes more bothersome or socially disabling, however, clomipramine 25 to 100 mg/day in one to two divided doses, protryptiline 2.5 to 5 mg/day in one to two divided doses, or fluoxetine 10 to 20 mg/day can be used to control cataplexy. Clomipramine seems to be the most effective.

The restless legs syndrome and disturbed night sleep may be seen in severe cases of narcolepsy and can be treated with clonazepam, 0.5 to 1.0 mg at bedtime, or gabapentin (Neurontin) 100 mg two or three times a day.

Supportive psychotherapy is needed to help the adolescent with narcolepsy cope with accepting the disorder, adapting to it, and making appropriate lifestyle changes. The Narcolepsy Network (Cincinnati) is a useful support group. It is important to counsel teenagers about avoiding driving and alcohol use. The REM-suppressant effect of alcohol is usually followed by a rebound increase in REM sleep, which exacerbates the patient's symptoms.

References

1. Gelineau J. De la narcolepsie. Gaz Hosp (Paris) 1880; 53:626–628.
2. Vogel G. Studies in the psychophysiology of dreams: III. The dream of narcolepsy. Arch Gen Psychiatry 1960; 3:421–428.
3. Rechtschaffen A, Wolpert EA, Dement WC, Mitchell SA, Fisher C. Nocturnal sleep of narcoleptics. Electroencephalogr Clin Neurophysiol 1963; 15:599–609.
4. Honda Y. Clinical features of narcolepsy: Japanese experiences. In: Honda Y, Juji T, eds. HLA in Narcolepsy. Berlin: Springer-Verlag, 1988: 24–57.
5. Dement WC, Carskadon M, Ley R. The prevalence of narcolepsy. Sleep Res 1973; 2:147.
6. Lavie P, Peled R. Narcolepsy is a rare disease in Israel. Sleep 1987; 10:608–609.
7. Yoss RE, Daly DD. Narcolepsy in children. Pediatrics 1960; 25:1025–1033.
8. Challamel M-J, Mazzola M-E, Nevsimalova S, Cannard C, Louis J, Revol M. Narcolepsy in children. Sleep 1994; 17(suppl 1):17–20.
9. Yoss R, Daly DD. Treatment of narcolepsy with Ritalin. Neurology 1959; 9:171–173.
10. Parkes JD, Baraister H, Harsden CF, Asselman P. Natural history, symptoms, and treatment of the narcoleptic syndrome. Acta Neurol Scand 1975; 52:337–353.
11. Passouant P, Billard M. The evolution of narcolepsy with age. In: Guilleminault C, Dement WC, Passouant P, eds. Narcolepsy. New York: Spectrum, 1976: 179–197.
12. Kotagal S. Narcolepsy in children. Semin Pediatr Neurol 1996; 3:36–43.
13. Matsuki K, Honda Y, Juji T. Diagnostic criteria for narcolepsy and HLA DR2 frequencies. Tissue Antigens 1987; 30:155–160.
14. ASDC (Association of Sleep Disorders Centers): Diagnostic classification of sleep and arousal disorders. Sleep Disorders Classification Committee, Chairman HP Roffwarg. Sleep 1979; 2:1–137.
15. Hublin C, Partinen M, Kaprio J, Kosenvuo M, Guilleminault C. Epidemiology of narcolepsy. Sleep 1994; 17(suppl 1):7–12.
16. Billiard M, Seignalet J, Besset A, Cadilhac J. HLA DR2 and narcolepsy. Sleep 1986; 9:149–152.
17. Langdon N, Lock C, Welsh K, Vergani D, Dorow R, Wachtel H, Palenschat D, Parkes JD. Immune factors in narcolepsy. Sleep 1986; 9:143–148.
18. Billiard M, Magnetto-Pasquie V, Heckman M, Carlander B, Besset A, Zachriev JF, Eliaou JF, Malafosse A. Family studies in narcolepsy. Sleep 1994; 17(suppl 1):54–59.
19. Orellana C, Villemin E, Tafti M, Carlander B, Besset A, Billard M. Life events in the year preceding the onset of narcolepsy. Sleep 1994; 17(suppl 1):50–53.
20. Mitler MM, Dement WC. Sleep studies on canine narcolepsy: pattern and cycle comparisons between affected and normal dogs. Electroencephalogr Clin Neurophysiol 1977; 43:691–699.

21. Foutz AS, Mitler MM, Cavalli-Sforza LL, Dement WC. Genetic factors in canine narcolepsy. Sleep 1979; 1:413–421.
22. Nishino S, Reid MS, Dement WC, Mignot E. Neuropharmacology and neurochemistry of narcolepsy. Sleep 1994; 17(suppl 1):S84–S92.
23. Mitler MM, Dement WC. Cataplectic-like behavior in cats after micro-injections of carbachol in the pontine reticular formation. Brain Res 1974; 68:335–343.
24. Pollack CP. The rhythms of narcolepsy. Network 1995; 8(2):1–7.
25. Montplaisir J, de Champlain J, Young SN, Missala K, Sourkes TL, Walsh J, Remillard G. Narcolepsy and idiopathic hypersomnia: biogenic and related compounds in CSF. Neurology 1982; 32:1299–1302.
26. Nevsimalova S, Roth B, Zouhar A, Zemanova H. Narkolepsie-kataplexie a periodicka hypersomnie se zacatkem v kojeneckem veku. Cs Pediatr 1986; 41(6):324–327.
27. Carskadon MA, Dement WC, Mitler MM, Roth T, Westbrook PR, Keenan S. Guidelines for the multiple sleep latency test (MSLT): a standard measure of sleepiness. Sleep 1986; 9:519–524.
28. Carskadon MA. The second decade. In: Sleeping and Waking Disorders: Indications and Techniques. Menlo Park: Addison-Wesley, 1982:99–125.
29. Lenn NJ. HLA-DR2 in childhood narcolepsy. Pediatr Neurol 1986; 2:314–315.
30. Wittig R, Zorick F, Roehrs T, Sichlesteel J, Roth T. Narcolepsy in a 7 year old. J Pediatr 1983; 102:725–727.
31. Kotagal S, Hartse KM, Walsh JK. Characteristics of narcolepsy in pre-teen aged children. Pediatrics 1990; 85:205–209.
32. Aldrich MS. Narcolepsy. N Engl J Med 1990; 323:389–394.
33. Zarcone V. Narcolepsy. N Engl J Med 1973; 288:1156–1166.
34. Young D, Zorick F, Cottig R, Roehrs T, Roth T. Narcolepsy in a pediatric population. Am J Dis Child 1988; 142:210–214.
35. Aldrich MS. The neurobiology of narcolepsy. Trends Neurosci 1991; 14:235–239.
36. Rogers AE, Rosenberg RS. Tests of memory in narcoleptics. Sleep 1990; 13:42–52.
37. Henry GK, Satz P, Heilbronner RL. Evidence of a perceptual encoding deficit in narcolepsy. Sleep 1993; 16:123–127.
38. Autret A, Lucas F, Henry-Lebras F, de Toffol B. Symptomatic narcolepsies. Sleep 1994; 17(suppl 1):21–24.
39. Tridon P, Montaut J, Picard I, Weber M, Andre JM. Syndrome de Gelineau et hemangioblastome kystique du cervelet. Rev Neurol 1969; 121:186–189.
40. Anderson M, Salmon MV. Symptomatic cataplexy. J Neurol Neurosurg Psychiatry 1977; 40:186–191.
41. Onofrj M, Curatola I, Ferraci F, Fulgente T. Narcolepsy associated with primary temporal lobe B-cell lymphoma in a HLA DR2 negative subject. J Neurol Neurosurg Psychiatry 1992; 55:852–853.
42. Schwartz WJ, Stakes JW, Hobson JA. Transient cataplexy after removal of a craniopharyngoma. Neurology 1984; 34:1372–1375.
43. Aldrich MS, Naylor MW. Narcolepsy associated with lesions of the diencephalon. Neurology 1989; 39:1505–1508.
44. Lankford DA, Wallman JJ, O'Hara C. Post-traumatic narcolepsy in mild to moderate closed head injury. Sleep 1994; 17(suppl 1):25–28.
45. Kandt RS, Emerson RG, Singer HS, Valle DL, Moser HW. Cataplexy in variant forms of Niemann-Pick disease. Ann Neurol 1982; 12:284–288.

46. Mamelak M. A model for narcolepsy. Canad J Psychol 1991; 45:194–220.
47. Carskadon MA, Harvey K, Dement WC. Multiple sleep latency tests during the development of narcolepsy. West J Med 1981; 135:414–418.
48. Swink TD, Kotagal S. Diagnostic considerations in childhood narcolepsy (abstr). Ann Neurol 1995; 38:548.
49. Kotagal S, Goulding PM. Characteristics of nocturnal sleep in children with narcolepsy. 9th Annual Meeting of the Association of Professional Sleep Societies, Nashville, TN, June 4, 1995.
50. Rechtschaffen A, Kales A, eds. A manual of standardized terminology, techniques, and scoring system for sleep stages of human subjects. Los Angeles: UCLA Brain Information Service/Brain Research Institute, 1968.
51. Dahl RE, Ryan ND, Perel J, Birmaher B, Al-Shabbout M, Nelson B, Puig-Anitch J. Cholinergic REM induction test with arecholine in depressed children. Psychiatry Res 1994; 51:269–282.
52. Roth B. Narcolepsy and hypersomnia: review and classification of 642 personally observed cases. Schweiz Arch Neurol Neurochir Psychiatr 1976; 119:31–41.
53. Recurrent Hypersomnia. In American Sleep Disorders Association. International Classification of Sleep Disorders, Revised: Diagnostic and Coding Manual. Rochester, MN: American Sleep Disorders Association, 1997: 43–46.
54. Bassetti C, Aldrich MS. Idiopathic hypersomnia: a series of 42 patients. Brain 1997; 120: 1423–1435.
56. Bruck D, Parkes JD. A comparison of idiopathic hypersomnia and narcolepsy-cataplexy using self-report measures and sleep diary data. J Neurol Neurosurg Psychiatry 1996; 60: 576–578.
57. Brown LW, Billiard M. Narcolepsy, Kleine-Levin syndrome and other causes of sleepiness in children. In: Ferber R, Kryger M, eds. Principles and Practice of Sleep Medicine in the Child. Philadelphia: Saunders, 1995: 125–134.
58. Thorpy MJ, Korman E, Spielman AJ, Golvinsky PB. Delayed sleep phase syndrome in adolescents. J Adolesc Health Care 1988; 9:22–27.
59. Marcus CL, Loughlin GM. Obstructive sleep apnea in children. Semin Pediatr Neurol 1996; 3:23–28.
60. Guilleminault C, Pelayo R, Leger D, Clerk A, Bocian RC. Recognition of sleep-disordered breathing in children. Pediatrics 1996; 98:871–882.
61. Takahashi Y. Clinical studies of periodic hypersomnolence: analysis of 28 personal cases. Psychiatr Neurol 1965; 853–889.
62. Ryan ND, Puig-Aintch J, Rabinovich H, Ambrosini P, Robinson D, Nelson B, Twomey J, Iyengar S. The clinical picture of major depression in children and adolescents. Arch Gen Psychiatry 1987; 44:854–857.
63. Lahmeyer HW, Poznanski EO, Bellur SN. EEG sleep in depressed adolescents. Am J Psychiatry 1983; 140:1150–1153.
64. Mitler MM. Evaluation of treatment with stimulants in narcolepsy. Sleep 1994; 17(suppl 1):103–106.
65. Billiard M, Besset A, Montplaisir J, Laffont F, Goldenberg F, Weill JS, Lubin S. Modafinil: a double-blind, multicentric study. Sleep 1994; 17(suppl 1):107–112.

16

Sleep Disorders in Children with Neurological Diseases

MARCO ZUCCONI

San Raffaele Institute
University of Milan
Milan, Italy

I. Introduction

Although sleep physiology and sleep-wake rhythm development are well documented in normal children, studies on sleep disorders in children with neurological impairment are relatively infrequent. In children with brain injuries and mental retardation, the development of regular sleep-wake rhythm as well as normal sleep architecture may be compromised. Children with prematurity, congenital diseases, chromosomal disorders, or primary brain diseases may be at risk for presence of sleep disorders. The lack of perception of external stimuli (such as light or sound) or difficulties in responding to them may be of crucial importance in determining altered circadian rhythms. Moreover, difficulties with social contacts and the eventual isolation are aggravating factors hindering normal development of time cues and therefore of regular sleep habits. Mentally retarded and brain-impaired children may also exhibit endogenous dysfunction in hormone release, some of them important in synchronizing circadian rhythms (i.e., the light-dark cycle) with sleep-wake alternation. Manifestations of this desynchronization are difficulty in falling asleep at a desired time, nocturnal awakenings, and difficulty maintaining sleep during the night. Some neurologically impaired children exhibit daytime sleepiness, finding it easy to sleep during the day and, in some cases, showing complete reversal of the night-day cycle for sleep. The interrelationship between neonatal pathologies and the sleep-wake cycle may lead to abnormal cyclic organization of active or rapid-eye-movement (REM) and quiet, non–rapid-eye-movement (NREM) sleep; abnormal characteristics of NREM and REM sleep with respect to respiratory pattern; heart rate, electromyographic (EMG) activity, ocular movements, and, in some cases, electroencephalographic (EEG) activity (i.e., the normal characteristics of the different stages of sleep are not present). Sleep disorganization and instability may worsen some disorders associated with brain pathologies such as seizure, EEG epileptiform abnormalities, respiratory disturbances, and daytime behaviors.

The impairment of cyclicity of NREM-REM (or quiet-active) sleep, with long periods of EEG stationarity in neonates, is an index of brain dysfunction. This may be associated with lack of normal rhythms in respiration, heart rate, motility, and EMG activity, which, together with poor sleep quality, are proportional to the severity of brain impairment. A lack of circadian rhythm of sleep-wake after 3 to 4 months of age has to be considered, in absence of environmental conditioning, a signal of brain dysfunction. Progression over time of sleep-wake rhythmicity may be considered a prognostic indicator of brain-impaired evolution. For example, in severely brain-impaired babies from perinatal insults, with no gaze, who are bedridden, have no response to stimulation, and are severely mentally retarded (acerebrate state), sleep disorders such as irregular sleep-wake pattern are very frequent (1). The Japanese group of Okawa extensively studied this kind of brain pathology and described several types sleep-wake rhythm alterations as follows: "monostage" sleep without the possibility to distinguish any sleep stage (in some cases not even quiet versus active sleep); "dispersed type" sleep without rhythmicity of REM sleep (not regularly distributed) but with two different type of NREM sleep (fast- and slow-wave stages); "polystage" sleep with differentiation of the classic four stages and with a consistent sleep-wake pattern ("consolidated type" sleep). Moreover, acerebrate children exhibit EEG disorders, such as absence of vertex sharp waves or reduction in spindles, which make the sleep elements difficult to recognize and classify. These alterations of sleep patterns and rhythms may be due to the extensive lesions of both cerebral hemispheres, subcortical nuclei such as thalamus or hypothalamus (for sleep elements), and brainstem areas controlling the sleep-wake cycle (1).

Recently some authors reported delayed maturation of melatonin secretion patterns in preterm infants even after correction for gestational age or time at home (2), confirming the importance of normal neural maturation for the development of normal circadian rhythms. Probably not only brainstem but also rostral brain structures are important in sleep-wake rhythm organization, as suggested by the results of a study in infants with hydranencephaly. In this condition brainstem structures are preserved while there is a lack of development of cerebral hemispheres. In these cases circadian rhythms such as hormonal, temperature, and motor activity variations do not develop (3). In lyssencephaly (agyria-pachygiria), a congenital malformation resulting from a disturbance of neuroblastic migration, the classification of NREM and REM sleep was normal, although there was an increase in spindling ("extreme spindles"), hypsarrhythmia, and a decrease in REM percentage as well as a reduction in the number of REMs per minute (4). A recent longitudinal study on sleep problems in children with severe mental handicap found that such problems were extremely common, including settling problems in 51%, waking problems in 67%, and nonrestorative sleep in 32% (5). On follow-up, these sleep problems were found to be very persistent and related to poor self-help skills, daytime behavior problems, incontinence, epilepsy, and to some family variables, although poor communication skills appeared to play the most important role.

Another condition not well studied in children is blindness, where, as in adults, sleep disorders are a very common complaint: unrefreshing sleep, difficulty in maintaining stable sleep-wake rhythms, excessive daytime sleepiness and sleep with, in some cases, an extremely irregular sleep-wake pattern. Such symptoms are frequently more prominent if blindness is congenital and associated with mental retardation (6), which makes it difficult to interpret social time cues (7). The melatonin-level curves of this type of patient are all phase-delayed and consecutive day measurements confirm a free-running melatonin rhythm corresponding to a free-running sleep-wake cycle without entrainment (8). Long-term treatment with melatonin may be a valuable tool in controlling disturbances of circadian rhythm in blind and mentally retarded children (8–11). However, these were clinical case observations where melatonin was given on a compassionate basis in open single-drug studies (8,10) or observations on a single subject (12). Placebo controlled studies on a much larger scale are needed to establish the short- and long-term efficacy and optimal dose and timing of administration (12).

II. Mental Retardation

In mental retardation there should be a deficiency in development of sleep-wake rhythm and of typical elements of sleep such as K-complexes, spindles, and the other phasic events, with characteristics different from normal children of the same age. Independent of the etiology of mental retardation, many sleep variables are often found to be abnormal, and a large proportion of mentally retarded children manifest sleep disturbances (13,14). From the first observation of Petre-Quadens and Jouvet in 1966 describing a reduction of REM sleep in mental retardation (15), sleep researchers focused on REM sleep in order to better understand the relationship between REM sleep and learning. Other authors confirmed early observations of an increase in first REM sleep latency, a decrease in REM period duration, and a decrease in the number of REM periods (16–20) underlying the relationship between REM sleep and immaturity of the brain. An important contribution to the argument came from Petre-Quadens, who reported that a decrease in the number of rapid eye movements and REM density in mentally retarded children correlated with level of intelligence (16,20). According to the Jouvet theory (21) on REM sleep as a sign of CNS plasticity and to the Petre-Quadens hypothesis on the relationship between oculomotor frequencies during REM sleep and learning organization, in mental retardation both handicaps should be present (low plasticity and low organization). The finding that rapid eye movements, spindles (22,23), and “undifferentiated sleep” (when sleep is difficult to classify in any classic stage) (20,24) can serve as indexes of a low-level of CNS organization confirmed the important role of REM sleep in brain development.

This pattern of sleep modifications has been confirmed in Down's syndrome by many authors (23–25) and, on the basis of the relationship between REM sleep and learning, several drugs were tested to evaluate their effects on REM sleep variables (duration, timing, percentage) and characteristics (eye movements). An increase in REM sleep may be associated with an increase in brain plasticity and learning abilities (25), but in general hypnotics decrease REM sleep. Butoctamide hydrogen succinate (BAHS), an organic bromide compound found in the cerebrospinal fluid of normal subjects (26) and known to increase REM sleep in animals (27) and volunteers (28), has been shown to significantly increase the percentage of REM sleep as well as to decrease undifferentiated sleep and the first REM latency (24,25,29), probably by a serotoninergic effect (28). In Down's syndrome children, intensive learning sessions resulted in increased oculomotor frequencies during REM sleep, although REM sleep duration and percentage were not modified (24).

III. Down's Syndrome

As pointed out above, in Down's syndrome children there are many reports indicating sleep modifications, including increase in wake after sleep onset (30), frequent body movements (31), a decrease in REM sleep with low REM sleep density (32,33), and fewer spindle bursts (32,33). Concerning hormone secretion, some reports indicate a decreased peak amplitude of GH release and altered timing in relationship to sleep structure (slow-wave sleep), although a certain pulsatility was evident (34,35). Regarding respiratory pattern during sleep, children with Down's syndrome have a high incidence of obstructive sleep apnea syndrome (OSAS) due to many predisposing factors such as midfacial and mandibular hypoplasia (36), macroglossia, glossoptosis and hypoplastic trachea (37), tonsillar and adenoid hypertrophy (38,39), obesity, and hypotonia. Several reports indicate a percentage of OSAS between 50% and 80% in this type of mental retardation (39–42). Recently, Ferri et al. emphasized the finding of central as opposed to obstructive apneas (89.4% versus 9.4%) in a series of ten Down's syndrome subjects without obesity or upper airway pathology (43). These central events were preceded by sighs, but they provoked significant oxygen desaturation. The authors hypothesized that brainstem abnormalities (ascribed to the specific syndrome and not to mental retardation or sleep disturbing factors) may be responsible for the centrally impaired control of respiration during sleep. This theory is supported by the existence of abnormalities in brainstem auditory evoked potentials in Down's syndrome children, suggesting a common brainstem dysfunction (44).

IV. Rett's Syndrome

Rett's syndrome is a peculiar form of severe mental retardation characterized by autistic tendencies during infancy associated with particular stereotyped behaviors, ventilatory abnormalities during wakefulness (alternating apnea and hyperventilation), and motor apraxia of unknown etiology. This unusual disorder is generally seen in females, but genetic and chromosomal studies are inconclusive. Irregular sleep-wake rhythms have been observed frequently (45–48), as well as breathing disorders during wakefulness consisting of intermittent hyperventilation and prolonged apnea associated with severe oxygen desaturation (49,50). During sleep, the respiratory pattern is usually normal (49), although some central or obstructive events were also reported (50), indicating an impairment of the behavioral (waking) respiratory control, while automatic ventilatory control is spared. EEG epileptiform abnormalities are common and typical but alterations in sleep have also been described, such as reduction of spindles and K-complexes (48,50) as well as sleep architecture modifications (decrease of REM sleep and of total sleep time) similar to those seen in other forms of mental retardation (50).

V. Autism, Fragile-X Syndrome, and Other Forms of Mental Retardation

Several authors have analyzed sleep in autistic children, in particular REM sleep, finding no alteration in the amount of REM sleep or the latency of the first REM period but observing modifications in other REM sleep components, including an increase in fast EEG components (10.5 to 15 Hz) and spindling, reduction in duration but not in number of the REM bursts, significantly greater average length of REM bursts, and a lower ratio between REM bursts to REMs out of bursts in autistic children (age up to 62 months) compared to normal controls (51,52). A recent study of Elia and coworkers evaluated sleep parameters and eye movements during sleep in a sample of four autistic children compared with normal age-matched controls (53). Most sleep parameters were not significantly different between the two groups except the proportion of stage 2 NREM sleep, which was significantly reduced in autistic subjects while REM sleep was similar (54). In contrast to data from children with Down's syndrome, these data suggest the potential in some autistic children of an unaffected ability of the brain to retain information (55). The same authors, contrary to previous literature, found higher values of REM density and oculomotor activity during REM sleep and a less evident tendency of REMs to cluster in bursts (53). These results indicate a deficit in inhibitory mechanisms controlling the redundancy of eye movements in REM sleep (probably located in the frontal cortex) or a dysregulation of the complex neurochemical mechanisms underlying REM sleep (56,57). The same research group, in a larger study, suggested that information processing (related to REM sleep) may be different in autistic mentally retarded subjects from subjects with mental retardation alone. Mentally retarded children seem to present a deficit in the production of REMs while autistic children show a deficit in the modulation of REMs (58).

Fragile-X syndrome, a genetic disorder caused by a mutation in a specific gene located on the X chromosome, is characterized (in the case of the full mutation) by mild to severe mental retardation, behavioral components such as social deficits with peers, abnormalities in language and communication, unusual responses to sensory stimuli, stereotypic behaviors and hyperactivity, cognitive dysfunction, and epilepsy. Recently an increased risk for OSA was shown in a group of male children and young adults (59). However, a subsequent report of seven fragile-X children, using polysomnography, found no obstructive apnea/hypopnea and only a few central respiratory events, preceded by sighs and without oxygen desaturation (60). Excluding the common risk factors for OSA in normal children, such as enlarged adenoids and tonsils, nasal septal deviation, and hypotonic oropharyngeal muscles, fragile-X syndrome children do not seem at particular at risk for OSA, which differs from the other genetic forms of mental retardation (Down's and Prader-Willi syndromes).

Concerning sleep neurophysiology, a study of nine fragile-X patients showed reduced total sleep time, decreased REM sleep percentage, and an increase in the first REM latency and in stage 3/4 NREM percentage (61). Moreover, in the same study an increase in twitch movements was observed during both stage 2 NREM and REM sleep. This may indicate a dysregulation of the cholinergic-monoaminergic system during sleep, leading to an imbalance between the two neurochemically different mechanisms, which is known to be involved in other clinical manifestations of this genetic syndrome (62).

Children with cerebral palsy exhibit significant sleep problems both with respect to sleep architecture and respiratory control. Nonspecific EEG findings such as an increase in arousals, increased first REM latency, and decreases in REM duration and gross body movements (30,63,64) as well as respiratory disturbances such as central apnea, obstructive apnea, and obstructive hypopnea were associated with brainstem dysfunction (65). Sleep apnea and a decreased ability to change body position may contribute to sleep disruption in cerebral palsy patients.

For other forms of mental retardation, studies of sleep are lacking and observations are limited to case reports or small groups of children. In Angelman syndrome, a genetic disorder characterized by severe mental retardation, epilepsy, and jerky limb movements, a sleep-wake rhythm disturbance with reduction of the nighttime sleep and frequent daytime naps has been pointed out in a single case report (66). Treatment with sleep hygiene, behavioral therapy, and reinforcing of the sleep-wake rhythm was documented to be as effective as hypnotic drugs (66).

In phenylketonuria, as expected, decreased REM sleep and increased undifferentiated sleep were reported (67). Increased spindling during NREM sleep in the absence of other sleep parameter modifications has also been reported (68). In Menkes' kinky hair disease (trichopoliodystrophy), characterized by kinky hair, epilepsy, and a disturbance in the copper metabolism (69), other than EEG alterations, some authors have reported a sleep-wake rhythm disorder with the increase in "undifferentiated" sleep and a reduction of quiet sleep typical of mental retardation (70,71). This finding might be correlated with the anatomical findings of thalamic degeneration (72). In hypothyroidism, besides the well-known EEG modifications with a decrease in amplitude and slowing in frequency, a pioneering study by Schultz and coworkers (73) showed an immature sleep pattern with a typical "tracé alternans" at 3 months of age with a reduction in spindles. Moreover they found a correlation between higher IQ level and the development of normal spindling activity.

In some other metabolic diseases—such as Leigh syndrome, Hunter syndrome (type 2 mucolysaccharidosis), and Riley-Day syndrome (familial dysautonomia)—sleep disturbances are mainly of respiratory origin, with obstructive (due to morphological upper airway modifications) or central (due to dysfunction of central chemosensitivity control) apneas/hypopneas. Sleep disorders have been described in neuronal ceroid-lipofuscinoses, a group of recessively inherited disorders due to the lysosomal storage of lipopigments and lipofuscin in neurons and other tissues. The clinical manifestations—myoclonic seizures, ataxia, dementia, and progressive visual loss—are often associated with sleep abnormalities such as disturbed sleep cycle (74,75) and respiratory and movement pattern disorders (76), both in the infantile and juvenile forms. A particular form of inherited mental retardation associated with a phakomatosis (tuberous sclerosis) has been extensively evaluated concerning the relationship between learning disability, epilepsy and sleep disorders. Hunt and coworkers (77) in a large sample of children with tuberous sclerosis, found a high percentage of sleep problems (more than 60%), which finding was confirmed in another study (78). These problems seem more likely to occur in children with ongoing seizures and a high level of behavioral problems. Seizures and interictal epileptiform discharges may play a crucial role in sleep disruption, fragmentation, and instability together with the distribution of cortical tubers in frontal and temporal lobes (79).

VI. Prader-Willi Syndrome

Prader-Willi syndrome—a congenital disease usually associated with a mutation on the chromosome 15q 11-13 and characterized by perinatal hypotonia, hyperphagia, hypogonadism, and learning difficulties (80)—is associated with some dysmorphic traits such as hypotelorism, high-arched palate, and down-turned mouth. These characteristics in association with weight gain lead to an increased risk for OSA, well documented by numerous authors (81–85). Daytime sleepiness is a very diffuse symptom associated with the syndrome and was recently listed, together with sleep apnea, as a minor characteristic in the consensus on diagnostic criteria (86). It was reported by several authors as a main behavioral characteristic of these children (82,87–89), increasing with the increase of age and weight and severe in cases with OSA or obesity hypoventilation. The presence of daytime somnolence in children with Prader-Willi syndrome was evaluated in two recent studies by Clift et al., and Hertz et al., focusing attention on sleep architecture, respiration, and the Multiple Sleep Latency Test (MSLT) (84,85). Clift et al. found daytime sleepiness to be present in 70% of children and young adults with the syndrome, severe in 50%, and in these cases related to OSA severity. In addition, they found atypical REM sleep with a short latency after sleep onset. Because of the presence of daytime sleepiness also in children without respiratory disturbances, they concluded that in Prader-Willi syndrome excessive daytime sleepiness it is mainly of central origin (hypothalamic involvement?) but that OSA may increase it, particularly in obese subjects. For this reason they recommended screening for sleep apnea independent of the subjective complaint of daytime somnolence (85). Hertz et al. studied developmental changes in sleep and respiration among a group of children and adults with the Prader-Willi syndrome and found little sleep apnea and frequent REM-related oxygen desaturation (only two out of nine children had overt OSA) that correlated with the degree of obesity. They described REM sleep abnormalities (both in children and adults) such as REM sleep fragmentation, variable REM latency, and sleep-onset REM periods (SOREMPs) on MSLT, but none of the patients had clinical symptoms of narcolepsy and cataplexy. Moreover, these sleep alterations appeared to be independent of disordered breathing, nocturnal oxygen desaturation, and daytime sleepiness, and the authors postulated a dysfunction in the posterior hypothalamus as responsible for sleep findings, while obesity was correlated with respiratory and oxygen saturation abnormalities (84). Concerning the REM sleep abnormalities, which are similar to those of narcolepsy, two recent reports exclude an association between HLA haplotype DR2(15) and DQ1(16) and the syndrome, even though these associations are typical for narcolepsy (90,91). Summarizing the literature, in Prader-Willi syndrome, somnolence during the day is a common symptom, becoming severe when associated with sleep-disordered breathing. There are no typical and consistent sleep architecture modifications but probably hypothalamic dysfunction acts on the central component of daytime sleepiness and obesity worsens the upper-airway obstruction during sleep.

Continuous positive airway pressure (CPAP) has been shown to be useful in the management of severe OSA and daytime sleepiness but is more difficult in children with mental retardation and behavioral-learning disabilities (83,85). However, with appropriate support from behavioral specialists, CPAP or bilevel positive airway pressure can be used successfully in this population (92).

VII. Achondroplasia

Achondroplasia is the most common form of dwarfism (with a prevalence between 1 in 25,000 and 1.5 in 10,000 live births). This autosomal dominant condition, due to a defect of endochondral bone formation, consists of short stature, lumbar lordosis, protuberant abdomen, short hands, and craniofacial deformities such as macrocephaly, frontal bossing, small foramen magnum, short cranial base, and severe midface hypoplasia. The bony modifications may lead to neurological problems like hydrocephalus or myelopathy. Recent literature describes a high prevalence of respiratory disturbances during sleep, both central and obstructive in origin, in children with achondroplasia (93–96). However, the relationship between respiratory events during sleep and upper-airway narrowing or neurological abnormalities (in particular of respiratory control centers located in the brainstem) has not been completely clarified. Our group recently observed a consecutive series of children with achondroplasia and evaluated sleep and respiration by polysomnography, correlating the results with clinical, magnetic resonance (MR), or computed tomography (CT) brain imaging and cephalometry (where possible) (97). Almost all the children studied had a history of habitual snoring and/or suspected sleep apnea and daytime symptoms predicting respiratory disturbances during sleep. As regards sleep parameters, they were normal for age and not different from a group of normally developed children with habitual snoring.

In 75% of the children with achondroplasia, we found breathing disorders during sleep ranging from obstructive sleep apneas with significant oxygen desaturation (to 66%), obstructive hypopnea, continuous and loud snoring with increased respiratory effort, brief (less than 8 sec in duration) obstructive events, and an increase of breathing rate during sleep (97). Twenty-five percent of the patients studied showed rare central apnea events during REM sleep, generally of short duration and without significant oxygen desaturation. There was no correlation between a reduction in size of the foramen magnum (showed by MRI or CT scan in 90% of examined children) and respiratory disturbances both of central and obstructive type. In particular there was no correlation between the size of the foramen magnum and the apnea-hypopnea index. These findings likely indicate that the morphological features of achondroplasia, such as craniofacial deformity, are more important in the pathogenesis of breathing disorders than any possible dysfunction of central respiratory control. Our results are not in accordance with previous studies (94,95), where a correlation between restricted foramen magnum and sleep-disordered breathing, especially central in type, was shown. However, our children did not exhibit respiratory complications during wakefulness. The importance of anatomic factors in the pathogenesis of respiratory problems during sleep was confirmed by the similar results found in the control group, which consisted of children with habitual snoring and OSA, and by cephalometric findings. The lateral cephalometric examination showed a defect in the sagittal and vertical growth, with posterior displacement of the maxilla and infraorbital rims and a class III occlusion with an open bite and labial incompetence. This particular facial conformation has been described in adult achondroplasia patients (98).

In conclusion, our results confirmed previous data concerning the degree of upper-airway obstruction during sleep in most patients (children and adults) with achondroplasia (96). The crucial role of craniofacial deformity with reduction in the sagittal dimension of the nasopharynx and probably an increase in upper-airway resistance seems to reduce the importance of the central control respiratory mechanism in the pathogenesis of sleep-disordered breathing. Nocturnal polysomnography is a useful tool to evaluate respiratory compromise during sleep.

VIII. Neuromuscular Diseases

Among the various types of diseases involving neuromuscular pathology, the more frequently encountered sleep-related findings are respiratory problems due to respiratory muscle weakness (diaphragm, intercostals and accessory respiratory muscles) and/or in central breathing control. Obstructive or central apneas together with hypoventilation are the more commonly described abnormalities during sleep in children with neuromuscular diseases. An important concept in this type of sleep-related respiratory problem is that if there is a problem with the respiratory neuromuscular system, respiratory insufficiency will be most marked in sleep and will first appear during periods of REM sleep (99). Upper airway obstruction may be due to anatomical factors independent of the disease or it may be provoked by the weakness of upper-airway muscles as a part of the neuromuscular disease. REM sleep is the crucial period during which sleep-disordered breathing occurs because there is a physiological inhibition of chest wall and accessory muscles involved in respiration, while diaphragm function is relatively spared. Usually, at least at the beginning of the disease, ventilation during NREM sleep is not compromised. When hypoventilation extends to NREM sleep, it is a sign of possible hypoventilation in the waking state too (with hypercapnia) and consequently a first step toward respiratory failure if left untreated. At this stage also the progression of the neuromuscular disease may play a role in increasing the hypoventilation during sleep and wakefulness by a worsening of muscle weakness.

If upper-airway obstruction is superimposed on sleep hypoventilation due to underlying weakness, the two overlap and worsen hypoventilation during sleep. Overnight oxygen saturation, static maximum inspiratory mouth pressure (Pimax), pulmonary function test during wakefulness, serial blood gas tensions, and full nocturnal polysomnography, together with clinical evaluation, seem to be the best parameters to determine the degree of respiratory disorder progression and to indicate the best treatment (99).

The neuromuscular disease associated with respiratory failure and sleep-related breathing disorders that has received the most study is Duchenne's muscular dystrophy. Both in children and in young adults, central and obstructive apneas/hypopneas, hypoventilation, and nocturnal oxygen desaturations have been observed in almost all the patients studied. Problems tend to be worse during REM sleep, with simple decreases of SaO_2 or apneas/hypopneas associated with significant O_2 desaturation (100). The magnitude of oxyhemoglobin desaturation appears to be significantly correlated with functional residual capacity (100), vital capacity (in supine versus the erect position if possible) as an index of diaphragm weakness, daytime PaO_2, $PaCO_2$ (101), or decreased maximum inspiratory pressure (102). Besides the inhibition of intercostal and accessory muscle activity and the relative preservation of diaphragm function in REM sleep, upper-airway obstruction in these patients may decrease chest wall motion sufficiently to produce apparent central apneas ("pseudocentral apnea") that is actually obstructive in origin (103–105). Disturbances of cardiac rhythm during sleep are also described (106) in these boys as well as a decrease of heart rate variability similar to that in adult Duchenne patients (107).

Myotonic dystrophy is another potential myopathy associated with sleep-related breathing problems that may present in the early stages of the disease. Besides the presence of frequent central apneas, not only in REM sleep but occurring throughout all the sleep stages (108), and less frequent obstructive events (109), there is an impairment of neural respiratory control indicated by the abnormal response to hypoxia and hypercapnia (99), which is due to the involvement of the CNS in the disease. The excessive daytime sleepiness often described in children with the initial stage of the myopathy (109) is probably independent from the apnea/hypopnea index, the oxygen desaturations, and the sleep fragmentation occurring because of the direct effect of the CNS lesions, as suggested by the cognitive and neuropsychological deficit (110,111).

IX. Epilepsy

The relationship between sleep and epilepsy is complex and appears to be multifactorial. Several studies have documented sleep disturbances in children with different forms of seizures or epilepsy, indicating sleep disruption associated with nocturnal seizures but also in relationship to the intercritical epileptiform discharges (IED). Conversely, sleep and sleep deprivation have an important activating role both in seizures and IED, depending on the type of epilepsy or seizures, the age of the child, and the degree of neurological impairment (i.e., the relationship between sleep disorders, seizures, and some forms of mental retardation was considered in the previous paragraphs).

With respect to sleep disorders in epileptic children, one of the major problems is the appearance and consequently the diagnosis of sleep parasomnias such as sleepwalking, night terrors, or, in some cases, nocturnal enuresis in children with a form of epilepsy. The main issue is when children have a type of nocturnal seizure [such as focal motor attacks in benign partial epilepsy with centrotemporal spikes (BECT) or in other idiopathic partial epilepsy such as nocturnal frontal lobe seizures and non-idiopathic partial forms]. Initially, because of similarities between epileptic and parasomnia attacks, suggested by the characteristics of the events, the prevalence of EEG epileptiform abnormalities, and the lack of memory for the episodes, a common origin was suggested by some authors (112,113). In the late sixties the Marseilles school denied the hypothesis of epileptic origin of nocturnal episodes emerging from NREM sleep on the basis of absent or rare interictal or ictal discharges in children with pavor nocturnus or somnambulisms (114–116). Until the mid-1980s, it was concluded that the night terrors, sleepwalking, and the majority of the forms of enuresis were of nonepileptic origin and not related to seizures. When the two types of phenomena coexisted they were considered to be independent of one another (117,118). However, recently, with the aid of videopolysomnographic recordings and extended EEG montages, some atypical clinical and electrophysiological patterns were described, suggesting a reevaluation of motor episodes during sleep, particularly in children (119–124). The identification of a form of nocturnal frontal lobe epilepsy (NFLE)—both sporadic and autosomal dominant, frequently starting in childhood or in infancy

(125–128), and with nocturnal attacks, similar to benign classical parasomnias—raises the problem of the differential diagnosis between the two types of motor phenomena during sleep (indistinguishable by history). This also raises the question of whether true parasomniac episodes (sleepwalking, sleep terrors, and other) really exist, especially if they persist from childhood into adolescence and adulthood (129–131).

As a general rule, based on nocturnal polysomnographic recording with videotape monitoring, detailed EEG, and motor behavior analysis, there are some differences between parasomnias and paroxysmal arousals with motor behaviors of epileptic origin (NFLE). NFLE is suggested by the following features: short-lasting episodes occurring in all sleep stages but predominantly in stage 2 NREM sleep, the repetitiveness and periodicity of attacks, the sudden and abrupt beginning of behaviors, and the stereotyped forms with two or three different types of event for each patients for NFLE. Parasomnias are different because of their longer duration, lower frequency (generally one or a few episodes per night), and the general characteristics of arising predominantly in the first part of the night during slow-wave sleep (119,129–134). We recently evaluated motor behaviors during sleep by videopolysomnography in 33 consecutive children (mean age 9.9 years) complaining of frequent nocturnal motor behaviors or motor agitation during sleep, with a mean age at onset of 5.1 years. Clinical evaluation showed an elevated mean frequency of the episodes (15 per month), with more than one-third of children exhibiting nightly attacks. Videopolysomnographic diagnosis, possible in all but seven cases, was of NFLE in 77% of children (both sporadic and genetic forms), with ictal and interictal discharges in 70% of NFLE children and male preponderance (16 out of 20 cases). The other diagnoses were sleep terrors (2 cases), rhythmic movement disorder (1 case), and nocturnal enuresis without arousal disorders (3 cases). These data indicated that also in children, the clinical evidence of motor parasomnia needs to be confirmed by videopolysomnography and that the criteria to identify classic benign parasomnias need to be revised (135). The differential diagnosis is important for treatment: drugs for a seizure disorder versus no treatment or at least a different pharmacological approach for classical child parasomnias (117).

Concerning nonspecific sleep disorders, both sleep and waking epilepsies may be characterized by sleep-structure modification, depending on the severity of the epileptic disorder and the number of seizures during sleep. Sleep abnormalities are more prevalent in generalized convulsive than focal epilepsies and when seizures are not well controlled (117,136,137).

Generalized symptomatic or cryptogenic epilepsy may be characterized by impairment of sleep phasic events such as spindles or K-complexes (like in mental retardation), reduction of REM sleep, and difficulties in staging sleep according to classic criteria. This means increase of "undifferentiated sleep" or indeterminate states in some disorders such as West and Lennox-Gastaut syndromes (138–140). In these disorders, poorly organized sleep-wake rhythms were observed and the co-occurrence of circadian disturbances with impaired melatonin rhythms raised the question of possible treatment by inducing a reorganization of melatonin normal rhythm (141). Otherwise, also in epileptic children and children with febrile convulsions, a phase advance with nocturnal melatonin peak appearing between 2400 and 0200 was found in the former, while a disappearance of the circadian rhythm of melatonin with only bursts throughout the light-dark cycle was demonstrated in the latter (142). The modifications of day-night melatonin levels, found also in partial epileptic patients, gave rise to the hypothesis that melatonin can have a inhibitory function on central nervous system activity (143). In conclusion, sleep abnormalities in epileptic children are frequent and consistent, depending on the type of disorder, the control of the seizures especially during the night, and the eventual neurologic impairment associated with the epilepsy. However, sleep fragmentation and instability due to arousals associated with seizures, IED, and frequent stage shifts may be better evaluated with microstructure analysis, taking into consideration arousal level oscillation related to epileptic phenomena (117,144–147).

Regarding the activation effect of sleep on seizures, NREM sleep has an interictal and ictal activation both for focal and generalized epilepsies, while in REM sleep the activation is predominant for focal IED. In epilepsies with seizures on awakening IEDs occur more prevalently in 1 to 2 NREM, while in epilepsies with sleep-related seizures (as mentioned before) both ictal attacks and IED are located throughout all NREM stages, with modulation or phasic-related arousal events. For partial epilepsy, a recent study (in adults) indicated that the level of NREM sleep depth may be important in activating foci, in terms of absolute log delta power, independently from arousal events, while REM sleep had the major relative suppression activity due to the absence of log delta power (148).

References

1. Okawa M, Sasaki H. Sleep disorders in mentally retarded and brain-impaired children. In: Guilleminault C, ed. Sleep and Its Disorders in Children. New York: Raven Press, 1987: 269–290.
2. Kennaway DJ, Stamp GE, Goble FC. Development of melatonin production in infants and the impact of prematurity. J Clin Endocrinol Metab 1992; 75:367–369.
3. Hashimoto T, Fukuda K, Endo S, Miyazaki M, Murakawa K, Tayama M, Kuroda Y. Circadian rhythm in patients with hydranencephaly. J Child Neurol 1992; 7:188–194.
4. Mori K, Hashimoto T, Tayama M, Miyazaki M, Fukuda K, Endo S, Kuroda Y. Serial EEG and sleep polygraphic studies on lissencephaly (agyria-pachygyria). Brain Dev 1994; 16:365–373.
5. Quine L. Sleep problems in children with mental handicap. J Ment Defic Res 1991; 35:269–290.
6. Okawa M, Nanami T, Wada S, Shimizu T, Hishikawa Y, Sasaki H, Nagamine H, Takahashi K. Four congenitally blind children with circadian sleep-wake rhythm disorder. Sleep 1987; 10:101–110.
7. Palm L, Blennow G, Wetterberg L. Correction of non-24-hour sleep-wake cycle by melatonin in a blind retarded boy. Ann Neurol 1991; 29:336–339.

8. Palm L, Blennow G, Wetterberg L. Long-term melatonin treatment in blind children and young adults with circadian sleep-wake disturbances. Dev Med Child Neurol 1997; 39: 319–325.
9. Jan JE. Head movements of visually impaired children. Dev Med Child Neurol 1991; 33:645–647.
10. Jan JE, Espezel H, Appleton RE. The treatment of sleep disorders with melatonin (see comments). Dev Med Child Neurol 1994; 36:97–107.
11. Sack RL, Lewy AJ, Blood ML, Stevenson J, Keith LD. Melatonin administration to blind people: phase advances and entrainment. J Biol Rhythms 1991; 6:249–261.
12. Camfield P, Gordon K, Dooley J, Camfield C. Melatonin appears ineffective in children with intellectual deficits and fragmented sleep: six "N of 1" trials (see comments). J Child Neurol 1996; 11:341–343.
13. Stores G. Sleep studies in children with a mental handicap. J Child Psychol Psychiatry 1992; 33:1303–1317.
14. Landesman-Dwyer S, Sackett GP. Behavioral changes in nonambulatory, profoundly mentally retarded individuals. Monogr Am Assoc Ment Defic 1978; 55–144.
15. Jouvet M, Petre-Quadens O. Paradoxical sleep and dreaming in the mentally deficient. Acta Neurol Psychiatr Belg 1966; 66:116–122.
16. Feinberg I. Sleep variables as a function of age in man. Acta Gen Psychiatry 1968; 18: 239–250.
17. Feinberg I, Braun M. Shulman E. EEG sleep patterns in mental retardation. Electroencephalogr Clin Neurophysiol 1969; 27:128–141.
18. Castaldo V, Krynicki V. Sleep pattern and intelligence in functional mental retardation. J Ment Defic Res 1973; 17:231–235.
19. Grubar JC. Le sommeil paradoxal de débiles mentaux. Enfance 1978; 2:165–172.
20. Grubar JC. Sleep and mental deficiency. Rev Electroencephalogr Neurophysiol Clin 1983; 13:107–113.
21. Jouvet M. Le comportement onirique. Pour la Science 1979; 25:512–527.
22. Shibagaki M, Kiyono S, Watanabe K, Hakamada S. Concurrent occurrence of rapid eye movement with spindle burst during nocturnal sleep in mentally retarded children. Electroencephalogr Clin Neurophysiol 1982; 53:27–35.
23. Colognola RM, Grubar JC, Gigli GL, Ferri R, Musumeci SA, Bergonzi P. Sleep in children with Down syndrome. In: Koella WP, Ruther E, Schulz H, eds. Sleep '84. Stuttgart-New York: Gustav Fischer Verlag, 1985:68.
24. Gigli GL, Grubar JC, Colognola RM, Amata MT, Pollicina C, Ferri R, Musumeci SA, Bergonzi P. Butoctamide hydrogen succinate and intensive learning sessions: effects on night sleep of Down's syndrome patients. Sleep 1987; 10:563–569.
25. Grubar JC, Gigli GL, Colognola RM, Ferri R, Musumeci SA, Bergonzi P. Sleep patterns of Down's syndrome children: effects of butoctamide hydrogen succinate (BAHS) administration. Psychopharmacology (Berl) 1986; 90:119–122.
26. Yanagisawa I, Yoshikawa H. A bromine compound isolated from human cerebrospinal fluid. Biochim Biophys Acta 1973; 329:283–294.
27. Otomo E, Araki G, Tomita T, Koga E. Effectiveness of N-(2-ethylhexyl)-oxybutyramide semisuccinate (M-2H) on sleep in insomniacs. Igaku No Ayumi 1975; 2:258–273.
28. Okudaira N, Torii S, Endo S. The effect of butoctamide hydrogen succinate on nocturnal sleep: all-night polygraphical studies. Psychopharmacology (Berl) 1980; 70: 117–121.

29. Grubar JC, Gigli GL, Colognola RM, Ferri R, Musumeci SA, Bergonzi P. Effects of Butoctamide (BAHS) on nocturnal sleep of Down's syndrome children. In: Koella WP, Ruther E, Schulz H, eds. Sleep '84. Suttgart-New York: Gustav Fischer Verlag, 1985: 420–422.
30. Prechtl HF, Theorell K, Blair AW. Behavioural state cycles in abnormal infants. Dev Med Child Neurol 1973; 15:606–615.
31. Goldie L, Curtis JA, Svendsen V, Roberton NR. Abnormal sleep rhythms in mongol babies. Lancet 1968; 229–230.
32. Fukuma E, Umezawa Y, Kobayashi K, Motoike M. Polygraphic study on the nocturnal sleep of children with Down's syndrome and endogenous mental retardation. Folia Psychiatr Neurol Jpn 1974; 28:333–345.
33. Clausen J, Sersen EA, Lidsky A. Sleep patterns in mental retardation: Down's syndrome. Electroencephalogr Clin Neurophysiol 1977; 43:183–191.
34. Castells S, Torrado C, Bastian W, Wisniewski KE. Growth hormone deficiency in Down's syndrome children. J Intellect Disabil Res 1992; 36:29–43.
35. Ferri R, Ragusa L, Alberti A, Elia M, Musumeci SA, Del Gracco S, Romano C, Stefanini MC. Growth hormone and sleep in Down syndrome. Dev Brain Dysfunct 1996; 9:114–120.
36. Allanson JE, O'Hara P, Farkas LG, Nair RC. Anthropometric craniofacial pattern profiles in Down syndrome. Am J Med Genet 1993; 47:748–752.
37. Aboussouan LS, O'Donovan PB, Moodie DS, Gragg LA, Stoller JK. Hypoplastic trachea in Down's syndrome. Am Rev Respir Dis 1993; 147:72–75.
38. Strome M. Obstructive sleep apnea in Down syndrome children: a surgical approach. Laryngoscope 1986; 96:1340–1342.
39. Southall DP, Stebbens VA, Mirza R, Lang MH, Croft CB, Shinebourne EA. Upper airway obstruction with hypoxaemia and sleep disruption in Down syndrome. Dev Med Child Neurol 1987; 29:734–742.
40. Marcus CL, Keens TG, Bautista DB, Von Pechmann WS, Ward SL. Obstructive sleep apnea in children with Down syndrome. Pediatrics 1991; 88:132–139.
41. Loughlin GM, Wynne JW, Victorica BE. Sleep apnea as a possible cause of pulmonary hypertension in Down syndrome. J Pediatr 1981; 98:435–437.
42. Stebbens VA, Dennis J, Samuels MP, Croft CB, Southall DP. Sleep related upper airway obstruction in a cohort with Down's syndrome. Arch Dis Child 1991; 66:1333–1338.
43. Ferri R, Curzi-Dascalova L, Del Gracco S, Elia M, Musumeci SA, Stefanini MC. Respiratory patterns during sleep in Down's syndrome: importance of central apnoeas. J Sleep Res 1997; 6:134–141.
44. Ferri R, Del Gracco S, Elia M, Musumeci SA, Stefanini MC. Age- and height-dependent changes of amplitude and latency of somatosensory evoked potentials in children and young adults with Down's syndrome. Neurophysiol Clin 1996; 26:321–327.
45. Hagberg B, Aicardi J, Dias K, Ramos O. A progressive syndrome of autism, dementia, ataxia, and loss of purposeful hand use in girls: Rett's syndrome: report of 35 cases. Ann Neurol 1983; 14:471–479.
46. Hagberg BA. Rett syndrome: clinical peculiarities, diagnostic approach, and possible cause. Pediatr Neurol 1989; 5:75–83.
47. Naidu S, Murphy S, Moser HW. Rett syndrome: natural history in 70 cases. Am J Med Genet 1983; 24:61.

48. Nomura Y, Segawa M, Hasegawa M. Rett syndrome—clinical studies and pathophysiological consideration. Brain Dev 1984; 6:475–486.
49. Lugaresi E, Cirignotta F, Montagna P. Abnormal breathing in the Rett syndrome. Brain Dev 1985; 7:329–333.
50. Glaze DG, Frost JDJ, Zoghbi HY, Percy AK. Rett's syndrome: characterization of respiratory patterns and sleep. Ann Neurol 1987; 21:377–382.
51. Ornitz EM, Ritvo ER, Brown MB, La Franchi S, Parmelee T, Walter RD. The EEG and rapid eye movements during REM sleep in normal and autistic children. Electroencephalogr Clin Neurophysiol 1969; 26:167–175.
52. Tanguay PE, Ornitz EM, Forsythe AB, Ritvo ER. Rapid eye movement (REM) activity in normal and autistic children during REM sleep. J Autism Child Schizophr 1976; 6:275–288.
53. Elia M, Ferri R, Musumeci SA, Bergonzi P. Rapid eye movement during night sleep in autistic subjects. Brain Dysfunct 1991; 4:348–354.
54. Ornitz EM, Ritvo ER, Walter RD. Dreaming sleep in autistic and schizophrenic children. Am J Psychiatry 1965; 122:419–424.
55. Grubar JC. Sleep and mental retardation: toward a synthesis. Brain Dysfunct 1989; 2:73–83.
56. Jeannerod M, Mouret J, Jouvet M. Etude de la motricité oculaire au cours de la phase paradoxale du sommeil chez le chat. Electroencephalogr Clin Neurophysiol 1965; 18:554–566.
57. Young JG, Kavanagh ME, Anderson GM, Shaywitz BA, Cohen DJ. Clinical neurochemistry of autism and associated disorders. J Autism Dev Disord 1982; 12:147–165.
58. Ferri R, Elia M, Musumeci MA, Candian C, Orviati S, Miano GM, Bergonzi P. Sleep rapid eye movement activity in autism: a Marcov-process approach. J Sleep Res 1994; 3(suppl 1):78.
59. Tirosh E, Borochowitz Z. Sleep apnea in fragile X syndrome. Am J Med Genet 1992; 43:124–127.
60. Musumeci SA, Ferri R, Elia M, Del Gracco S, Scuderi C, Stefanini MC. Normal respiratory pattern during sleep in young fragile-X syndrome patients (letter). J Sleep Res 1996; 5:272.
61. Musumeci SA, Ferri R, Elia M, Del Gracco S, Scuderi C, Stefanini MC, Castano A, Azan G. Sleep neurophysiology in fragile X patients. Dev Brain Dysfunct 1995; 8:218–222.
62. Brown WT, Jenkins E, Neri G, Lubs H, Shapiro LR, Davies KE, Sherman S, Hagerman R, Laird C. Conference report: Fourth International Workshop on the fragile X and X-linked mental retardation [published erratum appears in Am J Med Genet 1991 Dec 1; 41(3):391]. Am J Med Genet 1991; 38:158–172.
63. Hori T, Kodama M. Polygraphical study of sleep in cerebral palsied adults. Rinsho Noha 1975; 17:168–172.
64. Hayashi M, Inoue Y, Iwakawa Y, Sasaki H. REM sleep abnormalities in severe athetoid cerebral palsy. Brain Dev 1990; 12:494–497.
65. Kotagal S, Gibbons VP, Stith JA. Sleep abnormalities in patients with severe cerebral palsy. Dev Med Child Neurol 1994; 36:304–311.
66. Summers JA, Lynch PS, Harris JC, Burke JC, Allison DB, Sandler L. A combined behavioral/pharmacological treatment of sleep-wake schedule disorder in Angelman syndrome. J Dev Behav Pediatr 1992; 13:284–287.

67. Petre-Quadens O. Sleep in mental retardation. In: Clemente CD, Purpura DP, Mayer F, eds. Sleep and the Maturing Nervous System. New York: Academic Press, 1972: 384–417.
68. Schulte FJ, Kaiser HJ, Engelbart S, Bell EF, Castell R, Lenard HG. Sleep patterns in hyperphenylalaninemia: a lesson on serotonin to be learned from phenylketonuria. Pediatr Res 1973; 7:588–599.
69. Danks DM, Campbell PE, Stevens BJ, Mayne V, Cartwright E. Menkes's kinky hair syndrome: an inherited defect in copper absorption with widespread effects. Pediatrics 1972; 50:188–201.
70. Miles LE, Wilson MA. High incidence of cyclic sleep- wake disorders in the blind. Sleep Res 1977; 6:192.
71. Hashimoto T, Kwano N, Hiura K. Sleep polygraphic studies in Menkes' kinky hair disease: effect of copper administration. Rinsho Noha 1982; 24:418–422.
72. Anguilar MJ, Chadwick DV, Okuyama K. Kinky hair disease I. Clinical and pathological features. J Neuropathol Exp Neurol 1966; 25:507–522.
73. Schultz MA, Schulte FJ, Akiyama Y, Parmelee AHJ. Development of electroencephalographic sleep phenomena in hypothyroid infants. Electroencephalogr Clin Neurophysiol 1968; 25:351–358.
74. Santavuori P. Neuronal ceroid-lipofuscinoses in childhood. Brain Dev 1988; 10:80–83.
75. Santavuori P, Linnankivi T, Jaeken J, Vanhanen SL, Telakivi T, Heiskala H. Psychological symptoms and sleep disturbances in neuronal ceroid-lipofuscinoses (NCL). J Inherit Metab Dis 1993; 16:245–248.
76. Telakivi T, Partinen M, Salmi T. Sleep disturbance in patients with juvenile neuronal ceroid lipofuscinosis: a new application of the SCSB-method. J Ment Defic Res 1985; 29:29–35.
77. Hunt A. Development, behaviour and seizures in 300 cases of tuberous sclerosis. J Intellect Disabil Res 1993; 37:41–51.
78. Hunt A, Stores G. Sleep disorder and epilepsy in children with tuberous sclerosis: a questionnaire-based study. Dev Med Child Neurol 1994; 36:108–115.
79. Bruni O, Cortesi F, Giannotti F, Curatolo P. Sleep disorders in tuberous sclerosis: a polysomnographic study. Brain Dev 1995; 17:52–56.
80. Holm VA, Cassidy SB, Butler MG, Hanchett JM, Greenberg F, Whitmay BY, Greenswag LR. Diagnostic criteria for Prader-Willi syndrome. In: Cassidy SB, ed. Prader-Willi Syndrome and Other Chromosome 15q Deletion Disorders. Berlin: Springer-Verlag, 1992: 105–117.
81. Laurance BM, Brito A, Wilkinson J. Prader-Willi syndrome after age 15 years. Arch Dis Child 1981; 56:181–186.
82. Kaplan J, Frederickson PA, Richardson JW. Sleep and breathing in patients with the Prader-Willi syndrome. Mayo Clin Proc 1991; 66:1124–1126.
83. Sforza E, Krieger J, Geisert J, Kurtz D. Sleep and breathing abnormalities in a case of Prader-Willi syndrome: the effects of acute continuous positive airway pressure treatment. Acta Paediatr Scand 1991; 80:80–85.
84. Hertz G, Cataletto M, Feinsilver SH, Angulo M. Sleep and breathing patterns in patients with Prader-Willi syndrome (PWSD): effects of age and gender. Sleep 1993; 16:366–371.
85. Clift S, Dahlitz M, Parkes JD. Sleep apnoea in the Prader-Willi syndrome. J Sleep Res 1994; 3:12–26.

86. Holm VA, Cassidy SB, Butler MG, Hanchett JM, Greenswag LR, Whitman BY, Greenberg F. Prader-Willi syndrome: consensus diagnostic criteria. Pediatrics 1993; 91: 398–402.
87. Bray GA, Dahms WT, Swerdloff RS, Fiser RH, Atkinson RL, Carrel RE. The Prader-Willi syndrome: a study of 40 patients and a review of the literature. Medicine (Baltimore) 1983; 62:59–80.
88. Vela-Bueno A, Kales A, Soldatos CR, Dobladez-Blanco B, Campos-Castello J, Espino-Hurtado P, Olivan-Palacios J. Sleep in the Prader-Willi syndrome: clinical and polygraphic findings. Arch Neurol 1984; 41:294–296.
89. Cassidy SB, McKilloy JA, Morgan WP. Sleep disorders in the Prader-Willi syndrome. Proc Greenwood Centre 1990; 9:74–75.
90. Helbing-Zwanenburg B, Mourtazaev MS, D'Amaro J, Dahlitz M, vaughan R, Page G, Clift S, Parkes JD, Kamphuisen HA. HLA types in the Prader-Willi syndrome (letter). J Sleep Res 1993; 2:115.
91. Hertz G, Cataletto M, Feinsilver S, Angulo M. HLA typing in Prader-Willi syndrome: lack of evidence for narcolepsy. J Sleep Res 1994; 3:127.
92. Tirosh E, Tal Y, Jaffe M. CPAP treatment of obstructive sleep apnoea and neurodevelopmental deficits. Acta Paediatr 1995; 84:791–794.
93. Stokes DC, Phillips JA, Leonard CO, Dorst JP, Kopits SE, Trojak JE, Brown DL. Respiratory complications of achondroplasia. J Pediatr 1983; 102:534–541.
94. Nelson FW, Hecht JT, Horton WA, Butler IJ, Goldie WD, Miner M. Neurological basis of respiratory complications in achondroplasia. Ann Neurol 1988; 24:89–93.
95. Reid CS, Pyeritz RE, Kopits SE. Cervicomedullary cord compression in young children with achondroplasia: value of comprehensive neurologic and respiratory evaluation. In: Nicolletti B, Kopits SE, Askani E, McKusick VA, eds. Human Achondroplasia: A Multidisciplinary Approach. New York: Plenum Press, 1988: 199–206.
96. Waters KA, Everett F, Sillence D, Fagan E, Sullivan CE. Breathing abnormalities in sleep in achondroplasia. Arch Dis Child 1993; 69:191–196.
97. Zucconi M, Weber G, Castronovo V, Ferini-Strambi L, Russo F, Chiumello G, Smirne S. Sleep and upper airway obstruction in children with achondroplasia. J Pediatr 1996; 129:743–749.
98. Cohen MMJ, Walker GF, Phillips C. A morphometric analysis of the craniofacial configuration in achondroplasia. J Craniofac Genet Dev Biol Suppl 1985; 1:139–165.
99. Piper AJ, Sullivan CE. Sleep-disordered breathing in neuromuscular diseases. In: Saunders NA, Sullivan CE, eds. Sleep and Breathing, 2d ed. New York: Marcel Dekker, 1994: 761–786.
100. Manni R, Ottolini A, Cerveri I, Bruschi C, Zoia MC, Lanzi G, Tartara A. Breathing patterns and $HbSaO_2$ changes during nocturnal sleep in patients with Duchenne muscular dystrophy. J Neurol 1989; 236:391–394.
101. Bye PT, Ellis ER, Issa FG, Donnelly PM, Sullivan CE. Respiratory failure and sleep in neuromuscular disease. Thorax 1990; 45:241–247.
102. Calverley PM. Sleep-related breathing disorders: 7. Sleep and breathing problems in general medicine. Thorax 1995; 50:1311–1316.
103. Khan Y, Heckmatt JZ. Obstructive apnoeas in Duchenne muscular dystrophy (see comments). Thorax 1994; 49:157–161.
104. Smith PE, Calverley PM, Edwards RH. Hypoxemia during sleep in Duchenne muscular dystrophy. Am Rev Respir Dis 1988; 137:884–888.
105. Smith PE, Edwards RH, Calverley PM. Mechanisms of sleep-disordered breathing in

chronic neuromuscular disease: implications for management. Q J Med 1991; 81:961–973.
106. Carroll N, Bain RJ, Smith PE, Saltissi S, Edwards RH, Calverley PM. Domiciliary investigation of sleep-related hypoxaemia in Duchenne muscular dystrophy. Eur Respir J 1991; 4:434–440.
107. Ferini-Strambi L, Castronovo V, Zucconi M, Oldani A, Smirne S. Nocturnal oxygen desaturations and cardiac variability in X-linked muscular dystrophy. Sleep Res 1995; 24:389.
108. Cirignotta F, Mondini S, Zucconi M, Barrot-Cortes E, Sturani C, Schiavina M, Coccagna G, Lugaresi E. Sleep-related breathing impairment in myotonic dystrophy. J Neurol 1987; 235:80–85.
109. Guilleminault C. Sleep disorders in children. In: Berg BO, ed. Neurological Aspects of Pediatrics. Boston: Butterworth Heinemann, 1992: 617–626.
110. Broughton R, Stuss D, Kates M, Roberts J, Dunham W. Neuropsychological deficits and sleep in myotonic dystrophy. Can J Neurol Sci 1990; 17:410–415.
111. Ono S, Kurisaki H, Sakuma A, Nagao K. Myotonic dystrophy with alveolar hypoventilation and hypersomnia: a clinicopathological study. J Neurol Sci 1995; 128:225–231.
112. Popoviciu L, Szabo L. Polygraph study of sleep in nocturnal ambulatory automatism. Rev Roum Neurol 1970; 7:27–46.
113. Fuster B, Cstells C, Etcheverry M. Epileptic sleep terrors. Neurology 1954; 531–540.
114. Tassinari CA, Mancia D, Della Bernardina B, Gastaut H. Pavor nocturnus of non-epileptic nature in epileptic children. Electroencephalogr Clin Neurophysiol 1972; 33:603–607.
115. Fischer C, Byrne, Edward A, Kahn E. A psychophysiological study of nightmares. Am Psychoanal Assoc 1970; 18:747–782.
116. Gastaut H, Broughton R. A clinical and polygraphic study of episodic phenomena during sleep. Biol Psychiatry 1965; 7:197–221.
117. Shouse MN. Sleep, sleep disorders, and epilepsy in children. In: Guilleminault C, ed. Sleep and Its Disorders in Children. New York: Raven Press, 1987: 291–307.
118. Broughton RJ. Sleep disorders: disorders of arousal? Enuresis, somnambulism, and nightmares occur in confusional states of arousal, not in "dreaming sleep." Science 1968; 159:1070–1078.
119. Guilleminault C, Silvestri R. Disorders of arousal and epilepsy during sleep. In Sterman MB, Shouse MN, Passouant P, eds. Sleep and Epilepsy. New York: Academic Press, 1982: 513–531.
120. Fischer C, Kahn E, Edwards A, Davids DM. A psychophysiological study of nightmares and night terrors: I. Physiological aspects of the stage 4 night terror. J Nerv Ment Dis 1973; 57:75–98.
121. Pedley TA, Guilleminault C. Episodic nocturnal wanderings responsive to anticonvulsant drug therapy. Ann Neurol 1977; 2:30–35.
122. Peled R, Lavie P. Paroxysmal awakenings from sleep associated with excessive daytime somnolence: a form of nocturnal epilepsy. Neurology 1986; 36:95–98.
123. Montagna P, Procaccianti G, Lugaresi A, Zucconi M, Lugaresi E. Diurnal variability in cranial dystonia. Mov Disord 1990; 5:44–46.
124. Montagna P. Nocturnal paroxysmal dystonia and nocturnal wandering. Neurology 1992; 42:61–67.
125. Scheffer IE, Bhatia KP, Lopes-Cendes I, Fish DR, Marsden CD, Andermann F, Andermann E, Desbiens R, Cendes F, Manson JI. Autosomal dominant frontal epilepsy misdiagnosed as sleep disorder (see comments). Lancet 1994; 343:515–517.

126. Scheffer IE, Bhatia KP, Lopes-Cendes I, Fish DR, Marsden CD, Andermann E, Andermann F, Desbiens R, Keene D, Cendes F. Autosomal dominant nocturnal frontal lobe epilepsy: a distinctive clinical disorder. Brain 1995; 118:61–73.
127. Oldani A, Zucconi M, Ferini-Strambi L, Bizzozero D, Smirne S. Autosomal dominant nocturnal frontal lobe epilepsy: electroclinical picture (see comments). Epilepsia 1996; 37:964–976.
128. Oldani A, Zucconi M, Asselta R, Modugno M, Bonati MT, Dalpra L, Malcovati M, Tenchini ML, Smirne S, Ferini-Strambi L. Autosomal dominant nocturnal frontal lobe epilepsy: a video-polysomnographic and genetic appraisal of 40 patients and delineation of the epileptic syndrome. Brain 1998; 121:205–223.
129. Plazzi G, Tinuper P, Montagna P, Provini F, Lugaresi E. Epileptic nocturnal wanderings. Sleep 1995; 18:749–756.
130. Zucconi M, Oldani A, Ferini-Stramgi L, Smirne S. Arousal fluctuations in non-rapid eye movement parasomnias: the role of cyclic alternating pattern as a measure of sleep instability. J Clin Neurophysiol 1995; 12:147–154.
131. Zucconi M, Oldani A, Ferini-Strambi L, Bizzozero D, Smirne S. Nocturnal paroxysmal arousal with motor behaviors during sleep: frontal lobe epilepsy or parasomnia? J Clin Neurophysiol 1997; 14:513–522.
132. Kales A, Jacobson A, Paulson MJ, Kales JD, Walter RD. Somnambulism: psychophysiological correlates. I. All-night EEG studies. Arch Gen Psychiatry 1966; 14:586–594.
133. Kales A, Paulson MJ, Jacobson A, Kales JD. Somnambulism: psychophysiological correlates. II. Psychiatric interviews, psychological testing, and discussion. Arch Gen Psychiatry 1966; 14:595–604.
134. Mahowald MW, Schenck CH. Parasomnia purgatory: the epileptic/non-epileptic parasomnia interface. In: Rowan AJ, Gates JR, eds. Non epileptic seizures. Boston: Butterworth-Heinemann, 1993: 123–139.
135. Zucconi M, Ferini-Strambi L, Oldani A, Bizzozero D, Smirne S. Nocturnal motor behaviors in children: a video-polysomnographic study. Sleep 1998; 21(suppl):148.
136. Landau-Ferey J. A contribution to the study of nocturnal sleep in patients suspected of having epilepsy. In: Sterman MB, Shouse MN, Passouant P, eds. Sleep and Epilepsy. New York: Academic Press, 1982: 421–430.
137. Wolf P, Roder U. Sleep patterns in untreated epileptics with seizures during sleep or after awakening. In: Sterman MB, Shouse MN, Passouant P, eds. Sleep and Epilepsy. New York: Academic Press, 1982: 411–420.
138. Horita H, Kumagai K, Maekawa K, Endo S. Overnight polygraphic study of agenesis of the corpus callosum with seizures resembling infantile spasms. Brain Dev 1980; 2:379–386.
139. Hrachovy RA, Frost JDJ, Kellaway P. Sleep characteristics in infantile spasms. Neurology 1981; 31:688–693.
140. Rowan AJ, Veldhuisen RJ, Nagelkerke NJ. Comparative evaluation of sleep deprivation and sedated sleep EEGs as diagnostic aids in epilepsy. Electroencephalogr Clin Neurophysiol 1982; 54:357–364.
141. Laakso ML, Leinonen L, Hatonen T, Alila A, Heiskala H. Melatonin, cortisol and body temperature rhythms in Lennox-Gastaut patients with or without circadian rhythm sleep disorders. J Neurol 1993; 240:410–416.
142. Molina-Carballo A, Acuna-Castroviejo D, Rodriguez-Cabezas T, Munoz-Hoyos A. Effects of febrile and epileptic convulsions on daily variations in plasma melatonin concentration in children. J Pineal Res 1994; 16:1–9.

143. Molina-Carballo A, Munoz-Hoyos A, Rodriguez-Cabezas T, Acuna-Castroviejo D. Day-night variations in melatonin secretion by the pineal gland during febrile and epileptic convulsions in children. Psychiatry Res 1994; 52:273–283.
144. Terzano MG, Parrino L, Garofalo PG, Durisotti C, Filati-Roso C. Activation of partial seizures with motor signs during cyclic alternating pattern in human sleep. Epilepsy Res 1991; 10:166–173.
145. Terzano MG, Parrino L. Evaluation of EEG cyclic alternating pattern during sleep in insomniacs and controls under placebo and acute treatment with zolpidem. Sleep 1992; 15:64–70.
146. Terzano MG, Monge-Strauss MF, Mikol F, Spaggiari MC, Parrino L. Cyclic alternating pattern as a provocative factor in nocturnal paroxysmal dystonia. Epilepsia 1997; 38:1015–1025.
147. Shouse MN, Langer J, King A, Alcalde O, Bier M, Szymusiak R, Wada Y. Paroxysmal microarousals in amygdala-kindled kittens: could they be subclinical seizures? Epilepsia 1995; 36:290–300.
148. Malow BA, Kushwaha R, Lin X, Morton KJ, Aldrich MS. Relationship of interictal epileptiform discharges to sleep depth in partial epilepsy. Electroencephalogr Clin Neurophysiol 1997; 102:20–26.

17

Sleep in Children with Behavioral and Psychiatric Disorders

AMY R. WOLFSON and STEPHANIE V. TRENTACOSTE

College of the Holy Cross
Worcester, Massachusetts

RONALD E. DAHL

University of Pittsburgh Medical Center
Pittsburgh, Pennsylvania

I. Introduction

It is estimated that 15% to 20% of children and nearly 40% of adolescents experience a significant behavioral or emotional disorder sufficient to disrupt school, social, or family functioning (1,2). Difficulties related to behavioral and emotional control have become one of the leading sources of morbidity and mortality among youth in our nation. Problems related to depression, suicide, anxiety, attention-deficit disorders, alcohol and drug use, eating disorders, risk-taking behaviors/accidents, and aggression-related problems represent the leading causes of death and disability among children and adolescents in our nation (3). Many of these problems not only impair (and imperil) the lives of youth but also lead to lifetime adult disorders like depression and substance abuse and contribute to the soaring rates of incarceration among young adults.

For clinicians evaluating children with symptoms of possible sleep disorders, it is essential to underscore the overlap between sleep regulation and behavioral/emotional problems in children and adolescents. There is clearly two-way interaction between these systems. The development, regulation, and timing of sleep can be altered by behavioral/emotional disorders, while cognitive, behavioral, and emotional control during daytime hours can be influenced by the way children and adolescents sleep. Further, daytime activities, changes in the environment, and stressful events can have profound transient effects on children's sleeping patterns in the absence of any clear-cut psychopathology. Additionally, medications used to treat psychiatric disorders often affect sleep, and sleep loss can exacerbate mood and behavioral symptoms.

Clinically, it can be extremely difficult to tease apart the boundaries of these overlapping and interacting domains. For example, it can be impossible to retrospectively determine whether disturbed sleep symptoms antedated symptoms of depression or vice versa. Sleep interacts with both internalizing disorders (i.e., the primary symptoms are directed internally—such as depression or anxiety) as well as externalizing disorders [i.e., the primary symptoms are externally directed problems with behavior—such as attention-deficit/hyperactivity disorder (ADHD) and conduct problems]. This general classification (internalizing and externalizing disorders) forms the organization for the discussion below of the relationships to sleep in children and adolescents.

II. Sleep Alterations in Depression and Anxiety Disorders (Internalizing Disorders)

Many researchers believe that mood disorders in children and adolescents represent one of the most underdiagnosed emotional disorders in the mental health field. Population studies report prevalence rates of depression in children between 0.4% and 2.5% and in adolescents 4% and 8.5% (see review by Birmaher et al., Ref. 4). The epidemiological literature also reveals evidence for a secular increase in rates of depression among children over recent times. Further, the increased rates of depression seen in females appears to begin at midpuberty; rates of depression in boys and girls are similar until about midadolescence, when girls are twice as likely as boys to be diagnosed with depression (5).

Although mental health professionals recognize the existence of childhood depression, parents, teachers, and pediatricians often miss the disorder. Part of the problem is the *internalizing* nature of the symptoms—that is, children may not express complaints or symptoms unless questioned directly. Thus, it is critical for clinicians to actively probe about possible symptoms of depression—particularly in adolescents presenting with symptoms of insomnia. Symptoms are, in general, similar to those of adult depression, with some minor exceptions (see Table 1) (6). Depressed children/adolescents may also exhibit clinging behaviors, school refusal, exaggerated fears, and social withdrawal from family and/or peer activities. The evaluation of clinical symptoms of possible depression is best guided by the definition of major depressive disorder given by the *Diagnostic and Statistical Manual of Mental Disorders* (DSM-IV) (7). Typically, the presence of symptoms is evaluated by questionnaires such as the Beck Depression Inventory (BDI) or a structured interview such as the Schedule for Affective Disorders and Schizophrenia (K-SADS-PL) (8,9).

It is also important to emphasize that comorbidity with other disorders occurs frequently—particularly with anxiety disorders and with some externalizing disorders

Table 1 Symptoms of Depression

Depressed, unhappy, hopeless mood
Loss of pleasure/interest in usual activities
Disturbed appetite
Slowed or agitated movement and activity
Loss of energy or motivation
Feelings of worthlessness and guilt
Difficulties in thinking, concentrating, and/or remembering
Recurrent thoughts of death or suicide

Source: From Ref. 6.

including ADHD and conduct disorder. Consultation with a child psychiatrist or psychologist may be necessary to sort out complicated diagnostic issues in some cases with sleep symptoms and multiple behavioral and emotional symptoms.

Subjective sleep complaints are very common in children and adolescents diagnosed with major depressive disorder (MDD). Symptoms include insomnia (75% of cases) and hypersomnia (25%) (6). Hypersomnia difficulties are reported more frequently after puberty. Insomnia symptoms usually include difficulty falling asleep and a subjective sense of not having slept deeply all night. Early morning awakenings are less prevalent in children and adolescents than in adults with depression. Recently, clinicians and researchers have seen increasing numbers of adolescents with overlapping phase-delay disorders and/or other sleep-wake schedule disorders with depression (6,10). Depressed adolescents frequently have difficulty falling asleep, are unable to get up or refuse to go to school, sleep in late in the day, complain of extreme daytime fatigue and, over time, shift to increasingly more delayed sleep-wake schedules. Likewise, surveys in adolescents who obtain less than 6 ¾ hr of sleep each school night and/or report more than 2- hr differences between school night and weekend bedtimes reveal more complaints of depressed mood than adolescents getting more sleep and/or on more regular sleep-wake schedules (11). Clinicians experienced with these problems have pointed out that in many cases it is difficult to differentiate decreased motivation, school refusal/anxiety, delayed circadian phase, attention difficulties, and depressive symptomatology (10,12). Clearly, both sleep patterns and behavioral symptoms must be carefully assessed for prevention, accurate diagnosis, and/or treatment planning.

III. Sleep Studies in Depression

While electroencephalographic (EEG) studies in adult depression show a clear pattern of altered sleep regulation and *subjective* sleep complaints are quite prominent in depressed children and adolescents, *objective* (EEG) studies comparing depressed youth and normal controls have revealed a somewhat inconsistent pattern of findings.

In childhood depression (defined here as Tanner stage 1 or 2), increased sleep latency has been the most reliable finding associated with depression. Although reduced REM latency has been found in one controlled study (13), the majority of childhood studies these have been negative for differences in REM latency (14–17). However, in a follow-up study, where no baseline REM latency differences had been seen, a cholinergic challenge (with arecoline) resulted in reduced REM latency in depressed children compared to normal controls studied in the same environment (18).

The studies of depressed adolescents (ages 12 to 18 and Tanner stages 3, 4, and 5) have revealed a somewhat intermediate pattern between child and adult studies. Some studies have reported reduced REM latency in inpatient samples of depressed adolescents (19–21), while most outpatient studies have found negative or inconsistent results (21–23). With careful attention to sleep-wake schedule issues and adaptation to setting, reduced REM latency and prolonged sleep latency were detected in depressed adolescents (24). Increased REM density has also been seen in some studies, including a study that indicated increased REM density associated with increased recurrence of depressive episodes (25). Although these studies raised interesting questions regarding the pathophysiology and links between sleep changes and depression, it is important to emphasize that, from a clinical prospective, EEG sleep studies have not been found to contribute to diagnosis or treatment issues.

Treatment of sleep complaints and problems—including regularizing the sleep-wake schedule, cognitive behavioral therapy for insomnia, and/or short term medication treatment for severe insomnia—can have a positive impact on depressive symptoms in some cases (26). On the other hand, effective treatment of the depression can also be a critical aspect of improving the sleep.

A further area of overlap with adolescent insomnia, adolescent depression, and adolescent anxiety problems involves the tendency for adolescents to have distressing or negative cognitive ruminations at bedtime. Helping these patients to focus on positive images, relaxing thoughts, and engaging imagery associated with good positive emotions can be an important aspect of treatment. Similarly, careful attention to sleep-wake schedules (including consistency on weekends) and the frequent occurrence of delayed sleep-phase syndrome in adolescents must also be considered. Although anecdotal evidence suggests that melatonin has a role, controlled studies at this time indicate that cognitive and behavioral interventions around sleep schedules are probably of greater effectiveness.

IV. Sleep and Anxiety Disorders

The clinical picture for sleep changes in anxiety disorders largely parallels that described for depression, albeit with much less data on sleep. Anxiety disorders are quite common in children and adolescents, yet they often go undiagnosed. (For a review of anxiety disorders, see Ref. 27.) Subjective complaints of difficulty falling asleep and frequent nighttime awakening are common in children and adolescents with anxiety disorders. Increased fear and vigilance are in many ways antithetical to sleep, since sleep is in essence a behavioral cessation of vigilance. Feelings of danger or threat (emotional as well as physical) appear to interfere with the context of safety necessary to promote normal sleep onset and continuity. Adequate treatment of anxiety disorders, including cognitive behavioral interventions focused on the period proceeding sleep onset, can be an important component of treatment for these problems. The issues regarding sleep-wake schedules, sleep hygiene, and treatment of the primary disorder are very similar to those discussed in relation to depression.

V. Sleep in Externalizing Disorders: (Attention Deficit–Hyperactivity Disorder, Conduct Disorder, Oppositional Defiant Disorder)

Externalizing disorders is a general term that designates behavioral problems manifesting primarily in the expression of undesirable behaviors. These include ADHD (where inattentiveness and distractibility are core aspects of the problem), conduct disorder, and oppositional defiant disorder (where aggression and transgression of rules represent the core symptoms). (For a clinical overview and diagnoses of these disorders, see the review conducted by Corkum et al., Ref. 28.) Table 2 displays the symptoms associated with ADHD.

Most of the work addressing sleep changes with respect to externalizing disorders has been focussed on ADHD. Numerous clinicians and researchers have commented on the complex relationships between sleep and ADHD symptoms. There are four primary observations regarding this relationship: 1) children diagnosed with ADHD have high rates of subjective sleep complaints (and some evidence of sleep disturbances); 2) children obtaining insufficient sleep or with sleep disruption frequently show signs of inattentiveness (sometimes including hyperactivity); 3) stimulant medications used to treat ADDs can also interfere with sleep; and 4) behavioral problems associated with ADHD (as well as the other conduct disorder and oppositional defiant disorder) can interfere with bedtime organization and scheduling and thus can contribute to insufficient sleep from late and erratic bedtimes.

Table 2 Symptoms of Attention Deficit/Hyperactivity Disorder

Difficulty attending to details
Difficulty sustaining attention
Trouble listening when others are talking
Difficulty finishing tasks
Trouble organizing behaviors
Easily distracted and forgetful
Difficulty sitting still and engaging in quiet activities
Impulsive, interrupts, blurts out responses when others are talking
Difficulty waiting his or her turn

In addition to these general observations, there is some controversy regarding the degree of sleep disruption associated with ADHD. Although questionnaire and survey data of ADHD children and controls show very high rates of sleep problems and complaints, in general the more objective the study (including structured interviews and EEG studies), the weaker is the evidence for sleep abnormalities associated with ADHD (29,30). One apparent myth in this area is the suggestion that ADHD children *require* less sleep than normal age-matched children. The data in this regard indicate that ADHD children are more difficult to wake up on school mornings, suggesting that, if anything, ADHD children are getting less sleep than they require (30).

Two recent studies, however, have shown evidence for sleep disruption in some ADHD children. Recent studies reported increased rates of snoring as well as periodic limb movements in children with ADHD compared to controls (31,32). Clearly, better-controlled studies in these areas are necessary to understand the sleep changes associated with ADHD.

From a clinical perspective, children with ADHD should be thoroughly assessed for sleep problems (including clinical interview and sleep logs) addressing the presence of sleep symptoms and problems. The possibility of sleep apnea, periodic limb movements, narcolepsy, insufficient sleep secondary to behavioral or sleep-wake schedule problems, or other sleep disruptions should be assessed clinically. At this time it appears that the decision regarding a polysomnographic study should be made on an individual basis depending on the clinical assessment.

In addition, there is evidence for increased rates of ADHD symptoms in clinical populations of children with sleep disorders including children with obstructive sleep apneas (OSAS), periodic limb movement syndrome (PLMS), narcolepsy, and sleep-wake schedule disorders (30–34). Studies indicate that treating the primary sleep disorder can produce significant improvement in ADHD symptoms (35,36). Thus, additional recommendations for working with children and adolescents with ADHD symptoms and sleep problems include the following:

If there is any suggestion that the child with ADHD is obtaining insufficient sleep, behavioral interventions should be implemented to maximize sleep (including adequate time in bed and following a regular sleep-wake schedule).

Children who present with clinical evidence of sleep disorders (such as sleep apnea, narcolepsy, and PLMS) should receive optimal treatment for the primary sleep disorders.

Regarding sleep and the use of stimulant medications, stimulant medications used to treat ADHD can clearly show complex interactions with sleep patterns and problems. In some cases, stimulants or even a third dose of stimulant or long-acting stimulant seems to improve sleep by a more organized behavior in the evening, leading to an earlier bedtime and sleep onset. In other cases, stimulant medication does not seem to have any effect on sleep, whereas in some cases late dose stimulants or long-acting stimulants can clearly interfere with sleep onset (37–39). Once again, given the individual variation, decisions about medication affects must be considered on a case-by-case basis.

VI. Case Discussion

In the section below, cases are presented that highlight some of the complex issues that arise for children and adolescents that experience both depression and/or ADHD symptoms combined with problematic sleep behaviors and habits. These vignettes should give clinicians a sense of some of the issues and treatment approaches for these children and their families.

Case 1

J.S., a 14-year-old teenager, moved from the West Coast to a moderate-size northeastern city just before starting high school in ninth grade. She had a history of poor sleep habits (e.g., bedtimes past midnight, erratic sleep-wake schedule since about sixth grade, and described by her parents as a short sleeper prior to puberty). Her mother noted that J.S. rarely napped as a toddler and never seemed tired during her elementary school years. J.S.'s new high school started at 7:30 A.M. and she had a very difficult time getting up for school at that hour because her average bedtime was 2:00 A.M. Often she stayed up working on her computer and/or watching television. Before long she was sleeping through her alarm, missing school or arriving late, and/or finding friends' cars to nap in throughout the school day. J.S. started to fail classes and appeared increasingly more lethargic, subdued, and disinterested in school. Her school counselor referred her to a mental health clinic. Over the course of several months she was diagnosed with depression with some ADHD symptoms (e.g., difficulty finishing tasks, easily distracted, etc.). Later, a sleep specialist diagnosed J.S. with a circadian rhythm disorder, delayed sleep phase type, and worked with her to reset her circadian clock (e.g., combination of chronotherapy and light treatment). Although she continued psychotherapy for her depression and adjustment problems, treating and educating J.S. and her parents about sleep hygiene and the risks associated with delaying sleep were helpful. Throughout the course of treatment, J.S.'s parents and teachers reported that she was more motivated, less depressed and irritable, and more socially engaged when she remained on a more regular sleep-wake schedule.

Case 2

M.T., a 15-year-old boy, had a 2 year history of difficulty getting to sleep at night (usually falling asleep at 2 or 3 A.M.). He had trouble awakening in the morning, was distractible, had behavior problems at school. He also reported some symptoms of depression, including loss of interest in some activities, daytime fatigue, and worsening performance at school. M.T. had missed so much school (greater than 40 days in one school year) that his family was encountering legal difficulties with the school district. His mother complained that no one understood how hard the family had been struggling with M.T.'s sleep problems and how, despite all their efforts to send him to bed earlier and try to awaken him for school, this was an impossible pattern to change. After a lengthy evaluation, M.T. was not found to have a major depression. A trial of delayed-phase chronotherapy (successively delaying bedtime and rise time by 3 hr a night for six consecutive nights until sleep was realigned to an 11 P.M.–7 A.M. schedule) was initially successful. When M.T. was sleeping on his new schedule (for 2 weeks), he showed moderate improvement in many of his previous symptoms. However, he refused to comply with the schedule on weekends. Returning to a 3- to 4- A.M. bedtime on Friday and Saturday nights, he quickly reverted to his previous patterns despite several attempts to intervene. Eventually, he stated quite directly that his late-night activities and social life were too important to him, making him unwilling to give them up just to be able to wake up in time for school. Another clinician tried a trial of antidepressant medication, which was also unsuccessful in improving his problems.

Case 3

R.F., a 10-year-old boy, had difficulty getting to bed and to sleep at night, was difficult to awaken in the morning, and ADHD symptoms resulting in significant school and social difficulties. On a sleep log it was apparent that he was often obtaining less than 6 to 7 hr of sleep on school nights. He did not show daytime sleepiness (was hyperactive and distractible) but did often seem tired and irritable to his parents and was observed to fall asleep during car rides (if he did not have access to stimulating activities such as his hand-held video games). Following a behavioral intervention targeting bedtime behaviors and habits, his nighttime sleep increased to 8.5 hours and he showed significant improvement in many of his daytime symptoms of inattention, irritability, and emotional lability. He did, however, continue to show many ADHD symptoms and continued to require daytime stimulant medication for optimal functioning at school.

VII. Summary and Conclusions

This chapter reviewed the current research on sleep-wake patterns, sleep problems, and changes in sleep architecture associated with depression and other emotional disorders in child and adolescent populations. Children diagnosed with major depression, attention deficit-hyperactivity disorder, and other related emotional/behavioral disorders frequently have disrupted sleep-wake schedules and changes in sleep architecture. Similarly, children and adolescents with insufficient sleep, irregular sleep habits, and other sleep problems experience depressed mood, assorted behavioral difficulties, and generally difficulty functioning at school, on the job, and elsewhere. The recognition, investigation, and clinical care of sleep problems and emotional/behavioral symptoms span a number of disciplines—child psychiatry, developmental/child clinical psychology, pediatrics, neurology, and education. Clearly, children and adolescents' sleep needs to be given far more educational prominence in the professions concerned with the physical well-being, emotional welfare, and education of children.

References

1. Newman DL, Moffitt TE, Caspi A, Magdol L. J Consult Clin Psychol 1996; 64:552–562.
2. Institute of Medicine Report of Research on Child and Adolescents with Mental, Behavioral and Developmental Disorders. National Institute of Mental Health, U.S. Department of Health and Human Services. DHHS Pub. # (ADM901659), 1990.
3. Resnick MD, Bearman PS, Blum RW, Bauman KE, Harris KM, Jones J, Tabor J, Beuhring T, Sieving RE, Shew M, Ireland M, Bearinger LH, Udry JR. Protecting adolescents from harm: findings from the national longitudinal study on adolescent health. JAMA 1997; 278:10:823.
4. Birmaher B, Ryan ND, Brent DA, Williamson DE, Kaufman J, Dahl RE, Perel J, Nelson B. Childhood and adolescent depression: a review of the past ten years, Part I. J Am Acad Child Adolesc Psychiatry 1996; 35:11:1427–1439.
5. Birmaher B, Ryan ND, Brent DA, Williamson DE, Kaufman J. Childhood and adolescent depression: a review of the past ten years, Part II. J Am Acad Child Adolesc Psychiatry 1996; 35:1575–1583.
6. Dahl RE, Carskadon MA. Sleep in its disorders in adolescence. In: Ferber R, Kryger M, eds. Principles and Practice of Sleep Medicine in the Child. Philadelphia: Saunders, 1995: 19–27.
7. Diagnostic and Statistical Manual of Mental Disorders, 4th ed (DSM-IV). Washington, DC: American Psychiatric Association, 1994.
8. Beck AT, Ward C, Mendelson M, Mock J, Erbaugh J. An inventory for measuring depression. Arch Gen Psychiatry 1961; 4:561–571.
9. Chambers RD, Puig-Antich J, Hirsch M. The assessment of affective disorders in children and adolescents by semi-structured interview. Arch Gen Psychiatry 1985; 42:696–702.
10. Dahl RE. Sleep in behavioral and emotional disorders. In: Ferber R, Kryger M, eds. Principles and Practice of Sleep Medicine in the Child. Philadelphia: Saunders, 1995: 147–153.
11. Wolfson A, Carskadon M. Sleep schedules and daytime functioning in adolescents. Child Dev 1998; 69:875–887.
12. Ferber R. Clinical assessment of child and adolescent sleep disorders. In: Dahl R, ed. Child and Adolescent Psychiatric Clinics of North America: Sleep Disorders. Philadelphia: Saunders, 1996: 569–579.
13. Emslie GJ, Rush AJ, Weinberg WA, Rintelmann JW, Roffwarg HP. Children with major depression show reduced rapid eye movement latencies. Arch Gen Psychiatry 1990; 47:119–124.
14. Puig-Antich J, Goetz R, Hanlon C, Tabrizi MA, Davies M, Weitzmand E. Sleep architecture and REM sleep measures in prepubertal major depressives: studies during recovery from a major depressive episode in a drug free state. Arch Gen Psychiatry 1983; 40: 187–192.
15. Dahl RE, Ryan ND, Birmaher B, Al-Shabbout M, Williamson DE, Neidig M, Nelson B, Puig-Antich J. EEG sleep measures in prepubertal depression. Psychiatry Res 1991; 38:201–214.

16. Young W, Knowles JB, MacLean AW, Boag L, McConville BJ. The sleep of childhood depressives: comparison with age-matched controls. Biol Psychiatry 1982; 17:1163–1169.
17. Dahl RE, Ryan N, Birmaher B, Al-Shabbout M, Nelson B. Altered sleep/growth hormone in childhood depression. Sleep Res 1996; 25:158.
18. Dahl RE, Ryan ND, Perel J, Birmaher B, Al-Shabbout M, Nelson B, Puig-Antich J. Cholinergic REM induction test with arecoline in depressed children. Psychiatry Res 1994; 51:3:269–282.
19. Emslie GJ, Rush AJ, Weinberg WA, Rintelmann JW, Roffwarg HP. Sleep EEG features of adolescents with major depression. Biol Psychiatry 1994; 36:573–581.
20. Kutcher S, Williamson P, Szalai J, Marton P. REM latency in endogenously depressed adolescents. Br J Psychiatry 1992; 161:399–402.
21. Dahl RE, Puig-Antich J, Ryan ND, Cunningham S, Nelson B, Klepper T. EEG sleep in adolescents with major depression: the role of suicidality and inpatient status. J Affect Disorder 1990; 19:63–75.
22. Goetz R, Puig-Antich J, Ryan N, Rabinovich H, Ambrosini PJ, Nelson B, Krawiec V. Electroencephalographic sleep of adolescents with major depression and normal controls. Arch Gen Psychiatry 1987; 44:61–68.
23. Kahn AU, Todd S. Polysomnographic findings in adolescents with major depression. Psychiatry Res 1990; 33:313–320.
24. Dahl RE, Ryan ND, Matty MK, Birmaher B, Al-Shabbout M, Williamson DE, Kupfer DJ. Sleep onset abnormalities in depressed adolescents. Biol Psychiatry 1996; 39:6:400–410.
25. Rao U, Dahl RE, Ryan ND, Birmaher B, Williamson DE, Giles DE, Rao R, Kaufman J, Nelson B. The relationship between longitudinal clinical course and sleep and cortisol changes in adolescent depression. Biol Psychiatry 1996; 40:474–484.
26. Dahl RE, Ryan ND. The psychobiology of adolescent depression. In: Picchetti D, Toth SL, eds. Rochester Symposium on Developmental Psychopathology, Volume VII: Adolescence: Opportunities and Challenges. Rochester, NY: University of Rochester Press, 1996: 197–232.
27. Bernstein GA, Borchardt CM, Pervien AR. Anxiety disorders in children and adolescents: a review of the past 10 years. J Am Acad Child Adolesc Psychiatry 1996; 35:9: 1110–1119.
28. Corkum P, Tannock R, Moldofsky H. Sleep disturbances in children with attention-deficit/hyperactivity disorder. J Am Acad Child Adolesc Psychiatry 1998; 37:637–646.
29. Kaplan BJ, McNicol J, Conte RA, Moghadam HK. Sleep disturbance in preschool-aged hyperactive and nonhyperactive children. Pediatrics 1987; 80:839–844.
30. Dahl RE, Pelham WE, Greenslade KE, Cunningham SL. Sleep disturbances in children with attention deficit disorder. J Dev Behav Pediatr 1991; 11:4:217.
31. Chervin RD, Dillon JE, Bassetti C, Ganoczy DA, Pituch KJ. Pediatrics and sleep: symptoms of sleep disorders, inattention, and hyperactivity in children. Sleep 1997; 20: 1185–1192.
32. Picchietti DI, Walters AS. Restless legs syndrome and periodic limb movement disorder in children and adolescents: comorbidity with attention-deficit hyperactivity disorder. Child Adolesc Psychiatr Clin North Am 1996; 5:729–740.
33. Guilleminault C, Winkle R, Korobkin R, Simmons B. Children and nocturnal snoring—evaluation of the effects of sleep related respiratory resistive load and daytime functioning. Eur J Pediatr 1982; 139:165–171.

34. Ali NJ, Pitson D, Stradling JR. Sleep disordered breathing: effects of adenotonsillectomy on behaviour and psychological functioning. Eur J Pediatr 1996; 155:56–62.
35. Ali NJ, Pitson DJ, Stradling JR. Snoring, sleep disturbance, and behaviour in 4–5 year olds. Arch Dis Child 1993; 68:360–366.
36. Dahl RE, Pelham WB, Wierson MC. The role of sleep disturbance in attention deficit disorder symptomatology: a case study. J Pediatr Psychol 1991; 16:2:229–239.
37. Feinberg I, Hibi S, Braum M, Cavness C, Westerman G, Small A. Sleep amphetamine effects in MBDS and normal subjects. Arch Gen Psychiatry 1974; 31:723–731.
38. Chatoor I, Wells KC, Conners CK, Seidel WT, Shaw D. The effects of nocturnally administered stimulant medication on EEG sleep and behavior in hyperactive children. J Am Acad Child Psychiatry 1983; 22:337–342.
39. Dahl RE. Child and adolescent sleep disorders. In Dahl RE, ed. Child and Adolescent Psychiatric Clinics of North America: Sleep Disorder. Philadelphia: Saunders, 1996.

18

Gastroesophageal Reflux and Sleep

Does One Affect the Other?

JUDITH M. SONDHEIMER

University of Colorado Health Sciences Center
and The Children's Hospital
Denver, Colorado

I. Introduction

Does gastroesophageal reflux disease (GERD) have an impact upon the quantity and quality of sleep? Conversely, does sleep have an impact upon the frequency and duration of gastroesophageal reflux? Neither of these interrelated questions has been satisfactorily answered. In this chapter we will look at the data on these two important questions.

II. Effects of Sleep on Gastroesophageal Reflux

In 1974, Johnson and DeMeester published the results of the first prolonged recordings of distal esophageal pH in adults with symptomatic GERD (1). One of the observations from these original studies was that body position had a strong impact upon acid reflux episodes, with frequent short episodes occurring in the upright position and infrequent, but much longer episodes occurring while supine. It was assumed that body position was the key to this difference, and the fact that the patients were sleeping during supine recordings was all but ignored. Subsequent studies showed that all normal adults and children experience short reflux episodes in the upright position, especially after meals, but that reflux nearly disappears during sleep. In normal infants, reflux frequency decreases from 1.5 episodes per hour while awake to 0.4 episodes per hour during sleep. Acid clearance time (average duration of reflux episodes) increases from 1.5 min while awake to 5.4 min during sleep. Similar changes in episode frequency and duration while awake and asleep have been found in children with pathological reflux, though at a more abnormal level (2).

Probably the major mechanism by which sleep and/or recumbency decreases the frequency of reflux episodes is by reducing the frequency of transient lower esophageal sphincter relaxations (TLESR) (3,4). In adults, TLESRs are the most important mechanism permitting the reflux of gastric contents into the esophagus (5,6). The average frequency of TLESRs varies from study to study but is in the range of 8 per hour while awake. TLESRs are more frequent in the immediate postprandial period (6). During sleep, transient relaxations of the LES are suppressed, occurring primarily during periods of arousal. The suppression of TLESRs during sleep is independent of the volume or acidity of the gastric contents, both of which influence the frequency of TLESRs in awake subjects (7,8). It is reasonable to assume that there will be fewer reflux episodes when the number of TLESRs are decreased during sleep.

Other physiological changes during sleep affect the duration of reflux episodes. The frequency of swallowing is drastically diminished. Swallowing is the principal means by which GE reflux is cleared (9). In normal adults there is a wide range of swallowing frequencies during the day, depending upon activity and meals, with an overall rate of about 25 swallows per hour (10). During sleep, the frequency of swallowing is 5.3 per hour, with a fairly small standard deviation. Adults may experience periods of up to 30 min during sleep in which no swallows occur. Such prolonged swallow-free periods occur an average of seven times per night. Two-thirds of the swallowing during sleep occurs in short bursts of two to five swallows associated with movement arousal, an electroencephalographic (EEG) term indicating a lightening of sleep state associated with body movement (11). Movement arousals and swallowing bursts are most frequently seen during rapid-eye-movement (REM) sleep and sleep stages 1 and 2 (12). Orr and colleagues have shown that, in sleeping adults, acid clearance time decreases with increased arousal from sleep, probably as a result of the increased rate of swallowing during arousals (13). Studies of babies in our unit confirm the decrease in overall swallowing rate during sleep. Furthermore, infants with pathological levels of GE reflux fail to increase their swallowing rate in response to reflux during sleep. This is in contrast to the marked increase in swallowing that accompanies reflux occurring while awake (2).

Not only does the frequency of swallowing decrease during sleep but secretion of saliva necessary for buffering refluxed gastric acid is almost nil (14). Decreased swallowing and decreased salivary flow combine to cause a significant increase in the duration of reflux episodes occurring during sleep.

Although there are no studies of the mechanics of swallowing during sleep, it seems reasonable to assume, since swallows occurring during sleep involve very small boluses, that their characteristics would be those of “dry” swallows—i.e., having decreased pharyngeal propulsive force and often resulting in incomplete or failed esophageal peristalsis (15). These changes may also be expected to decrease the ability to clear the esophagus of refluxed gastric contents and thus increase the acid clearance time. The effect of sleep on esophageal peristalsis has only been tangentially investigated in children. Studies in awake adults indicate that esophageal peristaltic amplitude and velocity are the same either recumbent or upright (16). The effect of sleep independent of the recumbent position on esophageal peristalsis has not been evaluated.

There may be mechanisms of reflux onset during sleep independent of transient relaxation. Our observations of sleeping infants indicate that 50% of reflux episodes during sleep are not associated with sudden drops in esophageal pH or with relaxation of the lower esophageal sphincter (LES), either transient or swallow-related. These episodes occur gradually, with the esophageal pH drifting down gradually and then settling at a nadir that is a bit higher than that of standard reflux episodes. These episodes are characterized also by a total lack of movement arousal and by the very lowest swallowing frequency. They are terminated by swallow during movement arousal but often after a very long duration of reflux. The mechanisms that allow this gradual acidification of the esophagus are not known. What is clear is that these gradually developing episodes of sleeping reflux are most likely to occur in the deeper stages 3 and 4 of EEG-defined sleep rather than the active stages 1, 2, and REM (17).

In summary, sleep is a time when transient relaxations of the lower esophageal sphincter are reduced in number. Salivary secretion is reduced, as is swallowing frequency, swallowing force, and transmission of complete esophageal peristaltic waves. The recumbent position prevents gravity from assisting in esophageal clearance. This combination of events leads to fewer episodes of reflux but ones cleared less efficiently. The additional acid exposure that occurs during the sleeping state probably represents the major difference between those with pathological reflux and controls.

III. Effects of Gastroesophageal Reflux on Sleep

Gastroesophageal reflux has been credited for causing a wide variety of symptoms in childhood, including spitting and vomiting, failure to thrive, colic, cough, reactive airways, respiratory infection, and even apnea of infancy. Another common assumption is that acid reflux causes disturbance in the normal conduct of sleep. There is little proof for this assumption.

Careful studies in children and adults with reflux have identified no obvious disturbance of the overall conduct of sleep (18,19). Sleep efficiency—i.e., the amount of time with the lights out that the EEG actually shows a sleeping pattern, movement arousal frequency, and the distribution of sleep stages 1 through 4 and REM—is identical in neurologically normal patients with GERD and controls (18).

There is some evidence that acid reflux may produce awakening from sleep in infants. Studies by Kahn and associates (20) have shown that in infants, acidification of the proximal esophageal mucosa during reflux was associated with movement arousal to the awake state 75% of the time. The arousals were transient and, within 5 min of upper esophageal acidification, the character of sleep was back to its prereflux state with fewer than one-third of patients remaining awake. Kahn pointed out that 41% of all reflux episodes occurring at night actually started and ended while the subject was awake. Sacre and colleagues, in a study of infants with apparent life-threatening events (ALTE), noted that 75% of infants with "respiratory dysfunction" during sleep, a state defined as "unquiet disrupted sleep characterized by multiple irregularly repeated apneas," had GER. Furthermore, successful therapy of GER documented by pH probe was associated with disappearance of "respiratory dysfunction" (21). Ramet and colleagues experimentally simulated reflux in sleeping infants by infusing acid material into the esophagus or by distending the esophagus with a balloon. They noted movement arousal, prolonged RR interval on the electrocardiogram, and increased duration of the respiratory cycle following this manipulation (22).

The above studies notwithstanding, most evidence supports the notion that arousal from sleep precedes the onset of nighttime GER rather than reflux being the stimulus for arousal. Studies in infants have shown that 94.4% of GER episodes at night begin either during awake periods (30.7%) or during sleep stages 1 and 2 (33.0%) and REM (30.7%). These are the EEG stages most often associated with arousals. Only 5.7% of all reflux episodes start during stages 3 and 4 sleep when arousals and body movement are rare. In neonates, where sleep stage classification is based less upon EEG patterns and more upon clinical observations, the majority of GER episodes occur during active sleep which roughly correlates with REM sleep of older infants and adults. Body movement and brief arousal from sleep are frequently seen at the onset of GER in the sleeping infant and adult. Swallowing is more common during stages 1, 2, and REM than in the deeper stages of sleep, and, when associated with failed peristalsis, may permit reflux to occur. Onset of reflux rarely occurs in the deep stages 3 and 4 of sleep, during which swallowing and body movement are rare. These studies suggest that nighttime GE reflux does not cause arousal from sleep but that arousal allows nighttime reflux to occur and that falling back to sleep while the esophagus is acidified results in prolonged pathological reflux (18,23).

IV. Summary

There is no doubt that the sleeping state is accompanied by changes in gastrointestinal functions—e.g., decreased swallowing, decreased salivary flow, decreased LES relaxations, and changes in the propulsive force of swallowing—which reduce the frequency and prolong the duration of reflux episodes. It is these nighttime changes in reflux that are frequently the difference between the pH recordings of those with "physiological" reflux and those with "pathological" reflux. However, data are at present insufficient to determine whether the converse effect is true—i.e., whether GER occurring at night has an impact upon the quality and quantity of sleep. What is suggested by the few studies that have simultaneously evaluated sleep and reflux, is that much reflux occurring while a child is in bed actually begins during awake periods and then continues as the subject falls asleep. The one study suggesting that reflux during EEG-determined sleep causes arousal also suggests that most infants resume sleeping rapidly despite ongoing reflux. The number of arousals from sleep do not appear to be increased in patients with GER, and the partition of sleep stages appears normal. More studies will be necessary before one can support the commonly held suspicion that the sleep of the child with reflux is disturbed.

Since reflux during sleep may account for a significant proportion of the daily esophageal acid exposure time in the patient with pathological reflux, it will be important to develop therapeutic modalities that are effective during sleep. Although there is concern about recommending the prone sleeping position in young infants because of the association of prone sleeping with the sudden infant death syndrome, the effect of prone sleeping on reflux in older children deserves further study. Some small studies have demonstrated a particular effectiveness of prokinetic agents in reducing nighttime reflux frequency and duration (24). These preliminary studies should be further evaluated. The recent demonstration that continuous positive airway pressure reduces nighttime reflux in patients with sleep apnea should be further assessed for its efficacy in patients with pathological reflux (25).

References

1. Johnson LF, DeMeester TR. 24 hour pH monitoring of the distal esophagus. Am J Gastroenterol 1974; 62:325–332.
2. Sondheimer JM. Clearance of spontaneous gastroesophageal reflux in awake and sleeping infants. Gastroenterology 1989; 97:821–826.
3. Dent J, Dodds WJ, Friedman RH, Sekiguchi T, Hogan WJ, Arndorfer RC, Petrie DJ. Mechanism of gastroesophageal reflux in recumbent asymptomatic human subjects. J Clin Investigation 1980; 65:256–267.
4. Little AF, Cox MR, Martin CJ, Dent J, Franzi SJ, Lavelle R. Influence of posture on transient lower oesophageal sphincter relaxation and gastro-esophageal reflux in the dog. J Gastroenterol Hepatol 1989; 4:494–499.
5. Holloway RH, Dent J. Pathophysiology of gastroesophageal reflux—lower esophageal sphincter dysfunction in gastroesophageal reflux disease. Gastroenterol Clin North Am 1990; 19:517–535.
6. Mittal RK, McCallum RW. Characteristics and frequency of transient relaxations of the lower esophageal sphincter in patients with reflux esophagitis. Gastroenterology 1988; 95:593–599.
7. Orr WC, Robinson MG. The sleeping gut. Med Clin North Am 1981; 65:1359–1376.
8. Orr WC, Robinson MG, Johnson L. The effect of esophageal acid volume on arousals from sleep and acid clearance. Chest 1991 99:351–354.
9. Bremner RM, Hoeft SF, Costantini M, Crookes PF, Bremner CG, DeMeester TR. Pharyngeal swallowing—the major factor in clearance of esophageal reflux episodes. Ann Surg 1993; 218:364–370.
10. Lear CS, Flanagan JB, Moorrees CF. The frequency of deglutition in man. Arch Oral Biol 1965; 10:83–99.
11. Lichter I, Muir RC. The pattern of swallowing during sleep. Electroencephalogr Clin Neurophysiol 1975; 38:427–432.
12. Guilleminault C, ed. Sleep and Waking Disorders: Indications and Techniques. Menlo Park, CA: Addison Wesley, 1982.

13. Orr WC, Johnson LF, Robinson MG. Effect of sleep on swallowing, esophageal peristalsis and acid clearance. Gastroenterology 1984; 86:814–819.
14. Schneyer LH, Pigman W, Hanahan L, Gilmore RW. Rate of flow of human parotid, sublingual and submaxillary secretions during sleep. J Dental Res 1956; 35:109–114.
15. Dodds WJ, Hogan WJ, Reid DP, Stewart ET, Arndorfer RC. A comparison between primary esophageal peristalsis following wet and dry swallows. J Appl Physiol 1973; 35:851–856.
16. Orr WC, Shamma-Othman Z, Allen M, Robinson MG. Esophageal function and gastroesophageal reflux during sleep and waking in patients with chronic obstructive pulmonary disease. Chest 1992; 101:1521–1525.
17. Sondheimer JM, Hoddes E. Gastroesophageal reflux with drifting onset in infants: a phenomenon unique to sleep. J Pediatr Gastroenterol Nutr 1992; 15:418–425.
18. Sondheimer JM, Hoddes E. Electroencephalogram patterns during sleep reflux in infants. Gastroenterology 1991; 101:1007–1011.
19. Freidin N, Fisher MJ, Taylor W, Boyd D, Surratt P, McCallum RW, Mittal RK. Sleep and nocturnal acid reflux in normal subjects and patients with reflux oesophagitis. Gut 1991; 32:1275–1279.
20. Kahn A, Rebuffat E, Sottiaux M, Dufour D, Cadranel S, Reiterer F. Arousals induced by proximal esophageal reflux in infants. Sleep 1991; 140:39–42.
21. Sacre L, Vandenplas Y. Gastroesophageal reflux associated with respiratory abnormalities during sleep. J Pediatr Gastroenterol Nutr 1989; 9:28–33.
22. Ramet J. Cardiac and respiratory reactivity to gastroesophageal reflux: experimental data in infants. Biol Neonate 1994; 65:240–246.
23. Jeffry HE, Heacock HJ. Impact of sleep and movement on gastro-oesophageal reflux in healthy, newborn infants. Arch Dis Child 1991; 66:1136–1140.
24. Tucci F, Resti M, Fontana R, Novebre E, Lami CA, Vierucci A. Gastroesophageal reflux and bronchial asthma: prevalence and effect of Cisapride therapy. J Pediatr Gastroenterol Nutr 1993; 17: 265–270.
25. Kerr P, Shoenut JP, Steens RD, Millar T, Micflickier AB, Kryger MH. Nasal continuous positive airway pressure. A new treatment for nocturnal gastroesophageal reflux? J Clin Gastroenterol 1993; 17:276–280.

Part Four

ABNORMAL BREATHING DURING SLEEP

19

Breathing During Sleep in Infancy

ANDRÉ KAHN

Free University of Brussels
and University Hospital
for Children Queen Fabiola
Brussels, Belgium

JOSE GROSWASSER, BERNARD DAN, and SONIA SCAILLET

University Hospital
for Children Queen Fabiola
Brussels, Belgium

PATRICIA FRANCO

Eramus Hospital
Brussels, Belgium

IGOR A. KELMANSON

St. Petersburg State Pediatric
Medical Academy
St. Petersburg, Russia

INEKO KATO

Nagoya City University Medical School
Nagoya, Japan

I. Introduction

The major respiratory dysrhythmias observed during the first year of life are summarized in the present chapter. This review covers the standard recording techniques used to evaluate the ontogeny of breathing. The frequency of breathing dysrhythmias is then addressed, together with their potential clinical implications.

II. Definitions

A. Recording Techniques

Normative data depend on the selection of the subjects studied and on recording conditions. There has been a lack of agreement regarding the techniques to most reliably acquire and interpret data in infants. Some investigators use pneumograms, while others rely on more complex polysomnographic recordings. Some studies were conducted during 2- to 4-hr nap periods, whereas others were based on 7- to 9-hr nocturnal recordings. Data acquisition has been performed in well-controlled laboratory environments, hospital wards, or the children's home.

The most complete method for continuous recording of physiological variables is the polysomnogram. The recording is usually carried out in a sleep laboratory, in a quiet and darkened room, at an ambient temperature ranging between 20° and 23° and a humidity of 30%. The children sleep in their usual sleep position, without restraints, and care is taken to avoid neck flexion. The infants are observed continuously during recordings, and their behavior as well as nursing interventions are charted. Feeding is administered based on demand. The data are collected on standard polygraph recorders (paper speed 10 mm/sec) or by computerized systems. During standard recording sessions, the following variables are simultaneously recorded: scalp electroencephalogram (EEG), electro-oculogram; electrocardiogram; thoracic and abdominal respiratory movements; and airflow by thermistors taped under each nostril and on the side of the mouth. An actigram can be placed on one arm to measure gross body movements. Oxygen saturation is recorded from a transcutaneous sensor.

B. Data Analysis

Standard evaluation of the recordings is based on the analysis of 30-sec epochs. The tracings are analyzed visually by one or several independent scorers to ensure reliability. Interrater agreement is established, scoring discrepancies are discussed, and codes thus agreed upon are used in the data analysis. In appropriate study conditions, sleep recordings are reproducible from night to night. When sleep studies are repeated in normal infants during 3 successive nights, no significant difference is seen in the subject's sleep and cardiorespiratory characteristics from night to night (1).

Sleep States

The recordings are divided into three main sleep states according to the criteria recommended in the literature (2,3). *Quiet sleep*, also scored as non–rapid-eye-movement (NREM) sleep, is defined by regular cardiac and respiratory rates, associated with slow or absent eye and body movements. Quiet sleep is characterized by minimal movement except for irregularly occurring sudden generalized movements called "startles" that become rare after the newborn period. If the quiet state seems basal and regulated, the active state is highly activated physiologically. *Active sleep*, or rapid-eye-movement (REM) sleep, is defined by the presence of irregular heart rates and respiratory movements together with brisk eye and body movements. *Indeterminate sleep* is scored when the recording does not fulfill the criteria for either quiet or active sleep. Finally, wakefulness is defined by crying and opening of the eyes.

Respiratory Dysrhythmias

Several types of respiratory dysrhythmias are detected. A *central apnea* is scored when flat tracings are obtained simultaneously from the chest and abdominal wall sensors (e.g., strain gauges) and the thermistors. It is generally scored if it lasts 4 or more sec. *Periodic breathing* is defined as the succession of more than three central apneas separated from each other by less than 20 sec of breathing movements. An *obstructive apnea* is scored when continuous deflections are obtained from the strain gauges while a flat tracing is recorded from the thermistors. It is scored if it lasts 3 or more sec. *Mixed apneas* are defined as a central apnea directly followed by an obstructive episode. To avoid artifactual scoring of obstructive events due to displacement of the thermistors, any doubtful episodes, such as obstructed breathing preceded by a movement or a sigh, are rejected. The possibility thus exists that some obstructive events are unduly excluded from studies. *Increased airway resistance* is described in children as a form of partially obstructed airway without complete closure (4). For all forms of respiratory dysrhythmia, *apnea density* defines the number of apneas per hour.

III. Ontogeny of Respiratory Dysrhythmias

Breathing and sleep characteristics change as the child grows, from the early weeks of life to the end of the first year. At each stage of development, the density of respiratory dysrhythmias is closely linked to the sleep-wake characteristics.

A. Respiratory Dysrhythmia In Utero and at Birth

In Utero

The mechanisms that control breathing rhythms develop well before birth. In the human fetus, spontaneous movements can be identified by ultrasound visualization at approximately 10 weeks of gestation (5). Between 20 and 28 weeks, rhythmical cycling of activity is recorded in utero (6,7). The fetal rest-activity pattern is characterized by long silent periods, lasting minutes to hours, during which there are no respiratory movements. Cycle times tend to vary between 40 and 60 min (7). The periods of quiescence or sleep represent 53% of the time at 30 weeks conceptional age and increase to 60% near term.

B. Preterm Infants

In premature infants, after the 31st week of gestation, the percentage of active sleep is elevated and that of quiet sleep reduced when compared with later ages (8). Active sleep forms 90% of sleep at 31 weeks of gestation and only 50% at term. Irregular breathing patterns, such as respiratory pauses or irregular phasic relationships between thoracic and abdominal respiration, are frequent in premature infants and occur mainly during active (REM) sleep (9). When premature infants reaching 40 weeks of gestational age are compared with term infants at similar gestational ages, most respiratory differences vanish (10).

C. Respiratory Dysrhythmia from Birth to 12 Months of Life

Changes in Sleep-Wake Behavior

It takes several months before a regular circadian sleep-wake cycle is installed and before the infant sleeps through the night. By 1 month of age, sleeping periods are longer during the night and a sustained awakening begins to occur in the early evening hours. Long sleep periods shift to nighttime by 2 to 3 months of age (8,11,12).

The amount of quiet sleep increases with age as that of active sleep decreases. Quiet sleep is the dominant sleep phase in 60% of infants at 3 months and in 90% at 6 months (13), when the proportion of quiet sleep is twice as great as that of active sleep (14). By 1 year of life, active sleep occupies 40% of nocturnal sleep (1). These changes in sleep characteristics are accompanied by changes in the density of respiratory dysrhythmias.

Changes in Frequency and Types of Respiratory Dysrhythmias

Numerous studies have been conducted to collect information on the respiratory characteristics of healthy infants during sleep (6,15–31). The studies were done with different recording techniques, surveyed various types of subjects, and were analyzed with different criteria. Most studies were conducted with pneumograms. Those done with polysomnographic recording techniques usually included a limited number of subjects. Despite this apparent heterogeneity, most studies reported similar ontogenic changes in respiratory dysrhythmias—namely, a progressive decrease in density after the early weeks of life.

To collect normative data on a large population of healthy infants with the use of nighttime polysomnographic recordings, a multicenter prospective study was conducted from January 1988 to January 1994. Several sleep laboratories recorded infants polysomnographically over the course of one night. The studies were coordinated by the senior authors (A.K. and J.G.). The infants were of Caucasian origin, from all socioeconomic levels, and living mainly in urban areas. To enter the study, the infants had to fulfill the following criteria: they had to be younger than 12 months of age, be healthy, and be receiving no medication at the time of the study. There was no history of apnea or sudden infant death syndrome (SIDS) in the families. The infants were followed and had to suffer no sleep apnea event or unexpected death until the end of their first year of life. To fulfill technical standards, the sleep studies lasted at least 360 min, and total sleep time exceeded 240 min. Adequate information on oxygen saturation, heart rate, and respiratory movements was available for at least 85% of the total sleep time. Over 2500 infants were studied. Because they did not meet the inclusion criteria or because of poor recording quality, the data of 427 infants were excluded, leaving a total of 2073 infants for analysis. The study was based on one recording per child. The general characteristics of the infants who entered the study are shown in Table 1.

Table 1 Major Characteristics of the Population Studied[a]

Number of infants recorded	2073
Total recording time (min)	875 (520–1819)
Total sleep time (min)	456 (245–514)
Gender (M/F)	1041/1032
Gestational age (weeks)	38.5 (25–43)
Postnatal age (weeks)	17.1 (1–51)
Postconceptional age (weeks)	55.6 (34–91)
Birthweight (grams)	3127.8 (740–5160)
Weight at the study (grams)	5940.7 (2110–11,000)

[a]Major characteristics of the 2073 infants recorded. Figures represent absolute, median, and range values.

Sleep-Related Characteristics

As shown in Table 2, all types of apneas were seen, mainly during active sleep. Central apneas occurred frequently but rarely exceeded 15 sec and were infrequently associated with bradycardia or oxygen desaturation. The 90th percentile of the population studied had 5.8 apneas per hour in non-REM (NREM) sleep and 12.9 in REM sleep. Mixed and obstructive sleep apneas were less frequently seen and were also of short duration.

Table 2 Respiratory Dysrhythmias According to Sleep States[a]

Parameter	Quiet sleep	Active sleep	*p* Value (t-test)
Apneas (number per hour)			
Central apneas	2.6 ± 2.2	7.2 ± 5.7	.001
Mixed apneas	0.02 ± 0.12	0.13 ± 0.34	.001
Obstructive apneas	0.05 ± 0.23	0.46 ± 1.0	.001
Mean duration of apneas (seconds)			
Central apneas	6.4 ± 1.1	5.7 ± 0.4	.001
Mixed apneas	8.5 ± 3.2	8.0 ± 2.2	NS
Obstructive apneas	5.4 ± 2.6	5.2 ± 1.8	NS
Longest apneas (seconds)			
Central apneas	8.5 ± 2.3	9.3 ± 2.1	.001
Mixed apneas	8.7 ± 3.2	10.9 ± 4.6	.001
Obstructive apneas	5.9 ± 3.0	8.0 ± 4.7	.010
Blood oxygen saturation			
Mean SaO_2 (%)	94.9 ± 12.1	92.7 ± 12.3	.001

[a]Respiratory dysrhythmias in the 2073 infants studied, according to sleep state. Figures represent absolute, median, and range values.

The mean duration of the central apneas depended on sleep stage and was significantly longer in NREM sleep than in REM sleep. For the whole population, the 90th percentile of apnea length was 7.5 sec in NREM sleep and 6.2 sec in REM sleep. The longest central apnea did not exceed 20 sec.

Mean oxygen saturation was lower in REM than in NREM sleep ($p = .01$). The 90th percentile for SaO_2 was 99% in REM and 100% in NREM sleep. The values did not depend on the age of the infants.

Age-Related Characteristics: The First 6 Months of Life

Sleep Structure. With advancing age, from the 45th to the 66th week postconception, a significant decrease was seen in the time spent awake ($r = -.288$; $p = .001$) and in REM sleep ($r = .359$; $p = .001$); there was also an increase in the percentage of NREM sleep time ($r = .638$; $p = .001$). Between the 45th and the 66th week, the 90th percentile for wake time decreased from 24.5% of total recording time to 15%, and that of REM sleep from 74.3% to 63.5% of total sleep time, while that of NREM sleep increased from 36% to 53%.

Central Apneas. The frequency of central apneas, expressed as percentiles for postconceptional age, is shown in Table 3. The data are distributed according to sleep states (quiet or active sleep) and the gender of the infants.

Table 3 Frequency of Central Apneas[a]

	Girls			Boys		
Postconceptional age	P10	P50	P90	P10	P50	P90
<45 weeks						
Total sleep	2.9	8.1	22.3	2.8	7.6	26.8
Quiet sleep	0.1	2.3	9.1	0.9	2.9	7.8
Active sleep	3.5	8.7	24.8	3.2	9.2	29.1
45–46 weeks						
Total sleep	1.8	5.4	12.7	1.7	4.2	9.5
Quiet sleep	0.1	2.7	5.4	0	2.1	5.2
Active sleep	2.2	6.2	15.9	2.0	5.2	11.9
47–48 weeks						
Total sleep	1.8	5.9	14.8	1.5	4.9	10.8
Quiet sleep	0.4	2.8	7.8	0.5	2.7	6.2
Active sleep	1.7	7.1	19.0	1.6	5.9	12.6
49–50 weeks						
Total sleep	2.2	5.3	12.1	1.7	5.0	11.4
Quiet sleep	0.5	2.6	6.2	0.4	2.1	5.8
Active sleep	2.8	6.2	15.2	2.3	6.5	13.6
51–52 weeks						
Total sleep	1.7	5.1	10.2	1.7	4.5	9.5
Quiet sleep	0.3	2.5	5.8	0.4	2.3	5.8
Active sleep	2.1	6.5	14.1	2.2	5.9	11.7

Table 3 Continued

	Girls			Boys		
Postconceptional age	P10	P50	P90	P10	P50	P90
53–54 weeks						
Total sleep	2.0	5.2	10.2	1.8	4.1	11.2
Quiet sleep	0.4	2.1	5.3	0.4	1.8	5.4
Active sleep	2.5	6.6	13.6	2.6	5.4	12.9
55–56 weeks						
Total sleep	2.1	4.6	10.0	1.6	3.9	9.2
Quiet sleep	0.6	2.1	5.6	0.3	1.8	4.9
Active sleep	3.0	6.1	11.1	1.8	5.1	12.4
57–58 weeks						
Total sleep	1.5	3.8	7.9	1.2	4.1	7.8
Quiet sleep	0.3	1.3	4.4	0.3	1.8	4.9
Active sleep	1.9	5.3	10.6	1.8	5.8	11.1
59–60 weeks						
Total sleep	1.9	4.6	8.4	1.7	3.5	8.3
Quiet sleep	0.3	2.0	3.5	0.4	1.5	4.3
Active sleep	2.8	5.8	11.6	1.0	5.0	10.4
61–62 weeks						
Total sleep	1.8	5.2	10.8	1.4	3.9	7.3
Quiet sleep	0.4	2.4	3.5	0.3	1.6	4.4
Active sleep	2.4	7.5	15.1	2.3	4.8	8.8
63–64 weeks						
Total sleep	1.4	4.9	8.8	2.0	4.1	7.4
Quiet sleep	0.8	2.3	5.0	0.5	1.5	4.4
Active sleep	2.1	6.4	12.4	2.7	6.1	11.4
65–66 weeks						
Total sleep	1.4	5.1	7.5	1.5	4.2	7.4
Quiet sleep	0.2	1.9	3.6	0.2	1.4	4.3
Active sleep	2.1	7.3	11.8	2.7	6.1	10.3
>66 weeks						
Total sleep	1.5	4.1	7.9	1.3	3.4	6.5
Quiet sleep	0.4	1.7	3.8	0.3	1.8	4.0
Active sleep	2.4	6.2	12.0	1.8	4.6	9.2

[a]Density of central apneas per hour of sleep, according to sleep states and gender. Figures represent percentiles for age values.

The density of central apneas tended to decrease from the 45th postconceptual week to the end of the 65th week ($r = -.182$ in NREM sleep, and $-.168$ in REM sleep). The 90th percentile of apnea density was 12.7 at 45 weeks postconceptual age and 7.5 at 65 weeks.

No significant change in mean apnea duration was seen between the 45th and the 66th weeks of life, although in both sexes the mean apnea duration tended to increase during REM sleep and to decrease during NREM sleep. As a consequence, the time spent in central apnea tended to decrease with increasing age in both sleep stages and in both sexes. The changes were not statistically significant ($r = -.174$ in NREM sleep and $-.159$ in REM sleep).

Between the 45th and 66th weeks of postconceptual age, both the mean duration and the maximum duration of the central apneas tended to increase with age, but the trend was not statistically significant. There was no sex-related difference in the mean or maximum duration of the central apneas.

Some central apneas were associated with drops in heart rate and in oxygen saturation. Drops in heart rate or in oxygen saturation occurred with a frequency of 1.3 apneas per hour of sleep in both sexes. Both findings were more frequent with increasing apnea length but occurred with apneas as short as 4.5 sec in duration. The apnea-induced heart rate and oxygen saturation drops were both seen in all age groups, despite a slight tendency to decrease with increasing age ($r = -.102$ for heart rate drops and $-.251$ for oxygen desaturation).

At any age and in both sexes, three apneas per hour of sleep were immediately preceded by a sigh. There was a slight tendency for sigh-preceded central apneas to be less frequent with increasing age ($r = -.191$).

The 90th percentile for the time spent in periodic breathing was 3% of total sleep time at 45 weeks postconceptual age. In both sexes, the frequency of periodic breathing tended to decrease with advancing age ($r = -.196$) to reach 0.8% at 66 weeks.

Age-Related Characteristics: The Second 6 Months of Life

Few data are available on the frequency of respiratory dysrhythmia after the first 6 months of life. A multicenter prospective study was conducted between December 1991 and August 1993 on 385 children recorded in sleep laboratories. To enter the study, the children and their sleep recordings had to fulfill the criteria described previously on page 407. The children had a mean gestational age of 38.5 weeks. At the time of the study, these 212 boys and 173 girls were between 6 and 12 months old. As shown in Table 4, significantly more frequent central apneas were seen in active than in quiet sleep, but sleep states had little influence on apnea length.

IV. Polysomnographic Scoring: Confounding Factors

On the previously reported sleep studies, multivariate analysis was done to identify the factors that could influence the findings. MANOVA was used, utilizing birthweight, gestational age, weight at the time of study, and sex and postconceptional age as cofactors. Postconceptional age was found to be more significantly associated with most polygraphic variables than postnatal age, gestational age, or gender. Postconceptional age was classified with an F value of 5.234 (significant $F = .223$) in the determination of mean central apnea frequency, and with an F value of 4.481 (significant $F = .356$) in relation to obstructive apnea frequency.

Table 4 Respiratory Dysrhythmia According to Sleep State and Gender[a]

	Girls			Boys		
Central apneas	P3	P50	P97	P3	P50	P97
Number per hour						
Quiet sleep	<0.1	1.7	5.9	<0.1	1.6	5.3
Active sleep	1.3	6.4	21.0	1.0	5.1	12.0
Mean duration (seconds)						
Quiet sleep	4.7	6.2	8.2	4.7	6.3	8.7
Active sleep	5.0	5.8	6.8	4.9	5.8	6.9
Maximal duration (seconds)						
Quiet sleep	5.0	8.0	12.0	5.0	8.5	13.5
Active sleep	6.0	9.5	14.5	5.7	9.0	14.5
Periodic breathing						
Percent of total sleep time	0	0.2	3.3	0	0.2	2.4

[a]Central apneas and periodic breathing during total sleep time, expressed by sleep state and by gender. The results are presented as percentiles for age.

Postconceptional age had a statistically significant influence on the following variables: number of mixed and of obstructive apneas per hour of NREM sleep, mean length of central apneas during NREM sleep and of obstructive apneas during both NREM and REM sleep, mean length of mixed apnea during REM sleep, and heart rate variation during NREM sleep.

Gender had a significant effect on several variables. Higher values were seen in boys than in girls for the number of central apneas per hour of REM sleep and the coefficient of heart rate variation during REM sleep. Inversely, higher values were seen in girls than in boys for the following variables: the mean length of central apneas during REM and NREM sleep, mean heart rate during REM and NREM sleep, the percentage of periodic breathing during total sleep time, and the percentage of total wake time.

V. A Specific Issue: The Obstructive Sleep Apneas

A. Definition

Criteria and definitions for obstructive sleep apnea (OSA) patients vary with different investigators (32). The definition of OSA in infants is less stringent than that used in the older child or adult (32,33). OSA may be significantly shorter and less frequent in infants than in older children or in adults. The criteria used to define OSAs in adults may thus fail to identify infants with severe OSA (34). Most authors therefore admit that the criteria must be adapted according to the age of the patient (32–34). In infants, OSAs are usually scored if they last at least 3 sec.

B. Prevalence

There is a large amount of evidence that OSAs develop in young infants (31,33, 35–38). OSAs were reported to occur in up to 10% of randomly selected infants and are more frequently found in preterm than in term neonates (31,38).

The obstructions are mainly seen during active or light quiet sleep (33). OSA occurs more frequently in boys than in girls (33,38). The sex difference remains unexplained but could partly result from a protective role of female hormones (40) or from sex-related differences in the anatomy of the upper airway (41).

To evaluate the frequency of OSAs in otherwise healthy infants, we conducted a multicenter prospective survey between January 1992 and August 1993. The study was based on 1135 polygraphic recordings collected on 1053 healthy infants. The infants were all born at term (mean age of 39.5 ± 1.1 weeks) and were studied between the ages of 2 and 27 weeks. The inclusion criteria were similar to those already reported on page 407. The infants were divided according to postnatal age groups: 2 to 7 weeks, 8 to 11, 12 to 15, 16 to 19, 20 to 23, and 24 to 27 weeks.

The frequencies of both obstructive and mixed apneas were highest in the 2- to 7-week age group. The number of obstructive events decreased significantly after the seventh week of life. There was no significant difference in apnea frequency from the eighth to the twenty-seventh weeks of life. The general drop in apnea frequency was seen in both sleep stages, but the difference was significant in REM sleep only (Mann-Whitney $p = .030$).

Boys had significantly more frequent OSA than girls within the 8- to 11-week age group. There were no significant differences between the sexes in the other age groups.

The mean duration of the obstructive apneas did not change significantly between the different age groups. The mixed apneas were significantly longer in the infants aged 2 to 7 weeks than in those of the other age groups. The difference was seen during REM sleep only.

Subdividing the age groups by 2-week periods, the drop in apnea frequency after the seventh week of life was still present. In addition, a transient and significant increase in OSA was seen between 12 and 13 weeks of life. Similar findings have been reported by other authors (4). In the present study, the specific increase in apnea frequency was seen in boys only.

C. Mechanisms of OSA

In infants, OSAs are considered to be most frequently associated with anatomic abnormalities that reduce the patency of the upper airways. Such anatomic problems may be divided into three major groups: anatomic malformations, soft tissue infiltration, and neurological lesions (3,42).

The malformations frequently reported to induce OSAs in infants include craniofacial abnormalities, micrognathia, cleft palate, long soft palate, glossoptosis, small upper airways, Pierre Robin syndrome, and choanal atresia. Other conditions are also encountered, such as Down's syndrome (3,33,36,43–45).

Table 5 Obstructive Sleep Apneas in Full-Term Infants Between 1 and 27 Weeks of Age[a]

	Age groups (weeks)					
	2–7	8–11	12–15	16–19	20–23	24–27
Number of infants	55	502	288	194	67	29
Gender (M/F)	33/27	271/231	155/133	99/95	30/37	15/14
Gestational age (weeks)	39.3 ± 1.3	39.4 ± 1.2	39.4 ± 1.2	39.5 ± 1.1	39.1 ± 1.3	39.7 ± 0.9
Postnatal age (weeks)	5.3 ± 1.7	10.1 ± 0.9	13.4 ± 1.2	17.3 ± 1.1	21.1 ± 1.1	25.4 ± 1.1
Number of apneas per hour of total sleep						
Obstructive	0.1 (0–3.0)	0 (0–2.8)	0 (0–2.4)	0 (0–4.2)	0 (0–1.5)	0 (0–2.7)
Mixed	0 (0–1.7)	0 (0–4.4)	0 (0–2.1)	0 (0–0.7)	0 (0–1)	0 (0–0.3)
Combined	0.2 (0–3.9)	0 (0–5.1)	0 (0–3.1)	0 (0–4.9)	0 (0–1.8)	0.1 (0–2.8)
Number of apneas per hour of active sleep						
Obstructive	0.2 (0–4.6)	0 (0–4.0)	0 (0–3.4)	0 (0–4.9)	0 (0–2.7)	0 (0–3.3)
Mixed	0 (0–1.9)	0 (0–5.6)	0 (0–3.3)	0 (0–1.1)	0 (0–1.7)	0 (0–0.5)
Combined	0.3 (0–4.8)	0 (0–6.4)	0 (0–4.9)	0 (0–5.9)	0 (0–3.0)	0.2 (0–3.4)

[a]The number of apneas recorded per hour of sleep is classified under obstructive apneas, mixed apneas, or combined obstructive and mixed events. The figures represent absolute, mean ± SD, median, and range value.

Soft tissue infiltration may result from infection of the airways, allergy, supraglottic edema, adenotonsillar hypertrophy, mucopolysaccharide storage disease, laryngomalacia, subglottic stenosis, neck tumor, or hypothyroidism (43,46–48).

Abnormalities of the nervous system that induce airway obstruction include seizures, increased intracranial pressure (49), and brainstem compression, such as that associated with Chiari malformations type I or II or syringobulbia-myelia (50). Other neurological impairments limiting muscle contraction—such as recurrent laryngeal nerve palsy, palsies of the cranial nerves, or poliomyelitis—are also associated with obstructed breathing (3).

OSA is seen in infants suffering from autonomic dysfunction, such as familial dysautonomia, ganglioneuroma, Shy-Drager syndrome, or breath-holding spells (51). Atropine administration prevents the development of obstructive apneas in infants with breath-holding spells (52). Other factors that also contribute to the development of obstructive sleep apneas include neck flexion, sleep deprivation (53), excessive body weight (46,54), maternal cigarette smoking during gestation (55), or the administration of sedative drugs (56). In young infants, acid reflux in the esophagus may induce apneas (57), although such mechanisms have been questioned (58).

OSAs can also be seen in children without anatomic or neurological problems. Obstructive apneas could then result from abnormal timing between the upper airway muscles and the diaphragm contractions (59). Fluoroscopic studies show that the tongue and hypopharyngeal soft tissues approximate during inspiration, obliterating the hypopharyngeal air space, with intermittent and almost complete obstruction of airflow (60).

D. Clinical Implication of OSA in Healthy Infants

The potential short-term clinical consequences of OSA have not been assessed in otherwise healthy infants. The question of the long-term side effects, particularly on psychomotor development, of repetitive airway obstructions during sleep remains unanswered. The obstructive apneas usually disappear with age. It is not known whether a relationship exists between brief airway obstructions observed in early infancy and the sleep apnea syndrome described in childhood and adulthood.

E. OSA in Otherwise Healthy Infants: Risk Factor for the Sudden Infant Death Syndrome?

Some infants who eventually died of SIDS presented with symptoms associated with repeated obstructive apneas (while awake, difficulty in coordinating swallowing and respiration and breath-holding spells; while asleep, profuse sweating, noisy breathing, or snorting) (61).

Some future SIDS infants recorded polygraphically some weeks before death were characterized by the presence of repeated obstructive apneas during sleep. In a prospective multicenter case-control study conducted between January 1977 and January 1990, a total of 20,750 polygraphic studies were recorded, including those of 30 infants who eventually died of SIDS. The studies of the future SIDS victims were compared with those of 60 control infants matched for gender, age, gestational age, and birth weight (38).

Future SIDS victims tended to have fewer short central apneas than the control subjects. The median number of central apneas per hour of sleep was 9 (range: 3 to 56) in the future SIDS infants and 10 (range: 2 to 90) in the control subjects (not significantly different). The central apneas tended to be longer in the SIDS infants (median of 9 sec; range: 6 to 28) than in the control infants (median of 8 sec; range: 4 to 19). No difference was seen between the two groups for the frequency or the duration of periodic breathing (median number of periodic breathing episodes per hour: 0; range: 0 to 5).

Future SIDS victims presented significantly more frequent OSA events (both obstructive and mixed apneas) and less body movements than control subjects. Obstructed and mixed apneas were seen in 19 of the future 30 SIDS infants but in only 6 of 60 control subjects. The total number of obstructive respiratory events was significantly greater in the SIDS group. Of the 19 SIDS infants with obstructive apneas, 13 had at least three obstructive episodes, 11 more than five, and 3 more than twenty obstructions per night. In contrast, only 2 of the 60 control subjects had at least three obstructive episodes and only 1 infant had seven obstructive apneas per night. The obstructed and mixed apneas lasted longer in the SIDS than in the control infants. Of all obstructive and mixed apneas seen in the SIDS and control infants, 78.3% occurred during REM sleep. The obstructed breathing events were accompanied by drops in heart rates to 68 beats per minute and in SaO_2 to 75%. The level of bradycardia and desaturation was related to the duration of the obstruction. In the SIDS group, more boys than girls had obstructive apneas (13 of 19 boys, 6 of 11 girls; Fisher exact test: $p = .04$). Boys also had significantly more OSAs than girls (6.4 episodes per boy, range 0 to 25; 1.8 episodes per girl, range 0 to 6; Mann-Whitney test: $p = .04$).

In another study, the polysomnographic studies of 42 infants recorded some 2 to 6 weeks before death from SIDS were compared with those of a healthy control population of 1053 infants (Table 6). To enter the study, the children and their sleep recordings had to fulfill the criteria described previously (p. 407). Comparing the future SIDS infants with the control population by age, it was seen that within the 2- to 7-week age range there was no difference in the frequency of OSAs. Significant differences were found only for infants aged 8 to 15 weeks. In this age range, future SIDS victims had significantly more frequent OSAs than the control subjects. The differences disappeared in the 16- to 19-week age range. The findings support the possibility of a delay in the maturation of respiratory control in future SIDS victims.

VI. Factors That Influence Respiratory Dysrhythmia

Environmental factors may also alter significantly breathing characteristics and be potential confounding factors in the interpretation of studies on respiratory dysrhythmias. Such factors include feeding, body position during sleep, environmental temperature, or prenatal exposure to cigarette smoke.

Table 6 Frequency of Obstructive Sleep Apneas in Future SIDS Victims and Control Infants[a]

Age (weeks)		SIDS victims	Control infants	p
2–7	Mean ± SD	0.8 ± 0.6	0.5 ± 0.8	
	Median (range)	1.1 (0–1.5)	0.2 (0–3.9)	NS
8–11	Mean ± SD	0.5 ± 0.6	0.2 ± 0.4	
	Median (range)	0.6 (0–2.3)	0 (0–5.1)	.001
12–16	Mean ± SD	0.6 ± 0.5	0.2 ± 0.5	
	Median (range)	0.5 (0–1.4)	0 (0–3.1)	.003
16–19	Mean ± SD	0.3 ± 0.4	0.2 ± 0.5	
	Median (range)	0.3 (0–0.9)	0 (0–4.9)	NS

[a]Frequency of obstructive sleep apneas according to age, in future SIDS victims and in control infants. The figures represent mean ± SD values, median, and range values. p values were calculated using the Mann-Whitney test.

A. Feeding and Breathing Characteristics

Feeding increases the respiratory rate and modifies sleep architecture (62). Infants have a significantly greater probability of entering active sleep after feeding than after waking episodes without feeding (24). Thus, food intake may play a major role in entraining irregular breathing cycles and apneas. The type of feeding, whether breast- or bottle-feeding, does not significantly modify the breathing and sleep characteristics.

B. Body Position During Sleep

Premature and low-birth-weight neonates lain prone to sleep show greater respiratory efficiency, more regular breathing patterns, less frequent apneas (63,64), and a greater minute ventilation (65) than when lying supine. The effect of body position on respiratory characteristics is age-dependent. In 3- month-old infants, no difference in respiratory variables is seen when prone and supine sleep positions are compared (66). The prone body position is, however, associated with a significant increase in sleep duration and in the density of quiet sleep, together with a significant decrease in the number and duration of arousals (67). Ambient noise induces less central apnea in an infant sleeping prone rather than supine (68).

C. Exposure to Cigarette Smoke In Utero

Prenatal exposure to cigarette smoking by the mother increases the frequency of OSA in newborns and in 3-month-old infants (55). Cigarette smoking during gestation also elevates the arousal thresholds of the infants, increasing the risk for more frequent and longer apneas.

Autoregressive power spectral analysis of the R-R intervals showed a greater orthosympathetic activity both in the prone body position and in subjects with prenatal exposure to cigarette smoke than in control conditions (68). The mechanisms relating changes in autonomic control and in breathing control are not known.

VII. Conclusions

Infants' breathing characteristics and respiratory dysrhythmias depend largely on endogenous factors, such as age and sex. They are also dependent on environmental factors and recording conditions. Most studies, however, illustrated the importance of maturation processes on the control of sleep-wake states and breathing. The clinical implication of respiratory dysrhythmias is still the subject of intense research programs.

References

1. Rebuffat E, Groswasser J, Kelmanson I, Sottiaux M, Kahn A. Polygraphic evaluation of night-to-night variability in sleep characteristics and apneas in infants. Sleep 1994; 17:329–332.
2. Anders T, Emde R, Parmelee AH, eds. A Manual of Standardized Terminology, Techniques and Criteria for Scoring States of Sleep and Wakefulness in Newborn Infants. Los Angeles: UCLA Brain Information Service, NINDS Neurological Information Network, 1971.
3. Guilleminault C, Souquet M. Sleep states and related pathology. In: Korobkin R, Guilleminault C, eds. Advances in Perinatal Neurology. New York: Spectrum Publications, 1979: 225–247.
4. Guilleminault C. Obstructive sleep apnea syndrome in children. In: Guilleminault C, ed. Sleep and Its Disorders in Children. New York: Raven Press, 1987: 213–224.
5. Hoppenbrouwers T, Ugartechea JC, Combs D, Hodgman JE, Harper RM, Sterman MB. Studies of maternal-fetal interaction during the third trimester of pregnancy: I. Ontogenesis of the basic rest activity cycle. Exp Neurol 1978; 2:136–153.
6. Parmelee AH, Wenner WH, Akiyama Y. Sleep states in premature infants. Dev Med Child Neurol 1967; 9:70–77.
7. Sterman MB, Hoppenbrouwer T. The development of sleep-waking and rest-activity patterns from fetus to adult in man. In: Sterman MB, McGinty DJ, Adinolfi AM, eds. Brain Development and Behavior. New York: Academic Press, 1971: 203–225.
8. Parmelee AH, Stern E. Development of states in infants. In: Clemente CD, Purpura DP, Mayer FE, eds. Sleep and the Maturing Nervous System. New York: Academic Press, 1971: 199–228.
9. Curzi-Dascalova L. Phase relationships between thoracic and abdominal respiratory movements during sleep in 31–38 weeks CA normal infants: comparison with full-term (39–41 weeks) newborns. Neuropediatrics 1982; 13:15–20.
10. Curzi-Dascalova L, Lebrun F, Korn G. Respiratory frequency according to sleep states and age in normal premature infants: a comparison with full-term infants. Pediatr Res 1983; 17:152–156.
11. Coons S. Development of sleep and wakefulness during the first 6 months of life. In; Guilleminault C, ed. Sleep and Its Disorders in Children. New York: Raven Press, 1987: 17–27.

12. Hoppenbrouwers T, Hodgman JE, Arakawa K, Cabal LA, Durand M. Physiologic follow-up of preterm infants with apnea. Pediatr Res 1985; 19:346A.
13. Hoppenbrouwers T. Sleep in infants. In: Guilleminault C, ed. Sleep and Its Disorders in Children. New York: Raven Press, 1987: 1–16.
14. Sern E, Parmelee AH, Akiyama Y. Sleep cycle characteristics in infants. Pediatrics 1969; 43:65–70.
15. Richards JM, Alexander JR, Shinebourne EA, de Swiet M, Wilson AJ, Southall DP. Sequential 22-hour profiles of breathing patterns and heart rate in 110 full-term infants during their first 6 months of life. Pediatrics, 1984; 74:763–777.
16. Harper RM, Leak B, Hodgman JE, Hoppenbrouwers T. Developmental patterns of heart rate and heart rate variability during sleep and waking in normal infants and infants at risk for the sudden infant death syndrome. Sleep 1982; 5:28–38.
17. Gaultier C. Adaptation du controle de la ventilation. Prog Pediatr 1989; 6:69–79.
18. Rigatto H. Maturation of breathing control in fetus and newborn infant. In: Beckerman RC, Brouillette RT, Hunt CE, eds. Respiratory Control Disorders in Infants and Children. Baltimore: Williams & Wilkins, 1992: 61–75.
19. Kelly DH, Stellwagen LM, Kaitz E, Shannon DC. Apnea and periodic breathing in normal full-term infants during the first twelve months. Pediatrics 1985; 1:215–219.
20. Hunt CE, Brouillette RT, Hanson D, David RJ, Stein IM, Weissbluth M. Home pneumograms in normal infants. Pediatrics 1985; 106:551–555.
21. Stein IM, White A, Kennedy JL, Merisalo RT, Chernoff H, Gould JB. Apnea recordings of healthy infants at 40, 44, and 52 weeks postconception. Pediatrics 1979; 63:724–730.
22. Hoppenbrouwers T, Hodgman JE, Harper RM, Hofman E, Sterman MB, McGinty DJ. Polygraphic studies of normal infants during the first six months of life: III. Incidence of apnea and periodic breathing. Pediatrics 1977; 60:418–425.
23. Schechtman VL, Harper RM. The maturation of correlations between cardiac and respiratory measures across sleep states in normal infants. Sleep 1992; 15:41–47.
24. Harper RM, Leake B, Miyahara L, Hoppenbrouwers T, Sterman MB, Hodgman J. Temporal sequencing in sleep and waking states during the first 6 months of life. Exp Neurol 1981; 72:294–307.
25. Katona PG, Frasz A, Egbert J. Maturation of cardiac control in full-term and preterm infants during sleep. Early Hum Dev 1980; 4:145–159.
26. Gaultier C. Respiratory adaptation during sleep from the neonatal period to adolescence. In: Guilleminault C, ed. Sleep and Its Disorders in Children. New York: Raven Press, 1987: 67–98.
27. Coons S, Guilleminault C. Development of sleep-wake patterns and non-rapid eye movement sleep stages during the first six months of life in normal infants. Pediatrics 1982; 69:793–798.
28. Emde RN, Walker S. Longitudinal study of infant sleep: results of fourteen subjects studied at monthly intervals. Psychophysiology 1976; 13:456–461.
29. Anders TF, Keener M. Developmental course of nighttime sleep-wake patterns in full-term and premature infants during the first year of life. Sleep 1985; 8:173–192.
30. Lee D, Caces R, Kwiatkowski K, Cates D, Rigatto H. A developmental study on types and frequency distribution of short apneas (3 to 15 seconds) in term and preterm infants. Pediatr Res 1987; 22:344–349.
31. Flores-Guevara R, Plouin P, Curzi-Dascalova L, Radvanyi M-F, Guidasci S, Pajot N, Monod N. Sleep apneas in normal neonates and infants during the first 3 months of life. Neuropediatrics 1982; 13:21–28.

32. Krieger J. Obstructive sleep apnea: clinical manifestations and pathophysiology. In: Thorpy MJ, ed. Handbook of Sleep Disorders. New York: Marcel Dekker, 1990: 259–284.
33. Guilleminault C. Treatments in obstructive sleep apnea. In: Guilleminault C, Patinen M, eds. Obstructive Sleep Apnea Syndrome: Clinical Research and Treatment. New York: Raven Press, 1990: 99–118.
34. Rosen CL, DiAndrea L, Haddad GG. Adult criteria for obstructive sleep apnea do not identify children with serious obstruction. Am Rev Respir Dis 1992; 146:1231–1234.
35. Guilleminault C, Eldridge FL, Simmons FB. Sleep apnea in eight children. Pediatrics 1976; 58:23–31.
36. Diagnostic Classification Steering Committee, Thorpy MJ, Chairman: International Classification of Sleep Disorders: Diagnostic and Coding Manual. Rochester: American Sleep Disorders Association, 1990.
37. Brouillette RT, Fernbach SK, Hunt CE. Obstructive sleep apnea in infants and children. J Pediatr 1982; 100:31–40.
38. Kahn A, Groswasser J, Rebuffat E, Sottiaux M, Blum D, Foerster M, Franco P, Bochner A, Alexander M, Bachy A, Richard P, Verghote M, Le Polain D, Wayenberg JL. Sleep and cardiorespiratory characteristics of infant victims of sudden death: a prospective case-control study. Sleep 1992; 15:287–292.
39. Kahn A, Groswasser J, Sottiaux M, Rebuffat E, Sunseri M, Franco P, Dramaix M, Bochner A, Belhadi B, Foerster M. Clinical symptoms associated with brief obstructive sleep apnea in normal infants. Sleep 1993; 16:409–413.
40. Pickett CK, Regensteiner JG, Woodard WD. Progestin and estrogen reduce sleep-disordered breathing in postmenopausal women. J Appl Physiol 1989; 66:1656–1661.
41. Gunn TR, Tonkin SL. Upper airway measurements during inspiration and expiration in infants. Pediatrics 1989; 84:73–77.
42. Brouillette R, Hanson D, David R, Hunt CE. A diagnostic approach to suspected obstructive sleep apnea in children. J Pediatr 1984; 105:10–14.
43. Guilleminault C, Korobkin R, Winkle R. A review of 50 children with obstructive sleep apnea syndrome. Lung 1981; 59:275–287.
44. Guilleminault C, Powell N, Heldt G, Riley R. Small upper airway in near-miss sudden infant death syndrome infants and their families. Lancet 1986; 1:402–407.
45. Cozzi F, Pierro A. Glossoptosis-apnea syndrome in infancy. Pediatrics 1988; 8:836–843.
46. Kahn A, Mozin MJ, Rebuffat E, Sottiaux M, Burniat W, Shepherd S, Muller MF. Sleep pattern alterations and brief airway obstructions in overweight infants. Sleep 1989; 12:430–438.
47. Sullivan CE, Grunstein RR, Marrone O. Sleep apnea- pathophysiology: upper airway and control of breathing. In: Guilleminault C, Partinen M, eds. Obstructive Sleep Apnea Syndrome: Clinical Research and Treatment. New York: Raven Press, 1990: 49–69.
48. Thach BT. Neuromuscular control of the upper airway. In: Beckerman RC, Brouillette RT, Hunt CE, eds. Respiratory Control Disorders in Infants and Children. Baltimore: Williams & Wilkins, 1992: 47–60.
49. Jennum P, Borgesen SE. Intracranial pressure and obstructive sleep apnea. Chest 1989; 95:279–283.
50. Haponik EF, Givens D, Angelo J. Syringobulbia-myelia with obstructive sleep apnea. Neurology 1983; 33:1064–1069.
51. Kahn A, Rebuffat E, Sottiaux M, Muller MF, Bochner A, Grosswasser J. Brief airway obstructions during sleep in infants with breath-holding spells. J Pediatr 1990; 117:188–193.
52. Kahn A, Rebuffat E, Sottiaux M, Muller MF, Bochner A, Groswasser J. Prevention of air-

way obstructions during sleep in infants with breath-holding spells by means of oral belladonna: a prospective double-blind crossover evaluation. Sleep 1991; 14:432–438.
53. Canet E, Gaultier C, D'Allest AM. Effects of sleep deprivation on respiratory events during sleep in healthy infants. J Appl Physiol 1989; 66:1158–1163.
54. Mallory GB, Fiser DH, Jackson R. Sleep-associated breathing disorders in morbidly obese children and adolescent. J Pediatr 1989; 115:892–897.
55. Kahn A, Groswasser J, Sottiaux M, Kelmanson I, Rebuffat E, Franco P, Dramaix M, Wayenberg JL. Prenatal exposure to cigarettes in infants with obstructive sleep apneas. Pediatrics 1994; 93:778–783.
56. Kahn A, Hasaerts D, Blum D. Phenothiazine-induced sleep apneas in normal infants. Pediatrics 1985; 75:844–847.
57. Pickens DL, Schefft G, Thach BT. Pharyngeal fluid clearance and aspiration preventive mechanisms in sleeping infants. J Appl Physiol 1989; 66:1164–1171.
58. Kahn A, Rebuffat E, Sottiaux M, Dufour D, Cadranel S, Reiterer F. Lack of temporal relation between acid reflux in the proximal esophagus and cardiorespiratory events in sleeping infants. Eur J Pediatr 1992; 151:208–212.
59. Jeffries B, Brouillette RT, Hunt CE. Electromyographic study of some accessory muscles of respiration in children with obstructive sleep apnea. Am Rev Respir Dis 1984; 129: 696–702.
60. Felman AH, Loughlin GM, Leftridge CA. Upper airway obstruction during sleep in children. AJR 1979; 133:213–216.
61. Kahn A, Groswasser J, Sottiaux M, Rebuffat E, Sunseri M, Franco P, Dramaix M, Bochner A, Belhadi B, Foerster M. Clinical symptoms associated with brief obstructive sleep apnea in normal infants. Sleep 1993; 16:409–413.
62. Ashton R, Connolly K. The relation of respiration rate and heart rate to sleep states in the human newborn. Dev Med Child Neurol 1971; 13:180–187.
63. Hutchinson AA, Ross KR, Russell G. The effect of posture on ventilation and lung mechanisms in preterm and light-for-date infants. Pediatrics 1979; 64:429–432.
64. Masterson J, Zucker C, Schulze K. Prone and supine positioning effects on energy expenditure and behavior of low birth weight neonates. Pediatrics 1987; 80:689–692.
65. Fleming PJ, Muller NL, Bryan MH, Bryan AC. The effects of abdominal loading on rib cage distortion in premature infants. Pediatrics 1979; 64:425–428.
66. Orr WC, Stahl ML, Duke J, McCaffree MA, Toubas P, Mattice C, Krous HF. Effect of sleep state and position on the incidence of obstructive and central apnea in infants. Pediatrics 1985; 75:832–835.
67. Kahn A, Groswasser J, Sottiaux M, Franco P, Dramaix M. Prone or supine body position and sleep characteristics in infants. Pediatrics 1993; 91:1112–1115.
68. Franco P, Groswasser J, Sottiaux M, Broadfield E, Kahn A. Decreased cardiac responses to auditory stimulation during prone sleep. Pediatrics 1995; 97:174–178.

20

Apparent Life-Threatening Events

Pathogenesis and Management

MARTIN P. SAMUELS

Keele University and
North Staffordshire Hospital
Staffordshire, England

I. Introduction

The term *apparent life-threatening event* (ALTE) describes a clinical presentation involving a sudden, unexpected change in an infant's behavior that is frightening to the parents or caregivers but does not lead to death or persistent collapse. Thus an ALTE is an episode with a beginning and an end, the latter having come about either spontaneously or as a result of either vigorous stimulation or cardiopulmonary resuscitation. The infant will usually have been described by the observer of the event as having had a disturbance of at least two of the following: breathing, color, consciousness, movement, or muscle tone.

Although such episodes may occur in children older than 12 months, the majority of patients will be less than 1 year and predominantly under 6 months of age (1). This age distribution and the fear engendered in the observer provide support to the possibility that such episodes, if undetected, may lead to the sudden and unexpected death of the infant [cot death or sudden infant death syndrome (SIDS)].

Such episodes will be associated with the parent or caregiver being sufficiently concerned to take action at the time the infant was found. They will have thought the infant was at risk, in the process of dying, or actually dead, and their actions will usually reflect this. The emergency services will have been contacted and urgent admission to hospital arranged. The decision of parents or caregivers to resuscitate an infant is dependent on their perception of the situation as well as their knowledge and skills in performing resuscitative measures. When resuscitation has been instituted, it usually reflects a more severe event than one in which no resuscitation was given. However, it is possible that parents will react very differently to events of similar severity.

II. Relationship to Sudden Infant Death

The commonest category of death in infancy is that which is sudden and unexplained, despite a thorough autopsy, examination of the scene of death, and review of the case history (SIDS). It is probable that the mechanisms that cause sudden and unexpected death in an infant are similar in part to some of the mechanisms that cause ALTE. This is supported by the fact that, whereas most studies report survival in infants who have had an ALTE, a small proportion of infants who suffer recurrent ALTE progress to sudden and unexpected death (2). It has also been identified that a small proportion of infants who die of SIDS have a history of a previous ALTE or apnea: 7% in the National Institute of Child Health and Development Cooperative Epidemiological Study of SIDS in the U.S. (3) and 8.8% in an Australian series (4).

For these reasons, infants who suffer ALTE have been considered an "at risk" group (for sudden death), and their study has been of particular interest with regard to the mechanisms of SIDS. This approach helps our understanding of the pathophysiology of events in living infants that may produce sudden death and complements the approaches from pathological and epidemiological studies.

III. Definition

The National Institutes of Health Consensus Development Conference on Infantile Apnea (1987) defined an ALTE as an episode that is frightening to the observer and is characterized by a combination of apnea, skin color change, marked change in muscle tone, choking, and gagging (3). Such episodes were previously known as *near-miss SIDS*. However, the majority of infants who suffer an ALTE survive and are not at high risk of sudden death. This term has therefore been abandoned. The definition includes identification of the caregivers' reaction to the event; thus infants whose caregivers underreact may not come to the attention of health professionals or be characterized as having suffered an ALTE, even though they may have had some combination of these symptoms. Conversely, benign physiological events in babies may sometimes cause an overreaction by parents, particularly those who are anxious, are attention-seeking, or suffer a personality disorder. Such infants may thereby receive unnecessary hospital admission and investigations. Clinicians should be aware of this spectrum of parental reactions as these often determine management pathways, and it is important that the clinician maintain an objective view to avoid inappropriate investigations and treatment.

As well as the above situations, there are others in which it can be difficult to decide whether an infant is classified as having suffered an ALTE. For example, some infants with ALTE may recover only in part and thus continue to remain unwell when in hospital. In such infants, initial investigations and management will be guided by the ongoing symptoms and signs. In such cases, the finding of an abnormality (for example, a positive blood culture, a nasopharyngeal aspirate positive for respiratory syncytial virus, or an underlying metabolic disorder) will be followed by the diagnosis in the infant being reclassified from ALTE to a more specific illness or condition—for example, septicemia, bronchiolitis, or inborn errors of metabolism. Nevertheless, the parents may have as their greatest concern the presenting event. Such families may continue to require support along similar lines as if the infant had suffered an unexplained ALTE. There is also the scenario of an infant who collapses unexpectedly at home and who remains severely ill, sometimes without adequate explanation. In some cases recalcitrant shock and death follow, but the presentation may be akin to that of an ALTE. Conversely, the infant may spontaneously and fully recover, with the parents demonstrating less concern and reporting the event only at some later time to health professionals. The fear an event causes in parents or caregivers is assessed by their verbal reports and their actions. Whether such infants have had an ALTE is therefore debatable. Finally, infants who have recurrent ALTEs may be classified as suffering from apnea of infancy. This merely renames a clinical problem, does not define its cause, and confuses the definition, as not all ALTEs necessarily involve cessation of breathing.

IV. Review of Evidence Base

Most studies relating to ALTE, near-miss SIDS, or near-death episodes are at a low level of evidence; they involve a retrospective review of a series of cases and the results of usually selective investigations. Another group of studies examines the physiology of infants who have suffered ALTEs; they are often performed on the basis that these infants are a group at high risk for SIDS. Such studies aim to determine mechanisms of susceptibility in infants that may help to explain SIDS. However, these studies are difficult to compare because the populations of infants involved may differ widely. This is because 1) there is no single accepted definition by which infants may be included in studies and 2) clinical practices and diagnostic labeling differ even within a single health facility. The presentation and initial management of infants who present with ALTEs varies between regions and countries, partly as a result of different health care systems.

Most published case series of ALTE infants come from clinicians within specialist or teaching centers who have a special interest in the assessment of ALTE infants. Such data may not represent the pathophysiology or appropriate management pathways for infants presenting with ALTEs in other populations, particularly those that are community-based. Case series may also be biased, depending on whether the publications are from units that have a particular pediatric interest (e.g., gastroenterology or neurology). In addition to these biases in the published literature, there is a lack of adequate information on population-based measures, such as the incidence of ALTE and its outcome. There is wide variation between units, regions, and countries in the assessment, investigation, and management of such infants.

V. Epidemiology

Wennergren et al., in a prospective epidemiological multicenter study over 24 months, found an incidence of attacks of lifelessness of 0.46 per 1000 live births in Sweden (1). This was half the rate for SIDS (0.94 per 1000 live births). Studies have also shown that infants who suffer an ALTE are most likely to present in the daytime (1,5). If such episodes do occur at night, those infants who are unable to arouse or compensate may die and be classified as SIDS. The age distribution for ALTEs was similar in the Swedish study to that of SIDS cases, with a peak around 6 to 8 weeks of age. Such episodes may also occur in the neonatal period (6–8).

Myerberg et al. have estimated that 6 per 1000 full-term infants and 86 per 1000 preterm infants may suffer ALTE (a total of 11 per 1000 live births) (9). In South Australia, an episode of apnea or cyanosis resulted in hospital admission of 1.37% live births (14/100) (10); in North Staffordshire, England (population 480,000), with 6500 live births per year, a recent prospective study identified 30 infants presenting to hospital having suffered an ALTE in one year (4.6 per 1000) (personal observation). Thus, incidence rates for ALTEs vary roughly from 0.5 to 10 per 1000 live births, a 20-fold difference. This variability is likely to be related to different case definitions and ascertainment.

VI. Causes

Infants who present with ALTE are a varied group. In some cases their parents are overly concerned about a benign or physiological event, and in others the infant is truly in a life-threatening situation. Published case reviews have identified a large number of different causes for the clinical presentation of an ALTE (Table 1). Clinical management of such infants does not necessarily require an exhaustive list of investigations to find an abnormality, but rather a careful and focused clinical assessment of each case, commencing with history and examination and, usually, a period of inpatient observation.

It is important to appreciate that abnormal findings do not automatically imply that these were the cause of the infant's event. Abnormalities on investigation may be the result of the ALTE (particularly if it were severe) or simply represent homeostatic instability, autonomic dysfunction, or unrelated factors. Studies that have investigated large numbers of ALTE infants have shown that there is a failure to find a cause in 40 to 50% of cases (11,12). However, there is probably a wide variation in prac-

Table 1 Causes of Apparent Life-Threatening Events

Respiratory
Infection—e.g., respiratory syncytial virus, pertussis, pneumonia
Upper-airway obstruction—e.g., retrognathia (86,92,94–96)
Lower-airway obstruction or closure—e.g., tracheobronchomalacia
Intrapulmonary shunting—e.g., cyanotic breath-holding (12,49)
Neurological
Epileptic—seizure induced (21,97,98)
Intracranial hemorrhage—vitamin K deficiency, child abuse
Central hypoventilation—congenital, drugs, neurological disease
Neuromuscular disease
Infective
Septicemia, urinary tract infection, gastroenteritis
Meningoencephalitis
Autonomic
Vasovagal
Gastroesophageal reflux
Skin color changes
Child abuse (13,72,91)
Illness fabrication
Attempted suffocation
Poisoning
Cardiac
Tachyarrhythmias—Wolfe-Parkinson-White (90) and long-QT syndromes
Congenital heart disease
Inborn errors of metabolism (22)
Miscellaenous
Carbon monoxide poisoning (99)
Cat smothering (100)
Abnormal infant holding practices (101)
Hemorrhagic shock encephalopathy syndrome (102)
Unknown

tice, as some infants who present with ALTEs and in whom an investigation is found to be abnormal (e.g., nasal swab positive for pertussis) may be given a diagnosis of pertussis, rather than "ALTE—cause pertussis." Such issues confound the case ascertainment from one study to another.

VII. History and Examination

Health professionals should listen carefully to the parents' observations as well as their reactions or feelings. In this way, the professional may become more aware of the real and perceived risks of the episode.

A clear description of the event should be noted, including who was present, what each person observed, and what their actions were. The timing of the event should be noted, including whether the infant was awake or asleep and what activity he or she was performing. It may be of value to determine how it was discovered that the event was occurring. It is not uncommon that parents/caregivers discover such cases by chance.

A record of the infant's position should be made, whether there was movement and how the infant was holding itself. The color of the infant should be noted—this may be red, blue, purple, pale, gray, or white. It may be possible to clarify whether color change has occurred on the face as a whole (central cyanosis), just around the eyes and mouth, or in the limbs. The presence of vomit or blood from the nose and mouth should be recorded. This may be a marker for trauma and an event that is intentionally induced [from data of Southall et al.; odds ratio 41.0 (13)]. The presence or absence of breathing movements should be asked about, but it may be difficult for observers to report this finding reliably. Even a nurses's observations of the presence or absence of breathing in infants receiving hospital neonatal care may correlate poorly with recorded breathing patterns (14–16). In these studies, nurses failed to detect naturally occurring episodes in preterm infants on conventional bedside breathing movements and electrocardiographic (ECG) monitors: 46% to 67% of episodes documented on multichannel recordings went undetected.

The actions of the observers should be noted as well as the response of the infant to these. The time scale for these actions and the recovery of the infant should be noted and whether any similar event had occurred in the past.

A general pediatric history should be obtained of the mother's pregnancy and delivery as well as the infant's birth and neonatal progress. A history of feeding, weight gain, development, and recent minor symptoms should be noted. A detailed family medical history and social history should also be obtained. The latter should include who else is at home, other stresses and medical problems within the family, and any contact with psychiatric or social services.

Infants who are historically at particular risk of subsequent events or sudden death may be identified. These include those who were born prematurely, who may be suffering subclinical hypoxemia (17), and those who had bleeding from the mouth and nose, indicating trauma, child abuse or pulmonary hemorrhage (13).

A full clinical examination with the infant completely undressed should be performed. The height, weight, and head circumference should be recorded and plotted on a growth chart. Particular attention should be paid to examination of the upper airway and respiratory and cardiovascular systems. Neurodevelopmental assessment is important because a number of neurological conditions may present with apnea. To detect trauma, fundoscopy should be performed. All infants should undergo initial spot measurement of arterial oxygen saturation (Sp_{O_2}); in infants who were preterm or who may have a respiratory prodrome, a longer period of monitoring of Sp_{O_2} should be undertaken.

VIII. Initial Management and Investigations

Parents of an infant who has suffered an ALTE may be extremely anxious and may have been concerned that their infant was dying. For this reason alone, it is probably appropriate to admit all infants who have suffered a first ALTE. This allows time for a full assessment, a period of observation, and discussion with the family.

A recurrence rate for severe ALTE as high as 68% has been reported (18); for all ALTE, episodes are more likely to recur in the few days after the first event (1). These data provide further support for initial hospital admission. Some ALTEs may be recurrent within a short period of time (hours to days). These subsequent events, e.g., infantile spasms, may be observed and a diagnosis made by clinical observation. In addition, clinical physiological monitoring or recording allows documentation of any further events, and the findings from this may indicate a diagnosis (4,12,19). Both respiratory illnesses, such as respiratory syncytial virus (RSV) and pertussis (20), and epileptic seizures (21) may cluster in this way.

Some infants may initially be seen some days after the episode either in the pediatrician's office, admissions room, or outpatient clinic. In such cases, admission may not be required, if it is agreed the infant has had no further events and is clinically well.

No study has identified any single investigation as having a high positive predictive value for detecting an abnormality that will alter the outcome. There is thus much controversy as to which initial investigations should be undertaken in an infant presenting with a first ALTE. In most cases, it is not unreasonable to check serum sodium, potassium, calcium, renal and liver function, full blood picture, blood and urine cultures, throat/pharyngeal swabs, and chest x-ray (Table 2).

If the infant is seen very soon after the event, an arterial blood gas may help to provide documentation of the severity of the episode (13). Other markers of metabolic disturbance—such as blood glucose, lactate and ammonia—could also be measured at this time. Continued observation, particularly for the development of respiratory infection, fever, or other signs of sepsis, should be undertaken, with a low threshold for treating sepsis in infants under 4 weeks of age. Nose swabs/pharyngeal aspirates should be collected for viral immunofluorescence and culture and for pertussis culture. Urine should be collected for microscopy, bacterial culture, and antibiotic sensitivities and specimens also saved for urinary and blood metabolic screens (22). Urine and blood should be collected and held for toxicology screens. Parents/caregivers may not always provide complete information about medicines given to the infants, some of which may have been administered inadvertently and some deliberately.

A majority of infants suffer a single event only and survive. Adverse outcomes are more likely with infants who have had recurrent events or where there is a family history of SIDS. In the absence of these, investigations should be kept to a minimum in an otherwise well infant. However, if the infant remains unwell, develops new symptoms, has recurrent episodes, or there is a family history of SIDS, further

Table 2 Investigations in Infants Presenting with Apparent Life-Threatening Events

First-line investigations
- Hemoglobin
- White cell count
- Blood culture
- Urine culture
- Nasopharyngeal aspirate for viral immunofluorescence and culture
- Nasal swab for pertussis
- Chest x-ray
- Biochemical screen

Second-line investigations (severe/recurrent events)
- Multichannel physiological recordings/event recording[a]
- Blood sugar[b]
- Arterial blood gas[b]
- Lactate[b]
- Ammonia[b]
- Serum and urine metabolic studies (e.g., for amino/organic acids)
- Urinary toxicology screen
- Electroencephalography
- Cranial imaging (computed tomography, magnetic resonance imaging)
- Electrocardiography
- Esophageal pH monitoring
- Examination of the airway under anesthetic
- Echocardiography
- Skeletal survey
- Covert video surveillance

[a]Of particular value for documenting pathophysiology during subsequent event.
[b]If close to event/still unwell.

investigations should be undertaken. The most common diagnoses from some recent studies are shown in Table 3.

The role of multichannel physiological recording or esophageal pH recording as a routine in ALTEs is more complex and is discussed below.

IX. Physiology

Physiological studies in infants who have suffered ALTEs have not pointed to any particular test with a high positive predictive value for an adverse outcome. Studies have identified subgroups of infants who suffer from abnormal hypoxemia or

Table 3 Diagnostic Categories and Proportions of ALTE Infants in Each Category

		Proportions of infants with diagnosis (Reference and country of origin)					
Diagnostic category	Percentages of ALTE infants with diagnosis	Belgium (103)	Australia (4)	U.K. (12)	Others[a]		
Breathing problems	5–25	60/857	17/340	40/157	13/64 (53)		
Epilepsy	7–15	78/857	25/340	10/157	4/59 (53)	7/46 (89)	
Gastroesophageal reflux	24–62	263/857	211/340		12/50 (53)	72/117 (55)	9/17 (9,57)
Induced or fabricated illness	2–16		5/340	25/157			
Metabolic	2–8	14/857			5/65 (22)		
Vasovagal	11	95/857					
Unknown	33–55	281/857		80/157			

[a]Australia, Israel, United States, and France.

esophageal acidity; in these, recurrent events have reduced or stopped after intervention such as oxygen therapy (12) or treatment for reflux (23). Most physiological studies have looked at groups of infants suffering ALTEs and identified group differences from healthy controls. However, there is usually a large overlap between normals and ALTE infants, which limits the usefulness of physiological testing in identifying an individual's susceptibility to further events. Such studies, therefore, have little role in clinical management. That is, they do not help predict recurrence or risk for sudden death in individual patients.

Respiratory studies have identified the presence of increased apneic pauses (24–26), obstructive apnea (27), periodic breathing (28–29), higher heart and respiratory rates (30) and abnormalities in waking and ventilatory responses to carbon dioxide (31–33). These abnormalities have not always been borne out by other studies (34,35). Decreased specific airway conductance (36,37) and abnormalities in diaphragm strength (38) have also been identified in ALTE infants. Whether these are cause, effect, or associated phenomena in relation to the ALTE are unknown.

Studies suggest that there may be an abnormality in autonomic function in infants who have had an ALTE, as identified by increased sweating at night (39), abnormal heart rate variability (40), changes in sleep state (41), and blood pressure responses (42). Neurological studies such as brainstem auditory evoked responses (43,44) have not shown differences from controls.

X. Multichannel Recordings

Case series show an enormous variation in the proportion of infants who demonstrate abnormalities on pneumograms, sleep studies, or multichannel physiological recordings. Such studies have different methodologies and definitions of abnormality. They have not been found to be predictive of recurrence of events (30,45). Event recordings in infants during further events and in those who subsequently die of SIDS do not show apneic pauses (central apnea) to be a primary abnormality (46,47). Bradycardia has been identified in event recordings during death or near-death episodes (46), but this too may be secondary, for example, to hypoxemia (47). Event recordings that focuses on alarms based on apnea or bradycardia criteria have identified most events as being artifactual (48). However, when recordings are made of clinical events, hypoxemia has been identified as one of the main abnormalities (47).

This hypoxemia was due to varied causes, including respiratory events due to intrapulmonary shunting (49), epileptic seizure–induced events (21), and intentional attempted suffocation (13). The "shunt" events were manifest as hypoxemic episodes in association with chronic lung disease of prematurity, respiratory infections or cyanotic breath-holding. When recurrent, treatment with additional inspired oxygen helped reduce/stop events (12). The particular susceptibility of preterm infants to subclinical chronic lung disease and clinically undetected hypoxemia may put these infants at increased risk for hypoxemic episodes, ALTE, and sudden death. Additional oxygen therapy appeared to be therapeutic in reducing cyanotic-apnea episodes in this group of infants (17).

Although recognition and treatment of hypoxemia in infants who were born before term may be important in reducing subsequent events (50), standard recordings looking for apneic events (cessation or breathing/airflow) have been shown not to be predictive of future events (30,51). There is also no gain from routine multichannel recordings in subsequent siblings of ALTE infants (52).

XI. Gastroesophageal Reflux

Using a combination of 24-hr esophageal pH monitoring, barium swallow, and radionuclide milk scans, gastroesophageal reflux has been identified in up to 95% of infants who have suffered ALTE (53). Such reflux is particularly common during active sleep (54) and has been considered to act via reflex effects on central respiratory control (55,56) or, in some cases, to induce epileptic seizures (57). Initial reports of the finding of reflux suggested that it has a major role in producing life-threatening events; when found, its treatment should be mandatory (23,58). However, there is no "gold standard" for defining its presence; longer recordings of esophageal pH, or additional investigations such as milk scans have resulted in higher proportions of infants with this finding being identified (59,60). Whether esophageal reflux is a significant cause of hypoxemic episodes, a trigger in a susceptible infant, or, in fact, an associated manifestation is controversial. Studies that have aimed to correlate apneic pauses with falls in esophageal pH have failed to show a temporal relationship (61–64). One study has correlated hypoxemic episodes with acid reflux, but some falls in Sp_{O_2} may have been motion artifact, which may have occurred in association with movement and acid reflux (65). Interestingly, recordings of breathing movements and ECGs were normal in association with reflux.

Hypoxemia and apnea may occur in association with feedings but without evidence of gastroesophageal reflux (66). This may have arisen because of the effects of sucking and swallowing on breathing. Alternatively, gastroesophageal reflux may be a consequence of active expiratory muscle activity in infants prone to respiratory events. Infants may produce active expiratory activity to overcome decreased airway conductance (36,37) and thus increase intra-abdominal pressure. However, this has not been formally examined. When reflux is found in a patient, it may be of more relevance to determine whether it has a respiratory effect in terms of abnormal hypoxemic episodes, as it may be the infant's response to reflux that is responsible for the event rather than the reflux per se. The use of the modified Bernstein's test may be of value in throwing more light on the reflex physical and mechanical effects of stimulation within the esophagus or upper airway (67).

XII. Psychological Assessment

Families who have had infants with ALTEs see their infants more negatively than healthy infants, and mothers report feeling less attachment (68). Whether these are directly the result of the apnea or characterize the families whose infants present with ALTE is unknown. It is possible that some families present with infants with ALTE because they are more stressed or have different personality characteristics prior to the event. In view of the fact that parental anxiety, depression, and lack of parenting skills are detrimental to the emotional development of infants, close psychosocial assessment is warranted and support is provided where possible.

Mothers who present infants with recurrent ALTE episodes that are either fabricated or induced have adverse psychosocial backgrounds, mostly demonstrating personality disorders (13). Diagnosis may be aided by close examination of maternal and family responses to the infant, antecedent psychosocial history, and whether abnormal illness behavior exists within the family. Covert video surveillance may also be required to detect ALTE due to child abuse (13).

XIII. Discharge Planning and Home Monitoring

The plans for follow-up of infants and their families need to be individualized and depend on the underlying diagnosis, severity of the event, and views of parents, doctors and community staff. Infants with a single mild episode or definite diagnosis (e.g., bronchiolitis) require minimal follow up. This may, in turn, be reassuring to the families. Those with recurrent episodes require further investigation and follow-up. There is an increased risk of death for infants with subsequent events (69); therefore greater surveillance and more extensive investigation may be required to reach a diagnosis. This may include the longer-term use of hospital or home-based multichannel recordings (12). Because of the increased risk of death, special care must be taken in planning the discharge of infants who have had an ALTE and received cardiopulmonary resuscitation (69), in infants who were born very premature (70,71), and in those for whom there are possible child protection concerns (72).

The results of some studies suggest that home monitoring may prevent deaths in certain high-risk groups (2,18,73,74). However, there has been no randomized controlled trial showing that monitors reduce mortality, and they should not be provided on this basis.

Practices for offering home monitoring vary widely; some consider that home monitoring has no role to play while others offer it to all families. Cardiorespiratory monitors using impedance pneumography and electrocardiography has not been clinically validated to detect potentially severe apneic-hypoxemic episodes or ALTE; their use has thus been criticized (75). This is in contrast to monitors detecting abnormal oxygenation, which pick up 90% to 100% of serious hypoxemic apneic episodes (47,76). Cardiorespiratory monitors produce many false alarms (48) and may not detect ALTEs; deaths having occurred with such monitors (77,78). In the United Kingdom, apnea monitors that work by detecting body movements are used alone. These have a poor ability to detect potentially life-threatening, hypoxemic events (76), and deaths have occurred with these monitors too (79). There is also a theoretical risk in older infants of strangulation from such monitors (80). It does not seem appropriate to monitor for events due to upper- or lower-airway obstruction by using monitors that detect respiratory pauses. More appropriate monitors would involve the detection of hypoxemia by using pulse oximetry or transcutaneous P_{O_2} (76).

An advance in monitor technology in recent years has been the ability to record monitor use and the physiological signals prior to an alarm. Cardiorespiratory monitors have shown bradycardia rather than cessation of breathing movements to precede death/near- death episodes (81). Although oxygenation was not recorded in these studies, another study recording near-death episodes has shown hypoxemia to be the initial changing parameter (47).

Our own practice has been to offer home oxygen monitoring to infants with recurrent events, to those who have undergone cardiopulmonary resuscitation, or where there is increased anxiety—for example, because of prematurity or a previous baby who has died of SIDS (76). Such monitoring can record compliance and subsequent events (47). Our own event recorder stores 20 min of data on oxygenation, breathing movements, pulse waveform, ECG, and time around any clinically significant events (triggered by parents), whether or not an alarm has occurred. Alarms exist for detecting abnormal hypoxemia or sensor disconnection using transcutaneous P_{O_2}. This equipment allows the diagnostic process to continue at home and thus may avoid having an infant with recurrent events from spending weeks in a hospital setting.

Documented observations show variable compliance among parents using monitors (82,83). Furthermore, this procedure may both increase or lower parental anxiety (84,85). Ongoing support is likely to be required for many parents, particularly those who undergo home physiological monitoring. At the time of hospital discharge, parents require a clear account of what has happened; the observations, investigations, and results in the hospital; and the level of medical understanding of the infant's event. This may or may not include a diagnostic label, but health professionals should be cautious in applying diagnostic labels without good objective evidence. This will avoid the escalation of treatments for a recurrent condition that appears unresponsive to treatment. For example, infants with recurrent ALTE of unknown cause should avoid fundoplication (even if they have reflux) unless esophageal acidity has been objectively documented as the trigger for events. Similarly, infants with recurrent events should avoid being labeled as having epilepsy, and thus receiving escalating anticonvulsant therapy, unless objectively documented primary epileptic discharges have been captured on EEG during events (21).

If infants are discharged home without ongoing physiological monitoring, they should spend some time in hospital without monitors attached. Usually a period of observation of at least 24 hr while the infant is well will be required before discharge. This should be undertaken when the family feels confident and health professionals are happy with the infant's condition.

XIV. Specific Management for Recurrent ALTE

Specific treatments may be administered for those infants in whom a diagnosis of a specific condition has been found to account for their recurrent events; single events are less reliably categorized as being due to an associated medical problem, and early institution of treatments should be avoided.

Infants with recurrent events and findings of a small upper airway—due, for example, to retrognathia or Pierre Robin sequence—may benefit from continuous positive airway pressure (CPAP) (86). Hypoxemic-apneic episodes in infections such as RSV and pertussis may also benefit from lung-distending measures including CPAP or continuous negative extrathoracic pressure (87). In preterm infants with baseline hypoxemia, additional inspired oxygen may be effective therapy for recurrent cyanotic-apneic episodes (17) and may be of value in other episodes involving sudden intrapulmonary shunting (12). Oxygen therapy not only increases the baseline arterial P_{O_2} from which any respiratory event occurs, thus prolonging the time taken for the development of hypoxemia, but may also be therapeutic by improving airway conductance and pulmonary vasodilation (49).

For recurrent events that *begin* in the presence of a particular caregiver, consideration should be given to the possibility of imposed upper-airway obstruction or attempted suffocation (13,72). This is one manifestation of illness induction, and other abnormal illness behaviors may feature in the parent/caregiver or other children. Because this involves serious, life-threatening child abuse and is associated with emotional abuse, measures must be taken to investigate this possibility in a confidential manner. Working with parents who perform this abuse may not be possible and more extraordinary measures may be required to confirm the diagnosis, such as covert video surveillance (13). Such investigations should be undertaken in consultation with other agencies who have responsibility for child protection, such as the police and social services.

Apneic pauses and periodic breathing are reduced in term infants by the use of theophylline (26). However, treatment of these pneumographic findings probably has little clinical relevance; their presence does not predict sudden death (88). Furthermore, methylxantine medication increases the tendency to gastroesophageal reflux and lowers the seizure threshold. Such medications reduce alarms from monitors that detect apneic pauses, but these are of dubious pathological importance. Diagnosis and treatment of epilepsy will be important in infants and will require further neurological assessment to determine the underlying cause (89).

Pacemakers have been inserted into infants with profound bradycardia/sinus pauses in events (46), but it needs to be verified that these are primary cardiac electrophysiological abnormalities (90) and not secondary to hypoxemia from attempted suffocation (91), epileptic seizures (21), or sleep-related upper-airway obstruction (92).

XV. Outcome

The majority of infants survive and are normal at long-term follow-up (1,93). The families of infants who have had single mild events can usually be reassured that the likelihood of further events is extremely small. One study has reported a 13% risk for subsequent death in infants with recurrent episodes who have received resuscitation, particularly in association with either epilepsy or a previous history of SIDS (69). Infants with recurrent events require specialist assessment and follow-up, particularly with regard to the detection of causes that are either rarer (epileptic seizure–induced apnea) or more difficult to diagnose (attempted suffocation, which may be found by using covert video surveillance). In the latter category, there is a high mortality, thus increasing the need for early detection. Use of event recording and home oxygen monitoring in the group of infants who have received cardiopulmonary resuscitation—and awareness of the more difficult diagnoses—can be associated with a mortality of 2% (12). Some form of event capture is particularly important in diagnosing recurrent events.

References

1. Wennergren G, Milerad J, Lagercrantz H, Karlberg P, Svenningsen NW, Sedin G, Anderson D, Grögaard J, Bjure J. The epidemiology of sudden infant death syndrome and attacks of lifelessness in Sweden. Acta Paediatr Scand 1987; 76:898–906.
2. Kelly DH, Shannon DC, O'Connell K. Care of infants with near-miss sudden infant death syndrome. Pediatrics 1978; 61:511–514.
3. National Institutes of Health. Infantile Apnea and Home Monitoring. Report of a consensus development conference, 1987. NIH Publication No. 87-2905. Washington, DC: U.S. Department of Health and Human Services, Public Health Service,1987.

4. Rahilly PM. The pneumographic and medical investigation of infants suffering apparent life threatening episodes. J Paediatr Child Health 1991; 27:349–353.
5. Kahn A, Blum D, Hennart P, Sellens C, Samson-Dollfus D, Tayot J, Gilly R, Dutruge J, Flores R, Sternberg B. A critical comparison of the history of sudden death infants and infants hospitalised for near-miss for SIDS. Eur J Pediatr 1984; 143:103–107.
6. Grylack LJ, Williams AD. Apparent life-threatening events in presumed healthy neonates during the first three days of life. Pediatrics 1996; 97:349–351.
7. Burchfield DJ, Rawlings J. Sudden deaths and apparent life-threatening events in hospitalised neonates presumed to be healthy. Am J Dis Child 1991; 145:1319–1322.
8. Rodriguez-Alarcón J, Melchor JC, Linares A, Aranguren G, Quintanilla M, Fernandez-Llebrez L, de la Gandara A, Rodriguez-Soriano J. Early neonatal sudden death or near death syndrome: an epidemiological study of 29 cases. Acta Paediatr 1994; 83:704–708.
9. Myerberg DZ, Carpenter RG, Myerberg CF, Britton CM, Bailey CW, Fink BE. Reducing postneonatal mortality in West Virginia: a statewide intervention program targeting risk identified at and after birth. Am J Public Health 1995; 85:631–637.
10. Ponsonby AL, Dwyer T, Couper D. Factors related to infant apnoea and cyanosis: a population based study. J Pediatr Child Health 1997; 33:317–323.
11. Kahn A, Groswasser J, Sottiaux M, Rebuffat E, Franco P. Clinical problems in relation to apparent life-threatening events in infants. Acta Pediatr Suppl 1993; 389:107–110.
12. Samuels MP, Poets CF, Noyes JP, Hartmann H, Hewertson J, Southall DP. Diagnosis and management after life threatening events in infants and young children who received cardiopulmonary resuscitation. BMJ 1993; 306:489–492.
13. Southall DP, Plunkett MCB, Banks MW, Falkov AF, Samuels MP. Covert video recordings of life threatening child abuse: lessons for child protection. Pediatrics 1997; 100: 735–760.
14. Peabody JL, Volpe JJ. Episodes of apnea and bradycardia in the preterm infant: impact on cerebral circulation. Pediatrics 1985; 76:333–338.
15. Southall DP, Levitt GA, Richards JM, Jones RA, Kong C, Farndon PA, Alexander JR, Wilson AJ. Undetected episodes of prolonged apnea and bradycardia in preterm infants. Pediatrics 1983; 72:541–551.
16. Muttit SC, Finer NN, Tierney AJ, Rossman J. Neonatal apnea: diagnosis by nurse versus computer. Pediatrics 1988; 82:713–720.
17. Samuels MP, Poets CF, Southall DP. Abnormal hypoxemia after life threatening events in infants born before term. J Pediatr 1994; 125:441–446.
18. Ariagno RL, Guilleminault C, Korobkin R, Owen-Boeddiker M, Baldwin R. "Near miss" for sudden infant death syndrome infants: a clinical problem. Pediatrics 1983; 71: 721–730.
19. Guilleminault C, Ariagno RL. Why should we study the infant "near miss for sudden infant death"? Early Hum Dev 1978; 2/3:207–218.
20. Anas N, Boettrich C, Hall CB, Brooks JG. The association of apnea and respiratory syncytial virus infection in infants. J Pediatr 1982; 101:65–68.
21. Hewertson H, Poets CF, Samuels MP, Boyd SG, Neville BGR, Southall DP. Epileptic seizure induced hypoxemia in infants with apparent life threatening events. Pediatrics 1994; 94:148–156.
22. Arens R, Gozal D, Williams JC, Davidson Ward SL, Keens TG. Recurrent apparent life-threatening events during infancy: a manifestation of inborn errors of metabolism. J Pediatr 1993; 123:415–418.

23. Herbst JJ, Book LS, Bray PF. Gastroesophageal reflux in the "near miss" sudden infant death syndrome. J Pediatr 1978; 92:73–75.
24. Guilleminault C, Peraita R, Souquet M, Dement WC. Apneas during sleep in infants: possible relationships with sudden infant death syndrome. Science 1975; 190:677–679.
25. Haidmayer R, Kurz R, Kenner T, Wurm H, Pfeiffer KP. Physiological and clinical aspects of respiration control in infants with relation to the sudden infant death syndrome. Klin Wochenschr 1982; 60:9–18.
26. Hunt CE, Brouillette RT, Hanson D. Theophylline improves pneumogram abnormalities in infants at risk of sudden infant death syndrome. J Pediatr 1983; 103:969–974.
27. Guilleminault C, Ariagno R, Korobkin R, Nagel L, Baldwin R, Coons S, Owen M. Mixed and obstructive sleep apnea and near miss for sudden infant death syndrome: 2. Comparison of near miss and normal control infants by age. Pediatrics 1979; 64:882–891.
28. Kelly DH, Shannon DC. Periodic breathing in infants with near-miss sudden infant death syndrome. Pediatrics 1979; 63:355–360.
29. Brady JP, Ariagno RL, Watts JC, Goldman SL, Dumpit TM. Apnea, hypoxemia and aborted sudden infant death syndrome. Pediatrics 1978; 62:686–691.
30. Oren J, Kelly DH, Shannon DC. Pneumogram recordings in infants resuscitated for apnea of infancy. Pediatrics 1989; 83:364–368.
31. Anwar M, Marotta F, Fort MD, Mondestin H, Mojica C, Walsh S, Hiatt M, Hegyi T. The ventilatory response to carbon dioxide in high risk infants. Early Hum Dev 1993; 35: 183–192.
32. Haddad GG, Leistner HL, Lai TL, Mellins RB. Ventilation and ventilatory pattern during sleep in aborted sudden infant death syndrome. Pediatr Res 1981; 15:879–883.
33. McCulloch K, Brouillette RT, Guzzetta AJ, Hunt CE. Arousal responses in near-miss sudden infant death syndrome and in normal infants. J Pediatr 1982; 101:911–917.
34. Ariagno R, Nagel L, Guilleminault C. Waking and ventilatory responses during sleep in infants near-miss for sudden infant death syndrome. Sleep 1980; 3:351–359.
35. Parks YA, Paton JY, Beardsmore CS, MacFadyen UM, Thompson J, Goodenough PC, Simpson H. Respiratory control in infants at increased risk for sudden infant death syndrome. Arch Dis Child 1989; 64:791–797.
36. Kao LC, Keens TG. Decreased specific airway conductance in infant apnea. Pediatrics 1985; 76:232–235.
37. Hartmann H, Seidenberg J, Noyes JP, O'Brien L, Poets CF, Samuels MP, Southall DP. Small airway patency in infants with apparent life threatening events. Eur J Pediatr 1998; 157:71–74.
38. Scott CB, Nickerson BG, Sargent CW, Platzker AC, Warburton D, Keens TG. Developmental patterns of maximal transdiaphragmatic pressure in infants during crying. Pediatr Res 1983; 17:707–709.
39. Kahn A, Van de Merckt C, Dramaix M, Magrez P, Blum D, Rebuffat E, Montauk L. Transepidermal water loss during sleep in infants at risk for sudden death. Pediatrics 1987; 80:245–250.
40. Leistner HL, Haddad GG, Epstein RA, Lai TL, Epstein MA, Mellins RB. Heart rate and heart rate variability during sleep in aborted sudden infant death syndrome. J Pediatr 1980; 97:51–55.
41. Haddad GG, Walsh EM, Leistner HL, Grodin WK, Mellins RB. Abnormal maturation of sleep states in infants with aborted sudden infant death syndrome. Pediatr Res 1981; 15:1055–1057.

42. Fox GPP, Matthews TG. Autonomic dysfunction at different ambient temperatures in infants at risk of sudden infant death syndrome. Lancet 1989; 4:1065–1067.
43. Gupta PR, Guilleminault C, Dorfmann LJ. Brainstem auditory evoked potentials in near-miss sudden infant death syndrome. J Pediatr 1981; 98:791–794.
44. Lüders H, Orlowski JP, Dinner DS, Lesser RP, Klem GH. Far-field auditory evoked potentials in near-miss sudden infant death syndrome. Arch Neurol 1984; 41:615–617.
45. Hodgman JE, Hoppenbrouwers T, Geidel S, Hadeed A, Sterman MB, Haper R, McGinty D. Respiratory behavior in near-miss sudden infant death syndrome. Pediatrics 1982; 69:785–792.
46. Kelly DH, Pathak A, Meny R. Sudden severe bradycardia in infancy. Pediatr Pulmonol 1991; 10:199–204.
47. Poets CF, Samuels MP, Noyes JP, Hewertson J, Hartman H, Holder A, Southall DP. Home event recordings of oxygenation, breathing movements, and heart rate and rhythm in infants with recurrent life-threatening events. J Pediatr 1993; 123:693–701.
48. Weese-Mayer DE, Morrow AS, Conway LP, Brouillette RT, Silvestri JM. Assessing clinical significance of apnea exceeding fifteen seconds with event recording. J Pediatr 1990; 117:568–574.
49. Poets CF, Samuels MP, Southall DP. Potential role of intrapulmonary shunting in the genesis of hypoxemic episodes in infants and young children. Pediatrics 1992; 90:385–391.
50. Gray PH, Rogers Y. Are infants with bronchopulmonary dysplasia at risk for sudden infant death syndrome? Pediatrics 1994; 95:774–777.
51. Barrington KJ, Finer N, Li D. Predischarge respiratory recordings in very low birth weight newborn infants. J Pediatr 1996; 129:934–940.
52. Duke JC, Sekar KC, Toubas PL, McCaffree MA. Apnea in subsequent asymptomatic siblings of infants who had an apparent life-threatening event. J Perinatol 1992; 12: 124–128.
53. Jeffery HE, Rahilly P, Read DJC. Multiple causes of asphyxia in infants at high risk for sudden infant death. Arch Dis Child 1983; 58:92–100.
54. Jeffery HE, Reid I, Rahilly P, Read DJC. Gastro-oesophageal reflux in "near-miss" sudden infant death infants in active but not quiet sleep. Sleep 1980; 3:393–399.
55. de Bethmann O, Couchard M, de Ajuriaguerra M, Lucet V, Cheron G, Guillon G, Relier JP. Role of gastro-oesophageal reflux and vagal overactivity in apparent life-threatening events: 160 cases. Acta Paediatr Suppl 1993; 389:102–104.
56. Beyaert C, Marchal F, Dousset B, Serres MA, Monin P. Gastroesophageal reflux and acute life-threatening episodes: role of a central respiratory depression. Biol Neonate 1995; 68:87–90.
57. Tirosh E, Jaffe M. Apnea of infancy, seizures, and gastroesophageal reflux: an important but infrequent association. J Child Neurol 1996; 11:98–100.
58. Leape LL, Holder TM, Franklin JD, Amoury RA, Ashcraft KW. Respiratory arrest in infants secondary to gastroesophageal reflux. Pediatrics 1977; 60:924–928.
59. Graff MA, Kashlan F, Carter M, Rovell K, Ramos DG. Nap studies underestimate the incidence of gastroesophageal reflux. Pediatr Pulmonol 1994; 18:258–260.
60. MacFadyen UM, Hendry GMA, Simpson H. Gastro-oesophageal reflux in near-miss sudden infant death syndrome or suspected recurrent aspiration. Arch Dis Child 1983; 58:87–91.
61. Ariagno RL, Guilleminault C, Baldwin R, Owen-Boeddiker M. Movement and gastroesophageal reflux in awake term infants with "near miss" SIDS, unrelated to apnea. J Pediatr 1982; 100:894–897.

62. Rosen EL, Frost JD, Harrison GM. Infant apnea: polygraphic studies and follow up monitoring. Pediatrics 1983; 71:731–736.
63. Paton JY, Nanayakkara CS, Simpson H. Observations on gastro-oesophageal reflux, central apnea and heart rate in infants. Eur J Pediatr 1990; 149:608–612.
64. Newell SJ, Booth IW, Morgan MEI, Durbin GM, McNeish AS. Gastro-oesophageal reflux in preterm infants. Arch Dis Child 1989; 64:780–786.
65. See CC, Newman LJ, Berezin S, Glassman MS, Medow MS, Dozor AJ, Schwarz SM. Gastroesophageal reflux-induced hypoxemia in infants with apparent life-threatening event(s). Am J Dis Child 1989; 143:951–954.
66. Guilleminault C, Coons S. Apnea and bradycardia during feeding in infants weighing >2000 gm. J Pediatr 1984; 104:932–935.
67. Friesen CA, Streed CJ, Carney LA, Zwick DL, Roberts CC. Esophagitis and modified Bernstein tests in infants with apparent life-threatening events. Pediatrics 1994; 94: 541–544.
68. Jenkins RL. Indices for maternal/family anxiety and disruption related to infant apnea and home monitoring. Health Care Women Int 1996; 17:535–548.
69. Oren J, Kelly D, Shannon DC. Identification of a high-risk group for sudden infant death syndrome among infants who were resuscitated for sleep apnea. Pediatrics 1986; 77: 495–499.
70. Grether JK, Schulman J. Sudden infant death syndrome and birth weight. J Pediatr 1987; 114:561–567.
71. Wariyar V, Richmond S, Hey E. Pregnancy outcome at 24–31 weeks gestation: neonatal survivors. Arch Dis Child 1989; 64:678–686.
72. Meadows R. Suffocation, recurrent apnea and sudden infant death. J Pediatr 1990; 117: 351–357.
73. Kahn A, Blum D. Home monitoring of infants considered at risk for the sudden infant death syndrome. Eur J Pediatr 1982; 139:94–100.
74. Dufty P, Bryan MH. Home apnea monitoring in "near miss" sudden infant death syndrome (SIDS) and in siblings of SIDS victims. Pediatrics 1982; 70:69–74.
75. Hodgman JE, Hoppenbrouwers T. Home monitoring for sudden infant death syndrome: the case against. Ann NY Acad Sci 1988; 533:164–175.
76. Poets CF, Samuels MP, Noyes JP, Jones KA, Southall DP. Home monitoring of transcutaneous oxygen tension in the early detection of hypoxemia in infants and young children. Arch Dis Child 1991; 66:676–682.
77. Davidson Ward SL, Keens TG, Chan LS, et al. Sudden infant death syndrome in infants evaluated by apnea programs in California. Pediatrics 1986; 77:451–455.
78. Meny RG, Blackmon L, Fleischman D, Gutberlet R, Naumburg E. Sudden infant death and home monitors. Am J Dis Child 1988; 142:1037–1040.
79. Samuels MP, Stebbens VA, Poets CF, Southall DP. Deaths on infant "apnea" monitors. Matern Child Health 1993; 18:262–266.
80. Emery JL, Taylor EM, Carpenter RG, Waite AJ. Apnea monitors and accidental strangulation. BMJ 1992; 304:117.
81. Meny RG, Carroll JL, Carbone MT, Kelly DH. Cardiorespiratory recordings from infants dying suddenly and unexpectedly at home. Pediatrics 1994; 93:44–49.
82. Silvestri JM, Hufford DR, Durham J, Pearsall SM, Oess MA, Weese-Mayer DE, Hunt CE, Levenson SM, Corwin MJ. Assessment of compliance with home cardiorespiratory monitoring in infants at risk of sudden infant death syndrome. J Paediatr 1995; 127:384–388.

83. Gibson E, Spinner S, Cullen JA, Wrobel HA, Spitzer AR. Documented home apnea monitoring: effect on compliance, duration of monitoring, and validation of alarm reporting. Clin Pediatr 1996; 35:505–513.
84. Ahmann E. Family impact of home apnea monitoring: an overview of research and its clinical implications. Pediatr Nurs 1992; 18:611–615.
85. Noyes J, Stebbens V, Sobhan G, Samuels M, Southall D. Home monitoring of infants at increased risk of sudden death. J Clin Nurs 1996; 5:297–306.
86. Guilleminault C, Pelayo R, Clerk A, Leger D, Bocian RC. Home nasal continuous positive airway pressure in infants with sleep-disordered breathing. J Pediatr 1995; 127: 905–912.
87. Linney MJ, Marinaki T, Southall DP, Samuels MP. Negative pressure ventilation in severe bronchiolitis. Care Crit Ill 1997; 13:161.
88. Southall DP, Richards JM, Stebbens VA, Wilson AJ, Taylor V, Alexander JR. Cardiorespiratory patterns in 16 full term infants who suffered SIDS. Pediatrics 1986; 78:787–796.
89. Tirosh E, Jaffe M. Apparent life-threatening event: a neurologic perspective. J Child Neurol 1995; 10:216–218.
90. Keeton BR, Southall E, Rutter N, Anderson RH, Shinebourne EA, Southall DP. Cardiac conduction disorders in six infants with "near-miss" sudden infant deaths. BMJ 1977; 2:600–601.
91. Samuels MP, McClaughlin W, Jacobson RR, Poets CF, Southall DP. Fourteen cases of imposed upper airway obstruction. Arch Dis Child 1992; 67:162–170.
92. Guilleminault C, Heldt G, Powell N, Riley R. Small upper airway in near-miss sudden infant death syndrome infants and their families. Lancet 1986; 1:402–407.
93. Kahn A, Sottiaux M, Appelboom-Fondu J, Blum D, Rebuffat E, Levitt J. Long-term development of children monitored as infants for an apparent life-threatening event during sleep: a 10-year follow-up study. Pediatrics 1989; 83:668–673.
94. Gozzi DA, Bonanni M, Cozzi F, Villa MP, Polidori G. Recurrent apparent life-threatening event relieved by glossopexy. J Pediatr Surg 1996; 31:1715–1718.
95. Engelberts AC. The role of obstructive apnea in sudden infant death syndrome and apparent life threatening event. Int J Pediatr Otorhinolaryngol 1995; 32(suppl):S59–S62.
96. McMurray JS, Holinger LD. Otolaryngic manifestations in children presenting with apparent life-threatening events. Otolaryngol Head Neck Surg 1997; 116:575–579.
97. Aubourg P, Dulac O, Plouin P, Diebler C. Infantile status epilepticus as a complication of "near-miss" sudden infant death. Dev Med Child Neurol 1985; 27:40–48.
98. Singh B, Al Shahwan SA, Al Deeb SM. Partial seizures presenting as life-threatening apnea. Epilepsia 1993; 34:901–903.
99. Kahn A, Haesaerts D, Blum D. Carbon monoxide and near-miss cot death. Lancet 1985; 1:168–169.
100. Kearney MS, Dahl LB, Stalsberg H. Can a cat smother and kill a baby? BMJ 1982; 285: 777.
101. Byard RW, Burnell RH. Apparent life threatening events and infant holding practices. Arch Dis Child 1995; 73:502–504.
102. Levin M, Hjelm M, Kay JDS, Pincott JR, Gould JD, Dinwiddie R, Matthew DJ. Haemorrhagic shock and encephalopathy: a new syndrome with a high mortality in young children. Lancet 1983; 2:64–68.
103. Kahn A, Montauk L, Blum D. Diagnostic categories in infants referred for an acute event suggesting near-miss SIDS. Eur J Pediatr 1987; 146:458–460.

21

Sudden Infant Death Syndrome

Modifiable Risk Factors and the Window of Vulnerability

PETER J. FLEMING, PETER BLAIR, and ANDREW SAWCZENKO

Institute of Child Health
Royal Hospital for Sick Children
University of Bristol
Bristol, England

I. Historical Background

Sudden unexpected deaths in infancy have been recognized since antiquity. Prior to the present century, most babies in European and North American societies slept in bed with their parents, a practice that remains the norm in many parts of the world (1). Most unexpected infant deaths thus occurred in bed with an adult and were attributed to overlaying. In 1904, in his studies of sudden unexpected deaths in infancy in London, Willcox (2) observed that such deaths were particularly prevalent among the poorer families, and noted "... amongst the poorer classes of the crowded districts of London and many of our great towns the cradle or cot for the young infant is practically unknown." He concurred with Templeman (3), a decade earlier, in attributing the great majority of such deaths to overlaying by parents, and made a strong recommendation that parents be encouraged to use cribs for their babies to sleep in.

During the twentieth century, as more babies in Western countries slept in cribs and overall infant mortality rates fell, it became clear that certain infant deaths, unexpected by history, remained unexpected after detailed postmortem examination, and the term *cot death* or *crib death* became widely used to describe such deaths (4). While a small proportion of such deaths were (and remain) a result of deliberate parental actions, in most there is no suspicion of such actions, and the consistent epidemiological features of the condition (e.g., age incidence, seasonality) make such a cause inherently very unlikely for the great majority (5).

II. Definition of SIDS

For a proportion of sudden unexpected deaths in infancy, a complete explanation is forthcoming at postmortem examination or review of the circumstances of the death (6); but for the majority, no *sufficient* explanation is found for the death of an apparently healthy or mildly unwell infant. These latter infants are commonly identified as victims of the sudden infant death syndrome (SIDS). The study of sudden infant deaths has been hampered by the lack of a clearly identifiable marker that could be incorporated into a definition. The problem is further complicated by the wide variation both in the proportion of such deaths subjected to detailed postmortem examination between different countries and the variation in the quality and the interpretation of postmortem findings between pathologists.

In 1969 Beckwith drafted a definition of SIDS that has been widely used: "The sudden death of an infant or young child, which is unexpected by history, and in which a thorough post-mortem examination fails to demonstrate an adequate cause for death."

Many attempts have been made to improve upon this definition, particularly emphasizing the need for a review of the clinical history and the circumstances of death. At the third SIDS International Meeting in Stavanger in 1994, a modified definition was proposed, which, while retaining the inherent simplicity of the original definition, includes caveats to cover these concerns: "The sudden death of an infant, which is unexplained after review of the clinical history, examination of the circumstances of death, and post-mortem examination" (7).

In reviewing the epidemiological features of SIDS and their relationship to patterns of developmental physiology in infancy, it is important to identify which definition has been used in which study and to treat with caution findings based upon examination, however elegant, of samples or data from infants supposedly dying of SIDS. Unless the deaths have been thoroughly investigated [including a full pediatric autopsy and review of the clinical history and circumstances of death, and preferably a multidisciplinary case discussion meeting (8)] apparent differences in findings may be related to inclusion criteria rather than real physiological or epidemiological differences.

III. Incidence of SIDS and the Effects of Risk-Reduction Campaigns

The reported incidence of SIDS has varied widely between countries and over time. During the 1970s the incidence apparently rose in the United Kingdom and many other Western countries. This rise was attributed in the United Kingdom to diagnostic shift, in that the diagnosis of SIDS was not a registerable cause of death in the United Kingdom until 1971. Throughout the 1980s the incidence of SIDS in the United Kingdom and the United States remained relatively constant, at around 1.8 and 1.3 per 1000 live births, respectively. In some countries (e.g., New Zealand) the rates were consistently higher, at 3 to 4 per 1000 live births, and in others (e.g., Hong Kong) much lower, at 0.2 per 1000 live births or less. While part of this difference may be related to differences in definition, as noted above, the low incidence in Hong Kong Chinese was confirmed in a detailed study that included a 100% postmortem rate (9). The recognition in the late 1980s of the contributory role of prone sleeping position and the implementation in many countries of campaigns to reduce the risk of SIDS have led to a remarkable fall in incidence, to 0.7 in the United Kingdom and 1.4 in New Zealand. Similar falls have been reported from other countries in which risk reduction campaigns have taken place (e.g., Sweden, Norway, Denmark, and most recently the United States) (10–24).

The recognition that, by modifying a simple factor in routine child care, the incidence of SIDS could be reduced has led to an increased awareness and renewed investigation of the relationship between child-care practices, epidemiological risk factors, normal physiological development, and the risk of SIDS.

IV. The Epidemiological Features of SIDS and Other Sudden Unexpected Deaths in Infancy

A number of characteristic and consistent features of SIDS have emerged from studies in various countries over the past 30 years, notably a characteristic age distribution, with very few deaths in the first 2 weeks after birth, a peak at 2 to 3 months of age, and less than 10% of deaths occurring after 7 months of age; an excess of deaths in male babies; and (until recently) a marked seasonality, with more deaths in the winter months, particularly in temperate or colder regions. This excess of deaths in the colder months, when the incidence of viral upper respiratory tract infections is highest, has led to an interest in the role of infection in the etiology of SIDS. While most babies who die suddenly and unexpectedly have been apparently well in the preceding few days, an increased proportion compared to age-matched control infants have had signs or symptoms suggestive of minor viral infection (25,26). In a population-based case-control study of the role of viral infections in SIDS, Gilbert et al. (6) did not find a significant excess of viral infections in the infants who died but found that the combination of heavy wrapping and the presence of a viral infection was a major risk factor. A number of studies have found that recent immunization *reduced* the risk of SIDS (27).

The association between infant mortality and socioeconomic deprivation has been recognized since the nineteenth century, and the marked excess of SIDS in the most deprived groups in society has been noted in several epidemiological studies, though this pattern is not significantly different than that of other causes of infant mortality (28,29). SIDS occurs within all socioeconomic groups, but certain factors have consistently been found to be associated with increased risk, notably young maternal age, high parity, maternal smoking or drug abuse, short gestation, low birth weight for gestation, multiple births, and male sex. Such factors, while of value in identifying populations at increased risk of SIDS and thus potentially suitable for inclusion in studies of possible pathophysiological processes, are not (with the exception of smoking and drug abuse) within the power of the parents to change and are thus of limited value in any attempt to reduce the incidence of the condition.

In a large recent population-based study from the United Kingdom, almost all of the socioeconomic and related risk factors for SIDS were found to be as strongly associated with sudden but fully explained deaths of infants (30).

Certain other factors related to the risk of SIDS (e.g., breast or bottle feeding, maternal alcohol intake) may act as markers of lifestyle or socioeconomic status and have less consistently been found to have independent effects on the risk of SIDS (8,31,32).

While considerable attention has been focused on the subsequent siblings of SIDS victims as a group at increased risk of SIDS, large-scale population-based studies have not shown a greatly increased risk for such infants independent of environmental or parenting practices (which are likely to remain constant within families, and may thus lead to an apparently increased risk for successive infants in the same family) (33,34).

A family history of a previous unexplained infant death or of recurrent apparent life-threatening episodes may be suggestive of an underlying abnormality of physiology or a metabolic disorder but may also raise the question of imposed upper airway obstruction or other form of abuse (5,35) (see also Chap. 20).

V. Potentially Modifiable Risk Factors for SIDS

Over the past decade, attention has increasingly been given to a number of factors in the infant's pre- and postnatal environment that are associated with apparent effects upon the risk of SIDS and *are* potentially amenable to change, notably 1) sleeping position, 2) thermal environment (and minor viral infections), 3) parental smoking, 4) breast or bottle feeding, and 5) bed sharing.

Intervention campaigns aimed at reducing the risk of SIDS and directed at changing one or more of these factors have been followed by marked reductions in the incidence of SIDS (see above). Of these potentially modifiable risk factors, the one that has most consistently been a successful target of change has been infant sleeping position, for which the most clear evidence is now available of a causal link to SIDS. For other factors, notably smoking, although the evidence of causality is strong, campaigns have to date been largely ineffective. For other factors (e.g., breast-feeding, thermal environment, bed sharing), the evidence of causality remains inconclusive.

VI. Modifiable Risk Factors, Developmental Physiology, and the Effects of Patterns of Infant Care

A. Infant Sleeping Position

Over several hundred years, various recommendations have been made on the most appropriate sleeping position for infants; before the twentieth century, most were concerned rather more with the place in which the infant slept and with the perceived risk of overlaying than with the position in which the baby was placed. While the supine position was the most commonly recommended and by far the most commonly depicted in representations of babies in paintings and drawings, some mention was made in a number of books on the use of the side sleeping position, which was generally not recommended, as in a guide for nurses in 1729:

> ... so long as a Child takes no other nourishment but milk, 'tis better he should be laid to sleep on his back, than on either of his sides. For the back is, like the keel of a ship, the basis and foundation of the whole body, upon which the child may therefore rest with safety and ease. But if he be laid on either of his sides, there is danger that his rib-bones, which are as yet very soft and tender, and which are fastened by very slight ligaments, may give way, and bend inward, under the weight of the whole body ... (36).

The prone sleeping position was not mentioned (and certainly not recommended) prior to the 1930s or 1940s in the United States, and approximately 20 years later in the United Kingdom (37). Abramson, in 1944 (38), attributed the adoption of the prone sleeping position to certain perceived advantages, which included the idea that the baby was more comfortable, fell asleep more easily, and had a reduced incidence of flattening of the skull. At some point the suggestion was made that babies were less likely to inhale vomit if placed prone, but the origin of the observations upon which this claim was made are difficult to trace and are not cited by the authors who repeated it. In three (relatively recent) studies, in which attempts were made to test this hypothesis, the opposite conclusion was reached: namely that, while aspiration of gastric contents as a contributory factor in sudden unexpected death in infancy is rare, it is commoner among infants sleeping prone than those who are supine (39–41). We hypothesize that, during the 1940s and 1950s, as awareness of the importance of the "recovery position" for the unconscious patient became widely recognized and taught in the first-aid courses, the concept that the "immature" or vulnerable baby might be at similar risk became worthy of consideration. From such consideration, it was a relatively short jump to the categorical statement that such a risk existed.

Having been on the side of the traditionalists in 1955 in recommending the supine position, Dr. Benjamin Spock in the 1958 and subsequent editions of his book recommended avoiding this position partly in order to avoid the risk of choking on vomit and partly to avoid flattening of the head. He also recommended against the side sleeping position, which he regarded as inherently unstable: "I think it is preferable to accustom a baby to sleeping on his stomach from the start if he is willing" (42).

Idiopathic scoliosis in infancy was blamed on the side sleeping position, and was said to be rare in the United States because of the widespread use of the prone sleeping position (43).

During the 1960s and 1970s, as survival rates for preterm infants improved in neonatal intensive care units, a number of publications appeared showing the apparent benefits for the preterm infant of the prone sleeping position. Such benefits included better gastric emptying (44), better oxygenation (45), and more effective rib cage and abdominal coupling—with decreased work of breathing (46). While it is difficult to ascertain exactly which factors led to the rapid increase in prevalence of prone sleeping among babies in the United States, Europe, and Australasia during this period, it is likely that these publications, which influenced health care professionals' perceptions of the best positions for babies, had an impact. There was an assumption among the professions as well as among the general public that what seemed to be good for the preterm infant was also likely to be good for the term and older infant. Such an assumption was, with hindsight, clearly oversimplistic and potentially dangerous.

The possibility that the prone sleeping position might be a contributory factor in some cases of sudden unexpected death in infancy was raised in 1944 by Harold Abramson in New York (38), and his findings were taken up in a brief and, even then, somewhat controversial campaign by the New York State Department of Health in 1945 (47). He noted that 68% of infants found unexpectedly dead were in the prone position, and, attributing the deaths to mechanical suffocation, made the recommendation that "the routine nursing practice of placing infants in the prone position be avoided except during such times as the babies are constantly attended. The practice should, furthermore, be entirely done away with at night." Abramson's observations were reported to the U.K. medical profession in an editorial in the *British Medical Journal* in 1945, with an appeal that "perhaps it might be made an object for study by one of the new university departments of child health" (48). In 1947, in the *American Journal of Public Health*, Werne and Garrow disagreed with Abramson and suggested that the prone position may be advantageous: "... by placing the infant in this position, postural drainage of infected secretions from the tracheobronchial tree may lessen the likelihood of pneumonia" (49).

Studies from the United States in the 1950s showed a relatively high proportion of infants being found unexpectedly dead in the prone position (50), and the proportion of babies found dead in this position in the United Kingdom was higher than the proportion that usually slept in this position (37). However, the lack of controls in both studies limited their value.

In 1978, Susan Beal, a pediatrician from Adelaide, South Australia, suggested from the results of her visits to the homes of babies who had died of SIDS that the prone position was a contributory factor (51). In 1984, Saturnus published a study in Germany that supported Beal's suggestion, but this paper received very little attention (52). In 1985 Davies, in Hong Kong, noted that SIDS was an extreme rarity among the Chinese population, who routinely placed their babies supine to sleep, while among the European population, the incidence of SIDS was higher (53). These suggestions attracted considerable hostile criticism (54), as had those of Abramson over 30 years earlier, but in several countries case-control epidemiological studies were commenced to examine the possible role of sleeping position in the etiology of SIDS.

Between 1986 and 1996 a large number of case-control studies investigating the relationship between the risk of SIDS and infant sleeping position were published from Europe, Asia, North America, and Australasia (55–69). The great majority of these studies were retrospective in that information of the infants' sleeping positions was collected after the deaths occurred, but evidence from the Tasmanian study (65), in which prospective and a retrospective study were conducted simultaneously, showed that the information collected retrospectively was reliable. Information collected on the infants' sleeping positions at the time of discovery of the death in the Avon studies (6,63,66) showed close correlation with the information collected a few days later at the time of the parental interviews. With the exception of the study by Klonoff- Cohen (68), all of these case-control studies showed a significant excess of deaths among infants sleeping in the prone position. The odds ratios for the prone position varied from 3.2 (55) to 12.7 (56). In some studies, the parents were questioned about *usual* sleeping position (55,56,61,65,68), while in others the question related specifically to the position in the last sleep. In general the former studies found a lower odds ratio for prone sleeping (70). Because a greater proportion of babies who usually slept supine or on their side were placed prone during their last sleep, the studies of usual sleeping position would have consistently underestimated the real risk of prone sleeping (63). In the one study in which no significant association was found between sleeping position and the risk of SIDS (68), the information was collected many months after the deaths occurred; the authors therefore questioned parents of cases and controls about usual sleeping position only. They noted from information collected at the time of the death, that, while 66% of SIDS infants routinely slept prone, 80% did so during their final sleep. Unfortunately no comparable information was available for the controls. No studies have shown any evidence that for any population group the risk of SIDS is lower for those sleeping in the prone position.

The risk associated with the side sleeping position has been addressed in a number of studies. Mitchell and Engelberts estimated the odds ratio for the side position to be 2.2 (95% C.I., 1.5–3.1) compared with the supine position (71), and more recently Mitchell, in a prospective study, found an odds ratio of 6.57 (95% C.I., 1.71, 25.23) (72). In the CESDI study the multivariate odds ratio for the side sleeping position was 1.84 (95% C.I., 1.02, 3.31) when taking into account all other significant factors in the sleeping environment in a multivariate model (8). In the Nordic study the odds ratio was found to be 3.5 (95% C.I., 2.1, 5.7) (73).

Few babies under 6 months of age placed to sleep supine or prone turn over completely in bed, but for infants as young as 6 weeks, up to 40% of those put down to sleep on their side will be found in a different position, the great majority of these having rolled onto their back, with very few rolling prone (74). In contrast, Wigfield found in her study in Avon (66) that 18% of infants found dead in the prone position had rolled into that position after being put to sleep on their sides. Similarly, in the more recent CESDI study (8), among the control infants, only 3.8% had rolled from side to prone during the "reference" sleep, while among the infants who died of SIDS, 39% had done so. For infants put down on their sides but found prone, the univariate odds ratio was 21.69 (95% C.I., 8.84, 53.2). Despite anecdotal reports that putting babies to sleep on their sides with the lower arm extended reduced the risk of their rolling prone, no evidence was found of any such beneficial effects in this study (8).

There is no evidence of any benefit from the use of wedges, rolls, or other devices designed to keep babies in the side position. Many such devices carry the risk of preventing the baby from rolling into the supine position and increasing the risk of rolling into the prone position.

Studies of population groups in which the incidence of SIDS is consistently very low (e.g., Asian Indian families in Britain, Hispanics in the United States, Chinese in Hong Kong) have shown that among such populations the great majority of infants sleep supine (1,75,76), and there is no evidence of any increased incidence of other adverse health outcomes related to sleeping position among such infants.

While the pediatric, nursing, and child-care literature has contained many references to the apparently increased risk of aspiration pneumonia or inhalation of vomit among infants sleeping in the supine position (38,42,49), we have not been able to identify any studies showing this to be the case. In contrast, in those studies of SIDS in which the risk of aspiration in relation to sleeping position was investigated (39–41), the risk was very low, but in all three studies it was higher in the prone than the supine position. A prospective population based study of 14,000 infants born in Avon (U.K.) in 1991–1992 showed no evidence of any adverse health outcomes associated with the supine sleeping position and some evidence that respiratory and ear infections may be more common in infants who sleep prone (77,78).

Certain infants, notably those with abnormalities of the upper airway (e.g., Pierre Robin syndrome) are at risk of lethal upper airway obstruction if placed supine and should therefore be placed in the prone or possibly the side position for sleep.

Orenstein showed that for infants with moderate or severe symptomatic gastroesophageal reflux, the severity of the reflux was increased in the supine position (79). In a more recent study of the effect of sleeping position on gastroesophageal reflux, while the prone position was associated with the lowest prevalence of reflux, the left lateral position was found also to be associated with significantly less reflux than the supine position (80). Studies of the effects of position on sleep physiology (81) have shown that non–rapid-eye-movement (NREM) sleep was increased in infants sleeping prone, and Jeffery has shown that gastroesophageal reflux is reduced in NREM sleep compared to REM sleep (82). A reduction in reflux in the prone position may thus be at least partly an effect of sleep state. Gastroesophageal reflux is a very common condition, and, while severe reflux has been associated with apparent life-threatening events in infants, such episodes are more likely to be related to the potency of the laryngeal chemoreceptor apnea reflex rather than the severity of the reflux (82). For most infants with gastroesophageal reflux, the supine sleeping position would thus seem to be the safest, though the left lateral position may provide a compromise for infants with persisting symptomatic reflux, the prone position being used only for those with severe, symptomatic reflux and for those with recurrent apparent life-threatening events not responding to medical management.

B. What Is the Mechanism of Risk from the Prone Sleeping Position?

Infant sleeping position has effects on physiology, and a number of possible pathophysiological mechanisms for the increased risk of SIDS have been proposed, though evidence in favor of each is indirect. Clearly it is possible that more than one mechanism may be involved.

In the prone position the infant loses less heat than in the supine position, partly as a result of greater flexion of the legs on the body and partly because the face, a major site of heat loss, is potentially in contact with the bedding and thus effectively insulated. Studies of infant thermal physiology have been used to develop models of thermal balance in the infant (83–86), which support the contention that in the prone position the infant would potentially be at greater risk from the adverse effects of heat stress from a warm environment, or, more importantly, from heavy wrapping. Recordings of overnight baby and environmental temperatures have shown that, in the prone position, infants are slightly warmer and body temperature rises more rapidly during the latter part of the night than in the supine position (87). In the supine position, the adverse effects of heavy wrapping would thus be less important than in the prone position unless the head were completely covered. This is consistent with the findings from the Avon study of heavy wrapping and prone sleep position (63) as well as the more recent CESDI study (8). In Tasmania, Ponsonby found in a multivariate analysis that the risk of the prone position was potentiated by overnight heating, swaddling, recent infection, and soft mattress materials (88). Williams confirmed these findings in a study from New Zealand (89). The mechanism by which thermal imbalance might lead to death is not clear, though heat stress has been shown to have effects on the control of respiration (86), and studies in piglets by Galland (90) have shown that head covering could produce potentially lethal rises in brain temperature.

In the prone position babies are also potentially more vulnerable to the effects of rebreathing expired gases, particularly if sleeping on soft bedding. Kemp in the United States and Bolton in New Zealand have both shown that sleeping on soft bedding in the prone position could lead to potentially lethal rebreathing (91–93).

A further effect of the prone sleeping position is that in this position the arousal threshold is higher (94,95). Thus adverse events such as hypoxia, to which the normal responses might include arousal, may have more profound and possibly lethal effects in infants sleeping prone. Skadberg and Markestad (96) showed that, in the prone position, infants moved less, particularly during REM sleep, than in the supine position and had higher heart rates and peripheral temperatures.

Blackwell et al. (97) have suggested a possible mechanism by which the prone sleeping position, heavy wrapping, and the presence of a viral infection might predispose to the development of a secondary bacterial infection, with release of inflammatory mediators, particularly tumor necrosis factor, into the pharynx, leading to the rapid and potentially lethal development of shock.

C. Thermal Environment

Several studies have shown that SIDS victims were more heavily wrapped than controls and were more likely to have had heating on throughout the night (63). Gilbert found that the combination of a viral infection and heavy wrapping was associated with a very high relative risk of SIDS (6). In a study from Tasmania, Ponsonby found in a multivariate analysis that the risk of the prone position was potentiated by overnight heating, swaddling, recent infection, and mattress type (98). Williams confirmed these findings in a study from New Zealand and found a small additive effect if the mother smoked (89). Thermal stress could lead to death by direct hyperthermia (or hypothermia) or act via central control mechanisms by disruption of respiratory drive and the laryngeal closure reflex or depression of arousal mechanisms (86).

Parents vary greatly in the amount of insulation, bedding, and heating that they provide for their babies. Social class, maternal age, infant age, type of heating (if any), outside temperature, season, and cultural practices have been noted to be factors determining the amount of bedding used. Studies in England have shown that for the same environmental temperature, parents placed more insulation on babies in winter than in summer. Most parents added bedding appropriate to achieve conditions of predicted thermal neutrality, though poorer and social disadvantaged families were likely to add more bedding. Understanding how parents determine the nocturnal sleeping environment may therefore be relevant to SIDS (63,84,100).

A consistent feature of SIDS, most marked in temperate zones, has been an excess of deaths in the winter months, with a higher overall incidence and more marked seasonal variation in colder regions. The recent decline in the number of SIDS deaths has been greater in the winter than in the summer in Australia, New Zealand, and the United Kingdom. The prevalence of prone sleeping position does not change with season, though the relative risk of prone sleeping is higher in winter than in summer, suggesting an interaction with a seasonal factor, perhaps thermal environment or infection (101).

A decrease in environmental temperature was followed, after a 4- to 8-day lag, by an increase in SIDS in the United Kingdom and in Australia, despite higher average temperatures in Australia (102). Thus changes in temperature rather than absolute temperature may be etiologically important in some SIDS. Possible mechanisms for the association of SIDS and cold weather include hypothermia, reduced resistance to viral illness during a cold spell (possibly leading to overt or covert infection after a time lag) and altered child-care practices during colder weather (e.g., paradoxical overheating).

The newborn baby is particularly vulnerable to the effects of cold stress, but increasing evidence has accumulated that heavy wrapping or a high environmental temperature, perhaps accompanied by infection or other factors that affect thermoregulation, may be contributory factors in some SIDS. Thus there may be a developmental shift in vulnerability to thermal stress during early infancy (86).

There is an increase in daytime and a decrease in nighttime rectal temperature with increasing age during early infancy. Rectal temperature changes little during nighttime sleep in the newborn period, but around the age of 8 to 16 weeks a characteristic pattern appears, with a relatively abrupt fall to below 36.5 °C soon after sleep followed by a plateau and then a gradual rise in the early morning prior to waking. This "mature" pattern develops earlier in infants who are breast fed, female, firstborn, and from more affluent families; infants gaining weight most rapidly mature later (103).

The insulation provided by bedding and clothing does not influence infant rectal temperature during nocturnal sleep, and room temperature has a minimal effect. Bottle feeding or parental smoking individually did not affect rectal temperature, but in combination, bottle-fed babies exposed to smoke had rectal temperature 0.1°C higher for the entire night. In infants sleeping at home, the prone position is associated with an increased rectal temperature for some or all of the night (104).

Daytime metabolic rate increases rapidly during early infancy (105,106), but little is known about nocturnal maturation during this period. Metabolic rate is higher in growth-retarded babies, perhaps because of their relatively larger brains (107).

Many parents report that they have found their infant's head completely covered by bedding on at least one occasion, and prone sleeping appears to make it easier for infants to slip under bedding (8). Head covering may cause death by the effects of thermal imbalance. In a recent U.K. study, although few babies wore a hat, 18% of SIDS compared to 2% of controls had their head covered, and total covering emerged as the most potent of all risk factors (8). Night waking is more common in the most heavily dressed infants in warmer rooms (108). Failure of infants to attract parental action (for whatever reason), when thermally challenged may therefore be a behavioral risk factor for SIDS.

Thermal modeling of clothed infants over a wide range of environmental temperatures suggests that the most important determinant of heat loss is not the quantity of insulation (unless extreme) but the area of exposed skin, particularly that of the head (85,109). Rectal and peripheral temperature rises in infants when the head is covered even if there is a drop in metabolic rate (110). Rectal temperature falls more slowly during the initial part of the night in prone compared to nonprone infants, suggesting a reduced ability to lose heat in this position, probably because when infants are prone a greater proportion of body surface area is insulated by contact with the mattress (87).

In animal models, a period of mild hyperthermia during or shortly after an ischemic has similar effects on brain pathology to prolonging ischemia (111). The mechanism of the adverse effects of mild brain hyperthermia is unclear but may relate to increased release of peptide excitotoxins (112). There is growing evidence to suggest that interleukin-1 and tumor necrosis factor are central brain mediators of normal sleep and that changes in their activity may account for the increased sleep seen in ill or pyrexial patients (113). This work may therefore link viral illness, thermal stress, and sleep state/arousal.

In a prospective study of normal infants, we found variation with age, during viral respiratory tract infection, of daytime sleeping metabolic rate. In infants less than 3 months of age, the metabolic rate commonly fell at the time of an infection and fever was unusual, while in older infants the metabolic rate usually increased and fever was more common (114). In infants of all ages there are changes in nighttime temperature 3 to 7 days before obvious signs of illness, rectal temperature "rises" from that expected, despite the absence of pyrexia. During this prodrome, parents often reported that their infants were "not right." When they became obviously unwell, rectal temperature dropped back to that expected for age, and few were pyrexial (115).

These observations suggest changes of body temperature (and possibly metabolic rate) occur in the absence of significant clinical signs of illness and may fit with the concept of SIDS occurring in the prodromal phase of infection. Although evidence of recent infection (particularly viral upper respiratory infection) is commonly found in SIDS victims, Gilbert found only a slightly (nonsignificantly) increased incidence of viral infection in SIDS victims compared to age- and season-matched controls. The incidence of recent minor symptoms was slightly higher in the SIDS victims, and more had been seen by a doctor than the controls (6). Thus it seems that infection must interact with other factors to be a significant risk factor in the majority of SIDS.

There are many changes that occur around the peak SIDS age of 3 months, including the development of slow wave sleep, the waning of passive immunity, and rectal temperature "maturation." No SIDS risk factor lowers rectal temperature, but a number of factors are associated with small increases. If infant brain temperature falls during nocturnal sleep, then the question arises as to whether there are similar developmental patterns and variations as are seen in rectal temperature. Evidence is accumulating that absolute or *relative*, localized or generalized, brain overheating can occur in the absence of overt body pyrexia.

D. Parental Smoking

The increased risk of SIDS in infants born to mothers who smoke has been reported in a large number of studies. Of 30 case control studies in the world literature over the period from the early 1960s until the mid-1990s in which this relationship was investigated, an increased risk was identified in 29, of which only 2 were not statistically significant (6,25,27,59,116–141). The weighted pooled summary estimate of the odds ratio was highly significant [O.R. = 3.16 (95% C.I., 2.25–4.42)]. Notably, the risk associated with this factor appears to have risen from O.R. 2.92 (95% C.I., 2.07–4.08) before the fall in SIDS rate, to O.R. = 4.93 (95% C.I., 3.52–6.92) (27,138–140) after the fall. Results from the multivariate analyses of these four studies show that the risk associated with maternal smoking during pregnancy remained significant when controlled for several other factors, including low socioeconomic status and birthweight. The relationship with paternal smoking is also strong, all 8 reported studies (27,61,121,125,134,138,142,143) in which the relationship was examined showing an adverse effect, statistically significant in 6. In the CESDI study (31), this effect was shown to be independent of the effect of maternal smoking.

In the study by Blair, a highly significant effect of postnatal exposure to tobacco smoke was shown. The risk of SIDS increased by almost 100% for each hour of the day in which the infant was routinely in a room in which people sometimes smoked (31). In this study the population-attributable risk for SIDS from parental smoking was estimated to be over 60%—i.e., in the absence of parental smoking, the SIDS rate would be predicted to fall by over 60%.

The mechanism by which exposure to tobacco smoke increases the risk of SIDS is not clear, though there are several possibilities. Tobacco smoke affects infant apnea rates and may contribute to deficient hypoxia responses (144). Williams (89) showed an interaction between smoking and prone sleep position with SIDS, and Tuffnell (104) showed an interaction between smoking, bottle feeding, and rectal temperature. Exposure to tobacco smoke before or after birth may impair the development of autonomic function (as assessed by the infant's blood pressure response to changes in position from horizontal to a 60% head up tilt) (145) and increases the prevalence of respiratory infections throughout childhood (146).

Whatever the mechanisms, the strength and consistency of the adverse effects of exposure to tobacco smoke on the risk of SIDS is sufficient to suggest that, as for sleeping position, the relationship is one of causation rather than just association.

E. Breast or Bottle Feeding

Two prospective cohort studies have reported on the relationship between breast feeding and the risk of SIDS: the U.S. National Collaborative Study (147) and the Oxford record linkage study (120). While the former showed a lower prevalence of breast feeding among the SIDS victims, multivariate analysis suggested this was mainly an effect of socioeconomic factors, maternal education, and preterm delivery. No adjustment was made for maternal smoking. In the Oxford study, after adjusting for maternal age, parity, social class, and marital status, there was no difference in the prevalence of breast feeding between cases and controls.

While breast feeding was found to be strongly protective against SIDS in the New Zealand case-control study (64), a striking feature of this study was the very high prevalence of breast feeding, and an alternative interpretation might be that bottle feeding in this population might be a marker for other, less easily defined differences in parenting practices. Three studies from the United Kingdom (8,32,148) failed to show any protective effect of breast feeding in a multivariate model adjusted for the effects of maternal smoking. A recent prospective study from New Zealand, in which data were collected on all births over a 2-year period that started after the national risk-reduction campaign, showed no protective effect of breast feeding, either in univariate or multivariate analysis (72), while in the Nordic epidemiological study of SIDS (22) an apparent increase in protective effect over the years of the study was noted for breast feeding on multivariate analysis. No significant adverse effects of bottle feeding were noted for infants dying in 1991–1993 (which included the times of risk reduction campaigns) (O.R. = 1.6; 95%: C.I., 0.7, 3.3), but after that time a significant effect was apparent (O.R. = 4.6; 95% C.I., 1.4, 14.7).

While the benefits of breast feeding are multiple and important, current data do not show clear evidence of protection against SIDS.

F. Bed Sharing ("Cosleeping")

McKenna has pointed out that for most of the history of our species and over most of the world, the question of the position in which the infant was put down to sleep was to some extent irrelevant, since the infant would have been in close and more or less continuous contact with the primary caregiver, usually the mother (1). Studies of communities in which this traditional approach to infant care is still practiced, such as the Bangladeshi population in the United Kingdom, have shown that when the infant is put down to sleep it is almost invariably in the supine position (76). In such populations, the mother usually sleeps very close to the baby, very often in the same bed, and the incidence of SIDS is very low (1,53,75,76).

In New Zealand, the incidence of SIDS is particularly high in the Maori population, many of whom live in conditions of socioeconomic disadvantage. Among the Maori population smoking and high alcohol intake are relatively common, and bed sharing is a culturally accepted practice. In the initial reports of the results of the New Zealand cot death study, bed sharing was identified as a major risk factor for cot death (149), but on subsequent analysis of the data it became clear that this risk applied only to the Maori population and not to the infants of European or Pacific Island Polynesian origin (150). In a further multivariate analysis, the increase in risk of SIDS associated with bed sharing was found to apply only to infants of parents who smoked (151), and this has subsequently been confirmed in a prospective study of infants born after the risk-reduction campaign in New Zealand (72). In a study from California, Klonoff-Cohen found no evidence of any adverse effects of bed sharing (152), and in the CESDI study from the United Kingdom, bed sharing, while appearing as a major risk factor in the multivariate analysis, was only a significant risk factor for infants of parents who smoked (8). In this study parental alcohol intake was strongly associated with smoking and with increased risk of SIDS. In the New Zealand study, sharing a room with a parent seemed to have a protective effect (153), while in the analysis of data from the first 2 years of the CESDI study (8) no such effect was identified. Subsequent analysis of the data from the full 3 years of the CESDI study has confirmed the apparent protective effects of room sharing and lack of any adverse effects of bed sharing among nonsmoking families. The close relationship between bed sharing and breast feeding complicates the interpretation of these data (154).

VII. Summary

Many studies have shown consistent and strong links between certain epidemiological factors and the risk of SIDS. Some of these factors are potentially modifiable, and for at least one factor, sleeping position, changes in practice have been followed by a marked fall in SIDS rate in many countries. The physical and possible pathophysiological mechanisms by which such factors may have their effects have been reviewed and the relationship with known aspects of infant developmental physiology explored.

A major question remains: If other potentially modifiable risk factors (e.g., parental smoking) can be changed in a population in which the SIDS rate has already fallen after a change in infant sleeping position, will there be a further fall? The evidence suggests that, for exposure to tobacco smoke at least, this is likely to be true, while for other factors the evidence is less clear.

References

1. McKenna JJ, Thoman E, Anders T, Schechtman V, Glotzbach S. Infant-parent cosleeping in evolutionary perspective: implications for understanding infant sleep development and SIDS. Sleep 1993; 16:263–282.
2. Willcox WH. Infantile mortality from "overlaying." BMJ 1904; September 24:1–7.
3. Templeman C. Two hundred and fifty eight cases of suffocation of infants. Edinburgh Med J 1892; 38:322–329.
4. Limerick SA. Sudden infant death in historical perspective. J Clin Pathol 1992; 45(suppl):3–6.
5. National Advisory Body for CESDI. Annual Report for 1994. London: Department of Health, 1996.
6. Gilbert R, Rudd P, Berry PJ, Fleming PJ, et al. Combined effect of infection and heavy wrapping on risk of sudden unexplained infant death. Arch Dis Child 1992; 67:171–177.
7. Rognum TO, Willinger M. The story of the "Stavanger definition." In: Rognum TO, ed. Sudden Infant Death Syndrome: New Trends in the Nineties. Oslo: Scandinavian University Press, 1995: 21–25.
8. Fleming PJ, Blair P, Bacon C, et al. The environment of infants during sleep and the risk of sudden infant death syndrome: results of 1993–5 case-control study for confidential enquiry into stillbirths and deaths in infancy. BMJ 1996; 313:191–195.
9. Lee N, Chan YF, Davies DP, et al. Sudden infant death in Hong Kong: confirmation of low incidence. BMJ 1989; 298:721.
10. Fleming PJ, Blair PS. Role of sleeping position in the aetiology of the sudden infant death syndrome. In: McIntosh N, ed. Current Topics in Neonatology, No. 2. London: Saunders, 1997.
11. Stewart AJ, Mitchell EA, Tipene Leach D, Fleming PJ. Lessons from the New Zealand and United Kingdom Cot Death Campaigns. Acta Paediatr Scand 1993; 389(suppl): 119–123.

12. Mitchell EA, Ford RPK, Taylor BJ, et al. Further evidence supporting a causal relationship between prone sleeping position and SIDS. J Paediatr Child Health 1992; 28(suppl 1):S9–S12.
13. Fleming PJ. The Implementation of Risk Reduction for SIDS in the UK. Proc R Coll Physicians Edinburgh 1995; 25:213–220.
14. Dwyer T, Ponsonby AL, Blizzard L, et al. The contribution of changes in the prevalence of prone sleeping position to the decline in sudden infant death syndrome in Tasmania. JAMA 1995; 273:783–789.
15. Markestad T, Skadberg B, Hordvik E, et al. Sleeping position and sudden infant death syndrome: effect of an intervention programme to avoid prone sleeping. Acta Paediatr 1995; 84:375–378.
16. Irgens L, Markestad T, Baste V, et al. Sleeping position and sudden infant death in Norway 1967–91. Arch Dis Child 1995; 72:478–482.
17. McKee M, Fulop N, Bouvier P, et al. Preventing sudden infant deaths—the slow diffusion of an idea. Health Policy 1996; 37:117–135.
18. Willinger M, Hoffman HJ, Hartford RB. Infant sleep position and risk for sudden infant death syndrome: report of a meeting held January 13 and 14, 1994, National Institutes of Health, Bethesda, MD. Pediatrics 1994; 93:814–819.
19. Infant sleep position and sudden infant death syndrome in the United States: joint commentary from the American Academy of Pediatrics and selected agencies of the federal government. Pediatrics 1994; 93:820.
20. Wigfield R, Fleming PJ. The prevalence of risk factors for SIDS: impact of an intervention campaign. In: Rognum TO, ed. Sudden Infant Death Syndrome: New Trends in the Nineties. Oslo: Scandinavian University Press, 1995: 124–128.
21. Sudden Infant Deaths 1990–94. OPCS Monitor (DH3 95/3). London: Office of Population Censuses and Surveys, September 28, 1995.
22. Wennergren G, Alm B, Oyen N, Helweg-Larsen K, Milerad J, Skjaervven R, Norvenius SG, et al. The decline in the incidence of SIDS in Scandinavia and its relation to risk-intervention campaigns. Acta Paediatr 1997; 86:963–968.
23. Weese-Mayer D. Modifiable risk factors for sudden infant death syndrome: when will we ever learn? J Pediatr 1998; 132:197–198.
24. Daltveit AK, Oyen N, Skjaerven R, Irgens L. The epidemic of SIDS in Norway 1967–93: changing effects of risk factors. Arch Dis Child 1997; 77:23–27.
25. Gilbert RE, Fleming PJ, Azaz Y, Berry PJ, White DG, Orreffu V, Rudd PT. Signs of illness in babies preceding sudden unexpected infant death. BMJ 1990; 300:1237–1239.
26. Cole TJ, Gilbert RE, Fleming PJ, Morley CJ, Rudd PT, Berry PJ. Baby check and the Avon Infant Mortality Study. Arch Dis Child 1991; 66:1077–1078.
27. Mitchell EA, Stewart AW, Clements M, Ford RPK. Immunisation and the sudden infant death syndrome. BMJ 1995; 310:88–90.
28. Spencer N. Poverty and Child Health. Oxford, England: Radcliffe Medical Press, 1996.
29. Taylor JA, Sanderson M. A re-examination of the risk factors for the sudden infant death syndrome. J Pediatr 1995; 126:887–891.
30. Bacon C, Blair P, Leach CEA, Fleming PJ, Smith I, Ward-Platt M, Hall D. Sudden infant deaths other than SIDS. In: Report on CESDI, 1998. London: The Maternal and Child Health Research Consortium, 1998.
31. Blair P, Fleming PJ, Bensley D, et al. Smoking and sudden infant death syndrome: re-

sults of the 1993–5 case-control study for the confidential enquiry into stillbirths and deaths in infancy. BMJ 1996; 313:195–198.
32. Gilbert RE, Wigfield RE, Fleming PJ, et al. Bottle feeding and theSudden Infant Death Syndrome. BMJ 1995; 310:88–90.
33. Irgens LM, Oyen N, Skjaervan R. Recurrence of sudden infant death syndrome among siblings. Acta Paediatr 1993; 389(suppl 82):23–25.
34. Oyen N, Skjaerven R, Irgens L. Population-based recurrence risk of sudden infant death syndrome compared with other infant and fetal deaths. Am J Epidemiol 1996; 144:300–305.
35. Southall D, Plunkett MCB, Banks MW, Falkov AF, Samuels MP. Covert video recordings of life-threatening child abuse: lessons for child protection. Pediatrics 1997; 100:735–760.
36. Abramson H. Accidental mechanical suffocation in infants. J Pediatr 1944; 25:404–413.
37. An "Eminent Physician." The Nurse's Guide, or, the Right Method of Bringing Up Young Children. London: 1729.
38. Hiley C. PhD thesis, University of Cambridge, 1995.
39. Beal S, Porter C. Sudden infant death syndrome related to climate. Acta Paediatr Scand 1991; 80:278–287.
40. Tonkin S. Infant sleeping position and cot death. Aust Paediatr J 1989; 25:376–377.
41. Fleming PJ, Stewart A. What is the ideal sleeping position for infants? Dev Med Child Neurol 1992; 34:916–919.
42. Spock B. Baby and Child Care. London: New English Library, 1973.
43. Dickson RA. Idiopathic scoliosis. BMJ 1989; 298:906–907.
44. Martin RJ, Herrell N, Rubin D, Fanaroff A. Effect of supine and prone positions on arterial tension in the preterm infant. Pediatrics 1979; 63:528–531.
45. Yu V. Effect of body positioning on gastric emptying in the neonate. Arch Dis Child 1975; 50:500–504.
46. Fleming PJ, Muller N, Bryan MH, Bryan AC. The effects of abdominal loading on ribcage distortion in premature infants. Pediatrics 1979; 64:425–428.
47. Mechanical suffocation: leading cause of accidental death in early infancy. Health News. New York State Department of Health, 1945; vol. 22, no. 9 (Feb 26).
48. Accidental suffocation of infants (editorial). BMJ 1945; 524–525.
49. Werne J, Garrow I. Sudden deaths of infants allegedly due to mechanical suffocation. Am J Public Health 1947; 37:675–687.
50. Adelson L, Roberts Kinney E. Sudden and unexpected death in infancy and childhood. Pediatrics 1956; 17:663–697.
51. Beal S, Blundell H. Sudden infant death syndrome related to position in the cot. Med J Aust 1978; 2:217–218.
52. Saturnus KS. Plotzlicher Kindstod—eine Folge der Bauchlage? In: Festschrift Professor Leithoff. Heidelberg: Kriminalstatistik, 1985: 67–81.
53. Davies DP. Cot death in Hong Kong: a rare problem? Lancet 1985; 2:1346–1349.
54. Nicholl JP. Cot deaths in Hong Kong. Lancet 1986; 1:214.
55. Cameron MH, Williams AL. Development and testing of scoring systems for predicting infants with a high risk of SIDS in Melbourne. Aust Pediatr J 1986; (suppl):37–45.
56. Senecal J, Roussey M, Defawe G, et al. Procubitus et mort subite inattendue du nourrisson. Arch Francais Pediatr 1987; 44:131–136.

57. Nicholl JP, O'Cathain A. Sleeping position and SIDS. Lancet 1988, 2:106.
58. Beal SM. Sleeping position and sudden infant death syndrome. Med J Aust 1988; 149: 562.
59. De Jonge GA, Engelberts AC, Koomen-Liefting AJM, Kostense PJ. Cot death and prone sleeping in the Netherlands. BMJ 1989; 298:722.
60. Lee N, Chan YF, Davies DP, et al. Sudden infant death in Hong Kong: confirmation of low incidence. BMJ 1989; 298:721.
61. McGlashan N. Sudden infant deaths in Tasmania 1980–86. A seven year prospective study. Soc Sci Med 1989; 29:1015–1026.
62. Bouvier-Colle MH, Varnoux V, Hausherr E. Revue bibliographique des etudes sur la mort subite en relation avec la position de sommeil chez le nourrisson. Proceedings of Reunion du Groupe d'Etudes de langue Francais sur la mort subite du nourrisson. Nice, France, 1990.
63. Fleming PJ, Gilbert RE, Azaz Y, Berry PJ, Rudd PT, Stewart A, Hall E. The interaction between bedding and sleeping position in sudden infant death syndrome: a population-based case-control study. BMJ 1990; 301:85–89.
64. Mitchell EH, Scragg R, Stewart AW, et al. Results from the first year of the New Zealand cot death study. NZ Med J 1991; 104:71–76.
65. Dwyer T, Ponsonby AL, Newman NM, Gibbons LE. Prospective cohort study of prone sleeping and sudden infant death syndrome. Lancet 1991; 337:1244–1247.
66. Wigfield RE, Fleming PJ, Berry PJ, Rudd PT, Golding J. Can the fall in Avon's sudden infant death rate be explained by the observed sleeping position changes? BMJ 1992; 304:282–283.
67. Gormally S, Matthews TG. Sleep position and SIDS in Irish infants. Irish Med J 1994; 87:58.
68. Klonoff-Cohen HS, Edelstein SL. A case-control study of routine and death scene sleep position and sudden infant death syndrome in Southern California. JAMA 1995; 273: 790–794.
69. Taylor JA, Krieger JW, Reay DT, et al. Prone sleep position and the sudden infant death syndrome in King County, Washington: a case-control study. J Pediatr 1996; 128: 626–630.
70. Beal SM, Finch CF. An overview of retrospective case control studies investigating the relationship between prone sleeping position and SIDS. J Paediatr Child Health 1991; 27:334–339.
71. Mitchell EA, Engelberts AC. Sleeping position and cot deaths. Lancet 1991; 338:192.
72. Mitchell EA, Tuohy PG, Brunt JM, Thompson JMD, Clements MS, Stewart AW, Ford RPK, Taylor BJ. Risk factors for sudden infant death following the prevention campaign in New Zealand: a prospective study. Pediatrics 1997; 100:835–840.
73. Oyen N, Markestad T, Skjaerven R, Irgens L, Helweg- Larsen K, Alm B, Norrvenius G, Wennergren G. Combined effects of sleeping position and prenatal risk factors in sudden infant death syndrome: the Nordic epidemiological study. Pediatrics 1997; 100: 613–621.
74. Golding J, Fleming PJ, Parkes S. Cot deaths and sleep position campaigns. Lancet 1992; 339:748–749.
75. Beal SM. Sudden infant death syndrome: epidemiological comparisons between South Australia and communities with a different incidence. Aust Paed J 1986; 22(suppl): 13–16.

76. Gantley M, Davies DP, Murcott A. Sudden infant death syndrome: links with infant care practices. BMJ 1993; 306:16–20.
77. Gannon MM, Haggard MP, Golding J, Fleming PJ. Sleeping position—a new environmental risk factor for otitis media. In: Lim D, Bluestone C, eds. Recent Advances in Otitis Media. 1995.
78. Hunt L, Fleming PJ, Golding J. Does the supine sleeping position have any adverse effects on the child? (I) Health in the first 6 months. Pediatrics 1997; 100:1:11 (electronic pages). http://www.pediatrics.org/cgi/content/full/100/1/11.
79. Orenstein SR, Whittington PF. Positioning for prevention of gastroesophageal reflux. J Pediatr 1983; 103:534–537.
80. Tobin JM, McCloud P, Cameron DJS. Posture and gastro-oesophageal reflux: a case for left lateral positioning. Arch Dis Child 1997; 76:254–258.
81. Kahn A, Grosswasser J, Kelmanson I. Risk factors for SIDS: Risk factors for ALTE? In: Rognum TO, ed. Sudden Infant Death: New Trends in the Nineties. Oslo: Scandinavian University Press, 1995.
82. Jeffrey HE, Page M, Post EJ, Wood AKW. Physiological studies of gastro-oesophageal reflux and airway protective responses in the young animal and human infant. Clin Exp Pharmacol Physiol 1995; 22:544–549.
83. Azaz Y, Fleming PJ, Levine M, et al. The relationship between environmental temperature, metabolic rate, sleep state and evaporative water loss in infants from birth to three months. Pediatr Res 1992; 32:417–423.
84. Wigfield RE, Fleming PJ, Azaz Y, et al. How much wrapping do babies need at night? Arch Dis Child 1993; 69:181–186.
85. Nelson EAS, Taylor BJ, Weatherall IL. Sleeping position and infant bedding may predispose to hyperthermia and the sudden infant death syndrome. Lancet 1989; 1:199–201.
86. Fleming PJ, Levine MR, Azaz Y, Wigfield R. The development of thermoregulation and interactions with the control of respiration in infants: possible relationship to sudden infant death. Acta Paediatr Scand 1993; 389(suppl):57–59.
87. Tuffnell C, Petersen S, Wailoo M. Prone sleeping infants have a reduced ability to lose heat. Early Hum Dev 1995; 43:109–116.
88. Ponsonby AL, Dwyer T, Gibbons LE, et al. Factors potentiating the risk of sudden infant death syndrome associated with the prone position. N Engl J Med 1993; 329: 377–382.
89. Williams S, Taylor B, Mitchell E. Sudden infant death syndrome: insulation from bedding and clothing and its effect modifiers. Int J Epidemiol 1996; 25:366–375.
90. Galland BC, Peebles CM, Bolton DP, Taylor BJ. The micro-environment of the sleeping newborn piglet covered by bedclothes: gas exchange and temperature. J Paediatr Child Health 1994; 30:144–150.
91. Kemp JS, Nelson VE, Thach BT. Physical properties of bedding that may increase risk of sudden infant death syndrome in prone sleeping infants. Pediatr Res 1994; 36:7–11.
92. Bolton DP, Taylor BJ, Campbell AJ, Galland BC, Cresswell C. Rebreathing expired gases from bedding: a cause of cot death? Arch Dis Child 1993; 69:187–190.
93. Kemp J, Livne M, White DK, Arfken CL. Softness and potential to cause rebreathing: differences in bedding used by infants at high and low risk for SIDS. J Pediatr 132: 234–239.
94. Franco P, Groswasser J, Sottiaux M, et al. Decreased cardiac responses to auditory stimulation during prone sleep. Pediatrics 1996; 97:174–178.

95. Franco P, Pardou A, Hassid S, Lurquin P, Groswasser J, Kahn A. Auditory arousal thresholds are higher when infants sleep in the prone position. J Pediatr 1998; 132:240–243.
96. Skadberg BT, Markestad T. Behavior and physiological responses during prone and supine sleep in early infancy. Arch Dis Child 1997; 76:320–324.
97. Blackwell CC, Weir DM, Busuttil A, et al. Infection, inflammation and the developmental stage of infants: a new hypothesis for the aetiology of SIDS. In: Rognum TO, ed. Sudden Infant Death Syndrome: New Trends in the Nineties. Oslo: Scandinavian University Press, 1995: 189–198.
98. Ponsonby A, Dwyer T, Gibbons L, Cochrane J, Wang Y. Factors potentiating the risk of sudden infant death syndrome associated with the prone position. N Engl J Med 1993; 329:377–382.
99. Williams S, Taylor B, Mitchell E. Sudden infant death syndrome: insulation from bedding and clothing and its effect modifiers. Int J Epidemiol 1996; 25:366–375.
100. Bacon CJ, Bell SA, Clulow EE, Beattie AB. How mothers keep their babies warm. Arch Dis Child 1991; 66:627–632.
101. Douglas A, Allan T, Helms P. Seasonality and the sudden infant death syndrome during 1987–9 and 1991–3 in Australia and Britain. BMJ 1996; 312:1381–1383.
102. Campbell MJ. Sudden infant death syndrome and environmental temperature further evidence for a time-lagged relationship. Med J Aust 1989; 151:365–367.
103. Lodemore MR, Petersen SA, Wailoo MP. Factors affecting the development of night time temperature rhythms. Arch Dis Child 1992; 67:1259–1261.
104. Tuffnell CS, Petersen SA, Wailoo MP. Factors affecting rectal temperature in infancy. Arch Dis Child 1995; 73:443–446.
105. Azaz Y, Fleming PJ, Levine M, McCabe R, Stewart A, Johnson P. The relationship between environmental temperature, metabolic rate, sleep state, and evaporative water loss in infants from birth to three months. Pediatr Res 1992; 32:417–423.
106. Davies P, Clough H, Bishop N, Lucas A, Cole J, Cole T. Total energy expenditure in small for gestational age infants. Arch Dis Child 1996; 74:F208–F210.
107. Abdulrazzaq Y, Brooke O. Is the raised metabolic rate of the small-for-gestation infant due to his relatively large brain size? Early Hum Dev 1984; 10:253–261.
108. Wailoo MP, Petersen SA, Whitaker H. Disturbed nights and 3–4 month old infants: the effects of feeding and thermal environment. Arch Dis Child 1990; 65:499–501.
109. Jardine D. A mathematical model of life-threatening hyperthermia during infancy. J Appl Physiol 1992; 73:329–339.
110. Marks K, Devenyi A, Bello M, Nardis E, Seaton J, Ultman J. Thermal head wrap for infants. J Pediatr 1985; 107:956–959.
111. Dietrich W, Busto R, Valdes I, Loor Y. Effects of normothermic versus mild hyperthermic forebrain ischaemia in rats. Stroke 1990; 21:1318–1325.
112. Takagi K, Ginsberg M, Globus M, Martinez E, Busto R. Effect of hyperthermia on glutamate release in ischaemic penumbra after middle cerebral artery occlusion in rats. Am J Physiol Heart Circ Phys 1994; 36:H1770–H1776.
113. Krueger JM, Takahashi S, Kapas L, et al. Cytokines in sleep regulation. Adv Neuroimmunol 1995; 5:171–188.
114. Fleming PJ, Howell T, Clements M, Lucas J. Thermal balance and metabolic rate during upper respiratory tract infection in infants. Arch Dis Child 1994; 70:187–191.
115. Jackson JA, Petersen SA, Wailoo MP. Body temperature changes before minor illness in infants. Arch Dis Child 1994; 71:80–83.

116. Naeye RL, Ladis B, Drage JS. Sudden infant death syndrome: a prospective study. Am J Dis Child 1976; 130:1207–1212.
117. Steele R, Langworth JT. The relationship of antenatal and postnatal factors to sudden unexpected death in infancy. Can Med Assoc J 1966; 94:1165–1171.
118. Protestos CD, Carpenter RG, McWeeny PM, Emery JL. Obstetric and perinatal histories of children who died unexpectedly (cot death). Arch Dis Child 1973; 48:835–841.
119. Froggatt P. Epidemiological aspects of the Northern Ireland study. In: Bergman AB, Beckwith JB, Ray GC, eds. Sudden Infant Death Syndrome. Seattle: University of Washington Press, 1970: 32–46.
120. Fedrick J. Sudden unexpected death in infants in the Oxford Record Linkage area: the mother. Br J Prev Soc Med 1974; 28:93–97.
121. Fedrick J. Sudden unexpected death in infants in the Oxford Record Linkage area: an analysis with respect to time and space. Br J Prev Soc Med 1973; 27:217–224.
122. Getts AG, Hill HF. Sudden infant death syndrome: incidence at various altitudes. Dev Med Child Neurol 1982; 24:61–68.
123. Buck GM, Cookfair DL, Michalek AM, Nasca PC, Standfast SJ, Sever LE. Assessment of in utero hypoxia and risk of sudden infant death syndrome. Paediatr Perinat Epidemiol 1989; 3:157–173.
124. Standfast SJ, Jereb S, Janerich DT. The epidemiology of sudden infant death syndrome in upstate New York: birth characteristics. Am J Public Health 1980; 70:1061–1067.
125. Nicholl JP, O'Cathain A. Antenatal smoking, postnatal passive smoking and sudden infant death syndrome. In: Poswillo D, Alberman E, eds. Effects of Smoking on the Fetus, Neonate and Child. Oxford, England: Oxford Medical Publications, 1992.
126. Sunderland R, Emery JL. Febrile convulsions and cot death. Lancet 1981; 176–178.
127. Hoffman HJ, Hunter JC, Ellish NJ, Janerick DT, Goldberg J. Adverse reproductive factors and the sudden infant death syndrome. In: Harper RM, Hoffman HJ, eds. Sudden Infant Death Syndrome: Risk Factors and Basic Mechanisms. New York: PMA Publishing, 1988: 153–175.
128. Hoffman HJ, Hillman LS. Epidemiology of the sudden infant death syndrome: maternal, neonatal, and postneonatal risk factors. Clin Perinatol 1992; 19:717–737.
129. Hoffman HJ, Hunter JC, Damus K, Pakter J, Peterson DR, van Belle G, Hasselmeyer EG. Diphtheria-tetanus-pertussis immunization and sudden infant death: results of the National Institute of Child Health and Human Development co-operative epidemiological study of sudden infant death syndrome risk factors. Pediatrics 1987; 79:598–611.
130. Wagner M, Samson-Dolellfus D, Menard J. Sudden unexpected infant death in a French county. Arch Dis Child 1984; 59:1082–1087.
131. Alessandri LM, Read AW, Stanley FJ, Burton PR, Dawes VP. Sudden infant death syndrome and infant mortality in Aboriginal and non-Aboriginal infants. J Paediatr Child Health 1994; 30:242–247.
132. Einspieler C, Widder J, Holzer A, Kenner T. The predictive value of behavioural risk factors for sudden infant death. Early Hum Dev 1988; 18:101–109.
133. McLoughlin A. Sudden infant deaths in Tameside. Health Visitor 1988; 61:235–237.
134. Wierenga H, Brand R, Geudeke T, van Geijn HP, van der Harten H, Verloove-Vanhorick SP. Prenatal risk factors for cot death in very preterm and small for gestational age infants. Early Hum Dev 1990; 23:15–26.
135. Karagas MR, Hollenbach KA, Hickock DE, Daling JR. Induction of labor and risk of sudden infant death syndrome. Obstet Gynecol 1993; 81:497–501.

136. Beal S, Porter C. Sudden infant death syndrome related to climate. Acta Paediatr Scand 1991; 80:278–287.
137. Scragg RKR, Mitchell EA, Stewart AW, Ford RPK, Taylor BJ, Hassall IB, et al. Infant room-sharing and prone sleep position in sudden infant death syndrome. Lancet 1996; 347:7–12.
138. Ford RPK, Mitchell EA, Scragg R, Stewart AW, Taylor BJ, Allen EM. Factors adversely associated with breastfeeding in New Zealand. J Paediatr Child Health 1994; 30:483–489.
139. Wilson CA, Taylor BJ, Laing RM, Williams SM, Mitchell EA. Clothing and bedding and its relevance to sudden infant death syndrome: further results from the New Zealand Cot Death Study. J Paediatr Child Health 1994; 30:506–512.
140. Scragg R, Stewart AW, Mitchell EA, Ford RPK, Thompson JMD. Public health policy on bed sharing and smoking in the sudden infant death syndrome. NZ Med J 1995; 108:218–222.
141. Flahaut A, Messiah A, Jougla E, Bouvet E, Perin J, Hatton F. Sudden infant death syndrome and diphtheria/tetanus toxoid/pertussis/poliomyelitis immunisation (letter). Lancet 1988; 582–583.
142. Carpenter RG, Gardner A, Pursall E, McWeeny PM. Identification of some infants at immediate risk of dying unexpectedly and justifying intensive study. Lancet 1979; 343–346.
143. Taylor EM, Emergy JL. Family and community factors associated with infant deaths that might be preventable. BMJ 1983; 287:871–874.
144. Lewis KW, Bosque EM. Deficient hypoxia awakening response in infants of smoking mothers: possible relationship to sudden infant death syndrome. J Pediatr 1995; 127:691–696.
145. White M, Beckett M, O'Regan M, Matthew T. The effect of maternal smoking in pregnancy on autonomic function in infants. In: Rognum TO, ed. Sudden Infant Death Syndrome: New Trends in the Nineties. Oslo: Scandinavian University Press, 1995: 174–176.
146. Difranza JR, Lew RA. Morbidity and mortality in children associated with the use of tobacco products by other people. Pediatrics 1996; 97:560–568.
147. Kraus JF, Greenland S, Bulterys M. Risk factors for sudden infant death syndrome in the US Collaborative Perinatal Project. Int J Epidemiol 1989; 18:113–120.
148. Brooke H, Gibson A, Tappin D, Brown H. Case-control study of sudden infant death syndrome in Scotland 1992–5. BMJ 1997; 314:1516–1520.
149. Mitchell EA, Taylor BJ, Ford RPK, et al. Four modifiable and other major risk factors for cot death: the New Zealand study. J Paediatr Child Health 1992; 28(suppl 1):S3–S8.
150. Mitchell EA, Stewart AW, Scragg R, et al. Ethnic differences in mortality rate from sudden infant death syndrome in New Zealand. BMJ 1993; 306:13–16.
151. Scragg R, Mitchell EA, Taylor B, et al. Bed sharing, smoking and alcohol in the sudden infant death syndrome. BMJ 1993; 307:1312–1318.
152. Klonoff-Cohen H, Edelstein SL. Bedsharing and the sudden infant death syndrome. BMJ 1995; 311:1269–1272.
153. Scragg RKR, Mitchell EA, Stewart AW, et al. Infant room sharing and prone sleep position in sudden infant death syndrome. Lancet 1996; 347:7–12.
154. McKenna JJ, Mosko S, Richard C. Bedsharing promotes breastfeeding. Pediatrics 1997; 100:214–219.

22

Environmental Stressors and Sudden Unexpected Infant Death

JAMES S. KEMP

St. Louis University School of Medicine
St. Louis, Missouri

I. Introduction

Epidemiological, physiological, and pathological research findings support a triple-risk model for SIDS (1,2): susceptible infants, at a developmentally precarious time, and in an *environment* imposing a stressor that they are unable to overcome, die suddenly and unexpectedly. In this review we consider selected environmental stressors that have been investigated or implicated as contributing to the sudden infant death of infants less than 1 year of age.

We do not review deaths by drugs given intentionally (3–5) but consider accidental inhalation of smoke from crack cocaine. We review how beds and bedding may be dangerous in subtle ways but do not consider deaths in dangerous positions in patently dangerous beds (6,7). We review how bedding can cause thermal stress or rebreathing of exhaled gases.

These topics have been chosen because they are controversial. We do not review an equally important topic, that of passive exposure to cigarette smoke and its by-products, because its association with SIDS, if not the exact site of action, seems unequivocal (8–11).

It now is widely believed that investigating the scene of infant death, the environment of SIDS, will yield insights into the mechanism or reason for death. A death-scene investigation is a suggested requirement for the diagnosis of SIDS (12). Death-scene investigations and subsequent physiological studies based on scene findings have led to a fundamental reconsideration (13) of why infants die suddenly. New understanding of the role of sleep microenvironment (14–16) has, in fact, added to what is meaningful at the death scene (17,18). For example, counselors of grieving parents were once advised to ignore that the infant was found prone, with nose and mouth down into soft bedding (17). The implicit message was that some innate susceptibility that was ultimately unavoidable caused the death. This message may have served both counselors and parents, but it is based on outmoded thinking about the interaction between a prone victim and the sleep microenvironment.

Thus, below, we reexamine the role of environmental factors, or stressors, such as airborne lead, analyzed by earlier SIDS investigators but overshadowed by a decade or more of studies of infant susceptibility. Our purpose is not to diminish developmental or physiological explanations for sudden death but to balance them with a review of possible environmental components of the triple-risk model (2).

II. Air Pollution and Environmental Stressors Arising Outside the Sleep Environment

A. The Approach in the SIDS Literature to Pollutants and Toxins

Most environmental agents such as toxins (19) have been given little attention as causes of sudden death in the SIDS era. Studies of toxins in the environment of infants dying suddenly may have been discouraged by early interpretations of SIDS epidemiology. Influential writers believed that the epidemiological findings of age distribution, occurrence during sleep, seasonal "epidemicity," and financial impoverishment pointed away from toxins as a cause of death. However, in retrospect it is not clear why "the epidemiological facts would ... exclude such general categories as ... toxins" as causes for sudden death (20). In fact SIDS is consistently more common in winter in locales that have more air pollution in winter (e.g., Los Angeles, Taiwan) (21,22).

The dearth of case reports suggests that carbon monoxide poisoning and agents causing anaphylaxis are not frequent causes of sudden death (23,24). Occasional case reports describing scenes of death mention old furnaces that could produce much CO (25), but the determinations of carboxyhemoglobin levels have not been reported to prove CO poisoning. Most reports of toxins in sudden infant death (26–28) have involved pharmacological agents given intentionally. When environmental toxins are mentioned in forensic texts (29–31), it is first recommended that toxicological studies be based on death-scene findings suggesting exposure to noxious gases, etc. Much more commonly, however, forensic SIDS protocols and published guidelines for investigations of sudden death in children do not even mention a possible role for environmental toxins (32–36).

B. Outdoor Air Pollution and Sudden Unexpected Infant Death

Knoebel et al. have recently claimed that their "findings suggest that air pollution is linked to SIDS, and thus (should cause experts to) re-open the discussion" of this association (22). Knoebel et al. used visibility of reference objects in air as an optimetric proxy for the amount of air pollution. The less the visibility in Taiwan for 1 to 9 days before death, the greater was the relative risk for SIDS. Their results are provocative but hard to interpret: 1) Only 3% of cases had autopsies performed; 2) the correlations between visibility and the more standard, gravimetric measures of important pollutants were significant but not terribly strong ($r = -.41$ and $r = -.53$, respectively for SO_2 and CO); 3) their techniques cannot be used where fog causes reduced visibility; and, 4) the authors do not relate the levels measured to a mechanism for death from pollutants.

Another epidemiological study makes a stronger case for an important relationship between SIDS and air pollution. Hoppenbrouwers et al. (21) analyzed the seasonal incidence of SIDS in the Los Angeles basin between 1974 and 1977; their series included 693 SIDS deaths. Mean daily airborne levels of SO_2, NO_2, CO, hydrocarbons, and lead were measured. A single annual winter peak occurred in the frequency of SIDS as well as in the levels of SO_2, NO_2, CO, hydrocarbons, and lead. The peaks in the five air pollutants, including lead, were superimposed on one another and occurred consistently 7 weeks before the peak incidence of SIDS. Victims born during low-pollution months died 4 weeks later than those born in high-pollution months. The authors believe that their findings are "indirect evidence that the temporal relationship was also a functional one." They also state that the levels of CO they measured are similar to those causing increases in fetal carboxyhemoglobin levels and the levels of NO_2 are close to those causing respiratory epithelial injury. They thus proposed that chronic hypoxemia and increased susceptibility to respiratory infections might offer mechanisms for death associated with air pollutants.

The findings of Hoppenbrouwers et al. were later criticized by Carpenter and Gardner because the confounding effects of seasonal respiratory illness per se had not been characterized. Carpenter and Gardner, in their own work, found no significant relationship between SIDS incidence and the amount of dry sulfur in the air of England and Wales (23). Nevertheless, the elegant work of Hoppenbrouwers et al. done 20 years ago provides some evidence for a link between air pollutants and SIDS.

C. Indoor Air Pollution and Sudden Unexpected Infant Death: Lead, Cocaine

Although we will discuss more controversial indoor pollutants, it must be reemphasized that there is a consensus that cigarette smoke exposure, both transplacentally and passively after birth, has an association with SIDS that is causal (8). The mechanism of nicotine's effects and the site of its action relevant to SIDS have received much attention; the reader is referred to several recent manuscripts (8–11).

Erickson et al. (37) measured lead in tissues from 66 SIDS victims from St.

Louis, Missouri, and compared the results to levels from 23 control infants. Lead levels in lung, liver, renal cortex, and ribs were measured. The levels were corrected for age, because lead accumulates over time. Liver and rib tissue from SIDS victims contained significantly more lead than control tissues. Also, the age-corrected rate of increase in lung lead was higher in the SIDS victims. The increased rate of lung lead accumulation suggests that airborne lead was one important source of exposure in infants (4 to 26 weeks of age in this study), who were not likely to ingest lead paint chips. Erickson et al. speculate that the infants inhaled airborne lead arising from dried, flaking paint, automobile and industrial emissions, and smoke from coal fires used for heating. They recognized that tobacco smoke might also be a source of lead as well as cadmium, but their SIDS victims did not have increased cadmium levels. Although matching for socioeconomic status was not rigorous in this study, SIDS victims from the inner city had higher levels of lead in their tissues than did inner-city controls. This suggests that lead exposure per se, rather than poverty alone, could add to SIDS risk among these high-risk infants.

In a study designed to investigate effects of heavy metals and pesticides in human milk, Kleeman et al. (38), from Hanover, Germany, found no increase in lead levels in the blood and kidneys of SIDS victims. Their conclusions were limited, however, by small sample size, failure to calculate confidence limits of their negative results, and failure to explain why the controls had much higher levels for all substances measured.

Passive inhalation by infants of crack cocaine smoke was considered in a study done in Philadelphia of 600 sudden deaths between 1 week and 24 months of age (39). The death scene was visited in all cases. Sixteen of the infants had measurable levels of cocaine, or its metabolite benzoylecgonine, in postmortem toxicological studies done on blood, urine, kidney, and brain. The infants with apparent cocaine exposure were 2 weeks to 10 months of age at death. The blood levels of cocaine (0.0016 to 0.03 mg/dL) were similar to those recorded in other human and animal studies where cocaine had direct lethal effects (40). Scene investigations showed that just before death, all the infants had been in rooms that contained smoke from crack (39).

Many published reports document immediate toxicity from cocaine (40,41). Myocardial dysfunction and tachydysrhythmias, without demonstrable postmortem abnormalities, have been reported in humans, including infants. Thus, in addition to the well-known effects of transplacental cocaine on SIDS risk and on ventilatory control (42–44), cocaine may also cause unexpected infant death through direct toxic effects. In St. Louis, levels of cocaine in blood are measured after all possible SIDS. Though once common, the frequency here of antemortem cocaine exposure among infants dying suddenly may be less than it was 5 or 10 years ago (personal communication, Michael Graham, MD, Medical Examiner for the City of St. Louis).

III. Sleep Position and Environmental Stressors

Within the last 10 years it has been established that being placed prone to sleep or turning to the prone position during sleep increase SIDS risk. Furthermore, avoiding the prone position reduces the number of SIDS deaths as well as overall infant mortality (45–56). The second, momentous finding of a preventative role for nonprone and supine sleep indicates that prone sleeping or something almost inextricably linked to prone sleeping causes some sudden deaths that were previously inexplicable (57,58). Below, we consider at length possible deleterious interactions between sleep position and environmental stressors and whether the interactions are less dangerous for supine sleepers.

There are, of course, nonenvironmental explanations for the increased rate of prone deaths, including retropositioning of the mandible (59) and nasal occlusion (60). Both cause upper airway obstruction and are made much less likely by supine sleep (61,62). Kahn and colleagues have also shown that prone-sleeping infants arouse spontaneously from sleep less often than supine infants and are less sensitive to, for example, auditory stimuli that provoke arousal (63,64).

A. Thermal Stress as a Mechanism for Prone SIDS: Case-Control Studies and Case Series

Infants lying naked and prone on a firm surface have less skin surface available for heat dissipation—about 6% less area than when supine (65). This and information about overwrapping led to the development of the theory that thermal stress in the prone position causes lethal hyperthermia (discussed below) (66). Interest in this theoretical model of thermal stress was enhanced in particular by the seminal findings from New Zealand (46–48) linking prone sleep and SIDS and by a case-control study from Avon Country in the United Kingdom. Fleming et al. (67) assessed the interaction between prone sleep and thermal insulation of bedding in units called *togs* (A sheet provides thermal resistance of about 1 tog, a heavy comforter about 10 togs.) One tog unit is the thermal resistance of a fabric when the temperature differences between its faces is 0.1 °C for a flow of heat equivalent to 1 W/m^2 (68). In the Avon study (67), the relative risk (RR) for prone sleep alone was 8.8. However, if the thermal resistance of bedding was > 10 tog, the RR for prone sleep increased dramatically, to 25.2 [95% confidence intervals (CI) for RR, 3.7–169.0]. Later analyses from New Zealand have also shown this specific interaction between prone sleep and extra thermal insulation (69). A related case-control study by Ponsonby et al. (70), from Hobart, Tasmania, showed that the odds ratio (OR) for prone sleep alone was 4.5 (95% CI, 2.1–9.6); but heating the room to maintain a temperature of 15° to 29°C (59° to 84°F) significantly increased the OR for SIDS (6.9, 1.3–37.0).

In interpreting these findings, one should be aware of apparent differences in sleep practices between North America and, for example, England, New Zealand, and Tasmania. Although detailed descriptions of sleep thermal environment are lacking for infants from the United States, it is likely that most infants here sleep in rooms that are heated at night in winter. However, in New Zealand, it is common for infants to sleep all night during winter in rooms without heat. Infants there often wear hats, mittens, and several layers of clothing to bed. One report from the New Zealand Cot Death Study (69) showed that only 27% of 1985 infants slept in heated rooms. In contrast, during visits to the homes of nearly 100 SIDS victims or infants at high risk for SIDS in St. Louis, Missouri, we have not encountered a single home that lacked heat during a previous winter night (14,71,72). It is possible that groups of infants in the United States [such as Native Americans or those living in public housing (25)] sleep in cold rooms in winter. If so, their sleep practices deserve careful documentation.

There are thus three epidemiological studies linking potential thermal stress to increased risk of prone death: two implicating thermal insulation by bedclothes and one thermal stress from room heating. Many other reports suggest that thermal stress could play a part in sudden death. However, a specific harmful interaction between prone sleep and thermal stress was not discussed in these other studies. For example, without reference to sleep position or position found, infants dying suddenly have been shown to be hyperthermic by direct measurement of rectal temperature (73,74), to have been palpably warm or sweaty (46,73,75), or to have died in rooms that were as hot as 40°C (25,73). Perhaps more important in terms of number of affected infants, published reports also show that infants often die with their heads covered by bedding (25,46,54,76–79). However, the strength of an association, if any, among prone sleep, death with head covered, and thermal insulation has not been reported.

B. Case Series and Case-Comparison Studies Showing That Prone Infants Die Suddenly in Microenvironments Permitting Rebreathing of Exhaled Gases

Physiological studies done over the past 10 years have shown that infants dying with their noses and mouths into bedding, particularly those prone and face down, would rebreathe exhaled gases for some period before death (13,14,80–84). At least seven large case series reports dating back to the 1940s suggest the relevance of these physiological studies by showing that 20% to 52% of infants dying suddenly and unexpectedly are found dead with their noses and mouths into bedding (20,50,85–89). From the United States, the fraction has been consistently near 30% (86,89).

One of the first publications addressing this issue in detail was by Abramson, from New York City (85). In 1944 he showed that 68% of 139 infants dying unexpectedly were prone and "46% (of prone infants) were discovered with nose and mouth in occluding contact with ... soft pillows, mattresses, or mattress coverings." In criticizing Abramson's findings that up to 43 of 139 deaths were preventable, Werne and Garrow (90) in 1947 claimed that he had erroneously overlooked such causes of death as otitis media (20 cases) and unspecified congenital heart disease (4 cases). It is not clearly stated, however, why the infants with otitis died or what the occult heart defects were. The paper by Werne and Garrow as well as one by Wooley (91) claiming that infants will not suffocate in ordinary bedding deserve careful rereading and are germane to this discussion because they influenced subsequent interpretations of death-scene information and theories for sudden death (92). By current standards, however, their findings seem anecdotal and their conclusions questionable.

A recent case-comparison study by Scheers et al. (89) showed that 29% of 206 SIDS victims were found with their external airways covered by bedding. The death scene was visited and an infant mannequin used to recreate the scene. Of these 206 infants, 71% were prone; of 59 with airways covered, 57 were prone. Not surprisingly, being placed prone for the last sleep significantly increased the risk for being found dead in a rebreathing microenvironment—i.e., with nose and mouth covered (adjusted OR = 2.86, $p < .05$). Scheers et al. thus link prone sleep to an environmental stressor, created by a combination of bedding and sleep practices, that might be lethal.

Death-scene investigations using a mannequin for reconstruction have been useful in documenting the prevalence of the prone position with nose and mouth covered first reported by Abramson over 50 years ago (14,85,89).

IV. Prone Sleep and Toxins Arising from Beds and Bedrooms

Chemical toxins are rarely sought at postmortem unless the death-scene investigation suggests an obvious potential toxic exposure. As noted previously, the forensic literature offers little guidance regarding a search for toxins not apparent to the senses at the scene. In England and New Zealand, a group of chemists raised concerns that fire retardants in bedding posed a particular risk to infants directly exposed to them by sleeping prone (93). Trihydrides of phosphorus, arsenic, and antimony, produced by a fungus (*Scopulariopsis brevicaulis*) in damp, warm bedding, were hypothesized to be lethal. Particular concern was raised about antimony and its trihydride, stibine. The proponents of this mechanism, which remains largely hypothetical, were gratified when fewer infants in England died because they were no longer prone and thus, presumably, exposed to less stibine. However, as Fleming et al. point out in reviewing this controversy, there is no delineation of a mechanism for sudden death, no evidence for a dose effect, and no estimate of risk created by prone sleep on bedding treated with phosphorus, arsenic, or antimony (94).

There is, then, no direct physiological or epidemiological evidence supporting a role for toxic fire retardants in prone deaths (and there is little published evidence for a role for chemicals in bedding in any infant deaths). Nevertheless, the British thought it prudent to remove them from infant bedding in favor of less toxic retardants. One more observation on possible exposure to lethal toxins seems appropriate. If foul play can be reasonably ruled out, intense exposure to environmental chemicals might be considered in particular when two small infants, such as twins, die simultaneously in the same bed, a finding that is not uncommon in published reports, particularly when the infants are prone (95,96).

V. How Thermal Stress Might Cause Sudden Unexpected Death

A. Hyperthermia and Sudden Infant Death

(My collaborators and I have focused our research on rebreathing of exhaled gases and believe that this theory is the most straightforward explanation for a substantial fraction of prone deaths. Nevertheless, the components of a strong competing theory merit careful attention and thus are presented in detail.)

Hyperthermia is an elevation in body temperature due to thermoregulatory failure. Fever, by contrast, occurs in the context of "intact homeostatic responses" (97). Mammals dissipate heat by 1) evaporative water loss through sweating and panting; 2) vasomotor adjustments to increase thermal conductivity; and 3) movement into a cooler locale or changes in posture (98). Hyperthermia occurs as a result of excessive heat production (e.g., excessive exertion), diminished heat dissipation (e.g., overwrapping, anticholinergic drugs), and hypothalamic abnormalities [e.g., after central nervous system (CNS) trauma]. In fever there is an increase in the hypothalamic set point, but in hyperthermia the hypothalamic set point is normal.

Heat stroke, with death or neurological sequelae, is described in children who are overwrapped in warm environments (99,100). Death due to hyperthermia with heat stroke is associated with secondary shock, cardiac dysrhythmia, myocardial ischemia, renal failure, and disseminated intravascular coagulation (DIC) (97). A lethal syndrome of encephalopathy with hemorrhage has also been described in children exposed to severe thermal stress (101).

Some case series of "cot deaths," particularly from the United Kingdom, have a high prevalence of elevated postmortem rectal temperatures. Sunderland and Emery (74) found that 10 of 24 cot-death victims in Sheffield had rectal temperatures > 38°C several hours after death, and 5 were > 40°C. Stanton (73), in Yorkshire, reported 6 of 15 victims with postmortem temperatures ranging from 37° to 42°C and documented premortem circumstances that included "an unusually warm environment" and "excessive clothing or overwrapping." Bass et al. (25), described many infants who had died in hot environments (e.g., room temperatures from 39.5 ° to 41.0°C), and one of their victims had a rectal temperature of 41.5°C. Bass et al. explained that in New York City some apartments are not supplied with heat in winter between 10:00 P.M. and 6:00 A.M. They speculate that some infants dressed warmly for the cold night became hyperthermic when the heat was turned on in the morning.

Pathological findings consistent with heat stroke—e.g., rhabdomyolysis, acute myocardial or renal injury, or stroke—have not been reported in SIDS victims with postmortem temperature elevations. Reasons for death in the absence of pathological findings of heat stroke remain obscure in these cases. They have been attributed by Bacon to "febrile apnea," CNS ischemia, and unobserved seizures (102).

An important question about postmortem temperature elevations is raised in a paper by Hutchins (103). He measured pre- and postmortem rectal temperatures within 3 hr of death in 11 adult patients dying in the hospital. Several had postmortem temperatures 2 hr after death that were higher than those recorded just before death. None were heavily wrapped postmortem. Hutchins speculates that his findings were due to "continuing tissue and bacterial metabolism in the absence of the usual heat dispersal mechanisms," such as vasodilatation and sweating, that would, of course, be absent after death. Although postmortem temperature elevation would seem to be convincing evidence for premortem pyrexia, this remains an unproved assumption based on Hutchins's work.

Careful thermal balance studies done by Stothers and Warner (65) showed that the effective surface area for insensible heat loss in infants differed with sleep position. Supine infants had 15% of their total surface in contact with a mattress. Prone infants lying flat had 21% in contact with the mattress, a net reduction of 6% in surface available for heat loss. Stothers and Warner calculated that the loss in total capacity for heat dissipation would be small, however; < 3%, for prone infants compared to those supine under thermoneutral conditions.

A theoretical model was developed by Nelson et al. (66) to predict thermal stress leading to hyperthermia and prone SIDS. Nelson et al. speculated that hyperthermia per se or through an effect on ventilatory pattern could cause sudden death. Their model of thermal balance in infants incorporated estimates of metabolic heat production as well as body surface area available for dissipation, insulation from coverings, and skin and ambient temperatures. Nelson et al. validated their model by comparison to published results; they developed a table of thermoneutral temperatures and proposed ranges of ambient temperature within which an average 3-month-old infant could thermoregulate normally (thermoneutrality is the range of temperature that minimizes metabolic rate as estimated by measuring O_2 consumption). In their analyses, they included many different permutations of thermal insulation and sleep position. They simulated thermal balance in an infant who was lightly or heavily dressed and sleeping either prone, supine, prone and face down, lateral, or lateral with head covered. They calculated, for example, that the thermoneutral point for ambient temperature for a heavily dressed supine infant would be similar to that for one prone (14° versus 13°C); but if the prone infant was also face down, the thermoneutral point would be much lower, 10°C (57°, 55°, and 52°F, respectively). They calculated that the highest ambient temperature tolerated by the heavily wrapped prone infant would be 30°C; for the supine and heavily wrapped, 35°C; and for the prone, face-down, and heavily wrapped, 24°C (86°, 95°, and 75°F respectively). Beyond those highest temperatures, they predicted that a 3-month-old would be unable to thermoregulate during sleep and would become hyperthermic (66).

The results from the work by Nelson et al. have been presented in detail because the model has had great influence on thinking about mechanisms for prone death. However, work done "in the field," in the bedrooms of sleeping infants, seems to challenge the hyperthermia model.

Studies from England by Wailoo et al. in Leicester (68,104–106) and Wigfield et al. (107) in Avon seem to show that infants are able to avoid hyperthermia, even when prone, and overwrapped, in contradiction to the model developed by Nelson et al. Wailoo et al. have studied infants sleeping at home, with position and bedding chosen by the parents. On the study night, they recorded rectal and skin temperatures as well as room temperatures at the side of the infant's bed. They have shown that on a typical night infants thermoregulate so that their rectal temperature falls within the first hour of being put to sleep from near 37.0°C to a temperature, on average, 0.8°C lower (Fig. 1) (106).

In addition to describing normal patterns of thermoregulation during sleep in infants at home, Wailoo et al. have analyzed the impact of sleep position and thermal

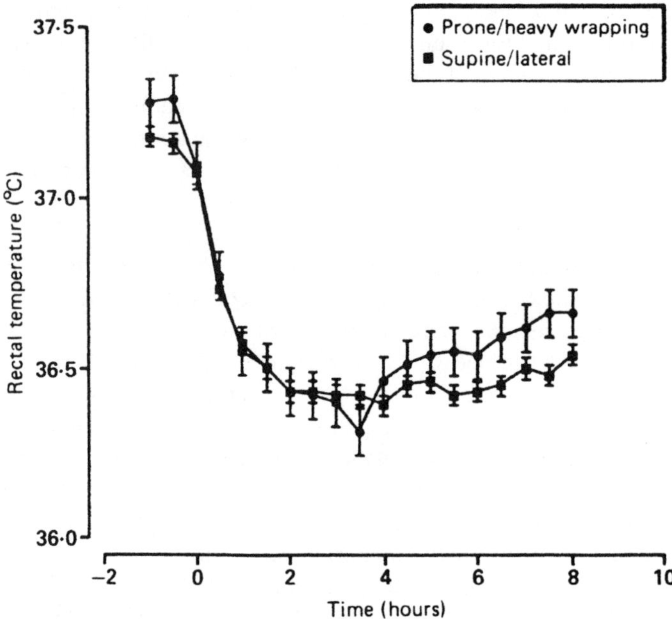

Figure 1 The rectal temperature of babies aged 12 to 22 weeks sleeping in the prone position covered with more than 15 tog units in rooms where the average temperature exceeded 18°C, compared with that of babies sleeping supine. Points show mean (SEM) of observations from 11 babies sleeping prone and 29 sleeping supine or lateral. Times are normalized to bedtime. (From Ref. 106.)

insulation on thermoregulation during sleep in a series of studies again done in infants' homes. In all studies they monitored rectal and skin temperature and ambient temperature near the bed. In one study of 115 infants, they found that prone infants slept in rooms where the average maximal nighttime temperatures were 20.2° ± 0.4°C. Prone infants were covered with up to 22.5 togs of insulation (mean, 12.3). As shown in Fig. 1, heavily wrapped prone infants were able to avoid hyperthermia and were able to thermoregulate; their overnight temperatures followed the patterns of supine infants and infants who were not heavily wrapped (106). The prone infants who were also heavily wrapped did tend to become slightly warmer than the supine infants, but only after about 6 hr in bed.

It is again worth emphasizing for North American readers that infants at home in England are kept in chilly bedrooms. Wailoo et al. (68) report that from December to March, among 74 homes in Leicester, in only 26% was the heat kept on all night in the infant's room. On average, *room temperature* during winter fell by 4.4°C (7.9°F) overnight to an average temperature of 14.0°C (57.2°F !!!). Room temperatures such as these must be extremely rare during winter in the cooler temperate regions of North America.

In response to these cool environmental temperatures, it was hypothesized (46) that infants would be overdressed by parents who overestimated their thermal needs. Although this may occur, studies by Wigfield et al. show that, on average, the thermal insulation placed by parents around infants at night during winter in Avon "allows them to remain in thermoneutral conditions throughout the night" (107).

These and other studies make it "*difficult to see how the prone position, even interacting with warm conditions, could induce lethal hyperthermia in otherwise normal babies*" (106) (italics mine).

B. Thermal Stress Without Hyperthermia: Interactions Between Thermoregulation and Ventilatory Control and Their Relevance to Sudden Infant Death

Prone sleeping in chilly rooms with all but the most extreme overwrapping (46) does not predictably cause hyperthermia (66,106). It appears, in England at least, that most infants, when exposed at home to the thermal stress that was predicted to cause hyperthermia, are able to thermoregulate normally (Fig. 1). Perhaps the challenge to thermoregulation imposed by prone sleep with extra thermal insulation is not via failure of heat dissipation leading to hyperthermia. It is conceivable that the extra thermal insulation found around SIDS victims (average excess 1.1 tog) causes thermal stress that alters ventilatory pattern or other life-sustaining functions, without hyperthermia (67,108).

Background in Sleep Physiology

The general topic of interactions among thermoregulation and sleep and ventilatory control is reviewed in detail elsewhere (98,109–111). The control of brain temperature and sleep pattern are so closely intertwined that some contend that one purpose of sleep is to accomplish thermoregulation—that is, allow the brain to cool. Kreuger and Takahashi (110) argue for the ultimate separateness of thermoregulation and control of sleep state and duration, but they concede, for example, that even single hypothalamic neurons appear to be involved in both regulation of sleep state (REM versus NREM) and thermoregulation.

The regulation of body temperature during sleep in normal adults and children is precise and robust. Adults who sleep normally, for example, invariably have a "sleep-evoked temperature fall with sleep onset." This occurs even when they fall asleep during the day. The fall in temperature "evoked" by sleep onset is not dependent only on diminished activity, because it occurs in subjects at bed rest (109). The fall is small but very predictable, about 0.5°C. Day (112) has demonstrated a similar fall in rectal temperature in children associated with activity of peripheral mechanisms to dissipate heat—i.e., increased evaporative water loss and elevated skin temperatures.

Warming of adult humans alters the ratio of REM/NREM sleep duration, but the effect depends on whether the warming occurs before or after the adult goes to sleep. Stages 3 and 4 of slow-wave sleep (SWS) are increased by an antecedent "waking heat load" in humans. That is, if an adult with a normal sleep pattern has, for example, a warm bath in the afternoon, several studies have shown that the amount of SWS increases during the ensuing night. Increase in body temperature by about 1.8°C by passively heating the awake subject, without exertion, both increases subsequent SWS and reduces REM time (113). In contrast, warming a sleeping subject who was in a thermoneutral environment tends to elicit arousal and further reduce the amount of REM sleep (98).

Thermoregulation is inhibited during REM sleep. In cool environments, shivering during sleep occurs only during NREM stages 1 and 2 and not during REM. In warm environments, sweating and evaporative water loss is much less in REM than NREM. It appears in general that changes in body temperature are passive in REM and that, during REM sleep, body temperature is much more dependent on ambient temperature.

Many other studies demonstrate the interaction between thermoregulation and sleep state, particularly studies of the putative centers controlling sleep and thermoregulation in the preoptic anterior hypothalamic hypnogenic system (POAH). In animals, direct electrical stimulation of the POAH elicits a thermoregulatory response during NREM but not during REM. There is also evidence from animal studies that heat exposure without changes in core temperature might affect sleep state. These findings are relevant to circumstances described above, where increased external insulation (bedding) is used by infants who are able to regulate their core temperature. A key component of this linkage is that the thermoregulatory center in the POAH receives "thermoafferents" from the skin. In the rat, warming the skin while cooling the brain POAH causes arousal, less total sleep time, and less REM. Thus the rat whose brain is cooled but whose skin is warmed behaves like the rat whose skin is passively warmed enough to increase brain temperature. Skin warming in the rat thus affects sleep and arousal states in a way that is at least partially independent of its effect on the temperature of the central thermoregulatory center. Again, this is analogous to an effect of thermal stress on sleep, without altering brain temperature, that is pertinent to our primary concern in this section. However, one obvious problem with these fascinating findings, in the context of a discussion of effects of thermal stress on infants, is that the changes are in the wrong direction if one is looking for a dangerous or lethal mechanism—i.e., less REM, more arousal.

Studies in Infants

Neonatologists recognized many years ago that "protecting premature infants against excessive heat loss improves their chances for survival" (114). However, observations made on infants who became apneic in servocontrolled isolettes raised concerns about "environmental manipulations [that] may also produce unfavorable conflicts with other homeostatic mechanisms" (114).

Using impedance monitors to detect apnea, Dailey and colleagues (115) studied 6 infants, aged 1 to 10 days, with birthweights of 1050 to 1572 g. They controlled the skin temperature at two levels: 36.0° and 36.8°C. They showed for paired 12 h periods that apnea > 20 sec was more common during the warmer (36.8°C) periods than the cooler periods (group mean number of apnea episodes per 12-h period, 7.2 versus 3.1, $p < .005$).

Perlstein and colleagues (114) analyzed the relationship between direction of change in incubator air temperature and apnea > 15 sec. They studied three premature infants using impedance monitors. The infants weighed 2013, 1600, and 1673 g and were studied between 1 and 10 days of age. Periods of apnea were much more likely to be associated with periods when the incubator temperature was increasing. Nonapneic control periods were more likely to occur when incubator temperature was decreasing. The average amplitude of ambient temperature change during on-off servocontrolled cycling was 1.5° ± 0.5°C. The lowest temperature at which apnea occurred was 34°C. Perlstein et al. emphasized the importance of these findings for prematures who were at high risk for apnea.

Steinschneider (116) reported the density of short apnea (> 2 sec) and longer episodes of apnea in five infants, four of whom were term. The infants ranged in age from 5 to 180 days at the time of study. A nasal thermistor and strain gauge were used to record breaths. The laboratory was heated to "90° ± 2°F" (32°C), so this paper described apnea in a warm laboratory. No results were reported at more conventional room temperatures. All subjects were sibs of infants dying suddenly or themselves had had episodes of cyanosis. The results suggested that apnea was common among infants believed to be at high risk for SIDS. However, in terms of understanding the effects of thermal stress, the interpretation of these results is difficult because the specific impact of room warming was not assessed, the sample size was small, and two of the five subjects appear to have had episodes of cyanosis at home that were not spontaneous (117).

Gozal et al. (118) studied respiratory control in a 6-month-old infant exposed accidentally to profound thermal stress by being very heavily dressed. Two weeks after the infant's presentation with respiratory failure, he had normal hypercapneic and hypoxic responses. This infant from Israel had presented with a rectal temperature of 41.2°C. His blood pressure was 90/55 and he was pale, sweaty, stuporous, and hypotonic. Following cooling to a rectal temperature of 37.7°C, he developed hypotension (BP = 60/35), became cyanotic (ABG, pH = 7.04; Pa_{CO_2} = 71.4; and Pa_{O_2} = 47.6), and required mechanical ventilatory support for 24 hr. An extensive evaluation for infectious causes was unrevealing. It was concluded as he recovered that his pyrexia was due to the many layers of clothing and bedding used before presentation. The importance of this case as evidence that thermal stress can alter ventilatory control is difficult to ascertain, however (69,108). Clear-cut evidence of a transient acquired abnormality in ventilatory control is lacking, both because no specific tests of ventilatory control could be done at the time of presentation and the infant presented in shock.

Glotzbach and Heller (98) have proposed the following hypothetical sequence linking thermal stress without hyperthermia to changes in ventilatory control: 1) an overbundled infant falls asleep in a warm room; 2) the onset of sleep is associated, as expected, with a reduction in the thermoregulatory set point; 3) because the infant cannot dissipate heat, it would be effectively hyperthermic to the central set point; 4) the skin would vasodilate; 5) an increase in REM sleep would follow in the presence of warm skin and a core temperature that is increased relative to the set point; and 6) the increase in REM would increase the risk of dangerous apnea with inadequate thermoregulatory responses during REM. Although thermal stress is well known to cause tachypnea, clinical physiology studies are needed to test this and related hypotheses for a more profound influence of thermal stress.

Fleming et al. (108) have taken an intriguing approach to understanding the interaction between thermoregulation and ventilatory control. They built on the concept of a "feed forward" component of the ventilatory control system that incorporates input from peripheral thermoreceptors in the skin. Using this conceptual framework, they have studied changes in breathing pattern following sighs at different temperatures within a plethysmograph (108,119) (Fig. 2). They have demonstrated that, after

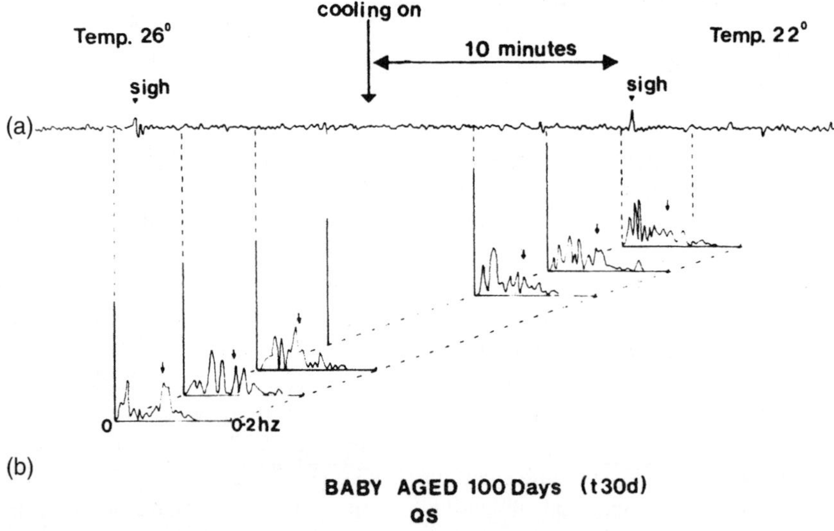

Figure 2 (a) A compressed, filtered plot of minute ventilation from an infant (t30d) aged 100 days in quiet sleep. The initial environmental temperature was 26°C, which is well within the metabolic thermoneutral range. At the point shown, the environment was cooled to 22°C, which is just below the lower critical temperature. The sigh that occurs at an environmental temperature of 26°C is followed by a prolonged oscillation of period, 12 sec. The second sigh, at an environmental temperature of 22°C, is followed by no identifiable oscillation in minute ventilation. (b) Fourier transforms of 3-m sections of (a), as shown. The peak at 0.08 Hz (arrowed), which is prominent in the three sections at higher environmental temperatures, is much less prominent at lower environmental temperatures. (From Ref. 108.)

sighs, the "oscillatory pattern" of breathing differs when infants are studied at 22°C versus 26°C. For infants near 3 months of age, the short-term oscillatory pattern after sighs is apparently accentuated by increasing and reduced by decreasing the environmental temperature. The relationship of this finding to ventilatory abnormalities leading to sudden death is the subject of ongoing studies. Published results available now are in an abstract and a review article, and it is not clear from these how many infants show these changes in postsigh oscillatory pattern.

The results of studies of thermal stress without hyperthermia may be summarized as follows: 1) increased rather than decreased, arousal, 2) apnea in nine premature infants at ambient temperatures ≥ 34.0°C, and 3) increases in oscillation of ventilatory pattern after sighs in an unspecified number of infants. There are few human data demonstrating an additive effect from overwrapping or from a warm room per se on the response to upper airway obstruction (120) or responses to hypoxia or hypercarbia (121,122). Thermal stress above the thermoneutral range would increase O_2 demand by definition, but the relative contribution of such increased O_2 demands to a lethal mechanism has not been reported.

VI. Selected Questions for Study About the Link Between Thermal Stress and Sudden Infant Death

The section above suggests some physiological issues for future study. Important questions about related child-care practices and epidemiology also remain.

It appears from several studies that infants who live in countries with inconsistent heating at night during the winter die with more bedding covering them. That is, too much bedding is used to overcompensate for a chilly room. Yet Wigfield et al. (107) have shown that, in general, parents in their part of England choose bedding that is much more likely to create a thermally neutral than a thermally stressful environment. Is there evidence that infant-care practices of the parents of SIDS victims are an aberration in this regard—i.e., do the extra togs found near SIDS victims actually create thermal stress?

Increased thermal insulation by bedding was associated with an increased prone risk in the New Zealand Cot Death Study but not in the case-control study in Tasmania (69,70). Conversely, perhaps, the perceived warmth of the room had little effect on SIDS in New Zealand (123), but having the heat on all night in the infant's room increased the risk for prone SIDS in Tasmania (70). Is there an explanation for these apparently discrepant findings? An explanation may be apparent when the relative importance of bedding versus room heating as thermal stressors is clarified.

In a recent report from the New Zealand Cot Death Study (69), the amount of bedding calculated to create a thermoneutral environment was used as the index of relative thermal stress. In addition to too much bedding, the New Zealand investigators also found that *too little* insulation relative to ambient temperature also increased SIDS risk for prone sleepers (OR = 2.63, 1.33–2.48). This finding is alone in the recent SIDS literature in suggesting that both cold and warm stresses are risk factors.

This finding appears problematic for those countries where infants' rooms are not heated, yet parents are cautioned, in particular, about keeping their infants cool by not putting too much bedding over them. Are there similar findings pending in epidemiological reports? Are there physiological hypotheses for these findings?

The importance of overwrapping within ethnic and sociodemographic high-risk groups is unclear (124,125). Maoris on the warmer North Island of New Zealand have a high rate of SIDS, but the relationship between togs of insulation and SIDS risk has not been reported for that group. Buve and Rodrigue (126), from London, have shown that in 1986 the higher rate of SIDS among the poor was more pronounced in summer than in winter. If, as it is assumed (46), the poor are more likely to overwrap their infants living in cold dwellings, should poor infants not be at even greater risk of death in winter? In addition, information is needed from the United States on thermal care practices among isolated high-risk groups, such as rural Native Americans and urban occupants of public housing (25).

Over a 3-year period, the New Zealand Cot Death Study has documented a remarkable fall in SIDS rate (from 4.2 per 1000 to 2.1 per 1000 live births), coincident with a reduction in the prevalence of prone sleeping from 43% to 5%. The contribution of reduced thermal stress to the success of this intervention is difficult to interpret. The New Zealand intervention did not actively discourage overwrapping, and the researchers there were unable to show that the mean thermal insulation of infants changed (127). In Avon, the fall in SIDS was also associated with a reduction in prone sleeping without a change in the thermal insulation over infants, despite a pointed message to reduce it (49). Does the extra 6% of surface area available for direct heat radiation (even if it is the head and face) in supine infants with comparable thermal insulation explain these findings from New Zealand and England? Are supine infants dying supine with their heads completely covered more likely to be overwrapped? (See Refs. 25, 46, 54, and 76–79.)

VII. Physiological Studies of Rebreathing Stress for Prone Infants Imposed by the Sleep Microenvironment

A. Studies Suggesting Rebreathing Is a Lethal Mechanism

The potential for lethal rebreathing of exhaled gases from bedclothes was described by Archibald in 1942 (128). He speculated "that a well baby might anesthetize himself by breathing back and forth into the mattress or pillow, or under the blanket, and then be unable to resist smothering." The potential of the resultant hypoxia and hypercarbia to cause asphyxia "from breathing in a confined space" was recognized. Archibald also noted that "In the cases of smothering the factors of mattress, pillow, or blankets are constant." Recently, we have measured the effective dead space for items of bedding on which infants have died face down, using techniques developed to measure the effective dead space of anesthesia equipment (129). We have studied sheepskins, polystyrene cushions, comforters, etc., and the imposed dead space ranged from about 600 to more than 1600 mL. Thus, as Archibald predicted, for a single breath to entrain fresh air when an infant is breathing only in these "spaces," it must be larger than any infant can muster.

Whether exhaled air trapped in bedding does create an environment of lethal hypoxia and hypercarbia was studied by Bolton et al. over 25 years ago (130). They used a mechanical model of infant respiration to show that CO_2 could accumulate about an infant on the mattress of a carry cot—a portable bassinet lined with plastic on the floor and sides. However, in this early work, Bolton et al. concluded that CO_2 accumulation would be significant only if the exhaled air was cooled.

Ryan, from Victoria, Australia, addressed the effect of cooling on the course of dispersal of exhaled air (131). Using a technique involving an infant model and a single-mirror Schlieren optical system, Ryan demonstrated visually that breaths exhaled over moist bedding in a cool room would tend to linger near the infant's face. He concluded that prone sleeping in a cool room could create a rebreathing microenvironment even when the infant's face was to the side and certainly when it was down. In later investigations, Bolton et al. confirmed that marked rebreathing could occur on sheepskins if an infant was prone with face to side as well as prone and face down (82).

In studies done in the laboratory of Bradley Thach, M.D., we have demonstrated that the posture shown in Fig. 3 could be associated with lethal rebreathing on a va-

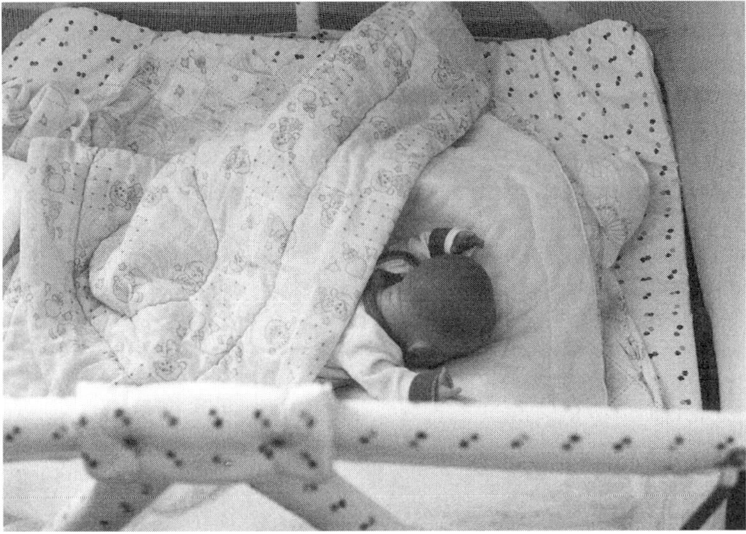

Figure 3 Thirty percent of SIDS deaths in the United States involved infants found face down when prone sleeping was more common. The photograph shows an infant mannequin as it was positioned by the mother of a 1-month-old boy found dead in this position on the bedding shown. The bed was a "playpen" with a plastic pad on its floor. The infant's face was into a comforter placed over a soft pillow.

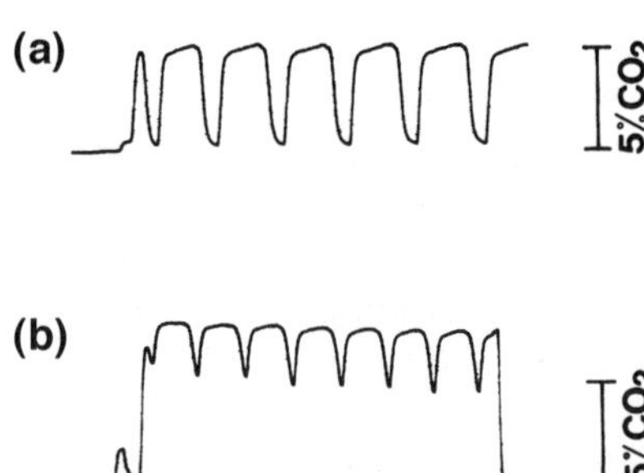

Figure 4 Carbon dioxide (CO_2) as measured through an endotracheal tube in rabbit 5. Exhalation causes an increase or plateau of percentage of CO_2 in the tube. Inspiration causes a decrease in percentage of CO_2 in the tube. (a) Baseline recording, with rabbit breathing through a mannequin's head alone. Percentage of inspiratory CO_2 was 0.21. (b) Recording after 5 min of breathing through a mannequin's head while face down on sheepskin. Bars indicate 5% CO_2. Note that the lowest percentage of inspiratory CO_2 rose to 4.4% in the face-down position, confirming marked rebreathing. (From Ref. 80.)

riety of sleep surfaces. The bedding was from case series and case-control studies of SIDS and included the bedding used by many infants dying prone with face down (14,81). Figure 4 shows capnometry tracings demonstrating that marked rebreathing occurs when a 4 kg rabbit breathes into a sheepskin (80). The rabbit, though sedated, mounted a brisk ventilatory response with a fourfold increase in $\dot{V}_E$. Nevertheless, profound hypoxemia, hypercarbia, and acidosis ensued (Fig. 5) with death in three of four rabbits. This physiological reconstruction was designed to be relevant to a case from the United States and to epidemiological findings from New Zealand, where many infants died prone and face down on sheepskins (88). Similar lethal abnormalities in gas exchange during rebreathing occurred in studies modeled after an outbreak of 22 deaths on infant cushions filled with polystyrene beads (13). In addition to bedding from other countries and bedding that is unusual in the United States, we have demonstrated that rebreathing and death occurred in rabbits breathing into "ordinary" bedding on which infants in St. Louis died face down (Fig. 3). [This finding, in particular, contradicts the claims made by Wooley 50 years ago (91) that infants would not smother in ordinary bedding.]

B. Studies in Infants

Several important publications (not reviewed here) show that a large subgroup of infants who are otherwise normal and able to maintain gas exchange during sleep appear nevertheless to have a blunted ventilatory and arousal response to hypercarbia and hypoxia when those conditions are created in their sleep environment (121,122,132). Furthermore, recent work presented below shows that it is quite plausible that normal infants may in general have limited ability to free their airways when the sleep environment imposes a rebreathing stressor.

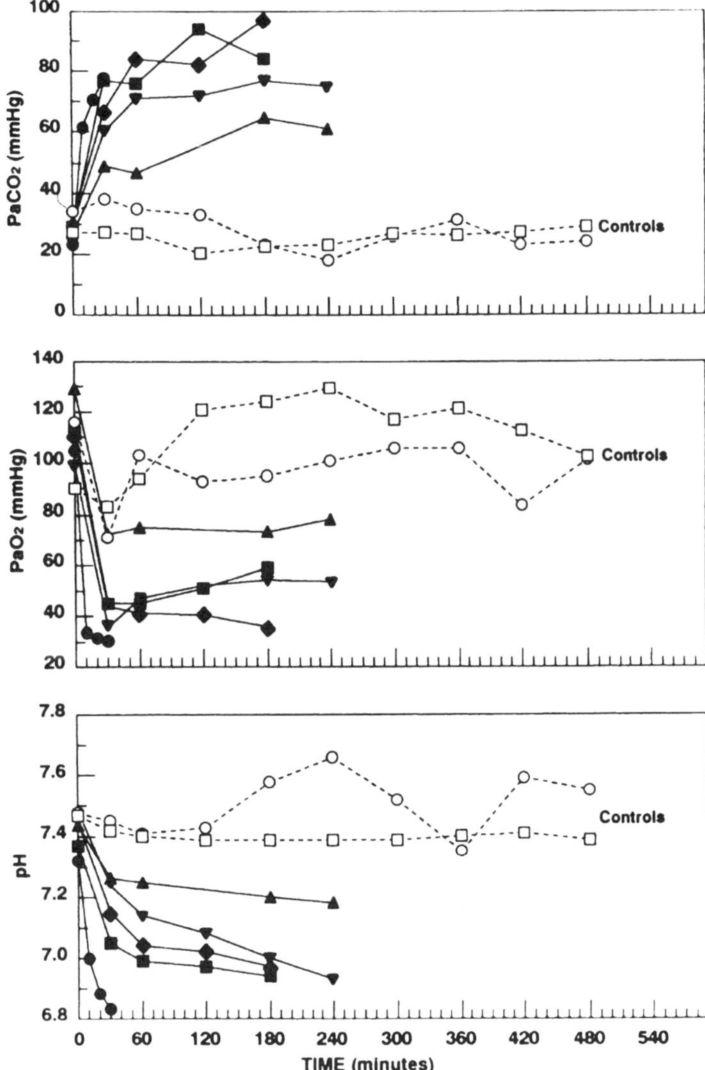

Figure 5 Levels of arterial blood gases for the five study rabbits and two controls. Solid lines indicate rabbits breathing into sheepskins; stippled lines, control rabbits. Squares, circles, triangles, and diamonds indicate individual rabbits. Blood gas levels at time 0 are baseline values that were obtained after 30 min of breathing through the mannequin's head alone. One rabbit (solid circles) was studied for only 30 min as part of a shorter protocol. Three of four rabbits studied for longer than 30 min died while breathing into the sheepskin. (From Ref. 80.)

Chiodini and Thach (133) used capnometry to show that prone, face-down infants would rebreathe in soft bedding. Percentage of inspired CO_2 increased to as high as 6.4% (mean 3.2%) among 11 infants on soft bedding. There was also a modest but significant increase in end-tidal percentage of CO_2 for the infants as a group.

Skadberg and Markestad (134) studied whether infants rebreathe in bedding and whether they are able to get access to fresh air after rebreathing begins. They studied both prone and supine infants ($n = 30$), at 2 ½ and 5 months of age. During the study, they covered the infants' heads with a heavy duvet (comforter, tog value, ~13), and recorded transcutaneous CO_2($_{tc}CO_2$) and O_2 and inspired percentage of CO_2. Within minutes, CO_2 accumulated in both sleep positions, with increases of inspired CO_2 to as high as 4.5% (typically to ~2%), and small but consistent increases in $_{tc}CO_2$. The increases in percentage of inspired CO_2 and $_{tc}CO_2$ were greater when the infants were prone. An important additional observation was that only one of the prone infants (4%) at 5 months was able to uncover its head to obtain fresh air, compared to 23% and 60% of the supine infants at 2 ½ and 5 months respectively. This work also demonstrates the obvious point that bedding which delivers much thermal insulation also can create a formidable rebreathing microenvironment within the space that it covers.

Skadberg and Markestad described infants' success in gaining access to fresh air when the head became covered while prone or supine. A related paper by Lijowska et al. (135) provides more detail about specific ventilatory and behavioral sequences elicited in response to rebreathing stressors within the sleep microenvironment. Lijowska et al. also show that the response sequence elicited by increased inspired CO_2 is similar to that seen with innate spontaneous arousals. They describe a sequence of sigh, startle, head lifting and turning, and rhythmic arm thrashing occurring both during rebreathing and exogenous CO_2 breathing as well as during spontaneous arousals (Fig. 6). They studied infants rebreathing when prone and face down into soft bedding and while supine with face and head covered. Face-down infants, by and large, gain access to fresh air by lifting and turning their heads (136). Supine infants with face covered by bedding gain access to fresh air with "flailing leg and arm movements" that include swiping near the face (135). During rebreathing, inspired CO_2 reached as high as 4.8% in prone infants, and was typically about 3.8% in the supine position. For the most part, arm thrashing in supine infants was less effective in ending rebreathing (40% of times) than was head lifting among prone infants face down. However, occasionally the prone infant's external airway was further compromised when a startle resulted in the infant's nose and mouth being turned deeper into the bedding, with greater increase in percentage of inspired CO_2. Lijowska et al., in showing several ways that prone and supine infants might curtail rebreathing, have developed a framework for studying whether infants at increased risk for SIDS are less able to complete the ventilatory and behavioral responses they described.

Lijowska et al. also noted that a rebreathing stressor is applied spontaneously when infants bring an arm near the face when sleeping prone with an arm over the head (135). Using an infant mannequin, Schmid (137) has shown that the time for CO_2 dispersal from near his model's face (138) increased by 25% just by reproducing this common arm-near-the-face prone position.

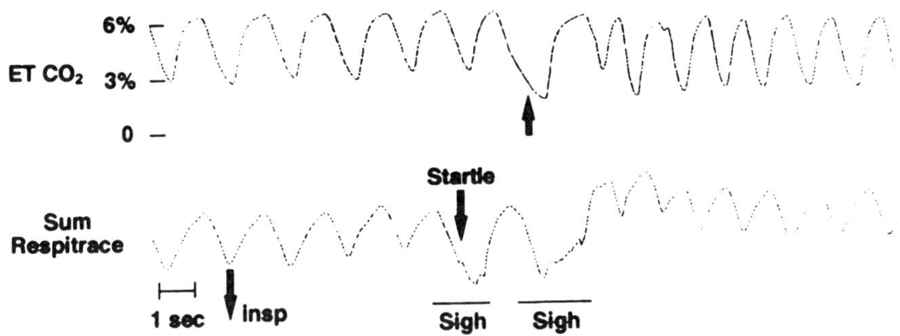

Figure 6 Polygraphic recordings of an airway-protective event in an infant sleeping in face-down position. Protective event begins with a sigh coupled with a startle [onset indicated by movement artifact in ECG trace (not shown)], with associated head lifting and turning. Sigh is indicated by Respitrace and long inspiratory time in CO_2 trace (arrow). During startle, head position changes from head straight down to head angled to the side, causing improved access to fresh air (i.e., inspired CO_2 is reduced). Respitrace tracing suggests that a second sigh follows the first. Lack of further movement following startle indicates minimal sleep disturbance. (From Ref. 135.)

How much an infant's spontaneous behavior and the bedding available might combine to compromise ventilation during sleep was demonstrated by Waters et al. (139) in video and polysomnographic studies done in infants' homes. They showed that infants frequently turn their noses and mouths down, with their arms near their faces. They also described one infant who pulled a mattress pad in front of her face, with presumptive rebreathing and a subsequent increase in ${}_{tc}CO_2$ by 37 torr, to 87. This critical anecdote shows that severe ventilatory compromise is possible when airway defenses fail to remove an imposed rebreathing barrier. We have also reported an investigation of the scene of a sudden infant death showing that a prone 2-month-old infant was found with a blanket between his flexed arm and face (140).

C. Physical Properties of Infant Bedding

Investigations of bedding that may cause lethal rebreathing have, for the most part, been based on the model of a prone, face-down infant (81). Detailed studies of physical properties of bedding causing face-up rebreathing are needed.

For the prone and face-down model, we have shown that the short-term dispersal of CO_2 from infant bedding can be described well by a single exponential equation (138) (Fig. 7). The $t_{1/2}$ for CO_2 dispersal, using tidal volumes and breathing rates appropriate for infants, correlates well with the changes in Pa_{CO_2} recorded during rebreathing in rabbits who were breathing into the same sheepskins, comforters, etc. This model assumes a variable volume that limits CO_2 dispersal and is more or less leaky. Our studies suggested that a threshold for lethal rebreathing is approximated when the time for CO_2 dispersal from bedding is 80% longer than when no rebreathing is occurring (12.5 versus 22.4 sec).

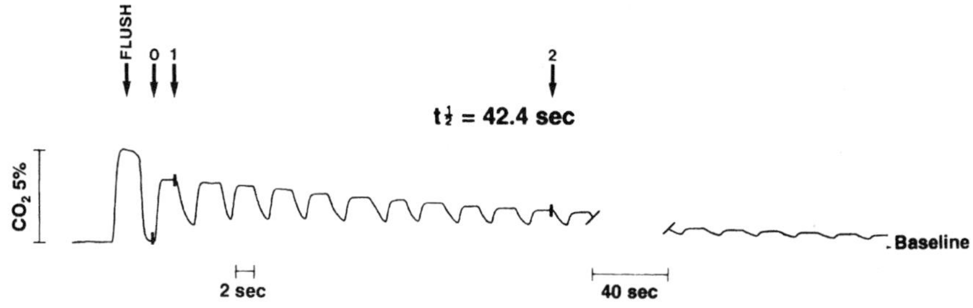

Figure 7 Representative washout curve study showing washout of CO_2 from mannequin's head face down on a sheepskin [halftime ($t_{1/2}$) = 42.4 sec]. This figure shows details of how curves were analyzed to estimate $t_{1/2}$. First wave corresponds to flushing of system volume with 5% CO_2. Arrow 0, beginning of washout; arrow 1, percent end-tidal P_{CO_2} (%PET_{CO_2}) (breath 1); arrow 2, % PET_{CO_2} that is one-half of breath 1. If the %CO_2 equal to one-half the %PET_{CO_2} of breath 1 occurred between two expirations, then $t_{1/2}$ was calculated by interpolation. Break consists of 40 sec; otherwise, time scale is as indicated by bar. (From Ref. 138.)

Items of bedding associated with prone SIDS and causing face-down rebreathing differ from standard firm bedding in their propensity to limit CO_2 dispersal (i.e., $t_{1/2}$) significantly longer. They also share other physical properties. They are of low resistance to airflow and thus are less likely to elicit an arousal due to resistive load. The items are also softer than standard hospital infant beds that have not been linked to face-down SIDS (81,89).

Finally, as pointed out above, bedding causing thermal stress when it covers the face and head is also likely to cause much rebreathing. It is plausible that the increases in CO_2 production and O_2 demand by the infant during thermal stress will be more problematic when an infant's airway is unavailable for either heat dissipation or optimal gas exchange.

D. Remaining Questions for Study About Rebreathing as a Mechanism for Sudden Infant Death

Capnometry has been used to demonstrate that rebreathing of CO_2 would occur before death with airways covered, particularly for infants in the prone position (82,83,134). However, much more remains to be understood about the details of deaths occurring in microenvironments causing rebreathing. Studies using prone, face-down or supine, head-covered models have not documented the degree of O_2 depletion of inspired air during rebreathing in bedding. This information is important because small closed environments or those with relatively small effective volumes compared to an infant's $\dot{V}_E$ would pose a much greater threat to the infant's reserve of oxygen than to its greater ability to compensate for respiratory acidosis. In this regard, it is also unclear whether certain bedding constituents—e.g., wool or polystyrene—could selectively trap CO_2 near an infant's external airway. Bedding that selectively traps or excludes O_2 or CO_2 would thus be more or less likely to cause hypoxemic or hypercapneic respiratory failure.

Lethal rebreathing has not been demonstrated using experimental animals in a face-up, head-covered model. Galland et al. (141) showed that covering the snouts and mouths of piglets with many layers of wool blankets and a comforter caused lethal hyperthermia but only modest increases in the percentage of inspired CO_2 (to 1.6%). Physiological reconstructions are needed of supine, face-covered deaths based on precise death-scene investigations.

Finally, it is not known whether one must postulate a deficit in arousal from sleep in infants dying while rebreathing. As pointed out by Lijowska et al. (135), infants may arouse to protect their airway, but their behavioral repertoire may not gain them access to fresh air. In general, more information is needed on the rate of success with which a sleeping and awakening infant deals with the rebreathing stressors within its sleep microenvironment (139).

VIII. Summary and Conclusions

Two scourges of the urban environment in the United States with known toxicity to infants—airborne lead and crack cocaine—should be reevaluated as possible contributing factors in sudden infant death. Over 20 years ago, Erickson et al., for example, showed that airborne lead accumulates in the tissues of SIDS victims more than it does in controls. Whether this is true since the introduction of lead-free gasoline may be of importance in understanding environmental factors in deaths occurring when all infants sleep on their backs. Levels of other air pollutants—including SO_2, NO_2, and hydrocarbons—have been linked to SIDS in convincing work that is also 20 years old. For similar reasons, these findings should be made current.

Two other environmental factors have been considered in detail because they might explain the critical association between prone sleep and sudden death. The role of thermal stress from bedding and heating is strongly supported by epidemiological data from England, New Zealand, and Australia. Prone infants are at even more risk if they use heavy bedding or sleep in a heated room. However, the relevance of these studies to North American infants, whose bedrooms are comfortable at night, is unclear. How thermal stress without resultant hyperthermia can cause death is also unclear. The role of rebreathing of exhaled gases is supported by reports of case series showing that infants often die suddenly and unexpectedly with nose and mouth covered by bedding. This scenario becomes more likely when infants are prone and on soft bedding that limits CO_2 dispersal (89). Animal studies show that rebreathing can be lethal to small mammals, but the specific lethal abnormality in gas exchange in each environment is unclear.

Recent research has added much to our understanding of the environmental components of the triple risk model for SIDS.

Acknowledgment

Supported by the National SIDS Alliance.

References

1. Panigraphy A, Filiano JJ, Sleeper LA, Mandell F, Valdes-Dapena M, Krous HF, Rava LA, White WF, Kinney HC. Decreased kainate receptor binding in the arcuate nucleus of the sudden infant death syndrome. J Neuropathol Exp Neurol 1997; 56:1253–1261.
2. Filiano JJ, Kinney HC. Perspective on neuropathologic findings in victims of the sudden infant death syndrome: the triple-risk model. Colloquium on Control of Breathing during Development and Apnea in the Newborn and in SIDS. Nancy, France: Université de Nancy, September 1, 1992.
3. Perrot LJ. Amitriptyline overdose versus sudden infant death syndrome in a two month-old white female. J Forensic Sci 1988; 33:272–275.
4. Smialek JE, Monforte JR. Toxicology and sudden infant death. J Forensic Sci 1978; 22: 757–762.
5. Merritt TA, Valdes-Sapena M. SIDS research update. Pediatr Ann 1984; 13:193–207.
6. Smialek JE, Smialek PZ, Spitz WU. Accidental bed deaths in infants due to unsafe sleeping conditions. Clin Pediatr 1977; 16:1031–1036.
7. Gilbert-Barness E, Hegstrand L, Chandra S, Emery JL, Barness LA, Franciosi R, Huntington R. Hazards of mattresses, beds, and bedding in deaths of infants. Am J Forensic Med Pathol 1991; 12:27–32.
8. Mitchell EA, Ford RPK, Stewart AW, Taylor BJ, Becroft DMO, Thompson JMD, Scragg R, Hassall IB, Barry DMJ, Allen EM, Roberts AP. Smoking and the sudden infant death syndrome. Pediatrics 1993; 91:893–896.
9. Blair PS, Fleming PJ, Bensley D, Smith I, Bacon C, Taylor E, Berry J, Golding J, Tripp J. Smoking and the sudden infant death syndrome: results from the confidential inquiry into stillbirths and deaths in infancy. BMJ 1996; 313:195–198.
10. Kinney HC, O'Donnell TJ, Kriger P, White WF. Early developmental changes in [3H] nicotine binding in the human brainstem. Neuroscience 1993; 55:1127–1138.
11. Milerad J, Larsson H, Lin J, Sundell HW. Nicotine attenuates the ventilatory response to hypoxia in the developing lamb. Pediatr Res 1995; 37:652–660.
12. Willinger M, James LS, Catz C. Defining the sudden infant death syndrome. Pediatr Pathol 1991; 11:677–684.
13. Kemp JS, Thach BT. Sudden death in infants sleeping on polystyrene-filled cushions. N Engl J Med 1991; 423:1858–1864.
14. Kemp JS, Kowalski RM, Burch PM, Graham MA, Thach BT. Unintentional suffocation by rebreathing: a death scene and physiological investigation of a possible cause of sudden infant death. J Pediatr 1993; 122:874–880.
15. Ponsonby A-L, Dwyer T, Gibbons LE, Cochrane JA, Jones ME, McCall MJ. Thermal environment and sudden infant death syndrome: case-control study. BMJ 1992; 304: 277–282.
16. Wilson CA, Taylor BJ, Laing RM, Mitchell EA. Clothing and bedding and its relevance to sudden infant death syndrome: further results from the New Zealand Cot Death Study. J Paediatr Child Health 1994; 30:506–512.
17. Emery JL. Sudden and unexpected deaths in infancy. Bedson Symposium, 1972.

18. Graham MA, Hutchins GM. Forensic pathology: sudden infant death syndrome. Clin Lab Med 1998; 18:252–254.
19. Guntheroth WG. Crib Death: The Sudden Infant Death Syndrome. 3rd ed. Armonk, NY: Futura, 1995: 78–80.
20. Bergman AB, Ray CG, Pomeroy MA, Wahl PW, Beckwith JB. Studies of the sudden infant death syndrome in King County, Washington: III. Epidemiology. Pediatrics 1972; 49:860–870.
21. Hoppenbrouwers T, Calub M, Arakawa K, Hodgman J. Seasonal relationship of sudden infant death syndrome and environmental pollutants. Am J Epidemiol 1981; 113: 623–635.
22. Knoebel HH, Chen C-J, Liang Y-K. Sudden infant death syndrome in relation to weather and optimetrically measured air pollution in Taiwan. Pediatrics 1995; 96:1106–1110.
23. Carpenter RG, Gardner A. Environmental findings and sudden infant death syndrome. Lung 1990; (suppl):358–367.
24. Valdes-Dapena M, Felipe RP. Immunofluorescent studies in crib deaths: absence of evidence of hypersensitivity to cow's milk. Am J Clin Pathol 1971; 56:412–415.
25. Bass M, Kravath RE, Glass L. Death-scene investigation in sudden infant death. N Engl J Med 1986; 315:100–105.
26. Sturner WQ. Some perspectives in cot death. J Forensic Med 1971; 18:96–107.
27. Smialek JE, Lambros Z. Investigation of sudden infant deaths. Pediatrician 1988; 15: 191–197.
28. Wigglesworth JS, Keeling JW, Rushron DI, Berry PJ. Pathological investigations in cases of sudden infant death. J Clin Pathol 1987; 40:1481–1483.
29. Platt MS. The differential diagnosis of child abuse: sudden infant death syndrome. In: Spitz WU, ed. Medicolegal Investigation of Death. Springfield, IL: Charles C Thomas, 1989:724–725.
30. Sturner WQ. Sudden, unexpected infant death. In: Tedeschi CG, Eckert WG, Tedeschi LG, eds. Forensic Medicine. Philadelphia: Saunders, 1977: 1015–1032.
31. Byard RW, Cohle SD. Sudden Death in Infancy, Childhood, and Adolescence. Cambridge, England: Cambridge University Press, 1993:36–39.
32. Jones AM, Weston JT. The examination of the sudden infant death syndrome infant: investigative and autopsy protocols. J Forensic Sci 1976; 21:833–841.
33. Taylor EM, Emery JL. Two-year study of the causes of postperinatal deaths classified in terms of preventability. Arch Dis Child 1982; 57:668–673.
34. Nelson EAS, Williams SM, Taylor BJ, Morris B, Ford RPK. Postneonatal mortality in south New Zealand: necropsy data review. Paediatr Perinatol Epidemiol 1989; 3: 375–385.
35. Valdes-Dapena M. The sudden infant death syndrome: pathologic findings. Clin Perinatol 1992; 19:701–715.
36. Iyasu S, Hanzlick R, Rowly D, Willinger M. Proceedings of Workshop on Guidelines for Scene Investigation of Sudden Unexplained Infant Deaths. J Forensic Sci 1994; 39: 1126–1136.
37. Erickson MM, Poklis A, Gantner GE, Dickinson AW, Hillman LS. Tissue mineral levels in victims of sudden infant death syndrome: I. Toxic metals—lead and cadmium. Pediatr Res 1983; 17:779–783.
38. Kleeman WJ, Weller J-P, Wolf M, Troger HD, Bluthgen A, Heeschen W. Heavy metals, chlorinated pesticides and polychlorinated biphenyls in sudden infant death syndrome. Int J Leg Med 1991; 104:71–75.

39. Mirchadani HG, Mirchandani IH, Hellman F, English-Rider R, Rosen S, Laposata E. Passive inhalation of free-base cocaine ("crack") smoke by infants. Arch Pathol Lab Med 1991; 115:494–498.
40. Mouhaffel AH, Madu EC, Satmary WA, Fraker TD. Cardiovascular complications of cocaine. Chest 1995; 107:1426–1434.
41. Bulbul ZR, Rosenthal DN, Kleinman CS. Myocardial infarction in the perinatal period secondary to maternal cocaine abuse. Arch Pediatr Adolesc Med 1994; 148:1092–1096.
42. Silvestri JM, Long JM, Weese-Mayer DE. Effect of prenatal cocaine on respiration, heart rate, and sudden infant death syndrome. Pediatr Pulmonol 1991; 11:328–334.
43. Davidson-Ward SL, Bautista DB, Woo MS, Chang M, Schuetz S, Wachsman L, Sehgal S, Bean X. Responses to hypoxia and hypercapnia in infants of substance-abusing mothers. J Pediatr 1992; 121:704–709.
44. Weese-Mayer DE, Barkov GA. Effect of cocaine in early gestation: physiological responses to hypoxia in newborn rabbits. Am Rev Respir Dis 1993; 148:589–596.
45. Davies DP. Cot death in Hong Kong: a rare problem? Lancet 1985; 1346–1348.
46. Nelson EAS, Taylor BJ, Mackay SC. Child care practices and the sudden infant death syndrome. Aust Paediatr J 1989; 25:202–204.
47. Mitchell EA, Scragg R, Stewart AW, Becroft DMO, Taylor BJ, Hassall IB, Barry DMJ, Allen EM, Roberts AP. Results from the first year of the New Zealand cot death study. NZ Med J 1991; 104:71–76.
48. Mitchell EA, Ford RPK, Taylor BJ, Stewart AW, Becroft DMO, Scragg R, Barry DMJ, Allen EM, Roberts AP, Hassall IB. Further evidence supporting a causal relationship between prone sleeping position and SIDS. J Paediatr Child Health 1992; 28(suppl 1): S9–S12.
49. Wigfield RE, Fleming PJ, Berry PJ, Rudd PT, Golding J. Can the fall in Avon's sudden infant death rate be explained by changes in sleeping position? BMJ 1992; 304:281–283.
50. Dwyer T, Ponsonby A-L, Newman NM, Gibbons LE. Prospective cohort study of prone sleeping position and sudden infant death syndrome. Lancet 1991; 337:1244–1247.
51. Dwyer T, Ponsonby A-L, Blizzard L, Newman NM, Cochrane JA. The contribution of changes in the prevalence of prone sleeping position to the decline of sudden infant death syndrome in Tasmania. JAMA 1995; 273:783–789.
52. Taylor JA, Krieger JW, Reay DT, Davis RL, Harruff R, Cheney LK. Prone sleep position and the sudden infant death syndrome in King County, Washington: a case-control study. J Pediatr 1996; 128:626–630.
53. Willinger M. Sleep position and sudden infant death syndrome. JAMA 1995; 273: 818–819.
54. Brooke H, Gibson A, Tappin D, Brown H. Case-control study of sudden infant death syndrome in Scotland, 1992–5. BMJ 1997; 314:1516–1520.
55. Oyen N, Markestad T, Skjaerven R, Irgens LM, Helweg- Larsen K, Alm B, Norvenius G, Wennergren G. Combined effects of sleeping position and prenatal risk factors in sudden infant death syndrome: the Nordic epidemiological SIDS study. Pediatrics 1997; 100:613–621.
56. Skadberg BT, Morild I, Markestad T. Abandoning prone sleeping: effect on risk of sudden infant death syndrome. J Pediatr 1998; 132:340–343.
57. Hill AB. The environment and disease: association or causation? Proc R Soc Med 1965; 58:295–300.

58. Mitchell EA. Cot death: should the prone sleeping position be discouraged? J Paediatr Child Health 1991; 27:319–321.
59. Tonkin S. Sudden infant death syndrome: hypothesis of a causation. Pediatrics 1975; 55:650–651.
60. Swift PGF, Emery JL. Clinical observations on response to nasal occlusion in infancy. Arch Dis Child 1973; 48:947–951.
61. Cross KW, Lewis SR. Upper respiratory obstruction and cot death. Arch Dis Child 1971; 46:211–213.
62. Thach BT, Davies AM, Koenig JS. Pathophysiology of sudden upper airway obstruction in sleeping infants and its relevance for SIDS. Ann NY Acad Sci 1988 533:314–328.
63. Kahn A, Groswasser J, Sottiaux M, Rebuffat E, Franco P, Dramaix M. Prone or supine body position and sleep characteristics in infants. Pediatrics 1993; 91:1112–1115.
64. Franco P, Pardou A, Hassid S, Lurquin P, Groswasser J, Kahn A. Auditory arousal thresholds are higher when infants sleep in the prone position. J Pediatr 1998; 132:240–243.
65. Stothers JK, Warner RM. Thermal balance and sleep state in the newborn. Early Hum Dev 1984; 9:313–322.
66. Nelson EAS, Taylor BJ, Weatherall IL. Sleeping position and infant bedding may predispose to hyperthermia and the sudden infant death syndrome. Lancet 1989; 1:199–200.
67. Fleming PJ, Gilbert R, Azaz Y, Berry PJ, Rudd PT, Stewart A, Hall E. Interaction between bedding and sleep position in the sudden infant death syndrome: a population-based case-control study. BMJ 1990; 301:85–89.
68. Wailoo MP, Petersen SA, Whittaker H, Goodenough P. The thermal environment in which 3–4 month old infants sleep at home. Arch Dis Child 1989; 64:600–604.
69. Williams SM, Taylor BJ, Mitchell EA. Sudden infant death syndrome: insulation from bedding and clothing and its effect modifiers. Int J Epidemiol 1996; 25:366–375.
70. Ponsonby A-L, Dwyer T, Gibbons LE, Cochrane JA, Wang Y-G. Factors potentiating the risk of sudden infant death syndrome associated with the prone position. N Engl J Med 1993; 329:377–382.
71. Kemp JS, Livne M, White DK, Arfken CL. Softness and potential to cause rebreathing: differences in bedding used by infants at high risk and low risk for sudden infant death syndrome. J Pediatr 1998; 132:234–239.
72. Kemp JS, White DK. Shared beds increase potential for rebreathing exhaled air in sleep microenvironments used by infants at high risk for SIDS. Pediatr 1998; 43:Abstract 1956.
73. Stanton AN. Overheating and cot death. Lancet 1984; ii:1199–1201.
74. Sunderland R, Emery JL. Febrile convulsions and cot death. Lancet 1981; ii:176–178.
75. Kahn A, Blum D. Phenothiazines and sudden infant death syndrome. Pediatrics 1982; 70:75–78.
76. Beal SM, Blundell H. Sudden infant death syndrome related to position in the cot. Med J Aust 1978; 2:217–218.
77. Fleming PJ, Blair PS, Bacon C, Bensley D, Smith I, Taylor E, Berry J, Golding J, Tripp J. Environment of infants during sleep and risk of the sudden infant death syndrome: results of the 1993–5 case-control study for confidential inquiry into stillbirths and deaths in infancy. BMJ 1996; 313:191–195.
78. Gilbert R, Rudd P, Berry PJ, Fleming PJ, Hall E, White DG, Oreffo VOC, James P, Evans JA. Combined effect of infection and heavy wrapping on the risk of sudden unexpected infant death. Arch Dis Child 1992; 67:171–177.

79. Ponsonby A-L, Dwyer T, Couper D, Cochrane J. Association between use of a quilt and sudden infant death syndrome: case-control study. BMJ 1998; 316:195–196.
80. Kemp JS, Thach BT. A sleep position-dependent mechanism for infant death on sheepskins. AJDC 1993; 147:642–646.
81. Kemp JS, Nelson VE, Thach BT. Physical properties of bedding that may increase risk of sudden infant death syndrome in prone-sleeping infants. Pediatr Res 1994; 36:7–11.
82. Bolton DPG, Taylor BJ, Campbell AJ, Galland BC, Cresswell CA. A potential danger for prone sleeping babies: rebreathing of expired gases when face down into soft bedding. Arch Dis Child 1993; 69:187–190.
83. Carleton JN, Donoghue AM, Porter WK. Mechanical model testing of rebreathing potential in infant bedding materials. Arch Dis Child 1998; 78:323–328.
84. Kemp JS. Rebreathing of exhaled gases: importance as a mechanism for the causal association between prone sleep and sudden infant death syndrome. Sleep 1996; 19: S263–S266.
85. Abramson H. Accidental mechanical suffocation in infants. J Pediatr 1944; 25:404–413.
86. Adelson L, Kinney ER. Sudden and unexpected death in infancy and childhood. Pediatrics 1956; 17:663–697.
87. Carpenter RG, Shaddick CW. Role of infection, suffocation, and bottle feeding in cot death: an analysis of some factors in the histories of 110 cases and their controls. Br J Prev Soc Med 1965; 19:1–7.
88. Taylor BJ. A review of epidemiological studies of sudden infant death syndrome in southern New Zealand. J Paediatr Child Health 1991; 27:344–348.
89. Scheers NJ, Dayton CM, Kemp JS. Sudden infant death with external airways covered: case comparison study of 206 deaths in the United States. Arch Pediatr Adolesc Med 1998; 152:540–547.
90. Werne J, Garrow I. Sudden deaths in infants allegedly due to mechanical suffocation. Am J Pub Health 1947; 37:675–687.
91. Wooley PV. Mechanical suffocation during infancy: a comment on its relation to the total problem of sudden death. J Pediatr 1945; 26:572–575.
92. Valdes-Dapena MA. Sudden and unexpected death in infancy: a review of the world literature 1954–1966. Pediatrics 1967; 39:123–138.
93. Richardson BA. Sudden infant death syndrome: a possible primary cause. J Forensic Sci Soc 1994; 34:199–204.
94. Fleming PJ, Cooke M, Chantler SM, Golding J. Fire retardants, biocides, plasticisers, and sudden infant deaths. BMJ 1994; 309:1594–1595.
95. Smialek JE. Simultaneous sudden infant death syndrome in twins. Pediatrics 1986; 77:816–821.
96. Beal S. Sudden infant death syndrome in twins. Pediatrics 1989; 84:1038–1044.
97. Simon HB. Hyperthermia. N Engl J Med 1993; 329:483–487.
98. Glotzbach SF, Heller HC. Temperature regulation. In: Kryger MR, Roth T, Dement WC, eds. Principles and Practice of Sleep Medicine. London: W.B. Saunders, 1994: 260–275.
99. Wadlington WB, Tucker AL, Fly F, Greene HL. Heat stroke in infancy. Am J Dis Child 1976; 130:1250–1251.
100. Bacon C, Scott D, Jones P. Heatstroke in well-wrapped infants. Lancet 1979; I:422–425.
101. Nelson EAS, Taylor BJ. Hemorrhagic shock encephalopathy syndrome. NZ Med J 1988; 10:167–169.

102. Bacon CJ. Overheating in infancy. Arch Dis Child 1983; 58:673–674.
103. Hutchins GM. Body temperature is elevated in the early postmortem period. Hum Pathol 1985; 16:560–561.
104. Wailoo MP, Petersen SA, Whittaker H, Goodenough P. Sleeping body temperatures in 3–4 month old infants. Arch Dis Child 1989; 64:596–599.
105. Tufnell CS, Petersen SA, Wailoo MP. Factors affecting rectal temperatures in infancy. Arch Dis Child 1995; 73:443–446.
106. Petersen SA, Anderson ES, Lodemore M, Rawson D, Wailoo MP. Sleeping position and rectal temperature. Arch Dis Child 1991; 66:976–979.
107. Wigfield RE, Fleming PJ, Azaz YEZ, Howell TE, Jacobs DE, Nadin PS, McCabe R, Stewart AJ. How much wrapping do babies need at night? Arch Dis Child 1993; 69:181–186.
108. Fleming PJ, Levine MR, Azaz Y, Wigfield R, Stewart AJ. Interactions between thermoregulation and the control of respiration in infants: possible relationship to sudden infant death. Acta Paediatr Scand 1993; 389:Suppl 57–59.
109. McGinty D, Szymusiak R. Neurobiology of sleep. In: Saunders NA, Sullivan CE, eds. Sleep and Breathing, 2nd ed. New York: Marcel Dekker 1993: 1–26.
110. Kreuger JM, Takahashi S. Thermoregulation and sleep: closely linked but separable. Ann NY Acad Sci 1997; 813:281–286.
111. Stothers JK. Head insulation and heat loss in the newborn. Arch Dis Child 1981; 56:530–534.
112. Day R. Regulation of body temperature during sleep. Am J Dis Child 1941; 61:734–746.
113. Horne JA, Reid AJ. Night-time sleep EEG changes following body heating in a warm bath. Electroencephalogr Clin Neurophysiol 1985; 60:154–157.
114. Perlstein PH, Edwards NK, Sutherland JM. Apnea in premature infants and incubator-air-temperature changes. N Engl J Med 1970; 282:461–466.
115. Daily WJR, Klaus M, Meyer HBP. Apnea in premature infants: monitoring, incidence, heart rate changes, and an effect of environmental temperature. Pediatrics 1969; 43:510–518.
116. Steinschneider A. Prolonged apnea and the sudden infant death syndrome: clinical and laboratory observations. Pediatrics 1972; 50:646–654.
117. Firstman R, Talan J. The Death of Innocents. New York: Bantam Books, 1997.
118. Gozal D, Colin AA, Daskalovic YI, Jaffe M. Environmental overheating as a cause of transient respiratory chemoreceptor dysfunction in an infant. Pediatrics 1988; 82:738–740.
119. Levine M, Fleming PJ, Azaz Y, McCabe R. Changes in breathing pattern accompanying environmental cooling in human infants (abstr). Early Hum Dev 1989; 19:216.
120. Fewell JE, Williams BJ, Szabo JS, Taylor BJ. Influence of repeated upper airway obstruction on the arousal and cardiopulmonary response to upper airway obstruction in lambs. Pediatr Res 1988; 23:191–195.
121. McCulloch K, Brouillette RT, Guzzetta AJ, Hunt CE. Arousal responses in near-miss sudden infant death syndrome and in normal infants. J Pediatr 1982; 101:911–917.
122. Van der Hal AL, Rodriguez AM, Sargent CW, Platzker ACG, Keens TG. Hypoxic and hypercapneic arousal responses and prediction of subsequent apnea in apnea of infancy. Pediatrics 1985; 75:848–854.
123. Schluter PJ, Ford RPK, Mitchell EA, Taylor BJ. Housing and sudden infant death syndrome. NZ Med J 1997; 110:243–246.

124. Mitchell EA, Stewart AW, Scragg R, Ford RPK, Taylor BJ, Becroft DMO, Thompson JMD, Hassall IB, Barry DMJ, Allen EM, Roberts AP. Ethnic differences in mortality from sudden infant death syndrome in New Zealand. BMJ 1993; 306:13–16.
125. Mitchell EA, Scragg R. Observations on ethnic differences in SIDS mortality in New Zealand. Early Hum Dev 1994; 38:151–157.
126. Buve A, Rodrigues LC. Sudden infant death syndrome: does winter affect poor and rich babies equally? J Epidemiol Community Health 1992; 46:485–488.
127. Mitchell EA, Brunt JM, Everard C. Reduction in mortality from sudden infant death syndrome in New Zealand: 1986–92. Arch Dis Child 1994; 70:291–294.
128. Archibald HC. Sudden unexplained death in childhood—can it be prevented? Arch Pediatr 1942; 59:57–61.
129. Nunn JF. Applied Respiratory Physiology, 3rd ed. Stoneham, MA: Butterworths, 1987: 166.
130. Bolton DPG, Cross KW, McKettrick AC. Are babies in carry cots at risk from CO_2 accumulation? BMJ 1972; iii:80–81.
131. Ryan EL. Distribution of expired air in carry cots: a possible explanation for some sudden infant deaths. Austr Phys Eng Sci Med 1991; 14:112–118.
132. Bolton DPG. The prevalence of immature respiratory control in a neonatal population. NZ Med J 1990; 103:89–92.
133. Chiodini BA, Thach BT. Impaired ventilation in infants sleeping facedown: potential significance for sudden infant death syndrome. J Pediatr 1993; 123:686–692.
134. Skadberg BT, Markestad T. Consequences of getting head covered during sleep in infancy. Pediatrics 1997; 100 (online).
135. Lijowska AS, Reed NW, Mertins-Chiodini BA, Thach BT. Sequential arousal and airway-defense behavior of infants in asphyxial sleep environments. J Appl Physiol 1997; 83:219–228.
136. Mograss MA, Ducharme FM, Brouillette RT. Movement/arousals: description, classification, and relationship to sleep apnea in children. Am J Respir Crit Care Med 1994; 150:1690–1696.
137. Schmid WR. Potential rebreathing danger of presumed "safe" sleep surfaces and a new approach to design (abstr). Pediatr Pulmonol 1996; 425.
138. Kemp JS, Thach BT. Quantifying the potential of infant bedding to limit CO_2 dispersal and factors affecting rebreathing in bedding. J Appl Physiol 1995; 78:740–745.
139. Waters KA, Gonzalez A, Jean C, Morielli A, Brouillette RT. Face-straight-down and face-near-straight-down in healthy, prone-sleeping infants. J Pediatr 1996; 128:616–625.
140. Kemp JS. Sudden infant death syndrome: the role of bedding revisited. J Pediatr 1996; 129:946–947.
141. Galland BC, Peebles CM, Bolton DPG, Taylor BJ. The micro-environment of the sleeping newborn piglet covered by bedclothes: gas exchange and temperature. J Paediatr Child Health 1994; 30:144–150.

23

Breathing and Sleep in Preterm Infants

HENRIQUE RIGATTO

University of Manitoba
Winnipeg, Manitoba, Canada

I. Introduction

Breathing and its modulation by sleep have unique characteristics in preterm infants. Our knowledge in this area is recent, having been developed over the past 40 years. There are two reasons for this late emergence: First, preterm infants rarely survived prior to 1950. Only during the second part of the century did survival improve to a point where studies on breathing were feasible. We must not forget that the first rudimentary neonatal intensive care unit was established only as recently as 1964 (1). Second, only after midcentury did the technology become adequate to measure breathing and sleep in these infants.

Prematurity profoundly affects breathing, making it highly irregular, with frequent pauses or apneas. We must be aware, however, of major differences in methodology when comparing preterm and term infants and adults. First, preterm and term infants have always been studied during sleep, since it is not possible to study them during wakefulness. This is relevant because most studies in adult subjects have been performed during wakefulness. Second, babies are almost invariably studied supine, whereas adults are more frequently studied seated. Third, babies are usually studied with a nose piece because they are nose-breathers; adults are usually studied using a mouthpiece. These methodological differences have made the comparison of breathing in preterm infants with that in adult subjects difficult to interpret. There is currently a major need for studies to be done using similar methodology.

In this chapter, we examine some of the important characteristics of breathing during sleep in preterm infants. Much of the data quoted relate to our own contribution over the last 30 years. An effort has been made to give a comprehensive view of how the knowledge in this area has evolved. Considerations regarding the added effect of sleep on the anatomical and functional limitations of the respiratory system at this age is also presented. Finally, the clinical implications of the effects of sleep on breathing is discussed.

II. History

Prematurity is probably as old as the history of humanity. Newton, for example, is known to have been premature, weighing 1600 g (2). The midwife told his parents that he would not survive; luckily, she was wrong. Accurate assessment of breathing in preterm infants began at the turn of the century. Studies were sporadic for the first half of the twentieth century and dealt mostly with simple measurements, such as respiratory frequency and tidal volume (3–7). A more focused investigational effort began in the late forties and early fifties, led by two major groups, the first in Britain with Kenneth Cross (8–12) and Geoffrey Dawes (13) and the second in the United States with Clement Smith and his group at Harvard (14,15). Subsequently, many other centers became interested in neonatal breathing, among them Babies Hospital in New York (Stanley James and colleagues), John Hopkins University (Mary Ellen Avery and colleagues), Vanderbilt University (Mildred Stahlman and colleagues)and the Cardiovascular Research Institute in San Francisco (Bill Tooley, John Clements, and colleagues). The initial studies had the objective of characterizing neonatal breathing both in preterm and term infants according to measurements being made in adult subjects. These measurements were primarily related to pulmonary function, such as vital capacity and its components, pulmonary compliance, airway resistance, alveolar ventilation, oxygen consumption, and pulmonary diffusion (14,16–27). At the same time, other investigations related to control of breathing were begun. Responsiveness to different concentrations of oxygen and carbon dioxide were measured, and a more meticulous analysis of breathing pattern emerged (28–32). The impact of respiratory muscle performance and pulmonary reflexes on breathing was evaluated (10,33–35). At first, all observations were made without regard to sleep state, even though Magnussen in 1944 (36) and Büllow in 1963 (37) had already outlined some of the effects of sleep on breathing. In 1965, Aserinsky (38) first reported the association of periodic breathing and rapid eye movement (REM) sleep in neonates. Today there is a vast literature on the modulatory effect of sleep on breathing in preterm infants (39–44). Two schools in particular, those of Prechtl in Groeningen (41) and Dreyfus-Brisac in Paris (45,46), have made significant contributions to our knowledge of sleep, behavior, and their relationship to breathing. As a result, today most studies on the characteristics of preterm breathing are standardized for sleep state.

III. Classification of Sleep in Preterm Infants

In order to understand how sleep affects breathing, we must first define sleep states in the preterm infant. Sleep has traditionally been divided into quiet, REM, transitional, and indeterminate states. Quiet sleep is characterized by the absence of rapid eye movements coupled with tracé alternans (45–48). REM sleep is defined by the presence of rapid eye movements and continuous, irregular low voltage on the electroencephalogram (EEG). Transitional sleep represents short epochs lasting 1 to 3 min, which are usually observed during the transition from quiet to REM or vice versa. Indeterminate sleep is defined as that state which cannot be described by other definitions. Twenty-nine percent (29%) of sleep time in neonates is spent in quiet sleep, 33% in REM, 7% in transitional sleep, and 31% in indeterminate sleep (49). Although breathing activity has been studied in all these states, the majority of physiological studies have been done in quiet and REM sleep.

IV. Anatomic and Functional Limitations of the Respiratory System in Preterm Infants

The central nervous system is immature in preterm infants and this has a profound influence on breathing. Purpura and Shade (50) have shown that the most significant feature of central nervous system immaturity is the lack of dendritic arborization and axodendritic synaptic connections. It is likely, therefore, that the synaptic excitatory drive exerted on respiratory neurons in both brainstem and spinal cord is much weaker in preterm infants than in either term infants or adult subjects. In addition, axosomatic synaptic connections tend to be inhibitory in nature rather than excitatory, and this induces a powerful suppression of neuronal cell activity (51). In preterm infants, this inhibition is enhanced because of the small size of the synaptic connections and rare arborizations. Because of these neuroanatomical constraints, it is difficult for the preterm infant to sustain a strong respiratory drive over time. REM sleep aggravates the situation, as it induces a strong inhibitory influence on the spinal motor neurons, including the respiratory neurons. This state of affairs makes breathing for preterm infants more difficult, particularly because these infants spend a larger percentage of their time in the REM sleep state.

Sleep state also influences the performance of the various components of the chest wall, which in the preterm infant are still unprepared for adequate respiratory activity.

The diaphragm in preterm infants has a relatively small apposition zone; that is, the zone that is in contact with the internal surface of the lower chest wall (52). Because of this, the ability to expand the lower rib cage during inspiration is limited. The compliant chest wall of these infants prevents the expanding influences of the lower rib cage on the upper rib cage unless there is intercostal muscle recruitment. During REM sleep, the intercostal muscles are inactivated, exaggerating the tendency of the upper rib cage to collapse during normal inspiration.

The intercostal muscles are also important for the normal respiratory activity (53). The external intercostal muscles raise the rib cage during inspiration and the internal intercostals lower it during expiration. In the newborn, the ribs are near horizontal, whereas in the adult they are angled caudally. This means that the increase in thoracic cross-sectional area induced by lifting the rib cage (the "bucket handle" mechanism) is less in the preterm infant than in the adult (54). The resulting mechanical disadvantage limits the contribution of the rib cage to tidal volume, leading to the common observation that newborns are "abdominal breathers" (55,56). This type of breathing appears to change at about 2 years of age. As alluded to above, the limited contribution of the external intercostal muscles to tidal volume and chest wall stability is lost during REM sleep (55–58).

The reduced outward recoil of the chest wall (59), which in the preterm infant is close to zero, is by far the most important feature of the immature respiratory apparatus (60). This is mainly due to lack of mineralization of the bones of the chest wall. Gehardt and Bancalari (61) found the chest wall compliance in the preterm infant at 32 weeks of gestation to be 6.4 $mL \cdot cmH_2O^{-1} \cdot kg^{-1}$, as opposed to 4.2 $mL \cdot cmH_2O^{-1} \cdot kg^{-1}$ in the term infant. Because the inward recoil of the lung is just slightly less than that in adult subjects, the functional residual capacity of small infants is only 10% of vital capacity. This is quite near the closing volume, resulting in significant atelectasis (62,63). On top of all these anatomic limitations, inactivation of intercostal muscles during REM sleep induces a 30% decrease in lung volume (57).

The contractile properties of immature respiratory muscles are also affected in preterm infants. Maxwell et al. (64) measured latent period, time-to-peak isometric tension, one-half relaxation time, and fatigue index (percent of maximal tension after a series of tetanic stimuli) in diaphragm muscle strips from both premature and adult baboons. Compared to the adult diaphragm, the latent period, time-to-peak isometric tension, and relaxation time were all longer in the premature muscle. These findings are consistent with the paucity of sarcoplasmic reticulum observed in the fetal diaphragm (64). The relevant clinical correlate of the physiological and histological observations is diaphragmatic fatigue (decreased tension generated by the muscle when at constant level of neuronal activation), which is not uncommonly observed in neonates, particularly in the preterm infant. Rib cage deformation increases diaphragmatic work, predisposing to fatigue (62). Muller and associates (34) demonstrated a shift in the electromyographic (EMG) power spectrum of the diaphragm during breathing with rib cage distortion in infants of 26 to 40 weeks gestational age. The shift was followed by either intercostal muscle recruitment or apnea (65), which suggest that changes in the power spectrum indicated diaphragmatic fatigue. Because chest distortion becomes more intense in REM sleep, fatigue is more likely to occur, and consequently the likelihood of apnea is increased. The highly unstable chest wall in association with diaphragmatic fatigue predisposes to apnea, although most apneas tend to be central. Knill and Bryan (66) have shown that rib cage deformation induced by airway occlusion or manual compression decreases inspiratory time and tidal volume in newborn infants. In exaggerated form, this reflex (the phrenic inhibitory reflex) may lead to apnea, although this has not been proven experimentally. The reflex is more prominent in REM than in quiet sleep.

The postinspiratory activity of the diaphragm is also affected by sleep state. This activity controls, in part, the duration of the expiratory time (67,68). In neonates, Reis et al. (42) observed that this activity was more pronounced in the lateral than crural part of the diaphragm, longer in quiet than in REM sleep, and more prolonged in preterm than in term infants (Fig. 1). The length and variability of this activity in preterm infants suggest that these infants use the postinspiratory diaphragmatic activity as a braking mechanism. The role of this mechanism in maintaining lung vol-

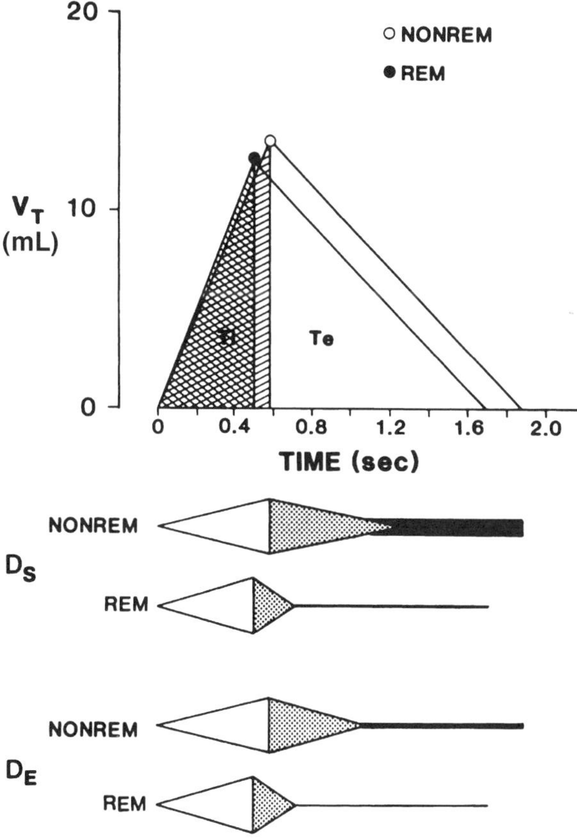

Figure 1 Diagrammatic changes in tidal volume (V_T), "timing" and diaphragmatic EMG in NREM (quiet) and REM (active) sleep. Note that total phasic activity diminishes from NREM to REM sleep. Also, in both sleep states, it is shorter in esophageal (D_E) than in surface EMG (D_S). Expiratory phasic activity as a proportion of total phasic activity decreases significantly from NREM to REM sleep. (From Ref. 42.)

ume by controlling expiratory time is much more important in preterms than in adults, because the former have a highly compliant chest wall.

Upper airway resistance is also affected by sleep. Harding et al. (69) have shown that the abductor muscle of the larynx (the posterior cricoarytenoid and cricothyroid) contract in phase with the diaphragm irrespective of sleep state. In contrast, the adductors (the thyroarytenoid, lateral cricoarytenoid, and intra-arytenoid) lose their phasic expiratory contraction during REM, resulting in an important increase in upper-airway resistance. Studies of the upper airway agree with clinical observations that obstructive apneas occur more frequently in REM than in quiet sleep (49,63). Finally, increased airway resistance, together with the chest wall factors described earlier, contribute to the decreased volumes observed in REM.

The work of breathing is also affected by sleep. REM sleep abolishes intercostal muscle activity and magnifies chest distortion. Luz et al. (70) found that the work of the diaphragm is 40% greater when the respiratory movements are out of phase, as occurs with distorted breathing in REM.

Pulmonary reflexes are also affected by sleep. Hering and Breuer (71) noted in 1868 that maintained distention of the lungs decreased the frequency of inspiratory effort in anesthetized animals. They showed this effect to be a reflex mediated by afferent vagal fibers (*Hering-Breuer reflex* or *inflation reflex*). The receptors for this reflex lie in the smooth muscle and epithelium of airways from trachea to bronchioles. The Hering-Breuer reflex is much more active in the newborn period than in adult life (10,72). Small increases in lung volume cause apnea. This response is so powerful in the newborn that many researchers have used this inflation to produce apnea and then study the mechanical properties of the respiratory system during the passive expiratory phase after apnea. The action of the stretch receptors is abolished during REM sleep. The irritant receptors use subepithelial chemoreceptors located in the trachea, bronchi, and bronchioles. They are designed to detect delicate deformations of the epithelial surface. The irritant receptors are poorly developed in preterm infants, and the reflexes mediated by them are also abolished during REM sleep (33). The airway mechanisms responsible for clearing, therefore, such as cough, are impaired during REM sleep.

The paradoxical reflex was described by Head in 1889 (73,74). He observed that in some rabbits, while warming the vagus, inflation of the lung produced a paradoxical effect—a further inspiration rather than inhibition of inspiration. This reflex is one of the earliest examples of physiology of positive feedback. Its function seems to be to provide a deep inspiration and further allow opening of the alveoli. The paradoxical reflex of Head is commonly observed in the neonate in the form of a sigh (75,76). Many attribute the high prevalence of sighs to the greater need for lung recruitment at this age (44). Sighs are more frequent in REM than in quiet sleep and also more frequent during periodic than regular breathing (75). Efforts to discover the mechanisms triggering sighs have been fruitless. Asphyxia is important but does not appear to be the only stimulus (75,76).

V. Breathing Pattern at Rest

The preterm infant breathes irregularly during sleep. Compared with the term infant and the adult subject, there is a great breath-to-breath variability as well as long stretches of periodic breathing, in which breathing intervals and apneic intervals alternate (77). We have found that the coefficients of variation in minute ventilation decrease with age (36%, 23%, and 10% in preterm, term, and adult subjects, respectively). The greater variation in the preterm infants was related to an increased variability in tidal volume (29% versus 13%) and respiratory frequency (27% versus 17%). The major determinant of frequency in preterm infants was expiratory time (71% variability); inspiratory time varied much less (18% variability). Inspiratory flow (V_T/T_i), a measure of central respiratory output, was lower in preterm infants. The "effective" respiratory timing (T_i/T_{tot}) was also lower in preterm infants, inspiratory time occupying only one-third of the duration of the breath in preterm infants versus half the duration of the breath in adult subjects.

Haldane has said that "the surprising fact is not that we breathe regularly but that we do not breathe periodically most of the time"; this observation applies more at this age than at any other (78). This irregularity of breathing is present also during brief episodes of wakefulness, such as those around feeding time, but sleep greatly enhances it. Quiet sleep becomes definable only after 32 weeks of gestation, and wakefulness occurs only 6 to 8 hr per day in the newborn (46).

VI. Periodic Breathing and Apnea

Periodic breathing is the alternation between breathing periods and 5- to 10-sec apnea. It is commonly seen in preterm infants, occurring in all three states (wakefulness, REM, and quiet sleep) but more commonly in REM sleep (9,79–85). It is a frequently stated misconception that in quiet sleep, the infant's breathing is regular. Prechtl (41) and ourselves, however, have clearly shown that periodic breathing is common in quiet sleep (48,83,86). The key difference is that periodic breathing in quiet sleep is regular—that is, the breathing and apneic intervals remain almost constant, whereas periodic breathing is very irregular in REM sleep. The best defined periodic breathing in preterm infants is observed in quiet sleep during tracé alternans (Fig. 2). Therefore, breathing pattern cannot be used in defining sleep states in preterm infants, in contrast to the conventional criteria applied to sleep definition in adults (87).

Adult subjects normally do not breathe periodically but can be made to do so in quiet sleep with induced hyperventilation (88,89). In infants during sleep, the continuous oscillation in sleep state, from REM to quiet and vice versa, may increase respiratory instability. This would agree with our previous findings of maximum incidence of periodic breathing when the rate of change in ventilation was maximal (82). This almost continuous change in resting ventilation during sleep would lead to what Douglas and Haldane (78) called "the hunting of the respiratory center." Sleep can

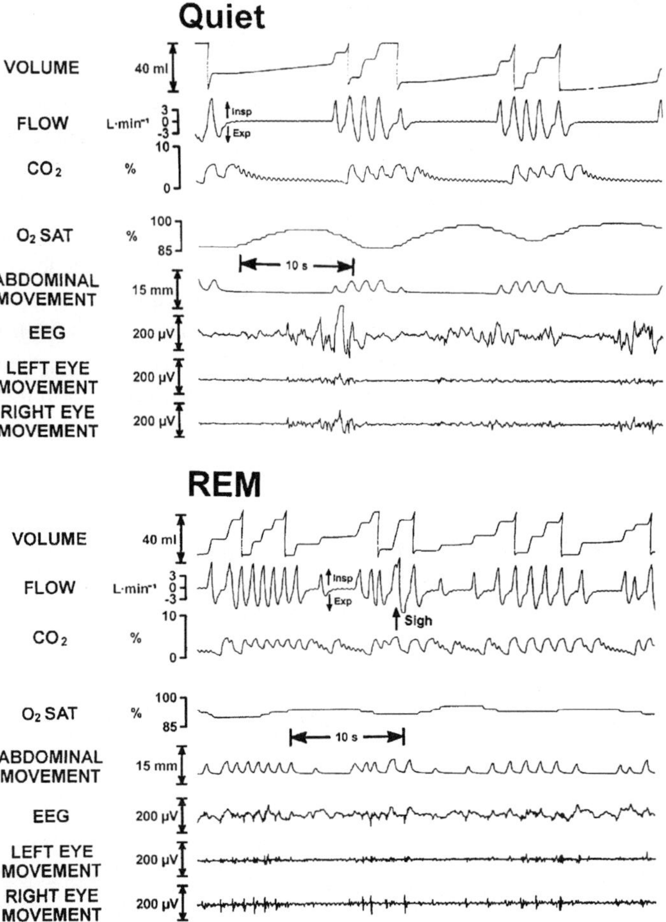

Figure 2 Periodic breathing in one preterm infant during quiet and REM sleep. Note that periodic breathing is more regular; that is, the apneas and breathing intervals are nearly constant, as opposed to the irregular periodicity observed in REM sleep. Also note the presence of sighs in REM sleep.

also contribute to periodic breathing and apnea through other mechanisms. For example, chest distortion during REM sleep may trigger a respiratory pause through the intercostal phrenic inhibitory reflex (66). The decrease in functional residual capacity during REM sleep decreases the buffering capacity for CO_2 and O_2 and predisposes to instability (57).

As with periodic breathing, apnea is common in preterm infants, yet we know little about its physiological mechanism. It is probably the most troublesome respiratory problem in preterm infants, now that hyaline membrane disease is largely preventable and treatable. There is mounting evidence that neonatal apnea is associated with brain damage.

Apnea means absence of respiratory movements. If apnea persists for five to 10 sec, alternating with normal breathing, the condition is defined as periodic breathing; when apnea is more prolonged, usually greater than 20 sec, the condition is known simply as apnea (81). Periodic breathing was thought to be a benign disorder because the respiratory pause is short, but our recent observations suggest that it can be associated with severe desaturation and may predispose to "apparent life-threatening events" (90,91). Apnea, however, has always been considered a serious condition and may lead to brain damage (92). Heart rate decreases substantially with apnea but only slightly or not at all with periodic breathing (93). With the advent of oxygen saturation monitors, it has become obvious that some apneas may reduce oxygenation dangerously without a major change in heart rate (94). This observation led to greater use of oxygen saturation monitors.

Approximately 40 to 50% of preterm infants breathe periodically during the neonatal period (3,95–98). The incidence increases dramatically with increased prematurity—90% at 28 to 29 weeks of gestation. Half of the infants with periodic breathing develop apnea at one time or another (93).

In early studies, apneas in preterm infants were considered a central event (81,82). Only in subsequent years did it become clear that obstruction of the airway was frequently present (99–103). Apneas have since been classified into central, obstructive, and mixed types. Central apneas are those without associated respiratory efforts; obstructive apneas are those with respiratory efforts; while mixed apneas are those with efforts for part of the apnea. By definition, therefore, airway obstruction occurs only in obstructive and mixed apneas but not in central apneas. Some investigators, however, by directly visualizing the upper airway or measuring the point in the tidal cycle where apnea starts, have suggested that the airway frequently closes during central apnea (99,104). They found that this closure occurs at the beginning of the apnea, raising the possibility that occlusion of the airway per se may be the cause for the apnea. Because respiratory efforts are absent, these apneas are central with "silent obstruction."

Extrapolating from the work of Milner et al. (99,104), we have devised a new method of classifying apneas based on the presence or absence of an amplified cardiac oscillation waveform observed in the respiratory flow tracing (105). Using this new method, we define *central apneas* as those with the oscillation present, *obstructive* as those with the oscillation absent, and *mixed* as those with the oscillation absent during part of the apnea (Fig. 3). The new method is more accurate than the traditional method because it relies on an airway signal that disappears if obstruction is present and not on respiratory efforts occurring elsewhere in the body. More importantly, because the amplitude of the oscillation signal is related to airway diameter, it is possible to time changes in airway diameter with precision.

This new method has provided us with some interesting observations not possible to obtain with the traditional method. First, it allowed us to determine the exact

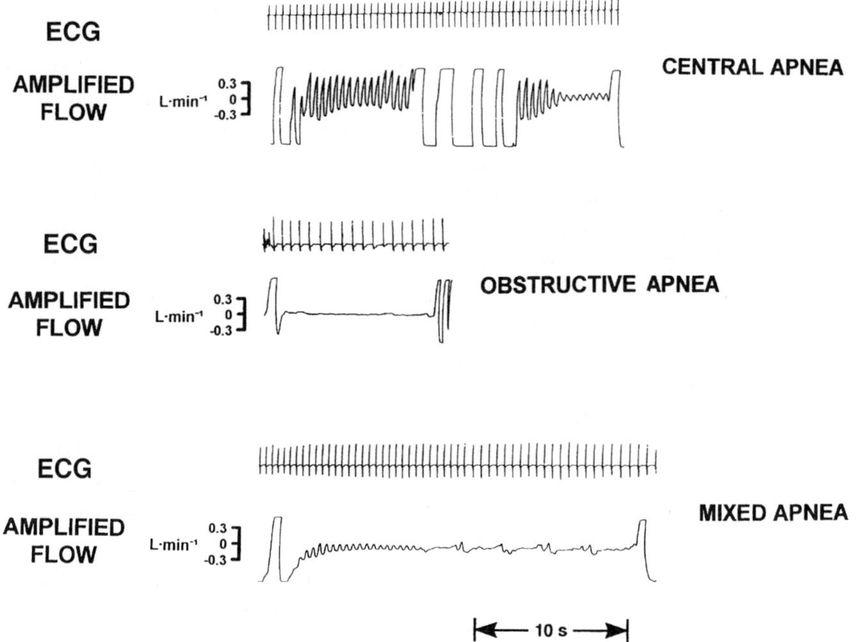

Figure 3 Classification of neonatal apneas according to the cardiac oscillation method. Central apneas are those in which the oscillation is present in the airflow tracing (top), obstructive apneas are those in which oscillations are absent (middle), and mixed apneas are those in which oscillations are present only during part of the apnea (bottom). (From Ref. 105.)

timing of airway closure during apnea. We found that 87% of mixed apneas are associated with an open airway initially, which then closes; in 13%, closure of the airway appears first. Second, based on the amplitude of the cardiac oscillation signal, we found that 13% of central apneas are associated with airway narrowing due to instability of the airway (102). This instability appears approximately 1 sec after the onset of apnea. This critical period is similar for apneas of different durations, and the maximal narrowing of the airway lumen always occurs a few seconds after the critical period, usually within 9 sec of the onset of apnea. Such knowledge has important implications in the treatment of apneas, since those with an obstructive component may respond better to continuous positive airway pressure (CPAP). Third, we found that in mixed apneas, airway obstruction can occur in the absence of respiratory efforts, suggesting that diaphragmatic contractions are not an essential initial event. In many cases diaphragmatic activity occurred after airway closure (106). Fourth, we found that purely obstructive apneas were almost nonexistent (107). In an analysis of more than 4000 apneas distributed according to length, we found that apneas became predominantly mixed when they were longer than 10 sec. Central apneas predominated, with durations of less than 10 sec. Purely obstructive apneas were extremely uncommon with apneas of any duration. These findings lend support to the idea that obstruction of the airway may be primarily a central phenomenon resulting in loss of tone of the upper airway musculature.

There has been controversy in the literature on whether periodic breathing and apnea are mechanistically different or whether long apneas are just a step further in the basic respiratory disturbance that induces the short apneas of periodic breathing. In a study carried out in our laboratory we were able to show 1) that a prolonged apnea almost never occurred in the absence of preceding short apneas and 2) that the risk of a prolonged apnea occurring increased significantly when the preceding period contained an increased number of apneic episodes, increased duration of the longest apneic interval, or increased duration of the apneic time (108). We believe that periodic breathing is a marker for apnea, since apneas never occur abruptly in infants breathing regularly but only in infants whose respiratory pattern is characterized by significant periodicity.

Apneas are more common, longer, and more frequently associated with profound bradycardia during REM sleep than during quiet sleep (39,84,85,95,109–112). This is true for apneas of all types: central, mixed, and obstructive. Both in infants with and without BPD the prevalence of obstructive apneas was found to be higher in REM than in quiet sleep (49) (Fig. 4). In our analysis of over 4500 apneas, the proportion of central apnea was greater in quiet sleep than in REM or indeterminate sleep (107) (Fig. 5). Although the reason for a higher prevalence of apnea during REM is not entirely clear, the inhibition of spinal motor neurons that occurs in this sleep state, acting on a background of poor dendritic arborization and axodendritic synaptic connections, may be very important (50,84). The more inhibitory axosomatic action combined with limited synaptic connections in the preterm infant constitute an ideal set-

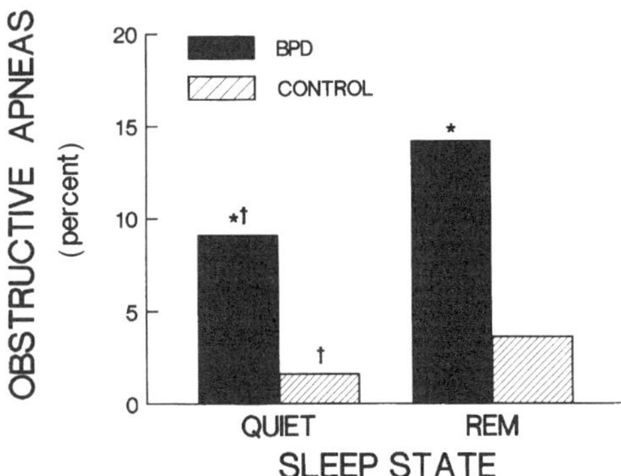

Figure 4 The incidence of obstructive apneas increased in REM sleep in preterm infants with and without BPD (control) († $p \leq .05$ between sleep states). The incidence of obstructive apneas was higher in the BPD group than in the control group in quiet and REM sleep, but this was of marginal significance (* $p \leq .05$ in relation to control). (From Ref. 49.)

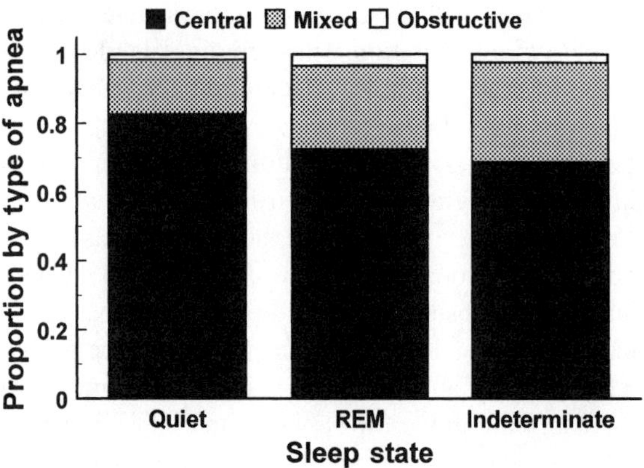

Figure 5 Proportion of central, obstructive, and mixed apneas in the various sleep states. Note that central apneas predominate in quiet sleep and its prevalence decreases toward indeterminate sleep. Concomitantly the prevalence of mixed apneas increased, in a mirror image. Purely obstructive apneas are extremely rare and their prevalence does not change in the various sleep states. (From Ref. 107.)

ting for the inhibitory action of REM sleep on the respiratory neurons in otherwise "healthy" preterm infants (84).

VII. Sighs

Sighs are frequent in preterm infants. On the respiratory tracing they look like a "breath on top of a breath." The increased frequency of sighs in these infants relates both to the highly compliant chest wall and also to sleep state. Because of the compliant chest wall, lung volume (functional residual capacity) is low. As mentioned earlier, during REM sleep, this volume decreases even further. Apneas, common in REM sleep, also contribute to a decrease in lung volume (31). In an attempt to maintain or recover lung volume, sighs are then generated. This situation is much more dramatic in the small preterm infant (< 1500 g) than in larger infants. In previous studies we found that the frequency of sighs was 0.23 ± 0.03 (preterm) and 0.13 ± 0.03 (term) sighs per minute during quiet sleep and 0.44 ± 0.05 (preterm) and 0.30 ± 0.05 (term) during REM sleep (75). The findings illustrate the approximate twofold increase in the prevalence of sighs in preterm versus term infants and in REM versus quiet sleep. During periodic breathing or apnea, the prevalence of sighs was equally distributed before and after apnea, indicating that their function is to recruit volume and not to trigger apnea, as suggested by some authors (113). In the studies we conducted using airway occlusion, in which the presence of a Head reflex was detected by deflections on an esophageal pressure catheter, sighs were more frequent on 15% inspired O_2 than on 21% O_2, suggesting that the chemical drive to breathe is also important to induce sighs. The overall findings suggest that, in addition to a decrease in lung volume during REM sleep, the relative hypoxemia of this sleep state plays a role in triggering sighs (75).

VIII. Ventilation

As with adult subjects, minute ventilation is higher during REM than during quiet sleep in preterm infants (42,47,49,83,114). This higher ventilation in REM sleep is due to a proportionally higher respiratory frequency with no significant change in tidal volume. Alveolar P_{CO_2} decreases also, indicating alveolar hyperventilation in REM sleep. Oxygen consumption is increased during REM. Arterial oxygen tension and O_2 saturation are lower in REM sleep (47,48). Baseline oscillations in arterial blood gases and O_2 saturation are also greater in REM sleep (83,115). These changes are likely consequences of the loss of intercostal muscle tone, upper-airway tone, and decreased functional residual capacity. As the lung partially collapses in REM sleep, ventilation is maintained via a faster respiratory rate. The decreased lung volume induces greater intrapulmonary shunt, with decreased oxygenation.

IX. The Response to CO_2

The newborn infant responds to inhaled CO_2 by increasing ventilation. Per unit body weight, the response of neonates is similar to that of adult subjects, about 0.035 $L{\bullet}min^{-1}{\bullet}kg^{-1}$ per torr increase in alveolar P_{CO_2} (81). The position of the CO_2 response curve in neonates (i.e., minute ventilation versus inspired CO_2 concentration) is shifted to the left of that of adult subjects by about 4 torr. This has been traditionally explained on the basis of a lower bicarbonate level in neonates (17,81).

Within the newborn population, preterm infants respond less markedly to CO_2 than term infants (25,116,117). It is not clear whether the decreased response to CO_2 in preterm infants is due to less responsive central chemoreceptors, poor performance of the respiratory "pump," or both. To elucidate this problem, we compared a group of preterm infants with a group of term infants using the rebreathing technique (48). Minute integrated diaphragmatic activity ($EMG_{di} \times f$), an index of central output, increased less in response to inhaled CO_2 in preterm than in term infants. However, indices of mechanical effectiveness, such as minute ventilation divided by mean inspiratory diaphragmatic activity ($\dot{V}_E/EMG_{di}/T_I$) were not different in preterm and term infants, suggesting that the respiratory pump effectively transduces the central output into negative intrapleural pressure or volume. It seems, therefore, that the decreased response is likely to be centrally mediated.

Using the steady-state method, we were unable to detect a difference in response to CO_2 in REM versus quiet sleep (47). Our observations using the rebreathing technique, however, suggested that during the "phasic" part of REM sleep, the respiratory system is less responsive to CO_2 (48) (Fig. 6). This is in accordance with studies in dogs in which the response to CO_2 was also less in REM than in quiet sleep (118,119). The explanation for the discrepancy between steady-state and rebreathing

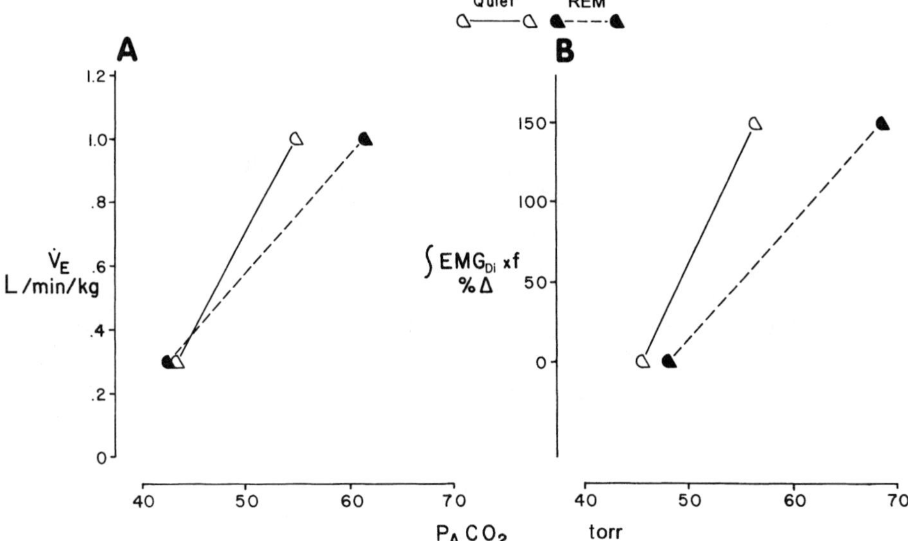

Figure 6 The ventilatory response to CO_2 rebreathing in neonates. Note that preterm infants show a decreased response to CO_2 in phasic REM as compared with quiet sleep. $\int EMG_{DI} \times f$ = integrated electromyography of the diaphragm times respiratory frequency. (From Ref. 48.)

is that it is difficult to do a steady-state response in REM sleep, since the epochs of "phasic" REM are too short. The response always includes some tonic REM, which obscures the differences.

Since the chest wall of preterm infants distorts with great ease, particularly during the phasic periods of REM sleep, it has been suggested that this distortion may contribute to the altered CO_2 response curve. However, we have found that if the response to CO_2 in quiet sleep is standardized by fixing the duration of distorted and nondistorted breaths, the response to CO_2 becomes indistinguishable in both states (70). These findings suggest that the decreased CO_2 response in REM as compared to quiet sleep is not due to the possible mechanical disadvantage of chest distortion during REM sleep. It is more likely that the combination of a high and variable respiratory frequency and small tidal volumes in REM sleep are less effective in generating an increase in ventilation during inhaled CO_2.

Considerable interest has been generated by the notion that behavioral activity, such as phonation, can override, within limits, the chemical control of breathing. Phillipson et al. (120) have shown that the response to inhaled CO_2 during speech mimics that seen in active sleep: it is quite scattered and decreased. We have found that the ventilatory response to CO_2 was reduced during suckling. The decreased response was related primarily to changes in "effective" respiratory timing—i.e., inspiratory time as a fraction of total respiratory cycle (T_I/T_{tot}), rather than in mean inspiratory flow (V_T/T_I) (121).

In summary, the response of neonatal ventilation to CO_2 is affected by sleep and behavior. These factors may be important in the response to chemical stimuli, especially when the ability to arouse is impaired.

X. The Response to Low O_2

In response to low O_2, preterm infants ultimately decrease their ventilation (8,12,82,122). This decrease in ventilation is primarily related to a decrease in frequency with no change or slight increase in tidal volume (82). The inability of these infants to better sustain hyperventilation in response to hypoxia remains an interesting peculiarity of the respiratory control system in the neonatal period (8,12,82,123). It is now clear that even the adult subject has a similar response, although ventilation is far better sustained than it is in the newborn infant (124,125). This biphasic response has also been demonstrated in rabbits, kittens, and monkeys (126–131). Like human neonates, anesthetized kittens respond biphasically with an initial increase in ventilation followed by a decrease when inspired O_2 concentrations were reduced from 21% to 6%–12%. The initial increase in ventilation is due to an increase in tidal volume and frequency, while the late (5–10 min) decrease in ventilation is due primarily to a decrease in frequency. In the unanesthetized kitten, studied in quiet sleep, the late decrease in ventilation was due primarily to a decrease in tidal volume—a fact that illustrates the differences that may occur due to anesthesia. The peripheral chemoreceptors were active during hypoxia, since we observed a steady increase in carotid body single-fiber firing. Despite the increase in carotid body activity, diaphragmatic activity decreased toward the end of hypoxia (5 min).

In acute experiments in which the phrenic nerve and diaphragm were recorded simultaneously, there was an initial increase in activity to a peak level at about 1 min, followed by a decrease, usually in frequency, but at times in peak activity as well (112). There was no distinction between the phrenic and diaphragmatic electrical activity. These latter findings together with those showing an increase in carotid nerve firing, which was maximal at the time respiratory efforts were about to stop, suggest that the late decrease in ventilation during hypoxia is due to inhibition at the central level, as originally suggested by Cross (8). This line of thinking is consistent with the inhibition of breathing present in the fetal sheep and released by midcollicular section (132).

Cross et al. (8,12) suggested that a decrease in metabolism could be the basis for the ultimate decrease in ventilation. Many studies have demonstrated a decrease in metabolism during hypoxia, both in animals (133,134) and in humans (12). A decrease in metabolism could induce a corresponding decrease in ventilation mediated through a decrease in CO_2 production (129). This decrease in metabolism is present in various species at various ages (128). It appears to be a uniform defense mechanism that mammals rely upon to compensate for the reduced availability of O_2 in the atmosphere. This decrease in metabolism was present in preterm infants in studies performed in our laboratory during quiet sleep, although it did not affect the biphasic shape of the response to hypoxia (131).

The argument for a central inhibitory effect of hypoxia following initial hyperventilation is compelling if one considers the following lines of evidence. First, there is a clear ontogenetic evolution in the response to hypoxia with maturation: hypoxia invariably abolishes breathing in the fetus (135), stimulates and depresses it in the neonate (8,12,82,97), and also stimulates and depresses it in the adult, but less so than in the neonate (125,136). The evolution is therefore one of gradually diminishing the magnitude of depression. Second, although adult subjects clearly show a biphasic response to hypoxia, the ventilatory depression lasts longer than the duration of hypoxia (125). This has been attributed to the release of inhibitory neurotransmitters, of which adenosine (137), endothelin (138), endorphins (139), and gamma aminobutyric acid (98) are good potential candidates. Third, in the paralyzed piglet model, the central neural output in response to hypoxia was not sustained despite a constant end-tidal P_{CO_2}, suggesting that it is not the metabolic rate that determines the late decrease in ventilation (140). The findings of Fung et al. (141) in paralyzed newborn rats also suggest that the ventilatory decrease during hypoxia is mediated via its action upon brainstem mechanisms. Fourth, central sites responsible for this depression have been suggested to exist in the upper medulla by Cross et al. (11) or above the midcolliculi by Dawes et al. (132). In the experiments of Dawes et al. (132), hypoxia stimulated breathing in the midcollicular transected fetal sheep, suggesting the possibility of an inhibitory action of hypoxia on a center located rostral to the section level. Finally, Gluckman and coworkers (142,143) have localized a specific area in the rostral lateral pons, in the region of the lateral parabrachial and Kölliker-fuse nuclei, which appears to be involved in the central inhibition of breathing during hypoxia in the fetal lamb. After electrolytic lesions of this area, hypoxemia stimulated rather than abolished breathing in the fetus. This appears likely to be the site of action for neurotransmitters that inhibit breathing and are released by hypoxia. Lesions of the red nucleus (144) and cooling of the locus ceruleus (145) have also been shown to block the fall in respiratory output with hypoxia.

We and others have speculated on the possible release of neuromediators during hypoxia as the primary mechanism for the late decrease in ventilation. Endogenous opiates have been suggested as mediators. In the newborn rabbit, Grunstein et al. (146) were able to prevent the late decrease in ventilation by administration of naloxone, an endogenous opiate antagonist. Hazinski et al. (147) showed an increase in ventilation of anesthetized rabbits in response to naloxone during the first 4 days of life. Observations in the newborn infant suggest that naloxone inhibits, at least in part, the late decrease in ventilation during hypoxia (139). Observations in the fetus are conflicting, with some studies showing a response and others no response to naloxone (148).

Adenosine has been considered a candidate in the newborn as it decreases ventilation mainly through changes in respiratory frequency. Adenosine has a depressant action on neural activities in many areas of the central nervous system (149). Even brief exposure to hypoxia is known to increase brain adenosine concentrations (150). Because of its respiratory depressant activity and increased concentration during hypoxia, adenosine is a potential mediator of late ventilatory depression during hypoxia. Since aminophylline pretreatment only attenuates but does not completely eliminate hypoxic ventilatory depression, adenosine may not be the predominant neurotransmitter responsible for late hypoxic ventilatory depression in adults (136).

Sleep affects the response to low oxygen. The increase in ventilatory response to hypoxia is better sustained during quiet sleep than during REM sleep or wakefulness (83) (Fig. 7). Jeffery and Read (148) also found a more sustained increase in ventilation during quiet as compared to REM sleep in calves. The results imply that the biphasic response to hypoxia is altered, in part, by behavioral influences on breathing, which are more pronounced during REM sleep and wakefulness.

Because the fetus stops breathing in response to hypoxia (135) and the neonate has a poorly sustained initial hyperventilation with a late decrease in ventilation, we

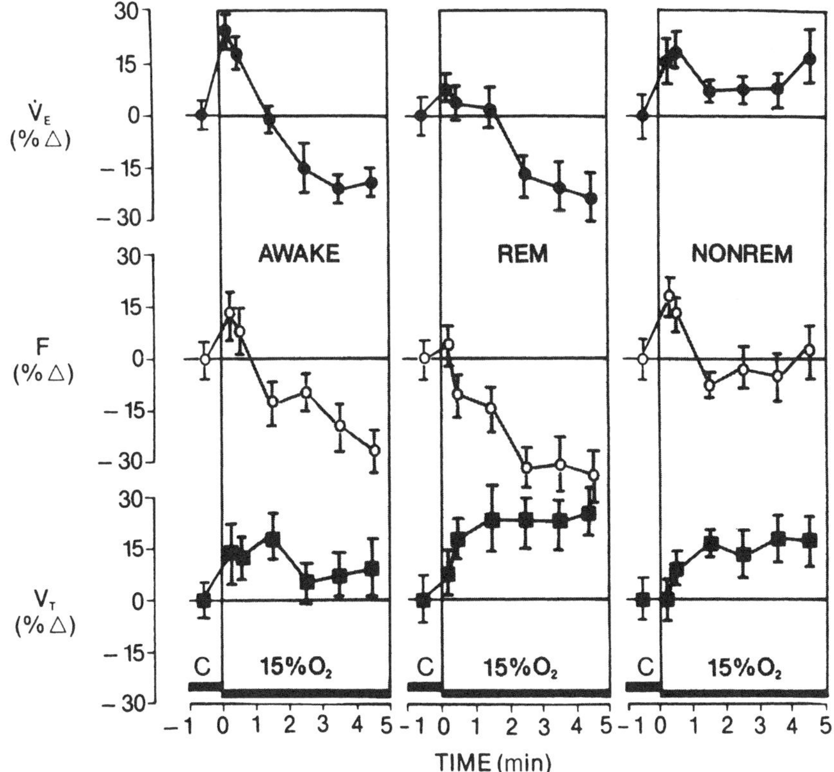

Figure 7 The ventilatory responses to 15% O_2 in preterm infants during wakefulness, REM, and NREM sleep; in NREM sleep or quiet sleep, hyperventilation is more sustained. This more sustained ventilation was related primarily to a more sustained respiratory rate in quiet sleep. (From Ref. 83.)

hypothesized that perhaps low-birth-weight infants (< 1500 g) would hypoventilate only in response to hypoxia (115). This was true in both sleep states, although the response was more pronounced in REM sleep. The decrease in ventilation was primarily related to a decrease in frequency, tidal volume remaining practically unchanged.

In summary, the biphasic ventilatory response to mild hypoxia in preterm infants is significantly affected by sleep state, being more sustained in quiet sleep. This effect is likely mediated through the action of a specific neuromediator. Since many of these mediators are presently unknown, the discovery of how sleep modulates this response may give us interesting insights into the manner in which the respiratory system is controlled during hypoxia.

XI. The Overall Clinical Implications

There is an important drive to breathe associated with wakefulness. During sleep, this drive ceases. Breathing is then more vulnerable, sustained primarily by brainstem structures and becoming prone to "oscillation." The following is a description of some clinical conditions in the preterm infant that are affected by sleep.

A. Periodic Breathing and Apnea

Although prematurity per se, with its inherent physiological limitations, is crucial to induce respiratory periodicity and apnea, respiratory instability is exaggerated by REM. Medications like theophylline increase central respiratory drive and muscular contractility (142,153,154). Although usually overlooked, theophylline also affects sleep state, making it lighter and much closer to wakefulness. In general, all medications or maneuvers that tend to wake the infant tend to be effective in reducing apnea, since breathing tends to become more regular with the increased drive produced by arousal.

B. Respiratory Disease and Ventilatory Strategy

The modern use of ventilators, with major efforts toward completely synchronized ventilation, involves great knowledge of the respiratory pattern under baseline conditions. Because this baseline pattern is profoundly affected by sleep, the corresponding effects of sleep must be thoroughly understood. We now know, for example, that the best ventilation in these tiny infants is provided with short inspiratory times of the order of 0.25 to 0.35 sec. Previously these infants were being ventilated with inspiratory times equal to or greater than 0.5 sec. Interfering with the normal pattern of ventilation in the nonparalyzed state increases the risk of pneumothorax and intraventricular bleeding (155,156). Furthermore, because of the low functional residual capacity in these infants, particularly in REM sleep, it is important to ventilate them with positive end expiratory pressures, which are known to recruit lung volume and retain the distal alveolar units open. Usually 4 to 6 cmH_2O is used for this purpose. Lower pressures are frequently associated with collapse and poor oxygenation.

C. Respiratory Insufficiency of Prematurity

Even "healthy" preterm infants present an interesting profile of high CO_2 tension and lower arterial P_{O_2} during the neonatal period. Burnard (157) called this "the respiratory insufficiency of prematurity." This was seen more dramatically in the era preceding the use of respiratory stimulants. Today it is still present, but such infants are usually receiving respiratory stimulants, and thus the abnormalities in arterial gas tensions appear less dramatic. The respiratory insufficiency is due to lung immaturity, stiffness, and residual lung disease, the effects of which are greatly aggravated during REM sleep. With the absence of intercostal muscle activity, the lung collapses and baseline arterial gases deteriorate. Depending on the severity of the condition, measures such as the use of methylxanthines (theophylline, caffeine), doxapram, or continuous positive airway pressure (CPAP) may not suffice, and the infant may need to be intubated and ventilated. If there is residual airway disease, as in bronchopulmonary dysplasia, the lack of response of the pulmonary irritant reflexes during REM sleep may further compromise clearing of the airway. This is particularly true in situations where there is chronic airway infection, repeated aspiration, or both.

D. The Long-Term Developmental Perspective

We now know that approximately one-third of small preterm infants who survive and are intact at 2 years of age will show some degree of neurological impairment at school age (158). The mechanism for these late sequelae is not known, but the problem is of major significance (159). Many feel that these late sequelae may be the consequence of the unphysiological brain development occurring during the premature days in hospital (159,160). If so, it may not be easy to correct. The nursery environment is likely to alter the sleep pattern and consequently the physiological processes involved in the development of the brain. It seems probable that a thorough understanding of the baseline physiology at this age, together with the possible effects of factors like the unusual length and type of sleep, are going to be important in minimizing complications. In the past, the challenge was to make preterm infants survive. We overcame that challenge and they now survive. It will be the task of the generations that will follow us to improve the quality of life of those survivors.

E. Sleep and SIDS

The incidence of sudden death in the preterm infant is low only because these infants remain in hospital and are intensively monitored. In the premonitoring era, before 1967, sudden death was common in these infants even in the "healthy preterm infant." Infants used to die during sleep, as is the case with classic SIDS victims who die at about 3 to 4 months of age. Because SIDS infants die during sleep, it has been assumed that the vulnerability of sleep is an important factor in their death, although there is no definitive proof that this is so. It is the view of the majority of investigators in this area [at least in those cases in which parental abuse has been ruled out

(161)], that SIDS has something to do with the inability to arouse during periods of suffocation, when the face is buried in soft mattresses or pillows. Arousal under these circumstances, allowing the infant to move its head and breathe fresh air, becomes a more important defense mechanism than any possible chemical stimulus to breathe. Preterm infants with bronchopulmonary dysplasia (BPD) have a more than twofold increase in incidence of SIDS (162,163). It is likely that compromised sleep-related defense mechanisms are present in these infants since birth.

F. Sleep and Central Congenital Hypoventilation

In no other neonatal problem is the importance of sleep more dramatic than in the syndrome of central congenital hypoventilation ("Ondine's curse") (164). In this syndrome, infants are born with the inability to sustain breathing, particularly during sleep. Respiration is overall vulnerable, but usually these infants have some ability to sustain ventilation while awake. This is lost during sleep, and breathing becomes ineffective. Ventilatory support is frequently necessary until phrenic pacing can be instituted. The success of this treatment is somewhat limited, though. The cause of this syndrome is unknown, and all investigative procedures, including imaging of the brain, have not shed light on the matter. In the last few years we have isolated cells from the upper medulla in the fetal rat, located 2 mm rostral to the obex, which have a respiratory phenotype (165). These are pacemaker cells uniquely responsive to CO_2 (Fig. 8). Although work needs to be done in order to define the respiratory specificity of these cells, we suggest that these cells are responsible for the generation of breathing. It may prove that central hypoventilation syndrome is the result of a mutation or an abnormality of these cells which, for some reason, partially lose their ability to respond to CO_2.

XII. Conclusion

The history of the influence of sleep on breathing is relatively young (36,37). Only 33 years ago, the relationship of REM sleep and periodic breathing was first reported (38). Since then, numerous studies have tried to determine the influence of the various states of sleep on breathing. The fact that the fetus has breathing activity only during REM and not quiet sleep shows how powerful this influence can be (44).

The effects of sleep on breathing in preterm infants are many. REM sleep increases the incidence of periodic breathing and apnea (40,47,83–85,111), increases minute ventilation (47,83,166–168), decreases the ventilatory response to CO_2 (48,118), enhances the late decrease in ventilation with hypoxia (83,148), increases the rate of sighs (75), increases chest distortion leading to muscle fatigue and increased oxygen consumption (34,47,65,70), inhibits pulmonary reflexes (33,75,169), and decreases upper-airway tone and postinspiratory activity of the diaphragm leading to partial lung collapse during expiration (42,69,70). Sleep is also likely to have a very important role in conditions such as SIDS (159,160) and congenital central hypoventilation syndrome (161).

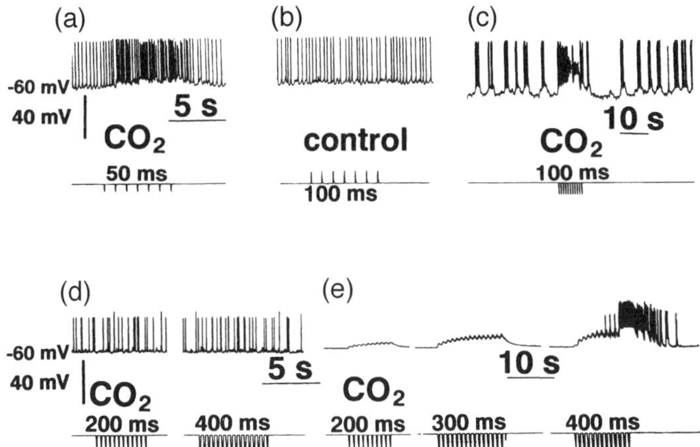

Figure 8 Representative tracing illustrating the changes in electrical activity of a pacemaker-like cell in response to administration of trains of pulses of medium equilibrated with high CO_2 and low pH. (a) Single beating cell responded to pulses of CO_2 of 50 and 100 ms with an increase in frequency and a decrease in amplitude. (b) Administration of a control solution had no effect on spontaneous electrical activity. (c) A bursting neuron also responded to CO_2 pulses of 50 to 100 ms with an increase in spike frequency and a decrease in amplitude; some degree of depolarization was also seen. (d) An irregular beating cell did not respond to high pulses of CO_2. (e) A silent cell shows some depolarization, but firing activity was only present with very high CO_2 pulses of 400 ms. (From Ref. 165.)

Little is understood presently on exactly how sleep interacts with breathing. Efforts to elucidate this are likely to have priority during the first part of the next century. Unraveling this mechanism may hold the key to understanding how breathing is generated and regulated.

Acknowledgments

We are indebted to Marie Meunier for helping in the typing and preparation of this chapter. Don Cates and Zalman Weintraub provided valuable comments and criticisms. Claudio Rigatto proofread the chapter and made valuable corrections. Our research cited in this chapter was supported over the years by the Medical Research Council of Canada, the Children's Hospital of Winnipeg Foundation, and the Manitoba Lung Association.

References

1. Comroe JH Jr. Premature science and immature lung: Part III. The attack on immature lungs. In: Retrospectroscope—Insights into Medical Discovery. Menlo Park, CA: Von Gehr Press, 1983: 173.

2. Newton I. In: Debus AG, ed. World Who's Who in Science. Chicago: Marquis—Who's Who, 1968: 1252.
3. Bouterline-Young HJ, Smith CA. Respiration of full-term and of premature infants. Am J Dis Child 1953; 80:753–766.
4. Deming J, Hanner JP. Respiration in infancy: II. A study of rate, volume and character of respiration in healthy infants during the neonatal period. Am J Dis Child 1936; 51: 823–831.
5. Deming J, Washburn AH. Respiration in infancy: method of studying rates, volume and character of respiration with preliminary report of results. Am J Dis Child 1935; 49: 108–124.
6. Murphy DP, Thorpe ES Jr. Breathing measurements on normal newborn infants. J Clin Invest 1931; 10:545–558.
7. Shaw LA, Hopkins FR. The respiration of premature infants. Am J Dis Child 1931; 42: 335–341.
8. Cross KW, Oppé TE. The effect of inhalation of high and low concentrations of oxygen on the respiration of the premature infant. J Physiol (Lond) 1952; 117:38–47.
9. Cross KW. Respiratory patterns. In: Wolfe H, ed. Mechanisms of Congenital Malformation: Proceedings of the Second Scientific Conference. New York: Association for the Aid of Crippled Children, 1954: 99–105.
10. Cross KW, Klaus M, Tooley WH, Weisser K. The response of the newborn baby to inflation of the lungs. J Physiol (Lond) 1960; 151:551–565.
11. Cross KW, Hooper JMD, Lord JM. Anoxic depression of the medulla on the new-born infant. J Physiol 1954; 125:628–640.
12. Cross KW, Tizard JPM, Tryhall DAH. The gaseous metabolism of the new born infant breathing 15% oxygen. Acta Pediatr 1958; 47:217–237.
13. Dawes GS. Foetal and Neonatal Physiology. Chicago: Year Book, 1968.
14. Nelson NM, Prod'hom LS, Cherry RB, Lipsitz PJ, Smith CA. Pulmonary function in the newborn infant: I. Methods—ventilation and gaseous metabolism. Pediatrics 1962; 30:963–974.
15. Smith CA, Nelson NM. The Physiology of the Newborn Infant, 4th ed. Springfield, IL: Charles C Thomas, 1976: 1–281.
16. Bryan MH. The work of breathing during sleep in newborns. Am Rev Respir Dis 1979; 119(suppl):137–138.
17. Avery ME, Chernick V, Dutton RE, Permutt S. Ventilatory response to inspired carbon dioxide in infants and adults. J Appl Physiol 1963; 18:895–903.
18. Chu JS, Dawson P, Klaus M, Sweet AY. Lung compliance and lung volume measured concurrently in normal full term and premature infants. J Pediatr 1964; 34:525–532.
19. Cook CD, Sutherland JM, Segal S, Cherry RB, Mead J, McIlroy MC, Smith CA. Studies of respiratory physiology in the newborn infant: III. Measurements of the mechanics of respiration. J Clin Invest 1957; 36:440–448.
20. Doershuk CF, Matthews LW. Airway resistance and lung volume in the newborn infant. Pediatrics 1969; 3:128–134.
21. Howard PJ, Bauer AR. Irregularities of breathing in the newborn period. Am J Dis Child 1949; 77:592–609.
22. Howard PJ, Bauer AR. Respiration of the newborn infant. Am J Dis Child 1950; 79: 611–622.
23. Koch G. Alveolar ventilation, diffusion capacity and A-a P_{O_2} difference in the newborn infant. Respir Physiol 1968; 4:168–192.

24. Krauss AN, Klain DB, Dahms B, Auld PAM. Vital capacity in premature infants. Am Rev Respir Dis 1973; 108:1361–1366.
25. Krauss AN, Klain DB, Waldman S, Auld PAM. Ventilatory response to carbon dioxide in newborn infants. Pediatr Res 1975; 9:46–50.
26. Nelson NM. Neonatal pulmonary function. Pediatr Clin North Am 1966; 13:769–799.
27. Wohl ME, Stigol L, Mead J. Resistance of the total respiratory system in healthy infants and infants with bronchitis. Pediatrics 1969; 43:495–509.
28. Graham BD, Reardon HS, Wilson JL, Tsao MU, Baumann MI. Physiologic and chemical response of premature infants to oxygen-enriched atmosphere. Pediatrics 1950; 6: 55–71.
29. Stahlman M. Ventilation control in the newborn: carbon dioxide tension and output. Am J Dis Child 1961; 101:216–227.
30. Stahlman M, Shepard F, Gray J, Yong W. The effects of hypoxia and hypercapnia on the circulation in newborn lambs. J Pediatr 1964; 65:1091–1092.
31. Thibeault DW, Wong MM, Auld PAM. Thoracic gas volume changes in premature infants. Pediatrics 1967; 40:403.
32. Wilson JL, Long SB, Howard PJ. Respiration of premature infants: response to variation of oxygen and to increased carbon dioxide in inspired air. Am J Dis Child 1942; 63: 1080–1085.
33. Fleming PJ, Bryan AC, Bryan MH. Functional immaturity of pulmonary irritant receptors and apnea in newborn preterm infants. Pediatrics 1978; 61:515–518.
34. Müller N, Gulston G, Cade D, Whitton J, Froese AB, Bryan MH, Bryan AC. Diaphragmatic muscle fatigue of the newborn. J Appl Physiol 1979; 46:688–695.
35. Polgar G, Weng TR. The functional development of the respiratory system: from the period of gestation to adulthood. Am Rev Respir Dis 1979; 120:625–695.
36. Magnussen G. Studies on the Respiration During Sleep. London: Lewis, 1944.
37. Bülow K. Respiration and wakefulness in man. Acta Physiol Scand 1963; 59(suppl 209):1
38. Aserinsky E. Periodic respiratory pattern occurring in conjunction with eye movement during sleep. Science 1965; 150:763–766.
39. Cruzi-Dascalova L, Christove GE. Respiratory pauses in normal prematurely born infants: a comparison with full-term newborns. Biol Neonate 1983; 44:325–332.
40. Guilleminault C, Ariagno R, Korobkin R, Nagel L, Balowin R, Coons S, Owen M. Mixed and obstructive sleep apnea and near miss for sudden infant death syndrome: 2. Comparison of near miss and normal control infants by age. Pediatrics 1979; 64:882–891.
41. Prechtl H. The behavioural states of the newborn infant (review). Brain Res 1974; 76: 185–212.
42. Reis FJC, Cates DB, Vandriault LV, Rigatto H. I. Diaphragmatic activity and ventilation in preterm infants—the effects of sleep state. Biol Neonate 1994; 65:16–24.
43. Stern E, Parmelee AH, Akiyama Y, Schultz MA, Wenner WH. Sleep cycle characteristics in infants. Pediatrics 1969; 43:65–70.
44. Rigatto H. Control of breathing during sleep in the fetus and neonate. In: Ferber R, Kryger MH, eds. Principles and Practice of Sleep Medicine in the Child. Philadelphia: Saunders, 1995: 29–43.
45. Dreyfus-Brisac C. Ontogenesis of brain bioelectrical activity and sleep organization in neonates and infants. In: Falkner F, Tanner JM, eds. Human Growth. Vol. 3. London: Plenum, 1979: 157.
46. Dreyfus-Brisac C. Ontogenesis of sleep in human prematures after 32 weeks of conceptional age. Dev Psychobiol 1970; 3:91–121.
47. Davi M, Sankaran K, MacCallum M, Cates D, Rigatto H. Effect of sleep state on chest

distortion and on the ventilatory response to CO_2 in neonates. Pediatr Res 1979; 13: 982–986.

48. Moriette G, Van Reempts P, Moore M, Yorke K, Rigatto H. The effect of rebreathing CO_2 on ventilation and diaphragmatic electromyography in newborn infants. Respir Physiol 1985; 62:387–397.
49. Fijardo C, Alvarez J, Wong A, Kwiatkowski K, Rigatto H. The incidence of obstructive apneas in preterm infants with and without bronchopulmonary dysplasia. Early Hum Dev 1993; 32:197–206.
50. Purpura DP, Schade IP. Growth and maturation of the brain. In: Progress in the Brain Research, Vol. 4. Amsterdam: Elsevier, 1964.
51. Eccles IC. The Inhibitory Pathways of the Central Nervous System. Liverpool: Liverpool University Press, 1969: 101–104.
52. Hershenson MB. The respiratory muscles and chest wall. In: Bekerman RC, Brouillette RT, Hunt CE, eds. Respiratory Control Disorders in Infants and Children. Baltimore: Williams & Wilkins, 1992: 28.
53. Hagan RAC, Bryan CA, Bryan MH, Gulston MH. The effect of sleep state on intercostal muscle activity and rib cage motion. Physiologist 1976; 19:214.
54. Oppenshaw P, Edwards S, Helms P. Changes in rib cage geometry during childhood. Thorax 1984; 39:624–627.
55. Hershenson MB, Stark AR, Mead J. Action of the inspiratory muscles of the rib cage during breathing in infants. Am Rev Respir Dis 1989; 139:1207–1212.
56. Hershenson MB, Colin AA, Wohl MEG, Stark AR. Changes in the contribution of the rib cage to tidal breathing during infancy. Am Rev Respir Dis 1990; 141:922–925.
57. Henderson-Smart DJ, Read DJ. Reduced lung volume during behavioral active sleep in the newborn. J Appl Physiol 1979; 46:1081–1085.
58. Thach BT, Abroms IF, Frantz ID, Sotrel A, Bruce EN, Goldman MD. Intercostal muscle reflexes and sleep breathing patterns in the human infant. J Appl Physiol 1980; 48: 139–146.
59. Agostoni E, Mead J. Statics of the respiratory system. In: Fenn WO, Rahn H, eds. Handbook of Physiology: 3. Respiration. Washington, DC: American Physiological Society, 1964: 387–409.
60. Agostoni E. Volume-pressure relationships of the thorax and lung in the newborn. J Appl Physiol 1959; 14:909–913.
61. Gerhardt T, Bancalari E. Chest wall compliance in full-term and premature infants. Acta Paediatr Scand 1980; 69:359–364.
62. Heldt GP, McIlroy MB. Distortion of the chest wall and work of the diaphragm in preterm infants. J Appl Physiol 1987; 62:164–169.
63. Kosch PC, Stark AR. Dynamic maintenance of end-expiratory volume in full-term infants. J Appl Physiol 1984; 57:1126–1133.
64. Maxwell IC, McCater RJ, Kuehl TJ, Robotham JL. Development of histochemical and functional properties of baboon respiratory muscles. J Appl Physiol 1983; 54: 551–561.
65. Lopes JM, Muller NL, Bryan MH, Bryan AC. Synergistic behavior of inspiratory muscles after diaphragmatic fatigue in the newborn. J Appl Physiol 1981; 51:547–551.
66. Knill R, Bryan AC. An intercostal-phrenic inhibitory reflex in human newborn infants. J Appl Physiol 1976; 40:352–356.
67. Remmers JE, Bartlett JR. Reflex control of expiratory airflow and duration. J Appl Physiol 1977; 42:80–87.

68. Remmers JE, DeGroot WJ, Sauerland EK, Auch AM. Pathogenesis of upper airway occlusion during sleep. J Appl Physiol 1978; 44:931–938.
69. Harding R, Johnson P, McClelland ME. Respiratory function of the larynx in developing sheep and the influence of sleep state. Respir Physiol 1980; 40:165–179.
70. Luz J, Winter A, Cates D, Moore M, Rigatto H. Effect of chest breathing and abdomen uncoupling on ventilation and work of breathing in the newborn during sleep. Pediatr Res 1982; 16:296A.
71. Hering E, Breuer J. Dir Selbsteurung der athmung durch den nervus vagus-sitzber akad-wiss wien 1868; 57:672–677.
72. Olinsky A, Bryan AH, Bryan AC. Influence of lung inflation on respiratory control in neonates. J Appl Physiol 1974; 36:426–429.
73. Head H. On the regulation of respiration: II. Theoretical. J Physiol (Lond) 1889; 10: 279–290.
74. Head H. On the regulation of respiration: I. Experimental. J Physiol (Lond) 1889; 1: 1–70.
75. Alvarez JE, Bodani J, Fajardo CA, Kwiatkowski K, Cates DB, Rigatto H. Sighs and their relationship to apnea in the newborn infant. Biol Neonate 1993; 63:139–146.
76. Thach BT, Tauesch HW. Sighing in human newborn infants: role of inflation-augmenting reflex. J Appl Physiol 1976; 41:502–507.
77. Al-Hathlol K, Idiong N, Hussain A, Kwiatkowski K, Alvaro R, Cates D, Rigatto H. A developmental study of the undisturbed breathing pattern in human subjects. Pediatr Res 1998; 43:272A.
78. Douglas CG, Haldane JS. The causes of periodic or Cheyne-Stokes breathing. J Physiol (Lond) 1980–1909; 38:401.
79. Fenner A, Schalk V, Hoenicke H, Wendenburg A, Roehling T. Periodic breathing in premature and neonatal babies: Incidence, breathing pattern, respiratory gas tensions, response to changes in the composition of ambient air. Pediatr Res 1973; 7:174–183.
80. Hornbein TF. The puzzle of periodicity. Pediatrics 1972; 50:183–185.
81. Rigatto H, Brady JP. Periodic breathing and apnea in preterm infants: I. Evidence for hypoventilation possibly due to central respiratory depression. Pediatrics 1972; 50: 202–218.
82. Rigatto H, Brady JP. Periodic breathing and apnea in preterm infants: II. Hypoxia as a primary event. Pediatrics 1972; 50:219–228.
83. Rigatto H, Kalapesi Z, Leahy F, MacCallum M, Cates D. Ventilatory response to 100% and 15% O_2 during wakefulness and sleep in preterm infants. Early Hum Dev 1982; 7: 1–10.
84. Gabriel M, Albani M, Schulte FJ. Apneic spells and sleep state in preterm infants. 1976; 57:142–147.
85. Schulte FJ, Busse C, Eichhorn W. Rapid eye movement sleep, motoneurone inhibition, and apneic spells in preterm infants. Pediatr Res 1977; 11:709–713.
86. Kalapesi Z, Durand M, Leahy FAN, Cates DB, MacCallum M, Rigatto H. Effect of periodic or regular respiratory pattern on the ventilatory response to low inhaled CO_2 in preterm infants during sleep. Am Rev Respir Dis 1981; 123:8–11.
87. Rechtshaffen A, Kales A. A Manual of Standardized Terminology Techniques and Scoring System for Sleep Stages in Human Subjects. NIH Publ. #204. Washington, DC: U.S. Government Printing Office, 1978.
88. Dempsey JA, Skatrud JB. A sleep-induced apneic threshold and its consequences. Am Rev Respir Dis 1986; 133:1163–1170.

89. Younes M. The physiologic basis of central apnea and periodic breathing. Curr Pulmonol 1989; 10:265–365.
90. Hussain A, Idiong N, Lin Y-J, Kwiatkowski K, Cates D, Rigatto H. The profile and significance of periodic breathing in preterm infants. Pediatr Res 1997; 41:255A.
91. Lin Y-J, Idiong N, Kwiatkowski K, Cates D, Rigatto H. Periodic breathing in term infants—is it benign? Pediatr Res 1997; 41:161A.
92. Bacola E, Behrle FC, Deschweinitz L, Miller HC, Mira M. Perinatal environmental factors in late neurogenic sequelae: I. Infants having birth weight under 1500; and II. Infants having birth weight from 1500 to 2500 grams. Am J Dis Child 1966; 112:359–369.
93. Daily WJR, Klaus M, Meyer HBP. Apnea in premature infants: monitoring incidence, heart rate, changes, and an effect of environmental temperatures. Pediatrics 1969; 43: 510–518.
94. Peabody JL, Schneider H, Huch A, Huch R. Clinical experience with transcutaneous PO_2 monitoring in neonatology and pediatrics. In: Fetal and Neonatal Physiological Measurements. Oxford, England: Department of Pediatrics, 1979: 92.
95. Glotzbach SF, Ariagno RL. Periodic breathing. In: Beckerman RC, Brouillette RT, Hunt CE, eds. Respiratory Control Disorders in Infants and Children. Baltimore: Williams & Wilkins, 1992:142–160.
96. Rigatto H. Apnea—symposium on the newborn. Pediatr Clin North Am 1982; 29: 1105–1116.
97. Rigatto H. Control of breathing in the fetus and newborn. In: Spitzer AR, ed. Intensive Care of the Fetus and Newborn. St. Louis: Mosby–YearBook, 1995: 458–469.
98. Young RSK, During JM, Donnelly DF, Aquila WJ, Perry VL, Haddad GG. Effect of anoxia on excitatory amino acids in brain slices of rats and turtles: in vitro microdialysis. Am J Physiol 1993; 264:716–719.
99. Milner AD, Boon AW, Saunders RA, Hopkin IE. Upper airway obstruction and apnoea in preterm babies. Arch Dis Child 1980; 55:22–25.
100. Thach BT. The role of pharyngeal airway obstruction in prolonging infantile apneic spells. In: Tilden JT, Roeder LM, Steinschneider A, eds. Sudden Infant Death Syndrome. New York: Academic Press, 1983: 279–292.
101. Dransfield DA, Spitzer AR, Fox WW. Episodic airway obstruction in premature infants. Am J Dis Child 1983; 137:441–443.
102. Lemke RP, Idiong N, Al-Saedi S, Kwiatkowski K, Cates DB, Rigatto H. Evidence of a critical period of airway instability during central apneas in preterm infants. Am J Respir Crit Care Med 1998; 157:470–474.
103. Thach BT, Stark AR. Spontaneous neck flexion and airway obstruction during apneic spells in preterm infants. J Pediatr 1979; 94:275–281.
104. Ruggins NR, Milner AD. Site of Supper airway obstruction in preterm infants with problematical apnoea. Arch Dis Child 1991; 66:787–792.
105. Lemke RP, Al-Saedi S, Alvaro R, Kwaitkowski K, Cates D, Rigatto H. Use of a magnified cardiac waveform oscillation to diagnose infant apnea: a theoretical and clinical evaluation. Am Rev Respir Crit Care Med 1996; 154:1537–1542.
106. Idiong N, Lemke R, Lin Y-J, Hussain A, Kwaitkowski K, Cates D, Rigatto H. Airway closure during mixed apneas in preterm infants: is respiratory effort necessary? Pediatr Res 1997; 41:302A.
107. Idiong N, Cates DB, Lemke RP, Alvaro RE, Kwaitkowski K, Rigatto H. Profile and significance of the various types of apnea in preterm infants. Pediatr Res 1996; 39:328A.
108. Al-Saedi SA, Lemke RP, Haider AZ, Cates DB, Kwaitkowski K, Rigatto H. Prolonged apnea in the preterm infant is not a random event. Am J Perinatol 1997; 14:195–200.

109. Albani M, Bentele KHP, Budde C, Schulte FJ. Infant sleep apnea profile: preterm vs term infants. Eur J Pediatr 1985; 143:261–268.
110. Flores-Guevara R, Plouin P, Curzi-Dascalova L, Radvanyi M-F, Guidasci S, Pajot N, Monod N. Sleep apneas in normal neonates and infants during the first 3 months of life. Neuropediatrics 1982; 13(suppl):21–28.
111. Hoppenbrouwers T, Hodgman JE, Harper RM, Hofmann E, Sterman MB, McGinty D. Polygraphic studies of normal infants during the first six months of life: III. Incidence of apnea and periodic breathing. Pediatrics 1977; 60:418–425.
112. Rigatto H. Control of ventilation in the newborn. Ann Rev Physiol 1984; 46:661–674.
113. Ardila R, Yunis K, Bureau MA. Relationship between infantile sleep apnea and preceding hyperventilation event. Clin Invest 1986; 9:A151.
114. Krieger J, Turlot J-C, Mangin P, Durtz D. Breathing during sleep in normal young and elderly subjects: hypopneas, apneas, and correlated factors. Sleep 1983; 6:108–120.
115. Alvaro R, Alvarez J, Kwiatkowski K, Cates D, Rigatto H. Small preterm infants (≤ 1500 g) have only sustained decrease in ventilation in response to hypoxia. Pediatr Res 1992; 32:403–406.
116. Frantz ID III, Adler SM, Thach BT, Taeusch HW Jr. Malnutritional effects on respiratory response to carbon dioxide in premature infants. J Appl Physiol 1976; 41:41–45.
117. Rigatto H, Brady JP, de la Torre Verduzco R. Chemoreceptor reflexes in preterm infants. I. The effect of gestational and postnatal age on the ventilatory response to inhalation of 100% and 15% O_2. Pediatrics 1975; 55:604–613.
118. Phillipson EA, Kozar LF, Rebuck AS, Murphy E. Ventilatory and waking responses to CO_2 in sleeping dogs. Am Rev Respir Dis 1977; 115:251–259.
119. Sullivan CE, Murphy E, Kozar LF, Phillipson EA. Ventilatory responses to CO_2 and lung inflation in tonic versus phasic REM sleep. J Appl Physiol 1979; 47:1304–1310.
120. Phillipson EA, McLean PA, Sullivan CE, Zamel N. Interaction of metabolic and behavioral respiratory control during hypercapnia and speech. Am Rev Respir Dis 1978; 117:903–909.
121. Durand M, Leahy FAN, MacCallum M, Cates DB, Rigatto H, Chernick V. Effect of feeding on the chemical control of breathing in the newborn infant. Pediatr Res 1981; 15: 1509–1512.
122. Brady JP, Ceruti E. Chemoreceptor reflexes in the newborn infant. Effects of varying degrees of hypoxia on heart rate and ventilation in a warm environment. J Physiol (Lond) 1966; 184:631–645.
123. Miller HC, Smull NW. Further studies on the effects of hypoxia on the respiration of newborn infants. Pediatrics 1955; 16:93–103.
124. Weil JV, Zwillich CW. Assessment of ventilatory response to hypoxia: methods and interpretation. Chest 1976; 70(suppl 1):124–128.
125. Easton PA, Slykerman LJ, Anthonisen NR. Ventilatory response to sustained hypoxia in normal adults. J Appl Physiol 1986; 61:906–911.
126. Schwieler GH. Respiratory regulation during postnatal development in cats and rabbits and some of its morphological substrate. Acta Physiol Scand 1968; 304(suppl):1–123.
127. Woodrum DE, Standaert TA, Mayock DE, Guthrie RD. Hypoxic ventilatory response in the newborn monkey. Pediatr Res 1981; 15:367–370.
128. Haddad GG, Gandhi MR, Mellins RB. Maturation of ventilatory response to hypoxia in puppies during sleep. J Appl Physiol 1982; 52:309–314.
129. Mortola JP, Matsuoka T. Interaction between CO_2 production and ventilation in the hypoxic kitten. J Appl Physiol 1993; 74:904–910.

130. Rigatto H, Wiebe C, Rigatto C, Lee DS, Cates D. Ventilatory response to hypoxia in unanesthetized newborn kittens. J Appl Physiol 1988; 64:2544–2551.
131. Rehan V, Haider AZ, Alvaro R, Nowaczyk B, Cates DB, Kwiatkowski K, Rigatto H. The biphasic response to hypoxia in preterm infants is not solely due to a decrease in metabolism. Pediatr Pulmonol 1996; 22:287–294.
132. Dawes GS, Gardner WN, Johnston BM, Walker DW. Breathing in fetal lambs: the effect of brainstem transection. J Physiol (Lond) 1983; 335:535–553.
133. Gershan WM, Forster HV, Lowry TF, Korducki MJ, Forster AL, Forster MA, Ohtake PJ, Aaron EA, Garber AK. Effect of metabolic rate on ventilatory roll-off during hypoxia. J Appl Physiol 1994; 76:2310–2314.
134. Mortola JP, Rezzonico R, Lanthier C. Ventilation and oxygen consumption during acute hypoxia in newborn mammals: a comparative analysis. Respir Physiol 1989; 78:31–48.
135. Boddy K, Dawes GS, Fisher R, Pinter S, Robinson JS. Fetal respiratory movements, electrocortical and cardiovascular responses to hypoxaemia and hypercapnia in sheep. J Physiol (Lond) 1974; 243:599–618.
136. Easton PA, Anthonisen NR. Ventilatory response to sustained hypoxia after pretreatment with aminophylline. J Apply Physiol 1988; 64:1445–1450.
137. Lopes JM, Davis GM, Mullahoc K, Aranda JV. The role of adenosine on the hypoxic ventilatory response of the newborn piglets. Pediatr Pulmonol 1994; 17:50–55.
138. Dreshraj IA, Haxhiu MA, Miller MJ, Martin RJ. Endothelin-1 (ET1) acting on central chemosensitive areas causes respiratory depression in piglets. Pediatr Res 1993; 33: A1923.
139. DeBoeck C, Van Reempts P, Rigatto H, Chernick V. Naloxone reduces decrease in ventilation induced by hypoxia in newborn infants. J Apply Physiol 1984; 56:1507–1511.
140. Lawson EE, Long WA. Central origin of biphasic breathing pattern during hypoxia in newborns. J Appl Physiol 1983; 55:483–488.
141. Fung ML, Kang W, Darnall RA, St John WM. Characterization of ventilatory responses to hypoxia in neonatal rats. Respir Physiol 1996; 103:57–66.
142. Gluckman PD, Johnston BM. Lesions in the upper lateral pons abolish the hypoxic depression of breathing in unanesthetized fetal lambs in utero. J Physiol (Lond) 1987; 382: 373–383.
143. Johnston BM, Gluckman PD. Peripheral chemoreceptors respond to hypoxia in pontine-lesioned fetal lambs in utero. J Apply Physiol 1993; 75:1027–1034.
144. Waites BA, Ackland GL, Noble R, Hanson MA. Red nucleus lesions abolish the biphasic respiratory response to isocapnic hypoxia in decerebrate young rabbits. J Physiol (Lond) 1996; 495:217–225.
145. Moore PJ, Ackland GL, Hanson MA. Unilateral cooling in the region of locus coeruleus blocks the fall in respiratory output during hypoxia in anesthetized neonatal sheep. Exp Physiol 1996; 81:983–994.
146. Grunstein MM, Hazinski TA, Schlueter MA. Respiratory control during hypoxia in newborn rabbits: implied action of endorphins. J Apply Physiol 1981; 51:122–120.
147. Hazinski TA, Grunstein MM, Schlueter MA, Tooley WH. Effect of naloxone on ventilation in newborn rabbits. J Apply Physiol 1981; 50:713–717.
148. Moss IR, Scarpelli EM. Generation and regulation of breathing in utero: fetal CO_2 response test. J Appl Physiol 1979; 47:527–532.
149. Phillis JW, Wu PH. The role of adenosine and its nucleotides in central synaptic transmission. Prog Neurobiol 1981; 16:187–239.

150. Winn HR, Rubio R, Berne RM. Brain adenosine concentration during hypoxia in cats. Am J Physiol 1981; 241:H235–H242.
151. Jeffery HE, Read DJC. Ventilatory responses of newborn calves to progressive hypoxia in quiet and active sleep. J Apply Physiol 1980; 48:892–895.
152. Shannon DC, Gotay F, Stein IM, Rogers MC, Todres ID, Moylan FMB. Prevention of apnea and bradycardia in low birth weight infants. Pediatrics 1975; 55:589–594.
153. Davi M, Rigatto H. Apnea. In: Nelson NM, ed. Current Therapy in Neonatal-Perinatal Medicine. B.C. Decker Inc. (Toronto/Philedelpia), 1985–86:147–149.
154. Uauy R, Shapiro DL, Smith B, Warshaw JB. Treatment of severe apnea in prematures with orally administered theophylline. Pediatrics 1975; 55:595–598.
155. Greenough A, Morley CJ. Pancuronium prevents pneumothoraces in ventilated premature babies who actively expire against positive pressure inflation. Lancet 1984; 1:1–3.
156. Perlman JM, McMenamin JB, Volpe JJ. Fluctuating cerebral blood flow velocity in respiratory distress syndrome: relationship to the development of intraventricular hemorrhages. N Engl J Med 1983; 309:209–213.
157. Burnard ED, Grattan-Smith P, Picton-Warlow CG, Graung A. Pulmonary insufficiency in prematurity. Aust Paediatr J 1965; 1:12–38.
158. Escobar GJ, Littenberg B, Petitti DB. Outcome among surviving very low birthweight infants: a meta-analysis. Arch Dis Child 1991; 66:204–211.
159. Volpe JJ. Subplate neurons-missing link in brain injury of the premature infant? (editorial) Pediatrics 1996; 97:112–113.
160. Roffwarg HP, Muzio JN, Dement WC. Ontogenetic development of the human sleep-dream cycle. Science 1966; 152:604–617.
161. Southall DP, Plunkett MCB, Banks MW, Falkov AF, Samuels MP. Covert video recording of life-threatening child abuse: lesions for child protection. Pediatrics 1997; 100: 735–760.
162. Shannon DC, Kelly DH. SIDS and near-miss SIDS. N Engl J Med 1982; 306:959–1028.
163. Kelly DH, Shannon DC. Periodic breathing in infants with near-miss sudden infant death syndrome. Pediatrics 1979; 63:355–360.
164. Mellins RB, Balfour HH, Turino GM, Winters RW. Failure of the automatic control of ventilation (Ondine's curse). Medicine 1970; 49:487–504.
165. Rigatto H, Fitzgerald SF, Willis MA, Yu C. Search of the central respiratory neurons: II. Electrophysiologic studies of medullary fetal cells inherently sensitive to CO_2 and low pH. J Neurosci Res 1992; 33:590–597.
166. Aizad T, Bodani J, Cates D, Horvath L, Rigatto H. Effect of a single breath of 100% oxygen on respiration in neonates during sleep. J Appl Physiol 1984; 57:1531–1535.
167. Alvaro RE, DeAlmeida V, Kwiatkowski K, Cates D, Kryger M, Rigatto H. A developmental study of the dose response of the upper airway reflex to CO_2. Am Rev Respir Dis 1993; 148:1013–1017.
168. Lee DS, Caces R, Kwiatkowski K, Cates D, Rigatto H. A developmental study on types and frequency distribution of short apneas (3 to 15 secs) in term and preterm infants. Pediatr Res 1987; 22:344–349.
169. Phillipson EA, Bowes G. Control of breathing during sleep. In: Fishman AP, Cherniack NS, Widdicombe JG, Geiger SR, eds. Handbook of Physiology—The Respiratory System II. American Physiological Society. Baltimore: Williams & Wilkins, 1986: 649–689.

24

Syndromes Affecting Respiratory Control During Sleep

THOMAS G. KEENS

University of Southern California
Keck School of Medicine
Children's Hospital Los Angeles
UCLA School of Medicine
and Mattel Children's Hospital at UCLA
Los Angeles, California

SALLY L. DAVIDSON WARD

University of Southern California
Keck School of Medicine
and Children's Hospital Los Angeles
Los Angeles, California

I. Introduction

Once upon a time, there was a mermaid named Ondine. Mermaids are the daughters of Poseidon (Neptune), the God of the Sea. They are immortal, but they lose their immortality if they marry a mortal. One day, Ondine fell in love with a knight named Hans, and she married him, losing her immortality. As time passed, Hans tired of Ondine, and he left her for another woman. Poseidon was so infuriated with Hans that he placed a curse upon him so that none of his automatic bodily functions would occur unless he consciously willed them. The story ends as Hans is about to fall asleep, knowing that he will die because he will "forget to breathe." In 1962, Severinghaus first used the term *Ondine's curse* to describe three adults who lacked ventilatory responsivity of CO_2 following surgery to the brainstem (1). Thus, this name from the legend has persisted. However, the term has been most frequently used to describe a rare disorder where infants appear to breathe reasonably well while awake but severely hypoventilate and/or become apneic during sleep. Interestingly, the legend predicts that this disorder would not be confined to abnormal control of breathing but might also include other autonomic nervous system dysfunction. This chapter describes some of the disorders in infants and children known to cause hypoventilation during sleep.

II. Congenital Central Hypoventilation Syndrome

The classic example of a disorder of ventilatory control, as described in the legend, is congenital central hypoventilation syndrome (CCHS). CCHS is defined as the failure of automatic control of breathing, present from birth, of unknown etiology (2–13). Since breathing during non–rapid-eye-movement (NREM) sleep is neurologically controlled almost entirely by the automatic system, ventilation is most severely affected during quiet sleep in this disorder (5,13,14). However, breathing is also abnormal during active sleep and wakefulness, though usually to a milder degree (3,5,8–10). Disordered ventilatory control may range in severity from relatively mild hypoventilation during quiet sleep with adequate ventilation during wakefulness to complete apnea during sleep and severe hypoventilation during wakefulness. Other signs of brainstem dysfunction may be present but are not essential to make the diagnosis of CCHS (1,2,9–13). The incidence of CCHS is unknown, but it is generally considered to be rare.

A. Etiology

The cause or causes of CCHS are unknown. It is likely that this is a generalized disorder of the central and/or autonomic nervous system, which affects more than just control of breathing (15–17). Hirschsprung's disease is associated with CCHS in about 15% to 20% of cases (9,18,19). Multiple mediastinal and adrenal ganglioneuromas (16) and other tumors of neural crest origin (19) have been described. Ophthalmological abnormalities—especially those of neural control of eye movement, pupillary response, etc.—are frequently seen in CCHS (20). These all suggest that CCHS may be a more generalized neurological disorder, possibly due to abnormal embryonic development and/or nerve cell migration during development of the central nervous system.

Although it is also possible that CCHS is an inherited disorder (21–23), there are large families with only one affected child. Ventilatory control in parents and siblings of CCHS patients shows normal hypoxic and hypercapnic ventilatory responses, suggesting that there are no subtle decreases in ventilatory control in potential heterozygotes for CCHS (24). However, there have been reports of CCHS in siblings and in twins, suggesting the possibility of an inherited basis for CCHS. One female CCHS patient has given birth to a child who also has CCHS (personal communication). Weese-Mayer and colleagues found a suggestion of multifactorial inheritance in CCHS patients with Hirschsprung's disease, but this was less strong in CCHS without Hirschsprung's (21). She also found an increased familial incidence of sudden infant death syndrome (SIDS) in CCHS families (21). Although CCHS is not likely to be due to a simple inherited pattern (i.e., one gene), it is possible that CCHS has a complex hereditary origin. It is also possible that CCHS has a number of causes and that some may be hereditary but others are not. Further research is required to investigate this. However, it appears that the CCHS recurrence risk for subsequent children in a family with a CCHS child is generally low.

B. Physiological Pattern of Respiratory Control Abnormality

CCHS was initially thought to be a disorder of central chemoreceptor (hypercapneic) responsiveness (1,2,4–6,25). Respiratory stimuli are sensed by central chemoreceptors (primarily CO_2) and peripheral chemoreceptors (primarily hypoxia). The ventilatory controllers receive input from the chemoreceptors and send commands to ventilatory muscles to perform breathing. Paton and coworkers found that children with CCHS have absent chemoreceptor responses to both hypercapnia and hypoxia, even while awake, when tested by the rebreathing technique (8). This could be explained either by two distinct lesions in two anatomically separate chemoreceptors or by one abnormality in the brainstem respiratory center, which receives chemoreceptor input. This latter hypothesis is more likely (8). Humans also have an arousal response to CO_2 and hypoxia. Because ventilatory and arousal responses to respiratory stimuli use different neural pathways, CCHS children who have a disorder of chemoreceptor input integration for ventilation may still arouse to respiratory stimuli. To test this, Marcus and coworkers performed hypoxic and hypercapnic arousal responses in CCHS children and showed that most children with CCHS arouse to hypercapnia under very controlled circumstances, indicating intact central chemoreceptor input (26). Because these children did arouse to hypercapnia, the most probable mechanism for CCHS is a brainstem lesion in the area where input from both chemoreceptors is integrated for ventilation (26,27).

If children with CCHS have absent rebreathing ventilatory responses to both hypercapnia and hypoxia (8), how are they able to sustain adequate ventilation during wakefulness? Gozal and coworkers hypothesized that the ability of CCHS patients to maintain waking ventilation was due to intact peripheral chemoreceptor function, which could stimulate the abnormal brainstem centers if the signal was strong enough (28). By testing with acute hypoxia, hyperoxia, or hypercapnia, they found that peripheral chemoreceptor function was present and intact in CCHS children who are able to sustain adequate ventilation during wakefulness (28). Thus, CCHS appears to represent a primary physiological abnormality of integration of chemoreceptor input to central respiratory controllers rather than abnormalities in the chemoreceptors themselves.

An interesting physiological finding in CCHS is the effect of body movement on ventilation. Chemoreceptors are thought to be important controllers of ventilation during exercise. Thus, one would predict that CCHS patients may have trouble with exercise. In fact, Silvestri and associates showed severe gas exchange abnormalities in full-time ventilatory-dependent CCHS patients during moderate exercise (29). However, Paton and coworkers showed that exercise-induced hyperpnea does occur in CCHS patients who require ventilatory assistance only during sleep (30). These patients showed only mild gas-exchange abnormalities (decrease in oxygenation and increase in P_{CO_2}), though not enough to limit exercise. These CCHS patients increased minute ventilation and tidal volume with increasing exercise, but not as much as normal subjects. Paton found that body movement during exercise entrained ventilation in the absence of chemoreceptor function (30). Gozal and coworkers showed that *passive* leg motion also increased alveolar ventilation in CCHS (31). They hypothesized that rhythmic entrainment of respiration plays a significant role in the modulation of breathing in CCHS children, and thus some may tolerate exercise well (31). The presumed mechanism for this stimulation is by mechanoreceptors in the extremities. This finding also suggests that CCHS patients may be at higher risk for hypoventilation when they are inactive, as when watching television, reading, or studying (30,31).

C. Diagnosis and Clinical Course

The clinical presentation of CCHS may vary, depending on the severity of the disorder (9). Most CCHS patients present with symptoms in the newborn period. Many will not breathe at birth and will require assisted ventilation in the newborn nursery. Many of these CCHS infants do not breathe at all during the first few months of life but may mature to a pattern of adequate breathing during wakefulness, while apnea or hypoventilation persist only during sleep. This apparent improvement is due to normal maturation of the respiratory system and does not represent a change in the basic disorder (8). Other infants, presumably with a milder form of CCHS, may present at a later age with cyanosis, edema, and signs of right heart failure as the first indications of CCHS (9). These infants have often been mistaken for cyanotic congenital heart disease patients. However, cardiac catheterization reveals only pulmonary hypertension. Still other CCHS infants may present with tachycardia, diaphoresis, and/or cyanosis during sleep. Presumably, these infants would develop right heart failure if the diagnosis were not made and treatment initiated. Finally, others may present with unexplained apnea or an apparent life-threatening event (9). All CCHS patients have abnormal ventilation both awake and asleep, but spontaneous breathing is always worse while asleep. Approximately one-third of CCHS patients have such severe spontaneous hypoventilation while awake that they will require full-time ventilatory support. The remainder of CCHS patients, though not normal while awake, breathe well enough that sleeping ventilatory support is all that is required to avoid pulmonary hypertension and central nervous system complications.

The diagnosis of CCHS depends on the documentation of hypoventilation during sleep that is not secondary to ventilatory muscle dysfunction, lung disease, or other known neurological or metabolic causes (12). Continuous noninvasive monitoring of the adequacy of ventilation during sleep is best performed by pulse oximetry, end-tidal P_{CO_2} monitoring, or transcutaneous P_{O_2}/P_{CO_2} monitoring (15). Intermittent blood-gas sampling by arterial puncture or arterialized capillary sampling is not adequate, as it will cause arousal and therefore may not represent ventilation during sleep. However, blood gases, which accurately reflect gas exchange during sleep, can be obtained through indwelling arterial catheters. Typically, CCHS infants have an absent ventilatory response to hypercapnia and hypoxia (8), but the ability to demonstrate these abnormalities depends on the methodology used for testing (28).

The diagnosis of CCHS implies that the etiology of the hypoventilation is unknown. Therefore, other causes of hypoventilation should be ruled out before making the diagnosis. It goes without saying that primary lung disease, ventilatory muscle weakness, and cardiac disease should be ruled out. Magnetic resonance imaging (MRI) and/or computed tomography of the brain and brainstem should be performed to rule out gross anatomic lesions, which are absent in CCHS (32). A variety of inborn errors of metabolism may cause apnea or hypoventilation. Thus, a metabolic screen should be performed. Similarly, patients should have a neurological evaluation to rule out known neurological conditions that may cause these symptoms.

CCHS is characterized by abnormal ventilatory control in the absence of obvious brainstem anatomic lesions (8,26,28,32). However, as the legend predicted, it is now clear that CCHS patients have other abnormalities in autonomic nervous system function. Woo and coworkers found that all CCHS patients showed decreased beat-to-beat heart rate variability, indicating a dysfunction in autonomic nervous system control of the heart (15). CCHS patients frequently exhibit ophthalmological abnormalities reflecting neural control of eye function (20). There are anecdotal reports that CCHS children have poor heat tolerance. One of our patients sweats on only one side of her body. Bradycardia is not uncommon in CCHS, especially during sleep, though it rarely necessitates implantation of cardiac pacemakers (10). Two studies have reported poor school performance and/or decreased intellectual function in CCHS patients (9,10,17). It is unclear whether this is due to hypoxia or a direct result of the primary neurological problem associated with CCHS. Approximately 15% to 20% of CCHS patients have Hirschsprung's disease (9,10,18,19). Thus, any CCHS patient with constipation should be evaluated for Hirschsprung's disease. Tumors of neural crest origin have been described in CCHS (16,19). These latter two associations suggest that abnormalities in central nervous system development and/or embryology may be associated with CCHS.

D. Clinical Management

The treatment of CCHS is to ensure adequate ventilation when the patient is unable to achieve adequate gas exchange by spontaneous breathing (7,9–11,17,18). This requires mechanical assisted ventilation, as no pharmacological respiratory stimulants have been shown to be effective (2,9,25,35). CCHS does not resolve spontaneously; therefore, chronic ventilatory support at home is necessary in order for these patients to leave the hospital (8). Positive-pressure ventilators via tracheostomy or nasal mask, bilevel positive airway pressure, negative-pressure ventilators (9,33,34,36,37), or diaphragm pacing (38,39) are options for these patients. Although oxygen administration improves the Pa_{O_2} and relieves cyanosis, this treatment is inadequate, as hypoventilation persists and pulmonary hypertension ensues (17). Details of home mechanical ventilation are described at the end of this chapter.

CCHS patients lack a very essential protective physiological response: the ventilatory response to hypoxia and CO_2. Trying to compensate for this in a child at all times is not easy. During the first years of life, CCHS infants may be very unstable. Even minor respiratory infections may cause complete apnea during both sleep and wakefulness. Patients frequently exhibit abrupt respiratory failure or full respiratory arrest. As they mature, the neurological condition does not change, but the other parts of the respiratory system (lungs, ventilatory muscles, chest wall) mature. Thus, these patients gradually become more stable. It should be noted that some CCHS patients will worsen at 2 to 5 years of age. We believe that is because at this age, they are increasing their time spent awake and therefore are receiving less time on assisted ventilation. Their inability to achieve adequate spontaneous ventilation during the increased hours of wakefulness may cause pulmonary hypertension or central nervous system compromise. Older children and adolescents are usually more stable. Respiratory infections usually do not cause the degree of ventilatory depression that was seen in the first few years of life. However, CCHS patients do not regain their ventilatory responses to hypoxia or CO_2 at any age.

It cannot be overemphasized that CCHS patients may suffer complete respiratory arrest or severe hypoventilation at sleep onset. Thus, they require continuous observation and/or monitoring so that ventilatory support can be initiated with each sleep episode. Apnea/bradycardia monitoring alone is not sufficient, as many patients hypoventilate but are not apneic. An impressive finding in CCHS is the complete absence of subjective or objective response to hypoxia or hypercapnia while awake or asleep (8). Clinicians usually recognize hypoxia or respiratory failure in a child by manifestations of intact ventilatory control. Hypoxia and hypercapnia ordinarily stimulate respiratory drive, which increases ventilation, retractions, nasal flaring, a sense of dyspnea, etc. However, in CCHS, respiratory drive is absent. Thus, hypoxia is detected only much later, when it has already caused central nervous system depression (lethargy), cyanosis, or other complications. Therefore, these children need to be monitored continually by trained observers in order to prevent significant and sustained hypoxia and its sequelae. CCHS children should not swim, for example, except when being directly and carefully observed. Even more important, they should never be permitted to engage in underwater swimming "contests," as they will invariably swim further and longer than their normal colleagues but may become quite hypoxic and lose consciousness underwater.

Progressive pulmonary hypertension and cor pulmonale are not uncommon in these patients and must be assumed to be due to inadequate ventilator settings until proven otherwise. Some infants will have progressive pulmonary hypertension even when ventilator settings during sleep are appropriate. This is usually due to hypoventilation during wakefulness. These patients will require ventilatory support during wakefulness as well (9). For such patients, diaphragm pacing is an optimal form of ventilatory support during wakefulness because it is portable and permits these children to participate in normal activities while receiving "assisted ventilation" (38,39).

E. Medical Complications and Outcome

In patients with CCHS, the most common problem is inadequate ventilation, which occurs both during sleep and wakefulness. Thus, if these patients have any unexplained problem (seizure, lethargy, etc.), they should be stabilized by hyperventilation with 100% oxygen until the source of the problem can be identified. In children with CCHS, the etiology of any such problem is likely to be hypoventilation until proven otherwise. A brief period of hyperventilation will not be harmful but may be lifesaving if the child has inadequate ventilation.

In our experience, most CCHS children ultimately achieve adequate growth and nutrition (9). The mean height and weight for the adequately treated CCHS child is between the 25th and 50th percentiles. However, many CCHS infants have swallowing difficulties, with up to half requiring gastrostomies in order to facilitate nutrition (9,18). These can usually be removed at an older age (9). Pulmonary hypertension, resulting from chronic hypoventilation with hypoxemia, is the commonest reported cause of morbidity and mortality in CCHS (9,10). With adequate ventilatory support, this can usually be prevented. Many children with CCHS have transient episodes of pulmonary hypertension associated with intercurrent infections or with hypoventilation due to inadequate ventilator settings. These episodes are generally reversible.

Seizures associated with acute hypoxemic episodes are seen and may progress to persistent seizures requiring anticonvulsant prophylaxis (7,9,18,32,38). In our experience, these children generally have severe CCHS requiring ventilatory support during wakefulness. Hypoxemic episodes are not infrequently associated with permanent neurological sequelae.

Children with CCHS are generally in the slow-learner range of mental processing abilities, compounded by significant learning disabilities. Neuropsychological function appears to correlate with the severity of CCHS. Children with the mildest form of CCHS may function in the above-average range. Children who function in the mentally retarded range often have severe forms of CCHS and may require ventilatory support during wakefulness as well as during sleep (9,17).

Most CCHS children we treat attend regular classes in regular schools. Some children have been identified by school systems as having learning disabilities, and they may attend special education classes at a regular school. Others attend special education classes at specialized schools. Children are encouraged to be mobile and to participate in all appropriate age-related activities with their peers (9,17).

There is no known cure for CCHS, which appears to be a lifelong disorder (8,9). No CCHS patients have been documented to outgrow this disorder. With modern techniques for home ventilation, most children with CCHS can have prolonged survival with a good quality of life (7,9). This is in contrast to the poor prognosis for CCHS reported earlier (18,19,38). Thus, in our experience, the mortality rate for CCHS is low in patients who are consistently treated (9). We currently care for a number of children with CCHS who attend regular school and have normal lives while awake (9). Some of our CCHS patients are now young adults, have married, and are employed.

III. Myelomeningocele with Arnold-Chiari Malformation

The Arnold-Chiari malformation (ACM) of the brainstem is a complex deformity of the central nervous system, bone, and soft tissues (40,41). There is herniation of the medulla and cerebellum, giving rise to obstruction of the cerebrospinal fluid flow at the fourth ventricular outlets. Thus, hydrocephalus is common. Type II ACM, commonly associated with myelomeningocele, is characterized by displacement of the cerebellar vermis, caudal brainstem, and fourth ventricle through the foramen magnum. It can be predicted that the Arnold-Chiari malformation of the brainstem should affect brainstem respiratory centers and thus affect the neurological control of breathing.

A. Etiology

There are two basic theories about the etiology of ACM in myelomeningocele. One group of theories suggests that the actual brain in ACM is normal but was deformed by one or both of two mechanical processes: 1) traction from the myelomeningocele, which tethers the spinal cord to the skin opening, pulling the brainstem down through the foramen magnum with growth, and 2) hydrocephalus and increased intracranial pressure, which causes reopening of the previously closed neural tube, pushing the brainstem down through the foramen magnum (41,42). The second theory suggests that the ACM represents a primary, unidentified insult to central nervous system tissue and that it is not secondary to other mechanical actions (41). This latter view is supported by the high incidence of brainstem nuclear hypoplasia noted in one study (41). Elements of both theories are probably correct, and ACM is associated with abnormal formation and/or destruction of brainstem nuclei.

B. Ventilatory Patterns During Sleep

Abnormal vocal cord motility and the resultant obstructive apnea in infants with myelomeningocele is a major manifestation of abnormal ventilation (42–47). It has been suggested that this is due to increased intracranial pressure and is often successfully treated when intracranial pressure is reduced. Infants have also been noted to have clinically significant sleep hypoventilation, obstructive apneas, and breath-holding spells (48). In some cases, these resolve following posterior fossa decompression surgery (48).

Infants with myelomeningocele, hydrocephalus, and Arnold- Chiari malformation have abnormalities in their ventilatory pattern during sleep (49). Davidson Ward and coworkers made two-channel pneumogram recordings in infants with ACM without clinically apparent apnea or hypoventilation, finding that 72% were abnormal (49). These abnormalities were not related to the level of the spina bifida lesion. Oren and coworkers also demonstrated central sleep apnea, hypoventilation, and hypoxia in infants with ACM (48). Encabo and coworkers performed polysomnograms on nine patients with syringomyelia and found that sleep abnormalities were a frequent finding in these patients, even in the absence of any sleep-related symptoms (50). It is important to emphasize that many of these infants were clinically asymptomatic, yet they still demonstrated abnormal ventilatory patterns during sleep.

C. Ventilatory Responses to Hypoxia and Hypercapnia

Swaminathan and coworkers found that hypercapnic ventilatory responses were significantly lower in ACM adolescents compared to controls (51). Hypoxic ventilatory responses were not significantly different between ACM and controls, but individual patients had blunted hypoxic ventilatory responses (51,52). Gozal and associates studied peripheral chemoreceptor function in ACM patients, using acute hypoxia, acute hypercapnia, and hyperoxia (52). They found that some patients had abnormally low hypoxic responses, while most were normal. These investigators speculated that central ventilatory controllers may be affected in some ACM patients, suggesting that the ACM interferes with central chemosensitivity and central integration of chemoreceptor output (51,52).

Worley and coworkers performed hypercapnic ventilatory responses on 31 patients with spina bifida and found 19 of them to be abnormal (53). The abnormal CO_2 response tests also correlated with clinical evidence of brainstem dysfunction such as stridor, apnea, and dysphasia (53).

Arousal is an important defense mechanism against danger-signaling stimuli during sleep. Arousal responses to respiratory stimuli, such as hypoxia or hypercapnia, are different than ventilatory responses. Some infants and children with ACM have a central hypoventilation syndrome, which results in clinical apnea and/or hypoventilation (48,54). Davidson Ward and coworkers studied hypoxic and hypercapneic arousal responses in six of these children and found abnormalities in their arousal response to both hypoxia and hypercapnia (54).

D. Physiological Pattern of Respiratory Control Abnormality

Swaminathan and coworkers (51) found that older children, adolescents, and young adults with ACM have abnormal ventilatory responses to hypercapnia, indicating persistent abnormalities of respiratory control in older patients. These findings suggest an abnormality in the area of the central chemoreceptors in the brainstem (51). Although the exact anatomic location of the central chemoreceptors has not been defined, it is believed to be in the ventrolateral medulla (55). This is compatible with the anatomic defect in Arnold-Chiari malformation. Swaminathan and Gozal also demonstrated depressed hypoxic ventilatory responses in some subjects with ACM, though as a group they were not significantly different from control values (51,52). This could indicate involvement of central integrating pathways and/or respiratory neurons in some patients with ACM (55).

E. Clinical Management

Hays and coworkers reported the outcome of 616 infants and children with ACM (56). Thirty-five children, or 5.7%, had evidence of central ventilatory dysfunction, which included apnea, bradycardia, aspiration, vocal cord paralysis, and stridor. Of these 35 patients, 24 died (69%) (56). Apnea, stridor, and/or aspiration were the primary causes of death in 14 of the 24. Two had sudden, unexplained deaths during sleep without previous clinical respiratory problems (3.2 per 1000 ACM). Six additional children died from acute apnea (9.7 per 1000 ACM). Three died from increased intracranial pressure (4.9 per 1000 ACM). Thus, infants and children with ACM have an increased incidence of sudden death, often presumably due to apnea (56). Other investigators have documented a high incidence of acute respiratory arrest in children with ACM, presumably due to increased intracranial pressure (57).

It cannot be determined whether these signs of abnormal ventilatory control are due to abnormal brainstem nuclei or to mechanical compression of the brainstem. Little can be done for abnormally developed nuclei. However, mechanical compression can be relieved. Therefore, infants with ACM should be evaluated for hydrocephalus, which will be present in nearly all of them. This should be corrected as soon as possible with a ventricular-peritoneal shunt. If symptoms persist after correction of the hydrocephalus, a posterior fossa decompression of the brainstem should be seriously considered (48,58). Kirk and coworkers reviewed treatment of sleep-disordered breathing in ACM from six centers and found that posterior fossa decompression was only effective in 4 of 13 patients (31%) (58). However, we are given few clinical details. If performed, posterior fossa decompression must be performed as soon as possible to prevent progressive brainstem damage. It is possible that once significant respiratory symptoms are clinically evident, irreversible brainstem damage has already occurred. On the other hand, having a high clinical suspicion for sleep-disordered breathing in ACM infants, early investigation, and early treatment may improve the clinical outcome of these and other therapeutic interventions (58). Infants with apnea should be monitored with home apnea-bradycardia monitoring.

Upper airway obstruction from vocal cord paralysis during wakefulness and/or sleep develops commonly in ACM patients. Signs of obstruction should be investigated by laryngoscopy. If vocal cord paralysis is present, a tracheostomy is usually required. Again, surgical treatment of hydrocephalus and posterior fossa decompression should be performed promptly.

Some infants and children with myelomeningocele and ACM will develop inadequate ventilation during sleep or during both sleep and wakefulness. This central hypoventilation syndrome requires chronic ventilatory support. Again, surgical treatment of hydrocephalus and posterior fossa decompression should be performed promptly to prevent deterioration (58). Some children will do well with home mechanical ventilation. Those who require only sleeping ventilatory support may be able to attend school and have a reasonable quality of life while off the ventilator during wakefulness. Progressive neurological problems, such as syrinx formation and hydrocephalus, may occur but can be effectively treated with shunts. Thus, one should have a high level of suspicion for these complications in patients who show neurological deterioration. On the other hand, infants and myelomeningocele children with severe neurological damage, who also require assisted ventilation, have a poor prognosis because of progressive neurological deterioration, and many will die despite mechanically assisted ventilation (59). Therefore, the benefits and burdens of home mechanical ventilation should be weighed individually for each child, considering the current neurological condition, the child's overall function, and expected benefits (59).

IV. Prader-Willi Syndrome

Prader-Willi syndrome is characterized by obesity, hyperphagia, hypogonadism, mental retardation, hypotonia, and behavioral and sleep disorders. One of the most remarkable features is an apparently insatiable appetite, resulting in obesity. Reduced life expectancy is probably related to complications of morbid obesity. The prevalence of this disorder is estimated at 1 per 10,000 to 1 per 25,000 live births. Prader-Willi syndrome is associated with a deletion of the long arm of the paternally derived chromosome 15 (15q11-q13) in approximately 50% to 70% of patients. It is believed that a primary hypothalamic dysfunction leads to the typical clinical and behavioral manifestations of Prader-Willi syndrome.

A. Sleep-Disordered Breathing

Patients with Prader-Willi syndrome often exhibit sleep-disordered breathing. This is characterized by snoring, obstructive sleep apnea, restless movements during sleep, hypoventilation, hypoxia, excessive daytime sleepiness, and abnormalities of sleep architecture (60). However, it is unclear how much of this is related to obesity alone versus an intrinsic disorder of ventilatory control.

B. Ventilatory and Arousal Responses

Arens and coworkers measured rebreathing ventilatory responses to hypercapnia and hypoxia in obese and nonobese patients with Prader-Willi syndrome (61). They found that the ventilatory responses to hypercapnia were normal in nonobese Prader-Willi patients but blunted in obese patients. Thus, abnormalities in response to CO_2 are probably explained by obesity rather than a primary disorder of ventilatory control (61). It is also possible that obesity could be a marker for severity of the ventilatory control disturbance in these patients. Conversely, rebreathing ventilatory responses to hypoxia were completely absent in about one-third of patients and blunted in the remainder. This finding was consistent in all Prader-Willi subjects whether or not they were obese. Thus, hypoxic ventilatory responses were decreased in both obese and nonobese Prader-Willi patients, suggesting a primary ventilatory control abnormality in peripheral chemoreceptor function (61). Gozal and coworkers studied peripheral chemoreceptor function specifically with hyperoxia and acute hypoxic and hypercapnic challenges and found absent or depressed peripheral chemoreceptor function in all Prader-Willi syndrome patients (62).

Arens and coworkers tested hypoxic arousal responses (P_{IO_2} 80 torr) in Prader-Willi patients versus controls (63). They found that Prader-Willi patients compared to control subjects rarely aroused from quiet sleep in response to hypoxia. Similarly, the increase in heart rate stimulated by hypoxia was blunted in Prader-Willi patients compared to controls (63). Since peripheral chemoreceptor function is required for intact hypoxic arousal, this finding supports the hypothesis that Prader-Willi syndrome patients have absent peripheral chemoreceptor function (63). Livingston and coworkers measured hypercapnic arousal responses in Prader-Willi syndrome (64). Although all patients and controls aroused from quiet sleep in response to a hypercapnic challenge, the level of P_{CO_2} at which arousal occurred was significantly higher in Prader-Willi subjects than in controls (64). Since ventilatory responses to hypercapnia appear to be intact, this increased CO_2 arousal threshold may also reflect abnormal peripheral chemoreceptor function (decreased tonic stimulation). Brainstem dysfunction in areas of integration and/or reticular activating system may also be present.

C. Physiological Pattern of Respiratory Control Abnormality

Obesity has an effect on respiratory control and is associated with obstructive sleep apnea syndrome (see below). Thus, this may explain some of the sleep-disordered breathing seen in these patients. Further, rebreathing ventilatory responses to hypercapnia were depressed in obese Prader-Willi patients but not in nonobese patients (61). However, ventilatory responses to hypoxia were depressed in both obese and nonobese Prader-Willi patients, suggesting a primary disorder of ventilatory control independent of obesity. These findings suggest a peripheral chemoreceptor dysfunction (61–63).

Prader-Willi syndrome is thought to represent a primary hypothalamic dysfunction. Altered hypothalamic function may lead to abnormal ventilatory responses (65). The hypothalamus may modulate both hypercapnic and hypoxic ventilatory responses (66,67). Thus, the hypothalamic dysfunction in Prader-Willi syndrome may contribute to the ventilatory control abnormality seen in these patients.

D. Clinical Management

In Prader-Willi patients, the main clinical problem related to ventilatory control appears to be sleep-disordered breathing. One can reduce the severity of this problem with avoidance of obesity. Unfortunately, this is difficult in Prader-Willi syndrome, because patients have an insatiable appetite on the one hand and mental retardation on the other. The mental retardation makes it difficult to motivate these patients to decrease caloric intake. Obstructive sleep apnea should be treated as in other patients and may require nasal continuous positive airway pressure (CPAP), bilevel positive airway pressure, or upper airway surgery. In our experience, it is uncommon for Prader-Willi patients to require home mechanical ventilation. However, we did care for a child through the first 3 years of life who required chronic ventilatory support from infancy. As she lost weight, her ventilatory requirements decreased and she was able to be off mechanical assisted ventilation during some portions of wakefulness. Since the primary defect is peripheral chemoreceptor dysfunction, one should be especially concerned about situations where the patient's inadequate response to hypoxia may be health- or life-threatening.

V. Achondroplasia and Other Skeletal Dysplasias

Achondroplasia is an autosomal disorder characterized by inhibition of endochondral bone formation. Affected individuals have disproportionate shortening of the proximal limbs, a small thoracic cage, and a large head with a depressed nasal bridge. Achondroplasia is caused by mutations in the fibroblast growth factor receptor 3 gene. The base of the skull is involved and there is midfacial hypoplasia. Thus, obstructive sleep apnea is common and may be severe. However, the membranous bones of the skull grow normally. This results in a large skull resting on a small base with spinal stenosis. Therefore, compression of the medullary and cervical cord and hydrocephalus are common. These abnormalities lead to a high risk for abnormalities of central respiratory control, such as hypoventilation, apnea, and sudden death.

Further complicating the respiratory system in achondroplasia is the presence of restrictive lung disease due to the abnormally shaped chest. Thus, the evaluation of sleep-disordered breathing in achondroplasia may require a multisystem approach, including imaging of the head and neck for hydrocephalus and cord compression, assessment of gas exchange during wakefulness, polysomnography, and pulmonary function testing.

Mogayzel and colleagues have characterized sleep-disordered breathing in a series of 88 infants and children with achondroplasia (68). Nearly half of the subjects had abnormalities documented by overnight polysomnography. The most common abnormality was hypoxemia. The majority did not have significant obstructive or central apnea or hypoventilation, but a small number of subjects were severely affected. The authors comment on the contribution of restrictive lung disease and diminished pulmonary reserve to severity of gas exchange abnormalities during sleep (68).

Treatment options include ventriculoperitoneal shunt for hydrocephalus, cervicomedullary decompression for central respiratory control abnormalities and other neurological dysfunction, oxygen for hypoxemia, adenotonsillectomy for obstructive sleep apnea syndrome (OSAS), or bilevel positive airway pressure for hypoventilation and/or OSAS. Some infants and children with achondroplasia will require tracheostomy for severe OSAS, and a few will need positive-pressure ventilation via tracheostomy for central hypoventilation complicated by restrictive lung disease. Despite these difficulties, children with achondroplasia have normal intelligence and will do well with appropriate therapy (68–71).

Other skeletal dysplasias may also affect the brainstem area and/or cause thoracic restriction. In skeletal dysplasias, the latter may occur prior to birth, restricting growth of the rapidly developing lungs and causing structural hypoplasia of the lungs. Even with subsequent growth of the thoracic cage or attempted surgical reconstruction, the hypoplastic lungs may not be reversible. Thus, the presence of hypoplastic lungs is an important prognosticator for these patients.

VI. Leigh's Disease

Leigh's disease, also called subacute necrotizing encephalomyelopathy, is a group of inherited disorders in infancy and childhood characterized by a progressive clinical course of deterioration in brainstem function (72–76). Patients may appear normal during infancy but develop progressive neurological symptoms later. Clinical symptoms include poor feeding, vomiting, apnea, alveolar hypoventilation, and regression of development. Occasionally, hypoventilation can precede other neurological symptoms. Brainstem symptoms may include nystagmus, bizarre eye movements, pupillary changes, hypotonia, seizures, and sleep/wakefulness disturbances. Brainstem lesions are bilateral but not necessarily symmetrical. There is preferential gray-matter involvement with vascular proliferation, endothelial swelling, and progressive neuronal destruction. There is also loss of myelin. Changes are predominantly seen in the midbrain, pons, periaqueductal gray matter, posterior colliculi, medulla, floor of the fourth ventricle, and posterior olive. CT or MRI of the brainstem often show changes suggesting this diagnosis. Leigh's disease was once thought to be an autosomal recessive disorder. It is now clear that it is a syndrome with many etiologies, presumably all due to inborn errors of metabolism (75,76).

Recently, mitochondrial ATPase deficiency has been identified as the cause of Leigh's disease in a patient we follow. This has a cytoplasmic inheritance pattern and so is passed from mother to offspring. The previously healthy child presented with acute respiratory failure requiring mechanically assisted ventilation at the age of 4 years, accompanied by generalized severe neurological dysfunction. He required full-time home mechanical ventilation, which was rapidly weaned to sleep only. His subsequent clinical course has been characterized by marked fluctuations with alternating improvement and deterioration in neurological symptoms. His mother was diagnosed only after he presented, though she had relatively milder symptoms and has no clinically apparent respiratory control problem.

There is no specific treatment for Leigh's disease. Chronic ventilatory support is the only treatment for chronic respiratory failure, but it is not offered to some of these patients because of their poor prognosis due to neurological deterioration (74).

VII. Joubert Syndrome

Joubert syndrome is due to agenesis of the cerebellar vermis, with associated episodes of tachypnea (as high as 100 to 200 breaths per minute) alternating with prolonged apneas (77,78). Patients also exhibit abnormal eye movements, hypotonia, and severe psychomotor retardation. Tachypnea and apnea may occur during sleep or wakefulness. The tachypnea spontaneously resolves after infancy. We provide medical care for one patient who has moderate hypoventilation in addition to the apneas (P_{CO_2} 50 to 55 torr). The child also has significant obstructive apnea and vocal cord paralysis, which are presumed to be nonspecific signs of brainstem involvement. The disorder is often progressive, and the abnormalities in ventilatory pattern can cause death.

VIII. Acquired Central Hypoventilation Syndromes

Abnormalities in neurological control of breathing can be acquired, usually due to damage to relevant areas of the brainstem. When sufficient damage occurs, it can result in a central hypoventilation syndrome with attendant hypoxia and hypercapnia. In less severe cases, intermittent apnea may occur with adequate baseline ventilation. Causes of acquired central hypoventilation syndrome can include brain tumors (79), infections (encephalitis) (74,80), trauma, congenital vascular malformations (such as rupture of aneurysms), neurological surgery, central nervous system (CNS) radiation, and cerebrovascular accidents (74). In our experience, these conditions are uncommon and are often associated with other severe neurological damage. While damage to the brainstem can cause a disorder in neurological control of breathing, there is no characteristic pattern of the abnormality, as this will depend on the specific area of injury and extent of damage. However, because peripheral chemoreceptors are anatomically distinct from the brainstem, one is not likely to see dysfunction of a primary peripheral chemoreceptor. Rather, these patients usually have a combination of central chemoreceptor and central integration (ventilatory controller) dysfunction. In addition to a true disorder of neurological control of breathing, brainstem injury may also disrupt motor tracts leading to the ventilatory muscles. Thus, respiratory control dysfunction in these children is usually accompanied by ventilatory muscle weakness or paralysis from damage to motor tracts.

We have some experience in providing medical care for children with brainstem tumors and acquired central hypoventilation syndrome severe enough to require chronic ventilatory support. These children usually have signs of generalized severe neurological damage in addition to hypoventilation. In general, these patients require full-time ventilatory support. We have also seen a number of children after resection of craniopharyngioma. In addition to multiple endocrine problems from panhypopituitarism, many of these children are obese and have OSAS, which also includes elements of central hypoventilation syndrome. We have treated these patients with bilevel positive airway pressure using a backup rate.

IX. Obesity Hypoventilation Syndrome

Obesity affects ventilation primarily through mass loading of the respiratory system (81). Increased adipose tissue causes mass loading of the abdomen and thorax, reducing intrathoracic volume and diaphragm descent (82). Thus, work of breathing and resting metabolic rate are increased in obesity (81). There is also increased deposition of adipose tissue in the upper airway, decreasing upper airway caliber (83). In obesity, this increases pharyngeal resistance (84). These factors predispose to obstructive sleep apnea in obese patients during sleep (81,85). In general, these findings have been documented in obese adults, but comparable studies in children are lacking. Despite these respiratory abnormalities, most obese children do not exhibit sleep-disordered breathing (81,86). Mallory reported that only 15 of 46 (33%) morbidly obese older children and adolescents (mean 208% ideal body weight) had abnormal overnight polysomnograms, and only two were severe enough to require clinical intervention (86). Thus, hypoventilation and severe obstructive sleep apnea are uncommon, even in significantly obese children. On the other hand, Marcus and coworkers found that 10 of 22 obese children and adolescents (46%) had abnormal polysomnograms, with more obese children having more apneas (87). Five of the children (23%) had severe sleep-disordered breathing with arterial oxygen saturations ranging from 48% to 80% and end-tidal P_{CO_2} ranging from 52 to 66 torr (87).

There have been reports of children with severe obesity hypoventilation syndrome, often associated with severe obstructive sleep apnea, hypoxia, hypercapnia both awake and asleep, hypersomnolence, and cor pulmonale (85,88–97). These patients exhibit severe and life-threatening symptoms. Obstructive apneas occur and can be severe. However, continuous partial upper airway obstruction with persistent hypoxia and hypercapnia are seen more commonly in children than in adults (85). Hypersomnolence can be so severe that patients fall asleep in the middle of a sentence. These patients often have hypoxia and hypercapnia during wakefulness, but they are worse during sleep. Cor pulmonale is due to pulmonary hypertension from hypoxia and hypercapnia during sleep. In one patient we followed, rebreathing hypercapnic ventilatory responses were nearly absent and did not return to normal for several weeks following tonsillectomy and adenoidectomy. The fact that it did return to normal suggests that blunted hypercapnic responsivity is secondary to the mechanical effects of obesity on the respiratory system and severe obstructive sleep apnea rather than a primary abnormality in neurological control of breathing. Ventilatory responses to hypoxia and hypercapnia were not decreased in nonobese children with OSAS, suggesting that the propensity for OSAS is not due to primary neurological respiratory control dysfunction in children (98). However, there was a subtler finding that the ventilatory response to repeated hypercapnic challenges was diminished in OSAS children compared to controls (99). This has not been studied in obese children. Thus, obesity hypoventilation syndrome in children is probably due primarily to the mechanical loading of the respiratory system due to extreme obesity, which causes sleep-disordered breathing and severe obstructive sleep apnea, resulting in chronic hypoxia and hypercapnia. The respiratory control dysfunction probably represents habituation of brainstem centers.

The aim of treating obesity hypoventilation syndrome in children is to attempt to eliminate the obstructive sleep apnea (81,85). Removal of the tonsils and adenoids is the initial therapeutic procedure (85). For some patients, this will significantly reduce OSAS, improve gas exchange, and eliminate cor pulmonale and serious complications. Even if the tonsils and adenoids are normally sized, they cause a disproportionate obstruction to upper airway flow because they are situated in a small airway. It should be emphasized that patients with significant hypoxia and hypercapnia may not breathe in the immediate postoperative period following removal of tonsils and adenoids because of habituation to hypoxia and hypercapnia. Therefore, ventilatory support may be required for some time postoperatively. Some patients will require therapy in addition to tonsillectomy and adenoidectomy. CPAP or bilevel positive airway pressure by nasal mask are also useful in reducing obstructive sleep apneas (100). A tracheostomy will relieve the upper airway obstruction but is usually used only in the most severely affected patients. Mechanically assisted ventilation, via nasal mask or tracheostomy, may be required for such patients. Supplemental oxygen can be used as interim therapy while awaiting more definitive treatment (101). Supplemental oxygen not only reduces hypoxia but also decreases the number and severity of obstructive apneas (101). Hypercapnic patients should be carefully monitored with end-tidal P_{CO_2} during the introduction of supplemental oxygen to be sure that hypoventilation does not worsen. Of course, weight loss is the best treatment. However, this is often difficult to accomplish and will not happen quickly even if successful.

X. Management of Respiratory Failure in Children With Respiratory Control Disorders

There is usually little that can be done to augment central respiratory drive in children with respiratory control disorders. However, central respiratory drive can be further inhibited by metabolic imbalance, such as chronic metabolic alkalosis. Thus, serum chloride concentrations should be maintained above 95 mEq/dL and alkalosis avoided. Pharmacologic respiratory stimulants are not helpful (8,9,25,35). Sedative medications should be avoided.

A. Candidates for Chronic Ventilatory Support at Home

Children with respiratory control disorders are generally good candidates for chronic home mechanical ventilation (33,34). Any coexisting pulmonary disease must be sufficiently stable that the child does not require frequent adjustments in ventilator settings to maintain adequate gas exchange. In general, children with chronically elevated P_{CO_2} greater than 55 to 60 mmHg due to decreased central respiratory drive will develop progressive pulmonary hypertension. Although oxygen administration improves the Pa_{O_2} and relieves cyanosis, this treatment alone is inadequate, as hypoventilation persists, with resulting pulmonary hypertension. Thus, these children require home mechanical ventilation.

To achieve successful home mechanical ventilation, the FI_{O_2} that maintains Sp_{O_2} at or above 95% should be 40% or less. The requirement for peak inspiratory pressures (PIP) to achieve adequate ventilation should be less than 40 cmH_2O. If possible, the child should be weaned from positive end-expiratory pressure (PEEP), since home ventilators do not provide continuous flow of gas, and the technique for providing PEEP decreases portability of the ventilator (33,34).

B. Philosophy of Chronic Ventilatory Support

For most children going home with chronic ventilatory support, weaning from the ventilator is not a realistic goal. In order to optimize quality of life, these children must have energy available for other physical activities. Thus, ventilators are adjusted to meet the ventilatory demands of these children completely, leaving much of their energy available for other activities. For children with respiratory control disorders, ventilators are adjusted to provide a $P_{ET_{CO_2}}$ of 30 to 35 mmHg and Sp_{O_2} greater than 95% (33,34). Optimal ventilation also avoids atelectasis and the development of coexisting lung disease. Children who are hyperventilated at night have better spontaneous ventilation while awake than those who are ventilated to higher P_{CO_2} levels (102). It has also been our experience that children with respiratory control disorders have fewer complications, and generally do better clinically, with hyperventilation during assisted ventilation.

For the child requiring home mechanical ventilation, mobility and quality of life are maximized if the child can breathe unassisted for portions of the day (33,34). In our experience, the weaning of daytime assisted ventilation at home is best accomplished by sprint weaning (33,34). From the patient, parent, and caregiver standpoint, it is preferable to have a child who can be free of the ventilator for several hours a day than a child who must remain on the ventilator at all times, even if the ventilator rate or other settings are lower (9,33,34). *Sprint weaning* is performed by first adjusting the ventilator settings to completely meet the child's ventilatory demands. The child is then removed from the ventilator for short periods of time during wakefulness two to four times per day. In some cases, these initial sprints may last only a few minutes. Supplemental oxygen may be required during sprinting. The child is carefully monitored noninvasively during sprints to prevent hypoxia or hypercapnia. Guidelines for terminating sprints, such as Sa_{O_2} less than 95% or $P_{ET_{CO_2}}$ greater than 45 to 50 torr, should be provided as written orders. In addition, if the child develops signs of distress, tachypnea, retractions, diaphoresis, tachycardia, hypoxia, or hypercapnia, the sprint should be stopped. However, the child with a respiratory control disorder may *not* exhibit these signs of distress. The length of each sprint is increased daily or every few days as tolerated. The results of noninvasive monitoring of gas exchange and the child's clinical status during sprinting should be documented. Physicians should avoid the temptation to increase the sprint length too rapidly, as this often hinders the progress of weaning. Initially, sprinting should be performed only during wakefulness, when central respiratory drive is more intact (9,33,34). It should be emphasized that patients with some types of respiratory control disorders, such as severe CCHS, are not candidates for sprinting.

C. Modalities of Home Mechanical Ventilation

The ideal ventilators for home use are different from those used in hospitals for the treatment of acute respiratory failure (33,34). Because children with respiratory control disorders usually do not have severe lung disease, they have the greatest number of options for different techniques to provide chronic ventilatory support at home. These include 1) portable positive-pressure ventilator via tracheostomy, mask, or bilevel positive airway pressure (33,34,36); 2) negative-pressure chest shell (cuirass) (37); wrap or portable tank ventilator; or 3) diaphragm pacing (38,39).

Portable Positive Pressure Ventilator via Tracheostomy

Portable positive-pressure ventilators are the most common method of providing home mechanical ventilation for infants and children (7,9,33,34). Commercially available electronic portable positive-pressure ventilators can be battery operated, are relatively portable, and thus maximize mobility. Positive-pressure ventilators powered by compressed air are considerably less portable and not desirable for home use. Portable positive-pressure ventilators are not as powerful, technologically sophisticated, or versatile as traditional hospital ventilators. Consequently, when infants and children acquire an intercurrent illness, portable ventilators may not be capable of adequately ventilating them and hospitalization may be required (9,33,34). A tracheostomy is required for positive-pressure ventilator access to most patients. While this may appear to be a disadvantage, most infants and small children are subject to frequent respiratory infections, which often require hospitalization and assisted ventilation with higher rates and/or pressures. Since the tracheostomy provides ready access to the airway without the need for endotracheal intubation, a tracheostomy is not always a major disadvantage in young children (33,34). We prefer to maintain a small tracheostomy in ventilator assisted children for two reasons: 1) the small tracheostomy is less likely to cause tracheomalacia and 2) the small tracheostomy allows a large expiratory leak, so that the child may speak. While use of the small tracheostomy necessitates a large leak around the tracheostomy, using the home ventilator in a pressure plateau mode allows us to compensate for this leak.

Most commercially available portable positive-pressure ventilators are volume-preset ventilators. In traditional hospital practice, a delivered tidal volume of 10 to 15 mL/kg is used for mechanically assisted ventilation in infants, children, and adults. However, ventilator-assisted children generally have uncuffed tracheostomies. Therefore, a significant portion of the ventilator-delivered breath escapes in the leak around the tracheostomy (103). In some older children and adolescents, this leak is relatively constant and a higher tidal volume setting can be used to compensate for the leak and achieve adequate ventilation at home. However, this tidal volume setting must be derived empirically, as there is no way to predict the portion of a ventilator delivered breath that escapes through the tracheostomy leak. In infants and smaller children, the tracheostomy leak is large and variable and can rarely be compensated for by a single tidal volume setting (103). In this situation, the tracheostomy leak can be compensated for by using the ventilator in a pressure-limited modality, also known as *pressure plateau ventilation* (33,34,103). Some commercially available portable positive pressure ventilators have a high-pressure limit adjustment which is separate from the high-pressure alarm, while others offer an external pressure-limit valve. The pressure limit is adjusted to the desired PIP and a very large tidal volume setting is dialed in. The ventilator now functions as a pressure preset ventilator. When the pressure limit is reached, the pressure "plateaus" at that level. The remainder of the ventilator's tidal volume is delivered to the room rather than to the patient. For a small tracheostomy leak, the desired pressure limit will be achieved quickly, and a relatively large portion of the breath escapes through the ventilator. For a large tracheostomy leak, it will take longer to achieve the desired pressure limit, but the lungs will still be inflated to the same peak inspiratory pressure. In either case, the lungs will be inflated to the desired PIP, corresponding to a constant tidal volume. This technique is very successful in home ventilation of infants and small children (9,33,34,103) and has allowed us to ventilate infants and young children without the use cuffed tracheostomy tubes, PEEP, or continuous gas flow (9). It is also useful in older children or adolescents who have large or variable tracheostomy leaks.

The use of bilevel positive airway pressure and positive pressure ventilation by mask is discussed in Chap. 36 of this text.

Negative Pressure Ventilation

Negative pressure ventilators apply a negative pressure outside the chest and abdomen during inspiration to generate ventilation. A chest shell ventilator uses a dome-shaped shell that is fitted over the anterior chest and abdomen (37). The negative pressure wrap ventilator is a "jumpsuit" that fits snugly around the neck, wrists, and ankles to minimize leaks. A metal "cage" inside the jumpsuit creates a space where negative pressure can be generated during inspiration. A portable tank is a negative pressure ventilator, and an infant or child may fit inside. Negative inspiratory pressure is generated inside the chest shell, wrap, or portable tank, which expands the chest and upper abdomen. The ventilator rate and the negative pressure developed inside the chest shell, wrap, or portable tank can be selected. The negative pressure is proportional to the tidal volume but may be limited by leaks around the chest shell or wrap. These ventilators can provide effective ventilation in children and adolescents, sometimes without a tracheostomy (37). However, with negative pressure ventilation, there is no synchronous activation of the upper airway muscles, as normally occurs during spontaneous breathing. Thus, airway occlusion can occur when breaths are generated by a negative pressure ventilator during sleep. Therefore, infants and young children may require a tracheostomy. Since the major potential benefit of negative-pressure ventilators is that a tracheostomy may not be needed in older children, this technique may offer little advantage over positive pressure ventilation in the infant or young child.

In order for negative pressure chest shell ventilators to provide adequate ventilation, the chest shell needs to be closely fitted to the chest to avoid large leaks. Chest shells need to be changed and refitted as the child grows. The adequacy of gas exchange produced by negative-pressure chest shell ventilation needs to be checked frequently to assure that the chest shell fit and ventilator settings are optimal. Negative pressure wrap ventilators or portable tanks need not conform exactly to the chest configuration. Thus, they are better suited for small children or some children with scoliosis or chest wall deformities. However, the effectiveness of negative pressure ventilation depends on the ability to move the chest wall. Thus, children with marked scoliosis or chest wall deformities, which restrict chest wall motion, are not good candidates for negative pressure ventilation.

Negative pressure ventilators are not as portable as electronic positive pressure ventilators, nor are they battery-operated. Some patients have difficulty sleeping in the supine position necessitated by the chest shell or wrap. The portable tank does permit sleeping on the back or side. Skin irritation may occur when the chest shell rubs on the skin, although this can usually be avoided by having the child sleep with a T-shirt under the chest shell and with the use of baby powder or cornstarch on the skin. In general, children complain that negative pressure ventilators are quite cool because of the continuous movement of air. Thus, wearing a warm shirt is sometimes necessary for comfort, even during warm weather.

Negative pressure ventilation may permit decannulation of a tracheostomy. We have successfully transitioned CCHS children from positive pressure ventilation via tracheostomy to negative pressure ventilation to be rid of the tracheostomy after 5 to 6 years of age. Upper airway obstruction can be minimized by tonsillectomy and adenoidectomy, which optimizes the size of the upper airway.

Diaphragm Pacing

Diaphragm pacing generates breathing using the child's own diaphragm as the respiratory pump and is well suited to infants and children with central hypoventilation syndrome (38,39). Because this technique can be portable, it is useful for daytime support of ambulatory children requiring full-time ventilatory support in combination with positive pressure ventilation via tracheostomy for nocturnal ventilation (9). In addition, it can be used without a tracheostomy, and we have successfully transitioned CCHS children from positive pressure ventilation via tracheostomy during sleep to diaphragm pacing without a tracheostomy. Again, upper airway obstruction may occur during diaphragm pacer-generated breaths because synchronous activation of upper-airway muscles does not occur. In our experience, upper-airway obstruction can be minimized by tonsillectomy and adenoidectomy, which optimizes the size of the upper airway. Diaphragm pacing is discussed in detail in Chapter 37 of this text.

D. Hospital Management in Preparation for Discharge

Although the decreased central respiratory drive necessitating home mechanical ventilation may not be reversible, improvement in pulmonary mechanics will reduce the work of breathing and may increase the patient's ability to breathe spontaneously (33).

Many children develop some degree of chronic lung disease with elements of bronchoconstriction, pulmonary edema, chronic inflammation of the airway, and impaired mucociliary clearance (33,34). Children should receive the routine immunizations and annual split-virion influenza vaccine. These approaches may allow weaning from assisted ventilation for some portion of the day, significantly improving mobility and quality of life.

Ventilators used in the home should be equipped with a disconnect or low-pressure alarm, so that inadvertent disconnection of the ventilator from the tracheostomy can be detected and remedied (33,34,103). However, in infants and small children, the tracheostomy tubes are small and may offer sufficient resistance that the low-pressure alarm does not sound, even if the child has been extubated. Therefore we recommend the use of apnea-bradycardia monitors, which sense chest wall movement (impedance), and electrocardiography as an additional precaution for infants and small children (33,34).

Respiratory status must be stable on the *child's home ventilator* for at least two weeks prior to initial discharge (33,34,103). It is important to emphasize that settings on a home ventilator do not provide the same ventilation as the same settings on a hospital ventilator. Therefore, the child must be managed on home equipment prior to discharge (33,34,103). Invariably, ventilator settings will need to be increased on the home ventilator to achieve the same level of gas exchange achieved on a hospital ventilator. In the hospital, it is important to use the actual ventilator and circuits the child will use in the home (33,34,103). Because it is difficult to deliver PEEP using presently available portable ventilators, the patient should be weaned from PEEP whenever possible. This can usually be accomplished by increasing the ventilator rate or other settings (33,34,103).

Prior to discharge from the hospital, the family must become familiar with all aspects of their child's care (33,34,103). They must demonstrate competency in equipment operation, tracheostomy care, pulmonary physiotherapy, administration of medications including aerosols, and cardiopulmonary resuscitation. Families need to become adept at recognizing signs of respiratory compromise. However, infants and children with respiratory control disorders often do not show classic signs of respiratory distress because they have insufficient central respiratory drive to increase ventilation. Thus, parents must be taught to look for more subtle signs of hypoventilation, such as edema, lethargy, pallor, and headache. For some patients, a pulse oximeter and/or end-tidal P_{CO_2} monitor may be helpful for use at home to assess the adequacy of ventilation.

E. Home Management of the Ventilator-Assisted Child

Routine evaluation on ventilator settings should be performed on a regular basis so that ventilation meets the changing requirements of the growing child (33,34,103). During the first year of life, settings should be checked every 3 to 4 months. In the second through fourth years of life, settings should be checked every 4 to 6 months. After the fourth year of life, ventilator settings still need to be checked every 6 to 12 months. Following any change in the respiratory system (severe infection, hospitalization, etc.), settings should also be checked and readjusted (33).

Some ventilator-assisted children will also require supplemental oxygen during spontaneous breathing and/or during mechanically assisted ventilation. Oxygen requirements need to be assessed at regular intervals using noninvasive monitoring of oxygenation. Supplemental oxygen is not a replacement for home ventilation in children with chronic hypoventilation due to respiratory control disorders.

Because mechanical ventilation may not completely meet the ventilatory requirements at all times, even the most successfully managed patients may be exposed to periods of alveolar hypoxia and hypoventilation. Thus, all ventilator-assisted children with respiratory control disorders are at risk for the development of pulmonary hypertension and cor pulmonale. The usual clinical findings of right heart failure may not be present until late in the course. Echocardiography is a more sensitive method for following right heart function. Echocardiography to measure right ventricular dimensions, pulmonic valve systolic time intervals, septal morphology, pulmonic valve *a* dip, pulmonic valve early systolic closure, and acceleration time of pulmonary artery flow (Doppler) should be obtained at least every 1 to 2 years and more often if clinically indicated. When signs of pulmonary hypertension are discovered, it should be assumed that the level of mechanical ventilation is inadequate until proven otherwise (33,34,103). The patient may require hospitalization for continuous noninvasive monitoring of gas exchange and ventilator adjustments. Some patients requiring assisted ventilation only while sleeping may hypoventilate intermittently while breathing spontaneously during wakefulness. If this occurs frequently, pulmonary hypertension may result, even if mechanical ventilation at night is adequate.

Common childhood illnesses pose a unique threat to the ventilator-assisted child (33,34). Children with central hypoventilation syndromes will not increase respiratory effort, tidal volume, or respiratory rate even though a respiratory infection might be causing increased secretions and/or pneumonia, resulting in worsening P_{O_2} and P_{CO_2} levels. These children do not experience subjective dyspnea, and thus there will be no clinical evidence of increasing respiratory failure unless blood gases are measured or there is noninvasive monitoring of gas exchange. Despite the use of preventive and therapeutic measures directed at these problems, even a relatively trivial upper respiratory infection may compromise the ventilator-assisted child. Ventilator adjustments with an increased level of support are often needed. Young children ordinarily requiring ventilation only during sleep often need 24-hr-per-day support during illnesses. Because of these changes in the ventilatory requirements, these patients frequently require hospitalization for blood gas monitoring and frequent ventilator changes, though some may be safely managed at home, especially those over 4 years of age (33,34).

XI. Summary

There are no generally effective pharmacological treatments for true disorders of neurological control of breathing. Thus, therapeutic management usually requires mechanically associated ventilation or close monitoring of less severe clinical problems (apnea). The prognosis for children with syndromes affecting respiratory control during sleep depends primarily on associated neurological problems, the extent of central nervous system injury or involvement, whether the disorder is progressive, and the severity of hypoventilation. Some children with central hypoventilation syndromes, such as CCHS, can have prolonged survival associated with a good quality of life for them and their families by using mechanically assisted ventilation. For other children with progressive or severe neurological disorders the prognosis is poor and mechanically assisted ventilation may not be indicated. Complications in these children may result from delayed diagnosis and intermittent hypoxemia. We believe that early diagnosis of central hypoventilation and treatment of occult hypoxemia or hypoventilation will result in the best outcome. The level of treatment ultimately instituted must be individually tailored to the child and the specific respiratory control disorder.

References

1. Severinghaus J, Mitchell RA. Ondine's curse—failure of respiratory center automaticity while awake. Clin Res 1962; 10:122.
2. Mellins RB, Balfour HH Jr, Turino GM, Winters RW. Failure of automatic control of ventilation (Ondine's curse). Medicine 1970; 49:487–504.
3. Fishman LS, Samson JH, Sperling DR. Primary alveolar hypoventilation syndrome (Ondine's curse). Am J Dis Child 1965; 110:155–161.
4. Shannon DC, Marsland DW, Gould JB, Callahan B, Todres ID, Dennis J. Central hypoventilation during quiet sleep in two infants. Pediatrics 1976; 57:342–346.
5. Fleming PJ, Cade D, Bryan MH, Bryan AC. Congenital central hypoventilation and sleep state. Pediatrics 1980; 66:425–428.
6. Guilleminault C, McQuitty J, Ariagno RL, Challamel MJ, Korobkin R, McClead RE. Congenital central alveolar hypoventilation syndrome in six infants. Pediatrics 1982; 70:684–694.
7. Oren J, Kelly DH, Shannon DC. Long-term follow-up of children with congenital central hypoventilation syndrome. Pediatrics 1987; 80:375–380.
8. Paton JY, Swaminathan S, Sargent CW, Keens TG. Hypoxic and hypercapneic ventilatory responses in awake children with congenital central hypoventilation syndrome. Am Rev Respir Dir 1989; 140:368–372.
9. Marcus CL, Jansen MT, Poulsen MK, Keens SE, Nield TA, Lipsker LE, Keens TG. Medical and psychosocial outcome of children with congenital central hypoventilation syndrome. J Pediatr 1991; 119:888–895.
10. Weese-Mayer DE, Silvestri JM, Menzies LJ, Morrow-Kenny AS, Hunt CE, Hauptman SA. Congenital central hypoventilation syndrome: diagnosis, management, and long-term outcome in thirty-two children. J Pediatr 1992; 120:381–387.
11. Weese-Mayer DE, Hunt CE, Brouillette RT. Alveolar hypoventilation syndromes. In: Beckerman RC, Brouillette RT, Hunt CE, eds. Respiratory Control Disorders in Infants and Children. Baltimore: Williams & Wilkins, 1992: 231–241.
12. Keens T, Hoppenbrouwers T. Congenital central hypoventilation syndrome (770.81). In: Diagnostic Classification Steering Committee of the American Sleep Disorders Associ-

ation, eds. The International Classification of Sleep Disorders: Diagnostic and Coding Manual. Lawrence, KS: Allen Press, 1990: 205–209.
13. Gozal D, Gaultier C. Proceedings from the first international symposium on the congenital central hypoventilation syndrome, held in New Orleans, LA, on May 11, 1996. Pediatr Pulmonol 1997; 23:133–168.
14. Gaultier C, Trang-Pham H, Praud JP, Gallego J. Cardiorespiratory control during sleep in the congenital central hypoventilation syndrome. Pediatr Pulmonol 1997; 23: 140–142.
15. Woo MS, Woo MA, Gozal D, Jansen MT, Keens TG, Harper RM. Heart rate variability in congenital central hypoventilation syndrome. Pediatr Res 1992; 31:291–296.
16. Swaminathan S, Gilsanz V, Atkinson J, Keens TG. Congenital central hypoventilation syndrome associated with multiple ganglioneuromas. Chest 1989; 96:423–424.
17. Silvestri JM, Weese-Mayer DE, Nelson MN. Neuropsychologic abnormalities in children with congenital central hypoventilation syndrome. J Pediatr 1992; 120:388–393.
18. Haddad GG, Mazza NM, Defendini R, Blanc WA, Driscoll JM, Epstein MF, Epstein RA, Mellins RB. Congenital failure of automatic control of ventilation, gastrointestinal motility and heart rate. Medicine (Baltimore) 1978; 57:517–526.
19. Roshkow JE, Haller JO, Berdon WE, Sane SM. Hirschsprung's disease, Ondine's curse, and neuroblastoma—manifestations of neurocristopathy. Pediatr Radiol 1988; 19: 45–49.
20. Goldberg DS, Ludwig IH. Ocular signs in children with congenital central hypoventilation syndrome. Pediatr Pulmonol 1997; 23:150–151.
21. Weese-Mayer DE, Silvestri JM, Marazita ML, Hoo JJ. Congenital central hypoventilation syndrome: inheritance and relation to sudden infant death syndrome. Am J Med Gen 1993; 47:360–367.
22. Kinane TB, Burton MD. A genetic approach to congenital central hypoventilation syndrome. Pediatr Pulmonol 1997; 23:133–135.
23. Burton MD, Kinane TB. Studies of respiratory control in RET mutant mice. Pediatr Pulmonol 1997; 23:135–136.
24. Marcus CL, Livingston FR, Wood SE, Keens TG. Hypercapnic and hypoxic ventilatory responses in parents and siblings of children with congenital central hypoventilation syndrome. Am Rev Respir Dis 1991; 144:136–140.
25. Oren J, Newth CJL, Hunt CE, Brouillette RT, Bachand RT, Shannon DC. Ventilatory effects of almitrine bismesylate in congenital central hypoventilation syndrome. Am Rev Respir Dis 1986; 134:917–919.
26. Marcus CL, Bautista DB, Amihyia A, Davidson Ward SL, Keens TG. Hypercapneic arousal responses in children with congenital central hypoventilation syndrome. Pediatrics 1991; 88:993–998.
27. Davidson Ward SL, Keens TG. Ventilatory and arousal responses. In: Beckerman RC, Brouillette RT, Hunt CE, eds. Respiratory Control Disorders in Infants and Children. Baltimore: Williams & Wilkins, 1992: 112–124.
28. Gozal D, Marcus CL, Shoseyov D, Keens TG. Peripheral chemoreceptor function in children with congenital central hypoventilation syndrome. J Appl Physiol 1993; 74: 379–387.
29. Silvestri JM, Weese-Mayer DE, Flanagan EA. Congenital central hypoventilation syndrome: cardiorespiratory responses to moderate exercise simulating daily activity. Pediatr Pulmonol 1995; 20:89–93.
30. Paton JY, Swaminathan S, Sargent CW, Hawksworth A, Keens TG. Ventilatory response

to exercise in children with congenital central hypoventilation syndrome. Am Rev Respir Dis 1993; 147:1185–1191.

31. Gozal D, Marcus CL, Davidson Ward SL, Keens TG. Ventilatory responses to passive leg motion in children with congenital central hypoventilation syndrome. Am J Respir Crit Care Med 1996; 153:761–768.
32. Weese-Mayer DE, Brouillette RT, Naidich TP, McClone DG, Hunt CE. Magnetic resonance imaging and computerized tomography in central hypoventilation. Am Rev Respir Dis 1988; 137:393–398.
33. Keens TG, Davidson Ward SL. Ventilatory treatment at home. In: Beckerman RC, Brouillette RT, Hunt CE, eds. Respiratory Control Disorders in Infants and Children. Baltimore: Williams & Wilkins, 1992: 371–385.
34. Keens TG, Jansen MT, DeWitt PK, Davidson Ward SL. Home care for children with chronic respiratory failure. Semin Respir Med 1990; 11:269–281.
35. Swaminathan S, Paton JY, Davidson Ward SL, Sargent CW, Keens TG. Theophylline does not increase ventilatory responses to hypercapnia or hypoxia. Am Rev Respir Dis 1992; 146:1398–1401.
36. Beckerman RC. Home positive pressure ventilation in congenital central hypoventilation syndrome: more than twenty years of experience. Pediatr Pulmonol 1997; 23: 154–155.
37. Hartman H, Samuels MP, Noyes JP, Southall DP. Negative extrathoracic pressure ventilation in infants and young children with central hypoventilation syndrome. Pediatr Pulmonol 1997; 23:155–157.
38. Glenn WWL, Brouillette RT, Dentz B, Fodstad H, Hunt CE, Keens TG, Marsh HM, Pande S, Piepgras DG, Vanderlinden RG. Fundamental considerations in pacing of the diaphragm for chronic ventilatory insufficiency: a multi-center study. PACE 1988; 11:2120–2127.
39. Weese-Mayer DE, Hunt CE, Brouillette JR. Diaphragm pacing in infants and children. J Pediatr 1992; 120:118:1–8.
40. Schut L. The Arnold Chiari malformation. Orthop Clin North Am 1978; 19:913–921.
41. Gilbert JN, Jones KL, Rorke LB, Chernoff GF, James HE. Central nervous anomalies associated with meningomyelocele, hydrocephalus, and Arnold-Chiari malformation: reappraisal of theories regarding the pathogenesis of posterior neural tube closure defects. Neurosurgery 1986; 18:559–564.
42. Ruff ME, Oakes WJ, Fisher SR, Spock A. Sleep apnea and vocal cord paralysis secondary to type I Arnold-Chiari malformation. Pediatrics 1987; 80:231–234.
43. Morley AR. Laryngeal stridor, Arnold-Chiari malformation and medullary hemorrhages. Dev Med Child Neurol 1969; 11:471–474.
44. Bluestone CD, Delevine AN, Samuelson GH. Airway obstruction due to vocal cord paralysis in infants with hydrocephalus and meningomyelocele. Ann Otol Rhinol 1972; 81:778–783.
45. Krieger AJ, Detwiler JS, Trooskin SJ. Respiratory function in infants with Arnold-Chiari malformation. Laryngoscope 1976; 86:718–723.
46. Hollinger PC, Hollinger LD, Reichert TJ, Hollinger PH. Respiratory obstruction and apnea in infants with bilateral abductor vocal cord paralysis, meningomyelocele, hydrocephalus and Arnold-Chiari malformation. J Pediatr 1978; 92:368–373.
47. Badr AI, McLone D, Seleny FL. Intraoperative autonomic dysfunction associated with Arnold-Chiari malformation. Childs Brain 1980; 7:146–149.
48. Oren J, Kelly DH, Todres ID, Shannon DC. Respiratory complications in patients with myelodysplasia and Arnold-Chiari malformation. Am J Dis Child 1986; 140:221–224.

49. Davidson Ward SL, Jacobs RA, Gates EP, Hart LD, Keens TG. Abnormal ventilatory patterns during sleep in infants with myelomeningocele. J Pediatr 1986; 109:631–643.
50. Encabo H, Gene R, Nogues MA. Polysomnographic findings in syringomyelia and syringobulbia. Sleep Res 1986; 15:474A.
51. Swaminathan S, Paton JY, Ward SLD, Sargent CW, Jacobs RA, Keens TG. Abnormal control of ventilation in adolescents with myelomeningocele. J Pediatr 1989; 115:898–903.
52. Gozal D, Arens R, Omlin KJ, Jacobs RA, Keens TG. Peripheral chemoreceptor function in children with myelomeningocele and Arnold Chiari malformation type 2. Chest 1995; 108:425–431.
53. Worley G, Oakes WJ, Spock A. The CO_2 response test in children with spina bifida. Am Acad Cereb Palsy Dev Med 1985; 40A.
54. Davidson Ward SL, Nickerson BG, van der Hal AL, Rodriguez AM, Jacobs RA, Keens TG. Absent hypoxic and hypercarbic arousal responses in children with myelomeningocele and apnea. Pediatrics 1986; 78:44–50.
55. Milhorn DE, Eldridge FL. Role of ventrolateral medulla in regulation of respiratory and cardiovascular systems. J Appl Physiol Respir Environ Exerc Physiol 1986; 61:1249–1263.
56. Hays RM, Jordan RA, McLaughlin JF, Nickel RE, Fisher LD. Central ventilatory dysfunction in myelodysplasia: an independent determinant of survival. Dev Med Child Neurol 1989; 31:366–370.
57. Tomita T, McLone DG. Acute respiratory arrest: a complication of malformation of the shunt in children with myelomeningocele and Arnold-Chiari malformation. Am J Dis Child 1983; 137:142–144.
58. Kirk VG, D'Andrea L, Marcus CL, Gozal D, Rosen C, Brouillette RT. Efficacy of treatments for sleep-disordered breathing (SDB) in patients with spina bifida/myelomeningocele (SB/MM). Am J Respir Crit Care Med 1998; 157:A534.
59. Woo MS, Jansen MT, Jacobs RA, Davidson Ward SL, Keens TG. Home mechanical ventilation for children with Arnold-Chiari malformation. Am J Respir Crit Care Med 1994; 149:A376.
60. Cassidy SB, McKillop J, Morgan W. Sleep disorders in Prader-Willi syndrome. Dysmorphol Clin Genet 1990; 4:13–17.
61. Arens R, Gozal D, Omlin KJ, Livingston FR, Liu J, Keens TG, Davidson Ward SL. Hypoxic and hypercapnic ventilatory responses in Prader-Willi syndrome. J Appl Physiol 1994; 77:2224–2230.
62. Gozal D, Arens R, Omlin KJ, Davidson Ward SL, Keens TG. Absent peripheral chemosensitivity in the Prader-Willi syndrome. J Appl Physiol 1994; 77:2231–2236.
63. Arens R, Gozal D, Burrell BC, Bailey SL, Bautista DB, Keens TG, Davidson Ward SL. Arousal and cardiorespiratory responses to hypoxia in Prader-Willi syndrome. Am J Respir Crit Care Med 1996; 153:283–287.
64. Livingston FR, Arens R, Bailey SL, Keens TG, Davidson Ward SL. Hypercapnic arousal responses in Prader-Willi syndrome. Chest 1995; 108:1627–1631.
65. Moskowitz MA, Fisher JN, Simpser MD, Streider DJ. Periodic apnea, exercise hypoventilation, and hypothalamic dysfunction. Ann Intern Med 1976; 84:171–173.
66. Dillon GH, Waldrop TG. Electrophysiological and morphologic properties of caudal hypothalamic hypoxic- and hypercapneic-sensitive neurons in vitro. Soc Neurosci Abstr 1992; 492:10A.
67. Waldrop TG. Posterior hypothalamic modulation of the respiratory response to CO_2. Pflugers Arch 1991; 418:7–13.

68. Mogayzel PJ, Carroll JL, Loughlin GM, Hurko O, Francomano CA, Marcus CL. Sleep disordered breathing in children with achondroplasia. J Pediatr 1998; 131:667–671.
69. Pauli RM, Scott CL, Wassman ER, Gilbert EF, Leavitt LA, Hoeve JV, Hall JG, Partington MW, Jones KL, Sommer A, Feldman W, Langer LO, Rimoin DL, Hecht JT, Lebovitz R. Apnea and sudden death in infants with achondroplasia. J Pediatr 1984; 104: 342–348.
70. Reid CS, Pyeritz RE, Kopits SE, Maria BL, Wang H, McPherson RW, Hurko O, Phillips JA, Rosenbaum AE. Cervicomedullary compression in young patients with achondroplasia: value of comprehensive neurologic and respiratory evaluation. J Pediatr 1987; 110:522–530.
71. Stokes DC, Phillips JA, Leonard CO, Dorst JP, Kopits SE, Trojak JE, Brown DL. Respiratory complications of achondroplasia. J Pediatr 1983; 102:534–541.
72. Friede RL. Mitochondrial diseases. In: Friede RL, ed. Developmental Neuropathology. New York: Springer-Verlag, 1989: 496–498.
73. Koch TK, Lo WD, Berg BO. Variability of serial CT scans in subacute necrotizing encephalomyelopathy (Leigh's disease). Pediatr Neurol 1985; 1:48–51.
74. Beckerman RC, Hunt CE. Neuromuscular disease. In: Beckerman RC, Brouillette RT, Hunt CE, eds. Respiratory Control Disorders in Infants and Children. Baltimore: Williams & Wilkins, 1992: 251–270.
75. Devivo DC, Hammond MW, Obert KA, Nelson JS, Pagliara AS. Defective activation of the pyruvate dehydrogenase complex in subacute necrotizing encephalomyelopathy (Leigh's disease). Ann Neurol 1979; 6:483–494.
76. Willem JL, Monnens LAH, Trijbels JMF, Veerkamp JE, Meyer AEFH, van Dam K, van Haelst U. Leigh's encephalomyelopathy in a patient with cytochrome c oxidase deficiency in muscle tissue. Pediatrics 1977; 60:850–857.
77. Joubert M, Eisenring JJ, Robb JP, Andermann F. Familial dysgenesis of the cerebellar vermis. Neurology 1969; 91:813–825.
78. Harmant van Rijckervorsel G, Aubert-Tulkens G, Moulin D, Lyon G. Le syndrome de Joubert. Etude clinique et anatomopathologique. Rev Neurol 1983; 139:715–724.
79. Kuna ST, Smickley JS, Murchison LC. Hypercarbic periodic breathing during sleep in a child with a central nervous system tumor. Am Rev Respir Dis 1990; 142:880–883.
80. Brouillette RT, Hunt CE, Gallemore GE. Respiratory dysrhythmia: a new cause of central alveolar hypoventilation (case report). Am Rev Respir Dis 1986; 134:609–611.
81. Mallory GB Jr, Beckerman RC. Relationship between obesity and respiratory control abnormalities. In: Beckerman RC, Brouillette RT, Hunt CE, eds. Respiratory Control Disorders in Infants and Children. Baltimore: Williams & Wilkins, 1992: 342–351.
82. Naimark A, Cherniack RM. Compliance of the respiratory system in health and obesity. J Appl Physiol 1960; 15:377–382.
83. Surratt PM, Dee P, Arkinson RL, Armstrong P, Wilhart SC. Fluoroscopic and computed tomographic features of the pharyngeal airway in obstructive sleep apnea. Am Rev Respir Dis 1983; 127:487–492.
84. White DP, Lombard RM, Cadieux RJ, Zwillich CW. Pharyngeal resistance in normal humans: influence of gender, age, and obesity. J Appl Physiol 1985; 5*:365–371.
85. Davidson Ward SL, Marcus CL. Obstructive sleep apnea in infants and young children. J Clin Neurophysiol 1996; 13:198–207.
86. Mallory GB Jr, Fiser DH, Jackson R. Sleep-associated breathing disorders in morbidly obese children and adolescents. J Pediatr 1989; 115:892–897.

87. Marcus CL, Curtis S, Koerner CB, Joffe A, Serwint JR, Loughlin GM. Evaluation of pulmonary function and polysomnography in obese children and adolescents. Pediatr Pulmonol 1996; 21:176–183.
88. Jenab M, Lade RI, Chiga M, Diehl AM. Cardiorespiratory syndrome of obesity in a child. Pediatrics 1959; 24:23–30.
89. Spier N, Karelitz S. The Pickwickian syndrome. Am J Dis Child 1960; 99:136–141.
90. Cayler GG, Mays J, Riley HD. Cardiorespiratory syndrome of obesity (Pickwickian syndrome) in children. Pediatrics 1961; 27:237–245.
91. Warel WA, Kelsey WH. The Pickwickian syndrome. J Pediatr 1962; 61:745–750.
92. Finkelstein JW, Avery ME. The Pickwickian syndrome. Am J Dis Child 1963; 106: 251–257.
93. Metzel K, Kertges P, Kantor J, Bordy M. The Pickwickian syndrome in a child. Clin Pediatr 1969; 8:49–53.
94. Riley DJ, Santiago TV, Edelman WH. Complications of obesity hypoventilation syndrome in childhood. Am J Dis Child 1976; 130:671–674.
95. Simpser MD, Strieder DJ, Wohl ME, Rosental A, Rochenmacher S. Sleep apnea in a child with the Pickwickian syndrome. Pediatrics 1977; 60:290–293.
96. Orenstein DM, Boat TF, Stern RC, Doershuk CF, Light MS. Progesterone treatment of the obesity hypoventilation syndrome. J Pediatr 1977; 90:477–479.
97. Bourne RA, Maltby CC, Donaldson JD. Obese hypoventilation syndrome in early childhood requiring ventilatory support. Int J Pediatr Otolaryngol 1988; 16:61–68.
98. Marcus CL, Gozal D, Arens R, Basinski DJ, Omlin KJ, Keens TG, Davidson Ward SL. Ventilatory responses during wakefulness in children with the obstructive sleep apnea. Am J Respir Crit Care Med 1994; 149:715–721.
99. Gozal D, Arens R, Omlin KJ, Ben-Ari JH, Aljadeff G, Harper RM, Keens TG. Ventilatory response to consecutive short hypercapnic challenges in children with obstructive sleep apnea syndrome. J Appl Physiol 1995; 79:1608–1614.
100. Marcus CL, Davidson Ward SL, Mallory GB, Rosen CL, Beckerman RC, Weese-Mayer DE, Brouillette RT, Trang HT, Brooks LJ. Use of nasal continuous positive airway pressure as treatment for childhood obstructive sleep apnea. J Pediatr 1995; 127:88–94.
101. Aljadeff G, Gozal D, Bailey-Wahl SL, Burrell B, Keens TG, Davidson Ward SL. Effects of overnight supplemental oxygen in obstructive sleep apnea in children. Am J Respir Crit Care Med 1996; 153:51–55.
102. Gozal D, Keens TG. Passive nighttime hypocapnic hyperventilation improves daytime eucapnia in mechanically ventilated children. Am J Respir Crit Care Med 1998; 157: A779.
103. Gilgoff IS, Peng R-C, Keens TG. Hypoventilation and apnea in children during mechanical assisted ventilation. Chest 1992; 101:1500–1506.

25

Epidemiology and Natural History of Snoring and Sleep-Disordered Breathing in Children

NABEEL JAWAD ALI

Kings Mill Hospital
Nottinghamshire, England

JOHN R. STRADLING

Oxford University
and Churchill Hospital
Oxford, England

I. Introduction

The epidemiology of sleep and breathing disorders in adults has been studied extensively in several populations in Europe (1–3), Australia (4), and North America (5). By comparison the epidemiology of these disorders in children has received much less attention and so far the only studies have been European. This despite the fact that many centers in Europe, North America, and Australia routinely evaluate, diagnose, and treat children with snoring and sleep-related breathing disorders. This is evidenced by the considerable number of clinical reports and series published each year describing the clinical features and treatment of sleep and breathing disorders in children.

II. Historical Review

The first account of sleep apnea and its treatment (by nasopharyngeal scarification—i.e., adenotonsillectomy) was reported in 1889 by Hill (6). After Hill and until the early 1980s, snoring and associated symptoms in children were the almost exclusive province of the otolaryngologist. For most of the first half of this century, rather surprisingly, it was symptoms of sleep and breathing disorders that became an accepted routine indication for adenotonsillectomy (7). This approach continued until the late 1950s, when performing adenotonsillectomy for reasons other than recurrent tonsillitis began to be questioned (8,9). Indeed, it was felt by some that the pendulum had swung too far and that now children with sleep apnea were being left untreated because of a general reluctance to perform adenotonsillectomy (10).

The modern era of studying sleep and breathing disorders in children may be said to have begun with the report in 1976, when Guilleminault et al. reported eight children with severe sleep apnea who were diagnosed using the relatively new clinical tool of polysomnography (11). In this early report and subsequently, techniques that had evolved to diagnose sleep apnea in adults were applied to children with little modification.

III. Diagnostic Methods and Definitions

Any discussion of epidemiology should properly start with definitions of the disorder under consideration, but there are no widely accepted definitions of what constitutes clinically significant disordered breathing during sleep in children. There is a spectrum of physiological disturbance to upper airway function during sleep, from simple quiet snoring at one end, to full-blown classic obstructive sleep apnea at the other. In between, there are degrees of disturbance whose clinical consequences and importance are uncertain.

Polysomnography-based definitions and diagnostic criteria have been adopted widely and have come to be regarded as definitive, although they have not been validated. Polysomnography is viewed by many as the "gold standard" investigation (12), but this is largely due to historical accident rather than because of any particular merit as a clinical or research tool. It is important to note here that the polysomnographic approach has not been subject to rigorous investigation. No studies have examined whether this approach accurately represents sleep and breathing disorders (in adults or children) in a way that provides thresholds for predicting the likely clinical consequences or indeed the likely response and benefits from treatment at any particular level of abnormality.

The deficiencies of conventional polysomnographic criteria to diagnose sleep and breathing disorders in children were apparent early on. In 1982 Guilleminault and coworkers reported on a group of children who snored and had symptoms identical to those with sleep apnea. Their polysomnographic sleep studies showed no evidence of sleep fragmentation or apneas by conventional criteria (13). The symptoms in these children were attributed to exhaustion from the effort of snoring (they improved after adenotonsillectomy). This paper should perhaps have prompted a more skeptical approach to polysomnography than has been the case. More recently Rosen and colleagues have shown that conventional polysomnographic criteria do not identify children with significant upper airway obstruction during sleep (14). The recently published American Thoracic Society (ATS) guidelines recommend polysomnography as the investigation of choice for children with suspected sleep and breathing disorders, but the authors were unable to give clear diagnostic guidelines to direct therapy (15). The question of what constitutes a clinically significant sleep and breathing disorder in children remains unanswered. Currently most clinicians use a combination of history, examination, and some sort of confirmatory sleep study to manage individual patients. In the future, diagnostic tests will need to be tested on their ability to predict outcomes, for example, response to treatment or long-term adverse effects.

The problem of which diagnostic tests to use and how to interpret them is further complicated because studies of children have to be viewed in the context of continued physical growth and neuropsychological development. A clear description of the natural history of sleep and breathing disorders and their consequences is therefore crucially important in formulating diagnostic criteria. Yet, only one study has reported on the natural history of snoring and associated symptoms in young children (16).

Various research groups have used different techniques to study children's sleep, making direct comparisons difficult, but none has been shown to be better than any other in any formal studies. As discussed above, polysomnography is not the gold standard against which other methodologies have to be compared. It is simply the oldest, and it will have to be evaluated alongside the newer approaches as regards their ability to predict outcome (in particular, response to treatment or long-term adverse effects on educational or behavioral measures). In the meantime we should view the different methodologies with an equally critical eye and design studies to evaluate them properly.

It is against this background of uncertain definitions that we review what is known about the epidemiology of snoring and sleep-disordered breathing in children. In this review, we have purposely avoided making a clear distinction between the epidemiology of snoring and what might be termed the *obstructive sleep apnea syndrome*. This is because we believe that these disorders lie on a continuum, and as yet we are unable to define thresholds to separate the normal from the pathological.

IV. Snoring

Snoring is produced by vibration of the soft palate and faucal pillars and indicates upper-airway narrowing during sleep. Snoring is a cardinal symptom of obstructive sleep and breathing disorders; as such, it can be a marker of obstructive sleep apnea. More importantly, however, it is increasingly accepted that snoring itself can be associated with sleep disturbance and daytime symptoms every bit as disabling as the full-blown obstructive apnea syndrome in children (13). Latterly, the term *upper airway resistance syndrome* (UARS) has been applied to symptoms in adults of sleep disturbance due to snoring without complete apnea or hypopnea. Used in its broadest sense, this term recognizes that the important initiating pathophysiological event is disturbed upper airway function during sleep and is a better term than apnea/hypopnea. Therefore, inasmuch as snoring is a sign of abnormal upper airway physiology during sleep, its epidemiology is of interest.

Table 1 Details of Six Studies That Have Reported Snoring Prevalence Determined by Questionnaire[a]

Author (ref.)	Age, years	Study population	Response rate %	Snoring prevalence (95% CI)	Comments
Corbo (17)	6–13	1615	97%	7.3% (6%–9%)	Excluded 747 children not sharing a bedroom.
Teculescu (22)	5–6	190	100% See comments	10% (7.8%–14.3%)	Excluded 124 children from original population of 314. Restricted social group. See text.
Ali (18)	4–5	996	79%	12% (9.7%–14.3%)	No exclusions. Reported snoring confirmed in one third of a sample studied at home.
Gislason (25)	0.5–6	555	81.8%	3.2% (1.7%–5.1%)	No exclusions.
Hulcrantz (26)	4	325	100%	6.2% (3.8%–9.3%)	Incomplete study, target population 500.
Owen (27)	0–10	260	See comments	11% (7.8%–16.5%)	Stratified sample from original population of 4005.

[a]See text for further details.

Six community-based questionnaire studies have reported on snoring prevalence in children. The studies have all been from Europe and have used different but comparable methodologies and questionnaires. The salient features of these studies are summarized in Table 1.

The first study to be published was a report by Corbo et al. (17) in 1989 from Abruzzi, Italy. All 2362 children aged 6 to 13 years attending school in two towns were surveyed by questionnaire, with a 97% response rate. It was found that children who slept alone had a lower prevalence of habitual snoring (3.6%) compared to those sharing a bedroom (7.3%). The authors considered this to be due to underreporting, due to absence of a witness, so excluded the 747 (31.6%) children who slept alone from further analysis. While this seems justified, it is not the only explanation for the difference in snoring prevalence. A child sharing a bedroom with its parents or siblings is likely to reflect important socioeconomic factors. Those sharing their bedroom are likely to live in more cramped conditions and so be exposed to more infections and passive smoking—the latter an important risk factor for snoring in children both in the latter authors' study and in ours (18). Strachan et al. have shown that passive smoke exposure in children is linked with poorer socioeconomic conditions (19). The effects of passive smoke exposure are discussed in more detail later in this chapter.

Snoring was defined in the study by Corbo on a four-point scale, "never," "only with colds," "occasionally apart from colds," and "often" (this was classified as "habitual" snoring). The study was designed to examine the relationship of snoring to respiratory symptoms and passive smoking exposure and so did not include questions about apneic episodes or nonrespiratory symptoms. In this study, snorers were younger than nonsnorers, but the prevalences reported were not stratified by age. Unfortunately, therefore, we cannot infer anything about the peak age for snoring. In common with most other studies (and in contrast to adults) there was no difference in snoring prevalence between the sexes.

The overall prevalence of habitual snoring ("often") was 7.3%, 95% confidence interval (CI) 6% to 9%, among the 1615 children included in the study. There were significant increasing trends across the snoring groups (from "never" snorers to "habitual" snorers) in the prevalence of rhinitis, cough, and phlegm production and, to a lesser degree, diagnosed asthma. "Habitual" snorers were 2.9 (95% CI 1.7 to 4.8) times more likely to have rhinitis than those who "never" snored, but asthma was not statistically significantly more common, despite the significant trend across all the groups noted above, and was thus only a weak effect. The relation between snoring and atopy is discussed below. One curious finding was that habitual snorers were 2.7 (95% CI 1.6 to 4.5) times more likely to have had a tonsillectomy than never snorers. The finding is surprising because tonsillectomy would be expected to relieve snoring in the majority of children (20). Perhaps parents were reporting their children's snoring historically rather than currently. Another possible though less likely explanation is that despite tonsillectomy, these children still had an abnormally narrowed upper airway. In the study of Stradling et al. on snoring children, the postadenotonsillectomy sleep studies had not returned to the level of the control subjects by 6 months (20). Hulcrantz and coworkers have reported facial remodeling toward a more normal shape after tonsillectomy (21), especially if performed before the age of 6 years. We have no information on the age at which tonsillectomy was performed in Corbo's study. In our repeat community survey of children aged 6 to 7 years, snoring had stopped in all the 24 of 507 children who had had a tonsillectomy (16) since they had been first surveyed 2 years before (18).

The next study to be published was a survey of French schoolchildren aged 5 to 6 years in the Nancy District by Teculescu et al. (22). The study was designed to examine the effects of urban pollution on respiratory function and included questions about snoring. Ten kindergartens were selected for study. The authors deliberately excluded kindergartens with a high immigrant population or with low socioeconomic status. Starting with a population of 314 children, various exclusions meant that results from only 190 (60.5%) were analyzed. The questionnaires were administered by one of the authors and all the children had an ear/nose/throat (ENT) examination. Medical records including height and weight were available to the authors. Detailed lung function measurements were recorded. Snoring was scored on a four-point scale similar to that of Corbo (17): "never," "only with colds," "sometimes without colds," and "often" (this last group being defined as "habitual" snorers).

Teculescu et al. found a prevalence of habitual snoring of 10% (95% CI 7.8 to 14%) and no difference between the sexes; 54% never snored. Like Corbo, they found that habitual snoring was associated with a history of adenotonsillectomy. After entering their data into a multiple logistic model, a history of exercise-induced bronchospasm [odds ratio (OR) 8.7, 95% CI 2.8 to 26], atopic disease in the child (OR 3.9, 95% CI 2.0 to 7.7) and its siblings (OR 2.4, 95% CI 1.1 to 5.2), and the finding of tonsillar hypertrophy on examination (OR 2.2, 95% CI 1.1 to 4.4) were all independently associated with habitual snoring. There were no significant differences between the lung function, weight, or height of snorers compared with nonsnorers. The relatively low response rate at 60.5% achieved, and the selection of the study population by excluding non-Caucasians and avoiding children from poor socioeconomic backgrounds, makes it difficult to generalize their findings. Nevertheless the results are in general agreement with that of Corbo and ourselves (see below).

We reported our first survey of snoring and associated symptoms in 1993. This was a postal questionnaire study of 996 children aged 4 to 5 years living in Oxford. They were identified from the records of the Community Paediatrics Department and included all children of the target age living in the city. A response rate of 79% (782 of 996) was achieved.

The questionnaire defined snoring along a four-point scale: "never," "rarely," "sometimes even without a cold," and "most nights" ("habitual" snoring). Twelve percent of these children were reported to snore on most nights (see Table 1). In this study, 9.8% of parents had been told at some time that their child had enlarged tonsils, yet only 9 (1%) children had had a tonsillectomy. In our subsequent study of these children 2 years later this tonsillectomy rate had risen to 4.8% (16). A history of enlarged tonsils was 8.8 (95% CI 4.2 to 22) times more common in the "habitual" snoring group compared to the "never" snoring group.

Other symptoms associated with snoring in this study were mouth breathing, frequent coughs and colds, and difficulties with sleep. Like Corbo (17), we examined the questionnaire data using chi-square trend analysis. Using this approach, we found that these associations showed a highly significant trend across the snoring groups. The dose-response relationship was that the prevalence of mouth breathing, coughs and colds, and sleeping difficulties increased across the snoring groups and was highest in the "habitual" snorers.

Uniquely among studies of snoring in children, the questionnaire responses were validated by home sleep studies. Of the 94 "habitual" snorers, 66 (70%) had a home video recording and oximetry. Of these 66 children, 22 (33%) snored on the night of study, while only one (1%) of 66 "never" snoring children studied in the same way snored. The questionnaire thus had high sensitivity but poor specificity. It seems, then, that snoring may be overreported by parents (at least on the basis of one night of monitoring) rather than the reverse, as suggested by Corbo and coworkers (17). This overreporting of symptoms compared to sleep study results has also been found in clinical studies with more highly selected groups referred for investigation. For example, in one study from the United Kingdom, only 50% snored on the night they were observed (23); similarly, only 75% did so in a study from the United States (24). Nevertheless, the results show that questionnaires have considerable validity as an epidemiological tool.

Gislason and Benediksdottir (25) surveyed all 555 children aged 6 months to 6 years living in the Icelandic town of Gardaber. They used a questionnaire designed to identify children with symptoms of sleep apnea, some of whom were later admitted for a formal sleep study. They achieved a response rate of 88.1% (489 of 555) after two reminders. The full questionnaire has not been published but included items about snoring as well as apneic episodes. Snoring was assessed on a five-point scale that was later compressed into three: "never/seldom" = nonsnorers, "occasional," "often/very often" = habitual snorers. Other items included in the questionnaire were upper respiratory symptoms, sleep disturbance, parental smoking, and adenotonsillectomy. The results are reported stratified by age.

Overall 14 of 454 (3.0%, 95% CI 1.7 to 5.1) snored habitually and another 3 snored and had apneic episodes "often" or "very often." Four children were reported to have apneas but not to snore habitually. The numbers in each age group were small, but looking at the sex distribution data, snoring was commoner in younger boys (mean age 20 months) and in older girls (mean age 46 months). Habitual snoring prevalence in this study at 3% is the lowest reported so far. While the 95% confidence interval overlaps with those from other studies reported, the low prevalence may either indicate that snoring is truly less common in Iceland or may reflect confounding factors. Apart from the generally younger age of this study group, one possible explanation is the high rate of adenoidectomy in this population. A particularly high 22.5% of boys and 14.4% of girls had had this operation, perhaps explaining both the low prevalence of snoring and the sex differences reported (the adenoidectomy prevalence increases with age and the surgery was apparently performed at an earlier age in boys). Curiously, this study, which found the lowest snoring prevalence, also reported the highest prevalence of apneic episodes in young children. This is discussed in a later section.

Two other questionnaire surveys of snoring have been reported. Hulcrantz et al. (26) published interim results of a continuing epidemiological survey in 1995. This study was designed to estimate the prevalence of sleep and breathing problems and to examine the effects on orthodontic development in a cohort of 500 four-year-old children from one dental district in Sweden. At the time of publication, the investigators had data on 325 children. They interviewed all the parents at the time of the dental examination. In this group snoring "every night" was reported in 6.2% of children and apneas every night in 1.5%. Ten children had detailed sleep studies in hospital, but beyond stating that the results of monitoring agreed with parental reports, no further information is provided.

Snoring was significantly associated with a history of tonsillitis and the use of oral pacifiers. Analysis of the dental casts obtained showed that snoring children had narrower maxillae and a shorter mandibular arch than nonsnorers. Snoring children were more likely to have a parent who had had an adenoidectomy or/and a tonsillectomy, hinting at possible genetic influences. These results are preliminary, and the data provided are inadequate for a thorough evaluation of the results. When published in full along with the 2 year follow up data, this study should shed important light on the natural history of snoring, apneas, and the effects of intervention on dental arch development.

Owen et al. (27) selected a random sample of 529 children up to the age of 10 years drawn from a population of 4005 living in the town of Frome in Somerset, England. The sample was stratified into 11 yearly groups from birth to 10 years, and an equal number of boys and girls were studied. In all, 260 of 529 agreed to be studied, but 15 were excluded because they had had a previous adenotonsillectomy; thus, 245 of 529 (46%) were actually studied. All the children were visited by a nurse and the parents completed a questionnaire about sleep, snoring, daytime behavior, ENT condition, and general health. Snoring was defined along a four-point scale, "never," "rarely," "sometimes," and "often." All 245 children had overnight oximetry; in 222, the results were interpretable. Overall habitual snoring (or "often") was reported in 27 children (10 male), giving a prevalence of 11%. A total of 154 of 245 (63%) never snored. Unfortunately the results of snoring prevalence are not stratified by age.

A. Natural History of Snoring and Related Symptoms

Our longitudinal study of the natural history of snoring in children was the first and, at the time of writing, the only one so far reported (16). Previously, Corbo had reported a cross-sectional study of children which suggested that snoring prevalence fell between the ages of 6 and 13 years (17). Although the results as published do not stratify snoring prevalence by age, snorers were slightly though significantly younger than nonsnorers (9.1 years versus 9.7 years). In the study of Icelandic children aged 6 months to 6 years, snoring prevalence increased with age in girls and fell in boys. These results have been discussed above, but it is notable that no other study has found a sex difference in snoring prevalence. Two factors may have been important; first, the low overall prevalence of snoring and, second, the higher rate of adenotonsillectomy in boys than girls (25). Both these studies were cross-sectional in design and inferences about natural history cannot be made with confidence.

We repeated our questionnaire survey of the children who had taken part in our original study (in 1989/90 at age 4 to 5 years) 2 years later in 1992 when they were 6 to 7 years of age (16). Responses were received from 507 of 782 (64.8%). There were no significant differences between the 507 who replied to the second survey and those who did not as regards their responses to the original questionnaire in 1989/90. Thus, on the whole, the 507 who responded were probably representative of the original group of 782 children.

The overall prevalence of snoring was the same at age 6 to 7 years (11.2%) as it had been at age 4 to 5 years. The prevalence of restless sleep and hyperactivity did not change either, although "sometimes" or "often" falling asleep during the day had become significantly less common, at 10.2% (compared to 20.7% in the same group 2 years earlier). Over this period of 2 years between the surveys, the adenotonsillectomy rate had increased from 1% to 4.7%.

More than half of the children who had snored habitually at age 4 to 5 no longer did so at age 6 to 7, yet there was a substantial number of children who had continued to snore habitually over the period of study. These persistent snorers appeared to be at greater risk of displaying behavioral problems (see Sec. V). It is clearly important to try to establish why snoring persists in some young children. It may be that genetic factors are important and determine a smaller upper airway, which is at risk of further narrowing during sleep. Perhaps adenotonsillar hypertrophy persists longer in these children (for genetic or environmental reasons such as passive smoking) and leads to alterations in dental arch and facial morphology, such that the pharyngeal airway remains smaller than average. In this respect the previously mentioned longitudinal studies of Hulcrantz et al. (26) will be very interesting. Longitudinal community studies of snoring children are crucially important in understanding the evolution and long-term consequences of sleep and breathing disorders. Long-term follow-up studies that include sleep monitoring and an assessment of educational achievement and social development are clearly needed.

V. Prevalence of Sleep-Disordered Breathing Determined by Sleep Monitoring

From the initial discussion, it is clear that the distinction between sleep apnea and lesser degrees of sleep and breathing is somewhat artificial. Snoring without apneas can be associated with restless sleep and daytime symptoms (see below). The purpose of epidemiological research to some extent is to define what constitutes abnormality by determining the impact of a particular factor (in this case snoring and disordered breathing during sleep) in unselected populations. There are no satisfactory definitions of abnormal breathing during sleep, as evidenced by the recently published ATS guidelines (15). To some extent the debate has been bogged down in arguments over what is the "gold standard" investigation. This has obscured the fact that we do not understand the pathophysiology of these disorders well enough to know which physiological signals best predict symptoms. We do not know whether we should measure respiratory variables such as apneas and snoring or whether restlessness or arousal from sleep registered by electroencephalography (EEG) better predict symptoms and response to treatment.

Despite this problem, there have been three studies which have attempted to determine the prevalence of significant sleep and breathing disorders by carrying out sleep studies on children and correlating the results with possible daytime consequences. Each used different techniques but some comparisons are possible.

The first was our study of 132 children drawn from an original population of 996 children initially surveyed by questionnaire, described above (18). A total of 66 were drawn from the "habitual" snorers with associated symptoms of sleep disturbance, and 66 from among "never" snorers. All 132 children were studied at home with video recording and overnight oximetry. Seven (0.7%, using 996 as the denominator) children both snored and had associated sleep disturbance (determined by measurement of movement arousals) that could be attributed to upper airway obstruction. Therefore, our estimate of the prevalence of detectable sleep and breathing disorder was at least 0.7% (95% CI 0.3 to 1.5). However, another four children from the 996 had by chance had a previous sleep study (which showed similar abnormalities) as part of an earlier study (20). They had since had adenotonsillectomies and were now normal. If they are included in our estimate of the prevalence of sleep-disordered breathing, we obtain a theoretical figure of 11/996 = 1.1% (95% CI 0.6 to 2.0).

If we apply different and less stringent criteria to this population—for example, using oximetry to identify children with more than 2.8 > 4% dips in Sa_{O_2} per hour—without review of the video, then another 9 children would have been classified as abnormal. This would inflate our estimate of the prevalence to 2% (95% CI 1.2 to 3.1). We did not include these children in our published estimate because review of the video recording did not convince us that these abnormalities were unequivocally due to upper airway obstruction.

Gislason and Benediktsdottir (25) estimated the lower limit of sleep apnea syndrome prevalence as 2.9% (95% CI 1.5 to 4.8) in children aged 6 months to 6 years. This is based on the assumption that the 7 children who refused sleep study had sleep apnea in the same proportion as the 11 who agreed to be monitored. Furthermore, the denominator used to make the estimate excludes 101 children who, for various reasons, were not included in the study. Including these children would lower the estimate to 2.3% (95% CI 1.5 to 4.8). Sleep apnea syndrome was defined as being present if a child had more than three > 4% dips in Sa_{O_2} per hour. As shown above, when we reanalyzed our data using a similar cutoff, our estimate of the prevalence is very close to theirs. Finally, of course, the age groups studied were different, which might have an important bearing on prevalence.

Owen and coworkers studied oximetry records of 222 children aged up to 10 years from a community sample (27). They reported that a quarter of their population had a > 4% Sa_{O_2} dip rate of more than 2 per hour (there was no difference between snorers and nonsnorers). These results are at odds with those reported by us, where none of the nonsnorers had a > 4% Sa_{O_2} dip rate of more than 2.8 per hour (18). One reason may have been the age of children studied. Oximetry recordings in very young children are prone to more artifact, and as Owen et al. did not carry out video recording, it is difficult to exclude awake movement artifact as the cause of these oximetric abnormalities.

In conclusion, the two major studies on the prevalence of sleep-related breathing disorders that included monitoring gave very similar estimates when reanalyzed using the same criteria to define abnormality. However, as we shall see in the subsequent discussion, associated symptoms rather than just sleep study abnormalities are probably more interesting and relevant as regards the epidemiology of sleep-related breathing disorders.

A. Risk Factors for Snoring in the General Population

All the studies of snoring prevalence discussed above have to some extent also included a search for related causal factors. As early as the late nineteenth century it was appreciated that snoring resulted from enlarged adenoids and tonsils (28), and the studies discussed above have generally found that a history (18) or finding of enlarged tonsils (26) is associated with snoring in the general pediatric population.

Mouth Breathing and Upper Respiratory Infections

Mouth breathing is commonly reported by parents of children who snore. As well as a higher prevalence of "habitual" snoring, we also found a higher prevalence of mouth breathing (17.5%) (18) when compared to the findings of Hulcrantz (26) (7.4%). In our questionnaire, mouth breathing was strongly linked to snoring. Mouth breathing usually reflects nasal obstruction, which itself can provoke snoring by further lowering the negative intraluminal pressures that tend to collapse the pharynx. Of more interest, perhaps, are the potential long-term consequences of mouth breathing on the dental arch and on facial development. In rhesus monkeys, experimentally occluding the nose and forcing mouth breathing leads to changes in neuromuscular control that lower the mandible, protrude and alter the shape of the tongue, and ultimately lead to consistent changes in facial morphology and dental crowding (29).

The long-term effects of adenotonsillar hypertrophy and mouth breathing in childhood may explain why some children with sleep apnea who are initially cured by adenotonsillectomy develop snoring and sleep apnea again during adolescence (30). To what extent this predisposition is acquired as a result of nasopharyngeal obstruction or is inherited (31) is unclear. Hulcrantz and coworkers have reported work suggesting that adenotonsillectomy reverses some of the dental arch abnormalities associated with adenotonsillar enlargement, particularly if surgery is performed before the age of 6 years (21), and they are currently engaged in a prospective study of this. In a different study, Hulcrantz (26) found that snoring children were more likely to have parents who had had adenotonsillectomy than nonsnorers. Perhaps a tendency for lymphoid tissue to hypertrophy is inherited, as well as other facial characteristics that reduce pharyngeal dimensions.

Snoring was associated with frequent upper respiratory infections in several studies. Corbo found a significant relation between snoring and "cough and phlegm" that was independent of the effects of passive smoking. We found a similar effect in our study (MD thesis, N. J. Ali, University of Southampton). Teculescu et al. did not find an association between snoring and lower respiratory infections. Some of the differences in results may be explicable on methodological grounds. The questions used by these studies to define respiratory infections were different and may have been measuring different pathologies. It is certainly plausible that frequent upper respiratory infections by causing tonsillar enlargement and nasal blockage could be associated with snoring.

Passive Smoking

Studies in adults have found that snoring is associated with smoking (32). It was reasonable, therefore, to look for a relation between snoring in children and passive smoking, particularly as adenotonsillectomy rates in children have been linked by Said and coworkers to passive smoke exposure (33). Four studies have examined this issue; two found a definite association, one was equivocal, and another did not find a relation.

In their study of Italian schoolchildren, Corbo and coworkers (17) showed a dose response effect between snoring in children and the number of cigarettes consumed by their parents. In our study of children in Oxford, we also found a dose-response effect linking snoring and passive smoking. Table 2 shows the parental smoking data in our study. As described above, from our original population of 996 children, two groups were selected for home sleep monitoring. One group (66 children) snored "habitually" and had other symptoms suggestive of sleep-disordered breathing and the other group (66 children) did not snore or have other relevant symptoms (18). Snoring and other symptoms of sleep-disordered breathing increased significantly with the amount of cigarettes consumed by the mother. The father's smoking habits had a weaker effect. Presumably, this is because young children spend more time with

Table 2 Passive Smoking and Snoring: Results of the Oxford Study[a]

	Number of cigarettes smoked per day			
Mother's smoking habits	None $n = 87$	1–9 $n = 12$	>9 $n = 33$	χ^2
Never-snoring group	60%	42%	27%	Trend = 10.2 $p = .001$
Habitual snoring group with sleep disturbance symptoms	40%	58%	73%	
	Number of cigarettes smoked per day			
Father's smoking habits	None $n = 93$	1–9 $n = 7$	>9 $n = 32$	χ^2
Never-snoring group	54%	43%	37%	Trend = 4.2 $p = .04$
Habitual snoring group with sleep disturbance symptoms	46%	57%	63%	

[a]Eight children came from a single-parent family. They are classified as having a nonsmoking father.

their mothers; therefore, her smoking habits have the greatest impact on their environment. After allowing for social class as a confounding factor, children whose mothers smoked were 4.4 (95% CI 1.5 to 13.1) times more likely to be in the "habitual" snoring group with symptoms than were those with nonsmoking mothers (18). In our study, the symptoms of sleep and breathing disorders were more common in lower socioeconomic groups. Multiple logistic regression analysis showed this to be entirely due to the fact that smoking was more common among women from the lower socioeconomic classes.

In the study of French schoolchildren, Teculescu et al. found an increased risk of snoring with passive smoking, but the relation did not reach statistical significance, which the authors ascribed to underpowering of the study (22). The low prevalence of snoring in the Gislason and Benediktsdottir (25) study of Icelandic children probably explains their failure to find an association with passive smoking.

In summary, the two largest studies to examine the effect of passive smoking found that it was associated with an increase in the prevalence of snoring. The demonstration of a dose-response effect in these two studies and the previous work of Said and coworkers (33) showing an effect on tonsillectomy rates makes a causal relationship biologically plausible.

Atopy

As discussed above, mouth breathing and rhinitis are frequently associated with snoring. Two separate but related questions arise. Are atopic children more likely to snore? If so, does atopy play a role in causing adenotonsillar hypertrophy?

A recently published study from Baltimore reported a 36% rate of allergic sensitization in 39 habitually snoring children referred for sleep study (34). Unfortunately, the study was uncontrolled and the expected atopy rate is unclear. Furthermore it was carried out in a tertiary center and the group studied are likely to have been highly selected and not representative of the normal population. The results are potentially interesting because they suggest that atopic children might be more susceptible to sleep-disordered breathing than nonatopics.

Unfortunately there are no good epidemiological studies of snoring and atopy, although two of the studies already discussed have contributed some data. Teculescu (22) used the ATS-DLD respiratory questionnaire (35) and found that atopy in the index child (OR 3.9, 95% CI 2.0 to 7.7) or in a sibling (OR 2.4, 95% CI 1.1 to 5.2) was independently and significantly associated with habitual snoring. Exercise-induced bronchospasm had an even more powerful effect (OR 8.7, 95% CI 2.8 to 26.4). No attempt was made to verify the history with skin testing, although the researchers did have access to the children's medical records.

In our study of 4- to 5-year-old children, we compared the prevalence of atopic history (eczema, asthma or rhinitis) in the 66 "habitual" snorers with symptoms of sleep disturbance versus the 66 "never" snorers with no symptoms. We did not find an excess of atopic history or prescription of medications used to treat atopic diseases (18) among the "habitual" snorers. We also attempted to carry out skin testing in these children using three allergens (Der p, cat dander, and grass pollen). Less than half the children agreed to skin testing. In the "habitual" snoring group, 8 of 34 had one or more positive skin tests compared with 5 of 26 from the "never" snoring group. Thus there was no support for a link to atopy in our study, but of course the low uptake greatly reduced the power of the study. It does, however, underline the difficulty of carrying out even minimally invasive tests on community samples of "normal" children.

Further studies are needed to clarify the role if any of atopy in snoring and sleep-disordered breathing, as it may allow new therapeutic approaches.

VI. Consequences of Snoring in the General Population

A. Restless Sleep

Two studies have examined the relation of snoring to restlessness at night. In our questionnaire study, there was a highly significant trend linking restlessness at night with snoring (18). Habitual snorers were twice as likely (RR 2.1, 95% CI 1.5 to 2.8) to be restless at night than those who never snored. Home video recording of a subgroup of children confirmed the questionnaire results: children who were reported to snore and be restless did indeed have more nocturnal movement assessed by automated analysis of video recording. This confirmed an earlier study of children going for adenotonsillectomy, in whom reported restlessness at night fell toward control levels, as did the results of video recording after surgery (20). Thus, in general, parental responses to this question are acceptably reliable for epidemiological purposes.

Very similar results were reported by Gislason and Benediktsdottir (25). In their study, snorers were 2.6 times (95% CI 1.8 to 3.7) more likely to be restless at night. These two studies show that snoring in "normal" children living in the community is associated with sleep disturbance. This adds physiological plausibility to studies suggesting that snoring in these children leads to measurable daytime symptoms of sleepiness and behavior problems (see next section).

Better methods of assessing sleep disturbance suitable for use at home need to be developed and validated. This would enable better studies of the relationship between snoring, sleep disturbance, and behavior.

B. Daytime Symptoms

Daytime symptoms associated with sleep and breathing disorders have been described in case reports and series from many centers. From these studies it is clear that snoring without apneas can be associated with significant daytime symptoms (13,20). In other studies, it has become obvious that criteria for the diagnosis of obstructive sleep apnea in adults miss significant sleep and breathing problems when applied to children (14). All of these studies have been in children referred for investigation of symptoms and who are therefore highly selected. In this context, the results of community studies that have examined the relationship between sleep-related breathing disorders and daytime symptoms are especially important in informing the debate about diagnostic criteria.

The first community-based study of the relation between daytime behavior and sleep-disordered breathing was a case-control study published in 1983. Weissbluth et al. (36) identified 71 children from a total of 2076 who had attended the offices of five independent pediatricians. Children with diagnosed neurological or metabolic disorders were excluded. The 71 children were selected on the basis that their parents had reported that they "currently have behavioral, developmental or academic problems." Five control children were randomly selected from the 2076 for each case. Snoring was 2.3 (95% CI 1.3 to 4.1) times more common among the problem group than controls, and "difficult or labored breathing asleep" was 2.6 (95% CI 1.1 to 6.2) times more common.

Our questionnaire survey of 782 children found that hyperactivity increased significantly with the severity of reported snoring (18). Daytime sleepiness also increased but was not statistically significant. Children who snored habitually were 1.7 (95% CI 1.4 to 3.2) times more likely to be considered hyperactive than nonsnorers. Hyperactivity was defined as an "often" response to the question "Is your child considered to be hyperactive?" In the more detailed examination of 132 children selected for sleep monitoring (66 "habitual" snorers with symptoms of sleep disturbance and 66 "never" snorers) we asked parents and teachers to complete the Conners Child Behavior Scale (37). This is a well-validated scale in child psychopathology (38–40). These were children drawn from a "normal" population and thus their results on this scale did not fall within the frankly pathological range; we therefore defined normality as the 95th centile score for the "never" snoring group. Thus any score above this was defined as abnormal for the purposes of this study. Using this analysis, about 30% of children who had symptoms of snoring and sleep disturbance had abnormally high scores on the hyperactivity and inattention subscales (both parents and teacher) (18) compared of course to about 5% in the control group. These behavior patterns may have an important bearing on the social development and academic achievement of children, but next to nothing is known about their natural history and consequences.

Our study of the natural history of snoring and other symptoms provides further supportive evidence of a link between poor daytime behavior and snoring (16). As discussed above in the natural history section, approximately half of the children who snored in the first survey in 1989/90 no longer snored in 1992. We were able, therefore, to reexamine the relationship between this symptom and daytime behavior in a substantially different group of children drawn from the same population and using the same questionnaire. The overall prevalence of hyperactive behavior did not change between the surveys, although this symptom had resolved in over half of the children who were originally thought to be hyperactive. We found substantially the same relationships between snoring and hyperactivity as we had in the original survey. Thus, snoring had resolved in a large proportion of children, and, with it, hyperactive behavior.

Because we had longitudinal questionnaire data, we were also able to examine the effects of chronicity of snoring on behavior. Would children who were reported to be habitual snorers at the ages of 4 and 5 as well as 2 years later, exhibit worse behavior than those who had stopped snoring? To do this we combined the results of the two surveys to define four groups of children:

1. Never snorers. Those who "never" or "rarely" snored in both 1989/90 and 1992.
2. Ex-snorers. Those who had snored "sometimes" or "most nights" in 1989/90 but "never" or "rarely" did 2 years later.
3. Recent snorers. Those had had "never" or "rarely" snored in 1989/90 but snored "sometimes" or "most nights" in 1992.
4. Persistent snorers. Children who snored "sometimes" or "most nights" in both 1989/90 and 1992.

The results of linear trend analysis and calculation of relative risk are shown in Table 3. There were significant increasing trends from never snorers to the persistent snorers in the proportion who displayed hyperactive behavior and daytime sleepiness. Children who snored persistently were 2.4 (95% CI 1.3 to 4.3) times more likely to be hyperactive than never snorers.

This longitudinal study of children supports clinical studies which have found that snoring and restless sleep are associated with behavioral problems (20). The finding that chronic snoring is associated with more behavioral problems is not unexpected but may be important in defining clinical abnormality. More work needs to be done in this area, with long-term follow-up to examine the effects of these relatively mild degrees of sleep-disordered breathing on behavior, academic achievement, and social development.

Only one other study has reported on the relation between daytime sleepiness and sleep-disordered breathing. The study of Icelandic children (25) found that "often" or "very often" being "irritable/tired" (RR 1.8, 95% CI 1.2 to 2.4), and "abnormally sleepy in the day" (RR 2.9, 95% CI 1.1 to 7.2) were significantly more common in the 18 children who snored and/or had apneic episodes than among the 436 children who did not. The relationship between snoring and abnormal daytime sleepiness was much stronger than that observed in our study (18). Despite the lower overall prevalence of snoring in the latter population, these 18 children had more severe sleep related breathing problems than in the children we had used to examine the relation of snoring with daytime sleepiness. Nevertheless the 95% confidence interval for their estimate overlaps ours (18).

C. Growth

Some clinical studies suggest that growth may be retarded by sleep-related breathing disorders (20,41). The mechanisms are unclear but may include excess energy ex-

Table 3 Relationship Between Persistent Snoring and Hyperactivity, Daytime Sleepiness, and Restless Sleep in Oxford Study

	Snoring category						
	Never-snorer (n = 242)	Ex-snorer (n = 79)	Recent snorer (n = 62)	Persistent snorer (n = 124)	χ^2 trend	Relative risk[a]	Relative risk[a] (95% CI)
Hyperactivity	11.4%	22%	21%	36%	28.2 ($p < .0001$)	1.7	1.1–2.4
Daytime sleepiness	7%	11%	8%	17%	8.9 ($p = .029$)	1.8	1.0–3.4
Restless sleep	26%	45%	47%	60%	39.7 ($p = .0001$)	1.3	1.0–1.6

[a]Relative risk calculated for persistent snorers versus ex-snorers and recent snorers.

penditure associated with upper airway obstruction during sleep (42) or reduced sleep entrained growth hormone secretion (41). So far only one study has included measurements of growth in children with snoring and sleep-disordered breathing. In their as yet incomplete study Hulcrantz (26) found no differences between snorers and nonsnorers in height at age 4 years. More data may be available in their follow up study. Measurements of growth velocity, energy expenditure during sleep (42), and urinary growth hormone may all prove useful avenues of research. It should be pointed out, that growth failure tends to occur in children with the most severe sleep-disordered breathing, a relative rarity in community studies. For this reason, the study of growth failure may be more fruitfully directed at children seen in referral centers.

VII. Conclusions

It is clear from the prevalence studies that habitual snoring in children is a common phenomenon, at around 10%. As with adults, a certain amount of pharyngeal narrowing during sleep is presumably unimportant, as it does not produce significant sleep fragmentation. However, the data we have reviewed show that in a subpopulation of snorers there are symptoms that it seems reasonable to ascribe to sleep fragmentation. Most of this association seems to be due to snoring and sleep disturbance, without frank sleep apnea, calling into question traditional diagnostic criteria.

The limited longitudinal data imply that children may move in and out of a small pool of snoring and usually mildly symptomatic subjects. The causes of this snoring are clearly mixed and relate to tonsillar enlargement, environmental factors (in particular passive smoking), and perhaps genetic influences on lower facial structure.

The implications of these studies for the treatment of snoring with fragmented sleep are not really clear. A small amount of sleep fragmentation with mild symptoms, which may pass off in a few months, is unlikely to justify a tonsillectomy. Conversely, a severely sleep-fragmented child with marked daytime symptoms may well justify surgery, even if there is a possibility that the tonsils will atrophy in a year or two. The best we can do at present for cases in the large gray area in the middle is, as with many decisions in medicine, to rely on clinical judgment of individual cases.

References

1. Lavie P. Sleep habits and sleep disturbances in industrial workers in Israel: main findings and some characteristics of workers complaining of excessive daytime sleepiness. Sleep 1981; 4:147–158.
2. Stradling JR, Crosby JH. Predictors and prevalence of obstructive sleep apnoea and snoring in 1001 middle aged men. Thorax 1991; 46:85–90.
3. Gislason T, Almqvist M, Eriksson G, Taube A, Boman G. Prevalence of sleep apnea syndrome among Swedish men—an epidemiological study. J Clin Epidemiol 1988; 41: 571–576.
4. Olson LG, King MT, Hensley MJ, Saunders NA. A community study of snoring and sleep disordered breathing: prevalence. Am J Respir Crit Care Med 1995; 152:711–716.

5. Young T, Palta M, Dempsey J, Skatrud J, Weber S, Badr S. Occurrence of sleep disordered breathing among middle aged adults. N Engl J Med 1993; 328:1230–1235.
6. Hill W. On some causes of backwardness and stupidity in children. BMJ 1889; 1:711–712.
7. Moore I. The Tonsils and Adenoids and Their Diseases. London: Heinemann, 1928.
8. Fry J. Are all "T's and A's" really necessary? BMJ 1957; 1:124–129.
9. Hendley JD. Tonsillectomy: justified but not mandated in special patients. N Engl J Med 1984; 310:717–718.
10. Check WA. Does drop in T and A's pose new issue of adenotonsillar hypertrophy? JAMA 1982; 247:1229–1230.
11. Guilleminault C, Eldridge FL, Simmons FB, Dement WC. Sleep apnea in eight children. Pediatrics 1976; 58:23–31.
12. Gaultier C. Obstructive sleep apnoea syndrome in infants and children: established facts and unsettled issues. Thorax 1995; 50:1204–1210.
13. Guilleminault C, Winkle R, Korbkin R, Simmons B. Children and nocturnal snoring: evaluation of the effects of sleep related respiratory resistive load and daytime functioning. Eur J Pediatr 1982; 139:165–171.
14. Rosen CL, D'Andrea L, Haddad GG. Adult criteria for obstructive sleep apnea do not identify children with serious obstruction. Am Rev Respir Dis 1992; 146:1231–1234.
15. American Thoracic Society. Standards and indications for cardiopulmonary sleep studies in children. Am J Respir Crit Care Med 1996; 153:866–878.
16. Ali N, Pitson D, Stradling J. The natural history of snoring and related behaviour problems between the ages of 4 and 7 years. Arch Dis Child 1994; 71:74–76.
17. Corbo GM, Fuciarelli F, Foresi A, De-Benedetto F. Snoring in children: association with respiratory symptoms and passive smoking [published erratum appears in BMJ 1990 Jan 27; 300(6719):226]. BMJ 1989; 299:1491–1494.
18. Ali NJ, Pitson DJ, Stradling JR. Snoring, sleep disturbance and behaviour in 4–5 year olds. Arch Dis Child 1993; 68:360–366.
19. Strachan D, Jarvis M, Feyeraband C. Passive smoking, salivary cotinine concentrations and middle ear problems in 7 year old children. BMJ 1989; 298:1549–1552.
20. Stradling JR, Thomas G, Warley ARH, Williams P, Freeland A. Effect of adenotonsillectomy on nocturnal hypoxaemia, sleep disturbance, and symptoms in snoring children. Lancet 1990; 335:249–253.
21. Hulcrantz E, Larson M, Hellquist R, Ahlquist Rastad J, Svanholm H, Jakobsson OP. The influence of tonsillar obstruction and tonsillectomy on facial growth and dental arch morphology. Int J Pediatr Otorhinolaryngol 1991; 22:125–134.
22. Teculescu DB, Caillier I, Perrin P, Rebstock E, Rauch A. Snoring in French preschool children. Pediatr Pulmonol 1992; 13:239–244.
23. Croft CB, Brockbank MJ, Wright A, Swanston AR. Obstructive sleep apnoea in children undergoing routine tonsillectomy and adenoidectomy. Clin Otolaryngol 1990; 15: 307–314.
24. Carroll JL, McColley SA, Marcus CL, Curtis S, Loughlin GM. Inability of clinical history to distinguish primary snorting from obstructive sleep apnea syndrome in children. Chest 1995; 108:610.
25. Gislason T, Benediktsdottir B. Snoring, apneic episodes, and nocturnal hypoxaemia among children 6 months to 6 years: an epidemiologic study of lower limit of prevalence. Chest 1995; 107:963–966.
26. Hulcrantz E, Lofstrand-Tidestrom B, Ahlquist-Rastad J. The epidemiology of sleep related breathing disorder in children. Int J Pediatr Otolaryngol 1995; 32(suppl):S63–S66.

27. Owen G, Canter R, Robinson A. Overnight oximetry in snoring and nonsnoring children. Clin Otolaryngol 1995; 20:402–406.
28. Wells WA. Some nervous and mental manifestations occurring in connection with nasal disease. Am J Med Sci 1898; 677–692.
29. Miller AJ, Vargervik K, Chierici G. Sequential neuromuscular changes in rhesus monkeys during the initial adaptation to oral respiration. Am J Orthodont 1982; 81:99–107.
30. Guilleminault C, Stoohs R. Obstructive sleep apnea syndrome in children. Pediatrician 1990; 17:46–51.
31. Redline S, Tosteson T, Tishler PV, Carskadon MA, Milliman RP. Studies in the genetics of obstructive sleep apnea: familial aggregation of symptoms associated with sleep-related breathing disturbances. Am Rev Respir Dis 1992; 145:440–444.
32. Bloom JW, Kaltenborn WT, Quan SF. Risk factors in a general population for snoring: importance of cigarette smoking and obesity. Chest 1988; 93:678–683.
33. Said G, Zalokar J, Lellouch J, Patois E. Parental smoking related to adenoidectomy and tonsillectomy in children. J Epidemiol Commun Health 1978; 32:97–101.
34. McColley S, Carroll J, Curtis S, Loughlin G, Sampson H. High prevalence of allergic sensitization in children with habitual snoring and obstructive sleep apnea. Chest 1997; 111:170–173.
35. Ferris B Jr. Recommended respiratory disease questionnaires for use with adults and children in epidemiological research. Am Rev Respir Dis 1978; 118:7–54.
36. Weissbluth M, Davis AT, Poncher J, Reiff J. Signs of airway obstruction during sleep and behavioral, developmental, and academic problems. J Dev Behav Pediatr 1983; 4:119–121.
37. Conners CK. A teacher rating scale for use in drug studies with children. Am J Psychiatry 1969; 126:884–888.
38. Trites RL, Blouin AGA, Ferguson HB, Lynch GW. The Conners teacher rating scale: an epidemiological inter-rater reliability and follow up investigation. In: Gadow K, Loney J, eds. Psychosocial Aspects of Drug Treatment for Hyperactivity. Boulder, Colorado: Westview Press, 1981.
39. Trites RL, Blouin AGA, Laprade K. Factor analysis of the Conners teacher rating scale based on a large normative sample. J Consult Clin Psychol 1982; 50:615–623.
40. Rapoport JL, Benoit M. The relation of direct home observations to the clinic evaluation of hyperactive school age boys. J Child Psychol Psychiatry 1975; 16:141–147.
41. Goldstein SJ, Wu RH, Thorpy MJ, Shprintzen RJ, Marion RE, Saenger P. Reversibility of deficient sleep entrained growth hormone secretion in a boy with achondroplasia and obstructive sleep apnea [published erratum appears in Acta Endocrinol (Copenh) 1987 Dec; 116(4):568]. Acta Endocrinol Copenh 1987; 116:95–101.
42. Marcus CL, Koerner CB, Pysik P, Loughlin GM. Determinants of growth failure in children with the obstructive sleep apnea syndrome. J Pediatr 1994; 125:506–511.

26

Obstructive Sleep Apnea in Childhood

Clinical Features

RAANAN ARENS

University of Pennsylvania School of Medicine
and The Children's Hospital of Philadelphia
Philadelphia, Pennsylvania

I. Introduction

Obstructive sleep apnea syndrome (OSAS) in children is characterized by recurrent events of partial or complete upper airway obstruction during sleep, resulting in disruption of normal ventilation and sleep patterns (1). OSAS is most frequently diagnosed in normal children between the ages of 2 and 6 in association with adenotonsillar hypertrophy. Children with craniofacial anomalies and/or neurological disorders affecting upper-airway configuration and collapsibility during sleep may present at any time from early infancy through childhood.

OSAS has a range of clinical presentations that are manifest in mild to severe forms. Childhood OSAS may have a tremendous impact on the health of a child, since it is presumed that, if left untreated, OSAS may cause profound neurobehavioral and cardiopulmonary consequences affecting a child's health and lifestyle.

OSAS is not a new disorder. Children with adenotonsillar hypertrophy associated with loud snoring, breathing pauses, and awakenings from sleep were noted in the nineteenth century by Hill (2) and Osler (3). It was not until the mid 1960s, with the development of polysomnography and the ability to simultaneously monitor the electroencephalogram (EEG), electrocardiogram (ECG), airflow, and thoracic impedance during sleep that an understanding of the link between obstructive events during sleep and daytime symptoms in adults was possible (4). Several reports had suggested an association between adenotonsillar hypertrophy and cor pulmonale in children (5,6). However, the relationship between the then unrecognized, disordered breathing during sleep and these findings was not considered. The first detailed description of 8 children (ages 5 to 14 years) with adenotonsillar hypertrophy and OSAS by nocturnal polysomnography was published by Guilleminault et al. in 1976 (7). That report, coupled with increasing awareness of OSAS among pulmonary and otolaryngology physicians, has resulted in a dramatic increase in publications on OSAS in children (8–12). This work clearly distinguishes OSAS in children from OSAS in adults with respect to etiology, age of presentation, clinical manifestations, complications, polysomnographic criteria for diagnosis, and treatment (1,8,9) (Table 1).

Table 1 Comparison of OSAS in Children and Adults

	Children	Adults
Population characteristics		
Estimated prevalence	2%	2–4%
Common age at presentation	2–6 years	30–60 years
Gender	M = F	M > F
Weight	Normal, decreased, increased	Overweight
Major cause	Obesity Adenotonsillar hypertrophy	Obesity
Associated conditions	Craniofacial anomalies Neurological disorders	Postmenopause
Polysomnography findings		
Gas exchange abnormalities	Frequent	Usually
Duration of obstructive apneas	Any duration is abnormal	Events > 10 sec are abnormal
Abnormal apnea index (AI)	AI > 1	AI > 5
Abnormal respiratory disturbance index (RDI)	No normative data	RDI > 10
Sleep architecture	Often normal	Usually altered
Movement/arousal	Occasional	Common
Complications		
Neurobehavioral	Hyperactivity Developmental delay Poor school performance EDS uncommon	Severe EDS,[a] cognitive impairment
Cardiopulmonary	Pulmonary hypertension Cor pulmonale	Systemic and pulmonary hypertension Arrhythmias
Treatment of choice	Adenotonsillectomy	CPAP

[a]EDS, excessive daytime somnolence; CPAP, continuous positive airway pressure.

II. Epidemiology

The incidence of OSAS in adults is estimated to be 4% in men and 2% in women (13). In adults, the incidence of OSAS was found to correlate with age, degree of obesity, and male gender (14). A significant rise in the incidence of OSAS in women occurs after menopause (15). Moreover, administration of androgens may induce OSAS in males who are hypogonadal (16), suggesting that hormonal differences between and within genders may play a role in the pathogenesis of OSAS in adults.

There are no large-scale studies in children assessing the prevalence of OSAS. In preschool children, the incidence of OSAS is estimated to be 2% (17), whereas habitual snoring is more common and is estimated to occur in 6% to 9% of school-aged children (18). OSAS occurs in children of all ages, including neonates. Children with underlying conditions affecting the structure of the upper airway, such as craniofacial anomalies, may present with symptoms of obstruction early in the neonatal period, while a later onset of symptoms may be found in obese children, associated with excessive weight gain or growth of the tonsils and adenoids. The peak incidence occurs between 2 and 6 years of age, paralleling the prominent growth of the lymphoid tissue during these years (19). Recent data suggest that OSAS may be more common in children with a family history of OSAS, in African-American children, and in children with chronic upper and lower respiratory tract diseases (20,21). It is not certain whether gender predisposes to OSAS during childhood. In one study of prepubertal children, the prevalence of OSAS was found to be equal among boys and girls (22). In another study of 413 children 15 years of age and younger with OSAS, the need for adenotonsillectomy and intervention with continuous positive airway pressure (CPAP) was greater among males (23), suggesting that a more severe form of OSAS may be present in males. It should be pointed out that neither study was population-based; thus conclusions regarding the role of gender in predisposing to childhood OSAS are premature.

III. Clinical Features

Although most cases of OSAS in children are secondary to enlarged tonsils and adenoids, many other medical conditions may lead to OSAS. Some of the more common reported conditions associated with OSAS during childhood are listed and referenced in Table 2 (24–63). Clinical features of OSAS in children can be divided into nocturnal and daytime signs and symptoms (Table 3).

The main physiological disturbance involves repetitive obstructive apneas and hypopneas leading to hypoxemia, hypercapnia, acidosis, and sleep disturbance (Figs. 1 and 2). Table 4 describes the breathing patterns associated with OSAS in children. The short- and long-term neurological, cardiovascular, and systemic complications found in children with OSAS are dependent on the severity and duration of these physiological aberrations.

Table 2 Medical Conditions Associated with OSAS in Children

	Refs.		Refs.
Craniofacial syndromes		Neurological disorders	
Midfacial hypoplasia		Cerebral palsy	40,41
Apert syndrome	24,25	Myasthenia gravis	42
Crouzon syndrome	24	Möbius syndrome	43
Pfeiffer syndrome	24,25	Arnold-Chiari malformation	44
Treacher-Collins syndrome	26	Miscellaneous disorders	
Macroglossia/glossoptosis		Obesity	45–47
Down syndrome	27–30	Prader-Willi syndrome	48,49
Beckwith-Wiedeman syndrome	31	Hypothyroidism	50
		Mucopolysaccharidosis	51,52
Pierre Robin sequence	32–34	Sickle cell disease	53–55
Other		Choanal stenosis	39
Achondroplasia	35	Laryngomalacia	56,57
Hallerman-Streiff syndrome	36	Airway papillomatosis	58
Klippel-Feil syndrome	37	Subglottic stenosis	59
Goldenhar syndrome	38	Face and neck burns	60
Marfan syndrome	39	Postoperative disorders	
		Pharyngeal flap	61,62
		Cleft lip repair	63

A. Nocturnal Symptoms

Breathing During Sleep

Snoring and difficulty breathing during sleep are the most common complaints of parents of children with OSAS. These symptoms are reported in more than 96% of cases (64,65). With the exception of young infants, children with OSAS often snore loudly and continuously. In the older child, snoring is often a low-frequency sound produced by vibration of the soft palate and tonsillar pillars. However, in a young child, the snoring sound may have a higher pitch if oversized adenoids and tonsils impede movement of the soft palate. Some children do not snore but have other forms of noisy breathing such as grunting, snorting, or gasping. Furthermore, infants may not produce sufficient flow to produce an easily audible snoring noise. Parents often describe episodes of retractions with increased respiratory effort. At times, absence of respiratory noise despite continued vigorous breathing may be noted. These episodes may be terminated by gasping, movement, or frequent awakenings. Breathing during sleep may be frightening to the parents, resulting in increased vigilance on the part of the family and the perceived need to intervene in order to improve breathing.

When possible, observation of the child during sleep is recommended. Snoring and labored breathing should be noted. This is manifest by visible supraclavicular, suprasternal, and subcostal retractions. Paradoxical rib cage movement has been de-

Table 3 Frequency of Signs and Symptoms in 23 Children with Obstructive Sleep Apnea Syndrome and in 46 Matched Controls

Sign/symptom	OSAS group, %	Control group, %	*p* Value
Difficulty breathing when asleep	96	2	.001
Snoring	96	9	.001
Mouth-breathes when awake	87	18	.001
Frequent upper respiratory tract infections	83	28	.001
Stops breathing when asleep	78	5	.001
Restless sleep	78	23	.001
Chronic rhinorrhea	61	11	.001
Sweating when sleeping	50	16	.007
Recurrent middle ear diseases	43	17	.019
Excessive daytime somnolence	33	9	.014
Poor appetite	30	9	.019
Frequent nausea/vomiting	30	2	.001
Difficulty swallowing	26	2	.002
Pathological shyness/social withdrawal	22	5	.027
Hearing problems	13	0	.014

Source: Modified from Ref. 65.

scribed as a marker of increased work of breathing. In the presence of complete or partial upper airway obstruction, inspiratory downward motion of the diaphragm will expand the abdominal wall; however, the sudden increase in negative intrathoracic pressure will cause a paradoxical inward movement of the highly compliant rib cage of the young child.

Children with OSAS are found to have both complete and partial upper-airway obstruction causing significant gas exchange abnormalities. Marcus et al., in a study of 50 healthy children 1 to 17 years of age, found that obstructive apnea was rare and was never longer than 10 sec, suggesting that obstructive apnea of any length is abnormal in children (11). Partial obstruction evidenced by snoring appears to dominate the respiratory pattern in children (8). Partial obstruction occurs continuously or it can be interrupted by periods of silence associated with continued vigorous respiratory effort (obstructive apnea). Variations in esophageal pressures as low as −50 and −70 cmH_2O and with significant abrupt changes in oxygenation have been reported (67,68). Although in some children partial obstruction may not result in hypoxemia or hypercarbia (69), Brouillette et al. showed that prolonged partial airway obstruction is often associated with more severe hypoxemia and hypercarbia than short events of obstructive apnea (69). Similar findings were noted by Rosen et al., who also reported more frequent occurrence of partial obstruction and profound hypoxemia than in children with predominant obstructive apneas (8).

Children with OSAS may have other abnormal breathing patterns in addition

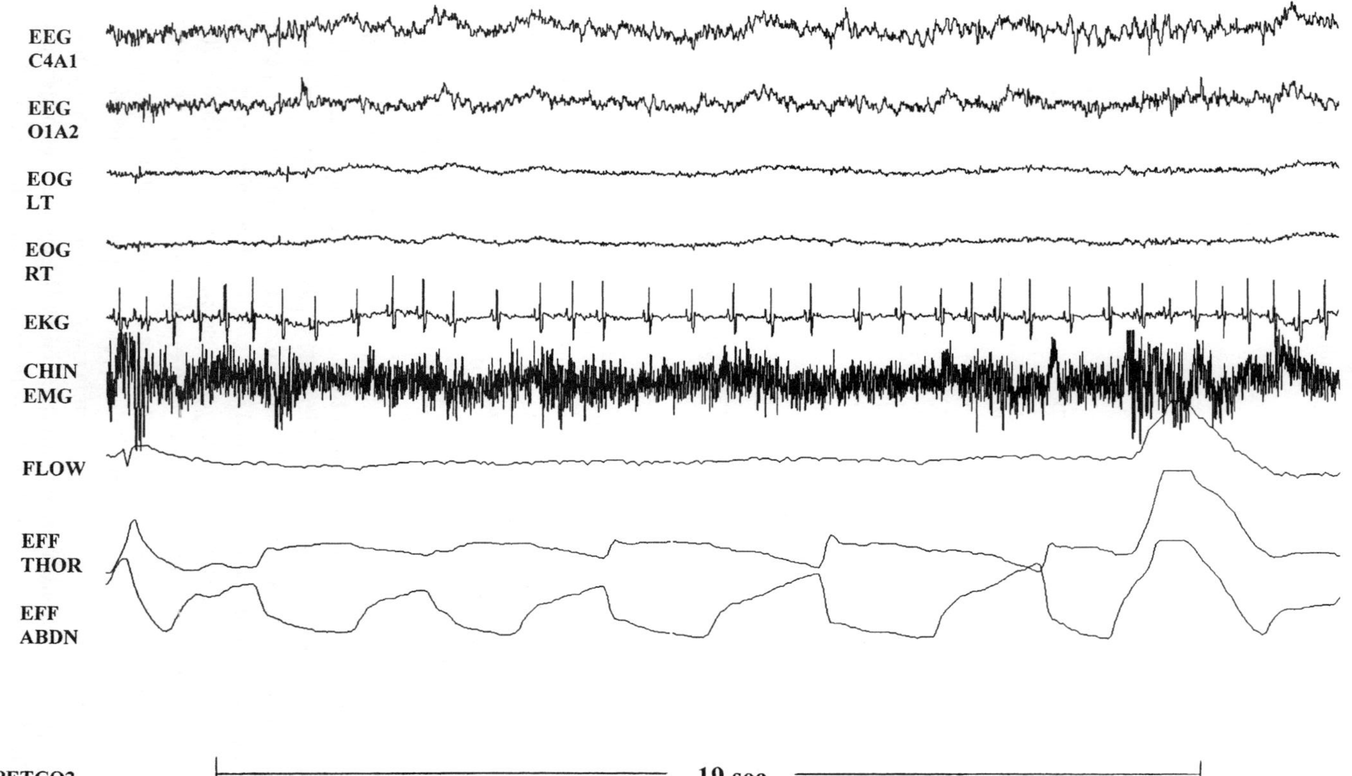

Figure 1 Polysomnography tracing showing an obstructive apnea lasting 19 sec and resulting in arterial oxygen desaturation. Paradoxical effort continues despite a cessation of flow seen on the nasal/oral flow and PET_{CO_2} channels.

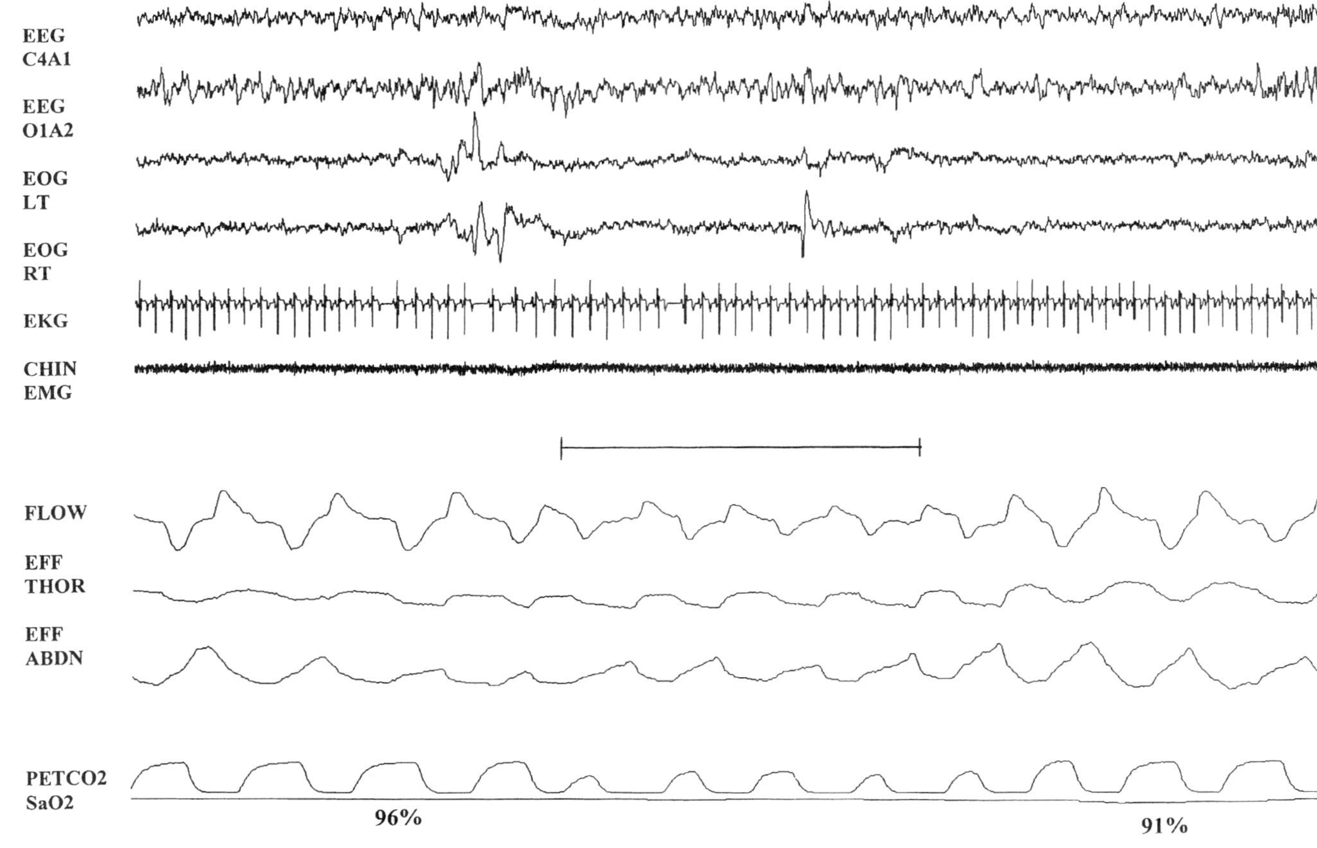

Figure 2 A 60-sec polysomnography tracing showing hypopnea followed by arterial oxygen desaturation. Note a 50% reduction in the nasal/oral flow as well as paradoxical breathing and a significant reduction in abdominal and thoracic effort channels.

Table 4 Patterns of Respiration

Obstructive apnea—Absence of oronasal airflow in the presence of continued respiratory effort lasting longer than two respiratory cycle times. Usually but not always associated with hypoxemia.

Central apnea—Cessation of respiratory effort lasting at least two respiratory cycle times.

Hypopnea—A 50% or greater decrease in the amplitude of the nasal/oral airflow signal, often accompanied by hypoxemia or arousal. Some have attempted to subtype hypopnea into obstructive and nonobstructive. Obstructive hypopnea is defined as a reduction in airflow without a reduction in effort. On the other hand, nonobstructive hypopnea is associated with a reduction in both airflow and respiratory effort by 50%.

Obstructive hypoventilation—Partial airway obstruction leading to a peak $P_{ETCO_2} > 55$ mmHg or $P_{ETCO_2} > 45$ mmHg for more than 60% of TST, or $P_{ETCO_2} > 55$ mmHg for more than 10% of TST (in the absence of lung disease).

Nonobstructive hypoventilation—Assuming CO_2 is measured, decreased breathing due to either a reduction in respiratory drive (central), decreased breathing caused by peripheral neural abnormalities or muscle weakness (neuromuscular), or decreased breathing secondary to decreased chest wall movements (restrictive).

to obstructive apnea and evidence of partial obstruction during sleep. Central and mixed apneas can coexist in these children and may account for 17% to 34% of the total number of apnea events, especially in infants and children with OSAS secondary to craniofacial or neuromuscular syndromes (64). In addition, a large number of children may present with increased work of breathing unassociated with gas exchange abnormalities. This condition is referred to as the *upper airway resistance syndrome* (12). Microarousals during sleep and impaired cognitive function are seen as a complication of this pattern (12,66).

Sleep Patterns

Restless sleep is commonly reported. Children may change sleep positions frequently, preferring positions promoting airway patency, such as lying prone or sideways. Unusual sleep positions—including sleeping sitting up or kneeling on the side of the bed with the head and shoulders resting on the mattress—have been reported by parents. The neck is often kept in a hyperextended position throughout sleep (70). Obese children with significant OSAS may prefer sleeping sitting upright or at least propped upon pillows (71).

Nocturnal Sweating

In a study of 50 children with OSAS, nocturnal profuse sweating was noted in 96% (64). In another study of 23 children with OSAS and 46 controls, 50% of children with OSAS had excessive sweating compared to 16% of controls ($p < .007$) (65). Night sweating is likely associated with the increased effort required to inspire against increased upper-airway resistance over the course of the night (66,72).

Nocturnal Enuresis

Nocturnal enuresis is a variable finding in children with OSAS. Frank et al. (73) reported that 33% of children older than 4 with OSAS had bed wetting, and Weider et al. (74) reported a 76% improvement in nocturnal enuresis after tonsillectomy and adenoidectomy. Guilleminault et al. reported that 6 of 8 children with severe OSAS, 5 to 14 years of age, had enuresis (7); in a second study on 50 children, 18% presented with secondary enuresis (64). However, in perhaps the best-controlled study, comparing 23 children with OSAS to 46 matched controls, Brouillette et al. (65), could not find a significant difference between the groups with respect to bed wetting.

Polyuria has been reported in adults with OSAS. Adults may make multiple trips to the bathroom during the night. In a recent study, six adults with polyuria and severe OSAS were found to have an increase level of atrial natriuretic peptide and catecholamines in the plasma. After initiation of CPAP treatment and resolution of apnea, these parameters were significantly reduced, and a 50% drop in nocturnal urine volume was noted (75). It is not known whether this mechanism also applies to children with OSAS, although there is some support that children with nocturnal enuresis in general may have alterations in diurnal antidiuretic hormone secretion (76).

Daytime Symptoms

Although respiration in children with OSAS is typically unremarkable during wakefulness, some children with severe OSAS may also experience difficulty breathing when awake, albeit this is less severe than when they are asleep. These symptoms are most likely due to adenoidal and tonsillar hypertrophy. The most common complaints reported by parents are mouth breathing, frequent upper respiratory tract infections, recurrent ear infections, as well as hearing and speech problems. Enlarged tonsils and adenoids may cause difficulty with swallowing. In addition, vomiting was also reported, although the link with OSAS is unclear.

In contrast to what has been reported in adults, excessive daytime somnolence (EDS) is thought to be uncommon in children with OSAS. However, there has been considerable variability in the reported frequency of this complication in children. In uncontrolled studies, parents and teachers of older children have observed EDS in between 9% to 84% of children with OSAS (64,66). However, in controlled studies (65), the reported frequency of this symptom is reduced considerably compared to that in adults with OSAS. Older children may complain of sleepiness, tiredness, and fatigue, but this may be difficult to distinguish from the usual school-week behavior of an average adolescent. Abnormal daytime behavior including hyperactivity and aggressiveness have been observed in 31% to 42% of children with OSAS (64,65,69), whereas pathological shyness and social withdrawal have been reported in 22% (65).

Children with an underlying genetic disorder, such as those with trisomy 21 or craniofacial malformation, may have an additional impairment in intellectual performance above and beyond that imposed by the underlying syndrome (64).

Morning headaches were reported in five of the eight patients originally described with OSAS by Guilleminault et al. (7). In a second report on 50 children with OSAS, Guilleminault et al. found that 16% of the children had the same complaint (64). However, a controlled study by Brouillette and coworkers failed to demonstrate an association between morning headaches and OSAS (65). A typical feature of these headaches was that they tended to dissipate completely by late morning. Possible mechanisms underlying these headaches include changes in cerebral blood flow secondary to hypoxia and hypercarbia or the effects of significant swings in intrathoracic pressure during obstructive events on cerebral blood flow and intracranial pressure. Pasterkamp et al. (77), described increased intracranial pressure associated with obstructive apnea in a 16-year-old girl with myelomeningocele and Arnold-Chiari malformation. After tonsillectomy, these elevations in intracranial pressure disappeared.

B. Physical Examination

Physical examination of the child with OSAS may be highly variable. Vital signs are typically normal. Occasionally, hypertension has been reported. Data on systolic hypertension in children is inconclusive, but Marcus and coworkers reported a pattern of diastolic hypertension associated with OSAS in children (78). Mouth breathing and a hyponasal voice quality suggest nasal obstruction, and a muffled voice is an indication of tonsillar enlargement. The lateral facial profile should be inspected for retrognathia and micrognathia as well as the angle of the mandible. In addition, as suggested by Guilleminault et al., a triangular face and midfacial hypoplasia are highly associated with OSAS (12). All can affect the nasopharyngeal and oropharyngeal passages and are key findings in identifying a high-risk population (12). The nose should be assessed for deviation of the septum, mucosal thickening, polyps, and patency of either vestibule by checking the airflow through one nostril while the opposite naris is occluded.

The oral cavity should be observed for tongue and soft palate size and appearance. A large tongue and/or a high-arched or elongated palate may predispose to sleep-disordered breathing. Integrity of the hard palate should be evaluated. Note that a bifid uvula may be associated with submucosal cleft palate. The size of the tonsils should be assessed. A scale from zero to a maximum of 4 if the tonsils meet in the midline is usually used. However, some children may have a normal examination with only mildly enlarged tonsils and adenoids. On the other hand, Guilleminault has identified a pattern of physical findings highly associated with OSAS. These include a small, steep mandibular plane, a high-arched hard palate and an elongated soft palate, retroposition of the mandible, and a long face (12). This facial pattern, especially if associated with large tonsils and adenoids, is highly correlated with OSAS. The size of the adenoids has recently been shown to correlate with the severity of obstructive apnea found on polysomnography (79).

The physical examination should also include an assessment of the child's growth pattern. Children with OSAS are typically of normal to mildly diminished height and weight. Severe failure to thrive was seen more commonly in the past. Increased awareness of OSAS in children has made this finding less common (80). Obesity, on the other hand, while not common, is a risk factor for developing OSAS (81).

The thoracic cavity usually has a normal configuration, although pectus excavatum has been reported in some patients (82). This would appear to be an acquired problem secondary to prolonged periods of rib cage paradox. The lungs are usually clear to auscultation except for transmitted upper-airway noises. The examination of the heart is typically normal; however, in advanced cases, evidence of pulmonary hypertension manifest by a loud pulmonary component of the second heart sound may be present. The prevalence of this finding is unknown. Systemic hypertension and clubbing have been reported but are uncommon findings. A neurological examination should focus on developmental status and evidence of neuromuscular dysfunction.

C. Physiological Consequences of OSAS

Hypoxemia

Marcus et al., in a study of polysomnography in normal children between 1 and 17 years, found the mean oxygen saturation nadir to be 96 ± 2%, with 1 child having a short desaturation to 89% during a central apnea event (11). However, desaturation events of > 4% from a baseline value during sleep were found more frequently, with a mean rate of 0.3 ± 0.7/hr. The maximal oxygen desaturation from peak to nadir value in these children was 4 ± 2%.

Repetitive oxygen desaturation events are frequent in most children with OSAS. Stradling et al. found that nearly two-thirds of 61 children referred for adenotonsillectomy but not OSAS were hypoxemic during sleep (70). Rosen et al. found significant oxygen desaturation to < 85% in 19 of 20 children referred for evaluation of OSAS, despite a relatively low apnea index of 1.9 + 3.2 (8). It is yet unknown how the degree and duration of hypoxemia relate to the outcome of children with OSAS in terms of their neurological or cardiopulmonary status. The point at which these hypoxemic events result in reversible versus permanent damage to these organ systems is also unknown. Hypoxemia can lead to permanent neurological disabilities in children with OSAS (83).

Hypercarbia

Obstructive apnea and hypopnea can be associated with hypoventilation. In healthy children, the partial pressure of CO_2 at the end of a tidal volume breath (PET_{CO_2}) is considered a reliable estimate of arterial CO_2 and thus of alveolar ventilation. Values of PET_{CO_2} > 45 torr during sleep have been by convention considered abnormal (83). More recently, normal values for PET_{CO_2} during sleep have been suggested for the pediatric age group. Based on data from 50 healthy infants and adolescents, hypoventilation may be described when peak PET_{CO_2} > 53 torr, or PET_{CO_2} > 50 torr more than 8% of sleep time, or when duration of hypoventilation (PET_{CO_2} . 45 torr) exceeds more than 60% of total sleep time (11).

Although the data on the number of children with nocturnal hypercarbia and the degree of hypercarbia are limited, hypercarbia during sleep in children with OSAS is not uncommon. Brouillette et al. (69) found hypercarbia (> 45 torr) during sleep in 12 out of 22 children with OSAS. Similarly, Rosen et al. found hypercarbia (> 50 torr) in 26 of 36 (72%) children who were referred for evaluation of OSAS (8).

Several groups are at high risk for developing hypercarbia and hypoventilation. Hypoventilation is the most common polysomnographic abnormality in children with Down syndrome and OSAS and was reported in 81% of 16 children studied by Marcus et al. (29). Obese children with OSAS were also found to develop hypoventilation during sleep. Silvestri et al. studied 32 obese children and found hypercarbia in 75% of them. Those who were morbidly obese, with an ideal body weight > 200%, were most at risk for the development of this abnormality (84).

Sleep and Sleep States

The effects of OSAS on sleep in children are poorly understood. In adults, OSAS is known to cause sleep fragmentation and alterations in sleep architecture due to multiple arousals. As a result, adults with OSAS have less rapid-eye-movement (REM) and slow-wave sleep and spend more time in light sleep of stages 1 and 2 (85). These alterations in sleep architecture are responsible for EDS, which is reported in more than 90% of cases (86). Several studies have found that children with OSAS have normal amounts of slow-wave sleep (73,74,87), and absence of sleep fragmentation was reported in children with hypopneas and OSAS (66). In contrast to this, significant alterations in sleep architecture were reported by Guilleminault et al. in all eight patients presenting with severe OSAS (7). In these children, normal progression to stages 3 and 4 non-REM (NREM) sleep was delayed or precluded due to the repetitive apneic events. In a second report on 50 children with OSAS, Guilleminault et al. reported complete disappearance of stage 3 NREM sleep in 86% of children, a 22% reduction in REM sleep, and an increase in percent of stage 1 NREM compared to controls. Moreover, movement time during sleep was higher than in controls by as much as 100% to 250% (64).

Movement/Arousals

Movement is a normal phenomenon during sleep. However, increased motor activity is frequently reported in subjects with OSAS. Movements may range from simple leg jerks to gross movements of extremities and trunk. Movements are usually associated with arousals or awakenings from sleep. In adults, movement/arousals were found to strongly correlate with the apnea-hypopnea index and were normalized with the use of CPAP (85).

Mograss et al. described three types of movement/arousals in children with OSAS in a sleep laboratory setting. They studied 15 children 2 to 11 years of age with a mean respiratory disturbance index of 7.5 ± 8.2 and classified movement/arousals as spontaneous, respiratory, and technician-induced (87). Of the total movement/arousals studied, spontaneous arousals were the most common and accounted for 51%. Respiratory arousals were found in 29.5% and technician-induced arousal in 19.5%. Nearly all obstructive events were terminated by a movement/arousal and had the effect of reestablishing airway patency in these children. In addition, the respiratory movement/arousal index was directly related to the respiratory disturbance index (RDI). However, these authors found that sleep stages were not altered and were similar to those reported in age-matched children. They have speculated that since movement/arousals were usually short (< 3 sec), children may have fragmented sleep without altered sleep architecture.

In a more recent study, McNamara et al. (88) reported that only a portion of the respiratory events in infants and children with OSAS were terminated by an EEG arousal, while the remaining events resolved spontaneously. 15 children (1 to 14 years of age), aroused following fewer than 40% of obstructive events and 20 infants (term to 21 weeks) aroused following only 8% of the obstructive events. These authors concluded that cortical arousal is not an important mechanism of termination of obstructive events during sleep in children and even less so in infants.

D. Sequelae

Cumulatively, OSAS may have adverse effects on neurological and cardiac function as well as on growth. Sequelae may be mild and reversible or become severe and progressive in untreated children. The various sequelae of childhood OSAS are the result of chronic nocturnal hypoxemia, acidosis, and sleep fragmentation.

Neurobehavioral and Neurocognitive Manifestations

Nocturnal hypoxemia and sleep fragmentation are considered to be the main causes of the neurobehavioral sequelae of OSAS. In adults, EDS, decreased ability to perform everyday tasks, impairment in memory and attention, and a reduction in general intellectual abilities have been reported (85,86,89,90). Sleep fragmentation may lead to personality changes, including irritability, anxiety, aggression, and depression.

EDS is less common in children with OSAS. However, there is some discrepancy in the prevalence of EDS reported in children with OSAS. Guilleminault et al. reported EDS in 84% of the 50 children with OSAS, and in 70% of the cases symptoms were noted by schoolteachers (64). However, Brouillette et al., in a controlled study, reported EDS in 33% of 23 children (65), and Frank et al. reported EDS as a significant problem in only 9% of the 32 children they studied (73). Carroll et al. reported a similarly low rate of EDS in a pediatric population (91). It is conceivable that fewer or shorter arousals and a more preserved sleep architecture seen in children with OSAS compared to adults with OSAS results in less daytime sleepiness (65,91). It is also possible that since EDS is a subjective complaint, it is underdiagnosed in young children, who may take daytime naps routinely.

Brouillette et al. reported significant neurological impairment related to OSAS in 7 of 22 children with OSAS (7). In 5 children, the dysfunction—which included

EDS, behavioral disturbances, and mild developmental delay—was reversible with treatment. However, two children, one of whom had a metabolic disorder, presented with permanent neurological dysfunction presumably related to asphyxia associated with obstructive events. Delays in referral and diagnosis were noted in most of these children and were considered the cause of some of the above sequelae. In another study, Guilleminault et al. reported abnormal behavior in 42% of children in schools, kindergartens, and day care centers. The most common behavioral abnormality described was hyperactivity; however, asocial behavior and disciplinary problems were also noted. A small group of patients were reported to have personality changes and bizarre withdrawn behavior suggestive of psychosis (64).

Learning difficulties, such as delayed language development and inadequate performance in school, are commonly reported, although only one report on neurocognitive function in children with OSAS has been published. Rhodes et al. studied 14 obese patients, of whom 5 had severe OSAS. The children with OSAS demonstrated significantly lower scores for learning, memory, and vocabulary tests. Moreover, the severity of OSAS, as measured by an apnea/hypopnea index, was found to be significantly and inversely correlated with the neurocognitive impairment (45). Recently, Gozal reported on the effects of sleep-related gas exchange abnormalities on school performance. His study demonstrated that correction of these abnormalities resulted in improved school performance among first- and second-grade students (92). These findings, although preliminary, may explain reports of poorer school performance and developmental delay in children with OSAS. However, it is still unknown whether the neurocognitive deficits in children result from chronic hypoxemia or sleep fragmentation and whether these deficits accumulate with time or are reversible. The extent to which recovery of function is possible may depend on the age of onset of OSAS, its severity, and the chronicity of the disorder. More studies of this type are clearly required to better define the effect of OSAS on neurobehavioral/cognitive function.

Cardiovascular Complications

In adults with OSAS, significant cardiovascular complications contribute to morbidity and mortality. These complications are associated with acute and/or chronic effects of hypoxemia, acidosis, and the hemodynamic effect of obstructive apnea on the cardiovascular system. Systemic hypertension is the most common chronic complication and is estimated to occur in 53% of middle-aged adult subjects (93). Acute cyclic changes in heart rate, blood pressure, intrathoracic pressures, and oxygen saturation may induce cardiac arrhythmia and various degrees of atrioventricular block. There is also evidence that adults with OSAS are at an increased risk for ischemic heart disease and cerebral infarction (94).

In contrast to adults with OSAS, systemic hypertension in children is reported only anecdotally (95,96). As noted, Marcus et al. found evidence of isolated diastolic hypertension in their study population (78). Pulmonary hypertension is the main cardiovascular complication described (97,98). If untreated, this complication may progress to cor pulmonale and heart failure. The prevalence of pulmonary hypertension and cor pulmonale in children with OSAS is unknown. Early reports of children with OSAS were strongly associated with this complication (5,6,97). However, several years after the recognition of OSAS in children, a significant number of children were still found to have cor pulmonale. In 1982, Brouillette et al. (69), found that 10 out of 22 (55%) children with OSAS had evidence of cor pulmonale. This finding was attributed to a significant delay in referral and diagnosis of these children. Nevertheless, each child who presented with cor pulmonale with or without cardiomegaly improved after surgical treatment of OSAS.

In 1988, Tal et al. performed a cardiac evaluation of 27 children with OSAS between 9 months and 7.5 years of age and found that 2 had evidence of cor pulmonale and heart failure. Clinical examination, chest x-ray, and ECG were negative in the others. However, a radionuclide heart scan demonstrated a significant reduction in right ventricular ejection fraction in 10 (37%) of the children (99). All children who underwent ventricular radionuclide scan before and after adenotonsillectomy showed normalization of heart function after surgery. This study demonstrated that a significant number of children with OSAS have unrecognized right ventricular dysfunction that is reversible after adenotonsillectomy.

Cor pulmonale has been reported in children with Down syndrome and associated congenital heart disease (100). The severity of pulmonary hypertension found in some of these children is at times out of proportion to the degree of left-to-right shunt, and it has been proposed that this may be related to the effects of sleep-disordered breathing (29,100).

Left ventricular function in children with OSAS is reported to be normal. Tal et al. did not demonstrate evidence of left ventricular dysfunction in 25 children with OSAS but nevertheless found an improvement of 10% in left ventricular ejection fraction in 5 of 11 patients with OSAS who were tested before and after adenotonsillectomy (99). Shiomni et al. studied six children with OSAS 3 to 14 years of age by M-mode two-dimensional echocardiography during sleep. In three of these children, periods of airway obstruction and progressive negative intrathoracic pressures were associated with decreased left ventricular end-diastolic dimension and leftward shift of the interventricular septum. These findings were completely reversed with treatment by nasal CPAP (101).

Cardiac arrhythmias during obstructive events have been observed in children with OSAS. Guilleminault et al. described sinus arrhythmia, second degree atrioventricular block, paroxysmal atrial tachycardia, and short periods of sinus arrest in a significant number of the 50 children who were studied (64). On the other hand, D'Andrea et al. studied 12 children with severe OSAS and found only modest changes in RR intervals, with no evidence of life-threatening arrhythmias or bradycardia during periods of severe oxygen desaturations to below 65% and extending 30 sec (102). In a recent study, Aljadeff et al. demonstrated alterations in heart rate variability in seven children with OSAS. These were most significant in the low heart rate range and were significantly higher than control subjects (103). Preoperative and postoperative cardiac related deaths have been observed in children with severe adenotonsillar hypertrophy and OSAS (104–106).

Growth Impairment

Growth impairment is one of the unique features of childhood OSAS. Early reports of children with severe OSAS were almost always associated with failure to thrive, especially when other complications such as cor pulmonale were present. Reports from the 1980s found failure to thrive in 27% to 56% of the children with OSAS, while obesity in the same populations was reported in about 10% of children (64,69). Williams et al. described 37 children between 6 and 36 months of age who underwent adenotonsillectomy for OSAS. The weight of these children was at or below the fifth percentile in 46% of the cases (107).

Adenotonsillectomy in children with OSAS has a significant impact on growth. Brouillette et al. found that relief of airway obstruction resulted in catch-up growth in all six children with failure to thrive (69). Williams et al. found that 65% of the 37 children with OSAS had at least a 15% increase in their weight after adenotonsillectomy (107). Moreover, Lind and Lundell described a group of 14 children with OSAS, 13 of whom had normal height and weight velocity prior to surgery and all of whom had significant increases in height and weight velocities after adenotonsillectomy (108).

Poor caloric intake may result in inadequate growth. Brouillette et al. reported poor appetite, difficulty swallowing, and nausea and vomiting in children with OSAS compared to controls (65). Similarly, Potsic et al. reported that 60% of children with OSAS were slow eaters and 37% had trouble swallowing (109).

Marcus et al. investigated the relation between growth, caloric intake, and energy expenditure during sleep before and after adenotonsillectomy in 14 children age 4 ± 1 years with moderate OSAS (72). Diagnosis was based upon an apnea index of 6 ± 3, an oxygen desaturation of $85 \pm 5\%$, and an increase in CO_2 during sleep. OSAS resolved in all cases following adenotonsillectomy. Caloric intake prior to intervention in these children was normal at 91 ± 30 kcal/kg per day and was the same after adenotonsillectomy. However, energy expenditure during sleep dropped from 51 ± 6 kcal/kg per day prior to surgery to 46 ± 7 kcal/kg per day after surgery ($p < .005$). This finding was associated with a significant increase in weight in all children. These findings suggest that poor growth described in some children with OSAS may be secondary to an increased energy expenditure from increased work of breathing during sleep rather than decreased caloric intake preoperatively.

Lind and Lundell (108) hypothesized that abnormal release of growth hormone may alter growth in children with OSAS. However, only one case report supports this hypothesis. Goldstein et al. reported a 9-year-old child with achondroplasia and OSAS with documented low levels of growth hormone during sleep (110). Following tracheostomy and resolution of OSAS, slow-wave sleep and growth hormone levels returned to normal. Bate et al. suggested that respiratory acidosis during sleep in children with OSAS may alter end-organ response to growth hormone (111). However, there are no studies to support a relationship between hypoventilation and lack of production of or response to growth hormone in children with OSAS.

The relationship between growth and childhood OSAS is still poorly understood. Many questions are still unanswered, such as the relationship between age, caloric intake, and growth impairment; the relationship between the severity of OSAS and growth; and finally the effect of sleep fragmentation on growth. (See also Chap. 6.)

IV. Course

The natural history of children with OSAS is variable. The time elapsed from initial symptoms to diagnosis and management is a significant factor in evaluating the outcome of children with long-standing OSAS. Today, with increased awareness of OSAS among physicians as well as parents, delays in diagnosis are seen less often. However, this was not the case 16 years ago, when Brouillette et al. reported an average delay of 23 months from presentation of symptoms to diagnosis of OSAS in children. They found that 16 (73%) of the 22 children had serious sequelae; 55% had cor pulmonale, 31% had neurological impairment, and 27% had failure to thrive at the time of diagnosis (69). It is difficult to predict the exact outcome of a child with OSAS diagnosed today. However, in severe cases and if untreated, children will probably progress, as in the past, to cor pulmonale and congestive heart failure and will encounter neurological deficits that may extend to permanent brain damage due to severe prolonged hypoxemia (69). The clinical course and long-term consequences of mild forms of OSAS are unknown. However, it is believed that most of the complications described in the pediatric literature—including cor pulmonale, behavioral problems, and growth impairments—are reversible once patients are treated.

Children with OSAS who also have craniofacial anomalies, neurological disorders, or systemic diseases are at increased risk to develop complications due to delay in diagnosis. In this group, history and clinical symptoms may be less apparent than in children with isolated adenotonsillar hypertrophy. Frequently, there is no evidence of tonsillar hypertrophy because these children often present well before the age when these tissues increase in size, and the significance of snoring is not often appreciated by parents and primary care physicians concerned with the more obvious underlying condition.

V. High-Risk Groups for Childhood OSAS

OSAS is associated with many pediatric conditions in addition to adenotonsillar hypertrophy. These fall mainly into the categories of craniofacial and neurological disorders affecting upper-airway anatomy and patency during sleep (Table 2). Children with craniofacial anomalies are prone to develop OSAS even in the absence of adenotonsillar hypertrophy, as these conditions may increase nasal or oropharyngeal resistance. Children who are neurologically impaired are at additional risk for developing OSAS due to one or more of the following: muscular hypotonia, abnormal control of ventilation, and poor arousal mechanisms.

A. Obesity

Obesity is a major risk in adults for developing OSAS (20), and an increased neck collar size is strongly associated with OSAS in this group (13). In contrast, the majority of children with OSAS are not obese. Normal weight and failure to thrive are seen more commonly. Nonetheless, there is evidence that obesity is also a risk factor for OSAS in children. Guilleminault et al. reported that 10% of the 50 children who were diagnosed with OSAS were obese (64), and a similar finding was reported by Brouillette et al., who studied 22 infants and children (69). A higher incidence of OSAS was reported when obese children were referred for evaluation of OSAS. Mallroy et al. reported abnormalities on polysomnography in 37% of 41 obese children (112), and Silvestri et al. found partial airway obstruction in 66% and complete airway obstruction in 59% of the 32 obese children (84).

The above studies were all performed on children who were referred for possible OSAS; therefore the prevalence of sleep-disordered breathing may have been overestimated in this group. To evaluate more precisely the prevalence of OSAS in the general obese population, Marcus et al. studied 22 obese children and adolescents aged 10± 5 years, with an ideal body weight of 184 ± 36% and no history of sleep-disordered breathing (47). They found that 10 children (46%) had abnormal polysomnography and in 6 (27%) abnormalities were moderate to severe. Moreover, a positive correlation between obesity and apnea index was found ($r = 0.47, p < .05$), and an inverse relation between obesity and oxygen saturation nadir ($r = 0.5, p < .01$). Asymptomatic obese infants also have a higher incidence of obstructive apnea events compared to controls (113), suggesting that OSAS is common in obese children of all ages.

Adenotonsillar hypertrophy is not always the cause of the development of OSAS in obese children (47,113). Several other factors may contribute to OSAS in this group. Upper airway narrowing may result from deposition of adipose tissue within the muscles and tissues surrounding the airway and result in increased pharyngeal resistance (114). Moreover, obese subjects have been shown to have decreased chest wall compliance and displacement of the diaphragm when in the supine position. This may result in decreased lung volumes and oxygen reserves during sleep and may increase the severity of OSAS in this group.

B. Prematurity

The association between prematurity and central apnea is well known. In addition, premature infants are predisposed to upper airway obstruction and oxygen desaturation during sleep due to poor airway stability and a highly compliant chest wall. Dransfield et al. found that of 76 premature infants presenting clinically with apnea, 52 (68%) of them had obstructive apnea and 24 (32%) had central apnea only (115). Milner et al. found that half of the apneic episodes associated with periodic breathing in eight premature infants were the result of upper airway obstruction and glottic closure (116). Spontaneous neck flexion was also found to cause upper airway obstruction in premature infants and was suggested to play a role in the pathogenesis of apnea in some preterm infants (117).

C. Infancy

Neonates are preferential nasal breathers and may develop upper-airway obstruction whenever a mild nasal obstruction, such as a respiratory infection, is present. Central nervous system immaturity, highly compliant chest wall, and reduced airway stability all predispose newborn infants to gas exchange abnormalities even during brief episodes of OSAS. OSAS in early infancy can coexist with central apnea and can sometimes be mistaken for central apnea. Guilleminault et al. found a peak incidence of obstructive and mixed apnea to occur at 6 weeks of age in 30 healthy infants. These events occur most commonly in NREM sleep and progressively declined by 6 months to a nonsignificant amount (118). Resolution of the events by 6 months may represent improved upper-airway stability with growth (119).

Several reports deal with the association between OSAS and apparent life-threatening events (ALTEs) during early infancy. Guilleminault et al. reported a higher number of mixed and obstructive sleep apneas in children with ALTEs (118). Moreover, a later report from the same group described five infants with ALTEs who subsequently developed severe OSAS. Polysomnography of the infants at the time of the initial ALTE (3 weeks to 6 months of age) demonstrated a high index of mixed and obstructive apnea. These infants became progressively more symptomatic by 6 to 10 months of age and improved only after adenotonsillectomy (120).

Similar findings have been observed in a few infants who had polysomnography and subsequently died of the sudden infant death syndrome. When compared to age matched controls, these infants showed a higher number of mixed and obstructive events (121,122).

VI. Mortality

Adults with OSAS have been reported to be at an increased risk of dying early, compared to the general population, mainly from respiratory and cardiovascular complications. Hypertension, obesity, age between 30 and 50 years, and a high apnea index increase the risk for early death in these patients (123). It has also been shown that when adults with OSAS were untreated, those with an apnea index > 20 had a significantly higher risk of dying than those with an apnea index < 20 (124). These reports indicate the need for early intervention in these high-risk groups.

The mortality rate in children with OSAS is unknown. Deaths thought to be secondary to OSAS in children occurred during a period when childhood OSAS was relatively unrecognized and were attributed to perioperative cardiorespiratory failure in children with associated craniofacial and neurological disorders (98,125–127). Deaths were also encountered in children who underwent surgical correction of velopharyngeal incompetence (i.e., from OSAS after surgery) (61). Sudden death in infancy attributed to OSAS has been reported by others (122,123). More data are needed on the morbidity and mortality, acute and long-term, associated with childhood OSAS.

References

1. American Thoracic Society. Standards and indications for cardiopulmonary sleep studies in children. Am J Respir Crit Care Med 1995; 153:866–878.
2. Hill W. On some causes of backwardness and stupidity in children. BMJ 1889; 2: 711–712.
3. Osler W. Chronic tonsillitis. In: The Principles and Practice of Medicine. New York: Appleton and Co., 1892: 335–339.
4. Gastuant H, Tassinari CA, Duron B. Polygraphic study of the episodic diurnal and nocturnal (hypnic and respiratory) manifestations of the Pickwick syndrome. Brain Res 1966; 2:167–189.
5. Menashe VD, Ferrehi F, Miller M. Hypoventilation and cor pulmonale due to chronic upper airway obstruction. J Pediatr 1965; 67:198–203.
6. Noonan JA. Reversible cor pulmonale due to hypertrophied tonsils and adenoids: studies in 2 cases. Circulation 1965; 32:164.
7. Guilleminault C, Eldridge FL, Simmons FB, Dement WC. Sleep apnea in eight children. Pediatrics 1976; 58:23–30.
8. Rosen CL, D'Andrea L, Haddad GG. Adult criteria for obstructive sleep apnea do not identify children with serious obstruction. Am Rev Respir Dis 1992; 146:1231–1234.
9. Carroll JL, Loughlin GM. Diagnostic criteria for obstructive sleep apnea syndrome in children. Pediatr Pulmonol 1992; 14:71–74.
10. Carroll JL. Sleep-related upper airway obstruction in children and adolescents. Child Adolesc Psychiatr Clin North Am 1996; 5:617–647.
11. Marcus CL, Omlin KJ, Basinski DJ, Bailey SL, Rachal AB, Von Pechmann WS, Keens TG, Ward SL. Normal polysomnogram values for children and adolescents. Am Rev Respir Dis 1992; 146:1235–1239.
12. Guilleminault C, Pelayo R, Leger D, Clerk A, Bocian RC. Recognition of sleep disordered breathing in children. Pediatrics 1996; 98:871–872.
13. Young T, Palta M, Dempsey J, Skatrud J, Weber S, Badr S. The occurrence of sleep disordered breathing among middle aged adults. N Engl J Med 1993; 328:1230–1235.
14. Block AJ, Boysen PG, Wynne JW, Hunt LA. Sleep apnea, hypopnea and oxygen desaturation in normal subjects. A strong male predominance. N Engl J Med 1979; 300: 513–517.
15. Redline S, Kump K, Tishler PV, Browner I, Ferrette V. Gender differences in sleep disordered breathing in a community based sample. Am J Respir Crit Care Med 1994; 149: 722–726.

16. Schneider BK, Pickett CK, Zwillich CW, Weil JV, McDermott MT, Santen RJ, Varano LA, White DP. Influence of testosterone on breathing during sleep. J Appl Physiol 1986; 61:618–623.
17. Ali NJ, Pitson DJ, Stradling JR. The prevalence of snoring, sleep disturbance, and sleep related breathing disorders, and their relation to day time sleepiness in 4–5 year old children. Arch Dis Child 1993; 68:360–366.
18. Corbo GM, Fuciarelli F, Foresi A, De Benedetto. Snoring in children: association with respiratory symptoms and passive smoking. BMJ 1989; 299:1491–1494.
19. Jeans WD, Fernando DC, Maw AR, Leighton BC. A longitudinal study of the growth of the nasopharynx and its contents in normal children. Br J Radiol 1981; 54:117–121.
20. Redline S, Tishler PV, Aylor J, Clark K, Burant C, Winters J. Prevalence and risk factors for sleep disordered breathing in children. Am J Respir Crit Care Med 1997; 155: A843.
21. Redline S, Tishler PV, Hans MG, Tosteson TD, Strohl KP, Spry K. Radial differences in sleep disordered breathing in African Americans and Caucasians. Am J Respir Crit Care Med 1997; 155:186–192.
22. Gozal D, Marcus CL, Keens TG, Ward SLD. Characteristics and polysomnographic abnormalities of children with obstructive sleep apnea syndrome. Pediatr Pulmonol 1991; 11:372.
23. Waters KA, Everett FM, Bruderer JW, Sullivan CE. Obstructive sleep apnea: the use of nasal CPAP in 80 children. Am J Respir Crit Care Med 1995; 152:780–785.
24. Lauritzen C, Lilja J, Jarlstedt J. Airway obstruction and sleep apnea in children with craniofacial anomalies. Plast Reconst Surg 1986; 77:1–6.
25. Mixter RC, David DJ, Perloff WH, Green CG, Pauli RM, Popic PM. Obstructive sleep apnea in Apert's and Pfeiffer's syndromes: more than a craniofacial abnormality. Plast Reconstr Surg 1990; 86:457–463.
26. Johnston C, Taussig LM, Koopmann C, Smith P, Bjelland J. Obstructive sleep apnea in Treacher Collins syndrome. Cleft Palate J 1981; 18:39–44.
27. Strome M. Obstructive sleep apnea in Down syndrome children: a surgical approach. Laryngoscope 1986; 96:1340–1342.
28. Donaldson JD, Redmond WM. Surgical management of obstructive sleep apnea in children with Down syndrome. J Otolaryngol 1988; 17:398–403.
29. Marcus CL, Keens TG, Bautista DB, von Pechmann WS, Ward SL. Obstructive sleep apnea in children with Down syndrome. Pediatrics 1991; 88:132–139.
30. Bower CM, Richmond D. Tonsillectomy and adenoidectomy in patients with Down syndrome. Int J Pediatr Otorhinol 1995; 33:141–148.
31. Smith DF, Mihm FG, Flynn M. Chronic alveolar hypoventilation secondary to macroglossia in the Beckwith Wiedemann syndrome. Pediatrics 1982; 70:695–697.
32. Abramson DL, Marrinan EM, Mulliken JB. Robin sequence: obstructive sleep apnea following pharyngeal flap. Cleft Palate Craniofac J 1997; 34:256–260.
33. Spier S, Rivlin J, Rowe RD, Egan T. Sleep in Pierre Robin syndrome. Chest 1986; 90: 711–715.
34. Cozzi F, Pierro A. Glossoptosis apnea syndrome in infancy. Pediatrics 1985; 75: 836–843.
35. Reid CS, Pyeritz RE, Kopits SE, Maria BL, Wang H, McPherson RW, Hurko O, Phillips JA, Rosenbaum AE. Cervicomedullary compression in young patients with achondroplasia: value of comprehensive neurologic and respiratory evaluation. J Pediatr 1987; 110:522–530.

36. Friede H, Lopata M, Fisher E, Rosenthal IM. Cardiorespiratory disease associated with Hallermann Streiff syndrome: analysis of craniofacial morphology by cephalometric roentgenograms. J Craniofac Genet Dev Biol 1985; 1:189–198.
37. Rosen CL, Novotny EJ, D'Andrea LA, Petty EM, Klippel. Feil sequence and sleep disordered breathing in two children. Am Rev Respir Dis 1993; 147:202–204.
38. Suzuki K, Yamamoto S, Ito Y, Baba S. Sleep apnea associated with congenital diseases and moderate hypertrophy of tonsils. Acta Otolaryngol 1996; 523:225–227.
39. Cistulli PA, Sullivan CE. Sleep disordered breathing in Marfan's syndrome. Am Rev Respir Dis 1993; 147:645–648.
40. Kosko JR, Derkay CS. Uvulopalatopharyngoplasty: treatment of obstructive sleep apnea in neurologically impaired pediatric patients. Int J Pediatr Otorhinolaryngol 1995; 32:2 41–246.
41. Cohen SR, Lefaivre JF, Burstein FD, Simms C, Kattos AV, Scott PH, Montgomery GL, Graham L. Surgical treatment of obstructive sleep apnea in neurologically compromised patients. Plast Reconst Surg 1997; 99:638–646.
42. Quera Salva MA, Guilleminault C, Chevret S, Troche G, Fromageot C, Crowe McCann C, Stoohs R, de Lattre J, Raphael JC, Gajdos P. Breathing disorders during sleep in myasthenia gravis. Ann Neurol 1992; 31:86–92.
43. Gilmore RL, Falace P, Kanga J, Baumann R. Sleep disordered breathing in Mobius syndrome. J Child Neurol 1991; 6:73–77.
44. Gozal D, Arens R, Omlin KJ, Jacobs RA, Keens TG. Peripheral chemoreceptor function in children with myelomeningocele and Arnold-Chiari malformation type II. Chest 1995; 108:425–431.
45. Rhodes SK, Shimoda KC, Waid LR, O'Neil PM, Oexmann MJ, Collop NA, Willi SM. Neurocognitive deficits in morbidly obese children with obstructive sleep apnea. J Pediatr 1995; 127:741–744.
46. Kudoh F, Sanai A. Effect of tonsillectomy and adenoidectomy on obese children with sleep associated breathing disorders. Acta Otolaryngol 1996; 523:216–218.
47. Marcus CL, Curtis S, Koerner CB, Joffe A, Serwint JR, Loughlin GM. Evaluation of pulmonary function and polysomnography in obese children and adolescents. Pediatr Pulmonol 1996; 21:176–183.
48. Arens R, Gozal D, Burrell BC, Bailey SL, Bautista DB, Keens TG, Ward SL. Arousal and cardiorespiratory responses to hypoxia in Prader Willi syndrome. Am J Respir Crit Care Med 1996; 153:283–287.
49. Hertz G, Cataletto M, Feinsilver SH, Angulo M. Developmental trends of sleep disordered breathing in Prader Willi syndrome: the role of obesity. Am J Med Genet 1995; 56:188–190.
50. Rajagopal KR, Abbrecht PH, Derderian SS, Pickett C, Hofeldt F, Tellis CJ, Zwillich CW. Obstructive sleep apnea in hypothyroidism. Ann Intern Med 1984; 101:491–494.
51. Shapiro J, Strome M, Crocker AC. Airway obstruction and sleep apnea in Hurler and Hunter syndromes. Ann Otorhinolaryngol 1985; 94:458–461.
52. Malone BN, Whitley CB, Duvall AJ, Belani K, Sibley RK, Ramsay NK, Kersey JH, Krivit W, Berlinger NT. Resolution of obstructive sleep apnea in Hurler syndrome after bone marrow transplantation. Int J Pediatr Otorhinolaryngol 1988; 15:23–31.
53. Maddern BR, Reed HT, Ohene Frempong K, Beckerman RC. Obstructive sleep apnea syndrome in sickle cell disease. Ann Otorhinolaryngol 1989; 98:174–178.
54. Derkay CS, Bray G, Milmoe GJ, Grundfast KM. Adenotonsillectomy in children with sickle cell disease. South Med J 1991; 84:205–208.

55. Halvorson DJ, McKie V, McKie K, Ashmore PE, Porubsky ES. Sickle cell disease and tonsillectomy: preoperative management and postoperative complications. Arch Otolaryngol Head Neck Surg 1997; 123:689–692.
56. McClurg FL, Evans DA. Laser laryngoplasty for laryngomalacia. Laryngoscope 1994; 104:247–252.
57. Marcus CL, Crockett DM, Ward SL. Evaluation of epiglottoplasty as treatment for severe laryngomalacia. J Pediatr 1990; 117:706–710.
58. Brodsky L, Siddiqui SY, Stanievich JF. Massive oropharyngeal papillomatosis causing obstructive sleep apnea in a child. Arch Otolaryngol Head Neck Surg 1987; 113:882–884.
59. Frankel LR, Anas NG, Perkin RM, Seid AB, Peterson B, Park SM. Use of the anterior cricoid split operation in infants with acquired subglottic stenosis. Crit Care Med 1984; 12:395–398.
60. Robertson CF, Zuker R, Dabrowski B, Levison H. Obstructive sleep apnea: a complication of burns to the head and neck in children. J Burn Care Rehab 1985; 6:353–357.
61. Kravath RE, Pollak CP, Borowiecki B, Weitzman ED. Obstructive sleep apnea and death associated with surgical correction of velopharyngeal incompetence. J Pediatr 1980; 96: 645–648.
62. Sirois M, Caouette Laberge L, Spier S, Larocque Y, Egerszegi EP. Sleep apnea following a pharyngeal flap: a feared complication. Plast Reconstr Surg 1994; 93:943–947.
63. Josephson GD, Levine J, Cutting CB. Septoplasty for obstructive sleep apnea in infants after cleft lip repair. Cleft Palate Craniofac J 1996; 33:473–476.
64. Guilleminault C, Korobkin R, Winkel R. A review of 50 children with obstructive sleep apnea syndrome. Lung 1981; 159:275–287.
65. Brouillette R, Hanson D, David R, Klemka L, Szatkowski A, Fernbach S, Hunt C. A diagnostic approach to suspected obstructive sleep apnea in children. J Pediatr 1984; 105:10–14.
66. Guilleminault C, Winkle R, Korobkin R, Simmons B. Children and nocturnal snoring: evaluation of the effects of sleep related respiratory resistive load and daytime functioning. Eur J Pediatr 1982; 139:165–171.
67. Miyazaki S, Itasaka Y, Yamakawa K, Okawa M, Togawa K. Respiratory disturbance during sleep due to adenoid tonsillar hypertrophy. Am J Otolaryngol 1989; 10:143–149.
68. Konno A, Togawa K, Hoshino T. The effect of nasal obstruction in infancy and early childhood upon ventilation. Laryngoscope 1980; 90:699–707.
69. Brouillette RT, Fernbach SK, Hunt CE. Obstructive sleep apnea in infants and children. J Pediatr 1982; 100:31–40.
70. Stradling JR, Thomas G, Warley AR, Williams P, Freeland A. Effect of adenotonsillectomy on nocturnal hypoxaemia, sleep disturbance, and symptoms in snoring children. Lancet 1990; 335:249–253.
71. Stool SE, Eavey RD, Stein NL, Sharrar WG. The "chubby puffer" syndrome: upper airway obstruction and obesity, with intermittent somnolence and cardiorespiratory embarrassment. Clin Pediatr 1977; 16:43–50.
72. Marcus CL, Carroll JL, Koerner CB, Hamer A, Lutz J, Loughlin GM. Determinants of growth in children with the obstructive sleep apnea syndrome. J Pediatr 1994; 125: 556–662.
73. Frank Y, Kravath RE, Pollak CP, Weitzman ED. Obstructive sleep apnea and its therapy: clinical and polysomnographic manifestations. Pediatrics 1983; 71:737–742.
74. Weider DJ, Sateia MJ, West RP. Nocturnal enuresis in children with upper airway obstruction. Otolaryngol Head Neck Surg 1991; 105:427–432.

75. Baruzzi A, Riva R, Cirignotta F, Zucconi M, Cappelli M, Lugaresi E. Atrial natriuretic peptide and catecholamines in obstructive sleep apnea syndrome. Sleep 1991; 14:83–86.
76. Norgaard JP, Rittig S, Djurhuus JC. Nocturnal enuresis: an approach to treatment based on pathogenesis. J Pediatr 1989; 114:705–710.
77. Pasterkamp H, Cardoso ER, Booth FA. Obstructive sleep apnea leading to increased intracranial pressure in a patient with hydrocephalus and syringomyelia. Chest 1989; 95: 1064–1067.
78. Marcus CL, Greene MG, Carroll JL. Blood pressure in children with obstructive sleep apnea. Am J Respir Crit Care Med 1998; 157:1098–1103.
79. Brooks LJ, Stephens BM, Bacevice AM. Adenoid size is related to severity but not the number of episodes of obstructive apnea in children. J Pediatr 1998; 132:682–686.
80. Marcus CL, Carroll JL. Obstructive sleep apnea syndrome. In: Loughlin GM, Eigen H, eds. Pediatric Lung Disease: Diagnosis and Management. Baltimore: Williams & Wilkins, 1995.
81. Marcus CL, Curtis S, Koerner CB, Joffe A, Serwint JR, Loughlin GM. Evaluation of pulmonary function and polysomnography in obese children and adolescents. Pediatr Pulmonol 1996; 21:176–183.
82. Fan L, Murphy S. Pectus excavatum from chronic upper airway obstruction. Am J Dis Child 1981; 135:550–552.
83. Brouillette RT, Weese-Mayer DE, Hunt CE. Disorders of breathing during sleep in pediatric population. Semin Respir Med 1988; 9:594–606.
84. Silvestri JM, Weese Mayer DE, Bass MT, Kenny AS, Hauptman SA, Pearsall SM. Polysomnography in obese children with a history of sleep associated breathing disorders. Pediatr Pulmonol 1993; 16:124–129.
85. Collard P, Dury M, Delguste P, Aubert G, Rodenstein DO. Movement arousals and sleep related disordered breathing in adults. Am J Respir Crit Care Med 1996; 154:454–459.
86. Partinen M, Guilleminault C. Daytime sleepiness and vascular morbidity at seven year follow up in obstructive sleep apnea patients. Chest 1990; 97:27–32.
87. Mograss MA, Ducharme FM, Brouillette RT. Movement/arousals: description, classification, and relationship to sleep apnea in children. Am J Respir Crit Care Med 1994; 150:1690–1696.
88. McNamara F, Issa FG, Sullivan CE. Arousal pattern following central and obstructive breathing abnormalities in infants and children. J Appl Physiol 1996; 81:2651–2657.
89. Greenberg GD, Watson RK, Deptula D. Neuropsychological dysfunction in sleep apnea. Sleep 1987; 10:254–262.
90. Findley LJ, Barth JT, Powers DC, Wilhoit SC, Boyd DG, Suratt PM. Cognitive impairment in patients with obstructive sleep apnea and associated hypoxemia. Chest 1986; 90:686–690.
91. Carroll JL, McColley SA, Marcus CL, Curtis S, Loughlin GM. Inability of clinical history to distinguish snoring from obstructive sleep apnea syndrome in children. Chest 1995; 108:610–618.
92. Gozal D. Sleep-disordered breathing and school performance in children. Pediatrics 1998; 102:616–620.
93. Shepard JW Jr. Hypertension, cardiac arrhythmias, myocardial infarction, and stroke in relation to obstructive sleep apnea. Clin Chest Med 1992; 13:437–458.
94. Koskenvuo M, Kaprio J, Telakivi T, Partinen M, Heikkila K, Sarna S. Snoring as a risk factor for ischaemic heart disease and stroke in men. BMJ 1987; 294:16–19.

95. Ross RD, Daniels SR, Loggie JM, Meyer RA, Ballard ET. Sleep apnea associated hypertension and reversible left ventricular hypertrophy. J Pediatr 1987; 111:253–255.
96. Serratto M, Harris VJ, Carr I. Upper airways obstruction, presentation with systemic hypertension. Arch Dis Child 1981; 56:153–155.
97. Luke MJ, Mehrizi A, Folger GM Jr, Rowe RD. Chronic nasopharyngeal obstruction as a cause of cardiomegaly, cor pulmonale, and pulmonary edema. Pediatrics 1966; 37:762–768.
98. Perkin RM, Anas NG. Pulmonary hypertension in pediatric patients. J Pediatr 1984; 105: 511–522.
99. Tal A, Leiberman A, Margulis G, Sofer S. Ventricular dysfunction in children with obstructive sleep apnea: radionuclide assessment. Pediatr Pulmonol 1988; 4:139–143.
100. Loughlin GM, Wynne JW, Victorica BE. Sleep apnea as a possible cause of pulmonary hypertension in Down syndrome. J Pediatr 1981; 98:435–437.
101. Shiomi T, Guilleminault C, Stoohs R, Schnittger I. Obstructed breathing in children during sleep monitored by echocardiography. Acta Paediatr 1993; 82:863–871.
102. D'Andrea LA, Rosen CL, Haddad GG. Severe hypoxemia in children with upper airway obstruction during sleep does not lead to significant changes in heart rate. Pediatr Pulmonol 1993; 16:362–369.
103. Aljadeff G, Gozal D, Schechtman VL, Burrell B, Harper RM, Ward SL. Heart rate variability in children with obstructive sleep apnea. Sleep 1997; 20:151–157.
104. Ainger LE. Large tonsils and adenoids in small children with cor pulmonale. Br Heart J 1968; 30:356–362.
105. Talbot AR, Robertson LW. Cardiac failure with tonsil and adenoid hypertrophy. Arch Otolaryngol 1973; 98:277–281.
106. Wilkinson AR, McCormick MS, Freeland AP, Pickering D. Electrocardiographic signs of pulmonary hypertension in children who snore. BMJ 1981; 282:1579–1581.
107. Williams EF, Woo P, Miller R, Kellman RM. The effects of adenotonsillectomy on growth in young children. Otolaryngol Head Neck Surg 1991; 104:509–516.
108. Lind MG, Lundell BP. Tonsillar hyperplasia in children. A cause of obstructive sleep apneas, CO_2 retention, and retarded growth. Arch Otolaryngol 1982; 108:650–654.
109. Potsic WP, Pasquariello PS, Baranak CC, Marsh RR, Miller LM. Relief of upper airway obstruction by adenotonsillectomy. Otolaryngol Head Neck Surg 1986; 94:476–480.
110. Goldstein SJ, Wu RH, Thorpy MJ, Shprintzen RJ, Marion RE, Saenger P. Reversibility of deficient sleep entrained growth hormone secretion in a boy with achondroplasia and obstructive sleep apnea. Acta Endocrinol 1987; 116:95–101.
111. Bate TW, Price DA, Holme CA, McGucken RB. Short stature caused by obstructive apnoea during sleep. Arch Dis Child 1984; 59:78–80.
112. Mallory GB Jr, Fiser DH, Jackson R. Sleep associated breathing disorders in morbidly obese children and adolescents. J Pediatr 1989; 115:892–897.
113. Kahn A, Mozin MJ, Rebuffat E, Sottiaux M, Burniat W, Shepherd S, Muller MF. Sleep pattern alterations and brief airway obstructions in overweight infants. Sleep 1989; 12: 430–438.
114. Horner RL, Mohiaddin RH, Lowell DG, Shea SA, Burman ED, Longmore DB, Guz A. Sites and sizes of fat deposits around the pharynx in obese patients with obstructive sleep apnoea and weight matched controls. Eur Respir J 1989; 2:613–622.
115. Dransfield DA, Spitzer AR, Fox WW. Episodic airway obstruction in premature infants. Am J Dis Child 1983; 137:441–443.

116. Milner AD, Boon AW, Saunders RA, Hopkin IE. Upper airways obstruction and apnoea in preterm babies. Arch Dis Child 1980; 55:22–25.
117. Thach BT, Stark AR. Spontaneous neck flexion and airway obstruction during apneic spells in preterm infants. J Pediatr 1979; 94:275–281.
118. Guilleminault C, Ariagno R, Korobkin R, Nagel L, Baldwin R, Coons S, Owen M. Mixed and obstructive sleep apnea and near miss for sudden infant death syndrome: 2. Comparison of near miss and normal control infants by age. Pediatrics 1979; 64:882–891.
119. Roberts JL, Reed WR, Mathew OP, Thach BT. Control of respiratory activity of the genioglossus muscle in micrognathic infants. J Appl Physiol 1986; 61:1523–1533.
120. Guilleminault C, Souquet M, Ariagno RL, Korobkin R, Simmons FB. Five cases of near miss sudden infant death syndrome and development of obstructive sleep apnea syndrome. Pediatrics 1984; 73:71–78.
121. Guilleminault C, Ariagno RL, Forno LS, Nagel L, Baldwin R, Owen M. Obstructive sleep apnea and near miss for SIDS: I. Report of an infant with sudden death. Pediatrics 1979; 63:837–843.
122. Kahn A, Blum D, Rebuffat E, Sottiaux M, Levitt J, Bochner A, Alexander M, Grosswasser J, Muller MF. Polysomnographic studies of infants who subsequently died of sudden infant death syndrome. Pediatrics 1988; 82:721–727.
123. Lavie P, Herer P, Peled R, Berger I, Yoffe N, Zomer J, Rubin AH. Mortality in sleep apnea patients: a multivariate analysis of risk factors. Sleep 1995; 18:149–157.
124. He J, Kryger MH, Zorick FJ, Conway W, Roth T. Mortality and apnea index in obstructive sleep apnea: experience in 385 male patients. Chest 1988; 94:9–14.
125. Brown OE, Manning SC, Ridenour B. Cor pulmonale secondary to tonsillar and adenoidal hypertrophy: management considerations. Int J Pediatr Otorhinolaryngol 1988; 16:131–139.
126. Massumi RA, Sarin RK, Pooya M, Reichelderfer TR, Fraga JR, Rios JC, Ayesterian E. Tonsillar hypertrophy, airway obstruction, alveolar hypoventilation, and cor pulmonale in twin brothers. Dis Chest 1969; 55:110–114.
127. Lauritzen C, Lilja J, Jarlstedt J. Airway obstruction and sleep apnea in children with craniofacial anomalies. Plast Reconstruct Surg 1986; 77:1–6.

27

Pathophysiology of OSAS in Children

CAROLE L. MARCUS

Johns Hopkins University School of Medicine
Baltimore, Maryland

I. Introduction

The pathophysiology of the childhood obstructive sleep apnea syndrome (OSAS) remains poorly understood. Unfortunately, little research has been done in children with obstructive sleep apnea, and much of our knowledge is extrapolated from studies in adults.

II. Normal Changes in Upper Airway Function with Sleep

The changes in upper airway function with sleep are described in detail elsewhere in this book. In order to understand the pathophysiology of OSAS, it is important to keep in mind the following principles:

1. Ventilatory drive is decreased during sleep. This applies not only to the overall ventilatory response to hypoxia and hypercapnia but also to the effect of the central ventilatory drive on augmenting upper airway tone.
2. Intercostal and upper airway muscle tone decreases during sleep, particularly during rapid-eye-movement (REM) sleep. This results in a decreased

functional residual capacity and therefore more rapid hypoxemia with apnea.

3. As a result of the decrease in upper airway tone, upper airway resistance increases during sleep. In adults, the upper airway resistance during sleep may be double that of wakefulness (1). Because the upper airway resistance makes up nearly half of the total pulmonary resistance (2), small increases in upper airway resistance can have a significant impact on breathing.
4. As a result of the above factors, there is relative hypoxemia and hypercapnia during sleep, particularly REM sleep, compared to wakefulness. This normal phenomenon is magnified in patients with underlying pulmonary or upper airway disease.

III. The Obstructive Sleep Apnea Syndrome

The normal upper airway is a complex area involving more than 30 pairs of muscles (3). The pharynx is collapsible in order to facilitate phonation and swallowing. However, other than the transient closure associated with the above functions, the pharynx normally remains patent.

A. Chain of Events in OSAS

Adult patients with OSAS have a narrowed upper airway (4–6). During wakefulness, they compensate for this by augmenting their upper airway tone (7). During sleep, the compensatory mechanism is lost (8) and airway closure occurs despite continuing respiratory effort. Hypoxemia and hypercapnia ensue. Arousal occurs, which results in increased upper airway tone and termination of the apnea, often by gasping. The trigger for arousal is thought to be the increased respiratory effort, because arousal secondary to isolated hypoxemia, hypercapnia or increased inspiratory resistance has all been demonstrated to occur at the same level of respiratory effort (9). The frequent arousals lead to sleep fragmentation, with resultant daytime sleepiness.

Does This Pattern of Events Differ in Children?

Like adults, children with OSAS tend to have a narrow upper airway. The site of obstruction in children tends to be more distal than in adults, typically involving the oropharynx and hypopharynx (10,11) (see Chap. 11 for more details).

Several studies have addressed the issue of electromyography (EMG) activation with obstructive apnea in children. Jeffries et al. showed that children with OSAS tended to have phasic inspiratory activity of their upper airway muscles throughout sleep (12). Praud et al. studied seven children with OSAS and found that the diaphragmatic and genioglossal EMG decreased at the onset of obstructive apnea in five patients, but did not decrease significantly for the group as a whole (13). During non–rapid-eye-movement (NREM) sleep, the abdominal EMG increased throughout the apnea (14). Roberts (15) studied infants with micrognathia and OSAS and found an increase in genioglossal EMG during investigator-induced episodes of nasal occlusion. In one study, respiratory muscle EMGs increased in response to OSAS-associated hypoxia and hypercapnia (12), whereas in another study it did not (13). Thus, most studies show that, in children, accessory respiratory muscles are activated during obstructive apnea. However, none of these studies compared muscle activity during sleep to that during wakefulness.

The pattern of arousal in response to OSAS in children clearly differs from that in adults. In children with OSAS, arousals occur less frequently than in adults (see below) and partial upper airway obstruction (obstructive hypoventilation) may therefore continue for long periods. The mechanism for apnea termination in children who do not have cortical arousals is unclear. However, evidence suggests that these children do have subcortical (movement) arousals.

B. Relationship Between Central and Obstructive Apneas

Central and obstructive apneas are not necessarily distinct entities. It is now recognized that pharyngeal occlusion often occurs during central apnea (16,17). If arousal does not occur, the central apnea may progress to a mixed apnea (16), perhaps because of the effort required to overcome mucosal adhesion forces. In addition, the presence of central apneas, with resultant fluctuations in chemical stimuli to the brain, can lead to central ventilatory system oscillations, which predispose to obstructive apnea (18,19). Upper airway narrowing may lead to central apnea in addition to obstructive apnea. Guilleminault et al. (20) reported a cohort of adults with central apnea who were found to have small upper airways on cephalometric evaluation. The central apnea resolved with continuous positive airway pressure (CPAP) therapy. Similarly, it has been shown that children with micro- or retrognathia have increased central apnea (21).

C. Polysomnographic Differences Between Children and Adults

The clinical picture of OSAS differs between children and adults, as described elsewhere in this volume. There are a number of polygraphic findings that are distinctive for childhood OSAS and demonstrate the differences in pathophysiology between children and adults. The main differences between children and adults are as follows:

Children appear to have clinical sequelae associated with milder forms of OSAS than adults; i.e., with fewer and shorter obstructive apneas. The reason for this is unclear, but may be due to the fact that significant desaturation may occur even with brief apneas. This is because children have a faster respiratory rate than adults and a smaller functional residual capacity.

Children are less likely to have cortical arousals in response to obstructive apnea. In general, children have a higher arousal threshold than adults; the younger the child, the fewer the arousals. This has been demonstrated using both nonrespiratory (acoustic) stimuli (22) and respiratory stimuli. McNamara and colleagues (23) studied children with OSAS ranging from birth to 14 years of age. They found that 51% of NREM and 35% of REM obstructive apneas were terminated by arousal. In infants, 18% of NREM and 12% of REM obstructive apneas were terminated by arousal. Respiratory-related arousals occurred most often in the older children.

Although cortical arousals are less common in children than adults, subcortical arousals probably occur frequently. Praud et al. (14) studied 10 prepubertal children and found that 12% of NREM obstructive apneas terminated in cortical arousals and 88% in movement arousals (defined as an increase in EMG in any channel accompanied by a change in pattern in any other channel). All REM obstructive apneas terminated in movement arousals. Thus, in this study, all obstructive apneas terminated in some type of arousal. The arousals were associated with a maximal increase in abdominal EMG, which suggests that the arousal played a role in respiratory muscle activation, and thus apnea termination. Mograss et al. (24) studied 15 children 2 to 11 years of age. They reported that "nearly all" apneas were terminated by movement arousals, with a close correlation between the respiratory disturbance index and the movement arousal index ($r = .99, p < .01$).

The arousal response to exogenous hypercapnia and hypoxemia has been studied in prepubertal children with OSAS (25). It was found that hypoxemia (Sp_{O_2} of 75%) was a poor stimulus to arousal in both children with OSAS and normal controls (children with OSAS aroused on 21% of trials versus 26% for controls; NS). Hypercapnia resulted in arousal in all subjects. However, the patients with OSAS aroused at a higher P_{CO_2} than controls (58 ± 2 versus 60 ± 5 mmHg, $p < .05$); those with the highest apnea index had the highest arousal threshold ($r = .52, p < .05$). The hypercapnic arousal threshold decreased following treatment, suggesting that the blunted arousal threshold was secondary to chronic nocturnal hypercapnia. Interestingly, hypoxic hypercapnia was a potent stimulus to arousal in this experimental setup, despite the fact that children with OSAS frequently have obstructive apneas associated with hypoxic hypercapnia and yet do not have cortical arousals.

The lack of frequent cortical arousals in children with OSAS may account for the low incidence of excessive daytime sleepiness compared to adults with OSAS. However, the presence of frequent movement arousals may play a role in the autonomic consequences of obstructive apnea in children, such as hypertension (26) and heart rate changes (27).

Children with OSAS have preserved sleep architecture, perhaps because of the lack of arousals (28,29). In contrast, adults with OSAS have sleep fragmentation, with decreased slow-wave and REM sleep (30,31). The normal sleep architecture in children with OSAS is another factor accounting for the reduced incidence of excessive daytime sleepiness compared to adults.

Children may show a pattern of persistent partial upper airway obstruction associated with hypercapnia and/or hypoxemia rather than cyclic discrete obstructive apneas. This has been termed *obstructive hypoventilation*. The decreased frequency of cortical arousals in response to obstructive apnea may permit this pattern of breathing to occur.

In children, obstructive apnea is predominantly a REM phenomenon. It is not unusual to see a child with severe REM-related obstructive apnea yet no obstruction during other stages of sleep. A recent study of children with severe OSAS showed that 56% of all obstructive apneas occurred during REM sleep (although REM sleep accounted for only 22% of total sleep time), 33% during stage 2 (48% of total sleep time), 3% during stage 1 (4% of total sleep time) and only 7% during slow-wave sleep (26% of total sleep time) (32). Furthermore, apneas were longer and more numerous during later REM periods than REM periods earlier in the night (32).

D. Upper Airway Collapsibility and the Starling Resistor Theory

The Starling resistor model, which describes the major determinants of airflow in terms of the mechanical properties of collapsible tubes, has been shown to be applicable to the upper airway in adults (33) and children (34) as well as other biological systems, such as blood vessels (35) and the lower airways (36). The model predicts that, under conditions of flow limitation, maximal inspiratory airflow is determined by the pressure changes upstream (nasal) to a collapsible locus of the upper airway and is independent of the downstream (hypopharyngeal and tracheal) pressure generated by the diaphragm. The upper airway can be represented as a tube with a collapsible segment, the resistance of which is zero (Fig. 1). The segments upstream (i.e., nasal) and downstream (i.e., hypopharyngeal) from the collapsible segment have fixed diameters and resistances (R_N and R_{HP}), and pressures (P_N and P_{HP}), respectively. For practical purposes, P_{HP} can be approximated by the esophageal pressure; P_N is represented by the nasal pressure.

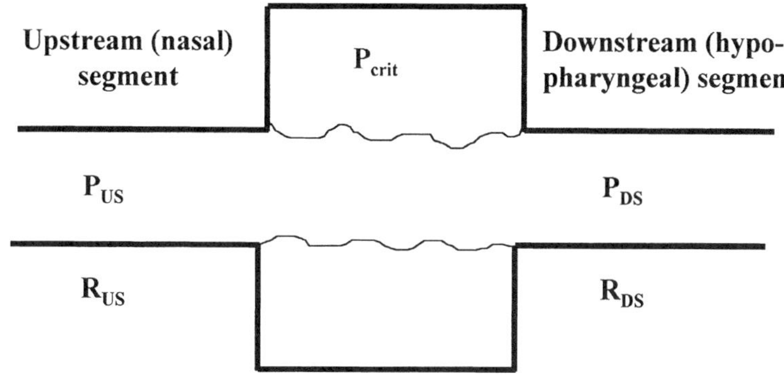

Figure 1 The Starling resistor model of the upper airway is shown. The upper airway is represented as a tube with a collapsible segment. The segments upstream (nasal) and downstream (hypopharyngeal) from the collapsible segment have fixed diameters and resistances (R_{US} and R_{DS}), and pressures (P_{US} and P_{DS}), respectively. Collapse occurs when the pressure surrounding the airway (P_{crit}) becomes greater than the pressure within the airway.

In this model of the upper airway, inflow pressure at the airway opening (the nares) is atmospheric and downstream pressure is equal to tracheal pressure. Collapse occurs when the pressure surrounding the collapsible segment of the upper airway (critical tissue pressure, P_{crit}) becomes greater than the pressure within the collapsible segment of the airway. In the normal subject with low upstream resistance or subatmospheric P_{crit}, P_{HP} never drops to P_{crit}; thus airflow is not limited and is largely determined by negative tracheal (inspiratory) pressure. However, if P_{HP} falls below P_{crit}, maximal inspiratory flow ($\dot{V}I_{max}$) reaches a maximum (inspiratory airflow limitation) and becomes independent of downstream pressure swings (Figs. 2 and 3). Under these circumstances, nasal resistance (R_N) and P_{crit} determine $\dot{V}I_{max}$ as described by the following equation: $\dot{V}I_{max} = (P_N - P_{crit})/R_N$. Airflow will become zero (i.e., the airway will occlude) when P_N falls below P_{crit}.

The measurement of P_{crit} has been a useful tool for studying upper airway function in OSAS. Measurements have been obtained by having the subject sleep while wearing a nasal mask. Airflow is measured via a pneumotachometer attached to the mask, upstream pressure via a transducer connected to the mask, and downstream pressure via a transducer connected to an esophageal balloon (34). The mask (upstream) pressure is then adjusted, either in a positive direction (using a CPAP device) or a subatmospheric direction (using a vacuum source). P_{crit} is determined by correlating the maximal inspiratory airflow with the level of mask pressure applied. The X intercept of the pressure-flow graph—i.e., the mask pressure at which zero flow occurs—represents P_{crit}.

P_{crit} provides an objective measure of upper airway collapsibility. In adults, P_{crit} is lowest in nonsnorers and increases progressively in subjects with snoring, hypopneas, and obstructive apneas. Gleadhill et al. (37) measured a P_{crit} of 2.5 ± 1.5 cmH_2O in adults with obstructive sleep apnea. This positive value indicates that the upper airway would collapse during sleep. Subjects with hypopnea had a marginally subatmospheric P_{crit} of −1.6 ± 1.4 cmH_2O, whereas subjects with primary snoring had a P_{crit} of −6.5 ± 2.7. This subatmospheric value indicates that the airway would remain patent. Similar results have been found in children. Marcus et al. (34), using the same technique as Gleadhill, showed that prepubertal school-aged children with OSAS had positive or only slightly subatmospheric P_{crit} values (1 ± 3 cmH_2O); this did not differ significantly from the values for adults (Fig. 4). Children with primary snoring had markedly subatmospheric P_{crit} values (−20 ± 9 cmH_2O). In the children with OSAS, P_{crit} correlated with the severity of sleep-disordered breathing, as demonstrated by the apnea index ($r = .83$), the arterial oxygen saturation nadir during sleep ($r = -.72$) and the peak P_{CO_2} during sleep ($r = .78$) (34). In adults with OSAS, P_{crit} has been demonstrated to decrease following successful treatment by either surgical (uvulopharyngopalatoplasty) (38) or medical (weight loss) (39) means. In three children, P_{crit} fell following tonsillectomy and adenoidectomy (from 2.1 ± 4.1 to −7.2 ± 4.0 cmH_2O), although it remained higher than in children with primary snoring (34).

Normal children snore less than adults and have fewer obstructive apneas (40). This suggests that normal children have less collapsible upper airways than normal

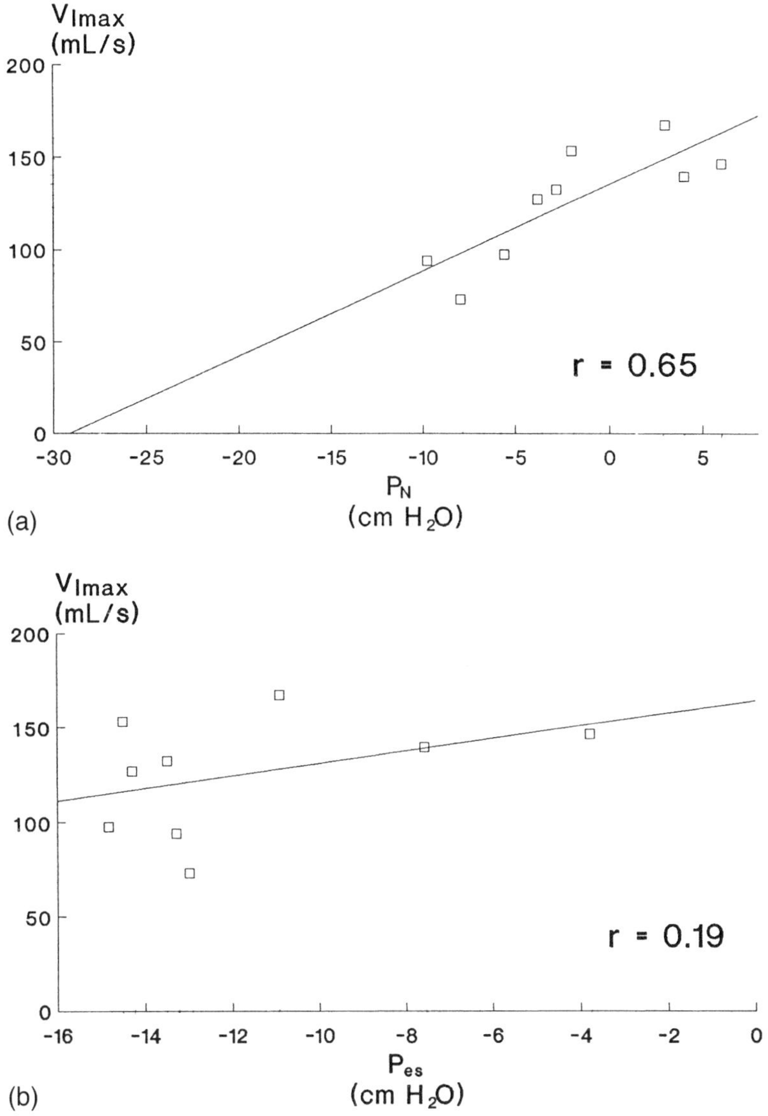

Figure 2 (a) Maximal inspiratory flow ($\dot{V}I_{max}$) versus nasal pressure (P_N) for a child with primary snoring. P_{crit} is represented by the level of P_N below which $\dot{V}I_{max}$ becomes zero (x-intercept). In this case, $P_{crit} = -29$ cm H_2O. $\dot{V}I_{max}$ varies in proportion to the level of P_N applied, with a correlation coefficient approaching significance ($r = 0.65$, $p = .06$). (b) $\dot{V}I_{max}$ versus esophageal pressure (P_{es}) for the same child. There is no correlation between inspiratory airflow and esophageal pressure ($r = .19$, $p = .62$). (From Ref. 34.)

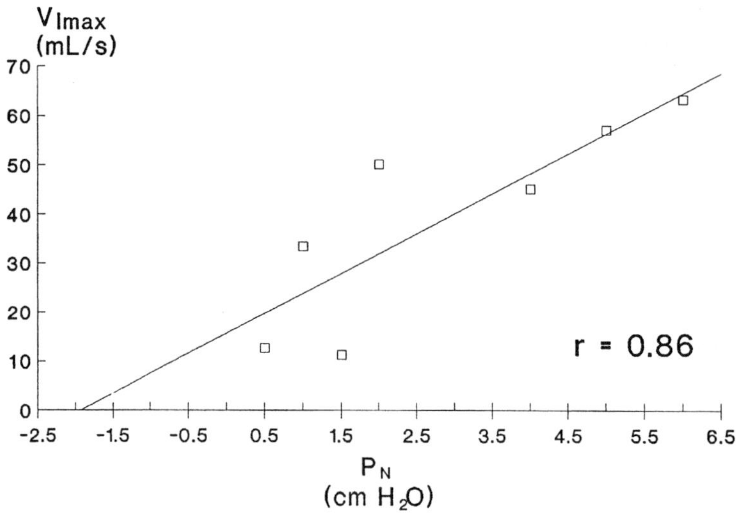

Figure 3 $\dot{V}I_{max}$ versus P_N for a child with obstructive sleep apnea syndrome. In this case, $P_{crit} = -1.9$ cmH_2O. $\dot{V}I_{max}$ is directly proportional to the level of P_N applied ($r = .86$, $p = .01$). (From Ref. 34.)

adults. This hypothesis has been confirmed by using the Starling resistor model to evaluate upper airway pressure-flow relationships. Children with primary snoring have a lower P_{crit} than adults with primary snoring (34,37). Preliminary evidence suggests that upper airway collapsibility is increased in adults as compared to children (41). This appears to be due to both increased body mass and decreased ventilatory drive to the upper airway with aging. In the living organism, P_{crit} reflects both upper airway neuromotor control and structural factors. The upper airway is not merely a passive conduit affected by mechanical forces but is also affected by activation of the upper airway muscles. Thus, closing pressures measured during wakefulness are markedly subatmospheric, even in patients with OSAS (42). Studies using denervated upper airway or postmortem preparations have shown that when upper airway muscle function is decreased or absent, the airway is more prone to collapse (43,44), whereas stimulation of the upper airway muscles by hypercapnia (45) or electrical stimulation (46) decreases collapsibility. One can therefore hypothesize that normal children compensate for a smaller upper airway by increasing the ventilatory drive to their upper airway muscles. This compensatory mechanism may be absent or diminished in children with OSAS.

Infants appear to have a more collapsible upper airway than school-aged children (preschool-aged children have not been studied). Upper airway closing pressures have been measured in infants, but by different techniques from those used in older children. Using a nasal occlusion technique, Roberts et al. (47) found the airway clos-

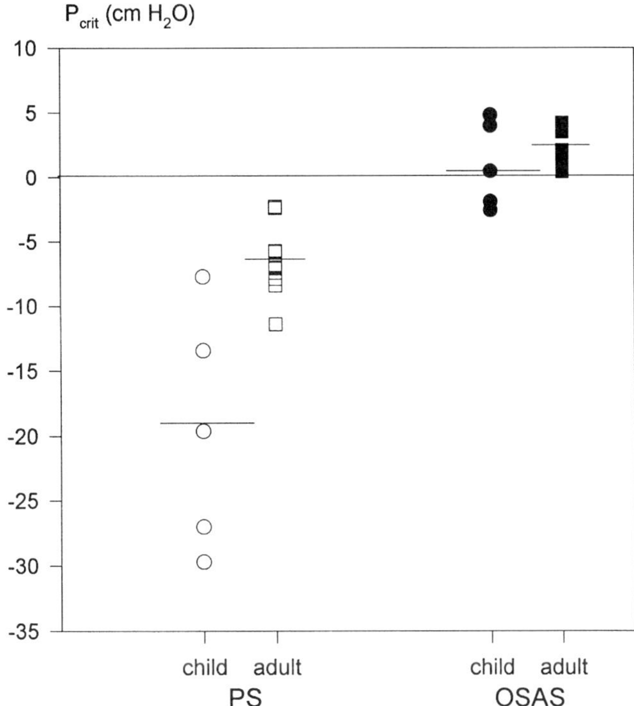

Figure 4 P_{crit} values for individual subjects with obstructive sleep apnea syndrome (OSAS) and primary snoring (PS) are shown. Group means are represented by bars. P_{crit} is significantly higher in children with OSAS versus PS ($p < .01$), and adults with OSAS versus PS ($p < .001$). P_{crit} is similar between children and adults with OSAS. However, P_{crit} is lower in children with PS than in adults with PS ($p < .01$). (Derived from Refs. 34 and 37.)

ing pressure in normal sleeping infants to be -3.8 ± 3.1 cmH_2O. Wilson et al. (48) demonstrated a closing pressure of 0.8 cmH_2O in postmortem infants. These data suggest that infants have more collapsible upper airways than older children, which is consistent with clinical findings. However, the different techniques used for these measurements make direct comparisons with other age groups difficult. The increased upper airway collapsibility noted in infants may be due to anatomic factors (see below) or differences in ventilatory control.

IV. Etiological Factors for Childhood OSAS

The etiology of OSAS is multifactorial. For OSAS to occur, there must probably be a combination of three factors (Fig. 5): 1) altered airway structure, 2) diminished neu-

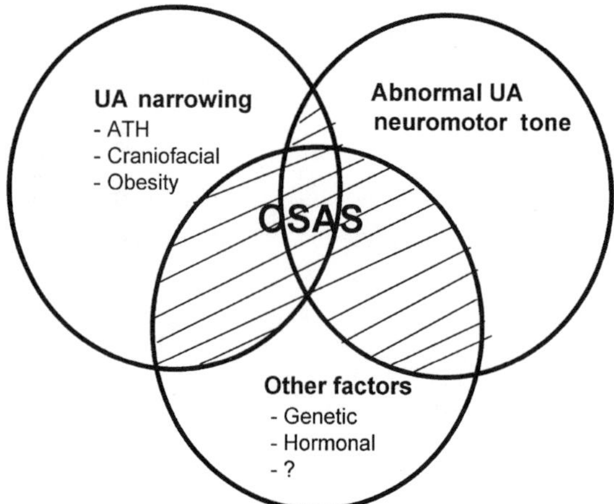

Figure 5 The etiology of the childhood obstructive sleep apnea syndrome (OSAS) is multifactorial. OSAS results from a combination of structural, neuromotor, and other factors. Structural factors, such as adenotonsillar hypertrophy (ATH), craniofacial anomalies, or obesity, result in upper airway (UA) narrowing. Subtle abnormalities in ventilatory drive or upper airway neuromotor control are probably present in all patients with OSAS; in some patients—e.g., those with cerebral palsy—abnormal neuromotor tone is a prominent factor. Other factors that may be important include a genetic predisposition, hormonal factors (particularly testosterone), and probably other, as yet unidentified, factors.

romuscular control, and 3) miscellaneous factors, such as genetic and hormonal influences. Thus, one child with a narrow airway due to adenotonsillar hypertrophy but with a high ventilatory drive may not develop OSAS, whereas another child with a similar degree of adenotonsillar hypertrophy but a lower ventilatory drive may have upper airway obstruction.

A. Structural Factors

Structural factors clearly play a large role in the majority of children with OSAS. Clinically, most children with OSAS have large tonsils and adenoids, and the OSAS resolves following tonsillectomy and adenoidectomy. However, adenotonsillar hypertrophy is not the sole cause of OSAS in these children, as they do not obstruct during wakefulness. Therefore, other factors must be present in addition to the structural component in order to produce airway obstruction during sleep.

Several studies have shown that adults with OSAS have narrow upper airways compared to controls (46). In addition, the shape of the upper airway is more elliptical, with the long axis oriented in the anteroposterior direction (5,49). As with adults, it seems as if most children with OSAS have some degree of structural narrowing of the upper airway, whether it be from adenotonsillar hypertrophy, craniofacial anomalies, or excess adipose tissue.

Adenotonsillar Hypertrophy

Adenotonsillar hypertrophy is the commonest condition associated with childhood OSAS. The lymphoid tissue in the upper airway increases in volume from birth to approximately 12 years of age (50). However, there is a concomitant increase in the size of the skeletal boundaries of the upper airway. Thus, the tonsils and adenoids are largest in relation to the underlying upper airway size between 3 and 6 years of age (51) (Fig. 6). This coincides with the peak incidence of childhood OSAS. In otherwise normal children with OSAS and adenotonsillar hypertrophy, tonsillectomy and adenoidectomy usually lead to resolution of OSAS (52). These facts suggest that adenotonsillar hypertrophy is a major contributing factor to OSAS. However, a number of factors suggest that associated abnormalities must be present—either abnormalities of neuromotor tone or additional structural factors: 1) As noted above, children with OSAS only obstruct during sleep. 2) Several studies have failed to show a correlation between upper airway/adenotonsillar size and OSAS. Radiological assessment of the adenoidal-nasopharyngeal ratio does not differentiate patients with OSAS from normals (53,54). Direct intraoperative measurements of the upper airway have had conflicting results. Laurikainen et al. (55) used the Static Charge Sensitive Bed

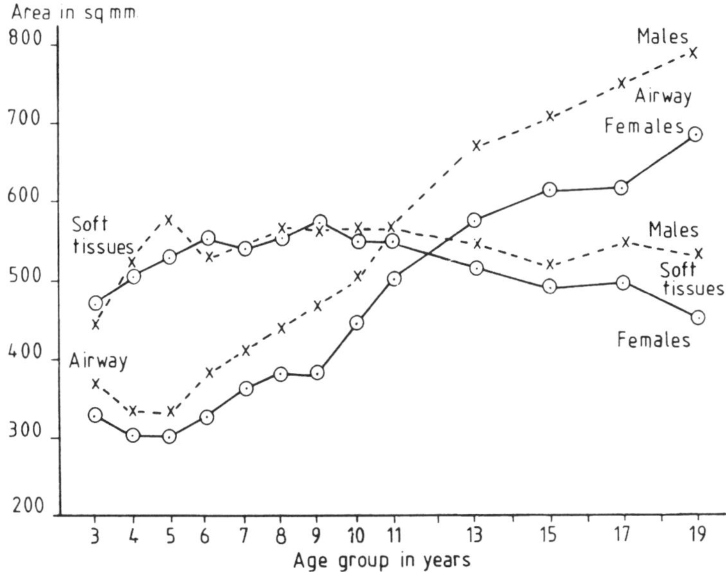

Figure 6 Changes in the mean areas of nasopharyngeal airway and soft tissues with age are shown for normal males and females. (From Ref. 51.)

to diagnose OSAS in young children and then compared upper airway measurements in these patients to controls. No difference was found between groups in the parameters of either the bony nasopharynx or the adenotonsillar volume. Brodsky et al. (56–58) performed similar studies in a number of experiments, and did not find consistent results between the different studies. This may be because no objective evaluation for sleep-disordered breathing was performed. Thus, there is no evidence that upper airway size correlates with obstructive apnea in children. 3) A small percentage of children without obvious additional risk factors for OSAS are not cured by tonsillectomy and adenoidectomy (52). Of the children requiring CPAP for OSAS at our institution, 20% are nonobese, otherwise healthy children in whom OSAS persisted following tonsillectomy and adenoidectomy. 4) Guilleminault and colleagues reported a cohort of children who were cured of their OSAS by tonsillectomy and adenoidectomy but developed a recurrence during adolescence (59).

The existence of otherwise healthy children with persistence or recurrence of OSAS following surgical treatment suggests two possibilities: 1) a discrete subset of children with OSAS associated with adenotonsillar hypertrophy have additional subtle abnormalities in upper airway structure or neuromotor control or 2) all children with OSAS and adenotonsillar hypertrophy have additional subclinical abnormalities that will lead to OSAS if additional risk factors (such as weight gain or testosterone secretion at puberty) are acquired.

Craniofacial Structure

OSAS occurs frequently in children with craniofacial anomalies due to narrowing of the upper airway. Some children with severe craniofacial anomalies require tracheostomies soon after birth because of fixed upper airway narrowing. However, less severely affected individuals may develop upper airway obstruction only during sleep, again suggesting that there must be some combination of structural and dynamic (neuromotor) factors for OSAS to occur. In some patients with craniofacial anomalies, OSAS begins or recurs during early childhood, in conjunction with adenotonsillar hypertrophy. OSAS has been reported to occur with a large number of syndromes (see Chap. 32 for details). It is most likely to occur when the patient has nasal obstruction, midfacial hypoplasia, micro- or retrognathia, macroglossia, or associated obesity or hypotonia.

The contributing role of craniofacial structure to OSAS is most obvious in children with known craniofacial syndromes. However, subclinical changes in craniofacial structure (such as minor degrees of retrognathia) probably play a role in the development of OSAS in other patients. This may explain why studies evaluating the degree of adenotonsillar hypertrophy without considering other anatomic factors such as mandibular size or position (60) do not show a direct correlation with OSAS.

Infants are predisposed to OSAS by virtue of their craniofacial structure. In infants, the mobile upper airway structures (such as the tongue and larynx) are large relative to the bony chambers that surround them. The larynx is displaced superiorly and anteriorly, such that the uvula almost approximates the epiglottis (61). The mandible is more horizontal and has a tendency to subluxate posteriorly along with the base of the tongue, particularly when the infant is supine. In addition, infants are prone to gastroesophageal reflux, which can cause upper airway edema and laryngomalacia.

Obesity

Most adults with OSAS are obese. In contrast, children with OSAS are often of normal weight or may even have failure to thrive. However, there is a subset of children with OSAS secondary to obesity (62–64), and asymptomatic, obese infants have been shown to have an increased frequency of obstructive apneas (65). In obese patients, upper airway narrowing results from deposition of adipose tissue within the muscles and soft tissue surrounding the airway (66,67) as well as external compression from the neck and jowls. Obesity causes restrictive lung disease, which can contribute to hypoxemia. In obese patients, the supine position alone may result in hypoxemia due to superior displacement of the abdominal contents. Additionally, obese patients may have a blunted central ventilatory drive (Pickwickian syndrome). Mallory et al. (63), studying obese children presenting to a clinic with symptoms of sleep-disordered breathing, found no correlation between the percentage of ideal body weight and the apnea hypopnea index ($r = .10$) or time with $Sp_{O_2} < 90\%$ ($r = -.02$). However, another study evaluating obese asymptomatic children from the community found a correlation between the percentage of ideal body weight and apnea index ($r = .47$, $p < .05$), Sp_{O_2} nadir ($r = -.60$, $p < .01$), and sleepiness on multiple sleep latency testing ($r = -.50$, $p < .05$) (62). Even in obese subjects, OSAS usually improves or resolves following tonsillectomy and adenoidectomy (62,68). Obstructive apnea results from the relative size and structure of the upper airway components; thus tonsillectomy and adenoidectomy may widen the airway of an obese patient sufficiently to result in clinical improvement. Alternatively, the postoperative improvement may be due to scarring, with subsequent stiffening of the upper airway.

Nasal Obstruction

Nasal obstruction can cause OSAS, the classic example being choanal stenosis. It had been thought that infants were *obligatory* nasal breathers, but current thinking is that they are *preferential* nasal breathers (69,70). Thus, it is not surprising that, in infants, mild nasal obstruction may result in OSAS. However, in all age groups, the nasal route for breathing is preferred over the oral route during sleep (71), and nasal obstruction (e.g., by nasal packing) can cause OSAS. In children, nasal obstruction secondary to adenoidal hypertrophy is a common cause of OSAS. Children with OSAS have a high prevalence of allergic sensitization (72); however, the role of allergic rhinitis in OSAS has not been studied in detail in children.

B. Neuromotor Factors

Neuromotor factors play an important role in the pathogenesis of OSAS. The fact that patients with OSAS breathe normally during wakefulness but obstruct during sleep indicates the presence of a neuromotor component in all patients with OSAS. However, this is most pronounced in patients with neurological or neuromuscular disease.

Role of the Central Ventilatory Drive

Adults with OSAS are thought to have a decreased ventilatory drive during wakefulness (73–76). In contrast, children with OSAS have normal hypoxic and hypercapnic ventilatory responses during both wakefulness (77) and sleep (25). There are several possible explanations for this discrepancy. First, a confounding factor in many of the adult studies was the presence of obesity and/or lung disease. These were not present in the pediatric subjects. Obstructive apneas are usually more frequent in adults, and of longer duration. Thus, it is possible that the depressed ventilatory drive in adults is acquired, secondary to chronic sleep-related hypoxemia and hypercapnia. This theory is supported by several studies showing an improvement in ventilatory drive following treatment by tracheostomy (78) or CPAP (79,80). Alternatively, pediatric OSAS and adult OSAS may be two distinct disease entities with different pathophysiologies.

Although children with OSAS have no overall decrease in their ventilatory responses, subtle abnormalities may be present. Gozal et al. (81) performed repetitive hypercapnic challenges in children with OSAS during wakefulness, early in the morning. Although OSAS subjects increased their minute ventilation during each individual hypercapnic challenge, they had a different pattern of breathing than controls. Control children had progressive increases in tidal volume and decreases in respiratory rate across the challenges resulting in a progressively increased minute ventilation, whereas OSAS subjects had a variable breathing response with no increase in minute ventilation. Responses normalized later in the day (two subjects) or after curative tonsillectomy and adenoidectomy (one subject). This study suggests that children with OSAS have a subtle, reversible abnormality in their hypercapnic ventilatory drive, which may be related to nocturnal hypercapnia. However, the exact mechanism for this abnormality is not known.

Role of the Upper Airway Muscles

The upper airway muscles are accessory muscles of ventilation and, as such, are activated by hypoxemia and hypercapnia. In adult patients with OSAS, the inhalation of CO_2 resulted in fewer obstructive apneas and an increased chin–chest wall EMG ratio, whereas inhaling O_2 resulted in increased obstruction and lower EMG tone (82). Similarly, the administration of exogenous CO_2 to children with OSAS resulted in a decrease in upper airway obstruction (Fig. 7) (25). Children with OSAS have been shown to have continued upper airway muscle activity during airway obstruction (12,13) and this muscle activity increases in proportion to the degree of hypercapnia and hypoxemia (12). However, it is not known whether children with OSAS augment

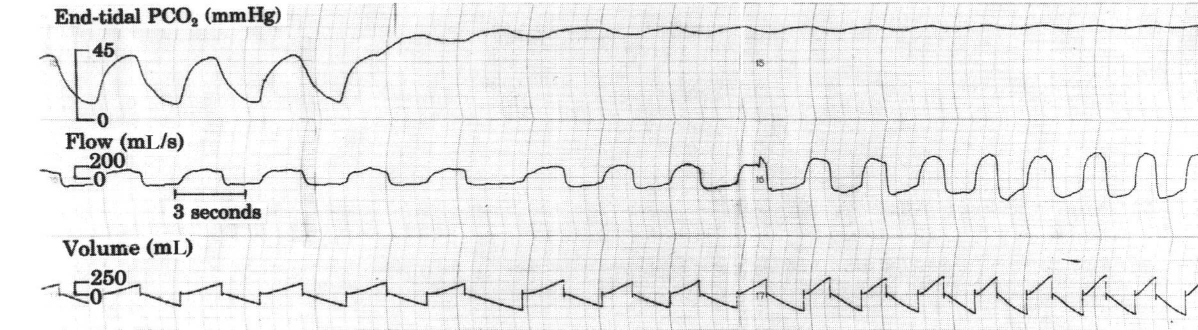

Figure 7 Portion of a tracing demonstrating a change from flow-limited breathing to non-flow-limited breathing in response to hypercapnia as a result of upper airway neuromotor activation. Prior to hypercapnia, flow limitation is present: i.e., airflow fails to increase despite increasing respiratory effort. The characteristic waveform pattern consists of increasing inspiratory flow followed by a mid-inspiratory plateau. As exogenous CO_2 is introduced, end-tidal Pco_2 increases and breaths become non-flow-limited. There is a simultaneous increase in flow (hence tidal volume) and respiratory rate. Arousal did not occur. Note that inspiration is represented by a downward deflection on the flow tracing. (From Ref. 25.)

their upper airway muscles in response to chemical stimuli or inspiratory loading to the same degree as normal children.

Disease States

Children with abnormal neuromotor control, such as those with hypotonia [e.g., muscular dystrophy (83)] or neuromotor incoordination [e.g., cerebral palsy (84)] often develop OSAS, even in the absence of adenotonsillar hypertrophy. Some of these patients improve after tonsillectomy and adenoidectomy, again demonstrating the interaction between structural and neuromotor factors.

C. Other Factors Contributing to the Development of OSAS

Genetic Factors

There is a familial tendency to OSAS (76,85–89). This appears to be due to a genetic influence on both ventilatory drive (76,90) and minor anatomic factors (85,89) and cannot simply be attributed to a familial tendency toward obesity (90). A report in a Japanese cohort described an association between OSAS and two HLA types (HLA-A2 and HLA B39) (91). Further research is needed in this area.

Racial/Ethnic Factors

Sleep-disordered breathing appears to be more common in African Americans than Caucasians. This has been demonstrated in both young (< 25 years of age) (92) and elderly (93) populations, although children have not been specifically evaluated.

Hormonal Factors

Hormonal factors clearly play a role in the pathogenesis of OSAS in adults. In adults, OSAS is twice as common in males as in females (94); the incidence increases in postmenopausal women (95). The administration of exogenous testosterone may result in OSAS (96–98). These facts suggest that androgens play a role in the pathophysiology of OSAS, either by altering upper airway morphology or by affecting ventilatory drive (99), and that female sex hormones may play a protective role, perhaps by enhancing ventilatory drive.

There are a number of potential explanations for the male propensity for OSAS. Clearly, there is a difference in the structure of the adult male upper airway compared to that of the female. This does not apply to children. With puberty, the male larynx enlarges, resulting in a deeper voice. However, in prepubertal children, there are only minimal differences in laryngeal anatomy (100) and upper airway size (by cephalometric measurements) (101) between the two sexes. The adult male distribution of body fat differs from the female, with a preponderance of fat deposition around the neck and central body. Thus, for a given body mass index, men are more likely to have OSAS than women (102). In adults, there appears to be a difference in the mechanical properties of the pharynx between males and females. Males have a greater sleep-related increase in upper airway resistance than females (103). In addition to the structural and mechanical differences between males and females, there are differences in upper airway neuromotor control and ventilatory drive. Popovic and White (104) demonstrated higher peak inspiratory and tonic expiratory genioglossal EMG activity during wakefulness in women than in men. The women had a sustained increase in EMG in response to inspiratory resistance loading, whereas the men had no significant response. This may be due to the stimulatory effect of progesterone on upper airway muscle activity (105,106), possibly through its role as a stimulant of central ventilatory drive.

Despite the apparent effect of sex hormones on upper airway function, the clinical relevance of hormonal factors is uncertain. The effects of therapeutic administration of female hormones (107–109) or androgen blockers (110) to patients with OSAS have been disappointing.

The gender-related prevalence of OSAS in prepubertal children remains unknown. In the past, it was frequently stated that OSAS occurred equally among male and female prepubertal children. However, we and others (personal communications) have noted a preponderance of boys presenting for evaluation for sleep-disordered breathing. To the best of our knowledge, there have been no population-based studies evaluating the prevalence of OSAS between the two genders during childhood. Thus, the role of sex hormones in childhood OSAS is unclear.

Drugs

OSAS may be caused or aggravated by drugs that affect the reticular activating system, reduce the central ventilatory drive, or directly depress upper airway muscle tone, such as sedatives, general anesthetics, and alcohol (111–114). Although chloral hydrate has been used to induce sleep for polysomnography without worsening of OSAS (115), it does depress genioglossal tone, and has been reported to precipitate obstructive sleep apnea in isolated cases (116).

V. Link Between Childhood and Adult OSAS

OSAS occurs in 1% to 3% of the pediatric population (117,118) and 2% to 4% of the adult population (94). Is this the same disease process recurring in adults initially treated by tonsillectomy and adenoidectomy during childhood, or are these two diverse diseases affecting discrete populations? Further study is needed. In one provocative report, Guilleminault and colleagues reevaluated adolescents who had been successfully treated during childhood by tonsillectomy and adenoidectomy (59). Of 49 potential cases, 31 could be located and 23 underwent polysomnography. Three patients (13% of those evaluated) were found to have obstructive sleep apnea. Interestingly, these were all males. This study suggests that patients with childhood OSAS may be at risk for recurrence.

It is possible that children at risk for OSAS, because of such factors as a small pharyngeal airway or decreased upper airway neuromuscular tone, develop OSAS when they reach the age of maximal adenotonsillar hyperplasia. This results in an increased mechanical load on a marginal upper airway, thus precipitating OSAS. Following surgical treatment, patients may become asymptomatic. While data are lacking on the natural history of the illness, it is possible that these high-risk children will develop a recurrence of OSAS during adulthood if they acquire additional risk factors, such as androgen secretion at puberty, weight gain, or excessive alcohol ingestion. Thus, childhood OSAS may be a precursor of adult OSAS.

VI. Conclusion

The pathophysiology of childhood OSAS remains poorly understood. However, it is thought to be caused by a combination of anatomic and neuromotor factors—i.e., by the superimposition of structural abnormalities upon an inherently more collapsible upper airway. Further study is needed to clarify the disease process.

Acknowledgments

Dr. Marcus was supported in part by the Pediatric Clinical Research Center #RR-00052, The Johns Hopkins Hospital, Baltimore, MD; and NHLBI grants #HL37379-09RO1 and HL58585-01.

References

1. Lopes JM, Tabachnik E, Muller NL, Levison H, Bryan C. Total airway resistance and respiratory muscle activity during sleep. J Appl Physiol 1983; 54:773–777.
2. Ferris BG, Mead J, Opie LH. Partitioning of respiratory flow resistance in man. J Appl Physiol 1964; 19:653–658.
3. van Lunteren E, Strohl KP. Striated respiratory muscles of the upper airways. In: Mathew OP, Sant'Ambrogio G, eds. Respiratory Function of the Upper Airway. New York: Marcel Dekker, 1988: 87–123.
4. Schwab RJ, Gupta KB, Gefter WB, Metzger LJ, Hoffman EA, Pack AI. Upper airway and soft tissue anatomy in normal subjects and patients with sleep-disordered breathing: significance of the lateral pharyngeal walls. Am J Respir Crit Care Med 1995; 152: 1673–1689.
5. Galvin JR, Rooholamini SA, Stanford W. Obstructive sleep apnea: diagnosis with ultrafast CT. Radiology 1989; 171:775–778.
6. Shelton KE, Woodson H, Gay S, Suratt PM. Pharyngeal fat in obstructive sleep apnea. Am Rev Respir Dis 1993; 148:462–466.
7. Mezzanotte WS, Tangel DJ, White DP. Waking genioglossal electromyogram in sleep apnea patients versus normal controls (a neuromuscular compensatory mechanism). J Clin Invest 1992; 89:1571–1579.
8. Mezzanotte WS, Tangel DJ, White DP. Influence of sleep onset on upper airway muscle activity in apnea patients versus normal controls. Am J Respir Crit Care Med 1996; 153:1880–1887.

9. Gleeson K, Zwillich CW, White DP. The influence of increasing ventilatory effort on arousal from sleep. Am Rev Respir Dis 1990; 142:295–300.
10. Gibson SE, Myer CM III, Strife JL, O'Connor DM. Sleep fluoroscopy for localization of upper airway obstruction in children. Ann Otol Rhinol Laryngol 1996; 105:678–683.
11. Felman AH, Loughlin GM, Leftridge CA, Cassisi NJ. Upper airway obstruction during sleep in children. AJR 1979; 133:213–216.
12. Jeffries B, Brouillette RT, Hunt CE. Electromyographic study of some accessory muscles of respiration in children with obstructive sleep apnea. Am Rev Respir Dis 1984; 129:696–702.
13. Praud JP, d'Allest AM, Delaperche MF, Bobin S, Gaultier CI. Diaphragmatic and genioglossus electromyographic activity at the onset and at the end of obstructive apnea in children with obstructive sleep apnea syndrome. Pediatr Res 1988; 23:1–4.
14. Praud JP, d'Allest AM, Nedelcoux H, Curzi-Dascalova L, Guilleminault C, Gaultier C. Sleep-related abdominal muscle behavior during partial or complete obstructed breathing in prepubertal children. Pediatr Res 1989; 26:347–350.
15. Roberts JL, Reed WR, Mathew OP, Thach BT. Control of respiratory activity of the genioglossus muscle in micrognathic infants. J Appl Physiol 1986; 61:1523–1533.
16. Badr MS, Toiber F, Skatrud JB, Dempsey J. Pharyngeal narrowing/occlusion during central sleep apnea. J Appl Physiol 1995; 78:1806–1815.
17. Sanders MH, Rogers RM, Pennock BE. Prolonged expiratory phase in sleep apnea. Am Rev Respir Dis 1985; 131:401–408.
18. Longobardo GS, Gothe B, Goldman MD, Cherniack NS. Sleep apnea considered as a control system abnormality. Respir Physiol 1982; 50:311–333.
19. Dempsey J, Smith CA, Harms CA, Chow C, Saupe KW. Sleep-induced breathing instability. Sleep 1996; 19:236–247.
20. Guilleminault C, Quera-Salva MA, Nino-Murcia G, Partinen M. Central sleep apnea and partial obstruction of the upper airway. Ann Neurol 1987; 21:465–469.
21. Guilleminault C. Obstructive sleep apnea syndrome and its treatment in children: areas of agreement and controversy. Pediatr Pulmonol 1987; 3:429–436.
22. Busby KA, Mercier L, Pivik RT. Ontogenetic variations in auditory arousal threshold during sleep. Psychophysiology 1994; 31:182–188.
23. McNamara F, Issa FG, Sullivan CE. Arousal pattern following central and obstructive breathing abnormalities in infants and children. J Appl Physiol 1996; 81:2651–2657.
24. Mograss MA, Ducharme FM, Brouillette RT. Movement/arousals: description, classification, and relationship to sleep apnea in children. Am J Respir Crit Care Med 1994; 150:1690–1696.
25. Marcus CL, Lutz J, Carroll JL, Bamford O. Arousal and ventilatory responses during sleep in children with obstructive sleep apnea. J Appl Physiol 1998; 84:1926–1936.
26. Marcus CL, Greene MG, Carroll JL. Blood pressure in children with obstructive sleep apnea. Am J Respir Crit Care Med 1998; 157:1098–1103.
27. Aljadeff G, Gozal D, Schechtman VL, Burrell B, Harper RM, Ward SL. Heart rate variability in children with obstructive sleep apnea. Sleep 1997; 20:151–157.
28. Marcus CL, Carroll JL, Koerner CB, Hamer A, Lutz J, Loughlin GM. Determinants of growth in children with the obstructive sleep apnea syndrome. J Pediatr 1994; 125:556–562.
29. Frank Y, Kravath RE, Pollak CP, Weitzman ED. Obstructive sleep apnea and its therapy; clinical and polysomnographic manifestations. Pediatrics 1983; 71:737–742.

30. Weitzman ED, Kahn E, Pollak CP. Quantitative analysis of sleep and sleep apnea before and after tracheostomy in patients with the hypersomnia-sleep apnea syndrome. Sleep 1980; 3:407–423.
31. Bradley TD, Phillipson EA. Pathogenesis and pathophysiology of the obstructive sleep apnea syndrome. Medical Clinics of North America 1985; 69:1169–1185.
32. Goh DYT, Marcus CL. Changes in obstructive sleep apnea characteristics in children through the night (abstr). Am J Respir Crit Care Med 1998; 157:A533.
33. Smith PL, Wise RA, Gold AR, Schwartz AR, Permutt S. Upper airway pressure-flow relationships in obstructive sleep apnea. J Appl Physiol 1988; 64:789–795.
34. Marcus CL, McColley SA, Carroll JL, Loughlin GM, Smith PL, Schwartz AR. Upper airway collapsibility in children with obstructive sleep apnea syndrome. J Appl Physiol 1994; 77:918–924.
35. Permutt S, Riley RL. Hemodynamics of collapsible vessels with tone: the vascular waterfall. J Appl Physiol 1963; 18:924–932.
36. Pride NB, Permutt S, Riley RL, Bromberger-Barnea B. Determinants of maximal expiratory flow from the lungs. J Appl Physiol 1967; 23:646–662.
37. Gleadhill IC, Schwartz AR, Schubert N, Wise RA, Permutt S, Smith PL. Upper airway collapsibility in snorers and in patients with obstructive hypopnea and apnea. Am Rev Respir Dis 1991; 143:1300–1303.
38. Schwartz AR, Schubert N, Rothman W, Godley F, Marsh B, Eisele D, Nadeau J, Permutt L, Gleadhill I, Smith PL. Effect of uvulopalatopharyngoplasty on upper airway collapsibility in obstructive sleep apnea. Am Rev Respir Dis 1992; 145:527–532.
39. Schwartz AR, Gold AR, Schubert N, Stryzak A, Wise RA, Permutt S, Smith PL. Effect of weight loss on upper airway collapsibility in obstructive sleep apnea. Am Rev Respir Dis 1991; 144:494–498.
40. Marcus CL, Omlin KJ, Basinki DJ, Bailey SL, Rachal AB, Von Pechmann WS, Keens TG, Ward SL. Normal polysomnographic values for children and adolescents. Am Rev Respir Dis 1992; 146:1235–1239.
41. Marcus CL, Smith PL, Lutz J, Schwartz AR. Developmental changes in upper airway collapsibility (abstr). Am J Respir Crit Care Med 1998; 157:A533.
42. Suratt PM, Wilhoit SC, Cooper K. Induction of airway collapse with subatmospheric pressure in awake patients with sleep apnea. J Appl Physiol 1984; 57:140–146.
43. Smith PL, Schwartz AR, Gauda E, Wise R, Brower R, Permutt S. The modulation of upper airway critical pressures during sleep. Prog Clin Biol Res 1990; 345:253–258; discussion, 258–260.
44. Brouillette RT, Thach BT. A neuromuscular mechanism maintaining extrathoracic airway patency. J Appl Physiol 1979; 46:772–779.
45. Schwartz AR, Thut DC, Brower RG, Gauda EB, Roach D, Permutt S, Smith PL. Modulation of maximal inspiratory airflow by neuromuscular activity: effect of CO_2. J Appl Physiol 1993; 74:1597–1605.
46. Schwartz AR, Thut DC, Russ B, Seelagy M, Yuan X, Brower RG, Permutt S, Wise RA, Smith PL. Effect of electrical stimulation of the hypoglossal nerve on airflow mechanics in the isolated upper airway. Am Rev Respir Dis 1993; 147:1144–1150.
47. Roberts JL, Reed WR, Mathew OP, Menon AA, Thach BT. Assessment of pharyngeal airway stability in normal and micrognathic infants. J Appl Physiol 1985; 58:290–299.
48. Wilson SL, Thach BT, Brouillette RT, Abu-Osba YK. Upper airway patency in the human infant: influence of airway pressure and posture. J Appl Physiol 1980; 48:500–504.

49. Leiter JC. Upper airway shape. Am J Respir Crit Care Med 1996; 153:894–898.
50. Vaughn VC. Growth and development. In: Behrman RE, Vaughn VC, eds. Nelson Textbook of Pediatrics, 12th ed. Philadelphia: Saunders, 1983: 10–38.
51. Jeans WD, Fernando DCJ, Maw AR, Leighton BC. A longitudinal study of the growth of the nasopharynx and its contents in normal children. Br J Radiol 1981; 54:117–121.
52. Suen JS, Arnold JE, Brooks LJ. Adenotonsillectomy for treatment of obstructive sleep apnea in children. Arch Otolaryngol Head Neck Surg 1995; 121:525–530.
53. Fernbach SK, Brouillette RT, Riggs TW, Hunt CE. Radiologic evaluation of adenoids and tonsils in children with obstructive apnea: plain films and fluoroscopy. Pediatr Radiol 1983; 13:258–265.
54. Mahboubi S, Marsh RR, Potsic WP, Pasquariello PS. The lateral neck radiograph in adenotonsillar hyperplasia. Int J Pediatr Otorhinolaryngol 1985; 10:67–73.
55. Laurikainen E, Erkinjuntti M, Alihanka J, Rikalainen H, Suonpaa J. Radiological parameters of the bony nasopharynx and the adenotonsillar size compared with sleep apnea episodes in children. Int J Pediatr Otorhinolaryngol 1987; 12:303–310.
56. Brodsky L, Moore L, Stanievich JF. A comparison of tonsillar size and oropharyngeal dimensions in children with obstructive adenotonsillar hypertrophy. Int J Pediatr Otorhinolaryngol 1987; 13:149–156.
57. Brodsky L, Adler E, Stanievich JF. Naso- and oropharyngeal dimensions in children with obstructive sleep apnea. Int J Pediatr Otorhinolaryngol 1989; 17:1–11.
58. Brodsky L, Koch RJ. Anatomic correlates of normal and diseased adenoids in children. Laryngoscope 1992; 102:1268–1274.
59. Guilleminault C, Partinen M, Praud JP, Quera-Salva MA, Powell N, Riley R. Morphometric facial changes and obstructive sleep apnea in adolescents. J Pediatr 1989; 114: 997–999.
60. Shelton KE, Gay SB, Hollowell DE, Woodson H, Suratt PM. Mandible enclosure of upper airway and weight in obstructive sleep apnea. Am Rev Respir Dis 1993; 148: 195–200.
61. Tonkin S. Sudden infant death syndrome: hypothesis of causation. Pediatrics 1975; 55: 650–661.
62. Marcus CL, Curtis S, Koerner CB, Joffe A, Serwint JR, Loughlin GM. Evaluation of pulmonary function and polysomnography in obese children and adolescents. Pediatr Pulmonol 1996; 21:176–183.
63. Mallory GB, Fiser DH, Jackson R. Sleep-associated breathing disorders in morbidly obese children and adolescents. J Pediatr 1989; 115:892–897.
64. Silvestri JM, Weese-Mayer DE, Bass MT, Kenny AS, Hauptman SA, Pearsall SM. Polysomnography in obese children with a history of sleep-associated breathing disorders. Pediatr Pulmonol 1993; 16:124–129.
65. Kahn A, Mozin MJ, Rebuffat E, Sottiaux M, Burniat W, Shepherd S, Muller MF. Sleep pattern alterations and brief airway obstructions in overweight infants. Sleep 1989; 12: 430–438.
66. Horner RL, Mohiaddin RH, Lowell DG, Shea SA, Burman ED, Longmore DB,Guz A. Sites and sizes of fat deposits around the pharynx in obese patients with obstructive sleep apnoea and weight matched controls Eur Respir J 1989; 2:613–622.
67. Stauffer JL, Buick MK, Bixler EO, Sharkey FE, Abt AB, Manders EK, Kales A, Cadieux RJ, Barry JD, Zwillich CW. Morphology of the uvula in obstructive sleep apnea. Am Rev Respir Dis 1989; 140:724–728.

68. Kudoh F, Sanai A. Effect of tonsillectomy and adenoidectomy on obese children with sleep-associated breathing disorders. Acta Otolaryngol 1996; 523(suppl):216–218.
69. Harding R. Nasal obstruction in infancy. Aust Paediatr J 1986; 22(suppl 1):59–61.
70. Miller MJ, Martin RJ, Carlo WA, Fouke JM, Strohl KP, Fanaroff AA. Oral breathing in newborn infants. J Pediatr 1985; 107:465–469.
71. Olsen KD, Kern EB. Nasal influences on snoring and obstructive sleep apnea. Mayo Clin Proc 1990; 65:1095–1105.
72. McColley SA, Carroll JL, Curtis S, Loughlin GM, Sampson HA. High prevalence of allergic sensitization in children with habitual snoring and obstructive sleep apnea. Chest 1997; 111:170–173.
73. Benlloch E, Cordero P, Morales P, Soler JJ, Macian V. Ventilatory pattern at rest and response to hypercapnic stimulation in patients with obstructive sleep apnea syndrome. Respiration 1995; 62:4–9.
74. Kunitomo F, Kimura H, Tatsumi K, Okita S, Tojima H, Kuriyama T, Honda Y. Abnormal breathing during sleep and chemical control of breathing during wakefulness in patients with sleep apnea syndrome. Am Rev Respir Dis 1989; 139:164–169.
75. Garay SM, Rapoport D, Sorkin B, Epstein H, Feinberg I, Goldring RM. Regulation of ventilation in the obstructive sleep apnea syndrome. Am Rev Respir Dis 1981; 124: 451–457.
76. Bayadi SE, Millman RP, Tishler PV, Rosenberg C, Saliski W, Boucher MA, Redline S. A family study of sleep apnea. Chest 1990; 98:554–559.
77. Marcus CL, Gozal D, Arens R, Basinski DJ, Omlin KJ, Keens TG, Ward SL. Ventilatory responses during wakefulness in children with obstructive sleep apnea. Am J Respir Crit Care Med 1994; 149:715–721.
78. Guilleminault C, Cummiskey J. Progressive improvement of apnea index and ventilatory response to CO_2 after tracheostomy in obstructive sleep apnea syndrome. Am Rev Respir Dis 1982; 126:14–20.
79. Berthon-Jones M, Sullivan CE. Time course of change in ventilatory response to CO_2 with long-term CPAP therapy for obstructive sleep apnea. Am Rev Respir Dis 1987; 135:144–147.
80. Lin C. Effect of nasal CPAP on ventilatory drive in normocapnic and hypercapnic patients with obstructive sleep apnoea syndrome. Eur Respir J 1994; 7:2005–2010.
81. Gozal D, Arens R, Omlin KJ, Ben-Ari G, Aljadeff G, Harper RM, Keens TG. Ventilatory response to consecutive short hypercapnic challenges in children with obstructive sleep apnea. J Appl Physiol 1995; 79:1608–1614.
82. Hudgel DW, Hendricks C, Dadley A. Alteration in obstructive apnea pattern induced by changes in oxygen- and carbon-dioxide-inspired concentrations. Am Rev Respir Dis 1988; 138:16–19.
83. Khan Y, Heckmatt JZ. Obstructive apnoeas in Duchenne muscular dystrophy. Thorax 1994; 49:157–161.
84. Kotagal S, Gibbons VP, Stith JA. Sleep abnormalities in patients with severe cerebral palsy. Dev Med Child Neurol 1994; 36:304–311.
85. Guilleminault C, Partinen M, Hollman K, Powell N, Stoohs R. Familial aggregates in obstructive sleep apnea syndrome. Chest 1995; 107:1545–1551.
86. Pillar G, Schnall RP, Peled N, Oliven A, Lavie P. Impaired respiratory response to resistive loading during sleep in healthy offspring of patients with obstructive sleep apnea. Am J Respir Crit Care Med 1997; 155:1602–1608.
87. Redline S, Tishler PV, Tosteson TD, Williamson J, Kump K, Browner I, Ferrette V,

Krijci P. The familial aggregation of obstructive sleep apnea. Am J Respir Crit Care Med 1995; 151:682–687.
88. Strohl KP, Saunders NA, Feldman NT, Hallett M. Obstructive sleep apnea in family members. N Engl J Med 1978; 299:969–973.
89. Douglas NJ, Luke M, Mathur R. Is the sleep apnoea/hypopnoea syndrome inherited? Thorax 1993; 48:719–721.
90. Redline S, Leitner J, Arnold J, Tishler PV, Altose MD. Ventilatory-control abnormalities in familial sleep apnea. Am J Respir Crit Care Med 1997; 156:155–160.
91. Yoshizawa T, Akashiba T, Kurashina K, Otsuka K, Horie T. Genetics and obstructive sleep apnea syndrome: a study of human leukocyte antigen (HLA) typing. Intern Med 1993; 32:94–97.
92. Redline S, Tishler PV, Hans MG, Tosteson TD, Strohl KP, Spry K. Racial differences in sleep-disordered breathing in African-Americans and Caucasians. Am J Respir Crit Care Med 1997; 155:186–192.
93. Ancoli-Israel S, Klauber MR, Stepnowsky C, Estline E, Chinn A, Fell R. Sleep-disordered breathing in African-American elderly. Am J Respir Crit Care Med 1995; 152: 1946–1949.
94. Young T, Palta M, Dempsey J, Skatrud J, Weber S, Badr S. The occurrence of sleep-disordered breathing among middle-aged adults. N Engl J Med 1993; 328:1230–1235.
95. Block AJ, Wynne JW, Boysen PG. Sleep-disordered breathing and nocturnal oxygen desaturation in postmenopausal women. Am J Med 1980; 69:75–79.
96. Schneider BK, Picket CK, Zwillich CW, Weil JV, McDermott MT, Santen RJ, Varano LA, White DP. Influence of testosterone on breathing during sleep. J Appl Physiol 1986; 61:618–623.
97. Johnson MW, Anch AM, Remmers JE. Induction of the obstructive sleep apnea syndrome in a woman by exogenous androgen administration. Am Rev Respir Dis 1984; 129:1023–1025.
98. Cistulli PA, Grunstein RR, Sullivan CE. Effect of testosterone administration on upper airway collapsibility during sleep. Am J Respir Crit Care Med 1994; 149:530–532.
99. White DP, Schneider BK, Santen RJ, McDermott M, Picket CK, Zwillich CW, Weil JV. Influence of testosterone on ventilation and chemosensitivity in male subjects. J Appl Physiol 1985; 59:1452–1457.
100. Kahane JC. A morphological study of the human prepubertal and pubertal larynx. Am J Anat 1978; 151:11–20.
101. Gunn TR, Tonkin SL. Upper airway measurements during inspiration and expiration in infants. Pediatrics 1989; 84:73–77.
102. Young T. Analytic epidemiology studies of sleep disordered breathing—what explains the gender difference in sleep disordered breathing? Sleep 1993; 16:S1–S2.
103. Trinder J, Kay A, Kleiman J, Dunai J. Gender differences in airway resistance during sleep. J Appl Physiol 1997; 83:1986–1997.
104. Popovic RM, White DP. Influence of gender on waking genioglossal electromyogram and upper airway resistance. Am J Respir Crit Care Med 1995; 152:725–731.
105. Leiter JC, Doble EA, Knuth SL, Bartlett D. Respiratory activity of genioglossus: interaction between alcohol and the menstrual cycle. Am Rev Respir Dis 1987; 135:383–386.
106. St. John WM, Bartlett D, Knuth KV, Knuth SL, Daubenspeck JA. Differential depression of hypoglossal nerve activity by alcohol: protection by pretreatment with medroxyprogesterone acetate. Am Rev Respir Dis 1986; 133:46–48.
107. Cook WR, Benich JJ, Wooten SA. Indices of severity of obstructive sleep apnea syn-

drome do not change during medroxyprogesterone acetate therapy. Chest 1989; 96:262–266.

108. Orr WC, Imes NK, Martin RJ. Progesterone therapy in obese patients with sleep apnea. Arch Intern Med 1979; 139:109–111.

109. Cistulli PA, Barnes DJ, Grunstein RR, Sullivan CE. Effect of short term hormone replacement in the treatment of obstructive sleep apnoea in postmenopausal women. Thorax 1994; 49:699–702.

110. Stewart DA, Grunstein RR, Berthon-Jones M, Handelsman DJ, Sullivan CE. Androgen blockade does not affect sleep-disordered breathing or chemosensitivity in men with obstructive sleep apnea. Am Rev Respir Dis 1992; 146:1389–1393.

111. Kahn A, Hasaerts D, Blum D. Phenothiazine-induced sleep apneas in normal infants. Pediatrics 1985; 75:844–847.

112. Sahn SA, Lakshminarayan S, Pierson DJ, Weil JV. Effect of ethanol on the ventilatory responses to oxygen and carbon dioxide in man. Clin Sci Mol Med 1975; 49:33–38.

113. Berry RB, Bonnet MH, Light RW. Effects of ethanol on the arousal response to airway occlusion during sleep in normal subjects. Am Rev Respir Dis 1992; 145:445–452.

114. Krol RC, Knuth SL, Bartlett D. Selective reduction of genioglossal muscle activity by alcohol in normal human subjects. Am Rev Respir Dis 1984; 129:247–250.

115. Marcus CL, Keens TG, Ward SL. Comparison of nap and overnight polysomnography in children. Pediatr Pulmonol 1992; 13:16–21.

116. Hershenson M, Brouillette RT, Olsen E, Hunt CE. The effect of chloral hydrate on genioglossus and diaphragmatic activity. Pediatr Res 1984; 18:516–519.

117. Ali NJ, Pitson DJ, Stradling JR. Snoring, sleep disturbance and behaviour in 4–5 year olds. Arch Dis Child 1993; 68:360–366.

118. Gislason T, Benediktsdottir B. Snoring, apneic episodes, and nocturnal hypoxemia among children 6 months to 6 years old. Chest 1995; 107:963–966.

28

Obstructive Sleep Apnea Syndrome in Children

Diagnosis and Management

GERALD M. LOUGHLIN

Johns Hopkins University School of Medicine
Baltimore, Maryland

I. Introduction

Establishing a diagnosis and determining the most appropriate intervention for a child with obstructive sleep apnea syndrome (OSAS) has proven to be a more complicated process than was initially envisioned (1,2). What was considered to be the typical presentation of OSAS in children, obstructive apnea and hypoxemia, appears to be merely the tip of the iceberg (3–5). This has resulted in considerable uncertainty as to what constitutes the best practice in terms of the diagnosis and management of OSAS in children. This chapter focuses on some of these areas of controversy or confusion and attempts to clarify them.

Childhood OSAS appears to be a continuum (Fig. 1) that includes *primary snoring* (PS), a benign condition of snoring with few if any physiological abnormalities or complications; *upper airway resistance syndrome* (UARS), a subtype or variation of classical OSAS characterized by increased upper-airway resistance and work of breathing during sleep as well as associated snoring, frequent microarousal from sleep, and daytime symptoms of excessive sleepiness or diminished neurocognitive function; *obstructive hypoventilation* (OH), partial upper-airway obstruction evidenced by snoring and increased work of breathing, leading to a peak end-tidal P_{CO_2} $PET_{CO_2} > 55$ mmHg, $PET_{CO_2} > 45$ mmHg for more than 60% of total sleep time (TST), or $PET_{CO_2} > 50$ mmHg for more than 10% of TST (in the absence of lung disease),

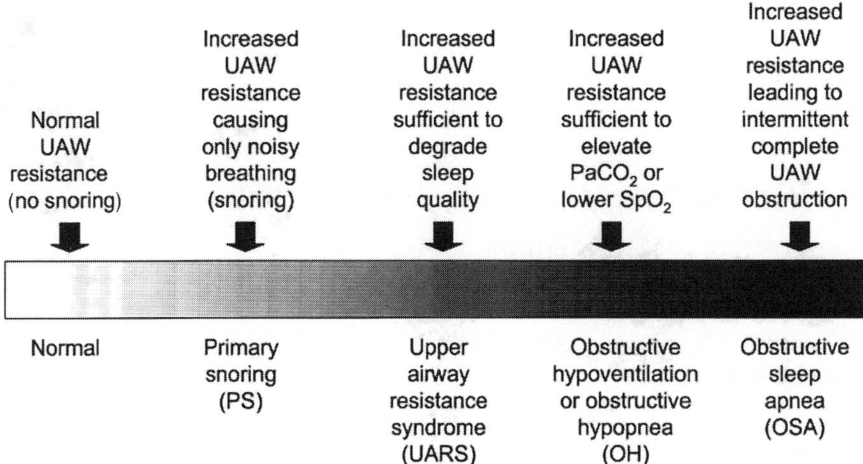

Figure 1 Continuum of sleep-related upper-airway obstruction (UAW) in children. (From Ref. 6.)

and finally, *obstructive sleep apnea syndrome* (OSAS), the classic presentation in which prolonged partial airway obstruction marked by snoring is interrupted by periods of total airway obstruction (obstructive apnea) resulting in hypoxemia, disturbed sleep and daytime symptoms. Of note in terms of approaching the diagnosis of OSAS is that snoring is common to all of these conditions. This observation, coupled with our limited ability to discriminate benign from pathological snoring clinically, has fueled much of the controversy and confusion surrounding the approach to diagnosis.

We have chosen to present these conditions on a continuous line (6) (Fig. 1), suggesting not only that they are linked, but also that a child can move from one state to another. Although this is an attractive hypothesis, the relationship between these states has not been established. There are limited data on the natural history of the spectrum of OSAS in children and even less on how these states are linked. For example, does a child pass from being normal through PS enroute to UARS or OSAS? What is the relationship between OSAS and UARS? It is simply a matter of severity, or are these two distinct clinical presentations influenced by different external or genetic factors? Can a child move back and forth along the continuum? If the answer to this question is yes, then what factors influence this movement positively and negatively? What is the natural history of this spectrum of breathing disorders? What becomes of the child who is diagnosed initially with primary snoring or, for that matter, mild OSAS and UARS? Marcus and coworkers followed a group of children referred for evaluation of snoring who, at baseline, had normal polysomnograms and were found, at follow-up polysomnography a year later, still to have a normal study (7). However, caution must be exercised in generalizing these data to children of different ages diagnosed with primary snoring. The study population was small, a number of subjects were lost to follow-up, and the mean age of the study population was 6 years. This is an age where one would anticipate little progression of OSAS, since tonsil and adenoid tissue is likely to be regressing rather than increasing. Whether or not the conclusion would be the same in a population of 2-year-olds or a group of preadolescents is unknown. In these populations risk factors that may aggravate OSAS may be increasing and it seems less likely that these patients would remain stable. Furthermore, although these children were felt to be normal in terms of daytime symptoms, it is possible that some of them may have had mild forms of the UARS (3,8). Longitudinal polysomnography studies coupled with appropriate outcomes research, including subjects of differing ages, are needed in order to resolve questions regarding the natural history of and the interrelationship among the various subtypes of OSAS.

II. Diagnostic Approach

Although the *International Sleep Disorders Coding Manual* lists excessive daytime sleepiness (EDS) and snoring with apnea as being essential diagnostic elements for OSAS in adults (9), EDS appears to be an uncommon and variable finding in children with equally severe OSAS (6,10,11).

Recognition of the signs, symptoms, and complications of OSAS in children is an essential role for the primary care provider. He or she should be aware of the risk factors for OSAS in children (Table 1) and include questions about potential sleep-related breathing problems in evaluating these patients. The primary care provider should also be aware of the potential clinical significance of snoring and restless sleep as well as the potential complications of disordered breathing during sleep. Table 2 summarizes a set of routine sleep questions and important elements of the physical examination that may help identify children who are at risk for disordered breathing during sleep.

Of all the features of OSAS in children, the most common reason that parents seek medical attention is their concern about their child's snoring and secondarily their concern about restless or disturbed sleep. The epidemiology of snoring is discussed in more detail in Chapter 25. Our focus is on its value in defining a diagnosis of the various subtypes of OSAS in children.

The clinical significance of habitual snoring of any duration or severity is still the subject of debate. Should snoring always be considered abnormal—just as one considers stridor and wheezing to be signs of upper-airway obstruction? As is presented in Chapter 25, snoring may be present in approximately 10% of children. This would put it at a frequency similar to that of asthma. Some would argue that snoring is always abnormal and that the failure to identify complications of snoring in some children merely reflects a lack of sensitivity of monitoring tools (8). Appreciation of the clinical significance of snoring in children has evolved from being largely ignored (13) to where, for some clinicians, its presence alone is considered sufficient indica-

Table 1 Risk Factors for Obstructive Sleep Apnea Syndrome

Risk factor
Factors influencing upper airway resistance or compliance
Nose
Chronic rhinitis (infectious, allergic)
Choanal stenosis
Nasal septal deviation
Fetal warfarin syndrome
Hematoma
Naso- and oropharynx
Adenotonsillar hypertrophy
Fat deposition—obesity
Macroglossia
Cystic hygroma
Velopharyngeal flap surgery
Larynx
Laryngomalacia
Craniofacial structures
Midface hypoplasia (Down syndrome, Crouzon syndrome, achondroplasia)
Mandibular hypoplasia (Pierre-Robin, Treacher-Collins, Shy Drager, Cornelia de Lange)
Mucopolysaccharidosis (Hunter's, Hurler's, and other syndromes)
Metabolic (osteopetrosis)
Factor influencing neural control
Generalized hypotonia (Down syndrome, neuromuscular disease)
Global central nervous system injury
Brainstem dysfunction
Arnold-Chiari malformation—brainstem dysplasia and/or compression
Foramen magnum stenosis (achondroplasia)
Brainstem lesions—tumors, hemangioma, anoxic injury
Idiopathic/genetic
Sedative medications
Alcohol consumption

tion for treatment. Although a history of snoring will at a minimum identify a group of patients at risk, a history of snoring alone is not diagnostic of OSAS (14–20). Historical information regarding snoring to define the problem is often inadequate largely because the parents' reporting of snoring, one of the major complaints with regard to OSAS in children, is a poor discriminator between benign and pathological conditions (14,16).

Regardless of whether one considers all snoring abnormal, the important question is whether the parents' report of snoring or the snoring sound itself can be used to diagnose a problem that needs therapy. Several factors limit the usefulness of parents' observations. Often, a parent may not go into the bedroom once the child is asleep. Thus, he or she may be unaware of the noise unless it is quite loud. Obtaining a history from a reliable sibling or peer who shares the room may be more helpful.

Table 2 Approach to the Child with Suspected Obstructive Sleep Apnea Syndrome

Sleep history: usual bedtime, behavior at bedtime, during sleep and upon awakening, duration of sleep, naps, sleep positions, restless sleep, enuresis
Snoring: frequency of nocturnal snoring (occasional, nightly, only with upper respiratory infection or allergy), onset, pitch, quality, loudness, presence of periods of silence, assessment of difficulty with breathing, parental concerns about their child's breathing
Findings awake:
History of recurrent adenotonsillar disease or chronic rhinitis, altered growth and development patterns
Functional status—developmental status, school performance, personality changes, behavior upon awakening, morning headaches or irritability
Associated cardiopulmonary or genetic syndromes
Physical examination:
Vital signs including height, weight, and blood pressure
Complete ear/nose/throat exam with emphasis on adenotonsillar hypertrophy
Craniofacial examination—small triangular chin, retroposition of the mandible, steep mandibular plane, long oval-shaped face, high-arched palate, elongated soft palate
Cardiac exam for evidence of cor pulmonale
Digital clubbing (rare)

Also, in infants and very young children, the amount of airflow may be insufficient to produce loud snoring. Even in older patients, some individuals may exhibit significant increases in airway resistance without obvious snoring (21). Thus, obstructed breathing may be easily overlooked, depending on the level of vigilance.

Other factors may affect the accuracy of parental reporting. If others in the family, especially the parents, snore, then snoring may be considered a family norm and be overlooked. We have also found that some parents have difficulty rating the significance of the snoring. Parents may report severe snoring, but only relatively unimpressive snoring may be found when the child is studied objectively.

Inclusion of other parts of a sleep history and physical examination—such as witnessed apneas, enuresis, tonsil size, and body weight—has not been shown to increase the diagnostic sensitivity and specificity of snoring (16,17). Goldstein and coworkers included an audiotape of breathing during sleep along with a history and physical examination, but that did not improve the diagnostic specificity (15). Despite these limitations, there are situations in which snoring must be taken seriously. A history of snoring and restless sleep in a child with failure to thrive, developmental delay, poor school performance, or excessive daytime sleepiness is highly suggestive of OSAS and demands that this diagnosis be ruled out by a primary care provider.

The physical examination complements the clinical impression and should be used to identify the "at risk" population (Table 2). Pertinent findings include hypertrophied tonsils and adenoids, craniofacial abnormalities associated with midface hypoplasia or micro- and retrognathia, and obesity. Guilleminault et al. have described a facial pattern that appears to improve the sensitivity of the physical examination in identifying an at-risk group (3). A small triangular chin, retroposition of the mandible, steep mandibular plane, high-arched palate, long, oval-shaped face, or a long soft palate were associated with OSAS, and the risk was increased in the presence of enlarged tonsils and adenoids (3). Additionally, blood pressure, growth, and development status and evidence of cor pulmonale can be used to assess disease severity.

III. Use of Clinical Scores

Since the history alone has not been shown to have sufficient diagnostic sensitivity, a number of individuals have proposed clinical scores as a way to identify a patient who should be treated for OSAS (22,23). The application of clinical scoring systems derived from parental questionnaire is discussed in detail in Chapter 35. However, experience with these tools has shown their value to be limited when applied to a group of children evaluated by a primary care provider and referred for snoring (14,20). Practically, a clinical scoring system may be useful for a primary care provider interested in screening referrals to a sleep center (22,23); however, it adds little to a careful history and physical examination in terms of clinical decision making for the specialist in pediatric sleep medicine. A child with a clearly negative score is unlikely to have a significant breathing disturbance. Routine care for the well child is all that is really needed. Conversely, a child with either a positive or indeterminate score needs a referral to a specialist in pediatric sleep medicine for additional workup in order to determine if the child has a clinically significant disturbance in breathing during sleep (14,16,17).

IV. Laboratory Evaluation

Laboratory studies that may be useful in the diagnosis and management of OSAS in children include studies that identify the location of the obstruction, assess the severity of the consequences of the disordered breathing during sleep, screen a population for OSAS, and finally establish a diagnosis (Table 3).

In the otherwise normal child, tests that identify the location of obstruction are limited to examination of the upper airway with an endoscope and radiological studies (24–28). Endoscopy of the upper airway has been proposed to evaluate adenoid size and rule out other causes of upper-airway obstruction that may cause obstructive sleep apnea (27,28). It is most useful as a way to determine options for therapy once a diagnosis of OSAS has been established. Although, fluoroscopy has been shown to be helpful in identifying the location of the collapse, it is difficult to perform routinely during natural sleep. It may have value in children who have had previous upper-airway pathology and when it is impossible to examine the upper airway completely (26). Computed tomography and lateral radiographs of the neck and upper airway are of limited value, since the airway collapse is a dynamic process easily missed by these nondynamic approaches. They are not needed routinely.

Table 3 Laboratory Evaluation

- **Tests to identify predisposing conditions**
  - Anteroposterior and lateral neck radiographs
  - Upper-airway fluoroscopy
  - Endoscopy
  - Brainstem magnetic resonance imaging or computed tomography
- **Tests to determine severity**
  - Hemoglobin and hematocrit—generally unaffected
  - Serum bicarbonate—usually within normal range
  - Echocardiogram
  - Neuropsychological evaluation
  - Polysomnography
- **Tests to determine diagnosis**
  - Screening studies
    - Clinical scoring systems
    - Audio- and/or videotaping
    - Cinefluorscopy of the upper airway
    - Nasal endoscopy during natural sleep (not practical for pediatrics)
    - Nocturnal oximetry
    - Nap studies
  - Diagnostic studies
    - Polysomnography (nap or nocturnal; see text)
      - Electroencephalography, electro-oculography, electromyography to stage sleep and detect arousal
      - Electrocardiography
      - Respiratory monitoring
        - Abdominal and chest wall movements: inductive plethysmography or strain gauges
        - Airflow: end tidal CO_2, nasal-oral thermistors, nasal pressure sensors
        - Ventilation: end-tidal or transcutaneous CO_2
        - Oxygenation: pulse oximetry (validate signal)
        - Respiratory effort: esophageal balloon; other methods including intercostal and diaphragmatic electromyography, phase angle measurement, and pulse transit time analysis are under investigation.

It is unclear whether all children need tests to assess for complications such as cor pulmonale, polycythemia, or behavioral and neurocognitive abnormalities. Generally, these studies are reserved either to help determine the need for therapy in patients with mild to moderately abnormal polysomnography or for children who are found to have severe apnea and hypoxemia. Although polycythemia and chronic CO_2 retention are uncommon in the modern era of OSAS, measurement of hematocrit as a marker of chronic hypoxemia or serum bicarbonate as a reflection of chronic CO_2 retention and evaluation of cardiac status by echocardiography may be helpful to the anesthesiologist in assessing risks for surgery and general anesthesia. It is not known how frequently these complications occur in children, although experience in adults with OSAS has shown that polycythemia occurs uncommonly (29,30). Assessment of behavioral disturbance and neurocognitive function may be most helpful after a diagnosis has been established in order to determine, especially when dealing with UARS, if therapy is indicated. However, the extent of the neurocognitive and behavioral complications secondary to UARS and OSAS are not known (see Chap. 29). This issue is further compounded by the fact that similar neurocognitive and behavioral symptoms may arise from other causes or underlying conditions.

The major area of controversy regarding the role of laboratory tests in the diagnosis of OSAS in children is the issue of whether laboratory confirmation of pathology is needed in all children with a history of snoring. If yes, then what tests should be done and for whom? What is the value and role of screening studies such as audio or videotaping and overnight pulse oximetry? Which children need polysomnography? What variables should be measured in order to achieve sufficient diagnostic sensitivity? These difficult issues are discussed below.

V. Screening Studies for OSAS

Several screening studies have been proposed to confirm a clinical impression and avoid the need for more expensive and time-consuming studies. If positive, a screening test can be helpful to the clinician. Difficulties arise when a child has a negative screening study yet has a history of snoring or risk factors for OSAS and/or complications that can be associated with OSAS. It is essential that the physician be aware of the sensitivity and specificity of the screening tool being used. A less sensitive or nonspecific test has limited value, and thus, when the results of such a screening study are normal, additional diagnostic studies will often be needed.

A. Direct Observation

A young or excessively sleepy child may fall asleep during a clinic visit. This brief period of observation may give the physician insight into what may be going on at night. Assuming that the observer understands the significance of the observations as well as the spectrum of findings associated with OSAS, these observations may even be diagnostic if the child is observed to have obvious obstructive apnea and oxygen desaturation confirmed by observation of cyanosis or by pulse oximetry. On the other hand, a finding of normal breathing during the daytime nap in a child with a history of snoring does not eliminate OSAS as a possible diagnosis. Marcus et al., using nap polysomnography under sedation, demonstrated that normal breathing during a nap does not preclude the finding of a significant breathing problem during extended nocturnal sleep, when the likelihood of rapid-eye-movement (REM) sleep is increased (31).

B. Audiotaping

Early studies reported success with use of a tape recording of the snoring sound as a diagnostic tool (32,33). However, subsequent work in other centers has not confirmed the diagnostic effectiveness of sound recordings alone as a screening study (15,16). Goldstein et al. demonstrated that a sound recording was positive when compared to polysomnography only about 50% of the time. Although they may detect obstructive apnea, sound recordings are limited by the inability to detect central apnea, obstructive hypoventilation, and the UARS. McCombe and coworkers used third-octave sound analysis to determine if the snoring of an adult patient with documented OSAS could be distinguished from simple snoring (34). An analysis of their data demonstrates that while both types of snoring contain a low-frequency content of linear sound, patients with OSAS also had a substantial high-frequency sound component. They suggest that with further development, analysis of this acoustic pattern could prove to be a useful screening tool for OSAS (34). Specific acoustic studies of snoring in children will be needed, since it is quite likely that the acoustic properties of the snoring noise made by a child will be different from that generated by an adult. Furthermore, age and gender may also influence the quality and components of the sound. Our clinical experience is that audiotaping can be useful diagnostically in the child with signs and symptoms of OSAS who has obstructive apnea followed by resumption of snoring. Its value diminishes in the patient with continuous partial obstruction, since it has not been demonstrated in controlled trials that it is possible to distinguish benign from pathological snoring simply by the sound the patient makes.

C. Videotaping

Since it is unlikely that a child will fall asleep in the presence of a physician, a videotape of the child during sleep can provide useful information. It can be used as a screening tool in the child's home, either by itself or as a part of a modified home sleep study (35–37). Videotaping affords the physician the opportunity to observe for disturbed sleep and qualitatively assess the work of breathing over an extended period (35,36). This is often impossible by direct observation, since the period of direct observation is brief. Videotaping is also an invaluable component of standard polysomnography, since it is unlikely that the physician interpreting an overnight polysomnography will be available to observe sleep activity and behavior. When videotaping is used as screening tool in the home, it is best to ask the parents to record the breathing pattern that worries them the most. Unless a sophisticated computer analysis system is available, it is unnecessary to record a full night of sleep, since it is unlikely that anyone will have the patience to review 8 hrs of videotape without use of a sophisticated computer-based analysis system. Sivan and coworkers asked parents to tape 30 min of their child's sleep. They developed a logistic regression based scoring system of the events found on the tape that had a sensitivity of 84% and a specificity of 65%. Video scores > 11 were highly predictive of OSAS, while a score < 5 was highly associated with normal PSG studies. Scores between 5 and 10 require polysomnography. The regression equation developed from the video score accurately predicted the PSG results in 49 of 58 patients (36). These authors conclude that the high sensitivity (abnormal video and PSG), the low false-negative rate (normal video with abnormal PSG), coupled with the relatively low specificity (normal video and PSG) make the video test an ideal screening tool. Work from the group in Montreal has demonstrated, both in a lab and a home environment, that sleep and wakefulness as well as obstructive apnea and hypopnea can be identified by a combination of a sophisticated computer-based video recording system and limited cardiorespiratory monitoring (35,37–49). However, readers must be aware that their success was dependent on a sophisticated system and one should not conclude that a parent with a home video recorder would have the same degree of success. Furthermore, the value of videotaping in screening children with UARS is yet to be determined. Nonetheless, these studies support the potential for development of a home-based video recording system as an effective way to screen for sleep-disordered breathing and to reduce the number of patients who need full PSG (36,39,40).

D. Continuous Pulse Oximetry

The finding of intermittent episodes of hypoxemia in a snoring child is highly suggestive of OSAS (41). In a study of patients scheduled to undergo adenotonsillectomy, Stradling and coworkers found an increased number of hypoxemic events during overnight oximetry in their study of snoring children scheduled for adenotonsillectomy for reasons other than OSAS (41). Similarly, Van Someren and coworkers studied 45 children scheduled to undergo adenotonsillectomy. Using a definition of hypoxemia that included a baseline sleeping oxygen saturation of < 90% or one dip in the percentage of oxygen saturation of at least 10% below baseline per hour, they identified 15 patients with abnormal findings. These patients could not be identified by history or physical examination, but a combination of mouth breathing, audible respiration at rest, and an awake oxygen saturation of less than 96% correctly identified 14 of 15 patients (93% sensitivity, 86% specificity) (42). Although oximetry may be useful diagnostically for the child who has classic OSAS with apnea and hypoxemia, it will miss the child with UARS and some children with obstructive hypoventilation (OH). Subsequent studies have shown that oximetry does not have sufficient sensitivity to be relied upon as a diagnostic study for the various presentations of OSAS (43–46). Several authors have suggested ways to improve the yield from nocturnal oximetry (43,47). Although these systems have value, they cannot compensate for the large number of children with snoring who have UARS without hypoxemia and yet have a significant disturbance of breathing and sleep. This is a serious limitation. Review of the experience at the Stanford Sleep Disorders Center suggests that UARS may be more common in children than previously thought. In a series of 411 children referred to the Stanford Sleep center for evaluation of breathing disorders during sleep, UARS was diagnosed in 259 (3). If others confirm the experience from the Stanford center, then the value of any screening tool unable to detect increased work of breathing and frequent arousal will be minimal (8,16,48). This is another area in need of more research.

VI. Diagnostic Studies

A. Direct Observation by a Trained Observer

As discussed above, direct observation of a sleeping child who has obvious upper airway obstruction has diagnostic value assuming that the individual making the observations appreciates their significance and recognizes that the absence of obstructive apnea in a snoring child does not mean that the child is normal (8,17). As discussed below, even in a child who is observed to have obstructive apnea, PSG may still be indicated in order to assess disease severity in order to provide appropriate postoperative care (17).

B. Polysomnography

The pediatric sleep lab and technical aspects of PSG in children are discussed in Chapter 34, and references (17,49). The reader is also referred to the recently published practice guidelines for cardiopulmonary sleep studies in adults (50,51). This section reviews some of the controversy surrounding current application of PSG in children. Although, practice guidelines have recently been published for children and adults (17,50,51). It is quite likely that the pediatric guidelines will need updating in the near future as more data are accumulated.

PSG, considered the "gold standard" for diagnosis, has never been subject to rigorous clinical study in children and, as suggested by Stradling, may be a tarnished standard (48). At the present time, many questions remain regarding its application to pediatric patients. Which children need it? When and how often should it be done? What are the sensitivity and specificity of PSG as a diagnostic tool? What are the essential parameters that need to be measured? What is the night-to-night variability of PSG in children? Is this variability influenced by the age of the child? Do we have reliable normative data that span the age range covered by pediatrics? Is PSG required in all children in order to establish a diagnosis? Is it required in all children prior to therapy, especially if the therapy involves surgery? Is the presence of a technician required for all PSG? What is the role of the computer in pediatric PSG? None of these questions has been answered. Clearly more work is needed in the area before definitive recommendations can be made.

Nonetheless, despite these questions and its limitations, PSG is at present considered the diagnostic study of choice for suspected abnormal breathing during sleep in children (17). The official recommendation of the American Thoracic Society is that PSG is indicated in all children in whom a diagnosis of OSAS cannot be made by direct observation of breathing during sleep (17). It is the only technique that allows comprehensive monitoring of both cardiorespiratory function and sleep in a relatively noninvasive way. In contrast to its widespread acceptance in adult sleep medicine, there has been considerable resistance to the routine application of PSG to children. Consequently, many parents and physicians have opted either not to test or to use less reliable methods to diagnose OSAS, in order to avoid the perceived inconvenience and expense of these studies. This reluctance among many primary care providers to use PSG is due in part to a lack of appreciation of the clinical significance of snoring coupled with concerns about expense, inconvenience, and a lack of readily available pediatric lab facilities.

Pediatricians, especially those in managed care organizations, need to be aware that the facility and staff of a sleep lab dedicated to adults is rarely conducive to studying the full range of pediatric patients. Our experience with young children studied in these facilities suggests that the studies are often of such poor quality that they must be repeated in a pediatric facility or are misinterpreted because adult diagnostic standards were applied (10). A child's age should never be a reason to forego a PSG, since a well-prepared pediatric sleep laboratory should be equipped to handle children of any age, from infants to adolescents.

If the indication for therapy is abnormal breathing during sleep, then it is incumbent on those involved in caring for the child to make a diagnosis before subjecting him or her to any therapy, especially surgery. Although it is impossible for an adult with OSAS to be put on continuous positive airway pressure (CPAP), a relatively innocuous therapy, without at least one and often two nocturnal PSGs, a child may be subjected to surgery without confirmation that the child has clinically significant OSAS to warrant surgery (C. Gaultier, personal communication).

PSG provides data on the severity of the breathing disorder and the response to therapy (11,17,52–54). Currently, no other study has emerged as a suitable substitute. Even in those diagnosed by direct observation, PSG can still play an important role in assessing severity (17,52). Current trends in managed care have made adenotonsillectomy an outpatient procedure, with the patient discharged from the hospital on the day of surgery. Work by McColley and coworkers and Rosen et al. has identified children who are at risk of postoperative complications (52,53). Included in this group are children with severe OSAS, whose disease severity would have been detected only by polysomnography.

The approach to PSG used in adults has largely been adapted for use in children (17,49–51). Although this adaptation has been reasonably successful, there are some peculiarities in terms of the approach and the interpretation of the data collected that are worthy of comment.

In spite of the fact that younger children may take daytime naps, polysomnography is best performed at night, during natural sleep. Nap studies can be useful if positive, but a negative nap study does not preclude a positive nocturnal study. Marcus et al. reported a positive predictive value of a daytime nap study of 100%, but a negative predictive value of less than 20% (31). Naps are limited because they may not include REM sleep. Furthermore, it is not uncommon to find that the sleep study is more abnormal in the latter part of the night (55). These abnormalities would be missed by a shorter monitoring period.

Sedative drugs and sleep deprivation should not be used to induce sleep. Sedatives such as chloral hydrate may depress upper-airway dilator muscle function and induce worse apnea in some patients predisposed to OSAS (56). Similar effects have been seen with sleep deprivation (57). Thus, a particular sleep study may be made more abnormal than it would have been during natural sleep, if it were performed under these conditions.

The variables that should be measured during PSG in a child are also somewhat controversial. Questions have been raised about the need to stage sleep, to measure CO_2, and the best way to measure respiratory effort in order to diagnose UARS.

Sleep Staging

Is sleep staging needed in all nocturnal PSG? The value of staging sleep stems largely from the need to be certain that a normal PSG in a child with a history of snoring includes at least one REM period, since REM sleep may be the period of the worst breathing and obstruction (58,59). In addition, identification of arousal from sleep, including microarousal, is essential to establish the diagnosis of the UARS (3–5,8,60). Practically, in the child with obvious obstructive apnea, the staging of sleep adds little to the diagnostic sensitivity of the nocturnal polysomnogram other than adding information on the adverse effects on sleep quality. However, in the child with a history of snoring without observed apnea, use of electroencephalography (EEG) to define sleep stages and identify increased numbers of microarousal is essential (3,5,8,60). Since there is no way of knowing which child may have OH or UARS prior to undertaking the study, sleep staging would appear to be necessary for the majority of PSG studies in children. Furthermore, the individual scoring the study must be aware of the limitations of staging sleep in epochs, since this may result in an underestimation of the number of microarousals in response to increased airways resistance (48).

Diagnosis of UARS

The debate over the need to monitor P_{CO_2} and respiratory effort continues to rage. This debate is fueled by the increasing awareness of the UARS and the conclusion drawn from the work of Rosen et al. and Guilleminault et al. that continuous partial airway obstruction, rather than frequent obstructive apnea, may be the most common presentation of disordered breathing during sleep in children (3,10). Rosen studied 20 patients and found that 80% of these children demonstrated a pattern consistent with obstructive hypoventilation rather than classic apnea (10). Similarly, Guilleminault, in his recent review of the data from the Stanford Sleep Center, suggests that the UARS is the most common presentation of disordered breathing during sleep in children of all ages (3). Consequently, the major challenge for those charged with diagnosing children suspected of having OSAS is how best to diagnose the UARS.

Although awareness of the physiological abnormalities and resultant complications of the UARS in children and adults is increasing (3,4,60), there is still much to be learned about this disorder in children (5,6,8). Moreover, not every child with increased work of breathing is found to have adverse consequences of that breathing pattern, either awake or asleep (5). Is a child who only demonstrates increased resistance to breathing at as great a risk for complications as the child who experiences gas exchange abnormalities as well? The need to make this diagnosis has profound implications in terms of what tests or components of tests are needed. What are the essential diagnostic features of the UARS in children versus adults? What abnormalities must be detected by PSG in order to make a diagnosis? If we are to avoid having to perform repeat PSG, as was required far too often in the report from the Stanford sleep program (3), it seems that the initial study needs to include techniques that allow identification of increased work of breathing and EEG arousal from sleep. Otherwise, polysomnography becomes a very expensive test of limited value.

Measurements of Respiratory Effort

There are a variety of approaches to measuring respiratory effort. Esophageal pressure measurements are considered by most to be the reference standard (61). The Stanford group recommends using a 1.6-mm-diameter pressure catheter. They report considerable success, with a $< 10\%$ need for repeat studies because of invalid data (3).

Reference data are limited. Esophageal pressure (PES) measurements ranging from -8 to -20 cmH_2O have been reported in normal children from 2 to 14 years (4,59). The Stanford group uses a value of < -10 cmH_2O as abnormal. It is considered clinically significant if found for $> 10\%$ of total sleep time (TST). These data are derived from unpublished internal controls from within the Stanford sleep research program. It is unclear whether there is a relationship between the degree and duration of increased negative inspiratory pressures and the severity of the daytime symptoms. Is there a dose-response curve for the amount of time spent breathing with excess negative inspiratory pressure? This concern is similar to that raised about the clinical significance of 1 or 2 obstructive apnea episodes per hour of sleep. This number of obstructive apneas has been shown to be *statistically* significant, but its *clinical* significance is yet to be determined (61). What is the clinical significance of minor increases in work of breathing for limited periods, such as might occur during REM sleep? Unfortunately, outcome data on the range of abnormalities are not available.

PES measurements have limitations. Placing an esophageal pressure catheter is more intrusive than one would like for a study that should aim to interfere as little as possible with a routine night of sleep. In adults, it has been shown to produce minor sleep disruption (63). In addition, for many parents who have reservations about the whole process of PSG itself, the need to insert an esophageal balloon may be viewed as being an unacceptable burden.

Other approaches to measuring respiratory effort include surface intercostal electromyography (EMG) (3), measuring flow limitation by a face mask connected to a pneumotachograph (64) or by nasal cannula/pressure catheter (65). Surface EMG recordings have not been shown to be effective in reliably detecting increased respiratory effort and appear to have limited value (3). Detection of flow limitation by a face mask is limited because it may disturb sleep, while the nasal cannula approach can be adversely affected, if significant mouth breathing is present (66,67). Other promising techniques that have been used to identify increased respiratory effort include measurement of the shift in phase angle with breathing (68) and measurement of pulse transit time (PTT) (69).

Measurement of the phase shift between the abdominal and rib cage components of breathing measured by a noncalibrated respiratory inductive plethysmograph has been used in infants and very young children (68). The study population consisted of infants with a mean age of 28 ± 15.3 months and demonstrated a correlation between abnormal nap PSG and measurement of the phase angle. This approach needs to be studied in older children. Another promising technique involves differentiating obstructive from central apnea by the use of PTT (69). PTT is the time taken for pulse pressure to travel from the aortic valve to the periphery. PTT has been shown to be inversely correlated with blood pressure and can be used to detect changes in respiratory effort through detection of changes in systemic blood pressure caused by increased pleural pressure swings associated with increased respiratory effort (70,71). In adults, this technique has been shown to have a high degree of sensitivity and specificity in differentiating obstructive from central apnea (69). However, it has not been studied extensively in children and it is not clear what role it may play in detecting UARS. Again additional research is needed.

Interpretation of any measurement of respiratory effort may be limited in infants and young children in whom paradoxical rib cage movements during REM sleep occur normally. Paradoxical inward rib cage movement (PIRCM) on inspiration occurs commonly during infancy (72,73). Infants and young children may have PIRCM during all stages of sleep, but it is more pronounced during REM sleep. By 3 to 4 years of age, PIRCMs are abnormal, and this finding may reflect upper airway obstruction during sleep (72,74).

Studies that look at the diagnostic sensitivity and specificity of these newer approaches correlated with sleep architecture as well as clinically significant adverse outcome measures are needed. The studies need to include children of all ages and the results compared to the gold standard, PES, as well as measures of ventilation. This is important, since it is unlikely that inclusion of esophageal pressure measurements in routine PSG will gain widespread acceptance. However, until other noninvasive techniques can be validated, it would seem that PES would remain the approach of choice in order to detect increased work of breathing.

CO_2 Monitoring

CO_2 can be detected noninvasively by either an end-tidal CO_2 (PET_{CO_2}) sampling catheter or by a transcutaneous CO_2 sensing electrode (17,75). The ATS consensus statement recommends the use of end-tidal recordings in order to detect hypoventilation during sleep (17). Several studies have reported hypercarbia associated with obstructive sleep apnea (2,3,10).

PET_{CO_2} recording is able to detect breath-to-breath changes in P_{CO_2}. Provided that there is a good waveform signal, the PET_{CO2} correlates well with the arterial P_{CO_2} except in situations of significant lung disease. PET_{CO_2} can provide information on obstructive breathing by detecting apnea and the effects on ventilation of airway obstruction. Some labs use end-tidal CO_2 recordings simply to detect airflow. Alternatively, the PET_{CO_2} value following obstructive apnea can be used to assess the consequences of both an individual apnea episode as well as the cumulative effects of the abnormal breathing pattern. The sensitivity of this approach is limited by the duration of an individual obstructive event. In children, who frequently have short apneas, significant hypercarbia following an individual episode may not be seen. However, the cumulative effect of frequent apnea and/or partial airway obstruction can be assessed with this technique (17). Several studies of children with OSAS have demonstrated elevated PET_{CO_2}. Brouillette and coworkers found PET_{CO_2} values greater than 45 mmHg in 11 of 22 patients (2). Similarly, Rosen et al. found peak PET_{CO_2} readings between 50 and 68 mmHg in children with OSAS, despite relatively normal readings when they were awake (10).

Use of end-tidal monitoring in a child is challenging. It requires meticulous attention to maintaining catheter patency and position throughout the study. Humidity accumulating in the cannula may interfere with readings. Despite these obstacles, in experienced hands, accurate readings can be accomplished routinely.

Transcutaneous CO_2 (Ptc_{CO_2}) recording has been recommended as a means to record ventilation, because it is technically less demanding and perhaps less sensitive to artifact (76). It provides a measurement of the duration of hypoventilation but is insensitive to transient elevations that may follow obstructive apnea. Other limitations include the lack of correlation between Ptc_{CO_2} and Pa_{CO_2}, the risk of burns from the heated sensor, and the need to change the sensor during the study—an activity that may disturb the patient. Placing two sensors at the beginning of the study and alternating the recording sites throughout the night may solve this problem, although even reattaching the sensor may disturb a light sleeper (R. Brouillette and C. Marcus, personal communication).

Morielli and coworkers suggested that simultaneous recording of both PET_{CO_2} and transcutaneous P_{CO_2} would provide a better and more consistent assessment of ventilation during PSG (76). Although simultaneous recording of both CO_2 measurements is optimal in terms of capturing the most complete assessment of ventilation, it is usually more data than are needed for most clinical settings. Practically, it is preferable to become skilled with the use of end-tidal CO_2 measurements, since this signal offers a considerable amount of information.

It is not clear how best to use these data. Recording the peak PET_{CO_2} and the duration of PET_{CO_2} readings greater than 45 or 50 mmHg have been proposed as the best ways to assess the severity of the disturbance in ventilation (11). However, it is not known if transient elevations of P_{CO_2} are harmful or what threshold in terms of duration of P_{CO_2} greater than 45 or 50 mmHg is associated with complications. Despite these limitations, there is still broad-based agreement that measurement of ventilation by P_{CO_2} offers considerable value in evaluating children with disordered breathing during sleep (17,75,76).

Table 4 Patterns of Respiration

Obstructive apnea—Absence of oronasal airflow in the presence of continued respiratory effort lasting longer than two respiratory cycle times. Usually but not always associated with hypoxemia.
Central apnea—Cessation of respiratory effort lasting at least two respiratory cycle times.
Hypopnea—A 50% or greater decrease in the amplitude of the nasal/oral airflow signal, often accompanied by hypoxemia or arousal. Some have attempted to subtype hypopnea into obstructive and nonobstructive. Obstructive hypopnea is defined as a reduction in airflow without a reduction in effort. On the other hand, nonobstructive hypopnea is associated with a reduction in both airflow and respiratory effort by 50%.
Obstructive hypoventilation—Partial airway obstruction leading to a peak $P_{ETCO_2} > 55$ mmHg or $P_{ETCO_2} > 45$ mmHg for more than 60% of TST, or $P_{ETCO_2} > 55$ mmHg for more than 10% of TST (in the absence of lung disease).
Nonobstructive hypoventilation—Assuming CO_2 is measured, decreased breathing due to either a reduction in respiratory drive (central), decreased breathing caused by peripheral neural abnormalities or muscle weakness (neuromuscular), or decreased breathing secondary to decreased chest wall movements (restrictive).

Breathing Patterns

Table 4 presents the currently accepted definitions of the various patterns of breathing found on cardiorespiratory PSG in children. Most of these definitions are reasonably straightforward; however, the concept of hypopnea deserves further discussion. *Hypopnea* refers to a reduction in breathing. In adult studies, several different definitions have been used (77–79). Some authors have defined it based on a 50% or greater reduction in either airflow or respiratory effort alone. Others require associated hypoxemia, and/or arousal in addition to a simple reduction in airflow. Not everyone considers that desaturation and/or arousal are needed in order to identify hypopnea. This term has been the source of some confusion because the methods used to define it are qualitative and yet the definition is based on a quantitative change in either airflow or respiratory effort. As pointed out by Redline and coworkers, this inconsistency limits the usefulness of this measurement in adults and most likely children as well (80).

The ATS Statement on the Standards and Indications for Cardiopulmonary Sleep Studies in Children defines hypopnea as a 50% or greater decrease in the amplitude of the nasal/oral airflow signal, often accompanied by hypoxemia or arousal (17). *Hypopnea* does appear to be a term frequently used in discussing pediatric sleep disorders. It may be particularly useful when P_{CO_2} is not being measured, since the reduction in effort or flow can be used as an indicator of hypoventilation. It may also be a marker of UARS. However, in order to improve its clinical and scientific usefulness, it is important to know how hypopnea was defined and whether desaturation or arousal was included in identifying events. Inclusion of oxygen desaturation in adult studies appears to improve the clinical correlation between hypopnea and complications of OSAS such as hypertension (81).

In contrast to adults, children can experience significant oxygen desaturation with apnea episodes that are not considered clinically significant by adult PSG scoring criteria (10). Recent work by Sanchez-Armengol and coworkers demonstrated the necessity of scoring these shorter episodes, since—despite their brevity—they can be associated with desaturation (82). Consequently, as is recommended in the consensus statement, all obstructive apnea episodes regardless of duration should be scored in children (17). Failure to do so will result in an underestimation of the degree of abnormality of PSG in a child (10,17,82).

As it is for studies in adults, computerized scoring of PSG in children is still in its infancy (83,84). Although computers can be used successfully for acquisition, transport, and storage of data, use of computerized scoring of apnea and sleep staging in children has not been studied. Considering the complexity and variability of the sleep and breathing patterns that can be associated with clinical abnormalities, it is unlikely that computer-based scoring will be available for pediatric studies in the near future.

VII. Management of OSAS in Children

Treatment options for OSAS in children are limited and are fairly straightforward. The various medical and surgical options are listed in Table 5. Although the choice of therapy for children with OSAS is well accepted, the question of who should be treated remains somewhat controversial. The threshold of PSG data or clinical findings that should trigger a referral for surgery is not clear. Do all children with certain abnormalities, either clinical or PSG, require therapy? What about children with study values outside the normal range, yet with no obvious clinical symptoms? Should they all be treated? Are parental concerns over snoring sufficient justification for surgery, es-

Table 5 Treatment Options

Medical management
Nasopharyngeal airway—acute, temporary
Mask positive airway pressure—continuous or bilevel
Weight loss for obese patients
Pharmacological therapy—respiratory stimulants not indicated; nasal steroids and alpha agonists may provide temporary relief of nasal edema
Surgical management
Adenotonsillectomy—most common surgical option
Tracheostomy—less common with advent of mask positive pressure
Maxillofacial plastic surgery
Uvulopalatopharyngoplasty (UPPP)—not recommended for children

pecially if lab data are normal or minimally abnormal? There is little argument that recurrent obstructive apnea and hypoxemia are harmful for the child and warrant intervention. However, it is not known whether any episode of desaturation, even for a brief period, is actually harmful. Similarly, the threshold for treating increased work of breathing and hypercarbia is undefined for children. Should treatment be based on the number of microarousals alone? Or should there be evidence of neurocognitive or behavioral problems? What threshold of work of breathing or growth impairment should serve as a clear indication for intervention? At the present time, with the exception of the child with severe apnea, nocturnal hypoxemia, and daytime symptoms, there are no clear guidelines for decision making regarding which children with OSAS or UARS should be treated. Children with mild OSAS on polysomnography or those diagnosed with UARS present a bigger challenge, since the natural history of either of these conditions as well as the limits of our ability to assess the daytime consequences of these disorders are unknown. The decision to treat or to follow clinically should be based on a combination of clinical and lab findings. This raises another question. Since excessive daytime sleepiness is an uncommon occurrence in children, what behaviors or cognitive dysfunction can be directly attributable to UARS to warrant therapy? This is an area in desperate need of outcomes research studies.

As mentioned, there are limited treatment options. If one encounters a child in severe distress, placement of a nasopharyngeal airway or use of nasal bilevel positive airway pressure or continuous positive airway pressure can provide temporary relief until more definitive therapy can be arranged. Patients with severe disease who are found to have severe hypoxemia during sleep, may be considered candidates for supplemental oxygen. However, clinical experience with these patients has shown that oxygen therapy may be dangerous because it may suppress respiratory drive (85,86). Increased CO_2 retention and prolongation of obstructive apnea may be seen. Supplemental oxygen can be used judiciously, but the patient needs to be monitored carefully by individuals who are aware of potential complications.

There is little argument that adenotonsillectomy is the treatment of choice for otherwise normal children with OSAS (5,85,87–91). In most instances, the overwhelming majority of otherwise normal children will have symptoms relieved following surgery (54). Similar recommendations can be made for treating UARS (3,88). Although these children are improved, whether or not they are cured is an entirely different question. Following surgery, some children are still at risk for OSAS. A preoperative history and physical examination cannot predict this risk, although polysomnography may help identify those at risk of postoperative persistence of OSAS (91). Guilleminault et al. reported a group of adolescents with a history of OSAS who had a recurrence of symptoms as teenagers (92). Similarly, we have encountered children who experience a recurrence of snoring associated with upper respiratory infections (URI) or nasal allergy and some in whom surgery does not correct the problem fully. Snoring and apnea symptoms are usually self-limited and improve with resolution of the URI or allergy. This experience suggests that, despite the dramatic improvement postoperatively, children may have an underlying predisposition to OSAS that may be brought out by other factors that either increase upper-airway resistance (obesity, allergic rhinitis) or decrease input to the pharyngeal dilator muscles (sedatives).

An additional concern with the decision of when and where to perform an adenotonsillectomy relates to the potential peri- and postoperative complications (93,94). As mentioned above, this is considered by some to be an outpatient procedure. Work by Reiner et al. suggests that even patients with OSAS can have surgery as outpatients (95). However, since the patients included in his study did not undergo PSG, the value of this study in terms of guiding clinical practice is limited, since there is no measure of disease severity. Severity is a risk factor for postoperative complications (52,53). In addition, age less than 3 years, presence of cor pulmonale, failure to thrive, and underlying conditions such as craniofacial disorders, neuromuscular disease, and morbid obesity have also been shown to predispose to postoperative respiratory complications; as such, these are indications for inpatient monitoring on the night of surgery (52–54). Postsurgical airway edema coupled with the lingering effects of anesthetic agents that may diminish neural control and most likely contribute to this increased risk (54).

In otherwise normal children, an adenotonsillectomy has been shown to be the most effective therapeutic intervention. A tracheotomy is rarely needed. However, in patients with severe craniofacial genetic syndromes or very young patients who may not have large tonsils and adenoids or may be difficult to treat with long-term bilevel positive-pressure nasal ventilation, a tracheotomy may be necessary. It is used more often in very young patients, children with genetic or neuromuscular syndromes, those who have not responded to tonsillectomy and adenoidectomy (T&A), and who cannot be managed with CPAP or bilevel positive-pressure nasal ventilation (see Chap. 36). These interventions are generally reserved for children who are not candidates for a T&A or who do not improve postoperatively (96). An aggressive craniofacial surgical approach to patients with craniofacial syndromes as well as children with cerebral palsy has been proposed. However results are fairly preliminary and long-term outcome studies are needed before these procedures can be recommended routinely (97–99). They are fairly invasive and future experience with the use of bilevel positive-pressure ventilation may eventually reduce the need for such surgery. Other therapies, such as uvulopalatopharyngoplasty and oral devices, have not been studied extensively in children and cannot be recommended at this time (11). There are limited if any data on the drug treatment of OSAS in children. Medications that reduce nasal resistance may provide transient relief, especially in a child whose symptoms may be exacerbated by allergy or a URI. There are no control studies to date. A recent review of pharmacological therapy of OSAS in adults suggests that drug treatment is currently experimental at best (100). Despite advertising claims regarding nasal dilator strips and their widespread use by NFL linemen, they have also not been fully evaluated in children. Scharf and coworkers studied the effects of nasal dilator strips in a small group of infants with and without nasal congestion (101). They reported a reduction in a respiratory disturbance index, especially in those infants with nasal congestion. Unfortunately, significant problems with research design and methods limit the value of the conclusions draw from this work (102). Additional studies of the role of nasal dilator strips in the treatment of OSAS in older children are needed before any recommendations can be made.

VIII. An Approach to Diagnosis and Management

In spite of the confusion and decided lack of outcome data to guide clinical practice, the clinician in both the primary care and sleep specialty setting must formulate a plan for approaching the diagnosis and management of the child with suspected disordered breathing during sleep. For the child with no risk factors (52,53) who has obvious signs and symptoms of OSAS and in whom a physician can confirm the presence of airway obstruction during sleep, referral to an otolaryngologist seems appropriate. However, in a child below 3 years of age or one who is at increased risk of complications, a diagnosis of disordered breathing during sleep must be made prior to recommending therapy, especially surgery. In 1999, the major obstacle to diagnosis and management facing parents and clinicians lies with the UARS and the inability of clinical history and routine diagnostic studies to distinguish or identify this common clinical presentation of disordered breathing during sleep. This experience demands that work continue aggressively on refining our ability to make the diagnosis. Recommendations in the otolaryngology surgical literature suggesting that sleep-disordered breathing in a child is a clinical diagnosis and that decisions regarding who needs surgery can be made without laboratory confirmation should be viewed cautiously by those responsible for their care (103).

References

1. Guilleminault C, Eldridge F, Simmons B, Dement WC. Sleep apnea in eight children. Pediatrics 1976; 58:23–30.
2. Brouillette RT, Fernbach SK, Hunt CE. Obstructive sleep apnea in infants and children. J Pediatr 1982; 100:31–40.
3. Guilleminault C, Pelayo R, Leger D, Clerk A, Bocian RCZ. Recognition of sleep disordered breathing in children. Pediatrics 1996; 98:871–882.
4. Guilleminault C, Winkle R, Korokin R, Simmons B. Children and nocturnal snoring: evaluation of the effects of sleep related respiratory resistive load and daytime functioning. Eur J Pediatr 1982; 139:165–171.
5. Gaultier C. Obstructive sleep apnoea syndrome in infants and children: established facts and settled issues. Thorax 1995; 50:1204–1210.
6. Greene MG, Carroll JL. Consequences of sleep-disordered breathing in childhood. Curr Opin Pulm Med 1997; 3:456–463.

7. Marcus CL, Hamer A, Loughlin GM. Natural history of primary snoring in children. Pediatr Pulmonol 1998; 26:6–11.
8. Guilleminault C, Pelayo R. Editorial: ... And if the polysomnogram was faulty? Pediatr Pulmonol 1998; 26:1–3.
9. Thorpy MJC, Diagnostic Classification Steering Committee. International Classification of Sleep Disorders: Diagnostic and Coding Manual. Rochester, MN: American Sleep Disorders Association, 1990.
10. Rosen CL, D'Andrea L, Haddad GG. Adult criteria for obstructive sleep apnea do not identify children with serious obstruction. Am Rev Respir Dis 1992; 146:1231–1234.
11. Carroll JL, Loughlin GM. Obstructive sleep apnea in children: diagnosis and management. In: Ferber R, Kryger M, eds. Principles and Practice of Sleep Medicine in the Child. Philadelphia: Saunders, 1995.
12. Carroll JL, Loughlin GM. Diagnostic criteria for obstructive sleep apnea in children. Pediatr Pulmonol 1992; 14:71–74.
13. Robin IG. Snoring. Proc R Soc Med 1968; 61:575–582.
14. Carroll JL, McColley SA, Marcus CL, Curtis S, Loughlin GM. Inability of clinical history to distinguish primary snoring from obstructive sleep apnea syndrome in children. Chest 1995; 108:610–618.
15. Goldstein NA, Sculerati N, Walsleben JA, Bhatia N, Friedman DM, Rapoport DM. Clinical diagnosis of pediatric obstructive sleep apnea validated by polysomnography. Otolaryngol Head Neck Surg 1994; 111:611–617.
16. Rosen CL. Obstructive sleep apnea syndrome (OSAS) in children: diagnostic challenges. Sleep 19:S274–S277.
17. Standards and indications for cardiopulmonary sleep studies in children. Am J Respir Crit Care Med 1996; 153:866–878.
18. Wang RC, Elkins TP, Keech D, Wauquier A, Hubbard D. Accuracy of clinical evaluation in pediatric obstructive sleep apnea. Otolaryngol Head Neck Surg 1998; 118:69–73.
19. Deagan PC, McNicholas WT. Predictive value of clinical features for the obstructive sleep apnea syndrome. Eur Respir J 1997; 9:117–124.
20. Nieminen P, Tolonen U, Lopponen H, Lopponen T, Luotenen J, Jokinen K. Snoring children: factors predicting sleep apnea. Acta Otolaryngol 1997; 529(suppl):190–194.
21. Stoohs R, Skrobal A, Guilleminault C. Does snoring intensity predict flow limitation or respiratory effort during sleep. Respir Physiol 1993; 92:27–38.
22. Brouillette R, Hanson D, David R, Klemka L, Szatkowski A, Fernbach S, Hunt C. A diagnostic approach to suspected obstructive sleep apnea in children. J Pediatr 1984; 105: 10–14.
23. Kahn A, Groswasser J, Sottiaux M, Rebuffat E, Sunseri M, Franco P, Dramaix M, Bochner A, Belhadi B, Foerster M. Clinical symptoms associated with brief obstructive sleep apnea in normal infants. Sleep 1993; 16:409–413.
24. Felman AH, Loughlin GM, Leftridge CA, Cassisi NJ. Upper airway obstruction during sleep in children. Am J Roentgenol 1979; 133:213–216.
25. Fernbach SK, Brouillette RT, Riggs TW, Hunt CE. Radiographic evaluation of adenoids and tonsils in children with obstructive sleep apnea: plain films and fluoroscopy. Pediatr Radiol 1983; 13:258–265.
26. Gibson SE, Myer CM III, Strife JL, O'Connor DM. Sleep fluoroscopy for localization of upper airway obstruction in children. Ann Otol Rhinol Laryngol 1996; 105:678–683.
27. Fan LL. Transnasal fiberoptic endoscopy in children with obstructive apnea. Crit Care Med 1984; 12:590–592.

28. Croft CB, Thompson HG, Samuels MP, Southall DP. Endoscopic evaluation and treatment of sleep associated upper airway obstruction in infants and young children. Clin Otolaryngol 1990; 15:209–216.
29. Hoffstein V, Herridge M, Mateika S, Redline S, Strohl KP. Hematocrit levels in sleep apnea. Chest 1994; 106:787–791.
30. Cahan C, Decker MJ, Arnold JL, Goldwasser E, Strohl KP. Erythropoietin levels with treatment of obstructive sleep apnea. J Appl Physiol 1995; 79:1278–1285.
31. Marcus CL, Keens TG, Ward SL. Comparison of nap and overnight polysomnography in children. Pediatr Pulmonol 1992; 13:16–21.
32. Marsh RR, Potsic P, Pasquariello PS. Reliability of sleep sonography in detecting upper airway obstruction in children. Int J Pediatr Otolaryngol 1989; 18:1–8.
33. Potsic WP. Comparison of polysomnography and sonography for assessing regularity of respiration during sleep in adenotonsillar hypertrophy. Laryngoscope 1987; 97:1430–1437.
34. McCombe AW, Kwok V, Hawke WM. An acoustic screening test for obstructive sleep apnoea. Clin Otolaryngol 1995; 20:348–351.
35. Morielli A, Laden S, Ducharme FM, Brouillette RT. Can sleep and wakefulness be distinguished in children by cardiorespiratory and videotape recordings? Chest 1996; 109: 680–687.
36. Sivan Y, Kornecki A, Schonfeld T. Screening obstructive sleep apnea syndrome by home videotape recording in children. Eur Respir J 1996; 9:2127–2131.
37. Mograss MA, Ducharme FM, Brouillette RT. Movement arousals: description, classification and relationship to sleep apnea in children. Am J Respir Crit Care Med 1994; 150: 1690–1696.
38. Jacob SV, Morielli A, Mograss MA, Ducharme FM, Schloss MD, Brouillette RT. Home testing for pediatric obstructive sleep apnea syndrome secondary to adenotonsillar hypertrophy. Pediatr Pulmonol 1995; 20:241–252.
39. Brouillette RT, Jacob SV, Morielli A, Mograss M, Lafontaine V, Ducharme F, Schloss M. There's no place like home; evaluation of obstructive sleep apnea in the child's home. Pediatr Pulmonol 1995; 11(suppl):86–88.
40. Brouillette RT, Jacob SV, Waters KA, Morielli A, Mograss M, Ducharme FM. Cardiorespiratory sleep studies for children can often be performed in the home. Sleep 1996; 19:S278–S280.
41. Stradling JR, Thomas G, Warley ARH, Williams P, Freeland A. Effect of adenotonsillectomy on nocturnal hypoxaemia, sleep disturbance, and symptoms in snoring children. Lancet 1990; 335:249–253.
42. Van Someren VH, Hibbert J, Stothers JK, Kyme MC, Morrison GAJ. Identification of hypoxemia in children having tonsillectomy and adenoidectomy. Clin Otolaryngol 1990; 15:263–271.
43. Vavrina J. Computer assisted pulse oximetry for detecting children with obstructive sleep apnea syndrome. Pediatr Otorhinolaryngol 1995; 35:239–248.
44. Owen GO, Canter RJ, Robinson A. Overnight pulse oximetry in snoring and non-snoring children. Clin Otolaryngol 1995; 20:402–406.
45. Owen GO, Canter RJ. Overnight pulse oximetry in normal children and in children undergoing adenotonsillectomy. Clin Otolaryngol 1996; 21:59–65.
46. Owen G, Canter R, Maw R. Screening for obstructive sleep apnoea in children. Int J Pediatr Otorhinolaryngol 1995; 32(suppl):S67–S69.

47. Lafontaine VM, Ducharme FM, Brouillette RT. Pulse oximetry: accuracy of methods of interpreting graphic summaries. Pediatr Pulmonol 1996; 21:121–131.
48. Stradling JR, Davies RJO, Pitson DJ. New approaches to monitoring sleep-related breathing disorders. Sleep 1996; 19:S77–S84.
49. Sheldon SH, Spire JP, Levy HB. Pediatric Sleep Medicine. Philadelphia: Saunders, 1992.
50. Indications for Polysomnography Task Force, American Sleep Disorders Association, Standards of Practice Committee. Practice parameters for the indications for polysomnography and related procedures. Sleep 1997; 20:406–422.
51. Chesson AL, Ferber RA, Fry JM, Grigg-Damberger M, Hartse KM, Hurwitz TD, Johnson S, Kader GA, Littner M, Rosen G, Sangal B, Schmidt-Nowara W, Sher A. The indications for polysomnography and related procedures. Sleep 1997; 20:423–487.
52. McColley SA, April MM, Carroll JL, Naclario RM, Loughlin GM. Respiratory compromise after adenotonsillectomy in children with obstructive sleep apnea. Arch Otolaryngol Head Neck Surg 1992; 118:940–943.
53. Rosen GM, Muckle RP, Mahowald MW, Goding GS, Ullevig C. Postoperative respiratory compromise in children with obstructive sleep apnea: can it be anticipated? Pediatrics 1994; 93:784–788.
54. Helfaer MA, McColley SA, Pyzik PL, Tunkel DE, Nichols DG, Baroody FM, April MM, Maxwell LG, Loughlin GM. Polysomnography after adenotonsillectomy in mild obstructive sleep apnea. Crit Care Med 1996; 24:1323–1327.
55. Goh DYT, Marcus CL. Changes in obstructive sleep apnea characteristics in children throughout the night. Am J Respir Crit Care Med 1998; 157:A533.
56. Biban P, Baraldi E, Pettenazzo A, Filippone M, Zacchello F. Adverse effects of chloral hydrate in two young children with obstructive sleep apnea. Pediatrics 1993; 92:461–463.
57. Canet E, Gaultier C, D'Allest AM, Dehan M. Effects of sleep deprivation on respiratory events during sleep in healthy infants. J Appl Physiol 1989; 66:1158–1163.
58. Praud JP, Gaultier C, Buvry M, Boule M, Girard F. Lung mechanics and breathing pattern during wakefulness and sleep in children with enlarged tonsils. Sleep 1984; 7:304–312.
59. Miyazaki S, Itasaka Y, Yamakawa K, Okawa M, Togawa K. Respiratory disturbance during sleep due to adenoid hypertrophy. Am J Otolaryngol 1989; 10:143–149.
60. Downey R, Perkin RM, MacQuarrie J. Upper airway resistance syndrome: sick, symptomatic, but under-recognized. Sleep 1993; 16:620–623.
61. Marcus CL, Omlin KJ, Basinski DJ, Bailey SL, Rachal AB, Von Pechmann WS, Keens TG, Davidson-Ward SL. Normal polysomnographic values for children and adolescents. Am Rev Respir Dis 1992; 146:1235–1239.
62. Baydur A, Berhakis PK, Zin M, Jaeger M, Millic-Emili J. A simple method for assessing the validity of the esophageal balloon technique. Am Rev Respir Dis 1982; 126:788–791.
63. Chediak AD, Demirozu MC, Nay KN. Alpha EEG sleep produced by balloon catheterization of the esophagus. Sleep 1990; 13:369–370.
64. Series F, Marc I. Accuracy of breath-by-breath analysis of flow volume loop in identifying sleep induced flow limited breathing cycles in sleep apnea-hypopnea syndrome. Clin Sci 1995; 88:707–712.
65. Hosselet JJ, Norman RG, Ayappa I, Rapoport DM. Detection of flow limitations with a nasal cannula/pressure transducer system. Am J Respir Crit Care Med 1998; 157:1461–1467.

66. Guilleminault C, Stoohs R, Duncan S. Snoring: daytime sleepiness in regular heavy snorers. Chest 1991; 90:40–48.
67. Montserrat JM, Farre R, Ballester E, Felez MA, Pasto M, Navajas D. Evaluation of nasal prongs for estimating nasal flow. Am J Respir Crit Care Med 1997; 155:211–215.
68. Sivan Y, Davidson Ward S, Deakers T, Keens TG, Newth JL. Rib cage to abdominal asynchrony in children undergoing polysomnographic sleep studies. Pediatr Pulmonol 1991; 11:141–146.
69. Argod J, Pepin JL, Levy P. Differentiating obstructive and central sleep respiratory events through pulse transit time. Am J Respir Crit Care Med 1998; 158:1778–1783.
70. Brock J, Pitson D, Stradling J. Use of pulse transit time as a measure of changes in inspiratory effort. J Ambul Monit 1993; 6:295–302.
71. Pitson D, Sandell A, Van de Hoot R, Stradling JR. Pulse transit time as a measure of respiratory effort in patients with obstructive sleep apnoea. Eur Respir J 1995; 8: 1669–1674.
72. Gaultier C. Respiratory adaptation during sleep in infants. Lung 1990; 168:905–911.
73. Gaultier C, Praud JP, Canet E, Delaperche MF, D'Allest AM. Paradoxical inward ribcage motion during rapid-eye movement sleep in infants and young children. J Dev Physiol 1987; 9:391–397.
74. Tabachnik E, Muller NL, Bryan AC, Levinson H. Changes in ventilation and chest wall mechanics during sleep in normal adolescents. J Appl Physiol 1981; 51:557–564.
75. Smith TH, Proops DW, Pearman K, Hutton P. Nasal capnography in children: automated analysis provides a measure of obstruction during sleep. Clin Otolaryngol Appl Sci 1993; 93:69–71.
76. Morielli A, Desjardins D, Brouillette RT. Transcutaneous and end-tidal carbon dioxide pressures should be measured during pediatric polysomnography. Am Rev Respir Dis 1993; 148:1599–1604.
77. Gould GA, Whyte KF, Rhind GB, Airlie AA, Catterall JR, Shapiro CM, Douglas NJ. The sleep hypopnea syndrome. Am Rev Respir Dis 1988; 137:895–898.
78. Whyte KF, Allen MB, Fitspatrick MF, Douglas NJ. Accuracy and significance of scoring hypopneas. Sleep 1992; 15:257–260.
79. Moser NJ, Phillips BA, Berry DTR, Harbison L. What is hypopnea, anyway? Chest 1994; 105:426–428.
80. Redline S, Sanders M. Hypopnea, a floating metric: implications for prevalence, morbidity estimates and case finding. Sleep 1997; 20:1209–1217.
81. Hla KM, Young TB, Bidwell T, Palta M, Skatrud JB, Dempsey J. Sleep apnea and hypertension: a population based-study. Ann Intern Med 1994; 120:382–388.
82. Sanchez-Armengol A, Capote-Gil F, Cano-Gomez S, Ayerbe-Garcia R, Delgado-Moreno F, Castillo-Gomez J. Polysomnographic studies in children with adenotonsillar hypertrophy and suspected obstructive sleep apnea. Pediatr Pulmonol 1996; 22:101–105.
83. Hirshkowitz M, Moore CA. Issues in computerized polysomnography. Sleep 1994; 17: 105–112.
84. White DP, Gibb TJ. Evaluation of a computerized polysomnographic system. Sleep 1998; 21:188–195.
85. Levin DL, Muster AJ, Pachman LM, Wessel HU, Paul MH, Koshaba J. Cor pulmonale secondary to upper airway obstruction: cardiac catheterization, immunologic and psychometric evaluation in nine patients. Chest 1975; 68:166–171.
86. Marcus CL, Carroll JL, Bamford OS, Pyzik P, Loughlin GM. Supplemental oxygen dur-

ing sleep in children with sleep-disordered breathing. Am J Respir Crit Care Med 1995; 152:1297–1301.

87. Potsic WP, Pasquariello PS, Baranak CC, Marsh RR, Miller LM. Relief of upper airway obstruction by adenotonsillectomy. Otolaryngol Head Neck Surg 1986; 94:476–480.
88. Guilleminault C, Korobkin R, Winkle R. A review of 50 children with obstructive sleep apnea syndrome. Lung 1981; 159:275–287.
89. Boudewyns AN, Van de Heying PH. Obstructive sleep apnea syndrome in children: an overview. Acta Otorhinolaryngol Belg 1995; 49:275–279.
90. Williams EF, Woo P, Miller R, Kellman RM. The effects of adenotonsillectomy on growth in young children. Otolaryngol Head Neck Surg 1991; 104:509–516.
91. Suen JS, Arnold JE, Brooks LJ. Adenotonsillectomy for treatment of obstructive sleep apnea in children. Arch Otolaryngol Head Neck Surg 1995; 121:525–530.
92. Guilleminault C. Treatments in obstructive sleep apnea. In: Guilleminault C, Patinen M, eds. Obstructive Sleep Apnea Syndrome. New York: Raven Press, 1990:99–108.
93. Wiatrak BJ, Myer CM, Andrews TM. Complications of adenotonsillectomy in children under 3 years of age. Am J Otolaryngol 1991; 12:170–172.
94. Price SD, Hawkins DB, Kahlstrom EJ. Tonsil and adenoid surgery for airway obstruction: peri-operative respiratory morbidity. Ear Nose Throat J 1992; 72:526–531.
95. Reiner SA, Sawyer WP, Clark KF, Wood MW. Safety of outpatient tonsillectomy and adenoidectomy. Otolaryngol Head Neck Surg 1990; 102:161–168.
96. Marcus CL, Ward SL, Mallory GB, Rosen CL, Beckerman RC, Weese-Mayer DE, Brouillette RT, Trang HT, Brooks LJ. Use of nasal continuous positive airway pressure as treatment of childhood obstructive sleep apnea. J Pediatr 1995; 127:88–94.
97. Cohen SR, Lafaivre JF, Burnstein FD, Simms C, Kattos AV, Scott PH, Montgomery GL, Graham L. Surgical treatment of obstructive sleep apnea in neurologically compromised patients. Plas Reconstr Surg 1997; 99:638–646.
98. Burnstein FD, Cohen SR, Scott PH, Teague GR, Montgomery GL, Kattos AV. Surgical therapy for severe refractory sleep apnea in infants and children: application of the airway zone concept. Plast Reconstr Surg 1995; 96:34–41.
99. Kefaivre JF, Cohen SR, Burnstein FD, Simms C, Scott PH, Montgomery GL, Graham L, Kattos AV. Down syndrome: identification and surgical management of obstructive sleep apnea. Plast Reconstr Surg 1997; 99:629–637.
100. Hudgel DW, Thanakitcharu S. Pharmacologic treatment of sleep disordered breathing. Am J Respir Crit Care Med 1998; 158:691–699.
101. Scharf MB, Berkowitz DV, McDonald MD, Stover R, Brannen DE, Reyna R. Effects of an external nasal dilator strip on sleep and breathing patterns in newborn infants with and without congestion. J Pediatr 1996; 129:804–808.
102. Givan DC, Eigen H. Breathing—what's the "right" answer? J Pediatr 1996; 129:781–782.
103. Messner AH. Evaluation of obstructive sleep apnea by polysomnography prior to pediatric adenotonsillectomy. Arch Otolaryngol Head Neck Surg 1999; 125:353–357.

29

Neuropsychological Consequences of Disordered Breathing During Sleep

CHRISTIAN GUILLEMINAULT and RAFAEL PELAYO

Stanford University
Stanford, California

I. Introduction

Daytime somnolence, declining school performance, mood and personality changes, morning headaches, and nocturnal enuresis were first reported as part of the obstructive sleep apnea syndrome in children in 1976 (1). Since this initial description, others have confirmed that neurological and behavioral symptoms are commonly seen in children with sleep-disordered breathing (2–8). Documented neurocognitive and behavioral disturbances include attention disorders, memory and learning disabilities, school failure, developmental delay, hyperactivity, aggressiveness, and withdrawn behavior (9–13). Improvement has been reported following successful treatment of obstructive sleep apnea syndrome (OSAS), suggesting a link between abnormal breathing during sleep and these neuropsychological problems (12,14). However, establishing a link between disordered breathing during sleep and certain neuropsychological or neurodevelopmental conditions has been hampered by a number of factors. Most of the reports lack adequate comparison groups. In many of the reports, formal testing was not performed and abnormalities were based largely on parental reporting. No studies to date have defined the spectrum of abnormalities associated with the various presentations of the childhood type of OSAS. Furthermore, the link between abnormalities found on polysomnography and specific neuropsychological disabilities has not been established. How much hypoxemia, hypercarbia, increase in work of breathing, or number of microarousals are needed to produce daytime symptoms? What is the relationship between complications such as failure to thrive and cor pulmonale and neurocognitive dysfunction? In addition, the limited awareness among clinicians of the role that sleep and breathing disorders may play in causing awake neurocognitive dysfunction and the fact that many of these neurological findings are not specific for sleep apnea also limit awareness. Recognition that a significant number of children may not present with the classic findings of recurrent obstructive apnea and hypoxemia and yet still have a significant disturbance in breathing during sleep further clouds the picture. This increased work of breathing appears to result in frequent arousal from sleep; it can be misleading to the clinician, whose attention may be focused on the more dramatic symptoms of airway obstruction and hypoxemia (15–17). This condition is referred to as the upper-airway resistance syndrome (UARS), and work from our lab suggests that it may be the most common presentation of disordered breathing during sleep in children (17). Despite this observation, UARS may be underdiagnosed in sleep labs unless aggressive attempts are made to record respiratory work and arousal (17,29).

II. Neurological and Behavioral Symptoms Associated with Sleep-Disordered Breathing

Symptoms reported by caregivers and observed by health professionals will vary depending on the age of the child.

A. Infancy

Sleep-disordered breathing has been diagnosed as early as 3 weeks of age (18–20). Most commonly, the infant is brought to clinical attention because of an apparent life-threatening event (ALTE). Often, this is a poorly explained event that occurs at home and is frightening to the parents. Polygraph recordings performed over 24 hr or for 12 hr at night may demonstrate abnormal respiratory events in some infants, but most studies have been within normal limits. Discrete symptoms may be present that will be uncovered by parental interviews. Unfortunately, the frequency of occurrence of the reported symptoms is often not indicated in the literature. For this chapter, we reviewed the last 100 children seen at Stanford for an ALTE. The clinical symptoms reported by parents during questioning are indicated in Table 1. Of the total, 41% of parents were unaware of the prior existence of any symptoms. Reports of infants being “lethargic,” have a “poor suck,” or being “delayed” were made by mothers who had had at least one previous child. Reports of “noisy breathing,” “mouth breathing,” and “snoring” were obtained independent of birth order.

B. Twelve Months to Kindergarten

This section contains data obtained from patients seen in our clinic. All children seen in this age range were referred for “snoring at night.” Once again, the literature does not provide much information on the distribution of neurological and behavioral

Table 1 Symptoms Indicated by Parents of 100 Infants with Apparent Life-Threatening Events and Abnormal Breathing Events During Sleep Recording[a]

Symptom	
Mouth breathing	29
Noisy breathing or snoring	26
Sweating during sleep	23
Abnormal "fuss"	19
Waking up frequently and disturbing the parents' sleep	19
Lethargy	17
Poor sucking	5
"Delayed" compared to peer or preceding siblings (late to roll over, hold up head, or sit)	8
"Colic"	2
No report by parents	41

[a]Parents may have reported more than one symptom.

symptoms. The collective data, however, suggest that abnormal behavior is commonly associated with polygraph findings of sleep-disordered breathing. The most common symptoms indicated by parents were pathological shyness, aggressive behavior, repetitive tantrums, continuous irritability, and repetitive nightmares. Table 2 outlines the frequency of symptoms reported by parents at interviews of the last 100 children seen in our clinic. The constellation of symptoms reported in these children included irritability, temper tantrums, aggressiveness against peers and siblings, and rebellious be-

Table 2 Symptoms Reported by Parents of 100 Children, Age 1 to 5 Years, with Sleep-Disordered Breathing at Polygraph Recording

Symptom	
Noisy breathing—chronic snoring	100
Mouth breathing during sleep	62
Rebellious behavior on a near daily basis	51
Abnormal sleep with awakening and crying	48
Nocturnal enuresis beyond 3 years of age	48
Aggressiveness against siblings and/or peers, violence	39
Falling asleep very easily during the daytime in quiet situations[a]	37
Abnormal sweating during sleep	33
Burst of irritability, tantrums recurring nearly daily	31
Frequent nightmares	26
Abnormal degree of shyness, absence of interactions with peers	24
Developmental delays (poor coordination, delayed walking or speech coordination)	22
Repetitive night terrors	18
Frequent sleepwalking	15
Fear of going to bed	12
Speech problems	12
Frequent report of nausea sometimes associated with vomiting	4

[a]Reported only in children 3 years of age or older.

havior. Similarly, pathological shyness, nightmares, and night terrors were also often described. Even if abnormal behavioral symptoms were the reason children were brought to the sleep clinic, daytime sleepiness was rarely a concern spontaneously expressed by parents.

C. Six Years and Older

All children were in school, and the most common cause for referral was for investigation of chronic heavy snoring, repetitive upper-airway infections, and/or repetitive earaches (55%). A pediatrician and an otolaryngologist made referrals. At the request of schoolteachers or school psychologists, 25% of the children were seen for "falling asleep in class," "being lethargic," "abnormal behavior with hyperactivity," and suspicion of attention deficit disorder. Pediatricians or parents initiated consultation for night terrors, sleepwalking, insomnia, or nocturnal awakening with difficulty falling back to sleep in 14% of the children, while 4% were referred by a psychiatrist or neurologist to rule out narcolepsy. Finally, 2% of the children were sent by orthodontists for bruxism or small mandibles with small upper airways. The nature of the referral corresponded with the emphasis placed by parents and physicians on a particular clinical symptom. However, clinical interviews revealed an association between the initial compliant that led to clinical attention and other behavioral symptoms suggestive of a breathing problem during sleep. It was in this age group that a large number of associated behavioral symptoms could be elicited at clinical interviews. Typically, complaints were reported in clusters. Excessive daytime sleepiness ("falling asleep in class," "being lethargic in class") was associated with reports of "being tired" and "refusing to participate in activities with peers, including pleasant ones." Parents also mentioned withdrawn behavior, avoidance of participation in sports, and the frequency of naps during travel to and from school or just after school. Some children were difficult to wake in the morning, leading to tardiness for school, or had awakenings associated with bursts of anger and/or verbal abuse against the parent in charge of getting the child out of bed. The daytime sleepiness also included early-morning confusion and disorientation or avoidance of going to bed despite obvious sleepiness. This may be due to the occurrence of hypnagogic hallucinations. Reports of daytime sleepiness were frequently associated with reports of learning difficulties and memory problems. Teachers complained of lack of attention, an impression of daydreaming, and a lack of interest in class activities associated with poor school grades. In some patients, parent interviews uncovered a recent decline in school performance compared to the previous years. At times, teachers complained more of hyperactivity in class that was disturbing to other students. It appears that rebellious behavior is encountered more often than frank sleepiness. Frequently, before referral to the sleep disorders clinic, the child has been seen by the school counselor; and concerns about attention deficit disorder, the need to be in special education classes due to difficulties participating or following in class or difficulty performing assignments had been raised. These constellations of complaints and symptoms may all be related to excessive daytime sleepiness. Parents may also report "bizarre behaviors" defined by "lapses," discontinuous thinking, "phasing out," being "absent," or being intermittently unresponsive to questions and environmental demands.

The clinical picture may first lead to consultation with a neurologist for suspicion of a complex partial seizure disorder. Aggressive and rebellious behavior will, in most cases, lead to early intervention; however, the withdrawn behavior of some children and their apparent refusal to interact with others may be tolerated longer by parents and teachers. Ultimately, this behavior may lead to concerns about a mood disorder.

A morning headache, seen frequently in patients with chronic obstructive pulmonary disease (COPD), is another symptom that may be difficult to define in children too young to articulate their complaints adequately. Headaches may vary in frequency, location, and severity but may also be the symptom that focuses attention on a breathing disorder. The child may initially be seen in a headache clinic, but other symptoms should orient the diagnosis. Rarely, headaches will wake the child in the middle of the night. In most cases, the headache dissipates shortly after the child wakes up, but it may sometimes last the whole morning (3–8,17,18,21–23) (Table 3).

III. Nocturnal Symptoms

The nocturnal behavior is usually abnormal; it is important to have it well defined. Restless sleep is common. The child or teenager may move in all directions, pulling the bedding apart, flailing the arms and more rarely the legs. Sometimes the child may fall out of the bed or sit up suddenly. The head may be held in hyperextension. Night sweats, varying in severity from profuse to mild, may also be reported. Drooling, with finding of wet pillows or traces of saliva on the cheek in the morning, as well as complaints of dry mouth and the need for a sip of water during the night are suggestive of mouth breathing. Dryness of the throat or mouth may be such that the child may keep a bottle next to his or her bed. Sleep talking is common. Nightmares, night terrors, and somnambulism can also be indicative of sleep-disordered breathing. Of 104 prepubertal school-age children with sleep-disordered breathing, Guilleminault et al. found that 31.7% had sleepwalking events and 26% had repetitive night terrors or nightmares (11). Somnambulism associated with sleep-disordered breathing has led to very serious self-inflicted injury in two of our teens.

In summary, behavioral symptoms in children may often be the primary clinical manifestation of sleep-disordered breathing. Furthermore, they should always be looked for in a child suspected of having OSAS or UARS.

IV. Laboratory Testing

If excessive daytime sleepiness is suspected, the multiple sleep latency test (MSLT) can be performed in children 8 years of age and older. It is a standardized test in which patients are asked to try to fall asleep while supine in bed in a dark, comfortable room

Table 3 Symptoms Reported at Interview in Prepubertal School-Age Children[a]

	Total group		OSAS		UARS	
Final diagnosis	*n*	(%)	*n*	(%)	*n*	(%)
Daytime tiredness or fatigue	90	86.5	20	83.3	56	91.8
Daytime sleepiness	76	73.0	17	70.8	45	73.8
Snoring or noisy breathing during sleep	72	69.2	23	95.8	48	78.7
Daytime mouth breathing	34	32.7	16	66.6	18	29.5
Nocturnal sweating	42	40.4	21	87.5	18	29.5
Nocturnal drooling (wet pillow)	36	34.6	20	83.3	16	26.2
Unexplained drop in school performance	19	18.2	5	20.8	12	19.7
Bruxism (and orthodontic referral)	18	17.3	5	20.8	13	21.3
Sleepwalking	33	31.7	14	58.3	9	14.8
Repetitive night terrors or nightmares	27	25.9	15	62.5	8	13.1
Aggressive behavior with hyperactivity	15	14.4	3	12.5	7	11.5
Secondary enuresis	8	7.6	1	4.2	4	6.6
Disturbed nocturnal sleep	21	20.2	10	41.6	6	9.8
Regular complaint of morning headache	11	10.5	8	33.3	3	4.9
Nausea and vomiting	6	5.7	2	8.3	2	3.3
Total	104	100	24	100	61	100

[a]Results of the investigation of 104 school-age children with sleep-disorderd breathing compared to 19 children observed during the same period, for other sleep disorders. One child may have had several symptoms.
OSAS, obstructive sleep apnea syndrome; UARS, upper-airway respiratory syndrome; SDB, sleep-disordered breathing (i.e., OSAS and UARS).
Source: From Ref. 17.

(24). The MSLT recording includes an electroencephalogram (EEG), chin electromyogram (EMG), right and left electrooculogram, and electrocardiogram. The MSLT must be performed after having a nocturnal polysomnogram executed the preceding night. It includes five naps administered every 2 hr, usually starting at 9 A.M. Each nap trial consists of a 20-min opportunity to fall asleep. If the patient falls asleep during those 20 min, the subject is allowed to sleep for 15 min more. During those 15 min of sleep, the patient is monitored for the appearance of rapid-eye-movement (REM) sleep. MSLT results are summarized by the average sleep latency and the number of REM-onset sleep periods that occur during the naps. The test is scored for sleep and wake in 30-sec epochs using the international atlas edited by Rechtschaffen and Kales (25). Carskadon has obtained normative data on individuals aged 8 and older (26). She has shown that the mean sleep latency is very long in children (Tanner stages 1 and 2), with sleep latency of 18.8 ± 1.8 min and 18.3 ± 2.1 min, respectively. With the onset of puberty, normal teenagers become sleepier. This is translated into a shorter

SDB			Other sleep pathologies			% of SDB and other sleep pathologies compared with total group by symptom	
n	(%)	Percentage of total group, *n* = 54	*n*	(%)	Percentage of total group, *n* = 54	SDB	Other
76	89.4	73.1	14	73.7	13.5	84.4	15.6
62	72.9	59.6	14	73.7	13.5	81.6	18.4
71	83.5	60.3	1	5.3	1	98.6	1.4
34	40.0	32.7	0	0	0	100	0
39	45.9	37.5	3	15.8	2.9	92.3	7.7
36	42.4	34.6	0	0	0	100	0
17	20.9	16.3	2	10.5	1.9	89.5	10.5
18	21.2	17.3	0	0	0	100	0
24	28.2	23.1	9	47.3	8.6	72.7	27.3
23	27.0	22.1	4	21	3.8	85.2	14.8
10	11.7	9.6	5	26.3	4.8	66.6	33.4
5	5.9	4.8	3	15.8	2.9	62.5	37.5
16	18.8	15.4	5	26.3	4.8	76.2	23.8
11	12.9	10.6	0	0	0	100	0
4	4.7	3.8	2	10.5	1.9	33.3	66.7
85	100	81.7	19	100	—	—	—

sleep latency. Teenagers at Tanner stage 3 presented a mean sleep latency of 16.5 ± 2.8 min, and those at Tanner stage 4 had a mean of 15.5 ± 3 min. Interpretation of results should, therefore, take into consideration the pubertal status of the child. Undoubtedly, a MSLT of 10 min or less is pathological. However, in a prepubertal child, a MSLT of 12 min after a good night of sleep is also abnormal. There are nap data on younger children but no validated studies (27).

None of the subjective scales used in adults for the evaluation of sleepiness has been validated in children. The maintenance of wakefulness test, also used as an objective test of alertness in adults, has not been validated for childhood.

V. Diagnosis

The initial presentation may not lead the physician to consider sleep-disordered breathing in the differential diagnosis of the child with behavioral or neurodevelopmental problems. Even if snoring is present, a child may be referred to a psychiatrist for behavioral problems and/or a mood disorder, or to a pediatric neurologist for migraine headaches, unexplained cephalgia, or suspicion of narcolepsy. Attention deficit disorder and abnormal nocturnal behavior may lead to a diagnosis of complex partial seizure rather than OSAS or UARS. Similarly, a history of nightmares or somnambulism may not lead to much scrutiny and search, since sleep-disordered breathing may not occur. However, a physician familiar with the clinical consequences of disordered breathing during sleep is likely also to include sleep-disordered breathing in the differential diagnosis. If a diagnosis of sleep-disordered breathing is considered, it can be confirmed in most instances by nocturnal polysomnography. As mentioned, one must also include the UARS in the differential, and the polysomnography lab should be equipped and prepared to identify this entity. Unfortunately, the 1996 standards of the American Thoracic Society have not addressed details related to detecting isolated increases in respiratory effort and associated microarousal during sleep (28). Specifically, the routine clinical application of esophageal pressure measurements, investigation of respiratory rate, and usage of intercostal-diaphragmatic EMG signal are not addressed (17,18,28). As discussed elsewhere, it is probable, based on new information, that these standards will need to be updated in the not too distant future. In difficult cases, monitoring of abnormal respiratory efforts during sleep with usage of esophageal pressure measurements may be needed in order to identify more subtle variants of UARS. This is particularly true since difficulties have been encountered identifying associated EEG microarousals (29).

VI. Conclusion

Behavioral and neurological symptoms are common in children with sleep-disordered breathing (30,31). This diagnosis may be difficult to make, since the symptoms are often nonspecific for a breathing disorder; thus an underlying respiratory cause may not be considered early in the course of the evaluation. Nonetheless, it is important to make this association, since, in most cases, appropriate treatment of the sleep-disordered breathing will improve the clinical picture. The recent report of Gozal et al. supports the value of early recognition of abnormal breathing during sleep and appropriate interventions (32). His work demonstrated, in a group of first-graders, that correction of sleep-associated gas exchange abnormalities was associated with improved school performance when compared to a control group with similar gas exchange abnormalities during sleep who were not treated with an adenotonsillectomy. On the other hand, Brouillette and coworkers described several patients in their 1982 series whose neurodevelopmental problems did not improve following successful therapy for the obstructed breathing, suggesting that in some patients with severe, protracted OSAS, failure to diagnose this condition soon enough may result in permanent neuropsychological deficits (4). It is also important to perform follow-up neurodevelopmental and psychological testing 3 to 4 months after resolution of the sleep-disordered breathing in order to identify persistent abnormalities. If the prior behavior or developmental abnormality attributed to sleep-disordered breathing has not resolved, specific treatment and counseling may be needed to resolve residual problems. Furthermore, persistence of symptoms also warrants repeat investigation of breathing during sleep to make certain that the abnormal breathing has resolved.

References

1. Guilleminault C, Eldridge F, Simmons F, Dement WC. Sleep apnea in eight children. Pediatrics 1976; 58:23–30.
2. Brouillette R, Hanson D, David R, Klemka L, Szatkowski A, Fernbach S, Hunt C. A diagnostic approach to suspected obstructive sleep apnea in children. J Pediatr 1984; 105: 10–14.
3. Frank Y, Kravath RE, Pollak CP, Weitzman ED. Obstructive sleep apnea and its therapy: clinical and polysomnographic manifestations. Pediatrics 1983; 71:737–742.
4. Brouillette RT, Fernbach SK, Hunt CE. Obstructive sleep apnea in infants and children. J Pediatr 1982; 100:31–40.
5. Carroll JL, McColley SA, Marcus CL, Curtis S, Loughlin GM. Reported symptoms of childhood obstructive sleep apnea syndrome (OSA) vs. primary snoring. Am Rev Respir Dis 1992; 145(part 2):A177.
6. Leach J, Olson J, Hermann J, et al. Polysomnographic and clinical findings in children with obstructive sleep apnea. Arch Otolaryngol Head Neck Surg 1992; 18:741–744.
7. Carroll JL, Loughlin GM. Diagnostic criteria for obstructive sleep apnea syndrome in children. Pediatr Pulmonol 1992; 14:71–74.
8. Weissbluth M, Davis AT, Poncher J, Reiff J. Signs of airway obstruction during sleep and behavioral, developmental, and academic problems. J Dev Behav Pediatr 1983; 4:119–121.
9. Rhodea SK, Shimoda KC, Wald LR, O'Neill PM, Oexmann MJ, Collop NA, Willi SM. Neurocognitive deficits in morbidly obese children with obstructive sleep apnea. J Pediatr 1996; 127:741–744.
10. Martin PR, Leibvre AM. Surgical treatment of sleep apnea associated psychosis. Can Med Assoc J 1981; 124:978–980.
11. Hecht JT, Thompson NM, Weir T, Patchell L, Horton WA. Cognitive and motor skills in achondroplastic infants: neurologic and respiratory correlates. Am J Med Genet 1991; 41: 208–211.
12. Ali NJ, Pitson D, Stradling JR. Sleep disordered breathing: effects of adenotonsillectomy on behavior and psychological functioning. Eur J Pediatr 1996; 155:56–62.
13. Greenberg GD, Watson RK, Deptula D. Neuropsychological dysfunction in sleep apnea. Sleep 1987; 13:960–964.
14. Chervin RD, Dillon JE, Bassetti C, Ganoczy DA, Pituch KJ. Symptoms of sleep disorders, inattention, and hyperactivity in children. Sleep 1997; 20:1185–1192.
15. Rosen CL. Obstructive sleep apnea syndrome (OSAS) in children: diagnostic challenges. Sleep 1996; 19:S274–S277.
16. Carroll JL, McColley SA, Marcus CL, Curtis S, Loughlin GM. Inability of clinical history to distinguish primary snoring from obstructive sleep apnea syndrome in children. Chest 1995; 108:610–618.
17. Guilleminault C, Pelayo R, Clerk A, Bocian RCZ. Recognition of sleep-disordered breathing in children. Pediatrics 1996; 98:871–882.
18. Guilleminault C, Winkle R, Korobkin R, Simmons B. Children and nocturnal snoring: evaluation of the effects of sleep related respiratory resistive load and daytime functioning. Eur J Pediatr 1982; 139:165–171.
19. Guilleminault C, Peraita R, Souquet M, Dement WC. Apneas during sleep in infants: possible relationship with SIDS. Science 1975; 190:677–679.

20. Guilleminault C, Souquet M. Sleep states and related pathology. In: Korobkin R, Guilleminault C, eds. Advances in Perinatal Neurology. New York: Spectrum Publications, 1979: 225–247.
21. Guilleminault C, Korobkin R, Winkle R. A review of 50 children with obstructive sleep apnea syndrome. Lung 1981; 159:275–287.
22. Goldstein NA, Sculerati N, Walsleven JA, Bhatia N, Friedman DM, Rapoport DM. Clinical diagnosis of pediatric obstructive sleep apnea validated by polysomnography. Otolaryngol Head Neck Surg 1994; 111:611–617.
23. Nieminen P, Tolonen U, Lopponen H, Lopponen T, Luotonen J, Jokinen K. Snoring children: factors predicting sleep apnea. Acta Otolaryngol Suppl 1994; 529:190–194.
24. Carskadon MA, Dement WC, Mitler M, Roth T, Westbrook P, Keenan S. Guidelines for the multiple sleep latency test (MSLT): a standard measure of sleepiness. Sleep 1986; 9: 519–524.
25. Rechtschaffen A, Kales A, eds. A Manual of Standardized Terminology: Techniques and Scoring Systems for Sleep Stages of Human Subjects. Los Angeles: UCLA Brain Information Service/Brain Research Institute, 1968.
26. Caraskadon C. The second decade. In: Guilleminault C, ed. Sleeping and Waking Disorders: Indications and Techniques. Menlo Park, NJ: Addison-Wesley 1982, appendix 1.
27. Weissbluth M. Naps in children: 6 months–7 years. Sleep 1995; 18:82–87.
28. American Thoracic Society. Standards and indications for cardiopulmonary sleep studies in children. Am J Respir Crit Care Med 1996; 153:866–878.
29. Guilleminault C, Black J, Carrillo O. EEG arousal and upper airway resistance syndrome (abstr). Electroencephalogr Clin Neurophysiol 1997; 103.
30. Ali NJ, Pitson DJ, Stradling J. Snoring, sleep disturbance, and behaviour in 4–5 year olds. Arch Dis Child 1993; 68:360–366.
31. Ali NJ, Pitson DJ, Stradling J. Natural history of snoring and related behaviour problems between the ages of 4 and 7 years. Arch Dis Child 1994; 71:74–76.
32. Gozal D. Sleep-disordered breathing and school performance in children. Pediatrics 1998; 102:616–620.

30

Effects of Breathing During Sleep in Children with Chronic Lung Disease

CLAUDE GAULTIER

University of Paris VII and
Hôpital Robert Debré
Paris, France

I. Introduction

The assessment of sleep-disordered breathing in infants and/or children with chronic respiratory disease should take into account the degree of maturation of sleep organization (see Chap. 3) and of cardiorespiratory adaptation during sleep (1). Alterations in breathing such as respiratory pauses, falls in oxygen saturation (Sa_{O_2}), and/or thoracoabdominal asynchrony decrease in frequency and amplitude throughout the first year of life (1). However, in children with lung disease and a limited pulmonary reserve, the normal effects of sleep on breathing can result in significant ventilatory and gas exchange abnormalities. Pediatricians and sleep specialists evaluating and caring for children should be aware of the effects of sleep on the pathophysiology and clinical course of chronic respiratory disease.

Bronchopulmonary dysplasia, also called chronic lung disease of prematurity and/or infancy (2–5), arises in infants and young children as a result of acute neonatal lung injury and its treatment. Asthma affects more than 10% of children in industrialized countries, and its prevalence and severity are increasing (6). Children with cystic fibrosis (CF), a genetically transmitted disorder affecting pulmonary and pancreatic exocrine function, now live longer lives, throughout which they experience chronic lung disease (7). Infrequent causes of chronic respiratory disease include chronic obstructive pulmonary disease (COPD), which in some cases is a consequence of a severe viral infection (8) or of ciliary dysfunction (9). Finally, chronic interstitial lung disease encompasses a heterogenous group of disorders seen infrequently in infants and children (10).

II. Bronchopulmonary Dysplasia

Bronchopulmonary dysplasia (BPD) was first described by Northway (2) in 1967 as a lung disease secondary to neonatal respiratory distress syndrome and defined based on radiological, clinical, and pathological criteria. Improvements in ventilatory support techniques achieved over recent years have translated into a reduced risk of chronic lung disease after neonatal respiratory distress syndrome. However, because of the increasingly successful use of ventilatory support at younger and younger gestational ages and of the introduction of replacement surfactant therapy at birth, BPD remains an important cause of mortality and morbidity, although the pathological changes are usually not as severe as when BPD was first described.

The clinical and functional criteria used to define BPD (and the age at which these criteria should be evaluated) have been modified since the seminal description by Northway (2–5). The term *BPD* is now often replaced by *chronic lung disease*, defined as a need for oxygen at 28 days of postnatal age in an infant with a birth weight of 1500 g or less. In the neonatal research study conducted in the United States by the National Institute of Child Health and Human Development, over 80% of infants weighing 800 g or less at birth developed chronic lung disease, compared to 29.7% of infants weighing 1001 to 1250 g and approximately 10% of infants weighing 1251 to 1500 g (11). In this chapter, the term *BPD* is used because it was widely employed until recently.

A. Cardiorespiratory Abnormalities During Sleep in BPD Infants

Several studies conducted starting in the late 1980s found that BPD infants experienced episodes of hypoxemia during sleep despite acceptable awake oxygen saturation (Sa_{O_2}) (12–16). Clinically unsuspected episodes of hypoxemia during sleep were documented by Garg et al. (16) in 14 BPD infants tested at a mean postconceptual age (PCA) of 41.0 ± 0.8 weeks. Episodes of desaturation with Sa_{O_2} values of less than 90% were more common during rapid-eye-movement (REM) sleep than during non-REM (NREM) sleep. Although abnormal pneumographic findings did not predict abnormal desaturation episodes, time spent with an Sa_{O_2} under 90% was correlated with airway resistance (16). The possibility that desaturation may be linked to impaired lung mechanics is of special importance, since hypoxic episodes in BPD infants may be potentiated by airway obstruction and by an inability to compensate for this abnormality (17). Furthermore, it has been suggested that a decrease in the inspired fraction of O_2 may worsen airway obstruction (18). Therefore, episodes of hypoxemia may of themselves worsen abnormalities of lung mechanics in BPD infants. On the other hand, high levels of oxygenation have been shown to decrease airway resistance in BPD infants (19).

Oxygen supplementation has been shown to be beneficial in BPD infants. Early studies found that the pulmonary vascular bed was responsive to oxygen in these patients (20,21). Sekar and Duke (14) reported that supplemental oxygen improved central respiratory stability in BPD infants, leading to decreases in central pauses and in periodic breathing episodes. Unsuspected marginal oxygenation during sleep in BPD infants, together with a limitation in pulmonary reserves, may divert energy away from growth. Moyer- Mileur et al. (22) showed that BPD infants with Sa_{O_2} values between 88% and 91% during sleep exhibited decreased growth. In contrast, BPD infants with Sa_{O_2} values greater than 92% during prolonged sleep showed better growth.

Hypoxemia during sleep can also occur in older infants and young children with a history of severe BPD. In a study of BPD patients aged 3 to 5 years, Loughlin et al. found marked, prolonged episodes of desaturation during sleep despite an awake Sa_{O_2}value greater than 93% (23). The most severe desaturation episodes occurred during REM sleep. The same finding was reported by Gaultier et al., who also noted REM sleep–related increases in transcutaneous partial pressure of CO_2 and thoracoabdominal asynchrony (24).

An abnormal sleep pattern with significantly reduced REM sleep has been reported in BPD infants (25,26). Harris and Sullivan (25) reported sleep fragmentation and decreased REM sleep in six BPD infants with baseline O_2 values greater than 90% during sleep. When supplemental oxygen was given, all six infants had an increase in sleep duration due largely to an increase in REM sleep.

The severity of abnormalities in lung mechanics as defined by Northway (2) correlated with the degree of thoracoabdominal asynchrony in BPD infants tested at a mean PCA of 49 ± 3.2 weeks during quiet sleep (27). Thoracoabdominal asynchrony, a well-known phenomenon during REM sleep in infants, is due to loss of rib cage stabilization as a result of inspiratory intercostal muscle inhibition (1,28). Rome et al. investigated whether residual BPD affects this phenomenon (29). BPD infants studied at a mean PCA of 41 ± 4 weeks experienced more asynchronous chest wall movements than normal preterm infants during both sleep states. The relationship between thoracoabdominal asynchrony and the severity of abnormalities in lung mechanics seems to override in large part the effect of sleep states on chest wall movements. In the group of infants with resolving BPD studied by Rome et al. (29), asynchronous chest wall movements throughout sleep were not associated with a significant difference in oxygenation between sleep states. Asynchronous chest wall movements during NREM and REM sleep were extensively studied in 14 young children (mean age, 32 months; range, 19 to 46 months) with severe BPD (30). During NREM sleep, thoracoabdominal asynchrony included paradoxical abdominal movement during early inspiration in the majority of these patients. Expiratory muscle activity was suggested as a potential mechanism for the paradoxical abdominal movement. The severity of paradoxical abdominal movement was significantly correlated with age between 2 and 4 years of age, suggesting that the change from the circular infant-type thorax with horizontal ribs to the elliptical adult-type thorax with oblique ribs, which occurs around 2 years of age in normal children (31), may result in patterns of thoracoabdominal asynchrony similar to those observed in adults with chronic lung disease. During REM sleep, the typical pattern of thoracoabdominal asynchrony included paradoxical rib cage movement during inspiration in the study young children with severe BPD (30).

The influence of sleep on cardiac function in severe BPD was assessed in five children aged 1.5 to 5 years (32). Left and right ventricular ejection fractions (LVEF and RVEF) were determined using equilibrium radionuclide ventriculography during the difference states of alertness assessed on the basis of neurophysiological criteria. During sleep, marked decreases in both LVEF and RVEF were seen in the two children with the lowest nocturnal Sa_{O_2} levels and the most prolonged paradoxical rib cage movements during inspiration (Fig. 1). These data suggest that sleep-related hypoxemia may lead to substantial impairment in right ventricular function and to mild impairment in left ventricular function. One study looked at heart rate variability during sleep in 10 oxygen-dependent patients with severe BPD aged 7 to 29 months (33). The patients were studied at normal Sa_{O_2} levels (greater than 95%) and at slightly decreased Sa_{O_2} levels (90% to 94%). Abnormalities in the autonomic control of heart rate variability suggesting long-term changes in autonomic heart rate control were

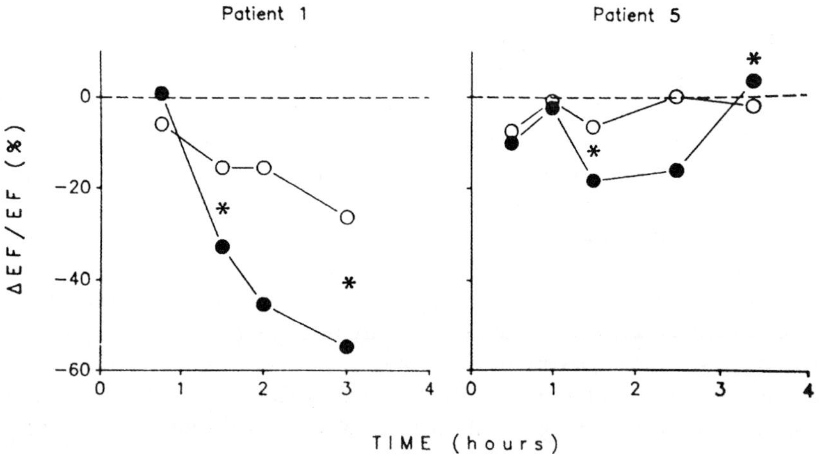

Figure 1 Variations in left ventricular ejection fraction (LVEF) (open circles) and right ventricular ejection fraction (REVF) (closed circles) during sleep in BPD patient 1 with oxygen desaturation and in BPD patient 5 without oxygen desaturation. On the abscissa, zero time is the time of ^{99m}Tc injection. Each LVEF and RVEF value is reported as the relative variation (DEF/EFw) from the value measured during wakefulness (Efw). Asterisks indicate data obtained during REM sleep. Note the larger decreases in LVEF and RVEF in BPD patient 1, who had lower Sa_{O_2} values during sleep than BPD patient 5. (From Ref. 32.)

found. The changes were more marked at slightly decreased Sa_{O_2} levels than at normal Sa_{O_2} levels, indicating that even mild hypoxemia occurring repeatedly may adversely affect autonomic heart rate control.

B. Sudden Infant Death Syndrome Risk in BPD Infants

An increased risk of mortality during the first year of life has been documented in BPD infants (34,35). Especially, it has been widely cited that infants with BPD are at high risk for sudden infant death syndrome (SIDS).

An association between BPD and SIDS was suggested by Werthammer et al. in the early 1980s (36). Neither pulse oximetry nor home oxygen therapy was available at the time. Werthammer et al. found that the incidence of SIDS was increased sevenfold in a group of 54 BPD outpatients versus a group of 65 control infants without BPD. Infants with BPD had Northway stage IV radiographic changes (2). Histological evidence of resolving BPD was found at autopsy in all the SIDS-BPD infants. The diagnosis of SIDS was based on the absence of any other cause of death at autopsy. This higher incidence of SIDS in BPD infants is at variance with a report by Sauve and Singhal (37). From 1975 through 1982, Sauve and Singhal studied the postdischarge death rate in 179 BPD infants and 112 controls. Of the 20 deaths recorded in the study group, only one was ascribed to SIDS (37).

During the early 1990s, two studies on the occurrence of an apparent life-threatening event (ALTE) and/or SIDS in BPD infants were published (38,39). Iles and Edmunds followed 35 infants with chronic lung disease of prematurity defined as oxygen dependency at 28 days of postnatal age or 36 weeks of PCA (38). There was no control group. ALTE occurred in seven cases, and one infant died unexpectedly. This infant was not receiving supplementary oxygen at the time of death; changes due to chronic lung disease were minimal and were not felt to be a significant factor in the infant's death. Gray and Rogers (39) reported follow-up data from 78 preterm infants of 26 to 33 weeks gestational age who were discharged following a diagnosis of BPD based on the clinical criteria of Bancalari (3). Twenty infants received home oxygen therapy. The control group comprised 78 infants matched with the study infants on birth-weight categories. None of the infants died during follow-up. Seven (8.9%) of the patients versus eight (10.5%) of the controls experienced an ALTE. None of the infants on home oxygen therapy had an ALTE. These findings suggest that BPD infants may not be at increased risk for SIDS if they receive appropriate management, including close attention to oxygenation. The treatment of BPD has changed considerably since the early 1980s, with far greater emphasis being placed on ensuring adequate oxygenation not only in the hospital but also after discharge.

However, the BPD infants who died of SIDS probably had clinically unrecognized periods of hypoxemia (16). Abnormal ventilatory and/or arousal responses during sleep may have contributed to their deaths. Garg et al. reported abnormal responses to a hypoxic challenge in BPD infants with a mean PCA of 41.4 ± 1.3 weeks (40). Twelve BPD infants weaned from supplemental oxygen breathed a hypoxic gas mixture (inspired partial pressure of O_2 equal to 80 mmHg) while asleep. Although 11 infants showed arousal in response to the hypoxic challenge, all the infants required vigorous stimulation and supplemental oxygen after this initial arousal response, suggesting an inability to recover from the hypoxia.

Ventilatory and arousal responses to hypoxia depend on the function of the peripheral chemoreceptors (41). These reset to a higher PO_2 level after birth (42). Hypoxia during the neonatal period has been shown to delay peripheral chemoreceptor resetting in newborn animals (43). Recent studies have sought to determine whether hypoxemic episodes in BPD infants result in altered responsiveness to chemoreceptor stimulation. Peripheral chemoreceptor function can be tested in isolation using either the hyperoxic test (HT) (44) or the alternating breath test (ABT) (45). The hyperoxic test induces "physiological chemodenervation" of the peripheral chemoreceptors. The ABT delivers a rapid hypoxic stimulus to the peripheral chemoreceptors by means of breath-by-breath alternations between a low and a normal inspired O_2 fraction. Both tests are reproducible under standardized conditions (46,47). Calder et al. (48) reported a reduced response to the ABT in eight BPD infants as compared to age-matched control infants. Katz-Salamon et al. designed a more extensive study involving an HT in 25 BPD infants and in 35 preterm infants without BPD (49). All infants were tested during the 40th week of PCA. Sixty percent of the BPD infants lacked a hyperoxic ventilatory response (Fig. 2). The intensity of the hyperoxic response was negatively correlated with the time spent on a ventilator and positively correlated with the time spent without supplemental oxygen. The degree of chemoreceptor activity was closely related to the severity of BPD, with none of the infants in the most severe BPD category (grade III) (4) showing a ventilatory response to hyperoxia. Thus, BPD infants may have deficient peripheral chemoreceptor function as a result of repeated and/or prolonged hypoxemia responsible for impaired postnatal peripheral chemoreceptor resetting.

The same group investigated whether peripheral chemoreceptor responsiveness returned to normal during recovery from BPD (50). Ten preterm infants with chronic lung disease and absence of a response to the HT were divided into subgroups based on disease severity (4). Episodes of desaturation were recorded during sleep despite supplemental oxygen therapy. However, these episodes decreased in number with advancing age. All the infants but two, who were in the category of maximum disease severity, developed a response to the HT within the first 4 months, at a mean postnatal age of 13 weeks (range 9 to 16). The two exceptions developed the response to hyperoxia at a much later postnatal age (6 and 8 months). Thus, the most severely affected infants lacked the HT response at the age of peak occurrence of SIDS. BPD infants who do not have functional peripheral chemoreceptors are unable to mount a protective response against hypoxemia and may therefore be at risk for ALTE and SIDS (51,52). Therefore, it may be suggested that peripheral chemoreceptor function should be tested in BPD infants at discharge and when cessation of supplemental oxygen therapy during sleep is considered. BPD infants with impaired peripheral

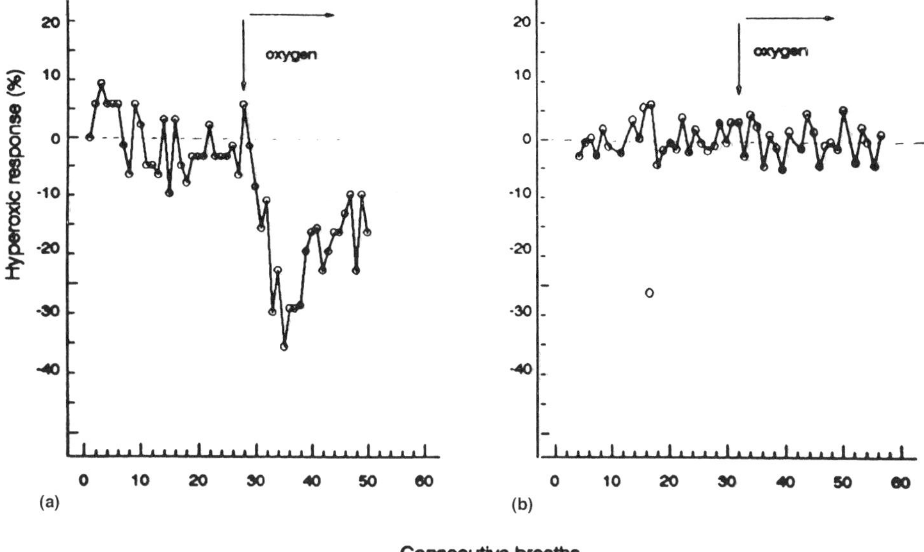

Figure 2 Percentage of deviations from mean resting ventilation during normoxic breathing and while breathing 100% oxygen for 30 sec. (a) An intact response in an infant with an initial diagnosis of respiratory distress syndrome that resolved without sequelae. (b) Data from a nonresponding BPD infant. Each dot represents one breath. (From Ref. 49.)

chemoreceptor function should be supervised closely. Preventing hypoxemic episodes in BPD infants is probably the most effective means of preventing SIDS (39).

C. Management of BPD Infants During Sleep

Awake Sa_{O_2} levels do not accurately predict hypoxemia during sleep (16,22). Sa_{O_2} should be measured during an extended period of sleep in BPD infants. Short-term Sa_{O_2} measurements are not sensitive indicators of Sa_{O_2} in patients breathing room air (22). Recording the plethysmographic waveform or the pulse amplitude modulation signals in addition to Sa_{O_2} is recommended to distinguish true drops in saturation from apparent drops due to movement artifacts or a weak pulse signal (53).

Studies have shown that maintaining Sa_{O_2} above 92% in infants with resolving BPD was associated with better growth (22,54). Criteria for determining when to discontinue oxygen therapy are not yet fully standardized. Recommendations on BPD from the American Thoracic Society ad hoc committee are currently under press (55). BPD infants who have been taken off O_2 supplementation should receive continuous monitoring during sleep if they develop polycythemia, cor pulmonale, failure to thrive, or sleep pattern disruption (56). In the most severe cases, oxygen supplementation alone may not be sufficient to maintain health. Nocturnal ventilatory support may be necessary and can be managed at home (57). A full polysomnography study can be of assistance in deciding when to discontinue the ventilatory support (58).

Pediatricians and families should be aware of the extreme vulnerability of BPD infants to common pediatric problems. Infectious agents usually responsible for mild disease can produce a life-threatening illness with impaired lung function and gas exchange (59). A full polysomnography study is in order if symptoms suggestive of upper-airway obstruction during sleep (e.g., snoring) occur at any time during recovery (56).

III. Asthma

A. Frequency of Nocturnal Asthma

Nocturnal cough and wheeze are common problems for patients with asthma. In a large survey of 7729 asthmatic adult patients conducted in Great Britain, 74% reported nocturnal awakening at least once a week and 64% at least 3 night a week (60). A good correlation was found between severity of asthma and frequency of nocturnal awakening (61). Some adult patients have primarily nocturnal symptoms. Recently, the phenotype of nocturnal asthma was shown to be associated with overrepresentation of the Gly 16 polymorphism of the β_2-adrenergic receptors as compared to adult patients with nonnocturnal asthma (62,63). In asthmatic children, less work has been performed on nocturnal symptoms (5,64–66). An entire school year of 8- to 9-year-old schoolchildren in Sheffield, England, were surveyed using a questionnaire (65) to assess the morbidity associated with diagnosed asthma (64). Of 5321 children surveyed, replies were obtained from 85.8%. A current diagnosis of asthma was reported in 10.3% ($n = 466$), and a further 6.4% reported symptoms compatible with significant undiagnosed asthma. Sleep disturbed at least once a week was reported in 32.6% of asthmatic children, and night cough at least once a week in 33.6%. In a hospital-based population of 796 asthmatic children (mean age 9 ± 4 years) (66), nocturnal symptoms were reported spontaneously by 38% of patients and on questioning by 47%. Cough was the most frequent nocturnal symptom (31%). Children with nocturnal asthma had lower forced expiratory volume in 1 sec (FEV_1) values, scored their asthma as more severe, and had more impairment of daytime activities than children without nocturnal asthma.

B. Death from Asthma

Several studies on asthma death in adult asthmatics have shown the greater incidence of respiratory arrests and death between 8 P.M. and 8 A.M. (67,68). Similar data were reported for deaths from asthma in children (69–71). Circumstances surrounding the deaths of 10 children due to asthma were investigated by Miller and Strunk (71). For the period more immediately surrounding the acute attack, 7 of 10 children had attacks starting during the night.

C. Circadian Variation of Airway Function

Normal lung function varies throughout the night; it is best around 4 P.M. and worst around 4 A.M. (72). In normal individuals, this variability is usually small. Greater variations in lung function levels have been shown in asthmatic adult patients (72).

Circadian rhythms of pulmonary function tests exploring airway patency [i.e., total pulmonary resistance (R_L) or peak expiratory flow rate (PEFR)] have been demonstrated and quantified in asthmatic children (73–75). We found that the mean amplitude of circadian variations of R_L, derived from cosinor analysis, was significantly greater in six children with stable asthma than in healthy children (74) (Fig. 3). Circadian rhythms were detected in both groups. The cosinor analysis of time series of asthmatic and healthy children showed that the R_L estimated acrophases (peak time) occurred at 04:04 A.M. and at 05:39 A.M., respectively (74). Diurnal variation of PEFR was demonstrated by Sly and coworkers in 73.5% of 66 children with clinically stable asthma whose ages ranged from 6 or 7 to 18.1 years (75). Mean amplitude of PEFR variations, derived from cosinor analysis, was 22.6 ± 13.2%. Spectral analysis confirmed that the major component of each child's variations in PEFR was due to a rhythm with a period of 24 hr. The amplitude of the PEFR variation was not related to the subject's age, sex, or medications but was inversely related to mean lung function. Similarly, in adult asthmatic patients, Martin and coworkers (76) found that the

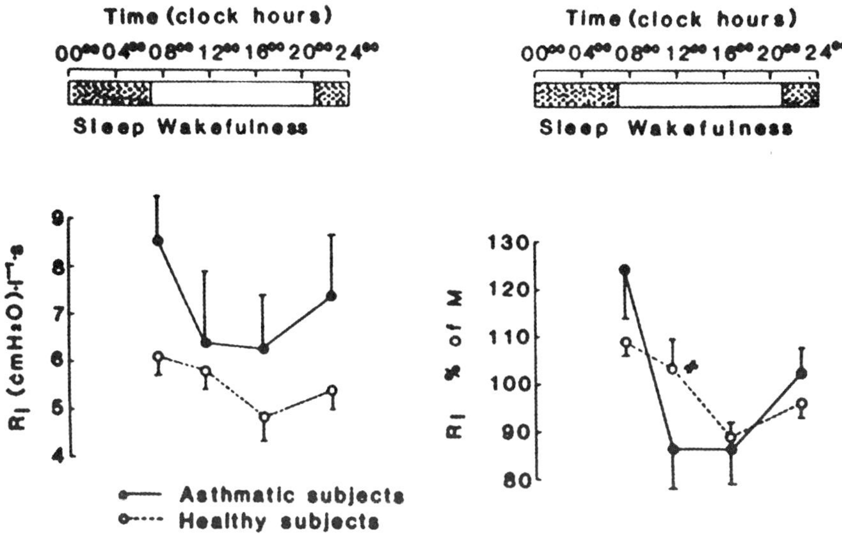

Figure 3 Circadian variations in total pulmonary resistance (R_L) in seven healthy children (dotted lines) and six asthmatic children (solid lines). Left: R_L is expressed as time point means (± SEM) in its unit of measurement. Right: R_L is expressed as a percentage of the individual circadian measure (24-hr adjusted average) (time point mean ± SEM); $p < .03$. (From Ref. 74.)

overnight decrement in lung function was related to the daytime measurements of airflow limitation.

D. Mechanisms Responsible for Nocturnal Asthma

Most of the studies looking at the mechanisms of nocturnal asthma were done in adult asthmatic patients. More than one mechanism is likely to be responsible for worsening of asthma at night (77). Nocturnal asthma represents an exaggeration of the circadian rhythm of airway function seen in normal people. This is reflected in an increased bronchial hyperresponsiveness, which is highest in the early hours of the morning (76). These changes have been shown to be associated with corresponding variations in autonomic function and hormonal levels (78,79). Bates and coworkers (79) showed, in 10 young adult asthmatic patients, that a circadian pattern in plasma cortisol was not associated with nocturnal asthma but that changes in plasma epinephrine contribute to nighttime airflow obstruction. Low circulating epinephrine levels were apparent in patients who experienced nocturnal asthma (79). A circadian rhythm in inflammatory cells in the lung has been observed in adult asthmatic subjects prone to nocturnal worsening (80).

There is some evidence that sleep itself is associated with deterioration in lung function independent of circadian rhythms (81,82). In a study by Ballard and coworkers, awake asthmatic patients exhibited a significant overnight increase in airflow resistance that was augmented when the patients were allowed to sleep (82). There was a twofold increase in airflow resistance during the sleep night, suggesting that sleep has an independent effect that is superimposed on the intrinsic circadian rhythm. Conflicting data have been reported on the effects of sleep stages. Initial observations in children showed that the majority of asthma attacks occur in stage 2 sleep, and no attacks were observed during the first third of the night (83). The role of REM sleep is controversial. In adult patients awakened in different sleep stages, FEV_1 and PEFR fell more during REM sleep than NREM sleep (84). However, Montplaisir and coworkers reported that asthma attacks were not proportionally more frequent during REM sleep than during NREM sleep (85). Bellia and coworkers (86) studied the interaction of sleep stages and asthma by recording the resistance of the lower respiratory tract in unstable asthmatic adult patients. They found that stages 3 to 4 were characterized by the highest peaks in airflow resistance and by longer episodes of bronchoconstriction.

The role of gastroesophageal reflux (GER) as a contributing factor of nocturnal asthma is unclear (87–90). Davis et al. (87) studied 9 children with nocturnal asthma and GER and found that acid infusion into the esophagus was associated with changes in respiratory pattern consistent with bronchoconstriction in the 4 children with a positive Bernstein test. However, Hugues and coworkers (88) found no association between GER and asthma symptoms in a group of adolescents with asthma. Furthermore, a possible reverse association between GER and asthma has been suggested (90). Asthma may cause GER and not vice versa. Through the effects of mechanical factors on the diaphragm, asthma could facilitate GER.

Upper-airway obstruction may also contribute to the pathogenesis of nocturnal asthma. Guilleminault and coworkers (91) studied 10 male adults with sleep apnea and asthma and 5 young asthmatics (mean age 17 ± 2.5 years) with frequent nocturnal asthma attacks and a history of snoring. They received nasal continuous positive airway pressure (CPAP) for a period of 6 to 9 months. Nasal CPAP eliminates snoring, obstructive apneas, and nocturnal asthma attacks. Chan et al. (92) similarly reported an improvement of nocturnal asthma in an adult asthmatic who snored and received nasal CPAP. The mechanisms by which nasal CPAP could improve nocturnal asthma in patients who snore is unclear. Martin et al. (93) studied nonapneic, nonsnoring asthmatic adults to determine the effects of nasal CPAP and found that it was associated with disrupted sleep architecture.

E. Functional Consequences of Nocturnal Asthma

Early study from Kales and coworkers (83) reported that children with asthma have abnormal sleep patterns. Ten asthmatic children from 5 to 15 years of age were studied. They were managed with chronic theophylline and epinephrine, but the treatment was stopped 6 hr before bedtime in most cases. In comparison to normal children of the same ages, the asthmatic children had a significant reduction in stage 4 of NREM sleep, frequent awakenings, and a significant decrease in the time spent asleep. Whereas, Hugues et al. (88) reported a normal sleep pattern in 9 asthmatic adolescents treated by short-acting β_2-agonists and/or theophylline. Similarly, Tabachnick and associates (94) found that sleep architecture was not affected in 8 adolescents in whom short-acting β_2-agonists were stopped 6 hours before sleep study. More recently, Avital et al. (95) studied sleep quality in 10 children, aged 10 to 17 years, with moderately severe asthma in a double-blind, crossover study that compared periods of treatment with cromolyn sodium or theophylline. Sleep efficiency was comparable during both periods, i.e., 94.1 ± 6% and 94.1 ± 3.3%, respectively. Sleep architecture was in the normal range (83) in both periods. During the cromolyn period, the number of awakenings from sleep > 1 min was 2.5 ± 1.4 and the number of central apneas ≥ 10 sec 6.7 ± 9.3 which is the normal range for age (96). Theophylline treatment did not significantly increase the number of awakening, but significantly decreased the number of central apneas to 2 ± 3.5 per night.

Hypoxemia in nocturnal asthma has been documented in asthmatic adults and children. Catterall and associates showed that adult stable asthmatics had greater and more frequent fall in Sa_{O_2} than age-matched healthy adults (97). Most hypoxemic episodes occurred in REM sleep and were associated with hypopnea or apnea. The severity of nocturnal hypoxemia was related to the level of Sa_{O_2} when the subjects were awake. Smith and Hudgel (98) reported the results of all-night monitoring of Sa_{O_2} in asthmatic children (Table 1). The children were awakened at 3 and 6 A.M. for FEV_1 measurements. In this study, the number and the severity of episodes of arterial oxygen desaturation correlated well with the extent of fall in FEV_1 during the night. Number of falls in Sa_{O_2} > 4% from baseline was reduced by optimizing theophylline treatment to prevent the nocturnal fall of FEV_1 (Table 1). Avital et al. (95) compared

Table 1 Lung Function Tests in Children and Adolescents with Asthma

Ref.	No. of subjects	Age (yr) mean ± SD	FEV_1 (%) mean ± SD	Treatment	Number of falls in Sa_{O_2}, mean ± SD	Maximal fall in Sa_{O_2}, mean ± SD	Minimal Sa_{O_2}, mean ± SD	VT	T_I/T_{TOT}	% Abd	% RC
99	8	12 ± 1.7	72 ± 30	T, A		5.1 ± 2.5					
98	16	11.4 ± 0.4	79.8 ± 2.8	$T^{(1)}$, A	4.1 ± 1.2*	8.9 ± 1.4					
				$T^{(2)}$, A	2.2 ± 1.1	3.9 ± 1.0					
94	8	13.6 ± 1.3	50 ± 12	T, A		3.9°	92 ± 2°	−15%	0.43°	+45	−43
						2.5^x	91.1 ± 2.5^x		0.35^x		
95	10	13.5 ± 2.4		CS	10.7 ± 27.3**						
				T	75.8 ± 10.6						

FEV_1 was measured during the daytime and just prior to sleep onset; T, theophylline treatment; A, short-acting β_2-agonist treatment; (1) 75% of the theophylline dose; (2) total theophylline dose; *fall in $Sa_{O_2} > 4\%$ from awake Sa_{O_2}; **fall in $Sa_{O_2} > 5\%$ from awake Sa_{O_2}; + and − indicate the changes in VT (tidal volume) and in the amplitude of abdominal movement (% Abd) and rib cage movement (% RC) in REM sleep as compared to NREM sleep; T_I/T_{TOT}, inspiratory time over total respiratory cycle duration; °, NREM sleep; ^{x}, REM sleep.

the effects of theophylline or cromolyn sodium on sleep oxygenation. The mean (± SEM) percentage of oxygen saturation for the entire night was slightly higher during the theophylline period than during the cromolyn period—i.e., 95 ± 2% and 94.2 ± 2.2, respectively. The time spent with Sa_{O_2} < 5% below the awake control value was significantly different between the two treatments, with longer periods of desaturation occurring during cromolyn treatment ($p < .05$) (Table 1). However, Chipps et al. (99) observed a significant fall in Sa_{O_2} during the night despite mean theophylline blood level of 15 ± 6 μg/mL in eight asthmatic children (Table 1). Tabachnik and associates studied the chest wall movements and pattern of breathing as well as sleep stages and Sa_{O_2} during sleep in eight asthmatic adolescents in whom bronchodilator therapy was withdrawn 12 hr before the start of the sleep study (94). The authors used a respiratory inductive plethysmograph and surface electromyogram (EMG) electrodes. During REM sleep, they observed a decrease in tidal volume associated with a decrease in intercostal EMG activity (Table 1) and paradoxical inward motion of the rib cage. Accompanying the abnormal chest wall mechanics there was an increase in diaphragmatic EMG activity. During REM sleep, there was a decrease in mean inspiratory flow rate and prolongation of the duty cycle (T_I/T_{TOT}) (Table 1). The mean minimal Sa_{O_2} was found during REM sleep (Table 1). Functional residual capacity (FRC) was not measured in this study. However, a study by Ballard and coworkers (100) in 10 asthmatic adults monitored overnight in a horizontal volume-displacement body plethysmograph demonstrated sleep-associated falls in FRC that were most marked during REM sleep. Data from Martin et al. (101) suggested that the fall in lung volume during sleep in the nocturnal asthmatic adult patients is a result, not a cause, of the overnight worsening of lung function. Furthermore, sleep-associated decrements in inspiratory muscle activity may contribute to sleep-associated reductions in FRC (102).

Hypoxemia during sleep may worsen airway obstruction. In fact, an increase in airway reactivity to methacholine was demonstrated following acute mild hypoxia in asthmatic adults (103,104). The potentiation of methacholine-induced bronchoconstriction by hypoxia appeared to be mediated via peripheral chemoreceptors (105). It follows that oxygen supplementation to patients with acute exacerbations of asthma may not only improve gas exchange but also reduce airway responsiveness to certain constrictor stimuli.

F. Management of Children with Nocturnal Asthma

In a recent workshop on pediatric asthma, it was stated that nocturnal asthma is underestimated and undertreated in pediatric practice (106). The Paediatric Asthma Quality of Life Questionnaire (PAQLQ), which includes an item on sleeping quality, should be incorporated into routine assessment of asthmatic children (107,108). Comprehensive management of asthmatic children must take into account the potential for significant variability in the severity of asthma during sleep. A detailed history of the timing and nature of nocturnal symptoms is essential in order to plan an appropriate therapeutic strategy. A diary may be useful for charting the night's events. Objective confirmation of patients' and parents' reporting can be obtained by use of home peak flow meter recordings. Measurements should be obtained at night, in the morning on waking up, and, if possible, when the patient wakes during the night with symptoms. Continuous documentation of oxygenation during sleep is infrequently needed in the routine management of children with asthma but should be considered for children with poorly controlled nocturnal asthma (56). Lung sound analysis for continuous monitoring of airflow obstruction during sleep has been shown to be effective. Wheeze quantification offers a possibility for noninvasive monitoring in nocturnal asthma (109). Advances in computer technology and improved methods for acoustical pattern recognition are likely to produce extended lung sound observations in clinical respiratory medicine, especially for nocturnal asthma.

The goal of asthma therapy in children is multiple, but control of nocturnal symptoms should be given equal weight to other aspects of management. Long-acting theophylline preparations may produce undesirable changes in temperament. Children may become hyperactive and restless. New long-acting inhaled β_2-agonists may provide prolonged protection against nighttime symptoms. Moore et al. recently reviewed data on long-acting β_2-agonists in asthma (110). Two recent studies reported experience in children with attention given to the improvement of nocturnal symptoms (111,112). The efficacy and safety of salmeterol have been assessed in a large multicenter study in children with mild to moderate asthma (111). Salmeterol 25 μg, salmeterol 50 μg, and salbutamol 200 μg were compared in two 3-month double-blind parallel-group studies, one using metered-dose inhalers (MDIs) and the other using dry powder inhalers (PDIs). Both studies were continued for a further 9 months. Children were eligible for inclusion if they had symptomatic asthma requiring an inhaled β_2-agonist and showed at least 15% reversibility of PEFR or FEV_1 following 200 μg of inhaled salbutamol. Children currently receiving inhaled glucocorticosteroids, sodium cromoglycate, nedocromil sodium, or ketotifen were allowed to continue with this treatment provided that the dose remained constant throughout the study period. After a 2-week run-in when all bronchodilator therapy was withdrawn, 279 patients received salmeterol 25 μg twice daily, 290 patients salmeterol 50 μg twice daily, and 278 patients salbutamol 200 μg twice daily. After 3 months of treatment, the change from baseline in daily morning and evening PEFR was significantly greater with salmeterol 50 μg than with salbutamol 200 μg ($p < .001$). Salmeterol 50 μg was significantly better than salmeterol 25 μg at improving mean morning PEFR ($p = .017$). Improvement in lung function was maintained throughout 12 months of treatment. Children receiving salmeterol 50 μg twice daily had significantly more symptom-free nights ($p < .01$). The improvements with salmeterol 50 μg twice daily were similar whether the drug was administered via a MDI or DPI. Adverse events—such as headache, tremor, palpitations and tachycardia—were not different across treatment groups or across age groups. In another double-blind parallel-group study, 67 children aged 6 to 16 years with mild to moderate asthma were treated for 1 year with salmeterol 50 μg or beclomethasone 400 μg twice daily (112). Asthma control and lung improvement were better with the inhaled corticosteroid than with the long-acting β_2-agonist given as monotherapy. Improvements in morning and evening PEFR were seen in both groups but were more marked in the beclomethasone group. The place of the long-acting β_2-agonists in the treatment of pediatric asthma remains unclear. Adding a long-acting β_2-agonist to an inhaled corticosteroid may deserve to be considered in children who remain symptomatic, particularly at night, despite inhaled corticosteroid therapy (113).

A recent exploratory study reported changes in sleep and daytime psychological function in 14 asthmatic children whose treatment was modified so as to place added emphasis on alleviating nocturnal symptoms (114). Home polysomnography, behavior, mood, and cognitive function were assessed before and 4 weeks after the treatment modification. Overall, improvements in nocturnal asthma symptoms provided by the treatment change were followed during the next few weeks by improvements in sleep efficiency and psychological function.

IV. Cystic Fibrosis

Cystic fibrosis (CF) is among the leading causes of airflow limitation in children and adolescents. Its incidence varies across geographic area and across ethic groups. In the United States, the incidence in live-born infants is about 1 in 3200 whites versus 1 in 15,000 blacks (115). The CF gene, or cystic fibrosis transmembrane conductance regulator (CFTR), has been mapped to chromosome 7. CF segregates as an autosomal recessive disorder and results from mutations in a single gene. The first CFTR mutation to be identified was ΔF508. Over 500 other CFTR mutations have now been reported (7). Recent studies suggest that the wide variability in the clinical expression of CF may reflect similar variability in the severity of the gene disruption caused by the different CFTR mutations (116,117).

In many instances, chronic lung dysfunction does not become obvious until late childhood or adolescence. Consequently, most of the data available on interactions between breathing and sleep in CF come from studies in older patients. In infants and younger children with CF, there is little published information on lung function (118) and virtually none on breathing during sleep.

A. Sleep-Related Disturbances

Starting with the earliest studies in the 1980s (119,122), research has been directed at characterizing the degree and mechanisms of nocturnal hypoxemia in CF. Recumbency may entail an increased risk of oxygen desaturation during sleep. Stokes et al. (122) found that the partial pressure of O_2 in arterial blood (Pa_{O_2}) decreased in the supine position in CF patients and that large declines were more likely to occur in patients whose obstructive lung disease was mild to moderate rather than severe. An increase in closing volume has been reported as contributing to postural hypoxemia in CF patients (122). The mechanisms underlying O_2 desaturation during sleep in CF patients during each sleep state have been investigated. REM sleep was associated with the largest saturation dips (119–121), seemingly as a result of alterations in ventilation-perfusion matching. Muller et al. noted that the transition from NREM to REM sleep was associated with a decrease in the tonic activity of intercostal and diaphragmatic muscles reflected by declines in baseline rib cage and abdominal magnetometer measurements, suggesting that the fall in oxygen saturation was preceded by a decrease in end-expiratory lung volume (121). This decrease may promote closure of the airways on dependent portions of the lung during tidal breathing, thereby worsening ventilation/perfusion mismatching (Fig. 4). The effects of decreased lung volume may be further exacerbated by episodes of hypoventilation responsible for an additional decrease in Sa_{O_2} (121). Tepper et al. used inductance plethysmography to study the effects of sleep on ventilation in six CF patients aged 10 to 16 years, with a mean ratio of FEV_1 over forced vital capacity equal to 0.52 (range 0.41 to 0.72) (124). During sleep, all subjects showed hypoventilation, oxygen desaturation episodes, and CO_2 retention. Mean Sa_{O_2} fell from 88 ± 3% during wakefulness to 82 ± 7% during tonic REM sleep and 76 ± 9% during phasic REM sleep. NREM sleep, in comparison to wakefulness, produced decreases in tidal volume and minute ventilation of 22% and 30%, respectively. There was a further depression in ventilation during phasic REM sleep. A recent study examined the effects of NREM sleep on ventilation and respiratory mechanics in five CF adults (29.6 ± 3.6 years, mean FEV_1: 42.2 ± 8.5% of predicted) (125). The patients were studied while sleeping in a horizontal body

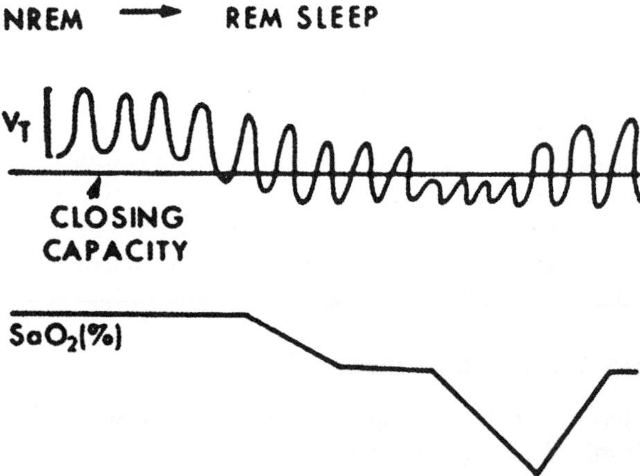

Figure 4 Diagrammatic representation of the presumptive mechanism of desaturation during rapid-eye-movement (REM) sleep. During REM sleep, a decrease in functional residual capacity causes the subject to breathe below the closing volume; consequently, some lung units remain closed throughout the tidal volume (V_T). This leads to a decrease in arterial O_2 saturation (Sa_{O_2}). (From Ref. 121.)

plethysmograph. Sa_{O_2} fell from 89.4 ± 1.5% during wakefulness to 88.3 ± 1.0% and 87.8 ± 1.2% during stages 2 and 3 to 4, respectively. The Sa_{O_2} decrease during NREM sleep was associated with decreases in tidal volume, minute ventilation, and mouth occlusion pressure. Airflow resistance and functional residual capacity remained unchanged during NREM sleep as compared to wakefulness.

Early studies in small group of CF patients (primarily adults) found that the magnitude of desaturation during sleep was related to the severity of the underlying lung disease (119–121). More recent studies in larger groups of CF patients, some of which were done during late childhood and adolescence, indicate that the degree of oxygen desaturation during sleep cannot be reliably predicted from clinical scores and/or awake pulmonary function (126–129). Coffey et al. examined associations among resting, awake, and exercise Sa_{O_2} in 21 adults and adolescents with CF, of whom 8 were hypoxemic (resting $Sa_{O_2} < 95\%$; FEV_1, 31.1 ± 12.4%) and 13 were not (FEV_1 of 59.1 ± 21.1%) (129). Overnight oximetry and treadmill exercise testing were performed. The most striking findings from this study were that nonhypoxemic CF patients experienced more severe desaturation during sleep than during exercise and that the magnitude of desaturation versus baseline during sleep could not be predicted from either awake Sa_{O_2} or the magnitude of exercise-related desaturation. However, arterial blood gas measurement during wakefulness may help identify those patients who should be screened for hypoxemia during sleep. CF patients with awake Pa_{O_2} values of less than 60 mmHg were found to spend over 80% of their sleep time with Sa_{O_2} values below 90%. Conversely, patients with awake Pa_{O_2} values above 70 mmHg spent less than 20% of their sleep time with Sa_{O_2} values below 90%.

Avital et al. reported overnight Sa_{O_2} measurements in 12 CF patients aged 7 to 17 years (130). Mean FEV_1 before bronchodilator administration was 62 ± 9% of predicted. Baseline Sa_{O_2} was 95.2 ± 1.7. During the overnight study, the percentage of time spent with a greater than 5% fall in Sa_{O_2} from baseline was 8.8 ± 3.6%.

Taken in concert, these data indicate that significant oxygen desaturation can be missed unless specifically looked for in CF patients. The American Thoracic Society made the following recommendations for overnight Sa_{O_2} monitoring in CF patients:

> Patients with CF who have an awake Pa_{O_2} < 70 mmHg or an equivalent Sa_{O_2} (< 95%) during a period of disease stability are at risk for worsening hypoxemia during sleep and should have continuous determination of Sa_{O_2} during nocturnal sleep (56). This study should be performed during a period of disease stability (generally at least 2 weeks following treatment for an acute pulmonary exacerbation) in order to determine the extent and severity of sleep-associated hypoxemia.

Montgomery et al. (127) evaluated the feasibility and reproducibility of home Sa_{O_2} measurement in 14 clinically stable CF patients (mean age 20 years; range 9 to 34 years). The difference between two measurements was 4 ± 2% (mean ± SEM) for the percent time with $Sa_{O_2} < 90\%$ and 3 ± 2% for the percent time with $Sa_{O_2} < 85\%$.

Sleep quality can be impaired in patients with CF. Spier et al. (123) found decreased sleep efficiency, more sleep-state changes, and more awakenings (> 5 min) per hour of sleep in patients with CF. The longer arousals often coincided with coughing paroxysms (123). Episodes of hypoxemia may conceivably contribute to sleep disturbances. However, an early study by Boysen et al. (131) found that arousals did not occur in response to hypoxemia in young adults with CF.

Episodes of obstructive and/or central apnea appeared to be uncommon in CF patients (123). However, nasal polyps are frequent in CF patients and may predispose to obstructive apnea during sleep. It follows that polysomnography may be required to rule out OSAS in CF patients with a history of snoring (56).

B. Sleep-Related Hypoxemia and Cor Pulmonale

Sleep hypoxemia may be a contributing factor to the development of cor pulmonale in CF patients, as it is in adults with chronic obstructive pulmonary disease. Furthermore, hypoxemia occurring during the growth period may impair the postnatal development of pulmonary blood vessels. Ryland and Reid reported a decreased number of arteries per unit of lung section surface area, with a correlation between this decrease and right ventricular hypertrophy (132). Moreover, in all their patients, pulmonary artery muscle was increased and extended further toward the periphery. Hypoplasia and remodeling of the pulmonary vasculature induced by chronic hypoxemia may play a role in the development of cor pulmonale (133).

However, the role of nocturnal hypoxemia in the pathogenesis of cor pulmonale in CF has not yet been clarified. One study investigated the relationship between hypoxemia during sleep and its role in reducing morbidity and mortality in 28 CF patients with a mean age of 23 ± 6 years (134). Mean awake Pa_{O_2} was approximately 60 mmHg. Of the total, 14 patients were assigned to nocturnal oxygen and 14 to air. Mean duration of O_2 therapy was 6.2 hr. Disease progression as assessed based on nutritional status, spirometry, blood gases, and maximal working capacity was not significantly different between air- and oxygen-treated patients over a 12-month period. Eight patients, four in each group, died after a mean follow-up of 26 ± 9 months. Right ventricular ejection fractions at rest and after exercise were not significantly different between survivors and decedents. However, because these findings were obtained in patients with advanced CF, they may not be generalizable to the overall CF population. The lack of a response to oxygen therapy may have been due to severe structural damage to the pulmonary vascular bed. The role for oxygen therapy in earlier stages of CF remains unclear, especially since right ventricular hypertrophy is sometimes present in patients with mild CF.

C. Nocturnal Oxygen Supplementation

The indications for supplemental oxygen during sleep in children and adolescents with CF remain ill defined. However, oxygen during sleep is clearly needed in patients with severe disease and a $Pa_{O_2} < 60$ mmHg during wakefulness. In patients with an awake $Pa_{O_2} > 60$ mmHg, the appropriateness of supplemental oxygen is still under investigation. The time at which oxygen therapy should be started is not agreed on.

The long-term consequences of brief episodes of oxygen desaturation during sleep are unknown. Conceivably, nocturnal oxygen supplementation may improve the quality of life (135) during the day by improving cognitive function. A noteworthy finding from the study by Zinman (134) is that the oxygen-treated patients continued to attend school or go to work, whereas the air-treated patients did not. Preliminary data have been reported on cognitive dysfunction in adults with CF (136). Neurophysiological abnormalities include deficits in working memory and/or visuospatial components. No such evaluation has been reported in children and/or adolescents with CF and mild to moderate oxygen desaturation during sleep.

The effect on sleep quality of oxygen supplementation during sleep were investigated in an unblinded crossover study in 10 CF patients in stable condition (123). Mean age was 22 ± 5 years (range, 16 to 31), mean awake Sa_{O_2} was < 92%, and FEV_1 was 22 ± 3% of predicted. As compared to air, oxygen supplementation during the night did not significantly improve the poor sleep quality of the patients. Oxygen therapy has been shown to be safe, with no excessive CO_2 retention, in most patients who are free from hypercapnia during the daytime (123,127,137).

D. Ventilatory Support During Sleep

Regnis and coworkers tested the benefits of nocturnal nasal CPAP in seven CF patients with severe lung disease (age range 14 to 39 years) (138). Nasal CPAP caused no changes in total sleep time or sleep efficiency but significantly reduced the number of respiratory events, most of which were observed during REM sleep. Nasal CPAP also improved Sa_{O_2} during both NREM and REM sleep.

Recent reports have provided data on the effects of nasal positive-pressure ventilation (NPPV) during sleep in CF patients with severe lung disease (139–142). With advancing lung disease, alveolar hypoventilation worsens during sleep. The potential benefits of NPPV include improved gas exchange, reducing both hypoxemia and hypercapnia; decreased work of breathing; and respiratory muscle resting. Granton and coworkers (139) tested the acute effects of NPPV in eight adult CF patients with severe airflow limitation (FEV_1 = 24 ± 3% of predicted, Pa_{O_2} = 67 ± 15 mmHg and Pa_{CO_2} = 50 ± 4 mmHg). Respiratory variables including tidal volume, respiratory rate, minute ventilation, and Sa_{O_2} were monitored over a 20-min period before and after NPPV application. In addition, esophageal pressure (Pes) was recorded in two patients. The acute effects of NPPV consisted of improved oxygenation and decreased minute ventilation. In the two patients who had Pes recordings, pressure swings decreased significantly, and in one of these two patients the ratio of Pes over inspiratory time was reduced, suggesting a reduction in the work of breathing. NPPV and supplemental oxygen during the night were compared by Gozal in six CF patients with moderate to severe lung disease (140). Mean age was 18.2 ± 3.6 years, mean FEV_1 was 29.4 ± 3.4% of predicted, mean Pa_{O_2} was 56.8 ± 6.8 mmHg, and mean Pa_{CO_2} was 44 ± 3 mmHg. Compared to the control night, both NPPV and supplemental oxygen significantly improved the overall nighttime Sa_{O_2}. NPPV markedly improved alveolar ventilation during all sleep states. Sleep architecture and arousals remained unchanged during both NPPV and supplemental oxygen therapy. Hill and coworkers reported their experience with long-term NPPV in 12 patients awaiting transplantation for hypercapnic respiratory failure (141). Mean age was 26 ± 4 years. Ten patients tolerated NPPV for 1 to 15 months (mean, 5.1 ± 1.4 months) and reported subjective improvements in headache and quality of sleep. After 3 months, there were significant improvements in forced vital capacity and Pa_{CO_2}. Baculard and coworkers used NPPV in six CF children aged 10 to 18 years previously treated for 6 months to 7 years with supplemental oxygen during 10 hr of every 24-hr cycle (142). Three patients were awaiting transplantation. Mean Pa_{O_2} was 57.1 ± 7.8 mmHg and mean Pa_{CO_2} was 44.8 ± 7.9 mmHg. In four patients, NPPV was given for 3 to 14 months.

Thus, available data on NPPV in moderate (140) and/or severe CF (141,142) suggest that NPPV may be a useful adjunct, especially in patients awaiting transplantation (143). However, prospective studies are required to determine the best time for starting NPPV. In addition to airflow and gas exchange measurements, noninvasive determination of the pressure-time index of inspiratory muscles may be useful (144). Impairment of inspiratory muscle function has been demonstrated in CF children who had a good nutritional status and only mild to moderate lung function test abnormalities (145). Conceivably, the pressure-time index may help to assess disease progression. Whether NPPV is effective in decreasing this index deserves to be determined.

V. Other Chronic Obstructive Pulmonary Diseases

Chronic obstructive pulmonary disease (COPD) other than CF can occur in children. Infections due to adenoviruses or parainfluenza viruses (8,146,147) can be followed by COPD. Children with postviral COPD have variable limitations in airflow and inspiratory muscle reserve (8,148). Some are hypoxemic during the daytime (8). During sleep, the hypoxemia can worsen, especially during REM periods (24). Another cause of COPD in children is abnormal motility of the cilia (9).

Sa_{O_2} monitoring during sleep is recommended in children with COPD who are hypoxemic during the daytime. In those with normal daytime Sa_{O_2}, close follow-up is in order to avoid unexpected falls in Sa_{O_2} during sleep. Children with severe COPD may need oxygen supplementation, or even NPPV, both of which can be given at home (57).

VI. Chronic Interstitial Lung Diseases

Chronic interstitial lung disease (CILD) is rare in children. CILD encompasses a broad spectrum of pulmonary disorders characterized by diffuse infiltrates, restrictive lung disease, and abnormal gas exchange (10,149). Children with CILD are sometimes hypoxemic during the daytime (150). The severity of the hypoxemia correlates with the increase in mouth occlusion pressure, suggesting that the drive to hyperventilation is due at least in part to hypoxemia (151).

Hypoxemia during sleep has been documented in adults with CILD. In two studies including some CILD patients who snored, severe oxygen desaturation was found during sleep, especially during the REM periods (152,153). In two other studies in which snoring was an exclusion criterion, moderate hypoxemia occurred during sleep (154,155). No sleep studies in children with CILD are available. CILD can induce progressive respiratory failure, and oxygen supplementation or even NPPV (57) are sometimes required in patients awaiting lung transplantation (156).

VII. Conclusion

Careful management of children with chronic lung disease should take into account the potential for deteriorations in lung function and gas exchange during sleep. The proportion of the 24-hr cycle spent sleeping is considerably longer in young children than in adults. Deterioration in lung function and gas exchange during sleep may adversely affect the overall development of children. Failure to thrive may result from an increase in the work of breathing during sleep. Repeated and/or prolonged episodes of hypoxemia may affect postnatal vascular lung growth. Finally, the development of neurocognitive functions may be compromised. Optimal treatment of children with chronic lung disease should cover the entire 24-hr cycle. It follows that pediatricians must be acutely aware of the affects of sleep on the pathophysiology of chronic lung disease.

References

1. Gaultier CL. Cardiorespiratory adaptation during sleep in infants and children. Pediatr Pulmonol 1995; 19:105–117.
2. Northway WH, Rosan RC, Porter DY. Pulmonary disease following respiratory therapy of hyaline membrane disease: bronchopulmonary dysplasia. N Engl J Med 1967; 276: 357–368.
3. Bancalari E, Abdenour GE, Feller R, Gannon J. Bronchopulmonary dysplasia: clinical presentation. J Pediatr 1979; 85:819–823.
4. Toce S, Farrel PH, Leavitt LA, Samuels PP, Edvards DK. Clinical and roentgenographic scoring systems for assessing bronchopulmonary dysplasia. Am J Dis Child 1984; 138: 581–585.
5. O'Brodovich HM, Mellins RB. Bronchopulmonary dysplasia: unresolved neonatal acute lung injury. Am Rev Respir Dis 1985; 132:694–709.
6. Lenney W, Wells NEJ, O'Neill BA. The burden of paediatric asthma. Eur Respir Rev 1994; 4:18:9–62.

7. Davis PS, Drumm M, Konstan MW. Cystic fibrosis. Am J Respir Crit Care Med 1996; 154:1229–1256.
8. Gaultier CL, Beaufils F, Boule M, Bompard Y, Devictor D. Lung functional follow-up in children after severe viral infection. Eur J Respir Dis 1984; 65:460–467.
9. Escalier D, Jouannet P, David G. Abnormalities of the ciliary axonemal complex in children: an ultrastructural and cinetic study in a series of 34 cases. Biol Cell 1982; 44: 271–282.
10. Fan LL, Langston C. Chronic interstitial lung disease in children. Pediatr Pulmonol 1993; 16:184–196.
11. Fanaroff AA, Wright LL, Stevenson DK, Shankaran S, Donovan EF, Ehrenkranz RA, Younes N, Korones SB, Stoll BJ, Tyson JE, Bauer CR, OH W, Lemons JA, Papile LA, Verter J. Very-low-birth-weight outcomes of the National Institute of Child Health and Human Development Neonatal Research Network, May 1991 through December 1992. Am J Obstet Gynecol 1995; 173:1423–1431.
12. Durand M, McEvoy C, MacDonald K. Spontaneous desaturations in intubated very low birth weight infants with acute and chronic lung disease. Pediatr Pulmonol 1992; 13: 136–142.
13. McEvoy C, Durand M, Hewlett V. Episodes of spontaneous desaturations in infants with chronic lung disease at two different levels of oxygenation. Pediatr Pulmonol 1993; 15: 140–144.
14. Sekar KC, Duke JC. Sleep apnea and hypoxemia in recently weaned premature infants with and without bronchopulmonary dysplasia. Pediatr Pulmonol 1991; 10:112–116.
15. Zinman R, Blanchard PW, Vachon F. Oxygen saturation during sleep in patients with bronchopulmonary dysplasia. Biol Neonate 1992; 61:69–75.
16. Garg M, Kurzner SI, Bautista DB, Keens TG. Clinically unsuspected hypoxia during sleep and feeding in infants with bronchopulmonary dysplasia. Pediatrics 1988; 81: 635–641.
17. Greenspan JS, Wolfson MR, Locke RG, Allen JL, Shaffer TH. Increased respiratory drive and limited adaptation to loaded breathing in bronchopulmonary dysplasia. Pediatr Res 1992; 32:356–359.
18. Teague WG, Pian MS, Heldt GP, Tooley WH. An acute reduction in the fraction of inspired oxygen increases airway constriction in infants with chronic lung disease. Am Rev Respir Dis 1988; 137:861–865.
19. Tay-Uybocco JS, Kwiatkowski K, Cates DB, Kavanagh L, Rigatto H. Hypoxic airway constriction in infants of very low birth weight recovering from moderate to severe bronchopulmonary dysplasia. J Pediatr 1989; 115:456–459.
20. Abman SH, Wolfe RR, Accurso FJ, Koops BL, Bowman M, Wiggins JW. Pulmonary vascular response to oxygen in infants with severe bronchopulmonary dysplasia. Pediatrics 1985; 75:80–84.
21. Halliday HL, Dumpit FM, Brady JP. Effects of inspired oxygen on echocardiographic assessment of pulmonary vascular resistance and myocardial contractility in bronchopulmonary dysplasia. Pediatrics 1980; 63:536–540.
22. Moyer-Mileur LJ, Nielson DW, Pfeffer KD, Witte MK, Chapman DL. Eliminating sleep-associated hypoxemia improves growth in infants with bronchopulmonary dysplasia. Pediatrics 1996; 98:779–783.
23. Loughlin GM, Allen RP, Pyzik P. Sleep related hypoxemia in children with bronchopulmonary dysplasia and adequate oxygen saturation awake. Sleep Res 1987; 16: 486.

24. Gaultier C, Praud JP, Clement A, Boule M, Khiati M, Tournier G, Girard F. Respiration during sleep in children with COPD. Chest 1985; 87:168.
25. Harris MA, Sullivan CE. Sleep pattern and supplementary oxygen requirements in infants with chronic neonatal lung disease. Lancet 1995; 345:831–832.
26. Sher MS, Richardson GA, Salemo DG, Day NL, Guthrie RD. Sleep architecture and continuity measures of neonates with chronic lung disease. Sleep 1992; 15:195–201.
27. Allen JL, Greenspan JS, Deoras KS, Keklikian E, Wolfson MR, Shaffer TH. Interaction between chest wall motion and lung mechanics in normal infants and in infants with bronchopulmonary dysplasia. Pediatr Pulmonol 1991; 11:37–43.
28. Gaultier C, Praud JP, Canet E, Delaperche MF, D'Allest AM. Paradoxical inward rib cage motion during rapid eye movement sleep in infants and young children. J Dev Physiol 1987; 9:391–397.
29. Rome ES, Miller MJ, Goldthwait DA, Osorio IO, Fanaroff AA, Martin RJ. Effect of sleep state on chest wall movements and gas exchange in infants with resolving bronchopulmonary dysplasia. Pediatr Pulmonol 1987; 3:259–263.
30. Goldman MD, Pagani M, Trang HTT, Praud JP, Sartene R, Gaultier C. Asynchronous chest wall movements during non-rapid-eye-movement and rapid-eye-movement sleep in children with bronchopulmonary dysplasia. Am Rev Respir Dis 1993; 147: 1175–1184.
31. Openshaw P, Edwards S, Helms P. Changes in rib cage geometry during childhood. Thorax 1984; 39:624–627.
32. Praud JP, Cavailloles F, Boulhadour K, De Recondo M, Guilleminault C, Gaultier C. Radionuclide evaluation of cardiac function during sleep in children with bronchopulmonary dysplasia. Chest 1991; 100:721–725.
33. Filtchev S, Curzi-Dascalova L, Spassov L, Kauffmann F, Trang HTT, Gaultier C. Heart rate variability during sleep in infants with bronchopulmonary dysplasia: effects of mild decrease in oxygen saturation. Chest 1994; 106:1711–1716.
34. Abman SH, Burchell MF, Schaffer MS, Rosenberg AA. Late sudden unexpected deaths in hospitalized infants with bronchopulmonary dysplasia. Am J Dis Child 1989; 143: 815–819.
35. Bhutani VK, Abbasi S. Long-term pulmonary consequences in survivors with bronchopulmonary dysplasia. Clin Perinatol 1992; 19:649–671.
36. Werthammer J, Brown ER, Neff RK, Taeusch HW Jr. Sudden infant death syndrome in infants with bronchopulmonary dysplasia. Pediatrics 1982; 69:301–303.
37. Sauve RS, Singhal N. Long-term morbidity of infants with bronchopulmonary dysplasia. Pediatrics 1995; 76:725–733.
38. Iles R, Edmunds AT. Prediction of early outcome in resolving chronic lung disease of prematurity after discharge from hospital. Arch Dis Child 1996; 74:304–308.
39. Gray PH, Rogers Y. Are infants with bronchopulmonary dysplasia at risk for sudden infant death syndrome? Pediatrics 1994; 93:774–777.
40. Garg M, Kurzner SI, Bautista D, Keens TG. Hypoxic arousal responses in infants with bronchopulmonary dysplasia. Pediatrics 1988; 82:59–63.
41. Fewell JE, Kondo CS, Ddascula F, Filyk SC. Influence of carotid denervation on the arousal and cardiopulmonary response to rapidly developing hypoxemia in lambs. Pediatr Res 1989; 25:473–479.
42. Hertzberg T, Hellström S, Lagercrantz H, Pequignot JM. Development of the arterial chemoreflex and turnover of carotid body catecholamines in the newborn rat. J Physiol 1990; 425:211–225.

43. Hanson MA, Kumar P, Williams BA. The effect of chronic hypoxia upon the development of respiratory chemoreflexes in the newborn kitten. J Physiol 1989; 411:563–574.
44. Hertzberg T, Lagercrantz H. Postnatal sensitivity of the peripheral chemoreceptors in newborn infants. Arch Dis Child 1987; 62:1238–1241.
45. Calder NA, Williams BA, Kumar P, Hanson MA. The respiratory response of healthy term infants to breath-by-breath alternations in inspired oxygen at two postnatal ages. Pediatr Res 1994; 35:312–324.
46. Bouferrache E, Krim G, Marbaix-Li Q, Freville M, Gaultier C. Reproductibility of the alternating breath test of fractional inspired O_2 in infants. Pediatr Res 1998; 44:239–246.
47. Bouferrache B, Filtchev S, Krim G, Marbaix-Li Q, Freville M, Gaultier C. The hyperoxic test in infants reinvestigated. Am J Respir Crit Care Med 2000; 161:160–165.
48. Calder NA, Williams BA, Smith J, Boon AW, Kumar P, Hanson MA. Absence of ventilatory responses to alternating breaths of mild hypoxia and air in infants who have had bronchopulmonary dysplasia: implications for the risk of sudden infant death. Pediatr Res 1994; 35:677–681.
49. Katz-Salamon M, Jonson B, Lagercrantz H. Blunted peripheral chemoreceptor response to hyperoxia in a group of infants with bronchopulmonary dysplasia. Pediatr Pulmonol 1995; 20:101–106.
50. Katz-Salamon M, Eriksson M, Jonsson B. Development of peripheral chemoreceptor function in infants with chronic lung disease and initially lacking hyperoxic response. Arch Dis Child 1996; 75:F4–F9.
51. Hanson MA, Calder N, Watanabe T, Kumar P. The drive to breathe and infant death syndrome. Acta Paediatr 1993; 92:47–49.
52. Hunt CE, McCulloch K, Brouillette RT. Diminished hypoxic ventilatory responses in near-miss sudden infant death syndrome. J Appl Physiol 1981; 50:1315–1317.
53. Lafontaine VM, Ducharme FM, Brouillette RT. Pulse oximetry: accuracy of methods of interpreting graphic summaries. Pediatr Pulmonol 1996; 21:121–131.
54. Hudak BB, Allen MC, Hudak NL, Loughlin GM. Home oxygen therapy for chronic lung disease in extremely premature infants. Am J Dis Child 1989; 143:357–360.
55. American Thoracic Society Committee on BPD. To be published.
56. American Thoracic Society: Standards and indications for cardiopulmonary sleep studies in children. Am J Respir Crit Care Med 1996; 153:866–878.
57. Fauroux B, Sardet A, Foret D. Home treatment for chronic respiratory failure in children: a prospective study. Eur Respir J 1995; 8:2062–2066.
58. Hermabessiere C, Monier B, Gaultier CL, Beaufils F, Benali K, Cathelineau L. Dysplasie bronchopulmonaire: devenir et traitement des formes sévères. Arch Franc Ped 1995; 2:628–635.
59. Chidekel AS, Bazz AR, Rosen CL. Rhinovirus infection associated with severe lower respiratory tract illness and worsening lung disease in infants with bronchopulmonary dysplasia. Pediatr Pulmonol 1994; 18:261–263.
60. Turner-Warnick M. Epidemiology of nocturnal asthma. Am J Med 1988; 85:6–8.
61. National Institutes of Health. Global initiative for asthma: global strategy for asthma management and prevention, NHLBI/WHO workshop report March 1993, Publication number 95-3659. Washington, DC: NHLBI/WHO, January 1995: 1–176.
62. Turki J, Pak J, Green SA, Martin RJ, Ligett SB. Genetic polymorphism of the β_2-adrenergic receptor in nocturnal and non-nocturnal asthma: evidence that Gly 16 phenotype correlates with the nocturnal phenotype. J Clin Invest 1995; 95:1635–1641.

63. Turki J, Green SA, Newman KB, Meyers MA, Liggett SB. Human lung cell β_2-adrenergic receptors desensitize in response to in vivo administered beta-agonist. Am J Physiol 1995; 269:L709–L714.
64. Powell CVE, Primhak RA. Asthma treatment, perceived respiratory disability and morbidity. Arch Dis Child 1995; 72:209–213.
65. Usherwood TP, Scrimgeour A, Barber JH. Questionnaire to measure perceived symptoms and disability in asthma. Arch Dis Child 1990; 65:779–781.
66. Meijer GG, Postma OS, Wempe JB, Gerritsen J, Knol K, Van Aalderen WMC. Frequency of nocturnal symptoms in asthmatic children attending a hospital out-patient clinic. Eur Respir J 1995; 8:2076–2080.
67. Hetzel MR, Clark TJH, Branthwaite MA. Asthma: analysis of sudden deaths and ventilatory arrests in hospitals. BMJ 1977; 1:808–811.
68. Robertson CF, Rufinfeld AR, Bowes G. Deaths from asthma in Victoria: a 12 months survey. Med J Aust 1990; 152:511–517.
69. Miller BD, Strunk RC. Circumstances surrounding the deaths of children due to asthma. Am J Dis Child 1989; 143:1294–1299.
70. Robin ED, Lewiston N. Unexpected, unexplained sudden death in young asthmatic subjects. Chest 1989; 96:790–793.
71. Carswell F. Thirty deaths from asthma. Arch Dis Child 1985; 60:25–28.
72. Hetzel MR, Clark TJH. Comparison of normal and asthmatic circadian rhythms in peak expiratory flow rate. Thorax 1980; 35:732–738.
73. Gaultier CL, Reinberg A, Girard F. Circadian rhythms in lung resistance and dynamic lung compliance of healthy children: effects of two bronchodilators. Respir Physiol 1977; 31:168–182.
74. Gaultier CL, Reinberg A, Motohashi Y. Circadian rhythm in total pulmonary resistance of asthmatic children: effects of a β-agonist agent. Chronobiol Int 1988; 5:285–290.
75. Sly PD, Hibbert ME, Sci MA, Landau LI. Diurnal variation of peak expiratory flow rate in asthmatic children. Pediatr Pulmonol 1986; 2:141–146.
76. Martin RJ, Cicutto LC, Ballard RD. Factors related to the nocturnal worsening of asthma. Am Rev Respir Dis 1990; 141:33–38.
77. Douglas NJ, Flenley DC. Breathing during sleep in patients with obstructive lung disease. Am Rev Respir Dis 1990; 141:1055–1070.
78. Barnes P, Fitzgerald G, Brown M, Dollery C. Nocturnal asthma and changes in circulating epinephrine, histamine and cortisol. N Engl J Med 1980; 303:263–267.
79. Bates ME, Clayton M, Calhoun W, Jarjour N, Schrader L, Geiger K, Schultz T, Sedgwick J, Swenson C, Busse W. Relationship of plasma epinephrine and circulating eosinophils to nocturnal asthma. Am J Respir Crit Care Med 1994; 149:667–672.
80. Martin RJ, Cicutto LC, Smith HR, Ballard RD, Szefler SJ. Airways inflammation in nocturnal asthma. Am Rev Respir Dis 1991; 143:351–357.
81. Catterall JR, Rhind GB, Stewart IC, Whyte KF, Shapiro CM, Douglas NJ. Effect of sleep deprivation on overnight bronchoconstriction in nocturnal asthma. Thorax 1986; 41: 676–680.
82. Ballard RD, Saathoff MC, Patel DK, Kelly PL, Martin RJ. Effect of sleep on nocturnal bronchoconstriction and ventilatory patterns in asthmatics. J Appl Physiol 1989; 67: 243–249.
83. Kales A, Kales JD, Sly RM, Scharf MB, Tan TL, Preston TA. Sleep patterns of asthmatic children: all-night electroencephalographic studies. J Allergy 1970; 46:300–308.

84. Shapiro CM, Catterall JR, Montgomery I, Raab GM, Douglas NJ. Do asthmatics suffer bronchoconstriction during rapid eye movement sleep? BMJ 1986; 292:1161–1164.
85. Montplaisir J, Walsh J, Malo JL. Nocturnal asthma: features of attacks, sleep and breathing patterns. Am Rev Respir Dis 1982; 125:18–22.
86. Bellia V, Cuttitta G, Insalaco G, Visconti A, Bonsignore G. Relationship to nocturnal bronchoconstriction to sleep states. Am Rev Respir Dis 1989; 140:363–367.
87. Davis RS, Larsen GL, Grunstein MM. Respiratory response to intraesophageal and infusion in asthmatic children during sleep. J Allergy Clin Immunol 1983; 72:393–398.
88. Hugues DM, Spier S, Rivlin J, Levison H. Gastroesophageal reflux during sleep in asthmatic patients. J Pediatr 1983; 102:666.
89. Tan WC, Martin RJ, Pandey R, Ballard RD. Effects of spontaneous and simulated gastroesophageal reflux on sleeping asthmatics. Am Rev Respir Dis 1990; 141:1394–1399.
90. Pack AI. Acid: a nocturnal bronchoconstrictor? Am Rev Respir Dis 1990; 141: 1391–1392.
91. Guilleminault C, Quera-Salva MA, Powell N, Romaker A, Partinen M, Baldwin R, Nino-Murcia G. Nocturnal asthma: snoring, small pharynx and nasal CPAP. Eur Respir J 1988; 1:902–907.
92. Chan CS, Woolcock AJ, Sullivan CE. Nocturnal asthma: role of snoring and obstructive sleep apnea. Am Rev Respir Dis 1988; 137:1502–1504.
93. Martin RJ, Pak J. Nasal CPAP in nonapneic nocturnal asthma. Chest 1991; 100: 1024–1027.
94. Tabachnik E, Muller NL, Levison H, Bryan AC. Chest wall mechanics and pattern of breathing during sleep in asthmatic adolescents. Am Rev Respir Dis 1981; 124:269–273.
95. Avital A, Steljes G, Pasterkamp H, Kryger M, Sanchez I, Chernick V. Sleep quality in children with asthma treated with theophylline or cromolyn sodium. J Pediatr 1991; 119: 979–984.
96. Carskadon MA, Harvey K, Dement WC, Guilleminault C, Simmons B, Anders TF. Respiration during sleep in children. West J Med 1978; 128:477–481.
97. Catterall JR, Douglas NJ, Calverley PMA, Brash HM, Brezinova V, Shapiro CM, Flenley DC. Irregular breathing and hypoxemia during sleep in chronic stable asthma. Lancet 1982; 1:301–304.
98. Smith TF, Hudgel DW. Arterial oxygen saturation during sleep in children with asthma and its relation to airway obstruction and ventilatory drive. Pediatrics 1980; 66:746–751.
99. Chipps BE, Mak H, Schuberth KC, Talamo JH, Menkes HA. Nocturnal saturation in normal and asthmatic children. Pediatrics 1980; 65:1157–1159.
100. Ballard RD, Irvin CG, Martin RJ, Pak J, Pandey R, White DP. Influence of sleep on lung volume in asthmatic patients and normal subjects. J Appl Physiol 1990; 68:2034–2041.
101. Martin RJ, Pak J, Irvin CG. Effect of lung volume maintenance during sleep in nocturnal asthma. J Appl Physiol 1993; 75:1467–1470.
102. Ballard RD, Clover CW, White DP. Influence of non-REM sleep on inspiratory muscle activity and lung volume in asthmatic patients. Am Rev Respir Dis 1993; 147:880–886.
103. Denjean A, Roux C, Herve P, Bonniot JP, Comoy E, Duroux P, Gaultier C. Mild isocapnic hypoxia entrances the bronchial response to methacholine in asthmatic patients. Am Rev Respir Dis 1988; 138:789–793.
104. Dagg KD, Thomson LJ, Clayton RA, Ramway SG, Thomson NC. Effect of acute alterations in inspired oxygen tension on methacholine induced bronchoconstriction in patients with asthma. Thorax 1997; 52:453–457.

105. Denjean A, Canet E, Praud JP, Gaultier C, Bureau M. Hypoxia-induced bronchial responsiveness in awake sleep: role of carotid chemoreceptors. Respir Physiol 1991; 83: 201–210.
106. Menardo JL. Assessing nocturnal asthma in children. Pediatr Pulmonol 1995(suppl) 11:38–39.
107. Juniper EF. How important is quality of life in pediatric asthma. Pediatr Pulmonol 1997; 15:17–21.
108. Juniper EF, Guyatt GH, Feeny DH, Ferrie PJ, Griffith LE, Townsend M. Measuring quality of life in children with asthma. Qual Life Res 1996; 5:35–46.
109. Baughman RP, Loudon RG. Lung sound analysis for continuous evaluation of airflow obstruction in asthma. Chest 1985; 88:365–368.
110. Moore RH, Khan A, Dickey BF. Long-acting inhaled β_2-agonists in asthma therapy. Chest 1998; 113:1095–1108.
111. Lenney W, Pedersen S, Boner AL, Ebbutt A, Jenkins MM, on behalf of an International Study Group. Efficacy and safety of salmeterol in childhood asthma. Eur J Pediatr 1995; 154:983–990.
112. Verberne AAPH, Frost C, Roorda RJ, Van Der Laag H, Kerrebijn KF, and the Dutch Paediatric Asthma Study Group. One year treatment with salmeterol compared with beclomethasone in children with asthma. Am J Respir Crit Care Med 1997; 156:688–695.
113. Verberne AAPH. Managing symptoms and exacerbations in pediatric asthma. Pediatr Pulmonol 1997; (suppl)15:46–50.
114. Stores G, Ellis AJ, Wiggs, Crawford C, Thomson A. Sleep and psychological disturbance in nocturnal asthma. Arch Dis Child 1998; 78:413–419.
115. Hamosh A, Fitzsimmons SC, Macek M, Knowles MR, Rosenstein BJ, Cutting GR. Comparison of clinical manifestations of cystic fibrosis in black and white patients. J Pediatr 1998; 132:255–259.
116. Hubert D, Bienvenu T, Desmazes-Defeu N, Fajac I, Lacronique J, Matran R, Kaplan JC, Dusser DJ. Genotype-phenotype relationships in a cohort of adult cystic fibrosis patients. Eur Respir J 1996; 9:2207–2014.
117. Corey M, Edwards L, Levison H, Knowles M. Longitudinal analysis of pulmonary function decline in patients with cystic fibrosis. J Pediatr 1997; 131:809–814.
118. Tepper RS, Montgomery GL, Ackerman V, Eigen H. Longitudinal evaluation of pulmonary function in infants and very young children with cystic fibrosis. Pediatr Pulmonol 1993; 16:96–100.
119. Francis PWJ, Muller NJ, Gurwitz D, Milligan DWA, Levison H, Bryan AC. Hemoglobin desaturation: its occurrence during sleep in patients with cystic fibrosis. Am J Dis Child 1980; 134:734–740.
120. Mansell AL. Sleep hypoxemia in patients with cystic fibrosis. Am J Dis Child 1980; 134: 133.
121. Muller NL, Francis PW, Gurwitz D, Levison H, Bryan AC. Mechanism of hemoglobin desaturation during rapid-eye-movement sleep in normal subjects and in patients with cystic fibrosis. Am Rev Respir Dis 1980; 121:463–469.
122. Stokes DC, Wohl MEB, Khaw KT, Strieder DJ. Postural hypoxemia in cystic fibrosis. Chest 1985; 87:785–789.
123. Spier S, Rivlin J, Hugues D, Levison H. The effect of oxygen on sleep, blood gases and ventilation in cystic fibrosis. Am Rev Respir Dis 1984; 129:712–718.
124. Tepper RS, Sktarud JB, Dempsey JA. Ventilation and oxygenation changes during sleep in cystic fibrosis. Chest 1983; 84:388–393.

125. Ballard RD, Sutanik JM, Clover CW, Suh BY. Effects of non-REM sleep on ventilation and respiratory mechanics in adults with cystic fibrosis. Am J Respir Crit Care Med 1996; 153:266–271.
126. Versteegh FGA, Neijens HJ, Bogaard JM, Stam H, Robijn RJ, Kerrebijn KF. Relationship between pulmonary function, O_2 saturation during sleep and exercise, and exercise responses in children with cystic fibrosis. Adv Cardiol 1986; 35:151–155.
127. Montgomery M, Wiebicke W, Bibi H, Pagtakhan RD, Pasterkamp H. Home measurement of oxygen saturation during sleep in patients with cystic fibrosis. Pediatr Pulmonol 1989; 7:9–34.
128. Pradal U, Braggion C, Mastella G. Transcutaneous blood gas analysis during sleep and exercise in cystic fibrosis. Pediatr Pulmonol 1990; 8:162–167.
129. Coffey MJ, Fitzgerald MX, McNicholas WT. Comparison of oxygen desaturation during sleep and exercise in patients with cystic fibrosis. Chest 1991; 100:659–662.
130. Avital A, Sanchez I, Holbrow J, Kryger M, Chernick V. Effect of theophylline on lung function tests, sleep quality, and nighttime Sa_{O_2} in children with cystic fibrosis. Am Rev Respir Dis 1991; 144:1245–1249.
131. Boysen PG, Block AJ, Wynne JW. Nocturnal pulmonary hypertension in patients with chronic obstructive pulmonary disease. Chest 1979; 76:536–540.
132. Ryland D, Reid L. The pulmonary circulation in cystic fibrosis. Thorax 1975; 30: 285–292.
133. Reid L. The pulmonary circulation: remodeling in growth and disease. Am Rev Respir Dis 1979; 119:531–546.
134. Zinman R, Corey M, Coates AL, Canny GJ, Connolloy J, Levison H, Beaudry PH. Nocturnal home oxygen in the treatment of hypoxemic cystic fibrosis patients. J Pediatr 1989; 14:368–377.
135. De Jong W, Kaptein AA, Van Der Schans CP, Mannes GPM, Aalderen WMC, Grevinck RG, Koeter GH. Quality of life in patients with cystic fibrosis. Pediatr Pulmonol 1997; 23:95–100.
136. Maddrey AM, Cullum CM, Prestidge C. Cognitive dysfunction in adults with CF. Pediatr Pulmonol 1997; 14(suppl):322.
137. Hazinski TA, Hansen TN, Simon JA, Tooley WH. Effect of oxygen administration during sleep on skin surface electrode oxygen and carbon dioxide tensions in patients with chronic lung disease. Pediatrics 1981; 67:626–630.
138. Regnis JA, Piper AJ, Henke KG, Parker S, Bye PTP, Sullivan CE. Benefits of nocturnal nasal CPAP in patients with cystic fibrosis. Chest 1994; 106:1717–1724.
139. Granton JT, Kesten S. The acute effects of nasal positive pressure ventilation in patients with advanced cystic fibrosis. Chest 1998; 113:1013–1018.
140. Gozal D. Nocturnal ventilatory support in patients with cystic fibrosis: comparison with supplemental oxygen. Eur Resp J 1997; 10:1999–2003.
141. Hill AT, Edenborough FP, Cayton RM, Stableforth DE. Long-term nasal intermittent positive pressure ventilation in patients with cystic fibrosis and hypercapnic respiratory failure (1991–1996). Respir Med 1998; 92:523–526.
142. Baculard A, Bedicam JM, Sardet A, Fauroux B, Tournier G. Ventilation mécanique par masque nasal en pression postivie intermittente chez l'enfant atteint de mucoviscidose. Ann Fr Pediatr 1993; 50:469–474.
143. Mendeloff EN, Huddleston CB, Mallory GB, Trulok EP, Cohen AH, Sweet SC, Lynch J, Sundaresan S, Cooper JD, Patterson GA. Pediatric and adult lung transplantation for cystic fibrosis. J Thorac Cardiovasc Surg 1998; 115:404–414.

144. Gaultier CL. Tension-time index of inspiratory muscles in children. Pediatr Pulmonol 1997; 23:327–329.
145. Hayot M, Guilleminault S, Ramonatxo M, Voisin M, Prefaut C. Determinants of the tension-time index of inspiratory muscles in children with cystic fibrosis. Pediatr Pulmonol 1997; 23:336–343.
146. Laraya-Cuasy LR, Deforest A, Huff D, Lischner H, Huang NN. Chronic pulmonary complications of early influenza virus infection in children. Am Rev Respir Dis 1977; 117:617–625.
147. Simila S, Linna O, Lanning P, Meikkinew E, Alahoulala M. Chronic lung damage caused by adenovirus 7: a ten-year follow-up study. Chest 1980; 80:27–131.
148. Gaultier CL, Boule M, Tournier G, Girard F. Inspiratory force reserve of the respiratory muscles in children with chronic obstructive pulmonary disease. Am Rev Respir Dis 1985; 131:811–815.
149. Fan LL, Mullan ALW, Brugman SM, Inscore SC, Parks DP, White CW. Clinical spectrum of chronic interstitial lung disease in children. J Pediatr 1992; 121:867–872.
150. Gaultier CL, Chaussain M, Boule M, Buvry A, Allaire Y, Perret L, Girard F. Lung function in interstitial lung diseases in children. Bull Eur Physiopathol Respir 1980; 16: 57–66.
151. Gaultier CL, Perret L, Boule M, Tournier G, Girard F. Control of breathing in children with interstitial lung disease. Pediatr Res 1982; 16:779–783.
152. Bye PTP, Issa F, Berthon-Jones M, Sullivan CE. Studies of oxygenation during sleep in patients with interstitial lung disease. Am Rev Respir Dis 1984; 129:27–32.
153. Perez-Padella R, West P, Lertzman M, Krieger MH. Breathing during sleep in patients with interstitial lung disease. Am Rev Respir Dis 1985; 132:224–229.
154. McNicholas WT, Coffey M, Fitzgerald MS. Ventilation and gas exchange during sleep in patients with interstitial lung disease. Thorax 1986; 41:77–782.
155. Midgren B, Hansson L, Ericksson L, Airikkala P., Elmquist D. Oxygen desaturation during sleep and exercise in patients with interstitial lung disease. Thorax 1987; 42:353–356.
156. Noyes BE, Kurland G, Orenstein DM. Lung and heart-lung transplantation in children. Pediatr Pulmonol 1997; 23:39–48.

31

Sleep and Breathing in Children with Neuromuscular Disease

DEBORAH C. GIVAN

Indiana University School of Medicine and
James Whitcomb Riley Hospital for Children
Indianapolis, Indiana

I. Introduction

All children with neuromuscular disease will eventually develop respiratory disturbances during sleep. Often these disturbances are the first evidence of respiratory muscle weakness. Sleep-disordered breathing and alveolar hypoventilation can occur even though minimal peripheral muscle weakness is present (1). Respiratory muscle weakness in neuromuscular disease is unmasked by the stress of sleep-induced changes in breathing control and respiratory muscle function. Childhood neuromuscular diseases associated with respiratory impairment are listed in Table 1.

II. Overview and Risk Factors for Sleep-Related Respiratory Muscle Dysfunction

A. Overview of Respiration During Wakefulness and Sleep

Respiration during wakefulness and sleep is dependent on central control and feedback mechanisms and muscle and chest wall mechanics. Ventilatory control during wakefulness is governed both volitionally by higher cortical centers and automatically by arterial chemoreceptors, metabolic activity, and intrapulmonary receptors. The latter have no known function during sleep (2). Hypercarbia is sensed and mod-

Table 1 Expected Impairment of the Respiratory System in Various Neuromuscular Diseases

Level	Disease	Respiratory abnormalities
Central–upper motor neuron	Cerebral palsy	Upper airway
Brainstem	Arnold-Chiari I & II	Upper airway, abdominals, central drive
Spinal cord	C1–C2	Upper airway
	C3–C5	Diaphragm, intercostal, abdominals
	Below C6	Intercostal, abdominals
Motor neuron	Spinal muscular atrophy	Generalized
	Poliomyelitis	Upper airway, abdominal, ± diaphragm
	Distal spinal muscular atrophy	Distal limb muscles, diaphragm
Peripheral nerve	Hereditary sensory motor neuropathies (Charcot-Marie-Tooth)	Upper airway, diaphragm
	Hereditary sensory autonomic neuropathy (Riley-Day)	Upper airway
	Phrenic nerve injury	Diaphragm
	Leukodystrophies	Generalized
	Guillain-Barré	Generalized
	Polyneuropathy	Generalized
Neuromuscular junction	Congenital myasthenia	Generalized
	Tetanus	Generalized
	Myasthenia gravis	Generalized
	Botulism	Generalized
Muscle (types)		
Dystrophinopathies	Duchenne MD, Becker MD	Generalized, myocardium
Nondystrophinopathies	Emery-Dreifuss (rigid spine?)	Generalized, myocardium, diaphragm
	Limb-girdle muscular dystrophy	Diaphram, intercostal, abdominals
	Fascioscapulohumeral, oculopharyngeal	Upper airway, neck, ± diaphragm
	Fukuyama type	Upper airway, generalized
	Merosin-deficient	Generalized, respiratory
	Merosin-positive	Upper airway
	Autosomal recessive distal MD	Rare respiratory, myocardium
Myotonic dystrophy	Myotonic dystrophy, congenital myotonic dystrophy	Upper airway, myocardium, diaphragm, decreased central drive?, apnea

Table 1 Continued

Level	Disease	Respiratory abnormalities
Congenital myopathies	Nemaline, central core, centronuclear, multicore, minicore, myotubular, congenital fibre-type disproportion	Generalized, diaphragm, upper airway
Metabolic myopathies	Acid maltase deficiency	Upper airway, diaphragm
Mitochondrial myopathies	Pyruvate dehydrogenase defect	Apnea, generalized
	Respiratory complex I defect	Generalized myocardium
	Respiratory complex IV defect	Generalized
Inflammatory myopathies	SLE, polymyositis, rhabdomyolysis	Generalized, diaphragm
Unclassified	Prader-Willi syndrome	Upper airway, generalized

MD, muscular dystrophy; SLE, systemic lupus erythematosus.

ulated by the carotid body and medullary chemoreceptors and hypoxemia by the carotid body chemoreceptors (3,4). The hypoxic response is hyperbolic, stimulating ventilation when the partial pressure of oxygen falls below 60 torr (3). The hypercapneic response is linear, with low levels of carbon dioxide inhibiting respiration and high levels initiating respiration (4).

Respiratory control is influenced by sleep and more specifically by the different stages of sleep. In non–rapid-eye-movement (NREM) sleep, chemoreceptor sensitivity is downregulated and ventilation is controlled by metabolic mechanisms (5). Behavioral (volitional) and arousal influences on respiration are virtually absent during NREM sleep. However, they may play an important role during rapid-eye-movement (REM) sleep, when metabolic and chemoreceptor sensitivity influences are markedly diminished (6).

Normal ventilatory changes during sleep include a decrease in tidal volume, decrease in alveolar ventilation, mild decrease in oxygen saturation, mild increase in carbon dioxide, and changes in respiratory rate and rhythm (increased rate in NREM and irregular rate in REM). The removal of wakefulness stimuli and associated reduction of chemosensitivity during sleep may be manifest at sleep onset as central apnea or waxing and waning of tidal ventilation (2). Arousal responses to hypoxemia and hypercarbia are depressed when compared to the wakefulness response. The hypercapneic ventilatory response is lowered by 20% to 50% during NREM sleep and by approximately 60% to 80% during REM sleep (2,5).

Several changes also occur in the respiratory muscles with sleep onset. There is generalized hypotonia of the dilating muscles of the upper airway during NREM sleep, which is associated with a marked loss of tonic activity of the tongue as well as the pharyngeal and laryngeal musculature (6,7). The intercostal muscles also lose tone during NREM sleep, with a consequent decrease in the functional residual capacity. During REM sleep, the cyclic inspiratory-related motor activity of the intercostal muscles disappears (6). The diaphragm maintains normal activity during NREM sleep. During REM sleep, diaphragm activity continues but is decreased and exhibits intermittent decremental activity during single breaths and clustered pauses (8,9).

Vulnerability to respiratory disturbances during sleep in children with neuromuscular disease is present throughout sleep but is most pronounced during REM. This is the consequence of three physiological factors: 1) marked deregulation of control of respiration, which occurs during REM sleep, 2) the atonia of the upper airway and intercostal muscles, and 3) the dependence of respiration on diaphragm function.

B. Control of Respiration

Respiratory drive, as measured by the response to hypoxia and hypercarbia, is normally diminished during sleep. This occurs primarily because of lowered sensitivity of the chemoreceptors and a higher threshold for stimulation in the arousal centers of the medulla and cortex, which is greatest during REM sleep (10–13). Factors, such as prior sleep deprivation, sedative medications, and a disturbed sleeping environment can also depress respiratory drive and the arousal response.

The respiratory drive is also depressed in patients with specific types of neuromuscular disease. Children with myelomeningocele and Arnold-Chiari malformation have abnormal hypercapneic ventilatory responses, suggesting a defect in central chemoreceptors (14–17). A central control problem in children with congenital myopathies and myotonic dystrophy has also been postulated (18,19), but it is difficult to distinguish an abnormality of respiratory drive from end-organ weakness. Subsequent researchers have been unable to confirm the presence of a central control problem in myopathies or myotonic dystrophy (20,21). More recent studies suggest that the respiratory drive in persons with neuromuscular disease is actually higher than in normals, albeit inadequate to overcome the poor strength and endurance of the respiratory muscles that cause hypoventilation (22). Measuring the mouth occlusion pressure (the negative pressure developed at the mouth in the first 0.1 sec of inspiration against a closed airway) may circumvent the difficulties in measuring respiratory drive separately from muscle strength. Using this technique, higher than normal mouth occlusion pressures have been measured in patients with neuromuscular disease, suggesting that most patients with neuromuscular disease possess a high rather than low ventilatory drive (23). Secondary changes in respiratory control may also occur with long-standing nocturnal hypoventilation from alteration of chemoreceptor sensitivity caused by ongoing hypoxemia and hypercarbia, metabolic alkalosis, and sleep fragmentation (18,20,23–25).

C. Muscle Atonia

Poor pharyngeal muscle tone, which occurs with sleep onset in normal subjects, leads to a rise in upper-airway resistance (26). This normal physiological response is superimposed on a system with a preexistent high resistance to airflow because of the small size and high compliance of airway structures in children. Resistance may be increased further by adenotonsillar hypertrophy, nasal congestion, and obesity. Children with cerebral palsy, myelomeningocele, hereditary motor and sensory neuropathies, and certain congenital myopathies may have selective bulbar involvement, with marked baseline weakness of the upper airway muscles.

A small cross-sectional area of the pharynx has been associated with sleep-disordered breathing in children and occurs more commonly in children with these neuromuscular disorders (27). These conditions are associated with a high incidence of upper-airway obstruction during sleep both because of these structural abnormalities of the airway and owing to the differential muscle involvement with the pharyngeal muscles, which are more severely affected than the accessory muscles or diaphragm. Partial airway obstruction is the most frequently seen abnormality in children with obstructive sleep apnea and is associated with a prolonged increase in upper airway resistance, hypoxemia, and eventually muscle fatigue. The respiratory muscle fatigue can be manifest as central apnea, with the muscles unable to generate a measurable response. Treating the obstruction usually alleviates this abnormality (24).

The atonia of the accessory and pharyngeal muscles has additional consequences. In children with neuromuscular disease, chest wall compliance is high and the diaphragm is horizontally placed, similar to that of an infant (28). Breathing is accomplished by the combined effort of the accessory muscles and diaphragm, while the abdominal muscles support and serve as a fulcrum for the diaphragm. These children have low tidal volumes and can increase minute ventilation only by raising their respiratory rate. Patients with neuromuscular disease also adopt a breathing strategy of alternating between using the diaphragm and then the other inspiratory muscles (29). The expiratory muscles are also recruited to improve the diaphragm's mechanical advantage and decrease the work of breathing by moving the diaphragm cephalad. Despite these strategies, these children become vulnerable to respiratory muscle fatigue with any additional breathing work. With the loss of accessory muscle tone and abdominal wall support that occurs during REM sleep, work of breathing can exceed the child's muscle energy stores and significant desaturation and hypoventilation can develop.

D. Diaphragmatic Function During Sleep

Because respiration is dependent on diaphragmatic function during REM sleep, there are special problems for the child with neuromuscular disorders characterized by diaphragm involvement. These disorders include distal spinal muscular atrophy, poliomyelitis, high cervical spinal cord injury, and certain mitochondrial, metabolic, and congenital myopathies. Diaphragm weakness is also present in Duchenne and Becker muscular dystrophies as the diseases progress. The tidal volume falls markedly when accessory muscles are paralyzed during REM sleep and respiration is solely dependent on the diaphragm. One study suggests that normal adults with isolated diaphragm paralysis exhibit only minor alterations of ventilation during sleep, even REM (30).

However, several authors have reported that patients with diaphragm paralysis have an elevated arterial carbon dioxide tension, which increases in the supine position. These patients then progressed to experience marked hypoventilation in REM sleep (31,32).

Infants with these problems are even more vulnerable. They have a highly compliant chest wall with low tidal volumes and normally sleep approximately 20 hr per day, with 40% to 80% of sleep time spent in REM sleep. Older children spend less than 30% of sleep time in REM. In normal infants, diaphragmatic work of breathing may be as high as 10% of the basal metabolic rate (33). Infants with diaphragm dysfunction have little metabolic reserve and a high morbidity and even mortality if diaphragmatic paralysis is not recognized and respiration is not supported (34).

Older children and adults with neuromuscular disease can also develop desaturation and hypercarbia during REM sleep because of the loss of accessory muscle support. As the muscle weakness progresses, accessory muscles of respiration are routinely enlisted during normal breathing to assist the diaphragm and, as noted previously, a pattern of respiration alternately favoring the diaphragm and then the accessory muscles develops (29). Compensation for muscle weakness may also be achieved by contraction of the abdominal muscles to produce expiration below functional residual capacity and then allowing passive inspiration with recoil of the chest wall (35). Without assistance from other inspiratory muscles, the diaphragm cannot maintain normal ventilation over time during REM sleep. Under these conditions, the diaphragm has little reserve and is unable to respond adequately to correct a metabolic abnormality such as acidosis, even with a greater respiratory drive.

E. Other Factors

A contributing factor to respiratory muscle failure with any neuromuscular disease is the development of scoliosis. This complication will occur in 60% to 85% of children with generalized muscle weakness and up to 90% of children with diseases such as Duchenne muscular dystrophy (36,37). With progression of scoliosis, lung volumes are reduced, with development of peripheral atelectasis and ventilation and perfusion abnormalities (38). For every 10-degree increase in curvature, the vital capacity will decrease by approximately 4% (37). The curvature of the chest wall and consequent torque placed on the inspiratory muscles results in mechanical problems when the chest wall moves with respiration. These altered length-tension relationships result in low tidal volumes, lessened diaphragmatic pressure generation, and more work of breathing. Lisboa and colleagues found that maximum transdiaphragmatic pressure was reduced to 48 ± 11 cmH_2O in nine adults with severe kyphoscoliosis (normal controls 110 ± 22 cmH_2O) (39). Still, recruitment of the accessory muscles of respiration can maintain normal ventilation during wakefulness and NREM sleep. However, the diaphragm is prone to fatigue during REM sleep, when respiration is totally dependent on this muscle. The low saturations and high carbon dioxide levels during REM in patients with scoliosis are undoubtedly related to these alterations in lung me-

Table 2 Consequences of the Normal Physiolgoical Changes During REM Sleep with Changes Associated with Neuromuscular Disease

Aspect of breathing	Changes with NMD	Normal REM changes	Consequences of combined defect
Respiratory drive			
Central drive	I/N/D[a]	D	Tachypnea, decreased tidal volumes, apnea, hypopnea
Chemosensitivity	N/D[a]	D	Hypoventilation
Muscle response to airway loading	D	D	Hypoventilation
Respiratory mechanics			
Accessory muscle contractions	D	Absent	Hypoventilation
Diaphragm strength	D	N	Hypoventilation
Muscle endurance	D	N	Hypoventilation
Upper-airway resistance	I	I	Obstructive apnea
Secretion clearance	D	D	Atelectasis, $\dot{V}/\dot{Q}$ mismatch
Work of breathing	I	I	Muscle fatigue

NMD, neuromuscular disease; N, normal; D, decreased; I, increased.
[a]Response depends on type of NMD.

chanics. The low lung volumes and decreased muscle strength characteristic of neuromuscular disease aggravate and, in turn, are aggravated by the scoliosis.

A summary of the abnormalities in respiration associated with neuromuscular disease is shown in Table 2. The table compares these abnormalities to normal changes during REM sleep, illustrating how these abnormalities become amplified and eventually result in hypercarbia and hypoxemia.

III. Progression of Sleep-Related Breathing Abnormalities in Neuromuscular Disease

Respiratory muscle dysfunction may first be noted with respiratory illnesses, anesthesia, or exercise. However, respiratory muscle dysfunction during sleep occurs at an even earlier stage of disease and is less likely to be recognized. Older adolescent and adult patients with neuromuscular disease typically follow a pattern of progressive respiratory dysfunction, with initial abnormalities noted almost exclusively during REM sleep (35). These findings may persist without progression for several years, depending on the natural history of the underlying disorder and the occurrence of complications (35). Following pneumonia, an asthma exacerbation, growth or weight gain, development of obstructive sleep apnea or chronic lung disease, or any condition that elevates work of breathing, the respiratory abnormalities often progress to involve

NREM sleep as well. Decreased awake oxygen saturation and expiratory reserve volume highly correlate with severity of sleep desaturation in patients with obstructive sleep apnea (40). In patients with neuromuscular disease, a low vital capacity and high level of disability seem to be more predictive of sleep desaturation (41–43). Unfortunately, these values can neither discriminate among patients who already have severe abnormalities nor predict which patients will have life-threatening events (43). As nocturnal hypoventilation progresses, daytime abnormalities such as hypercarbia, decreased mean oxygen saturation, or constitutional symptoms such as fatigue, morning headaches, or irritability may appear or worsen. Sleep fragmentation from hypercarbia, hypoxemia, and possibly obstruction is followed by decreased arousability and progressive sleep hypoventilation and daytime respiratory failure. This type of respiratory failure is partially reversible with intervention. Nocturnal nasal intermittent positive-pressure ventilation has been shown to improve daytime arterial saturations and relieve nocturnal hypoventilation and sleep apnea in patients with neuromuscular disease (25).

The progression of sleep abnormalities in infants and young children with neuromuscular disease is not as well defined as in adults. The type and extent of neuromuscular involvement plays a major role in determining whether the respiratory muscles will be involved early or later in the course of the disease. In particular, proximal or generalized muscle involvement has a worse respiratory prognosis. Still, respiratory muscles may be severely affected in some types of muscle disease characterized primarily by limb involvement (1,44). Diseases that cause diaphragm weakness are usually associated with early onset and severe sleep hypoventilation and respiratory failure (45). Additional factors affecting respiratory compromise include age of onset (respiratory muscle failure is more often fatal in infants), nutritional status (malnutrition reduces diaphragm muscle weight and strength), metabolic imbalances (acidosis, hypocalcemia, hypophosphatemia, and hypomagnesemia all impair diaphragmatic function), and whether mechanical ventilation is undertaken (1,46–53).

More subtle indications of sleep disturbances may be present before changes in oxygenation during REM sleep occur. One group of adolescents with Duchenne muscular dystrophy demonstrated moderate sleep disruption characterized by decreased REM sleep, increased arousals, and increased stage 1 sleep. Daytime intermittent elevation of the end-tidal carbon dioxide and restrictive lung disease, a vital capacity of 10% to 54% predicted, were the only daytime abnormalities (54). Sleep fragmentation or deprivation can precede and intensify the respiratory abnormality in obstructive sleep apnea (55). Sleep fragmentation has been identified as playing a similar role in neuromuscular disease (25). Efforts to support respiration using nocturnal noninvasive ventilation at an early stage of respiratory muscle fatigue have been made. Respiratory muscle strength and lung function do not always improve in adults with neuromuscular disease, despite improvement sleep hypoventilation and daytime blood gases (25).

Lung function in children and adolescents with nonprogressive or very slowly progressive neuromuscular disease may stabilize or even improve with ventilatory support (49,50). Noninvasive ventilatory support may also stabilize lung function in more rapidly progressive neuromuscular disease such as Duchenne muscular dystrophy (56). One collaborative study did find that noninvasive ventilation worsened respiratory muscle failure and possibly hastened death in some patients with Duchenne muscular dystrophy (57). It has been argued that problems with this study design and subject recruitment may have affected the outcome. These included factors that could have contributed to early death, such as selection of severely affected males, absence of monitoring of ventilator compliance and adequacy of support, and lack of screening for the presence of cardiomyopathy (56,58). The mechanisms postulated for the improvement seen with nocturnal noninvasive positive pressure have included resting the muscles (possibly enhancing endurance or strength), increasing lung compliance (possibly improving or preventing atelectasis), and reducing sleep fragmentation and improving nocturnal ventilation, resetting the chemoreceptors. Studies thus far have primarily found evidence to support the last of these theories (improvement of sleep fragmentation and resetting the chemoreceptors) (25,29,60).

IV. Respiratory Dysfunction in Specific Neuromuscular Conditions

A. Spinal Cord Injury

Traumatic spinal cord injury in children is relatively uncommon, with an incidence of 0.02 per 1000 children (61). The increased mobility of the spinal column, underdevelopment of the neck and paraspinous musculature, and horizontal orientation of the facet joints of the vertebrae account for this low risk of injury. However, these same factors and the large head-to-torso ratio contribute to the high rate of cervical and high thoracic cord injuries when trauma does occur (61). Automobile and sporting accidents cause the majority of spinal cord injuries in children and adolescents (62). Respiratory complications are frequently encountered and are the most common cause of death for patients with spinal cord injury of all ages (63).

Only one report has described the long-term outcome of children with a high spinal cord injury. In this study, 13 children, ages 9 months to 18 years, with injuries at C4 or above were initially ventilator-dependent (64). Of these children, 4 were treated with electrophrenic pacing, 2 others were successfully weaned from the ventilator, and 4 died, 2 from ventilator disconnection and 2 from unknown causes. Ventilator settings and assessment of nocturnal ventilation were monitored by arterial blood gases (64).

Spinal cord injuries in infants account for 11% of spinal cord trauma in children and primarily occur as a complication of delivery (65). Upper cervical lesions (C1–C3) occur predominantly with a cephalic presentation and attempted forceps rotation; cervicothoracic lesions (C4–T4) are seen more commonly with a breech presentation (66). MacKinnon described 9 infants with upper cervical cord injury, with 1 infant experiencing rapid, complete recovery, 2 infants dying, 4 infants who required long-term continuous ventilation, and 2 infants eventually requiring mechanical ventilation only during sleep (66). Details regarding the evaluation and reason for the nocturnal ventilatory dependence in these 2 infants were not available. Putative factors for the respiratory failure during sleep in neonatal spinal cord injury would include the infants' highly compliant chest wall, paralyzed intercostal muscles, and diaphragm weakness or paralysis from phrenic nerve root involvement.

In older children, nocturnal ventilatory dependence has been described in patients with C2 lesions (64,67). Daytime independence from ventilation can be achieved if the child has intact capital flexors, capital extensors, and cervical flexors and can be taught neck breathing or glossopharyngeal breathing (64,67). These methods of breathing cannot be continued during sleep.

Pulmonary function abnormalities may include a generalized restrictive defect, an elevated expiratory reserve volume from weakness of the abdominal and intercostal muscles, and a low negative inspiratory force that correlates with increased muscle tone (68). Studies performed in adults show decreased inspiratory muscle strength and endurance measured by maximum static inspiratory mouth pressure at functional residual capacity and the Hi:Lo frequency components of electromyography of the diaphragm in patients with lesions between C3 and T1 (69). Some 40% of adults with a C3 level injury or above remain dependent on continuous ventilation (70). Statistics regarding the number of patients with quadriplegia requiring only sleep support are not available. Reports of polysomnographic findings in children or adults with spinal cord injury are lacking, even though study of these patients by polysomnography during sleep is recommended to routinely assess them before and after ventilatory support is implemented (71–73).

Polysomnography is a valid tool for assessment of these children, since respiratory abnormalities are likely to vary from wakefulness to sleep and between NREM and REM sleep. The adequacy of glossopharyngeal or neck breathing can also be evaluated in this manner. Assessment of these children becomes especially important for attempts at weaning ventilator support, since it is clear that daytime blood gases are not adequate to assess nocturnal respiratory problems prospectively.

B. Myelomeningocele with Arnold-Chiari Malformation

Myelomeningocele is a neurodysplasia characterized by incomplete closure of the spinal canal at the occipital level or lower. Most lesions occur in the lumbosacral area with an incidence of 25% sacral, 29% lumbosacral, 34% lumbar, 4.5% thoracic, 9.5% cervical, and less than 1% occipital (74). The incidence of this disorder is approximately 1 per 1000 live births, though this frequency is diminishing (75). This lesion of the spinal cord is commonly associated with downward displacement of the medulla and cerebellar tonsils, with elongation and extension of the fourth ventricle into the spinal canal (Arnold-Chiari malformation type II). In addition to the Chiari malformation, other brain malformations can be present and include hydrocephalus (90% incidence) and, less commonly, hypoplasia of the cranial nerve nuclei, agenesis of the corpus callosum, syringobulbia, and syringomyelia (76). Vertebral abnormalities include absent or malformed vertebrae (76). Clinically, these abnormalities manifest themselves as abnormal respiratory drive with decreased or absent arousal responses, hypoventilation, central apnea, obstructive apnea (from vocal cord paralysis), aspiration, cor pulmonale, sudden death, and scoliosis (14,76–82).

Some infants with myelomeningocele were noted to have life-threatening, prolonged apneic pauses during periodic breathing episodes that occurred during the transition to REM sleep (14). Later work confirmed abnormal respiratory patterns during sleep in infants with myelomeningocele as well as impaired arousal responses to hypoxia and hypercapnia (15,80,83). As many as 60% of newborns with myelomeningocele can exhibit abnormal responsiveness to carbon dioxide (17). Apnea and cyanosis during sleep have also been documented in adolescents with myelomeningocele (16). Ventilatory responses to hypercapnia awake and asleep were depressed and the normal correlation between the hypoxic and hypercapnic ventilatory responses was not present (16).

The prevalence of sleep-disordered breathing in children with myelomeningocele was evaluated by polysomnography and was found to be present in 62% of 83 patients studied (82). Forty-two percent of these children had mild abnormalities with an apnea/hypopnea index of 1 to 4.9/hr; 20% had moderate to severe abnormalities defined as an apnea/hypopnea index greater than 5/hr and desaturation to less than 90%. Of those with severe abnormalities, 64% had a mean carbon dioxide level exceeding 53 torr. In the majority of these patients, abnormalities were worse during REM sleep. The authors found that symptoms of snoring, apnea, and hypersomnolence did not predict the presence of sleep-disordered breathing. Having restrictive lung disease identified by pulmonary function testing, scoliosis, thoracic-level lesion or higher, or brainstem malformations increased the risk of sleep-disordered breathing (82).

Carrey and coworkers studied the effects of nasal positive-pressure ventilation on diaphragmatic pressure in 9 patients with restrictive lung disease (51). Two of the patients, ages 25 and 33 years, had myelomeningocele, with a vital capacity of 33% and 15% respectively, and hypercapnia and hypoxemia at rest. Using esophageal balloons and diaphragmatic electromyograms, the investigators attempted to assess diaphragmatic effort. The patients as a group improved ventilation and decreased inspiratory effort, and therefore work of breathing, while using nasal ventilation. The authors speculated that resting the muscle improved daytime ventilation in these patients (51).

Abnormalities of the respiratory drive with hypoventilation will become worse in these patients during sleep, when regulatory drive is already depressed. Cranial nerve dysfunction can lead to symptomatic upper-airway dysfunction (vocal cord paralysis, pharyngeal muscle dysfunction) that becomes greater during sleep, especially REM sleep, and can result in apnea and cyanosis, as previously described. The high incidence of scoliosis and restrictive lung disease in this population also contributes to sleep hypoventilation and desaturation during REM sleep. This is because of low lung volumes from limited excursion of the rib cage, causing ventilation/perfusion imbalances and diffusion abnormalities (84).

Daytime problems that can complicate the neurological and respiratory status of these children have been described. A dysfunctional swallow with aspiration is present in some infants and can complicate the pulmonary abnormalities, although this problem may resolve with surgical decompression of the Chiari malformation (79,81,85,86). A malignant type of breath-holding spell has also been described. These spells occur during wakefulness and result in hypoxia, hypercarbia, and sudden death (79,81); they are not improved by tracheostomy and have not been described during sleep.

The data would indicate that sleep-disordered breathing and hypoventilation occur commonly in patients with myelomeningocele. The disordered breathing is not predictable on the basis of symptoms alone but can be detected with polysomnography. Obstructive apnea and sleep hypoventilation contribute significantly to the morbidity and mortality associated with this disorder. These problems have been successfully treated with positive pressure and nocturnal ventilatory support, respectively, improving both quality and quantity of life for these patients.

C. Spinal Muscular Atrophy

Spinal muscular atrophy (SMA) is an autosomal recessive congenital disease of the anterior horn cells and, frequently, the motor nuclei of cranial nerves V through XII (87–89). It is characterized by weakness of the distal muscles of the upper and lower extremities and progressive involvement of the chest wall muscles. The phrenic motor neurons are preserved in SMA and the diaphragm is usually uninvolved until the late stages of the disease (90). The disease is classified into three forms based on age of clinical presentation and level of maximum gross motor function: early infantile or type I (Werdnig-Hoffmann disease), late infantile form or type II (intermediate or Oppenheim's disease), and mild juvenile form or type III (Kugelberg-Welander disease) (89). The disease incidence is 1 per 25,000 births (88). All forms have been linked to DNA markers in the 5q 11–13 region of chromosome 5, with different mutations in the same or contiguous genes resulting in the three disease forms (89).

Infants with SMA I will have decreased movement and marked hypotonia noted soon after birth. The maximal function of these infants is sitting with support. The bulbar muscles are often affected, causing difficulty in sucking and swallowing and development of partial airway obstruction during sleep. The inspiratory and expiratory muscle weakness rapidly progresses, with an episode of respiratory infection often precipitating frank respiratory failure. Polysomnography performed in the early stages may show marked tachypnea with a decreased mean baseline saturation and hypocapnia (Fig. 1). Respiratory failure is progressive, with most children dying before the age of 2 to 3 years unless artificial mechanical respiratory support is undertaken. Respiratory and orthopedic management can change this outcome, achieving a survival time of greater than 40 years for some patients (49). The children with bulbar involvement cannot speak and rarely achieve any ventilator-free time. They func-

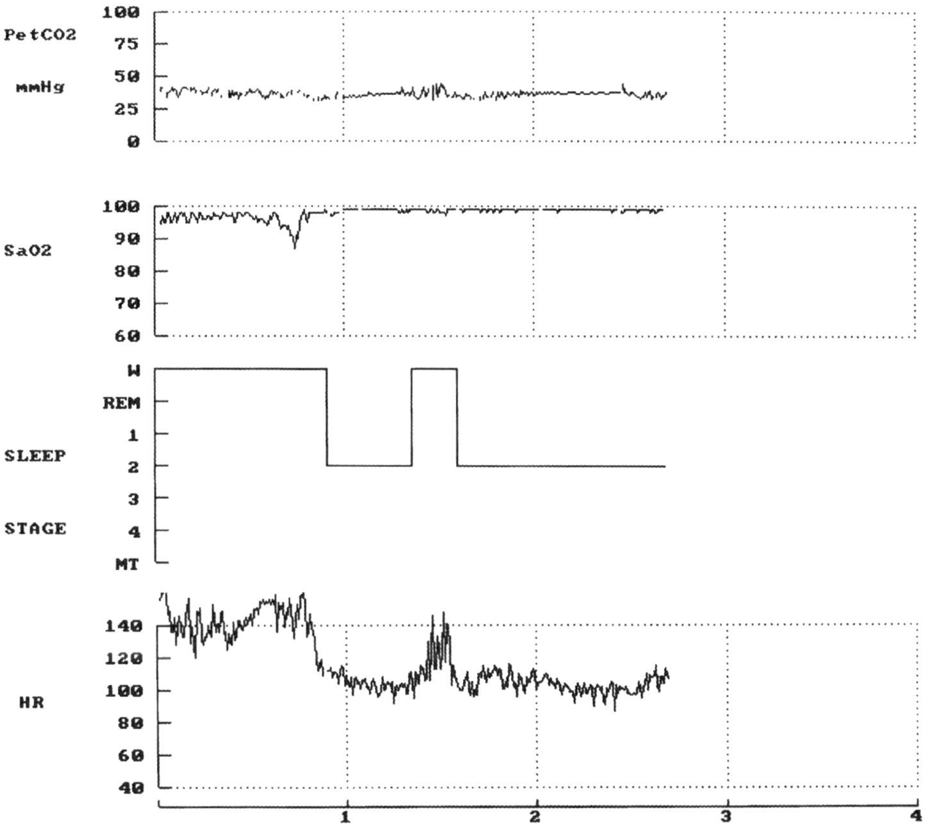

Figure 1 This is a graphic summary of a 3-hr polysomnogram of a 3-month infant with SMA 1. Each block represents 1 hr of recording time. Note the low end-tidal carbon dioxide level ($P_{ET_{CO_2}}$), normal oxygen saturation (Sa_{O_2}), and brief desaturation during wakefulness, associated with excessive secretions.

tion best with a tracheostomy, which allows suctioning and delivery of positive-pressure ventilation.

Children with SMA type II achieve a maximum gross motor function of sitting independently (91). In these children, the peripheral muscle weakness appears to stabilize, with respiratory musclcs only partially compromised. However, the high demands placed on the compromised respiratory muscles may lead to respiratory failure and, at times, to more generalized muscle deterioration (92,93). These children manifest problems with desaturation and hypoventilation during sleep that are rarely recognized before acute respiratory failure from a respiratory infection occurs (94). Using the criteria of daytime hypoxemia, daytime hypercarbia, and recurrent pneumonia as the indication for nocturnal ventilation, improvement in vital capacity and daytime ventilation has occurred following the initiation of nocturnal ventilation (95). In this study, 81% of the patients were maintained on nocturnal ventilation only for years (95). The authors postulated that these children remained stable because the nocturnal ventilation ensured adequate gas exchange during sleep; reversed atelectasis, thus decreasing inspiratory muscle work; and may have rested the respiratory muscles (95). It is likely, however, that this effect was achieved by correcting the metabolic abnormalities caused by chronic hypoventilation and resetting the central chemoreceptors and/or improving sleep fragmentation (25,59,60). Barois et al. have advocated undertaking ventilator support before the age of 4 years in these patients to improve rib cage development and foster lung growth (49).

One report assessing pulmonary function and polysomnographic findings in SMA recruited 8 patients, ages 10 to 37 years, with SMA types II and III (41). The patients included 4 children, ages 10 to 13 years. No patient noted any sleep difficulties or symptoms except for one child, who reported mild snoring. Daytime blood gases were normal in 6 patients and showed mild hypoxemia in 2 patients. All of the patients had decreased pulmonary volumes and maximal mouth pressures during wakefulness; 5 patients (2 children) had unsuspected prolonged central or mixed apnea and hypopnea and 4 patients (one child) had saturations less than 90% for 1% to 4% of total sleep time (nadir 68% to 95%). The lowest values were noted during REM sleep. These authors found an inverse correlation between the vital capacity and functional residual capacity and the percent of total sleep time with oxygen saturation less than 90% (41).

Canani et al. performed polysomnography on 5 children with SMA type II to assess for nocturnal hypoventilation before daytime clinical abnormalities occurred (50). One child had obstructive sleep apnea and all children had mild to moderate hypercarbia with a low mean oxygen saturation or desaturation during sleep. A predilection for abnormalities during REM sleep could not be assessed (50).

It is difficult to determine the ultimate prognosis for children with SMA until they reach their maximum gross motor function. If the disease develops in utero, SMA I can be diagnosed with assurance. However, the development of marked muscle weakness before age 6 months has been described with both type I and type II disease. Until the disease entity and therefore ultimate prognosis is determined, the option of respiratory support should be discussed with the parents. It has been suggested that early intervention with respiratory support may actually allow for greater lung growth and improved respiratory outcome (49). The quality of life is a subjective determination, and many of these children lead successful and productive lives despite their disability (64,95,96).

D. Distal Spinal Muscular Atrophy

Distal spinal muscular atrophy is a presumed autosomal recessive disease characterized by weakness of the distal muscles of the upper and lower extremities. The anterior horn cells of the distal muscles and in some cases the diaphragm are preferentially diminished in number (34). When phrenic motor neuron units are involved, the diaphragm becomes weak or paralyzed (34,97). The disease may present with respiratory failure before there is evidence of involvement of the muscles of the chest wall or extremities (34,97). There is no cranial nerve involvement and upper-airway obstruction and swallowing difficulties are not prominent features of this disease. Sleep hypoventilation from supine positioning and loss of intercostal muscle tone during REM sleep were postulated as causal factors in the death during sleep of one infant who had been active and without discernible respiratory distress in the hours before death (97). Nocturnal ventilatory support could potentially avoid sleep hypoventilation and allow these children with often minimal physical disability to remain active, as observed with a patient with this disorder followed at our institution.

E. Hereditary Motor and Sensory Neuropathies (Charcot-Marie-Tooth)

Children with hereditary motor and sensory neuropathy can present with ataxia, dysesthesia, progressive weakness of the distal muscles of the lower extremities, diminished to absent deep tendon reflexes, and hand and foot deformities (98,99). There are several genetic disorders with similar clinical findings, some associated with known gene defects (type I1a, Ib, III, and X-linked) and others with unknown genetic abnormalities (type I autosomal dominant, type I autosomal recessive, type II, and type III; some X-linked and some complex forms) (99). The prevalence of this disorder is 19 to 36 cases per 100,000 children (99). As many as 20% of adults with these disorders may have symptoms of nocturnal sleep disruption and approximately 7.5% have respiratory muscle weakness (100). Respiratory muscle weakness (as measured by a decreased vital capacity, postural changes in vital capacity, and a decreased maximal inspiratory force) had a high correlation with the presence of proximal muscle weakness. In this field study, these abnormalities also did not appear to be related to the patient's current age or age of disease onset (100). Respiratory muscle weakness was also documented in 10 adult patients (7 without pulmonary symptoms) with hereditary motor and sensory neuropathy recruited from a muscular dystrophy clinic for the purpose of assessing frequency of respiratory muscle abnormalities (101). All patients had a maximal expiratory pressure of less than 60% predicted. Three patients with dyspnea had significant restrictive defects (vital capacity 63% or less) and marked inspiratory and expiratory muscle weakness (101). The authors found a modest correlation between the severity of the respiratory muscle dysfunction and severity of the skeletal muscle abnormality (101).

Diaphragm weakness has been described most consistently in type I disease when disease designation was reported (101–103). Isolated cases of adults with hereditary motor and sensory neuropathy and respiratory muscle involvement resulting in respiratory failure have been documented. In a recent overview of Charcot-Marie-Tooth disease, phrenic nerve involvement was listed as rare, with only 1 of 95 patients with diaphragm paralysis requiring intermittent assisted ventilation (103). One elderly patient who presented in respiratory failure with absent phrenic nerve conduction was, reportedly, eventually maintained successfully on nocturnal ventilation (104). Another adult with Charcot-Marie-Tooth and suspected diaphragm involvement required continuous ventilation and eventually died of urosepsis (105). Two adult patients with hereditary motor and sensory neuropathy underwent pulmonary function testing and sleep studies for the evaluation of symptoms of dyspnea and orthopnea (106). Both had restrictive ventilatory defects with a fall in vital capacity when moving to the supine position and both had absent phrenic nerve conduction, consistent with diaphragm paralysis. The polysomnographic studies were unremarkable. Neither patient had desaturation less than 90% and both had only a mild increase in transcutaneous carbon dioxide of 3 to 7 mmHg going from wakefulness to sleep (106).

Despite the rarity of reports, phrenic nerve involvement in Charcot-Marie-Tooth disease may not be rare. In a recent study from Japan, 4 out of 5 unselected adult patients with hereditary motor and sensory neuropathy type I had abnormally long phrenic nerve latencies (102). In addition, 2 of these patients had restrictive lung disease with daytime hypoventilation. These 2 patients were studied during sleep and showed periodic desaturation and prolonged central apnea (102).

It is not known whether significant symptoms of sleep-disordered breathing occur in children with this disorder, but such children do tend to be more severely affected (107). Diaphragm involvement should be suspected in children with this disease who have sleep disruption or daytime or postural dyspnea, especially those who are severely affected and have proximal muscle weakness. The presence of respiratory muscle involvement is unrelated to age at onset of muscle symptoms, age of presentation, or duration of the disease and therefore may be genetically determined (100). If the condition is genetic, then absence of significant pathology on polysomnography should predict respiratory stability with further studies unnecessary, though this remains to be proven. Children with sleep hypoventilation have the most to gain from ventilatory support, with increased longevity and improved quality of life. Though this disease is classically associated with a normal life span, there are reports of early death secondary to respiratory problems (107). Further investigation of the pulmonary course in children with this abnormality is needed.

F. Duchenne Muscular Dystrophy

Duchenne and Becker muscular dystrophy are X-linked recessive disorders with a defective gene located at band p21 on the short arm of the X chromosome. Duchenne muscular dystrophy (DMD) is characterized by the complete or nearly complete absence of dystrophin, the protein transcribed at this locus, while Becker muscular dystrophy has either a defective or partially functioning gene (108). The incidence of this disease is approximately 1 per 3500 males and approximately 20 females are also reported with this disorder (108). Respiratory failure, which first occurs at an average age of 13 years, is the cause of death in 90% of individuals before the age of 20 years

(56,109). Many affected males have below normal intelligence and there is a high incidence of mental retardation in those with this disease. This is perhaps related to the altered dystrophin present in neural tissue (108). Involvement of cardiac muscle is a well-known phenomenon, and the extent of cardiac involvement and number of patients affected increases with age (110). Smooth muscle also contains dystrophin, and upper gastrointestinal muscle dysfunction has been reported (111).

Outcome measures that help predict when respiratory problems will occur are 1) the loss of ambulation (usual age 12 to 13 years), 2) decrease in vital capacity, and 3) the development of scoliosis (usually after age 11 years) (109). Reduction of lung volumes, flow rates, and muscle inspiratory and expiratory strength have been correlated with the functional class of the disease (112). These measurements appear to be maximal at functional class 3 (walks and climbs stairs slowly), then slowly decline (112). Pneumonia reportedly developed more frequently when the forced vital capacity decreased below 2 L (109). Several studies have failed to show that vital capacity can accurately predict either daytime hypercarbia or respiratory failure (21,112–114). Daytime arterial blood gases have been normal just prior to death, which often occurs during sleep (25,112,115,116).

The development of scoliosis precedes the loss of ambulation. Curves of greater than 35 degrees are noted only after loss of ambulation, but cause and effect are uncertain (109). Treatment of scoliosis before the vital capacity drops below 1 to 1.5 L or 40% predicted has resulted in either improvement or a slowing of the rate of deterioration of vital capacity and a longer life span (109,117–119). However, Miller et al. found no correlation between severity of scoliosis and vital capacity when the vital capacity had already declined below 35% to 40% of predicted before scoliosis developed (120). They also found that the rate of decline in vital capacity as a percentage of normal was not affected by surgery (120).

Breathing during sleep in DMD patients has been studied extensively. Redding et al. recorded sleep studies in 5 nonambulatory adolescents with DMD (54). All had restrictive lung disease with vital capacity 10% to 54% predicted and respiratory muscle weakness. Sleep was markedly disrupted with decreased sleep efficiency, an increased amount of stage 1 sleep, and decreased REM sleep. Intermittent hypoventilation was noted and some desaturation was present, but these were neither prolonged nor severe, according to the authors (54). The significance of the sleep fragmentation is not known but may lead to blunting of the arousal response or may increase the risk of sleep aspiration (25,54). Eleven children with DMD from Italy, ages 12 to 21 years, also with restrictive disease and respiratory muscle weakness, did not exhibit the sleep fragmentation described by Redding. Manni et al. reported that they found no significant sleep-disordered breathing in this group of patients (121). The data reported from this study did show that 4 patients had 5 to 15 episodes of desaturation to less than 90%, 6 subjects had frequent apneas, some exceeding 20 sec, and at least 1 subject had REM sleep desaturation not associated with apnea. Hypercapnia was not evaluated (121). Manni and coworkers also performed longitudinal sleep studies with these patients (122). The patients were asymptomatic at the time of the initial study and remained so at the repeat study 2 years later. None of the children had disturbed sleep, but 5 had NREM and REM sleep desaturation. REM sleep desaturation had worsened by the time of the second study, and one of the previously normal patients developed REM desaturation (122). Of these patients, who were not obese, none developed sleep apnea. All exhibited a worsening of their restrictive lung disease. The authors found a positive correlation between a low functional residual capacity and nocturnal desaturation (122).

Other studies have also described the prominent presence of REM desaturation in children with DMD. Fourteen patients, ages 15 years to 22 years, with normal daytime blood gases and no sleep-related symptoms were evaluated (123). All patients had severe restrictive lung disease and respiratory muscle weakness as measured by pulmonary function testing. Polysomnographic findings included apnea and hypopnea in all patients, and nine of the young men had significant oxygen desaturation most marked during REM sleep (123). This group of researchers later examined six subjects with REM sleep desaturation to better identify the cause of the breathing dysfunction. Using inductive plethysmography, they found that minute ventilation, which was normal during wakefulness, fell in NREM sleep and fell further in REM sleep (124). This fall was most marked in subjects with paradoxical breathing and decreased abdominal (presumably diaphragmatic) contribution to breathing noted with the plethysmograph (124).

This work was later confirmed by another group who studied six patients, ages 12 to 22 years, and performed pulmonary function testing, arterial blood gas measurements, and polysomnography (25). These patients were similar to the earlier group in age and severity of disability. Careful history revealed symptoms of sleep-disordered breathing such as snoring, sleepiness, morning headache, and insomnia. Five of the six patients had an apnea/hypopnea index greater than 5.0, with most apneas of the central type. Two patients had a history of snoring and had obstructive apnea. The most severe desaturation was noted during REM sleep, with many of the desaturation events following central or obstructive apneas. The severity of the restrictive defect did not predict the sleep-disordered breathing; however, the one patient with awake hypercapnia and hypoxemia also had the most severe polysomnographic abnormalities (25).

A prior study examined pulmonary function data and polysomnography data in 11 children with DMD, ages 4.5 to 16 years, and attempted to compare the polysomnographic data with eventual outcome (125). Two of the seven children less than 13 years of age had apnea and desaturation during REM sleep only. Three of the four children older than 13 years, including one with cardiomyopathy, had apnea and desaturation in both REM and NREM sleep. One 16-year-old male had normal polysomnography. The teenagers with abnormal studies had better sleep efficiency than the preteens (93% versus 87%). The three adolescents with REM and NREM sleep abnormalities died within 15 months of the initial study. In the 4 years following the initial polysomnogram, one 10-year-old with REM abnormalities subsequently developed NREM abnormalities at age 14 years (125). These data suggest that the development of NREM sleep abnormalities may signal impending respiratory failure and death.

Conservative care with pulmonary toilet and scoliosis stabilization were the only interventions made in the above studies. Some groups have undertaken assisted ventilation in an attempt to provide support for otherwise terminal patients. More recently, clinicians have intervened in an expectant manner to prevent progression to respiratory failure, as noted above.

Hill and coworkers studied the effects of nocturnal negative-pressure ventilation on 12 patients with DMD without cardiomyopathy, ages 16 years to 37 years, with severe restrictive lung disease and chronic hypoventilation (126). These patients were believed to be stable on the ventilator and underwent polysomnographic monitoring. Obstructive apnea and desaturation were found in most of the patients and increased arousals were present in some. Nasal continuous positive airway pressure (CPAP) or tracheostomy placement resolved these abnormalities. Treatment with supplemental O_2 improved saturations but prolonged the apneas (126). The obstruction was felt to be precipitated by the negative-pressure ventilation and presumably by the failure of the normal preinspiratory activation of upper-airway muscles (126,127).

Long-term nasal intermittent positive-pressure ventilation has been used to treat and possibly prevent nocturnal hypoventilation in DMD (56,128–132). A 2-year study of 10 patients, age 13 years to 27 years, compared pulmonary function testing and outcome of 5 nocturnally noninvasively ventilated patients with hypercarbia with 5 patients who had declined ventilation but received supportive care (128). The maximal voluntary ventilation declined in both groups, though by a greater amount in the untreated group, and the forced vital capacity declined in the untreated group only. Of the 5 untreated patients, 4 died within 15 months of the initial study. All ventilated patients were alive with normal awake blood gases and stable vital capacity measurements at the end of 24 months (128). Rideau and coworkers reported 14 patients with DMD where 8-hr nocturnal nasal ventilation was instituted at the beginning of decline in vital capacity measurements and before daytime hypercarbia occurred (56). In 71% of the patients, the predicted decline in vital capacity was significantly modified, with a loss of only 48 mL/year, versus a loss of 200 mL/year in untreated patients. However, 29% (4) of the patients failed to respond to treatment, with three eventually requiring tracheostomy and continuous ventilation and two dying of respiratory failure (56). The presence of cardiomyopathy in these patients was not addressed.

Respiratory failure tends to occur with a lower level of physical disability and higher vital capacity in DMD than in SMA II (42). The reason for this is not known, though it is possible that diaphragm muscle function is better preserved in SMA II (42,90). This contention is further supported by spirometric measurements showing depressed maximal inspiratory and expiratory pressures in preteens with DMD (112). Ultrasonographic studies also describe baseline diaphragm thickening in preteens with DMD with less than normal thickening during maximal contraction as compared to controls (133). Increased echogenicity of the diaphragm suggestive of fatty tissue infiltration and fibrosis has been described in adolescents (133). The diaphragm weakness may be obscured clinically by the absence of the usual symptoms of tachypnea and shallow breathing during the daytime and the sedentary lifestyle of most of these children (21,123,124).

Cardiac involvement without symptoms has been reported in 25% of patients less than 6 years of age with DMD and 59% of children aged 6 to 10 years (134). The severity of the involvement increases with age, to the point where 57% of patients over 18 years of age develop mitral valve prolapse, left ventricular dilatation, or conduction defects, reportedly from fibrous replacement of the cardiac muscle (110). Normally skeletal and cardiac tissue contain the highest levels of dystrophin, but dystrophin is absent in the heart muscle in DMD (108,135). The cardiac degeneration is progressive and cannot be predicted by the extent of dystrophin gene deletion, skeletal muscle involvement, vital capacity measurements, or respiratory status (110,136). It is possible that the cardiac dystrophin abnormality predisposes to the development of the progressive cardiac abnormalities when combined with nocturnal hypoxemia, hypercarbia, and acidosis. This theory is somewhat supported by the outcomes of 19 patients, ages 15 to 54 years, with advanced DMD, who were ventilated, first nocturnally, then some continuously, and who never developed significant cardiomyopathy (137). The findings of one longitudinal study of DMD suggested that children with more rapidly progressive muscle disease had a lower vital capacity for age and died of respiratory failure or pneumonia, while those with slower disease progression died from cardiac failure with relatively good lung function (109). Whether cardiac death in DMD decreases or disappears when early and adequate artificial ventilation is implemented is an area requiring further investigation.

All persons with DMD eventually have progression of the respiratory muscle weakness to a point where continuous ventilation is necessary to maintain normal daytime blood gases (137–140). There is a perception among some physicians and caregivers that quality of life is poor for patients who require ventilatory support (141). However, this is contrary to the documented feelings of the patients with the disability and to what is known regarding the quantity and quality of life for DMD patients (142). Counseling about ventilator support should be undertaken when vital capacity stabilizes and before it starts to decline. Participation of the informed patient and caretakers in the decision first for nocturnal ventilation and then for continuous ventilation is strongly recommended (95,143).

G. Myotonic Dystrophy

Myotonic dystrophy is the most common inherited muscle disorder affecting adults and children (144). This is a multisystem disease with variable expression and penetrance resulting in abnormalities of the muscle, brain, heart, pancreas, lens, testes, and gastrointestinal tract (145). It is an autosomal dominant muscle disease with an incidence of one per 3500 births. The defect is located on chromosome 19q13, where an expanded base triplet is involved in the encoding of the myotonin-protein kinase gene (146). The abnormal triplet sequence in the affected gene increases in length in successive generations and is responsible for the progressive severity of the phenotype, a phenomenon known as *anticipation* (147). The normal protein is believed to modulate ion channels and is not tissue-specific; therefore this gene defect alters function in many organ systems (145).

Congenital myotonic dystrophy is a biphasic disorder. The early presentation is characterized by a spectrum of severity from mild hypotonia and hip contractures to marked hypotonia, facial diplegia with sucking and swallowing dysfunction, and profound respiratory muscle weakness, often resulting in neonatal respiratory failure. Children born to mothers with myotonic dystrophy, themselves often only mildly affected, are most likely to present in this latter fashion. The myotonic dystrophy allele inherited from the mother is unstable, and the child tends to have a marked increase in number of triplet repeats (147). The increased triplet repeat alone does not fully explain the initial disease severity and later improvement (148). An intrauterine factor has been postulated, since depressed fetal breathing has been observed (149–151). Autopsy reports describe poorly developed diaphragmatic and pharyngeal muscles (150). Central nervous system abnormalities may also play a role in the respiratory depression at birth. Ventricular dilatation is a common feature in severe congenital myotonic dystrophy. Difficult and prolonged labor and intrauterine growth retardation suggest a prenatal or perinatal component of the birth depression (151). Respiratory insufficiency results in a perinatal mortality rate of 17% to 36% (150,151). A poor prognosis is reported for neonates requiring ventilation for more than 30 days (150). Other authors found that tracheostomy placement or the use of nasal positive pressure enabled children with long-term ventilation to be gradually weaned from support (151,152). The only complication after weaning was aspiration in one infant (152). This would suggest that upper-airway collapse contributes significantly to the persistent respiratory problems.

In the children who survive, muscle strength improves and the pattern of greater proximal than distal muscle weakness reverses (151,153). In fact, no correlation has been found with severity of disease in the neonatal period and severity of disease in adolescence (151). However, a high mortality rate from sudden unexplained death (5%), cardiac abnormalities (3%), and anesthetic-related deaths (3%) has been reported in young adults with congenital myotonic dystrophy (154).

Mental retardation occurs in virtually all children with congenital myotonic dystrophy (151,152,155). Long-term follow-up studies have found that the children acquire mobility, although at a delayed age. Complications are primarily related to the mental retardation, behavioral problems, speech and hearing deficits, and gastrointestinal problems—such as aspiration, reflux, and severe constipation—rather than the muscle weakness (151,153,154,156). No series of pulmonary function tests or sleep studies have been reported in children with this form of the disease. Sleep-disordered breathing and alveolar hypoventilation is likely in view of descriptions of sudden death and decreased survival into adulthood as well as symptoms of hypersomnolence and the occasional reports of hypercarbia in adolescents (150,154,157). The progression of cardiac problems may also be caused by sleep-related breathing abnormalities.

The classic form of myotonic dystrophy is caused by the same genetic abnormality but with fewer triplet repeats. This may first present in adolescence with muscle weakness, muscle wasting, and myotonia (delayed muscle relaxation after voluntary contraction or mechanical stimulation). Patients can demonstrate cardiac dysrhythmias, hypersomnia, psychiatric problems, endocrine dysfunction, and gastrointestinal abnormalities. These patients also exhibit marked sensitivity to anesthetic agents and are prone to develop malignant hyperthermia, sometimes resulting in postoperative respiratory failure or sudden death (144,154). Unlike the congenital variety of this disorder, cognitive function is usually normal, though psychiatric symptoms such as apathy and depression are common (155).

Sleep-related breathing dysfunction and alveolar hyperventilation have been recognized for several years. Kilburn et al. described nine patients, ages 22 to 58 years, with myotonic dystrophy, all ambulatory but with muscle weakness (19). Seven of these patients had respiratory symptoms such as mild cough, dyspnea on exertion, and recurrent respiratory infections, and four had decreased maximum voluntary ventilation. Only one patient also had a decreased vital capacity. Awake carbon dioxide levels were elevated to 48 to 59.8 torr in six patients and became higher with breathing 100% oxygen. Five had oxygen saturations less than 95%. The patients also had a depressed response to carbon dioxide inhalation. Two patients had Cheyne-Stokes respiration and documented pulmonary hypertension with hypoxemia that worsened during sleep (19).

Six men with myotonic dystrophy, ages 17 to 34 years, with mild to moderate peripheral muscular involvement were studied by pulmonary function testing, blood gas monitoring, and polysomnography (157). One patient had a restrictive defect, five of the patients had a decreased maximal expiratory flow rate, and all six patients demonstrated decreased maximal voluntary ventilation, consistent with respiratory muscle weakness. Polysomnographic monitoring showed a decreased amount of stage 3 and 4 sleep in two patients with the most severe daytime somnolence. Three of the patients had an increased apnea index and all patients had sleep desaturation with the lowest saturation values occurring during REM sleep in five patients. Four of the patient had abnormal electrocardiograms only during sleep (157).

Begin and coworkers argued that chemosensitivity was well preserved in 12 myotonic dystrophy patients, ages 11 to 26 years (20). These patients had normal levels of carbon dioxide with normal ventilatory function except for a markedly diminished maximal expiratory pressure. The authors noted that the occlusion pressures of these patients were similar to the controls during hypoxic and hypercarbic challenges, but the muscle response was much lower, consistent with respiratory muscle weakness (20). This finding was noted again in a second study (158). These patients with myotonic dystrophy also exhibited higher transdiaphragmatic pressure during normal breathing, suggesting a high impedance of the respiratory system. The authors postulated that this might be related to myotonia of the expiratory muscles (158). A subsequent study, however, found no evidence of respiratory muscle myotonia during quiet breathing in patients with myotonic dystrophy but noted that myotonia may occur at high ventilation levels (159).

Nineteen patients with myotonic dystrophy, ages 15 to 62 years, with mild to severe muscular disability were found to have moderate to severe respiratory muscle weakness characterized by decreased transdiaphragmatic pressures during maximal inspiratory efforts (160). In this study, no evidence for a central medullary defect was found. The authors suggested that abnormalities of the muscle spindle might impair afferent activity, causing decreased muscle response (160). However, when 12 patients with myotonic dystrophy, ages 30 to 61 years, were assessed for respiratory sensation, they exhibited no differences from controls in effort sensation, occlusion pressures, or ventilatory response to carbon dioxide (161). These findings were consistent with an intact central drive and a normal afferent limb (161).

No respiratory irregularity was found during slow-wave sleep in seven patients, ages 39 to 52 years, with myotonic dystrophy and awake breathing irregularity (162). Presumably, the breathing irregularity seen during wakefulness and light sleep did not originate in the medulla and therefore was not an indicator of central regulatory problems (162). These authors did find restrictive disease (vital capacity 50% to 93% and decreased inspiratory and expiratory pressures) and evidence of sleep-disordered breathing, with an increased apnea/hypopnea index in all patients (162).

The hypersomnolence in myotonic dystrophy has been attributed to both a central abnormality and to sleep-disordered breathing (157,163). The hypersomnolence has been reported to occur irrespective of alveolar hypoventilation (163–165). Other researchers have found hypersomnolence only in patients with sleep-disordered breathing (19,20,157,166,167). Hypersomnolence was initially described in four patients with myotonic dystrophy, one a 16-year-old female. In this patient, hypersomnolence was the initial presentation of the myotonic dystrophy (164). Coccagna et al. studied a patient with long-standing hypersomnolence who had a severe restrictive ventilatory defect on pulmonary function testing, daytime hypoxemia and hypercarbia, limited excursion of the diaphragm recorded by fluoroscopy, and myotonia of the intercostal muscles (165). Polysomnography revealed an irregular breathing pattern with central and obstructive apnea, alveolar hypoventilation that was worse during REM sleep, and elevation of the pulmonary and systemic arterial pressures. Several episodes of sleep-onset REM were also observed (165). The patient was treated with intermittent positive-pressure ventilation, which improved blood gases but had no effect on the hypersomnolence, suggesting that hypersomnolence was caused by a central defect (165). Evidence for a central defect causing hypersomnolence was also reported in a 38-year-old male with myotonic dystrophy and hypersomnolence for 20 years (168). This patient had normal ventilatory function and lung volumes but had diurnal hypoxemia and hypercarbia (168). A normal sleep pattern with increased central apnea and an apnea index of 9 was reported. Nocturnal oxygen and carbon dioxide levels were not recorded. Because the vital capacity was normal, the hypersomnolence was attributed to a central defect (168).

VanderMeche and coworkers described a patient with myotonic dystrophy who presented in acute respiratory failure with marked hypersomnolence (163). He had a markedly decreased maximal inspiratory pressure consistent with respiratory muscle weakness. His hypersomnolence did not improve with artificial ventilation, but over the next year, daytime blood gases and hypersomnolence did improve when treated with methylphenidate. A limited polysomnographic study during the acute illness showed snoring and prolonged apnea. Oxygen and carbon dioxide levels were not recorded (163). Daytime hypersomnolence in 17 patients with myotonic dystrophy was subsequently investigated and reported (169). Sleep apnea was noted in 3 of the patients who complained of daytime sleepiness. Methylphenidate improved 7 of the 11 patients who actually underwent testing, prompting the authors to conclude that the hypersomnolence was of central origin (169). Twelve patients, ages 27 to 70 years, with myotonic dystrophy were evaluated using polysomnography. The researchers attempted to correlate the nocturnal abnormalities with symptoms, physical findings, pulmonary function results, and daytime blood gases (166). Maximal expiratory pressures less than 42% were documented in all patients as well as carbon dioxide retention that worsened during sleep. Desaturation during sleep in 11 patients and significant sleep apnea in 5 patients was documented. The severity of the oxygen desaturation correlated best with a high body mass index. The only patient with hypersomnolence also had obstructive sleep apnea (166). Cirignotta et al. reported eight patients, ages 39 to 49 years, with myotonic dystrophy who were studied by polysomnography and with multiple sleep latency tests. All patients had severely disrupted sleep, with central and/or obstructive apnea and desaturation. Five patients complained of daytime sleepiness, but only two had multiple sleep latency tests consistent with diurnal hypersomnolence (170).

Begin and coworkers studied 134 patients, ages 22 to 60 years, and found a relationship between chronic hypercapnia and decreased maximal inspiratory pressure (167). Proximal muscle weakness and daytime hypersomnolence also correlated with sleep hypoventilation. Using multiple regression analysis, they determined that inspiratory muscle weakness played a major role in chronic hypercapnia, but did not fully explain the extent of the abnormality. They postulated a central defect or sleep apnea as an explanation for this discrepancy (167).

Sleep hypoventilation could also occur with a defect of the central and peripheral respiratory motor pathways in myotonic dystrophy (171). The integrity of the pathway in 25 patients, ages 21 to 68 years, was assessed using cortical and cervical magnetic stimulation, phrenic nerve conduction studies, and needle electromyography of the diaphragm and intercostal muscles (171). Magnetic stimulation of the cortical area to assess function of the corticospinal tracts produced decreased compound muscle action potentials in some patients and increased excitability thresholds in others, consistent with impairment of motor conduction (20% of patients). The diaphragmatic compound muscle action potential was decreased following stimulation of the phrenic nerve in an additional 20% of patients, a finding consistent with a myopathy. Nineteen patients exhibited myotonia of the respiratory muscles, primarily the diaphragm. Thirteen patients had normal findings except for myotonia (171).

The preponderance of evidence supports diaphragmatic dysfunction either from weakness or decreased corticospinal tract conduction as the cause of hypoventilation in myotonic dystrophy, especially when the disease is complicated by sleep apnea and other factors that increase the work of breathing. Sleep apnea is common in this disease, possibly because fetal and neonatal muscle weakness affects craniofacial and mandibular growth, creating a small upper airway (172). The data suggest that hypersomnolence may be a primary central nervous system disorder or be caused by sleep disruption from sleep-disordered breathing. It is also possible that sleep disruption or alveolar hypoventilation unmasks a genetic predisposition to develop disabling hypersomnolence.

The cardiac findings in myotonic dystrophy result from myocardial muscle involvement with abnormalities identical to those found in peripheral muscles (173). Sudden death during sleep and following anesthesia has been reported (173). Cardiac conduction abnormalities have been unmasked by sleep (157).

Treatment of myotonic dystrophy has not been widely reported. Isolated cases have been described where patients responded well to nocturnal ventilation. Improvements in symptoms, daytime oxygenation, nocturnal hypoventilation, and pulmonary function have been observed (50,174). It is highly likely that hypoventilation and sleep-disordered breathing play an important role in worsening of cardiac and neurological function and possibly sudden death. Significant respiratory abnormalities may occur in the absence of symptoms. Evaluation by polysomnography with the continuous measurement of carbon dioxide enables the physician to assess both the presence and severity of nocturnal respiratory abnormalities (175). Effective treatment of the respiratory insufficiency could improve quality of life and prolong survival in these otherwise minimally disabled individuals.

H. Congenital and Other Nonprogressive Myopathies

This group of muscle disorders includes several diseases characterized by nocturnal hypoventilation (1,176). These children can present with diaphragmatic weakness that is disproportionately greater than the weakness of the limb muscles. Specific conditions associated with this presentation include some of the nondystrophinopathic muscular dystrophies (Emery-Dreifuss muscular dystrophy, limb-girdle muscular dystrophy, fascioscapulohumeral muscular dystrophy), some of the congenital myopathies (nemaline, central core, multicore, minicore, and myotubular), metabolic myopathies such as acid maltase deficiency, and mitochondrial myopathies (176–179).

Emery-Dreifuss muscular dystrophy is an X-linked disorder mapped to distal part of chromosome Xq28 (148). Progressive development of muscle contractures of the Achilles tendon, elbow, and posterior cervical muscles, often appearing before the onset of muscle weakness, is typical in this disease. Most patients also develop atrial conduction defects that progress to heart block. Recurrent syncope and a sudden death rate as high as 40% have been reported (148,180). Rigid spine syndrome may be the same or a similar disorder (148,181). The missing protein, emerin, is similar to membrane proteins involved in the vesicular transport pathway (148). The diaphragm has been reported to demonstrate pathology similar to the limb muscles (182).

Ras et al. recorded respiratory muscle abnormalities in nine normally functioning, ambulatory patients, ages 13 to 39 years with rigid spine syndrome (182). Dyspnea on exertion was present in eight patients and cor pulmonale in three. Inspiratory and expiratory maximal pressures were less than 50% predicted for all patients. The presence of scoliosis was not associated with more severe respiratory muscle weakness. One adult had significant daytime hypercapnia and hypoxemia, two adolescents had hypercapnia, and the second adult developed nocturnal hypoventilation. One adult male required nasal continuous positive airway pressure during sleep, one adolescent and one adult required nocturnal positive pressure ventilation via tracheostomy. These patients also had the most severe respiratory muscle weakness. Sleep studies were not performed (182). The ventilatory response to hypercapnia was abnormal, possibly indicating a central control problem, but it was more likely secondary to the muscle weakness (158,182).

In a group of patients with nonprogressive neuromuscular disease and respiratory failure, Heckmatt et al. included two patients with Emery-Dreifuss muscular dystrophy (1). Both males, ages 11 and 24 years, were ambulatory and exhibited diurnal hypoxemia and marked hypercarbia. Both patients had a vital capacity less than 25% predicted and developed desaturation during sleep. Marked improvement in symptoms, daytime blood gases, and resumption of regular activity occurred following initiation of nocturnal ventilation with a cuirass. The older patient also required CPAP to treat sleep apnea (1).

Limb girdle muscular dystrophy is characterized by weakness of the trunk and proximal limb muscles and is diagnosed after other types of muscular dystrophy have been excluded (148). These patients develop chronic hypercapnia in the absence of precipitating factors, presumably as a consequence of respiratory muscle weakness (21,148). Gigliotti et al. described 15 patients ages 20 to 74 years, with limb girdle muscular dystrophy, 3 nonambulatory (178). All patients exhibited a mild to severe decrease in vital capacity to 37% to 87% predicted, mild to severe decrease in maximal inspiratory pressures to 23% to 84% predicted, and a moderate to severe decrease in maximal expiratory pressures to 13% to 41% predicted. Neural respiratory drive was increased, but ventilation was decreased, consistent with respiratory muscle weakness (178). Though sleep studies were not performed, these abnormalities are similar to those seen in patients who have developed sleep hypoventilation.

Newsom-Davis described three patients with limb girdle muscular dystrophy and severe diaphragmatic weakness or paralysis (21). One patient had normal daytime blood gases and two had chronic alveolar hypoventilation. Kilburn et al. examined eight patients with either limb girdle muscular dystrophy or fascioscapulohumeral muscular dystrophy, ages 22 to 64 years, all with decreased maximum breathing capacity and five with significant restrictive lung disease. Two patients had diurnal hypercarbia, but nocturnal studies were not performed (19).

Nocturnal desaturation was identified in three patients with limb girdle muscular dystrophy (25). One patient snored and two had daytime hypoventilation. All patients had a moderate restrictive defect with a decreased vital capacity, a decreased maximal inspiratory and expiratory pressure, and abnormal daytime blood gases.

Polysomnography evaluation revealed that two patients had a respiratory disturbance index greater than 10, all had increased stage 1 and 2 sleep, and all had desaturation during sleep. All patients benefitted from nocturnal nasal intermittent positive-pressure ventilation with improvement in the apnea index, nocturnal oxygen saturation, sleep fragmentation, and daytime blood gases. Symptoms resolved immediately following initiation of the ventilation (25).

Other nondystrophopathic muscular dystrophies have been associated with respiratory insufficiency, but the precise pathophysiology has not been described. Fukuyama-type congenital muscular dystrophy is a slowly progressive muscle disease, with respiratory failure resulting in death usually between the ages of 12 to 15 years (148). Merosin-deficient congenital muscular dystrophy is an autosomal recessive, slowly progressive disorder, with death before age 2 years from respiratory insufficiency (148). Fascioscapulohumeral muscular dystrophy, an autosomal dominant disease localized to chromosome 4q35, affects muscles of the face, neck, and shoulders, with progression to the muscles of the pelvis and lower extremity (183). This disease has been associated with respiratory symptoms such as cough and dyspnea (19). No reports of respiratory failure are available, but respiratory abnormalities from muscle weakness or upper airway obstruction can occur (19,21).

The congenital myopathies are a heterogeneous group of neuromuscular disorders that present in infancy or early childhood. They are usually hereditary, slowly progressive or nonprogressive, with morphological lesions identified by electron microscopy (184). Respiratory insufficiency, most likely from diaphragmatic involvement, has been described in many of these disorders. Skeletal deformities of the face and myopathic facies from the muscle disorder can predispose to upper airway obstruction (184).

Infantile nemaline myopathy is associated with a 90% mortality rate from respiratory failure before the age of 16 months (185). The less severe form can present with mild to moderate hypotonia and respiratory muscle involvement. It may, however, be associated with swallowing dysfunction and aspiration. Death during adolescence from sleep-related hypoventilation has been reported (185). Necropsy has shown nemaline rods in the diaphragm muscle fibers, compatible with significant involvement of this organ (185–187). Pulmonary function testing demonstrated a severe restrictive defect with vital capacity of 22% to 52% predicted and daytime hypercarbia in an 8-year-old, 13-year-old, 16-year-old, and 24-year-old with this disease (1,18,176). Oxygenation was studied during sleep by either oximetry or arterial blood gases. Sleep staging was not performed. All patients exhibited apnea and irregular breathing, marked desaturation, and elevation of carbon dioxide when it was measured (1,18,176). All patients experienced improvement in respiratory symptoms and daytime arterial blood gases following the initiation of nocturnal positive-pressure ventilation. Two of the studies documented decreased carbon dioxide responsiveness that improved after the initiation of ventilation. The technique used to assess carbon dioxide responsiveness could not distinguish between central drive abnormalities and end-organ responsiveness (18,176).

The remaining congenital myopathies associated with respiratory insufficiency include central core, multicore, minicore, and the desmin-related forms such as granulofilamentous myopathy and cytoplasmic body myopathy (184). Skeletal abnormalities of the face are also seen in the desmin-related myopathies (184). Pulmonary function testing performed on two subjects with multicore myopathy, ages 33 and 15 years, showed a low vital capacity, decreased maximal inspiratory and expiratory pressures, decreased transdiaphragmatic pressure, and hypercarbia (177). Polysomnography in the older patient showed no evidence of snoring, hypopnea, or apnea, but other details of the study were not available. The younger patient became wheelchair-dependent and developed severe orthopnea and died at age 19 years of cardiac and respiratory failure (177). Three children with minimal-change myopathy and minicore myopathy were studied after developing daytime hypoventilation (188). All had restrictive lung disease with vital capacity less than 30% predicted as well as a fall in vital capacity when assuming the supine position, consistent with diaphragmatic weakness. Observation of breathing movement and oxygen saturation during sleep showed frequent desaturation to 50% to 60%. All patients were started on nocturnal ventilation with either a cuirass ventilator or nasal positive-pressure ventilation with improvement in nocturnal oxygen saturation to greater than 95%, normal daytime blood gases, and resolution of symptoms (188).

A 24-year-old patient with congenital myopathy (type unknown), was studied by Riley and coworkers (18). The patient had orthopnea and severe hypercapnia at rest. Negative-pressure ventilation improved the daytime blood gases, but nocturnal hypercarbia occurred after the ventilator was weaned. Nocturnal ventilation was continued, resulting in normal daytime blood gases and return to activity until the patient died suddenly from pneumonia. Atrophy of the diaphragm was noted on autopsy (18).

Respiratory failure in the neonatal period has been described in centronuclear (myotubular) myopathy (189). O'Leary described a 2-year-old and a 17-year-old with this disorder who developed chronic alveolar ventilation that responded to nocturnal negative-pressure ventilation (190).

Disorders of glycogen, lipid, or mitochondrial metabolism affect the muscles by causing progressive weakness or acute, recurrent muscle dysfunction (191). The glycogen metabolism disorder, acid maltase deficiency, has been associated with respiratory insufficiency (191). The infantile form, Pompe disease, is characterized by profound hypotonia and weakness, macroglossia, cardiomegaly, and hepatomegaly. Death occurs before the age of 2 years from respiratory and cardiac failure (191). Childhood and adult forms of acid maltase deficiency appear as slowly progressive myopathies with eventual respiratory failure resulting in death in the second to fourth decade of life (191). Involvement of the respiratory muscles, particularly the diaphragm, is the presumed cause of the respiratory failure, which can be the presenting symptom (192).

Six patients with acid maltase deficiency were studied as part of a group of 53 patients with proximal myopathy (193). The patients with acid maltase deficiency were included in the group that demonstrated hypercapnia when respiratory muscle strength was less than 30% predicted and vital capacity was less than 55% predicted (193). Bellamy et al. described a 34-year-old male with alveolar hypoventilation and acid maltase deficiency (179). He had mild restrictive disease on pulmonary function testing, and electromyography of the diaphragm demonstrated a diffuse myopathic pattern. During sleep, he was noted to have bradypnea with a respiratory rate as low as one to two breaths per minute (179). Obstructive sleep apnea has also been described with this disease in a 55-year-old male (194). The subject presented with daytime somnolence and was placed on nasal positive pressure during sleep. He subsequently developed respiratory failure and died. Postmortem examination revealed macroglossia with infiltration of fatty tissue and fibrous tissue replacing the tongue muscle (194).

Mitochondrial myopathies are a heterogeneous group of disorders characterized by structural abnormalities of the muscle mitochondria and elevated levels of serum lactate (195). The myopathies vary in the age of onset, course, and severity and distribution of muscle weakness. Defects of substrate oxidation and defects of the respiratory chain peptides in the mitochondria have been associated with ventilatory disorders (191).

Defects of substrate oxidation, specifically pyruvate dehydrogenase complex, cause neonatal hypotonia, episodic apnea, seizures, lactic acidosis, agenesis of the corpus callosum, and death before 6 months of age. An infantile presentation also occurs, with hypotonia, episodic apnea, seizures, optic atrophy, and death by the age of 3 years (191). Syndromes associated with defects in the respiratory chain can present with ventilatory abnormalities. Complex I deficiency can cause a fatal infantile disease with the symptoms of hypotonia, weakness, lactic acidosis, psychomotor delay, cardiomyopathy, and cardiorespiratory failure, ending in death in the neonatal period (191). Patients with complex IV deficiency can present with profound weakness and respiratory distress at birth, with death from renal failure before the age of 1 year or may have severe weakness, ventilator dependency, and poor feeding with spontaneous improvement and return to normal by age 2 to 3 years (191). There are several descriptions of sudden unexplained death in childhood and SIDS in families with mitochondrial disorders (196).

Individuals with mitochondrial disorders and ventilatory muscle weakness treated with nocturnal ventilation have been described in the literature. Braun et al. included two adults with mitochondrial myopathy in their study of 53 patients with proximal myopathies (193). These patients as a group had severe respiratory muscle weakness and diurnal hypoventilation. Specific values for the patients with mitochondrial myopathies were not available. In another report, a 36-year-old female with mitochondrial myopathy demonstrated weakness of the respiratory muscles with vital capacity 61% predicted, decreased maximal inspiratory and expiratory pressures, and decreased transdiaphragmatic pressure (197). While the patient showed no desaturation or apnea during sleep, it is significant that she did not enter REM sleep (197). A 24-year-old with mitochondrial myopathy using nocturnal negative-pressure ventilation and then nasal positive-pressure ventilation presented with restrictive lung disease, daytime hypercapnia, and sleep hypoxemia. Saturations improved and daytime activity resumed with use of the nocturnal ventilation (188). A 23-year-old with mitochondrial encephalomyopathy and obesity who reported a 5-year history of snoring, daytime somnolence, and loss of ambulation has been described (198). Pulmonary function testing revealed a mild restrictive defect with normal daytime arterial blood gases. The sleep study was very abnormal, with sleep fragmentation, increased central and obstructive apnea, markedly decreased mean saturation, and elevated end-tidal carbon dioxide levels. A repeat polysomnogram 5 months after treatment with tracheostomy demonstrated improvement in all parameters, including resolution of sleep disruption, decreased apnea index, and improved mean saturation and end-tidal carbon dioxide levels. The patient's mood and energy level improved and she also resumed ambulation. The electroencephalogram, originally diffusely slow, become normal (198).

The metabolic myopathies vary considerably in the extent of pulmonary involvement. Even those myopathies associated with profound weakness and respiratory distress can improve with time. Children with identified respiratory abnormalities should be followed closely for signs of alveolar hypoventilation and obstructive sleep apnea. Care should be taken in families with this disorder to assess infants for apnea and hypoventilation and prevent sudden death. Polysomnography has potential for evaluating these infants and children to prevent sequelae attributable to hypoventilation. Nocturnal ventilatory support can improve quality of life for those with mild muscle disease and marked pulmonary muscle involvement.

V. Assessment

Physical examination of the infant with neuromuscular disease may show a bell-shaped chest, moderate tachypnea, intercostal retractions, and paradoxical breathing. Although these findings are not specific to respiratory muscle failure, they indicate significant distress and, in the child with respiratory muscle weakness, may predict impending failure. Older children may show no physical signs or symptoms despite nocturnal respiratory embarrassment. Rarely, as noted previously, the muscle disease may present as respiratory failure. Only as the disease progresses will signs and symptoms of nocturnal respiratory failure—such as morning headaches, irritability, hyperactivity, impaired learning, fatigue, and progressive muscle weakness—become apparent during wakefulness. Somnolence is an uncommon complaint in children. Some children will report insomnia or frequent awakenings. While snoring suggests upper airway obstruction, this may not be noticeable or a significant symptom, since this type of obstruction is caused by loss of pharyngeal muscle strength and tone rather than floppy tissue (24). Children with advanced respiratory failure may have orthopnea, difficulty awakening, vomiting, and cor pulmonale (1). Death during sleep has also been reported (1).

Evaluation of pulmonary function can reveal the presence of restrictive lung disease. Although a low vital capacity measurement does not predict respiratory failure, children with a vital capacity that has stabilized or is starting to decline should be considered at risk for the development of respiratory failure (199). A marked reduction in vital capacity of greater than 20% when the patient assumes the supine position is strongly suggestive of diaphragmatic weakness (31,197). Maximal inspiratory pressures are reduced most markedly with diaphragmatic weakness, and maximal expiratory pressures are reduced with abdominal muscle weakness. Children with low values are more likely to experience respiratory muscle fatigue and failure. No value is predictive of respiratory failure for a given age or disease.

The poor discriminating ability of pulmonary function testing for predicting respiratory muscle failure may be because the role of other factors such as upper-airway obstruction, ability to clear the airway, abdominal wall stability, obesity, malnutrition, and level of activity is difficult to assess. With the limitations of pulmonary function testing for respiratory muscle strength and endurance, it is not surprising that nocturnal hypoventilation can occur without significant abnormalities of daytime pulmonary dysfunction (1,18,117,197). Nonetheless, assessment of pulmonary function by obtaining a battery of tests that measure spirometry, respiratory muscle strength, and oxygen saturation every 6 months is helpful in determining the extent and progression of the pulmonary involvement.

Diaphragm movement and strength can also be assessed indirectly by fluoroscopy, but significant diaphragmatic dysfunction can be missed if the results are misinterpreted (31). A serum bicarbonate should be obtained at the first patient visit or in the patient suspected of hypoventilation. The invasiveness and discomfort associated with tests such as transdiaphragmatic pressure or phrenic nerve stimulation makes them impractical to use in children. In adults, these techniques have contributed to an understanding of the neuromuscular disorders.

The most conclusive way to assess nocturnal respiratory sufficiency is by polysomnography (72). Early findings may include sleep disruption and paradoxical breathing in all stages of sleep (Fig. 2). Mild tachypnea and a mean oxygen saturation less than 95% are also early findings. The level of carbon dioxide increases before significant changes in oxygen saturation occur; therefore carbon dioxide level should be routinely measured during polysomnography in children (Fig. 3). Ventilatory support may be considered and initiated at this time, since the elevation of carbon dioxide without evidence of intrinsic lung disease suggests impairment of the respiratory pump (22). If the study is normal, further testing is performed on a yearly basis or every 2 years unless there is an increase in symptoms, marked weight gain or loss, significant growth, change in pulmonary function parameters, or increased hospitalizations for pneumonia. Oxygen desaturation during REM sleep usually follows and indicates increasing diaphragmatic weakness. In our center, this is an indication for nocturnal ventilatory support, since the rapidity of progression of respiratory failure from this point cannot be predicted. Eventually desaturation and hypoventilation occur throughout sleep (Fig. 4). Daytime symptoms of headache, irritability, hypersomnolence, and fatigue are usually present, along with elevation of plasma bicar-

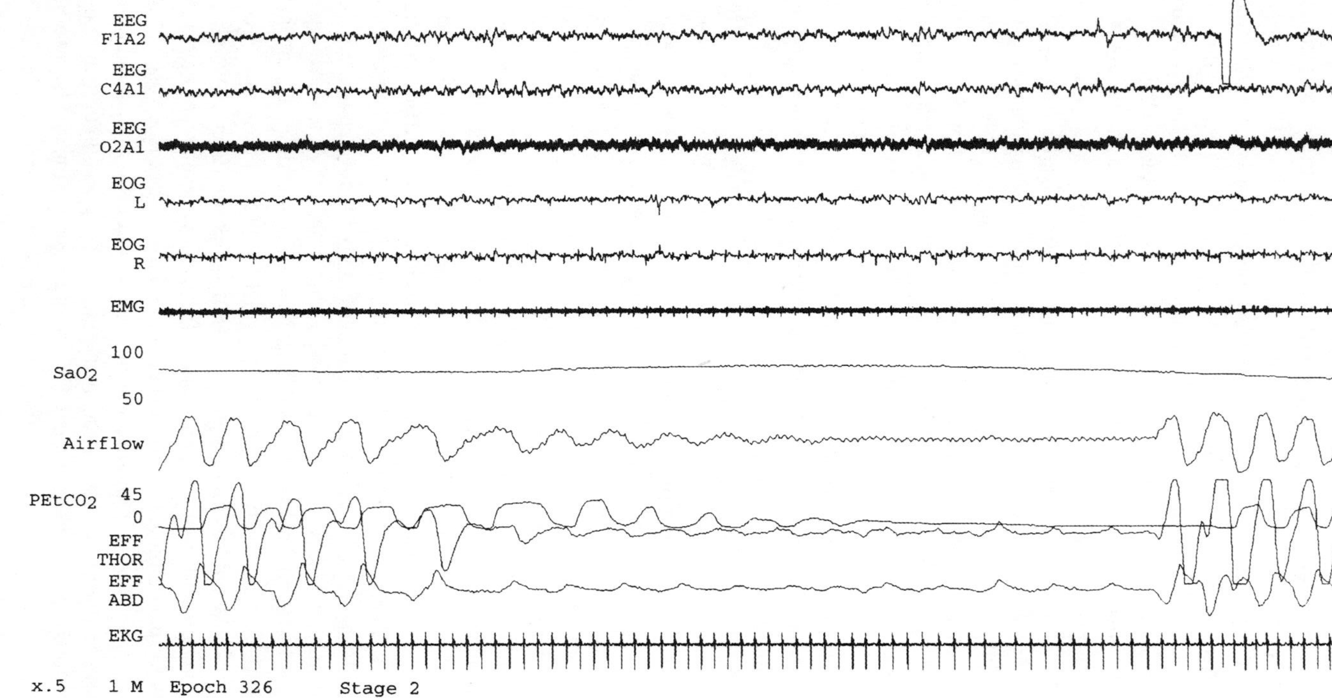

Figure 2 This is a 30-sec epoch of stage 2 sleep in a 10-year-old child with Duchenne muscular dystrophy. Note the paradoxical breathing, leading to an obstructive apnea.

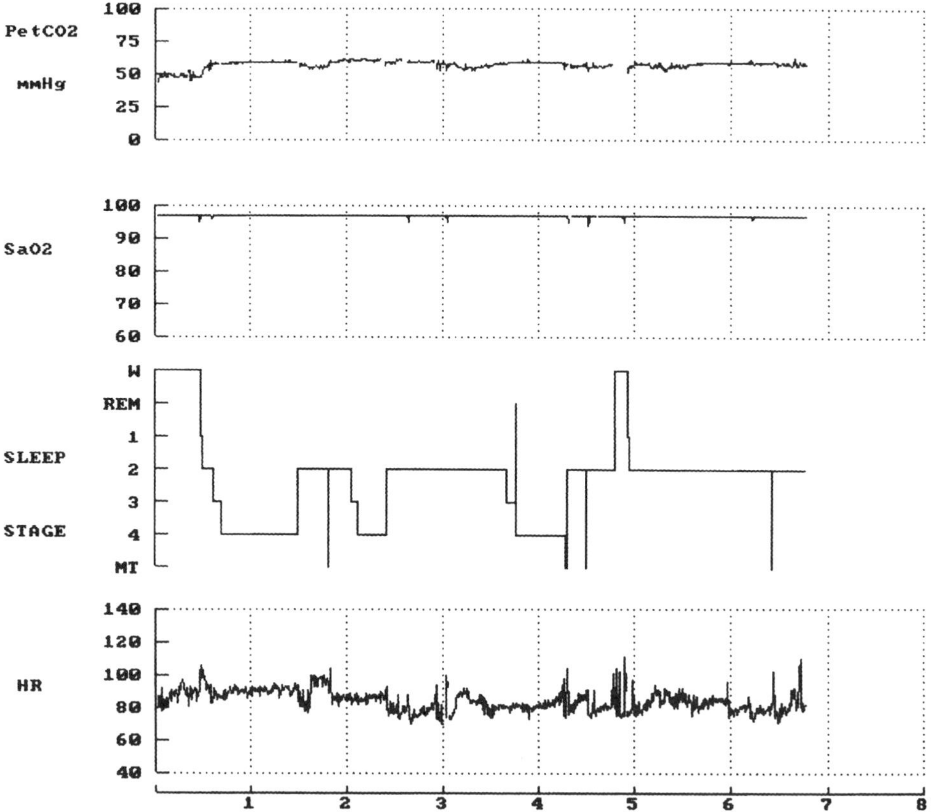

Figure 3 This is a 7-hr summary of a polysomnogram of a 10-year-old child with Duchenne muscular dystrophy. Note the elevation of end-tidal carbon dioxide ($P_{ET_{CO_2}}$) and low mean saturation (Sa_{O_2}).

bonate and daytime oxygen desaturation. These patients face a high risk of cor pulmonale, cardiac failure, and sudden death unless they are treated with mechanical ventilation.

VI. Treatment

The cornerstones of therapy for patients with neuromuscular disease include nutritional support for those with feeding problems and limitation of calories in the obese. Each child must have adequate calories to meet the high-energy demands of breathing. Children with diseases often associated with obesity need nutritional counseling to monitor for adequate caloric intake in the early stages and to avoid excessive in-

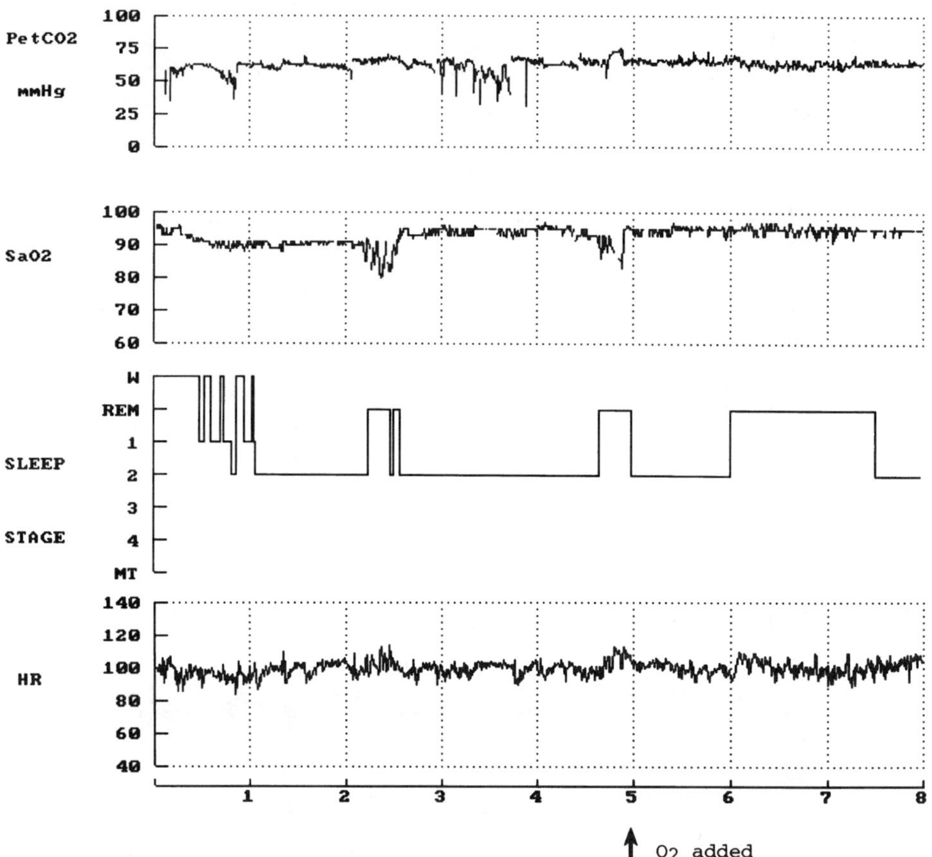

Figure 4 This is an 8-hr summary of a polysomnogram of a 14-year-old child with Duchenne muscular dystrophy. Note the elevation of end-tidal carbon dioxide (PET_{CO_2}) and desaturation, most marked during REM sleep periods.

take after becoming nonambulatory. Correction or stabilization of scoliosis is also important and should ideally be undertaken before significant loss of lung function occurs. Progressive respiratory muscle involvement with the eventual development of respiratory failure is the major cause for morbidity and mortality for almost all of these diseases. The development of respiratory failure can be forestalled by the use of nocturnal ventilator support (1,35,49,50,96,117,152). With the nonprogressive neuromuscular disorders, ventilatory support only during sleep may be all that is ever needed.

The adequacy of any device used to relieve nocturnal respiratory failure should be assessed in a suitable location, such as the sleep laboratory or intensive care unit, where the child can be fully monitored and measurements of both oxygen saturation and carbon dioxide can be obtained. Negative-pressure support devices such as the iron lung or cuirass ventilators are suitable for some children; however, the appropriateness of this type of intervention must be assessed. Problems associated with negative-pressure ventilation include worsening of upper-airway obstruction during sleep due to a lack of coordination of negative inspiratory pressure with upper-airway muscle function and the difficulty associated with assessing and delivering care to patients using the device (200). Nasal ventilation has become a popular and effective intervention for those patients requiring intermittent or nocturnal ventilation. Questions persist on whether the benefits of ventilation outweigh the disadvantages. While this has traditionally been decided by the physician, studies show that physically able individuals underestimate the level of life satisfaction attained by ventilator-dependent individuals (143). Discussion with the patient and caretakers of the consequences of withholding or starting ventilation is strongly recommended before the point of respiratory failure is reached (141,201).

VII. Summary

Sleep is a stressful activity and places a high demand on the muscles of respiration. This demand is often excessive in the face of weakened respiratory muscles, and these abnormalities of muscle function will be unmasked during sleep. The severity of the abnormality is both a function of the age of the child, the type of neuromuscular disease, and the degree of involvement of the upper-airway and respiratory muscles. There are no awake symptoms or signs that clearly predict early abnormalities during sleep. Mild hypercapnia and REM sleep desaturation are the first abnormalities noted and can be diagnosed only with an overnight sleep study. The polysomnography must include parameters to stage sleep and measure respiratory values, especially the level of carbon dioxide. Treatment is limited to supportive measures, though nocturnal ventilation can prolong the quantity and most importantly improve the quality of life in these patients.

References

1. Heckmatt JZ, Loh L, Dubowitz V. Nocturnal hypoventilation in children with nonprogressive neuromuscular disease. Pediatrics 1989; 83:250–255.
2. White DP. Ventilation and the control of respiration during sleep: normal mechanisms, pathologic nocturnal hypoventilation, and central sleep apnea. In: Martin RJ, ed. Cardiorespiratory Disorders During Sleep. Mount Kisco, NY: Futura, 1990: 53–108.
3. Weil J, Byrne-Quinn E, Sodal IE, Friesen WO, Underhill B, Filley GF, Grover RF. Hypoxic ventilatory drive in normal man. J Clin Invest 1970; 49:1061–1072.
4. Read DJC. A clinical method for assessing the ventilatory response to carbon dioxide. Australas Ann Med 1967; 16:20–32.
5. Douglas NJ. Control of ventilation during sleep. Clin Chest Med 1985; 6:563–575.

6. Phillipson EA. Control of breathing during sleep. Am Rev Respir Dis 1978: 909–939.
7. Skatrud JB, Dempsey JA. Airway resistance and respiratory muscle function in snorers during NREM sleep. J Appl Physiol 1985; 59:328–335.
8. Kline LR, Hendricks JC, Davies RO, Pack AI. Control of activity of the diaphragm in rapid eye movement sleep. J Appl Physiol 1986; 61:1293–1300.
9. Orem J. Neuronal mechanisms of respiration in REM sleep. Sleep 1980; 3:251–267.
10. Chokroverty S. Physiologic changes in sleep. In: Chokroverty S, ed. Sleep Disorders Medicine: Basic Science, Technical Considerations, and Clinical Aspects. Boston: Butterworth-Heinemann, 1994: 57–76.
11. Douglas NJ, White DP, Weil JV, Pickett CK, Martin RJ, Hudgel DW, Zwillich CW. Hypoxic ventilatory response decreases during sleep in normal men. Am Rev Respir Dis 1982; 125:286–289.
12. Douglas NJ, White DP, Weil JV, Pickett CK, Zwillich CW. Hypercapnic ventilatory response in sleeping adults. Am Rev Respir Dis 1982; 126:758–762.
13. Berry RB, Gleeson K. Respiratory arousal from sleep: mechanisms and significance. Sleep 1997; 20:654–675.
14. Wealthall SR, Whittaker GE, Greenwood N. The relationship of apnea and stridor in spina bifida to other unexplained infant deaths. Dev Med Child Neurol 1974; 16(suppl): 107–116.
15. Davidson Ward SL, Nickerson BG, van der Hal AL, Rodriguez AM, Jacobs RA, Keens TG. Absent hypoxic and hypercarbic arousal responses in children with myelomeningocele and apnea. Pediatrics 1986; 78:44–50.
16. Swamenathan S, Paton JY, Ward SLD, Sargent CW, Jacobs RA, Keens TG. Abnormal control of ventilation in adolescents with myelomeningocele. J Pediatr 1989; 115: 898–903.
17. Petersen MC, Wolraich M, Sherbondy A, Wagener J. Abnormalities in control of ventilation in newborn infants with myelomeningocele. J Pediatr 1995; 126:1011–1015.
18. Riley DJ. Santiago TV, Daniele RP, Schall B, Edelman NH. Blunted respiratory drive in congenital myopathy. Am J Med 1977; 63:459–466.
19. Kilburn KH, Eagan JT, Sieker HO, Heyman A. Cardiopulmonary insufficiency in myotonic and progressive muscular dystrophy. N Engl J Med 1959; 261:1089–1096.
20. Begin R, Bureau MA, Lupien L, Lemieux B. Control and modulation of respiration in Steinert's myotonic dystrophy. Am Rev Respir Dis 1980; 121:281–289.
21. Newsom Davis J. The respiratory system in muscular dystrophy. Br Med Bull 1980; 36: 135–138.
22. Baydur A. Respiratory muscle strength and control of ventilation in patients with neuromuscular disease. Chest 1991; 99:330–338.
23. Rochester DF. Respiratory muscles and ventilatory failure: 1993 perspective. Am J Med Sci 1993; 305:394–402.
24. Aldrich MS. Neurologic aspects of sleep apnea and related respiratory disturbances. Otolaryngol Clin North Am 1990; 23:761–769.
25. Barbe F, Quera-Salva MA, deLattre J, Gajdos P, Aguste AGN. Long-term effects of nasal intermittent positive-pressure ventilation on pulmonary function and sleep architecture in patients with neuromuscular diseases. Chest 1996; 110:1179–1183.
26. Tabachnik E, Muller NL, Bryan AC, Levison H. Changes in ventilation and chest wall mechanics during sleep in normal adolescents. J Appl Physiol 1981; 51:557–564.
27. Isono S, Shimada A, Utsugi M, Konno A, Nishino T. Comparison of static mechanical

properties of the passive pharynx between normal children and children with sleep-disordered breathing. Am J Respir Crit Care Med 1998; 157:1204–1212.
28. Papastamelos C, Panitch HB, Allen JL. Chest wall compliance in infants and children with neuromuscular disease. Am J Respir Crit Care Med 1996; 154:1045–1048.
29. Roussos C, Fixley M, Gross D, Macklem PT. Fatigue of inspiratory muscles and their synergistic behavior. J Appl Physiol 1979; 46:897–904.
30. LaRoche CM, Carroll N, Moxham J, Green M. Clinical significance of severe isolated diaphragm weakness. Am Rev Respir Dis 1988; 138:862–866.
31. Newsom-Davis J, Goldman M, Loh L, Carson M. Diaphragm function and alveolar hypoventilation. Q J Med 1976; 177:87–100.
32. Skatrud J, Iber C, McHugh W, Rasmussen H, Nicolas D. Determination of hypoventilation during wakefulness and sleep during diaphragm paralysis. Am Rev Respir Dis 1980; 121:587–593.
33. Guslits BG, Gaston SE, Bryan MH, England SJ, Bryan AC. Diaphragmatic work of breathing in premature human infants. J Appl Physiol 1987; 62:1410–1415.
34. Bertini E, Gadisseux JL, Palmieri G, Ricci E, DiCapua M, Ferriere G, Lyon G. Distal infantile spinal muscular atrophy associated with paralysis of the diaphragm: a variant of infantile spinal muscular atrophy. Am J Med Genet 1989; 33:328–335.
35. Piper AJ, Sullivan CE. Sleep-disordered breathing in neuromuscular disease. In: Saunders NA, Sullivan CE, eds. Sleep and Breathing, 2d ed. Vol. 71. New York: Marcel Dekker, 1994: 761–786.
36. Stricker U, Moser H, Aebi M. Predominantly posterior instrumentation and fusion in neuromuscular and neurogenic scoliosis in children and adolescents. Eur Spine J 1996; 5:101–106.
37. Kurz LT, Mubarak SJ, Schultz P, Park SM, Leach J. Correlation of scoliosis and pulmonary function in Duchenne muscular dystrophy. J Pediatr Orthop 1983; 3:347–353.
38. Shannon DC, Riseborough EJ, Valenca LM, Kazemi H. The distribution of abnormal lung function in kyphoscoliosis. J Bone Joint Surg 1970; 52A:131–144.
39. Lisboa C, Moreno R, Fava M, Ferretti R, Cruz E. Inspiratory muscle function in patients with severe kyphoscoliotic. Am Rev Respir Dis 1985; 132:48–52.
40. Bradley TD, Martinez D, Rutherford R, Lue F, Grossman RF, Moldofsky H, Zamel N, Phillipson EA. Physiologic determinants of nocturnal arterial oxygenation in patients with obstructive sleep apnea. J Appl Physiol 1985; 59:1364–136X.
41. Manni R, Cerveri I, Ottolini A, Zoia MC, Lanzi G, Tartara A. Sleep related breathing patterns in patients with spinal muscular atrophy. Ital J Neurol Sci 1993; 14:565–569.
42. Lyager S, Steffensen B, Juhl B. Indicators of need for mechanical ventilation in Duchenne muscular dystrophy and spinal muscular atrophy. Chest 1995; 108:779–785.
43. Labanowski M, Schmidt-Nowara W, Guilleminault C. Sleep and neuromuscular disease: frequency of sleep-disordered breathing in a neuromuscular disease clinic population. Neurology 1996; 47:1173–1180.
44. Vincken W, Elleker MG, Cosio MG. Determinants of respiratory muscle weakness in stable chronic neuromuscular disorders. Am J Med 1987; 82:53–58.
45. Sivan Y, Galvis A. Early diaphragmatic paralysis in infants with genetic disorders. Clin Pediatr 1990; 29:169–171.
46. Schmalbruch H, Kamieniecka Z, Arroe M. Early fatal nemaline myopathy: case report and review. Dev Med Child Neurol 1987; 29:800–804.
47. Szeinberg A, England S, Mendorff C, Fraser IM, Levison H. Maximal inspiratory and

expiratory pressures are reduced in hyperinflated, malnourished, young adult male patients with cystic fibrosis. Am Rev Respir Dis 1985; 132:766–769.

48. Lewis MI, Belman MJ. Nutrition and the respiratory muscles. Clin Chest Med 1988; 9: 337–347.
49. Barois A, Estournet-Methiaud B. Ventilatory support at home in children with spinal muscular atrophies (SMA). Eur Respir Rev 1992; 2:319–322.
50. Canani SF, Givan D, Weibke J, Eigen H. Does nasal positive pressure ventilation improve pulmonary function in patients with non-progressive neuromuscular disease? Am J Respir Crit Care Med 1997; 155:A709.
51. Carrey Z, Gottfried ST, Levy RD. Ventilatory muscle support in respiratory failure with nasal positive pressure ventilation. Chest 1990; 97:150–158.
52. McCool FD, Mayewski RF, Shayne DS, Gibson CJ, Griggs RC, Hyde RW. Intermittent positive pressure breathing in patients with respiratory muscle weakness. Chest 1986; 90:546–552.
53. Samuels MP, Southall DP. Negative extrathoracic pressure in treatment of respiratory failure in infants and young children. BMJ 1989; 299:1253–1257.
54. Redding GJ, Okamoto GA, Guthrie RD, Rollevson D, Milstein JM. Sleep patterns in nonambulatory boys with Duchenne muscular dystrophy. Arch Phys Med Rehabil 1985; 66:818–821.
55. Gothe B, Van Lunteren E, Dick TE. The influence of sleep on respiratory muscle function: the interaction between upper airway and chest wall muscles. In: Saunders NA, Sullivan CE, eds. Sleeping and Breathing, 2d ed. Vol. 71. New York: Marcel Dekker, 1994:239–256.
56. Rideau Y, Delaubier A, Guillou C, Renardel-Irani A. Treatment of respiratory insufficiency in Duchenne's muscular dystrophy in the initial stages. Monaldi Arch Chest Dis 1995; 50:235–238.
57. Raphael J, Chevret S, Chastang C, Bouvet F. Randomised trial of preventive nasal ventilation in Duchenne muscular dystrophy. Lancet 1994; 343:1600–1604.
58. Bach JR. Misconceptions about nasal ventilation. Lancet 1994; 344:752–753.
59. Bach JR, Robert D, Leger P, Longevin B. Sleep fragmentation in kyphoscoliotic individuals with alveolar hypoventilation treated by NIPPV. Chest 1995; 107:1552–1558.
60. Annane D, Quera-Salva MA, Vercken JB, Lesieur O, Fromageout C, Lofaso F, Clair B, Gajdos PH, Raphael JC. Mechanism underlying effects of nighttime ventilation on gas exchanges in neuromuscular disease. Am J Respir Crit Care Med 1998; 157:A779.
61. Hamilton MG, Myles ST. Pediatric spinal injury: review of 174 hospital admissions. J Nuerosurg 1992; 77:700–704.
62. Anderson JM, Schutt AH. Spinal injury in children. Mayo Clin Proc 1980; 55:499–504.
63. Devivo MJ, Kartus PL, Stover SL, Rutt RD, Fine PR. Cause of death for patients with spinal cord injuries. Arch Intern Med 1989; 149:1761–1766.
64. Splaingard ML, Frates RC, Harrison GM, Carter E, Jefferson LS. Home positive-pressure ventilation. Chest 1983; 84:376–382.
65. Rossitch E, Oakes WJ. Perinatal spinal cord injury: clinical, radiographic and pathologic features. Pediatr Neurosurg 1992; 18:149–152.
66. MacKinnon JA, Perlman M, Kirpalani H, Rehan V, Sauve R, Kovacs L. Spinal cord injury at birth: diagnostic and prognostic data in twenty-two patients. J Pediatr 1993; 122: 431–437.
67. Gilgoff IS, Barras DM, Jones MSJ, Adkins HV. Neck breathing: a form of voluntary res-

piration for the spine-injured ventilator-dependent quadriplegic child. Pediatrics 1988; 82:741–745.
68. Roth EJ, Lu A, Primack S, Oken J, Nussbaum S, Berkowitz M, Powley S. Ventilatory function in cervical and high thoracic spinal cord injury. Am J Phys Med Rehabil 1997; 76:262–267.
69. Gross D, Ladd HW, Riley EJ, Macklem PT, Grassino A. The effect of training on strength and endurance of the diaphragm in quadriplegia. Am J Med 1980; 68:27–35.
70. Wicks AB, Menter RR. Long-term outlook in quadriplegic patients with initial ventilator dependency. Chest 1986; 90:406–410.
71. Chervin RD, Guilleminault C. Diaphragm pacing: review and reassessment. Sleep 1994; 17:176–187.
72. American Thoracic Society. Standards and indications for cardiopulmonary sleep studies in children. Am J Respir Crit Care Med 1996; 153:866–878.
73. Weese-Mayer DE, Hunt CE, Brouillette RT, Silvestri JM. Diaphragm pacing in infants and children. J Pediatr 1992; 120:1–8.
74. Epstein BS. The Spine: A Radiologic Text and Atlas, 3d ed. Philadelphia: Lea & Febiger, 1969:195–200.
75. Badell A, Bender H, Dykstra DD, Easton JKM, Matthews DJ, Molnar GE, Noll SF, Perrin JCS. Pediatric rehabilitation: 3. Disorders of the spinal cord: spinal cord injury, myelodysplasia. Arch Phys Med Rehabil 1989; 70:S170–S174.
76. Liptak GS, Bloss JW, Briskin H, Campbell JE, Hibert EB, Revell GM. The management of children with spinal dysraphism. J Child Neurol 1988; 3:3–20.
77. Fitzsimmons JS. Laryngeal stridor and respiratory obstruction associated with meningomyelocele. Arch Dis Child 1965; 40:687–688.
78. Hesz N, Wolbraich M. Vocal cord paralysis and brainstem dysfunction in children with spina bifida. Dev Med Child Neurol 1985; 27:522–531.
79. Cochrane DD, Adderly R, White CP, Norman M, Steinbok P. Apnea in patients with myelomeningocele. Pediatr Neurosurg 1990–91; 16:232–239.
80. Ward SLD, Jacobs RA, Gates EP, Hart LD, Keens TG. Abnormal ventilatory patterns during sleep in infants with myelomeningocele. J Pediatr 1986; 109:631–634.
81. Oren J, Kelly DH, Todres ID, Shannon DC. Respiratory complications in patients with myelodysplasia and Arnold-Chiari malformation. Am J Dis Child 1986; 140:221–224.
82. Waters KA, Forbes P, Morielli A, Hum C, O'Gorman AM, Vernet O, Davis GM, Tewfik TL, Ducharme FM, Brouillette RT. Sleep disordered breathing in children with myelomeningocele. J Pediatr 1998; 132:672–681.
83. Gozal D, Arens R, Omlin KJ, Jacobs RA, Keens TG. Peripheral chemoreceptor function in children with myelomeningocele and Arnold-Chiari malformation type 2. Chest 1995; 108:425–431.
84. Carstens C, Paul K, Nuthard FU, Pfeil J. Effect of scoliosis surgery on pulmonary function in patients with myelomeningocele. J Pediatr Orthop 1991; 11:459–464.
85. Putnam PE, Orenstein SR, Pang D, Pollack IF, Proujansky R, Kocoshis SA. Cricopharyngeal dysfunction associated with Chiari malformations. Pediatrics 1992; 89: 871–876.
86. Bell WO, Charney EB, Bruce DA, Sutton LN, Schut L. Symptomatic Arnold-Chiari malformation: review of experience with 22 cases. J Neurosurg 1987; 66:812–816.
87. Lowe NL. Spinal muscular atrophy syndromes. Pediatr Ann 1977; 6:35–48.
88. Russman BS, Iannaccone ST, Buncher CR, Samaha FJ, White M, Perkins B, Zimmerman L,

Smith C, Burhans K, Barker L. Spinal muscular atrophy: new thoughts on the pathogenesis and classification schema. J Child Neurol 1992; 7:347–353.

89. Fidzianska A. Spinal muscle atrophy in childhood. Semin Pediatr Neurol 1996; 3:53–58.
90. Kuzuhara SD, Chou SM. Preservation of the phrenic motoneurons in Werdnig-Hoffman disease. Ann Neurol 1981; 9:506–510.
91. Russman BS, Buncher CR, White M, Samaha FJ, Iannaccone ST, DCN/SMA Group. Function changes in spinal muscular atrophy II and III. Neurology 1996; 47:973–976.
92. Iannaccone ST, Brone RH, Samaha F, Buncher CR, DCN/SMA Group. Prospective study of spinal muscular atrophy before age 6 years. Pediatr Neurol 1993; 9:187–193.
93. Samaha FJ, Buncher CR, Russman BS, White ML, Iannaccone ST, Barker L, Burhans K, Smith C, Perkins B, Zimmerman L. Pulmonary function in spinal muscular atrophy. J Child Neurol 1994; 9:326–329.
94. Bach JR, Wang T-G. Noninvasive long-term ventilatory support for individuals with spinal muscular atrophy and functional bulbar musculature. Arch Phys Med Rehabil 1995; 76:213–217.
95. Gilgoff I, Prentice W, Baydur A. Patient and family participation in the management of respiratory failure of Duchenne's muscular dystrophy. Chest 1989 95:519–524.
96. Frates RC, Splaingard ML, Smith EO, Harrison GM. Outcome of home ventilation in children. J Pediatr 1985; 106:850–856.
97. McWilliam RC, Gardner-Medwin D, Doyle D, Stephenson JBP. Diaphragmatic paralysis due to spinal muscular atrophy. Arch Dis Child 1985; 60:145–149.
98. Lütschug J, Müller HJ, Malik NJ. The value of family investigations in newly detected Charcot-Marie-Tooth disease in children. Eur J Pediatr 1995; 154:S40–S43.
99. Ouvrier RA. Hereditary neuropathies in children: the contribution of the new genetics. Semin Pediatr Neurol 1996; 3:140–151.
100. Nathanson BN, Ding-Guo Y, Chan CK. Respiratory muscle weakness in Charcot-Marie-Tooth disease. Arch Intern Med 1989; 149:1389–1391.
101. Eichacker PQ, Spiro A, Sherman M, Lazar E, Reichel J, Dodick F. Respiratory muscle dysfunction in hereditary motor sensory neuropathy, type-I. Arch Intern Med 1988; 148: 1739–1740.
102. Akiba Y, Kimura T, Kitaoka T, Toyoshima E, Fujuichi S, Osanai S, Nakano H, Ohsaki Y, Yahara O, Kikuchi K. Respiratory disorders in type-1 hereditary motor and sensory neuropathy. Nippon Kyobu Shikkan Gakkai Zasshi-Jpn J Thoracic Dis 1996; 34: 850–855.
103. Ionasescu VV. Charcot-Marie-Tooth neuropathies: from clinical description to molecular genetics. Muscle Nerve 1995; 18:267–275.
104. Chan CK, Mohsenin V, Lake J, Virgulto J, Sipski L, Ferranti R. Diaphragmatic dysfunction in siblings with hereditary motor and sensory neuropathy (Charcot-Marie-Tooth disease). Chest 1987; 91:567–570.
105. Dyer EL, Callahan AS. Charcot-Marie-Tooth disease and respiratory failure. Chest 1988; 92:221.
106. Laroche CM, Carroll N, Moxham J, Stanley NN, Courtenay Evans RJ, Green M. Diaphragm weakness in Charcot-Marie-Tooth disease. Thorax 1988; 43:478–479.
107. Hogan GR. Respiratory muscle dysfunction in hereditary neuropathy. Arch Intern Med 1988; 148:1707–1708.
108. Darras BT. Molecular genetics of Duchenne and Becker muscular dystrophy. J Pediatr 1990; 117:1–15.

109. Brooke MH, Fenichel GM, Griggs RC, Mendell JR, Moxley R, Florence J, King WM, Pandya S, Robison J, Schierbecker J, Signor L, Miller JP, Gilder BF, Kaiser KK, Mandel S, Arfken C. Duchenne muscular dystrophy: pattern of clinical progression and effects of supportive therapy. Neurology 1989; 39:475–481.
110. Ishikawa Y, Bach JR, Sarma RJ, Tamara T, Song J, Marra SW, Ishikawa Y, Minami R. Cardiovascular complications in the management of neuromuscular disease. Semin Neurol 1995; 15:93–108.
111. Staiano A, Del Giudice E, Romano A, Andreotti MR, Santoro L, Marsullo G, Rippa PG, Sovine A, Salvatore M. Upper gastrointestinal tract motility in children with progressive muscular dystrophy. J Pediatr 1992; 121:720–724.
112. Inkley SR, Oldenburg FC, Viguous PJ. Pulmonary function in Duchenne muscular dystrophy related to stage of disease. Am J Med 1974; 56:297–306.
113. Bye PTP, Ellis ER, Issa FG, Donnelly PM, Sullivan CE. Respiratory failure and sleep in neuromuscular disease. Thorax 1990; 45:241–247.
114. Canny GJ, Szeinberg A, Koreska J, Levison H. Hypercapnia in relation to pulmonary function in Duchenne muscular dystrophy. Pediatr Pulmonol 1989; 6:169–171.
115. Hapke EJ, Meek JC, Jacobs J. Pulmonary function in progressive muscular dystrophy. Chest 1972; 61:41–47.
116. Rideau Y, Gatin G, Bach J, Gines G. Prolongation of life in Duchenne muscular dystrophy. Acta Neurol (Napoli) 1983; 5:118–124.
117. Rideau Y, Glorion B, Delaubier A, Tarle O, Bach J. The treatment of scoliosis in Duchenne muscular dystrophy. Muscle Nerve 1984; 7:281–286.
118. Jenkins JG, Bohn D, Edmonds JF, Levison H, Barker GA. Evaluation of pulmonary function in muscular dystrophy patients requiring spinal surgery. Crit Care Med 1982; 10:645–649.
119. Galasko CSB, Williamson JB, Delaney CM. Lung function in Duchenne muscular dystrophy. Eur Spine J 1995; 4:263–267.
120. Miller F, Moseley CF, Koreska J, Eng P, Levison H. Pulmonary function and scoliosis in Duchenne dystrophy. J Pediatr Orthop 1988; 8:133–137.
121. Manni R, Ottolini A, Cerveri I, Bruschi C, Zoia MC, Lanzi G, Tartara A. Breathing patterns and $HbSa_{O_2}$ changes during nocturnal sleep in patients with Duchenne muscular dystrophy. J Neurol 1989; 236:391–394.
122. Manni R, Zucca C, Galimberti CA, Ottolini A, Cerveri I, Bruschi C, Zoia MC, Lanzi G, Tartara A. Nocturnal sleep and oxygen balance in Duchenne muscular dystrophy: a clinical and polygraphic 2-year follow-up study. Eur Arch Psychiatry Clin Neurosci 1991; 240:255–257.
123. Smith PEM, Calverley PMA, Edwards RHT. Hypoxemia during sleep in Duchenne muscular dystrophy. Am Rev Respir Dis 1988; 137:884–888.
124. Smith PEM, Edwards RHT, Calverley PMA. Ventilation and breathing pattern during sleep in Duchenne muscular dystrophy. Chest 1989; 96:1346–1351.
125. Kerr SL, Kohrman MH. Polysomnographic abnormalities in Duchenne muscular dystrophy. J Child Neurol 1994; 9:332–334.
126. Hill NS, Redline S, Carskadon MA, Curran FJ, Millman RP. Sleep-disordered breathing in patients with Duchenne muscular dystrophy using negative pressure ventilators. Chest 1992; 102:1656–1662.
127. Hyland RH, Hutcheon MA, Perl A, Bowes G, Anthonisen NR, Zamel N, Phillipson EA. Upper airway occlusion induced by diaphragm pacing for primary alveolar hypoventi-

lation: implications for the pathogenesis of obstructive sleep apnea. Am Rev Respir Dis 1981; 124:180–185.

128. Vianello A, Bevilaoqua M, Salvador V, Cardaioli C, Vincenti E. Long-term nasal intermittent positive pressure ventilation in advanced Duchenne's muscular dystrophy. Chest 1994; 105:445–448.
129. Segall D. Noninvasive nasal mask-assisted ventilation in respiratory failure of Duchenne muscular dystrophy. Chest 1988; 93:1298–1300.
130. Ellis ER, Bye PTP, Bruderer JW, Sullivan CE. Treatment of respiratory failure during sleep in patients with neuromuscular disease. Am Rev Respir Dis 1987; 135:148–152.
131. Baydur A, Gilgoff I, Prentice W, Carlson M, Fischer DA. Decline in respiratory function and experience with long-term assisted ventilation in advanced Duchenne's muscular dystrophy. Chest 1990; 97:884–849.
132. Bach JR. Mechanical exsufflation, noninvasive ventilation and new strategies for pulmonary rehabilitation and sleep disordered breathing. Bull NY Acad Med 1992; 68: 321–340.
133. DeBruin PF, Ueki J, Bush A, Khan Y, Watson A, Pride NB. Diaphragm thickness and inspiratory strength in patients with Duchenne muscular dystrophy. Thorax 1997; 52: 472–475.
134. Nigro G, Comi LI, Limongelli FM, Giugliano MA, Politano L, Pettretta V, Passamano L, Stefianelli S. Prospective study of x-linked progressive muscular dystrophy in Campania. Muscle Nerve 1983; 6:253–262.
135. Bies RD, Friedman D, Roberts R, Perryman MB, Caskey CT. Expression and localization of dystrophies in human cardiac Purkinje fibers. Circulation 1992; 86:147–153.
136. Backman E, Nylander E. The heart in Duchenne muscular dystrophy: a noninvasive longitudinal study. Eur Heart J 1992; 13:1239–1244.
137. Bach J, Alba A, Pelkington LA, Lee M. Long-term rehabilitation in advanced stage of childhood onset, rapidly progressive muscular dystrophy. Arch Phys Med Rehabil 1981; 62:328–331.
138. Bach JR, O'Brien J, Krotenberg R, Alba A. Management of end stage muscle failure in Duchenne muscular dystrophy. Muscle Nerve 1987; 10:177–182.
139. Mohr CH, Hill NS. Long-term follow-up of nocturnal ventilatory assistance in patients with respiratory failure due to Duchenne-type muscular dystrophy. Chest 1990; 97: 91–96.
140. Curran FJ, Colbert AP. Ventilator management in Duchenne muscular dystrophy and postpoliomyelitis syndrome: twelve years' experience. Arch Phys Med Rehabil 1989; 70:180–185.
141. Bach JR. Ventilator use by muscular dystrophy association patients. Arch Phys Med Rehabil 1992; 73:179–183.
142. Bach JR, Campagnolo DI, Holman S. Life satisfaction of individuals with Duchenne muscular dystrophy using long-term mechanical ventilatory support. Am J Phys Med Rehabil 1991; 70:129–135.
143. Bach JR, Barnett V. Ethical considerations in the management of individuals with severe neuromuscular disorders. Am J Phys Med Rehabil 1994; 73:134–140.
144. Alberts MJ, Roses AD. Myotonic muscular dystrophy. Neurol Clin 1989; 7:1–8.
145. Ptacek LJ, Johnson KJ, Griggs RC. Genetics and physiology of the myotonic muscle disorders. N Engl J Med 1993; 328:482–489.
146. Tsilfidus C, MacKenzie AE, Mettler G, Barcela J, Korneluk RG. Correlation between CTG trinucleotide repeat length and frequency of severe congenital myotonic dystrophy. Nat Genet 1992; 1:192–195.

147. Fu YH, Pizzuti A, Funwick RG, King J, Rajnarayan S, Duane PN, Dubel J, Nasser GA, Ashizawa T, DeJong P, Wieringa B, Korneluk R, Perryman MB, Epstein HF, Caskey CT. An unstable triplet repeat in a gene related to myotonic muscular dystrophy. Science 1992; 255:1256–1258.
148. Nonaka I, Kobayashi O, Osari S. Nondystrophinopathic muscular dystrophies including myotonic dystrophy. Semin Pediatr Neurol 1996; 3:110–121.
149. Harper PS. Congenital myotonic dystrophy in Britain: II. Genetic basis. Arch Dis Child 1975; 50:514–521.
150. Rutherford MA, Heckmatt JZ, Dubowitz V. Congenital myotonic dystrophy: respiratory function at birth determines survival. Arch Dis Child 1989; 64:191–195.
151. Roig M, Balliu P-R, Navarro C, Brugera R, Losada M. Presentation, clinical course, and outcome of the congenital form of myotonic dystrophy. Pediatr Neurol 1994; 11: 208–213.
152. Keller C, Reynolds A, Lee B, Garcia-Prats J. Congenital myotonic dystrophy requiring prolonged endotracheal and noninvasive assisted ventilation: not a uniformly fatal condition. Pediatrics 1998; 101:704–705.
153. Dodge PR, Gamstorp I, Byers RK, Russell P. Myotonic dystrophy in infancy and childhood. Pediatrics 1965; 35:3–19.
154. Reardon W, Newcombe R, Fenton I, Selbert J, Harper PS. The natural history of congenital myotonic dystrophy: mortality and long term clinical aspects. Arch Dis Child 1993; 68:177–181.
155. Tuikka RA, Laaksonen RK, Somer HVK. Cognitive function in myotonic dystrophy: a follow-up study. Eur Neurol 1993; 33:436–441.
156. O'Brien TA, Harper PS. Course, prognosis and complications of childhood onset myotonic dystrophy. Dev Med Child Neurol 1984; 26:62–67.
157. Guilleminault C, Cummisky J, Motta J, Lynne-Davies P. Respiratory and hemodynamic study during wakefulness and sleep in myotonic dystrophy. Sleep 1978; 1:19–31.
158. Begin R, Bureau M, Lupien L, Bernier JP, Lemieux B. Pathogenesis of respiratory insufficiency in myotonic dystrophy: the mechanical factors. Am Rev Respir Dis 1982; 125:312–318.
159. Rimmer KP, Golar SD, Lee MA, Whitelaw WA. Myotonia of the respiratory muscles in myotonic dystrophy. Am Rev Respir Dis 1993; 148:1018–1022.
160. Serisier DE, Mastaglia FL, Gibson GJ. Respiratory muscle function and ventilatory control in patients with motor neurone disease and in myotonic dystrophy. Am J Med 1982; 202:205–226.
161. Clague JE, Carter J, Coakley J, Edwards RHT, Calverley PMA. Respiratory effort perception at rest and during carbon dioxide rebreathing in patients with dystrophia myotonica. Thorax 1994; 49:240–244.
162. Veale D, Cooper BG, Gilmartin JJ, Walls TJ, Griffith CJ, Gibson GJ. Breathing pattern awake and asleep in patients with myotonic dystrophy. Eur Respir J 1995; 8:815–818.
163. VanderMeche FGA, Boogaard JM, VanderBerg B. Treatment of hypersomnolence in myotonic dystrophy with a CNS stimulant. Muscle Nerve 1986; 9:341–344.
164. Phemister JC, Small JM. Hypersomnia in dystrophia myotonica. J Neurol Neurosurg Psychiatry 1961; 24:173–175.
165. Coccagna G, Mantovani M, Parchi C, Mironi F, Lugaresi E. Alveolar hypoventilation and hypersomnia in myotonic dystrophy. J Neurol Neurosurg Psychiatry 1975; 38: 977–984.
166. Finnimore AJ, Jackson RV, Morton A, Lynch E. Sleep hypoxia in myotonic dystrophy and its correlation with awake respiratory function. Thorax 1994; 4:66–70.

167. Begin P, Mathieu J, Almirall J, Grassino A. Relationship between chronic hypercapnia and inspiratory muscle weakness in myotonic dystrophy. Am J Respir Crit Care Med 1997; 156:133–139.
168. Hansotia P, Frens D. Hypersomnia associated with alveolar hypoventilation in myotonic dystrophy. Neurology 1981; 31:1336–1337.
169. VanderMeche FG, Bogard JM, VanderSluys JC, Schemsheimer RJ, Ververs CC, Busch HF. Daytime sleepiness in myotonic dystrophy is not caused by sleep apnea. J Neurol Neurosurg Psychiatry 1994; 57:626–628.
170. Cirignotta F, Mondini S, Zucconi M, Barrot-Cortes E, Sturani C, Schiavina M, Coccagna G, Lugaresi E. Sleep-related breathing impairment in myotonic dystrophy. J Neurol 1987; 235:80–85.
171. Zifko VA, Hahn AF, Remtulla H, George CFP, Wihlidal W, Bolton CF. Central and peripheral respiratory electrophysiologic studies in myotonic dystrophy. Brain 1996; 119: 1911–1922.
172. Culebras A. Sleep and neuromuscular disorders. Neurol Clin 1996; 14:791–805.
173. Martin RJ. Neuromuscular and skeletal abnormalities with nocturnal respiratory disorders. In Martin RJ, ed. Cardiorespiratory Disorders During Sleep, 2d ed. Mount Kisco, NY: Futura, 1990:251–281.
174. Masa JF, Celli BR, Riesco JA, Sandhez de Cos J, Disdier C, Sojo A. Noninvasive positive pressure ventilation and not oxygen may prevent overt ventilatory failure in patient with chest wall diseases. Chest 1997; 112:207–213.
175. Barthlen GM. Nocturnal respiratory failure as an indication of noninvasive ventilation with neuromuscular disease. Respiration 1997; 64:35–38.
176. Maayan CH, Springer C, Armon Y, Bar-Yishay E, Shapira Y, Godfrey S. Nemaline myopathy as a cause of sleep hypoventilation. Pediatrics 1986; 77:390–395.
177. Rimmer KP, Whitelaw WA. The respiratory muscles in multicore myopathy. Am Rev Respir Dis 1993; 148:227–231.
178. Gigliotti F, Pizzi A, Duranti R, Gorini M, Iandelli I, Scano G. Control of breathing in patients with limb girdle dystrophy. Thorax 1995; 50:962–968.
179. Bellamy D, Newsom Davis JM, Hickey BP, Benatar SR, Clark TJH. A case of primary alveolar hypoventilation associated with mild proximal myopathy. Am Rev Respir Dis 1975; 112:867–873.
180. Dickey RP, Ziter FA, Smith RA. Emery-Dreifuss muscular dystrophy. J Pediatr 1994; 104:555–559.
181. Voit T, Krogman O, Lenard HG, Neuen-Jacob E, Wechsler W, Goebel HH, Rahif G, Lininger A, Nienaber C. Emery- Dreifuss muscular dystrophy: disease spectrum and differential diagnosis. Neuropediatrics 1988; 19:62–71.
182. Ras GJ, VanStaden M, Schultz C, Stübgen J-P, Lotz BP, vanderMerwe C. Respiratory manifestations of rigid spine syndrome. Am J Respir Crit Care Med 1994; 150:540–546.
183. Köhler J, Rupilius B, Otto M, Bathke K, Koch MC. Germline mosaicism in 4q 35 facioscapulohumeral muscular dystrophy (FSHD1A) occurring predominantly in oogenesis. Hum Genet 1996; 98:485–490.
184. Goebel HH. Congenital myopathies. Semin Pediatr Neurol 1996; 3:152–161.
185. Martinez BA, Lake BD. Childhood nemaline myopathy: a review of clinical presentation in relation to prognosis. Dev Med Child Neurol 1987; 29:815–820.
186. Wada H, Nishio H, Kugo M, Waku S, Ikeda K, Takada S, Murakami R, Itoh H, Matsuo M, Nakamura H. Severe nemaline myopathy with delayed maturation of muscle. Brain Dev 1996; 18:135–138.

187. Norton P, Ellison P, Sulaimon AR, Harb J. Nemaline myopathy in the neonate. Neurol 1983; 33:351–356.
188. Heckmatt JZ, Loh L, Dubowitz V. Night-time nasal ventilation in neuromuscular disease. Lancet 1990; 335:579–582.
189. Sandler DL, Burchfield DJ, McCarthy JA, Rojiani AM, Drummond WH. Early-onset respiratory failure caused by severe congenital neuromuscular disease. J Pediatr 1994; 124:636–638.
190. O'Leary J, King R, LeBlanc M, Moss R, Liebhaber M, Lewiston N. Cuirass ventilation in childhood neuromuscular disease. J Pediatr 1979; 94:419–421.
191. Tein I. Metabolic myopathies. Semin Pediatr Neurol 1996; 3:59–98.
192. Servidei S, DiMauro S. Disorders of glycogen metabolism of muscle. Neurol Clin 1989; 7:159–178.
193. Braun NM, Arora NS, Rochester DF. Respiratory muscle and pulmonary function in polymyositis and other proximal myopathies. Thorax 1983; 38:616–623.
194. Margolis ML, Howlett P, Goldberg R, Effychiadis A, Levine S. Obstructive sleep apnea syndrome in acid maltase deficiency. Chest 1994; 105:947–949.
195. Zeviani M, Bonilla E, Devivo DC, DiMauro S. Mitochondrial diseases. Neurol Clin 1989; 7:123–156.
196. Ogle RF, Christodoulou J, Fagan E, Blok RB, Kirby DM, Seller KL, Dahl H-HM, Thorburn DR. Mitochondrial myopathy with tRNA Leu (UUR) mutation and complex I deficiency responsive to riboflavin. J Pediatr 1997; 130:138–145.
197. White JES, Drinnan MJ, Smithson AJ, Griffiths CJ, Gibson GJ. Respiratory muscle activity and oxygenation during sleep in patients with muscle weakness. Eur Respir J 1995; 8:807–814.
198. Sembrano E, Barthlen GM, Wallace S, Lamm C. Polysomnographic findings in a patient with the mitochondrial encephalomyopathy NARP. Neurology 1997; 49: 1714–1717.
199. Rideau Y, Jankowski LW, Grellet J. Respiratory function in the muscular dystrophies. Muscle Nerve 1981; 4:155–164.
200. Hill NS. Noninvasive ventilation: does it work, for whom, and how? Am Rev Respir Dis 1993; 147:1050–1055.
201. Shneerson JM. Home mechanical ventilation in children: techniques, outcomes, and ethics. Monaldi Arch Chest Dis 1996; 51:426–430.

32

Genetic Syndromes Affecting Breathing During Sleep

LEE J. BROOKS

Robert Wood Johnson Medical School
University of Medicine and Dentistry of New Jersey and
The Children's Regional Hospital at Cooper Hospital/
University Medical Center
Camden, New Jersey

I. Introduction

Breathing efforts and the success of those efforts are both affected by genetic factors. Respiratory rhythms are generated in the medulla and pons and influenced by chemoreceptors in the central nervous system and carotid and aortic bodies as well as by mechanoreceptors in the chest wall, upper airway, tracheobronchial tree, lung parenchyma, and respiratory muscles (1). Normal sleep results in central hypoventilation but may also result in upper airway obstruction through relaxation of the muscles that maintain pharyngeal patency. Any factors that decrease the size and/or increase the floppiness of the upper airway increase the individual's risk for obstructive sleep apnea (OSA). Many genetic syndromes can therefore affect breathing during sleep, either through anatomic abnormalities affecting respiratory control or anatomic and/or physiological factors affecting the properties of the pharynx.

Genetic syndromes affecting breathing during sleep can be classified into one of four categories: those producing micrognathia, those producing midfacial hypoplasia, disorders of neuromuscular control, and miscellaneous disorders (Table 1). Some of the more common syndromes with these features are reviewed here.

Table 1 Classification and Some Examples of Genetic Syndromes Affecting Breathing During Sleep

Micrognathia	Pierre Robin sequence
	Treacher Collins syndrome
Midface hypoplasia	Achondroplasia
	Crouzon syndrome
	Apert syndrome
	Pfeiffer syndrome
Abnormal respiratory control	Arnold-Chiari malformation
	Prader-Willi syndrome
Multifactorial and miscellaneous	Mucopolysaccharidoses
	Down syndrome

II. Micrognathia

A. Treacher Collins Syndrome

This autosomal dominant syndrome is caused by mutations in the *TCOF1* gene in the region of 5q32–33.2 that codes for the treacle protein (2,3). Sixty percent of the cases represent fresh mutations. There is wide variability in expression, but the characteristic findings include mandibular hypoplasia (78% of cases), often with malar hypoplasia (81%), antimongoloid slanting palpebral fissures (89%), malformed auricles (77%), and coloboma of the eyelid (Fig. 1) (4). Conductive deafness is present in 40% of the patients. Mental deficiency has been reported in only 5% of cases (4). The overall prevalence and severity of OSA in these patients is not known, but individual case reports describe complete resolution of OSA following mandibular advancement (5,6). Nasal continuous positive airway pressure (CPAP) has also been used successfully in patients awaiting definite repair (7) and may minimize the need for tracheostomy.

B. Pierre Robin Sequence

The Pierre Robin sequence, consisting of micrognathia and posterior displacement of the tongue and soft palate, may occur singly or in association with other malformations such as trisomy 18, the Stickler syndrome, velocardiofacial/DiGeorge syndrome, or the cerebrocostomandibular syndrome (8). The single initiating defect may be hypoplasia of the mandibular area prior to 9 weeks in utero, allowing the tongue to be posteriorly located and thereby impairing closure of the palatal shelves that must grow over the tongue to meet in the midline (9). This posterior displacement of the tongue may impair the action of the genioglossus, an important upper airway dilating muscle (10). Significant airway obstruction can develop in the first few weeks of life, contributing to mortality as high as 30% (9). Although the obstruction may improve

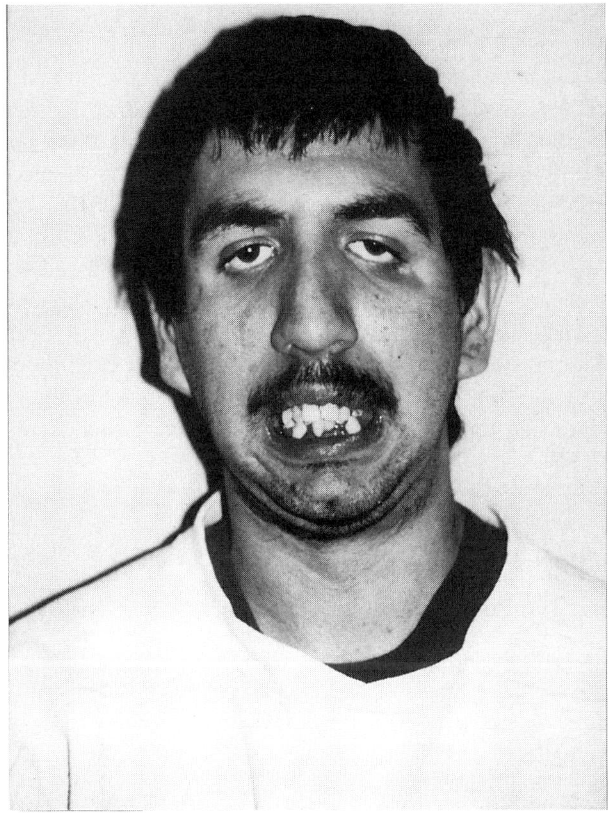

Figure 1 This 19-year-old man with Treacher Collins syndrome had severe obstructive sleep apnea with a respiratory disturbance index (RDI; apneas and hypopneas per hour of sleep) of 55.0. Nasal CPAP, 10 cmH_2O, resulted in normalization of his RDI to 0.8.

clinically, some degree of micrognathia often persists, which can contribute to OSA in later life. Sixty-five percent of teenagers and young adults with Pierre Robin sequence who responded to a questionnaire reported chronic snoring (11). Eight of the patients agreed to polysomnography (PSG) as well as electrocardiographic, echocardiographic, and cephalometric evaluation. These patients had more respiratory events during sleep and lower oxyhemoglobin saturation than did controls, and all had right ventricular end-diastolic dimensions greater than the 50th percentile for weight (11). Significant hypoxemia may be present without clinically apparent symptoms (12), but oximetry alone does not provide adequate assessment because obstructive episodes without desaturation will not be detected (12). Therefore, serial polysomnography is recommended (9,12,13). Fifteen percent of the patients in one series had gastroesophageal reflux (GER) contributing to the frequency and severity of respiratory events (12). Esophageal pH monitoring during PSG should be considered in any patient with symptoms suggestive of GER or who fails to thrive despite apparently appropriate treatment of the airway obstruction.

Treatment for OSA in patients with Pierre Robin sequence depends on the severity of obstruction and the presence of associated abnormalities. Prone positioning may be beneficial but it is rarely effective in the long term (10). Sher successfully managed 20 of 53 infants with nasopharyngeal intubation alone (10). Although oxygen and/or home monitoring have been suggested (12), oxygen does not ameliorate the obstructive events and standard impedance home monitors cannot detect obstruction unless it is associated with bradycardia. Adenotonsillectomy may enlarge the pharyngeal airway and lessen upper airway resistance in selected cases. A tongue-lip adhesion procedure may cause significant morbidity (12) but can improve airway patency sufficiently to allow the child to grow. Twenty percent of the patients in one series required tracheostomy (12), but nasal CPAP may be an alternative to surgical intervention (7,14).

III. Midfacial Hypoplasia

A. Apert Syndrome, Crouzon Syndrome, Pfeiffer Syndrome

Mutations in the fibroblast growth factor receptor (*FGFR-2*) gene, which map to chromosome 10q25–q26, are responsible for most Apert, Crouzon, and Pfeiffer syndromes. The latter may be genetically heterogenous, with some cases of Pfeiffer syndrome due to mutations in FGFR-1, mapping to chromosome 8p11.22–p12 and some cases of Crouzon syndrome due to mutations in *FGR-3*, mapping to *4p16.3*, the gene for achondroplasia. All are autosomal dominant, but the majority of cases represent fresh mutations (15). Common features of these syndromes include craniosynostosis, which limits anteroposterior growth of the cranium, producing maxillary hypoplasia (16) (Fig. 2). Cleft palate and mental retardation may also be associated. The prevalence of obstructive sleep apnea ranges from 24% to 88% (17,18). Abnormalities of the cartilaginous structures including the lower respiratory tree may lead to other complications in managing the airway (17,19); 11 of 12 patients reported by Mixter had laryngomalacia and/or trachomalacia (17). The trachea and mainstem bronchi may also be firm, without rings but rather a full cartilaginous sleeve (17,19).

In contrast to children with Pierre Robin sequence, patients with Apert, Crouzon, and Pfeiffer syndromes may have worsening of their OSA with growth. As the maxillary complex fails to grow, the mandible and other structures grow at a normal rate, resulting in further narrowing of the nasopharyngeal airway (20). Serial PSG is required to define the nature and extent of sleep-disordered breathing as well as the response to treatment. As with normal children (21), not all patients with a clinical history suggestive of sleep apnea had confirmation on PSG (17). Midface advancement by LeFort osteotomy has been described as "very effective in relieving apnea" (22),

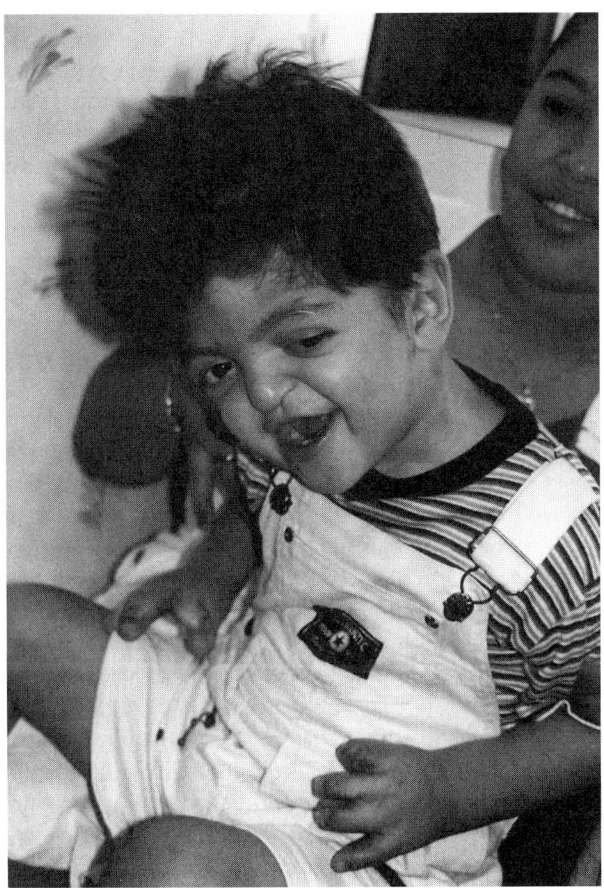

Figure 2 A 2-year-old boy with Apert syndrome and obstructive sleep apnea. His baseline respiratory disturbance index of 36.0 improved to 0.8 with 11 cmH_2O CPAP.

but Mixter et al. found little PSG improvement following the procedure (17); they found that prone positioning was equally effective. The procedure is not recommended in patients under 4 to 5 years of age (22). Tracheostomy has been suggested in young patients with severe OSA (22), but the high prevalence of tracheobronchial abnormalities can lead to severe complications (17); careful observation postoperatively is imperative. The tracheobronchial anatomy should be defined by bronchoscopy prior to surgery if tracheostomy is contemplated. Nasal CPAP is probably the safest treatment for OSA pending surgical repair (17,23), but particular skill and experience with children is necessary to obtain compliance (24). If the patient is obese, a weight-loss program should be instituted in addition to medical and surgical management.

B. Achondroplasia

Achondroplasia is an autosomal dominant skeletal dysplasia, primarily of endochondral bone. It occurs with a frequency of about one in 15,000 births. Virtually all cases demonstrate the same single base-pair substitution in the gene encoding *FGFR-3*, located at 4p16.3. About 90% of the cases represent a fresh mutation, often associated with greater paternal age (25). Defective endochondral ossification results in small stature with disproportionate shortening of the proximal limbs, short flared ribs, megalencephaly with a short cranial base, small foramen magnum, and midface hypoplasia (Fig. 3). These patients are at risk for several types of respiratory complications. Their abnormal rib cage results in a low functional residual capacity that may cause airway closure, atelectasis, hypoxemia, and/or alveolar hypoventilation (26). The abnormal skull base can result in spinal cord compression and central apnea (27), which may produce sudden unexpected death (28). Obstructive sleep apnea is the most common respiratory complication. Waters et al. reported on 20 patients with achondroplasia; all had a history of snoring, and 75% had more than five apneas per hour of sleep documented on PSG (29). A similar prevalence of OSA was found in other studies (30,31). Of 88 children studied by Mogayzel et al., 17 had at least one obstructive apnea per hour of sleep, but there were more frequent episodes of hypoxemia that might represent hypopnea (32). Therefore, all patients with achondroplasia warrant a thorough pulmonary evaluation including chest roentgenograms and overnight polysomnography, including measurement of exhaled CO_2 to evaluate central and obstructive apnea and hypoventilation (26). Electrocardiography and an echocardiogram may be needed to evaluate right heart strain from hypoxemia. Pulmonary function testing is helpful in patients old enough to cooperate. Although there appears to be no relationship between foramen magnum stenosis and sleep- disordered breathing (31), patients with respiratory problems not caused by OSA, restrictive pulmonary disease, or other primary pulmonary system disorders should undergo brainstem imaging studies (such as computed tomography with multiplanar reconstruction or magnetic resonance imaging flow studies) to evaluate the brainstem, since they may benefit from cervical cord decompression (27,33). Nasal CPAP may be the best treatment for OSA in patients with achondroplasia; adenotonsillectomy was effective in only 3 of the 10 patients in whom it was recommended (30). This is not surprising given the complex anatomic and physiological factors that interact to produce OSA in these patients.

IV. Abnormal Neuromuscular Control of the Upper Airway

A. Arnold-Chiari Malformation

The Arnold-Chiari malformation is a congenital abnormality of the hindbrain characterized by a downward elongation of the brainstem and cerebellum into the cervi-

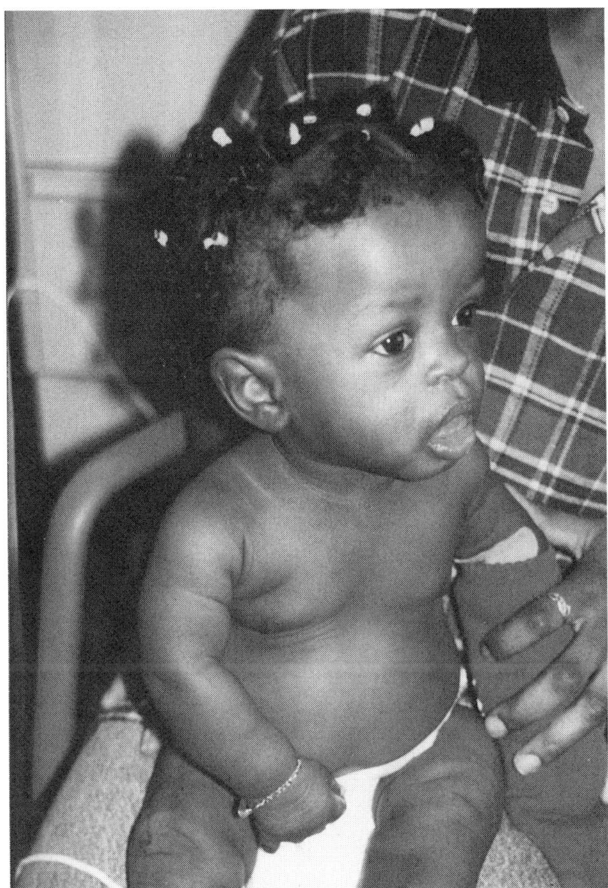

Figure 3 This 1-year-old girl with achondroplasia had snoring and apneas at home. Polysomnography revealed a respiratory disturbance index of 4.1 with oxyhemoglobin desaturation to 87%. She had prolonged episodes during REM sleep during which she had a slight drop in oxyhemoglobin saturation with an increase in end tidal CO_2 to 50 torr, suggesting obstructive hypoventilation.

cal portion of the spinal cord. It is commonly associated with spina bifida (34). The exact mechanism of the malformation is unclear; one family has been reported with an autosomal dominant inheritance (35), but teratogenic mechanisms have also been implicated. In the absence of meningomyelocele or hydrocephalus (Chiari I), patients may present with signs and symptoms of damage to the cerebellum, medulla, and lower cranial nerves. These may include oculomotor disturbance, syncope, torticollis, paralysis, or even sudden death (36). Compression of the brainstem may cause central apnea by reducing central response to hypercapnia or affecting peripheral response to hypoxia by compromising ninth cranial nerve afferents from the carotid body (37). OSA may result from abductor vocal cord paralysis (38) or a decrease in pharyngeal muscle dilator response (39) due to damage to the ninth or tenth cranial nerve.

Three of 11 patients described by Dure had apnea, but there was no differentiation between central and obstructive events (36). A larger, earlier study did not describe any respiratory symptoms in 71 patients with type 1 Arnold-Chiari malformation, although the authors noted that 14% of patients had "respiratory depression ... most marked at night" following posterior fossa decompression, and one additional patient died 36 hr postoperatively during an episode of sleep apnea (40). Waters et al. found that 17 of 83 children with meningomyelocele had five or more respiratory events per hour of sleep, but 34 of the 83 had had posterior fossa decompression and 8 had had adenoidectomy and/or tonsillectomy prior to the study (41).

There have been several case reports of central apnea in patients with Arnold-Chiari syndrome (37,42) that resolved with posterior fossa decompression. Results of neurosurgery for the patients with OSA have been variable; Shiihara et al. reported improvement in their patient's OSA following posterior fossa decompression, but this was not documented with polysomnography (43). The patient of Doherty et al. showed improvement in his OSA 3 months following decompression, but this worsened within 2 years and the patient died suddenly in his sleep 3 years after surgery (39). Another patient required tracheostomy when his vocal cord abductor paralysis did not resolve after posterior fossa decompression (38). Milerad et al. described two infants who responded well clinically to acetazolamide as a respiratory stimulant, although one of them still has frequent mixed and obstructive apneas during sleep (44). Nasal CPAP has been used successfully in some patients (7).

In summary, patients with Arnold-Chiari malformation may be at risk for both central and obstructive sleep apnea due to brainstem compression affecting respiratory drive and/or activation of the pharyngeal and laryngeal muscles that are enervated by the ninth and tenth cranial nerves. Full PSG is required to determine the nature and extent of any respiratory pauses as well as to ensure an adequate response to treatment. Although posterior fossa decompression is often the first treatment attempted, it may not completely ameliorate the respiratory problems, particularly when the apneas are obstructive in nature.

B. Prader-Willi Syndrome

Prader-Willi syndrome (PWS) is characterized by infantile hypotonia, obesity, hypogonadism, and mild to moderate mental retardation (Fig. 4). It occurs in about 1 in 15,000 births. Approximately 70% of affected individuals have a deletion of the long arm of chromosome 15 at q11q13. PWS occurs only if the deletion is in the paternal chromosome; a deletion in the same region of the maternally derived chromosome 15 results in Angelman syndrome (45). In another 20% of cases there is inheritance of

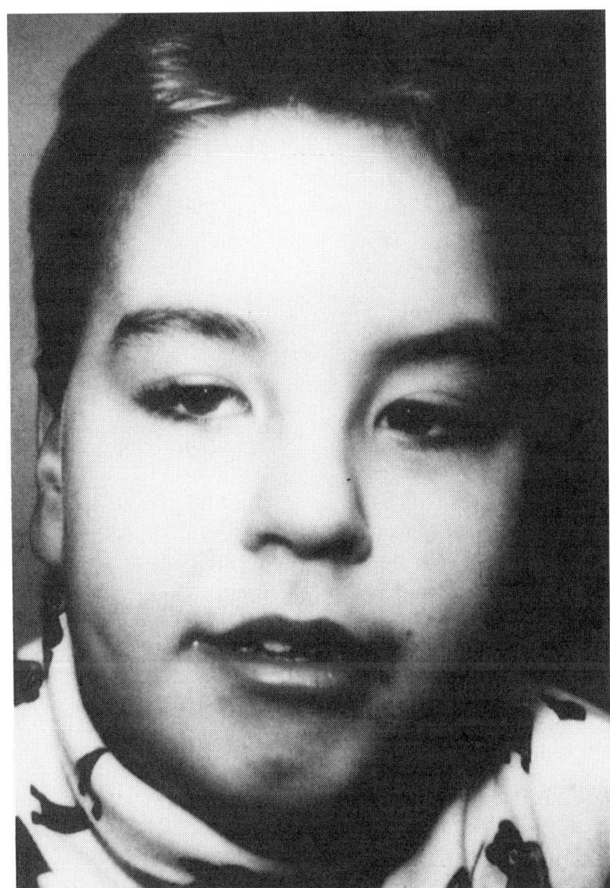

Figure 4 This 8-year-old boy has Prader-Willi syndrome with maternal uniparental disomy of chromosome 15. He is > 98th percentile for weight, 50th percentile for height. At age 4 years he had snoring and respiratory pauses at home; polysomnography revealed a respiratory disturbance index of 5.2 with oxyhemoglobin desaturation as low as 83%. His symptoms resolved completely after adenotonsillectomy.

both copies of chromosome 15 from the mother (maternal uniparental disomy) (46). Patients with PWS are at risk for both central and obstructive apneas due to their obesity, hypotonia, and possibly abnormal ventilatory control.

The prevalence of OSA in patients with PWS is only 10% to 15% (47,48). Although individuals may have severe OSA (49), the mean apnea-hypopnea index is usually less than 10 (49,50). Hypopneas and hypoventilation may be even more prevalent than obstructive events. The number of hypopneas and degree of oxyhemoglobin saturation is related to the level of obesity (47,50) and may be compounded by a restrictive pulmonary defect (52) and/or decreased chemoreceptor sensitivity (53–56). These respiratory events may result in sleep fragmentation and excessive daytime sleepiness (48). Patients with PWS may have a primary sleep disorder, as some studies have demonstrated a high prevalence of sleep onset REM independent of respiratory events (50,57) but this has not been a universal finding (47,51).

Early identification of sleep-disordered breathing can facilitate early therapeutic intervention, which may prevent or delay the onset of cor pulmonale. Weight control is extremely difficult in patients with PWS (58,59). Individual case reports have described good success treating hypoventilation with progesterone (60) and OSA with nasal CPAP (49).

V. Multifactorial and Miscellaneous

A. Mucopolysaccharidoses

The mucopolysaccharidoses (MPS) are a group of metabolic diseases caused by deficiencies of enzymes normally responsible for mucopolysaccharide degradation. The first to be described was Hunter syndrome, an X-linked recessive disorder, whose primary defect is a deficiency of iduronate sulfatase. The gene for Hunter syndrome has been mapped to Xq27–q28 (61). Hurler syndrome was described in 1919, two years after Hunter's report, and consists of a deficiency of α-L–iduronidase (IDUA), which is responsible for the degradation of the glycosaminoglycans, heparin sulfate, and dermatan sulfate. Inheritance is autosomal recessive, and the IDUA gene has been mapped to chromosome 4p16.3. Different mutations of the gene can lead to milder phenotypes such as Scheie's syndrome or Hurler-Scheie syndrome. Although these disorders share biochemical and clinical similarities, their phenotypic distinctions, natural histories, and prognoses depend in large part on the specific organ systems in which glycosaminoglycan catabolites accumulate and to what degree (62). Boys with Hunter syndrome have coarse facial features, macrocephaly, and macroglossia with a declining growth rate and mental and neurological deterioration. Patients with Hurler syndrome can have, in addition, hazy corneas and more rapid onset of pathological features (Fig. 5) (61). Both groups are at risk for airway obstruction due to instability of the cervical spine as well as macroglossia, a deformed pharynx, and a short, thick neck. Thickening of the epiglottis as well as tonsillar and adenoid tissues and tracheal narrowing occurs due to mucopolysaccharide accumulation (61). Semenza and Pyeritz described the respiratory complications of 21 patients with mucopolysaccharidosis, representing 21% of the 98 MPS patients followed at the time by the Johns Hopkins hospital (62). All patients had varying degrees of bony involvement that potentially affected respiratory function, including scoliosis, hyperkyphosis, thoracolumbar gibbus, and/or lumbar hyperlordosis. Of the 21 patients, 18 had a narrow upper airway; 9 patients underwent overnight PSG, and OSA was confirmed in 8 of those nine. Thus, the prevalence of OSA in patients with MPS is somewhere between 89% (8 of 9) and 8% (8 of 98). None of the patients had central apnea.

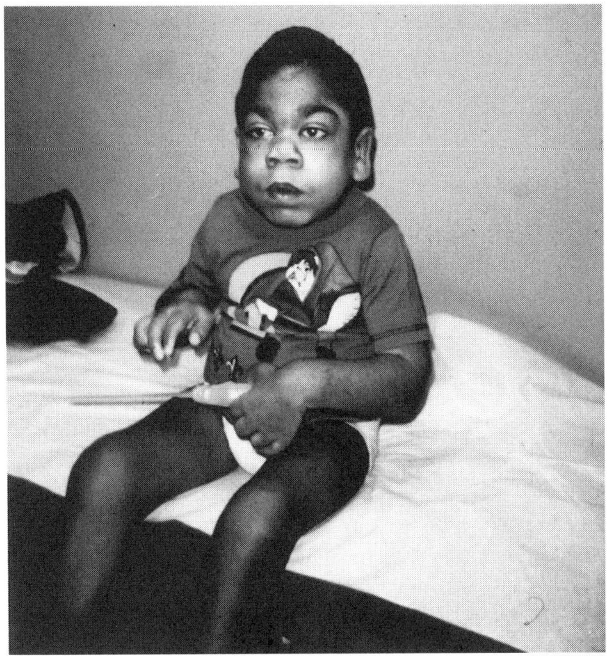

Figure 5 A 12-year-old boy with Hurler syndrome and obstructive sleep apnea. His baseline respiratory disturbance index of 24.4 improved to 0.5 with 12 cmH_2O CPAP.

Belani et al. described clinical OSA in 50% of 30 patients with MPS, although not all the patients underwent PSG (63).

Its complex multifactorial pathophysiology makes OSA difficult to treat in patients with MPS. Continued deposition of mucopolysaccharides in the airways and pharynx can result in progression of obstruction even after treatment. Removal of the tonsils and/or adenoids was not particularly helpful in the four patients described by Shapiro et al., and three went on to require tracheostomies (64). Even this may not be sufficient, since more than one-fifth of patients may have tracheomalacia and/or tracheal narrowing (63). Adachi and Chole described two children with Hurler syndrome who had continued airway obstruction despite tracheostomy and required repeated laser excision of mucopolysaccharide deposits from the trachea (65). Bone marrow transplantation resulted in marked improvement in symptoms suggestive of OSA in all children who underwent this therapy, but no PSG data were reported (63). Nasal CPAP might also prove useful for these patients (66).

In summary, patients with mucopolysaccharidoses are at risk for obstructive apnea due to anatomic airway abnormalities compounded by deposits of mucopolysacharides throughout the airway, including the tongue, pharynx, trachea, and bronchi. These patients can be difficult to intubate, and special care must be taken because of the likelihood of cervical spine abnormalities. Surgical treatment has met with limited success, but nasal CPAP and bone marrow transplantation to treat the underlying biochemical disorder offer promise.

B. Down Syndrome

Down syndrome is the most common pattern of malformation in humans, occurring in about 1 in 660 newborns. First described in 1866, the syndrome is the result of trisomy or mosaic trisomy for all or part of chromosome 21. Greater maternal age is an important risk factor; the syndrome occurs in 1 in 50 births to mothers over age 45 but only 1 in 1500 births to mothers between 15 and 29 years of age. The patients are hypotonic, with mental deficiencies. About 40% have congenital cardiac lesions, including endocardial cushion defect, ventricular septal defect, and patent ductus arteriosus, among others (67). They are at increased risk for obstructive sleep apnea because of their craniofacial structure (maxillary hypoplasia, small nose with low nasal bridge) (Fig. 6), likely compounded by poor neuromuscular activation of the pharynx due to hypotonia and/or mental deficiencies. Increased upper airway infections may lead to adenotonsillar hypertrophy (68). Respiratory difficulties may be compounded by spinal cord compression due to atlantoaxial instability.

Sleep-disordered breathing is common in patients with Down syndrome. One-third of the patients studied by Stebbens et al. had upper airway obstruction identified by a questionnaire and/or limited recordings during sleep (69). More than three-quarters of the 53 patients studied by Marcus et al. had abnormal nap PSG (70); 24 had obstructive apnea. However, hypoventilation was the most common abnormality, found in 35 children. The hypoventilation may be a result of pulmonary hypoplasia (71) and/or decreased respiratory drive. Nocturnal hypoxia may contribute to the high prevalence of pulmonary hypertension in children with Down syndrome (72,73), which seems to be out of proportion to any underlying congenital cardiac abnormalities.

Treatment of sleep-disordered breathing in children with Down syndrome is difficult, and those children with the lowest level of neurophysiological functioning seem to have the poorest response to all treatments (74). Respiratory stimulants such as medroxyprogesterone or protriptyline may be helpful in some patients (75), especially those in whom hypoventilation is the predominant feature. Adenotonsillectomy usually results in improvement but may not completely normalize OSA (70). Adenoidectomy under endoscopic guidance may be preferable to ensure maximal removal of tissue (76). A questionnaire survey of 21 parents of children with Down syndrome who had undergone adenotonsillectomy revealed that two-thirds of patients with OSA and half the patients with snoring were felt to be "cured." However, there was no PSG confirmation of the parents' impression (77). More extensive pharyngeal surgery has been suggested, ranging from uvulopalatopharyngoplasty (78) to an aggressive pro-

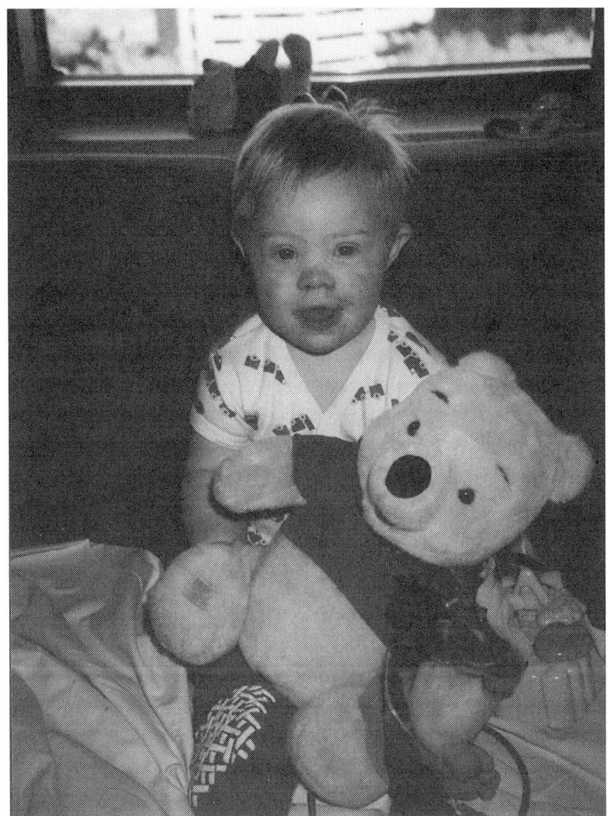

Figure 6 A 15-month-old boy with Down syndrome, snoring, and restless sleep. His respiratory disturbance index was markedly elevated at 31.2, with drops in oxyhemoglobin saturation to 84% and end-tidal CO_2 rising as high as 71 torr. His clinical symptoms improved markedly following adenotonsillectomy.

gram including uvulopalatopharyngoplasty, tongue reduction, and/or maxillary or midface advancement (68,79). Nasal CPAP is effective in the patients who tolerate it (7,74).

In summary, children with Down syndrome are at risk for sleep-disordered breathing due to anatomic factors (pulmonary hypoplasia, craniofacial structure) as well as poor neuromuscular activation of the pharynx. This may contribute to pulmonary hypertension and cor pulmonale. The diagnosis should be confirmed with nocturnal PSG, since nap studies may underestimate the severity of the disorder (70). Treatment is difficult due to the multifactorial origins of the disorder, and success should be confirmed with PSG.

VI. Summary

Many genetic syndromes may influence breathing during sleep through effects on pulmonary or pharyngeal anatomy and/or respiratory control. These syndromes can be classified into those that result in micrognathia, midface hypoplasia, abnormal respiratory control, or multifactorial effects. It is important to have a high index of suspicion for sleep-disordered breathing in these patients; overnight PSG is important to diagnose and confirm the severity of the abnormality and the response to treatment. Treatment is best directed at the underlying abnormality when possible.

Acknowledgments

The author thanks Arthur S. Brown, M.D., Scott R. Schaffer, M.D., and Rhonda E. Schnur, M.D. for helpful comments on the manuscript, and Jean Lee for expert secretarial assistance.

References

1. Berger AJ. Control of breathing. In: Murray JF, Nadel JA. Textbook of Respiratory Medicine. Philadelphia: Saunders, 1988:149–166.
2. Treacher Collins Syndrome Collaborative Group. Positional cloning of a gene involved in the pathogenesis of Treacher Collins syndrome. Nat Genet 1996; 12:130–136.
3. Wise CA, Chiang LC, Paznekas WA, Sharma M, Musy MM, Ashley JA, Lovett M, Jabs EW. TCOF1 gene encodes a putative nuclear phosphoprotein that exhibits mutations in Treacher Collins syndrome throughout its coding region. Proc Natl Acad Sci USA 1997; 94:3110–3115.
4. Jones KL. Smith's Recognizable Patterns of Human Malformation. Philadelphia: Saunders, 1997:250–251.
5. Johnston C, Taussig LM, Koopmann C, Smith P, Bjelland J. Obstructive sleep apnea in Treacher-Collins syndrome. Cleft Palate J 1981; 18:39–44.
6. Colmenero C, Esteban R, Albarino AR, Colmenero B. Sleep apnea syndrome associated with maxillofacial abnormalities. J Laryngol Otol 1991; 105:94–100.
7. Marcus CL, Ward SLD, Mallory GB, Rosen CL, Beckerman RC, Weese-Mayer DE, Brouillette RT, Trang HT, Brooks LJ. Use of nasal continuous positive airway pressure as treatment of childhood obstructive sleep apnea. J Pediatr 1995; 127:88–94.
8. Plotz FB, Van Essen AJ, Bosschaart AN, Bos AP. Cerebro-costo-mandibular syndrome. Am J Med Genet 1996; 62:286–292.
9. Jones KL. Smith's Recognizable Patterns of Human Malformation. Philadelphia: Saunders, 1997:234–235.
10. Sher AE. Mechanisms of airway obstruction in Robin sequence: implications for treatment. Cleft Palate Craniofac J 1992; 29:224–231.
11. Spier S, Rivlin J, Rowe RD, Egan T. Sleep in Pierre Robin syndrome. Chest 1986; 90:711–715.

12. Bull MJ, Givan DC, Sadove AM, Bixler D, Hearn D. Improved outcome in Pierre Robin sequence: effect of multidisciplinary evaluation and management. Pediatrics 1990; 86:294–301.
13. Freed GF, Pearlman MA, Brown AS, Barot LR. Polysomnographic indications for surgical intervention in Pierre Robin sequence: acute airway management and follow-up studies after repair and take down of tongue lip adhesion. Cleft Palate J 1988; 25:151–155.
14. Deegan PC, McGlone B, McNicholas WT. Treatment of Robin sequence with nasal CPAP. J Laryngol Otol 1995; 109:328–330.
15. Jones KL. Smith's Recognizable Patterns of Human Malformation. Philadelphia: Saunders, 1997:416–421.
16. Kaplan LC. Clinical assessment and multispecialty management of Apert syndrome. Clin Plast Surg 1991; 18:217–225.
17. Mixter RC, David DJ, Perloff WH, Green CG, Pauli RM, Popic PM. Obstructive sleep apnea in Apert's and Pfeiffer's syndromes: more than a craniofacial abnormality. Plast Reconstr Surg 1990; 86:457–463.
18. Kakitsuba N, Sudaoka T, Motoyama S, Fujiwara Y, Kanai R, Hayashi I, Takahashi H. Sleep apnea and sleep related breathing disorders in patients with craniofacial synostosis. Acta Otolaryngol 1994; 517(suppl):6–10.
19. Cohen MM, Kreiborg S. Upper and lower airway compromise in the Apert syndrome. Am J Med Genet 1992; 44:90–93.
20. McGill T. Otolaryngologic aspects of Apert syndrome. Clin Plast Surg 1991; 18:309–313.
21. Suen JS, Arnold JE, Brooks LJ. Adenotonsillectomy for the treatment of obstructive sleep apnea in children. Arch Otol Head Neck Surg 1995; 121:525–530.
22. Tajima S, Imai K. Obstructive sleep apnea attack in complex craniosynostosis. Acta Otolaryngol 1994; 517(suppl):17–20.
23. Hui S, Wing YK, Kew J, Chan YL, Abdullah V, Fok TF. Obstructive sleep apnea syndrome in a family with Crouzon's syndrome. Sleep 1998; 21:298–303.
24. Brooks LJ, Crooks RL, Sleeper GP. Compliance with nasal CPAP by children with obstructive sleep apnea. Am Rev Respir Dis 1992; 145:A556.
25. Jones KL. Smith's Recognizable Patterns of Human Malformation. Philadelphia: Saunders, 1997:346–351.
26. Stokes DC, Phillips JA, Leonard CO, Dorst JP, Kopits SE, Trojak JE, Brown DL. Respiratory complications of achondroplasia. J Pediatr 1983; 103:534–541.
27. Fremion AS, Garg BP, Kalsbeck J. Apnea as the sole manifestation of cord compression in achondroplasia. J Pediatr 1984; 104:398–401.
28. Pauli RM, Scott CI, Wassman ER, Gilbert EF, Leavitt LA, Hoeve JV, Hall JG, Partington MW, Jones KL, Sommer A, Feldman W, Langer LO, Rimoin DL, Hecht JT, Lebovitz R. Apnea and sudden unexpected death in infants with achondroplasia. J Pediatr 1984; 104:342–348.
29. Waters KA, Everett F, Sillence D, Fagan E, Sullivan CE. Breathing abnormalities in sleep in achondroplasia. Arch Dis Child 1993; 69:191–196.
30. Waters KA, Everett F, Sillence DO, Fagan ER, Sullivan CE. Treatment of obstructive sleep apnea in achondroplasia: evaluation of sleep, breathing, and somatosensory- evoked potentials. Am J Med Genet 1995; 59:460–466.
31. Zucconi M, Weber G, Castronovo V, Ferini-Strambi L, Russo F, Chiumello G, Smirne S. Sleep and upper airway obstruction in children with achondroplasia. J Pediatr 1996; 129:743–749.

32. Mogayzel PJ, Carroll JL, Loughlin GM, Hurko O, Francomano CA, Marcus CL. Sleep disordered breathing in children with achondroplasia. J Pediatr 1998; 131:667–671.
33. Reid CR, Pyeritz RE, Kopits SE, Maria BL, Wang H, McPherson RW, Hurko O, Phillips JA, Rosenbaum AE. Cervicomedullary compression in young patients with achondroplasia: value of comprehensive neurologic and respiratory evaluation. J Pediatr 1987; 110:522–530.
34. Greer M. Arnold-Chiari malformation. In: Rowland LP, ed. Merritt's Textbook of Neurology. Baltimore: Williams & Wilkins, 1995:528–532.
35. Coria F, Quintana F, Rebello M, Combarros O, Berciano J. Occipital dysplasia and Chiari type I deformity in a family. J Neurol Sci 1983; 62:143–158.
36. Dure LS, Percy AK, Cheek WR, Laurent JP. Chiari type I malformation in children. J Pediatr 1989; 115:573–576.
37. Keefover R, Sam M, Bodensteiner J, Nicholson A. Hypersomnolence and pure central sleep apnea associated with the Chiari I malformation. J Child Neurol 1995; 10:65–67.
38. Ruff ME, Oakes WJ, Fisher SR, Spock A. Sleep apnea and vocal cord paralysis secondary to type I Chiari malformation. Pediatrics 1987; 80:231–234.
39. Doherty MJ, Spence DPS, Young C, Calverley PMA. Obstructive sleep apnea with Arnold-Chiari malformation. Thorax 1995; 50:690–691.
40. Paul KS, Lye RH, Strang FA, Dutton J. Arnold-Chiari malformation: review of 71 cases. J Neurosurg 1983; 58:183–187.
41. Waters KA, Forbes P, Morielli A, Hum C, O'Gorman AM, Vernet O, Davis GM, Tewfik TL, Ducharme F, Brouillette RT. Sleep-disordered breathing in children with myelomeningocele. J Pediatr 1998; 132:672–681.
42. Balk RA, Hiller FC, Lucas EA, Scrima L, Wilson FJ, Wooten V. Sleep apnea and the Arnold-Chiari malformation. Am Rev Respir Dis 1985; 132:929–930.
43. Shiihara T, Shimizu Y, Mitsui T, Saitoh E, Sato S. Isolated sleep apnea due to Chiari type I malformation and syringomyelia. Pediatr Neurol 1995; 13:266–267.
44. Milerad J, Lagercrantz H, Johnson P. Obstructive sleep apnea in Arnold-Chiari malformation treated with acetazolamide. Acta Paediatr 1992; 81:609–612.
45. Jones KL. Smith's Recognizable Patterns of Human Malformation. Philadelphia: Saunders, 1997:202–205.
46. Mascari MJ, Gottlieb W, Rogan PK, Butler MG, Waller DA, Armour JAL, Jeffreys AJ, Ladda RL, Nicholls RD. The frequency of uniparental disomy in Prader-Willi syndrome. N Engl J Med 1992; 326:1599–1607.
47. Brooks LJ, Owens RP. Sleep and breathing patterns in patients with Prader-Willi syndrome. Sleep Res 1992; 21:285.
48. Hertz G, Cataletto M, Feinsilver SW, Angulo M. Sleep and breathing patterns in patients with Prader-Willi syndrome: effects of age and gender. Sleep 1993; 16:366–371.
49. Sforza E, Krieger J, Geisert J, Kurtz D. Sleep and breathing abnormalities in a case of Prader-Willi syndrome. Acta Paediatr Scand 1991; 80:80–85.
50. Hertz G, Cataletto M, Feinsilver SH, Angulo M. Developmental trends of sleep disordered breathing in Prader-Willi syndrome: the role of obesity. Am J Med Genet 1995; 56: 188–190.
51. Kaplan J, Fredrickson PA, Richardson JW. Sleep and breathing in patients with Prader-Willi syndrome. Mayo Clin Proc 1991; 66:1124–1126.
52. Hakonarson H, Moskovitz J, Daigle KL, Cassidy SB, Cloutier MM. Pulmonary function abnormalities in Prader-Willi syndrome. J Pediatr 1995; 126:565–570.
53. Orenstein DM, Boat TF, Owens RP, Horowitz JG, Primiano FP, Germann K, Doershuk CF. The obesity-hypoventilation syndrome in children with the Prader-Willi syndrome:

a possible role for familial decreased response to carbon dioxide. J Pediatr 1980; 97: 765–767.
54. Arens R, Gozal D, Omlin KJ, Livingston FR, Liu J, Keens TG, Ward SLD. Hypoxic and hypercapnic ventilatory responses in Prader-Willi syndrome. J Appl Physiol 1994; 77: 2224–2230.
55. Gozal D, Arens R, Omlin KJ, Ward SLD, Keens TG. Absent peripheral chemosensitivity in Prader-Willi syndrome. J Appl Physiol 1994; 77:2231–2236.
56. Livingston FR, Arens R, Bailey SL, Keens TG, Ward SLD. Hypercapnic arousal responses in Prader-Willi syndrome. Chest 1995; 108:1627–1631.
57. Vela-Bueno A, Kales A, Soldatos CR, Dobladez-Blanco B, Campos-Castello J, Espino-Hurtado P, Olivan-Palacios J. Sleep in the Prader-Willi syndrome. Arch Neurol 1984; 41: 294–296.
58. Bray GA, Dahms WT, Swerdloff RS, Fiser RH, Atkinson RL, Carrel RE. The Prader-Willi syndrome: a study of 40 patients and a review of the literature. Medicine 1983; 62:59–80.
59. Donaldson MDC, Chu CE, Cooke A, Wilson A, Greene SA, Stephenson JBP. The Prader-Willi syndrome. Arch Dis Child 1994; 70:58–63.
60. Orenstein DM, Boat TF, Stern RC, Doershuk CF, Light MS. Progesterone treatment of the obesity-hypoventilation syndrome in a child. J Pediatr 1977; 447–479.
61. Jones KL. Smith's Recognizable Patterns of Human Malformation. Philadelphia: Saunders, 1997:450–471.
62. Semenza GL, Pyeritz RE. Respiratory complications of mucopolysaccharide storage disorders. Medicine 1988; 67:209–219.
63. Belani KG, Krivit W, Carpenter BLM, Braunlin E, Buckley JJ, Liao JC, Floyd T, Leonard AS, Summers CG, Levine S, Whitley CB. Children with mucopolysaccharidosis: perioperative care, morbidity, mortality, and new findings. J Pediatr Surg 1993; 28:403–410.
64. Shapiro J, Strome MS, Crocker AC. Airway obstruction and sleep apnea in Hurler and Hunter syndromes. Ann Otol Rhinol Laryngol 1985; 94:458–461.
65. Adachi K, Chole RA. Management of tracheal lesions in Hurler syndrome. Arch Otolaryngol Head Neck Surg 1990; 116:1205–1207.
66. Ginzburg AS, Onal E, Aronson RM, Schild JA, Mafee MF, Lopata M. Successful use of nasal-CPAP for obstructive sleep apnea in Hunter syndrome with diffuse airway involvement. Chest 1990; 97:1496–1498.
67. Jones KL. Smith's Recognizable Patterns of Human Malformation. Philadelphia: Saunders, 1997:8–13.
68. Lefaivre JF, Cohen SR, Burstein FD, Simms C, Scott PH, Montgomery GL, Graham L, Kattos AV. Down syndrome: identification and surgical management of obstructive sleep apnea. Plast Reconstr Surg 1977; 99:629–637.
69. Stebbens VA, Dennis J, Samuels MP, Croft CB, Southall DP. Sleep related upper airway obstruction in a cohort with Down's syndrome. Arch Dis Child 1991; 66:1333–1338.
70. Marcus CL, Keens TG, Bautista DB, von Pechmann WS, Ward SLD. Obstructive sleep apnea in children with Down syndrome. Pediatrics 1991; 88:132–139.
71. Cooney TP, Thurlbeck WM. Pulmonary hypoplasia in Down's syndrome. N Engl J Med 1982; 307:1170–1173.
72. Rowland TW, Nordstrom LG, Bean MS, Burkhardt H. Chronic upper airway obstruction and pulmonary hypertension in Down's syndrome. Am J Dis Child 1981; 135:1050–1052.
73. Loughlin GM, Wynne JW, Victorica BE. Sleep apnea as a possible cause of pulmonary hypertension in Down syndrome. J Pediatr 1981; 98:435–437.

74. Brooks LJ, Bacevice AM, Beebe A, Taylor HG. Relationship between neuropsychological function and success of treatment for OSA in children with Down syndrome. Am J Resp Crit Care Med 1997; 155:A710.
75. Clark RW, Schmidt HS, Schuller DE. Sleep induced ventilatory dysfunction in Down's syndrome. Arch Intern Med 1980; 140:45–50.
76. Schaffer SR, Yoskovitch A. Transoral endoscopic adenoidectomy: operative techniques. Otolaryngol Head Neck Surg 1997; 8:52–55.
77. Kavanagh KT, Kahane JC, Kordan B. Risks and benefits of adenotonsillectomy for children with Down syndrome. Am J Ment Defic 1986; 91:22–29.
78. Strome M. Obstructive sleep apnea in Down syndrome children: a surgical approach. Laryngoscope 1986; 96:1340–1342.
79. Donaldson JD, Redmond WM. Surgical management of obstructive sleep apnea in children with Down syndrome. J Otolaryngol 1988; 17:398–403.

33

Sickle Cell Disease and Breathing During Sleep

CAROL J. BLAISDELL

Johns Hopkins University School of Medicine
Baltimore, Maryland

I. Introduction

Sickle cell disease is a serious, life-shortening autosomal recessive disorder most commonly affecting individuals of African descent. It is also found in people of Mediterranean descent. The prevalence of sickle cell disease is approximately 1 in 400 births. Average life span is into the fourth decade, with early mortality often due to end-organ damage. The occurrence of one of the most common manifestations of this disease—painful crises of the extremities, ribs, or chest—is not evenly distributed. Of 3578 patients with sickle cell disease studied over a 9-year period, 39% had no painful episodes requiring medical attention, whereas 1% had more than six episodes per year. A total of 5.2% of the patients accounted for 32.9% of all painful episodes (1). The spectrum of disease severity even in patients with similar hematological indices suggests that there may be genetic, cellular, physiological, and psychological modifying factors. It is clear that despite identification of the gene defect that causes sickle cell disease, we do not understand well the factors that lead to the significant morbidity and mortality associated with this disease. Many investigators have noted the frequent occurrence of arterial oxygen desaturation in patients with sickle cell disease and have suggested that deoxygenation is not only a marker of disease severity but also a risk factor for acute and chronic illness.

Polymerization of deoxygenated sickle hemoglobin is the primary event in the molecular pathogenesis of sickle cell disease. While the polymerization of deoxygenated sickle hemoglobin is for the most part reversible, repeated cycles of oxygenation/deoxygenation can lead to irreversible damage to red cell membranes. This results in distortion of the erythrocyte into a sickle shape, markedly decreasing its deformability as it passes through the capillary bed. Even with only partial deoxygenation, there can be sufficient quantities of hemoglobin S (HbS) polymer to alter the rheological properties of the sickle red blood cell. Irreversibly sickled cells, which cannot bind oxygen, are removed from the circulation (and reflect the degree of hemolytic anemia). Erythroid marrow hyperplasia results and stress reticulocytes are released into the circulation. These reticulocytes are associated with increased adhesion and contribute to vaso-occlusion. The major disability for individuals with sickle cell disease is related to painful vaso-occlusive crises and secondary end-organ damage as a result of sickling and occlusion of the microvasculature of the bones of the trunk and extremities, resulting in severe pain. When the vaso-occlusive (VOC) process occurs in other organs, the clinical syndromes include stroke, the acute chest syndrome, hepatic crisis, priapism, and acute renal papillary infarction. These VOC events increase the relative risk of chronic lung disease (1.6 times that over control patients with sickle cell disease but without VOC). Acute chest syndrome specifically increases that risk to 17 times control (2).

The process of HbS polymerization is influenced by factors such as red cell heterogeneity, intracellular HbS concentration, pH, osmolarity, and oxygenation/deoxygenation. Interestingly, polymers form in less than 20% of sickle erythrocytes because the transit time through the capillary bed is shorter than the time required to form polymer. Factors that increase the exposure of sickle hemoglobin to low oxygen tension (< 75 mmHg) will increase the likelihood of polymer formation. Therefore the ability to evaluate factors that lead to hypoxemia and predispose individuals with sickle cell anemia to vaso-occlusive crises is important.

II. Measurements of Oxygenation

In practice, the noninvasive measurement of oxyhemoglobin saturation with pulse oximetry is used as a means to predict Pa_{O_2}. Studies in healthy individuals have demonstrated a close agreement between hemoglobin oxygen saturation measurements by pulse oximetry and arterial blood gas values (3,4). However, there is greater error in these measurements in patients with sickle hemoglobin. Craft et al. found that pulse oximetry had a mean bias of 6.9% compared to arterial oxygen saturation measured by co-oximeter (5). This bias increased at pulse oximetry values less than 95% (mean bias 7.2%; 95% CI 3.0% to 11.4%). Carboxyhemoglobin accounted for most of this error. An oxygen saturation less than 90% implies a $Pa_{O_2} < 60$ mmHg. In patients with sickle hemoglobin, the oxyhemoglobin curve tends to be right-shifted and the upper portion of the dissociation curve is slow-rising. The Pa_{O_2} at which hemoglobin is 50% saturated with oxygen (P_{50}) is 42 to 56 mmHg in sickle cell patients (6), with HbS as compared with a P_{50} of 26.5 mmHg seen in the general population with HbA. Therefore, the partial pressure of oxygen in those patients could be normal (> 80 mmHg). This may explain why pulse oximetry is not a good predictor of hypoxemia and risk of acute vaso-occlusive crises. While patient monitoring may be more difficult, these data suggest that Pa_{O_2} is likely to be a better predictor of the VOC process, since the risk of polymerization of sickle hemoglobin is higher at $Pa_{O_2} < 75$ mmHg (7).

Low baseline Pa_{O_2} at rest and awake is a marker of chronic lung disease in patients with sickle cell disease (8). A Pa_{O_2} of ≤ 70 mmHg at rest indicates stage 3 chronic lung disease, defined as pulmonary fibrosis on chest radiograph, a restrictive pattern on pulmonary function testing, and right ventricular enlargement (2). Although data are limited, overnight monitoring of Pa_{O_2} might identify patients at risk for chronic lung disease before baseline awake values are abnormal. It is important to remember that nocturnal oxygen desaturation may not predict lung disease—since, as discussed, the oxyhemoglobin curve of any individual patient is usually not known, and an oxygen saturation of 90% could be associated with a Pa_{O_2} of > 80 mmHg rather than the expected 60 mmHg (9).

III. Nocturnal Hypoxemia

Obstructive sleep apnea syndrome (OSAS) and sleep-related disturbance in ventilation as seen in patients with chronic obstructive lung disease or interstitial lung disease may predispose the patient with sickle cell anemia to hypoxemia during sleep. Over the past decade, several investigators have suggested that VOC disease may result from undetected hypoxemia during sleep. Scharf et al. studied two patients with a history of recurrent VOC disease with overnight polysomnography including electroencephalography (EEG), electromyography (EMG), electro-oculography (EOG), nasal and oral thermistors, abdominal volumetric pressure transduction, pulse oximetry, and TcP_{O_2} monitoring (10). Episodes of desaturation to as low as 55% (average 65% to 70%) in a 10-year-old boy and hypoxemia to an average of 60 mmHg (measured by TcP_{O_2}) were not related to episodes of apnea or hypopnea. The second patient, a 39-year-old man, had profound desaturation events unrelated to apnea and awoke from sleep with painful crises requiring medical intervention. No TcP_{O_2} data were available for this patient. This study did not ascertain the minute ventilation or measure exhaled CO_2 with sleep in either of these patients to indicate if the desaturation events were due to hypoventilation. Although it is intriguing that these authors were able to demonstrate the onset of a VOC episode in one of their two patients during a period of profound hypoxemia, alveolar hypoxia has not been demonstrated to uniformly lead to VOC events (11).

To investigate whether or not sickle cell patients have more oxygen desaturation with sleep than during wakefulness, Castele et al. studied seven patients with moderately severe sickle cell disease (12). Four of these were recovering from sickle cell crises and were in hospital, three were stable and not hospitalized. All had a history of frequent admissions for sickle cell crises and were taking narcotic analgesics. It was hypothesized that a decrease in respiratory drive due to narcotic use would increase the risk of hypoxemia. Although this group of patients taking narcotics was not compared with patients with a similar history of frequent crises while they were not taking narcotics, the authors demonstrated that decreased tidal volumes—not respiratory rates—were associated with increasing hypoxemia (as measured by ear oximetry). As tidal excursions of the rib cage and abdomen decreased to less than 60% maximal, oxygen saturations dropped to less than 90%. With sleep, the patients had an average fall in oxygen saturation nadir by 3.5% to a mean of 86.5% ± 0.9%. Oxygen desaturations were distributed similarly in rapid-eye-movement (REM) and non-REM (NREM) sleep. Only one patient had any apneic episodes, and these were nonobstructive. End-tidal CO_2 (ET_{CO_2}) and minute ventilation were not measured. This study did not address whether changes in oxygen saturation with sleep predict risk of acute or chronic lung disease.

Brooks et al. found that nocturnal oxygen desaturation did not correlate with frequency of VOC episodes (13). Using overnight polysomnography, they studied 11 "severe" patients with two or more hospitalizations in the previous year for painful crises and eight "mild" patients with no hospitalizations in the preceding year. There was no difference in the median oxyhemoglobin saturation between the two groups (mild 90.5% ± 5.4, severe 93.4% ± 4.0), or oxyhemoglobin saturation nadir (mild 84.6% ± 4.0, severe 84.9% ± 6.8). While the numbers are small, the association of undetected nocturnal hypoxemia with severity of disease could not be found, and trends were actually in the opposite direction of what would be predicted. It is possible that the degree of hypoxemia recorded in these patients was too mild to be the cause of VOC events. Again, concern about the ability of the pulse oximeter to detect hypoxemia may explain the lack of correlation.

IV. Obstructive Sleep Apnea

Investigators have pursued OSA as an etiology for desaturation events during sleep, since young children with enlarged tonsils and adenoids can have profound hypoxemia as a result of OSA. Patients with sickle cell anemia may be at increased risk of airway obstruction due to a compensatory hyperplasia of tonsils and adenoids following splenic infarction, reactive enlargement due to repeated infections with encapsulated organisms, and increased hematopoietic needs because of the hemolytic anemia (14–17). In children with sickle cell disease, OSA with desaturation might then predispose these patients to vaso-occlusive crises. In 1988 Sidman et al. (18) reported the case of a 12-year-old girl with sickle cell disease who had been hospitalized 30 times for vaso-occlusive events since infancy. In the preceding 12 months she had been hospitalized every 2 weeks. She also snored and had episodes of apnea during sleep as well as daytime somnolence. Her overnight polysomnogram showed oxygen desaturations from 97% to 78%, associated with periods of paradoxical respirations and apnea. She had a tonsillectomy and adenoidectomy, and within 2 weeks of surgery, snoring ceased. A polysomnogram 3 months after surgery revealed normal oxygen saturations and no obstructive apneas. For 2 years following surgery, she had no VOC episodes and no hospitalizations. The authors speculated that the patient's frequent vaso-occlusive crises were due to repeated oxygen desaturations as a result of OSA. However, a study by Brooks et al. of 28 children with sickle cell disease found that there were no differences in the respiratory disturbance index or hemoglobin desaturation between the mild and severe sickle cell patients studied (13).

Of 400 patients followed in the Sickle Cell Center of Southern Louisiana, Maddern and his colleagues found 21 individuals with OSA, based on history, symptoms, physical exam, and polysomnography (ages 2 to 21 years) (14). Thirteen of these patients agreed to surgery. Following tonsillectomy and adenoidectomy, all had resolution of symptoms, including snoring, sleep disturbance, and restlessness. School attendance and performance also improved. By polysomnography, there was a decrease in ET_{CO_2} and number of apneas > 10 sec. However, while the mean number of apneas was 7.2/hr preoperatively, this did not change significantly postoperatively. In addition, neither oxygen saturation nor transcutaneous O_2 changed preoperatively to postoperatively. Of the four patients who refused surgery and had repeat polysomnograms more than 1 year later, three improved spontaneously, and one had worsening findings as defined by ET_{CO_2} measurements. There were no data regarding the frequency of VOC crises in the pre- or postoperative period for these patients.

The most complete study to date is that of Samuels et al. (19). They studied 53 children over 20 months old with sickle cell disease who were attending the Central Middlesex Hospital pediatric hematology clinic. All had a clinical assessment for upper-airway obstruction and a sleep study. They were compared to 50 age-matched controls, half of whom were Afro-Caribbean and half who were Caucasian. Of the 53 sickle cell patients, 29 (55%) had history and exams suggestive of obstructive sleep apnea. Of the sickle cell patients, 18 (36%) had sleep-related upper-airway obstruction, 14 were suspected to have OSA by screening, but 4 were from the 24 patients with sickle cell disease considered not to have OSA by history and physical (8%). Of the 18 patients, 13 with OSA had normal oxygen saturations during sleep. The remaining 5 had low baseline oxygen saturations (88% to 94%) asleep. Four of these had episodic desaturations from their baseline, which improved after tonsillectomy and adenoidectomy. Postoperatively, the mean baseline oxygen saturation improved in the 15 patients studied. This study provides useful data regarding the incidence of OSAS in children with sickle cell disease with a positive history and exam (34%). But it also demonstrates that routine screening may miss sickle cell individuals with OSAS (8%). Of importance, snoring and large tonsils in children with sickle cell disease do not predict who will have oxygen desaturation. As discussed previously, there are limitations of the pulse oximeter to adequately define hypoxemia ($Pa_{O_2} \leq 70$ mmHg). Unfortunately, the authors did not collect information regarding VOC episodes in their patients in an effort to correlate polysomnographic findings with frequency of crises or their resolution with surgical intervention for OSA.

The consequences of OSAS can be devastating to patients with sickle cell anemia; stroke has been reported in several cases in the literature (17,20), and it may contribute to recurrent VOC episodes (18). Diagnosis and treatment of OSAS are important in these patients, just as in otherwise healthy children, although data so far have not supported a strong correlation between OSAS and VOC events. Nonetheless, the possibility that OSAS and episodic hypoxemia are associated with painful crises and stroke in some patients with sickle cell disease makes it essential that we at least consider the diagnosis.

V. Interventions

OSA in patients with sickle hemoglobin should be treated surgically. Besides the benefits of relieving upper-airway obstruction, tonsillectomy may also reduce the incidence of complications from recurrent pneumococcal infections, since the tonsils of individuals with sickle cell anemia almost invariably harbor *Streptococcus pneumoniae* (15). Perioperative management is controversial. Because of the intraoperative risk of anemia and hypoxemia, some advocate preoperative transfusion to increase the hematocrit to a minimum of 35% and the ratio of HbA to HbS at least 60:40 (14,21). Halvorson et al. found that in 75 patients with sickle cell disease undergoing elective tonsillectomy, postoperative complications were increased if the preoperative HbS was greater than 40% or the patient was less than 4 years old (22). The requirement of transfusion therapy prior to adenotonsillectomy is by no means universal (21). One center has had success with perioperative attention to hydration, temperature, and oxygen monitoring without the need for exchange transfusion (19). Intravenous hydration and penicillin prophylaxis are also given (14,23). Postoperative management includes intravenous fluid, supplemental oxygen, pain medications, and sedation as needed. While narcotics may increase the risk of hypoventilation and thus hypoxemia, some authors suggest that adequate analgesia may actually decrease the risk of splinting due to pain and thus increase oxygen saturation (24).

There are no data to support the use of continuous nocturnal oxygen to decrease the risk of VOC crises in patients with episodic or baseline oxygen desaturation associated with sleep. Several studies have shown little correlation between frequency of sickle cell crises and oxygen desaturation (8,12,13). This may be more a reflection of poor predictability of the pulse oximeter to detect hypoxemia ($Pa_{O_2} < 75$ mmHg) in patients with sickle hemoglobin. Since too much oxygen can decrease the release of erythropoietin (25), supplemental oxygen may actually worsen the anemia. Supplemental oxygen therapy should not be initiated on the basis of pulse oximetry data alone. Further study of supplemental oxygen as a therapy for nocturnal oxygen desaturation is warranted to determine the risks/benefits to patients with sickle cell disease in the outpatient setting.

Promising new therapies to inhibit sickling and increase oxygen-carrying capacity in patients with sickle hemoglobin include induction of fetal hemoglobin synthesis, reduction of the intracellular hemoglobin concentration [high mean cell hemoglobin content (MCHC) is associated with increased polymerization], and chemical inhibition of HbS polymerization (26). The effect of these inhibitors of sickling on nocturnal oxygen desaturation or hypoxemia ($Pa_{O_2} < 75$ mmHg) has not been studied but would be important to evaluate.

VI. Future Directions

Although sickle cell disease is associated with severe acute and chronic respiratory illness, we clearly do not have sufficient information to correlate hemoglobin unsaturation that may occur during sleep with disease severity in individuals with sickle cell anemia. This may reflect the modifying influences of HbF concentrations, state of erythrocyte dehydration, or tissue bed acidosis. In addition, we are not able to directly measure tissue hypoxia, where polymerization of sickle hemoglobin is most likely to occur. Noninvasive measurement of arterial oxygen desaturation by pulse oximetry does not predict partial pressure of oxygen due to the right shift of the sickle oxyhemoglobin curve. It is the Pa_{O_2} that predicts polymerization of sickle hemoglobin, the development of chronic lung disease, and pulmonary hypertension. Studies are needed to measure Pa_{O_2} directly as a means to better predict those patients at risk. The benefits of supplemental oxygen therapy to prevent sickling crises based on a low baseline oxygen saturation have not yet been demonstrated. Since oxygen therapy could worsen anemia, further study of the benefits and risks of this therapy is required before it can be recommended in the outpatient setting.

As with all children, the presence or absence of snoring and large tonsils in children with sickle cell disease does not predict who will have obstructive sleep apnea (19). Polysomnography is therefore necessary to confirm OSA. Certainly, individuals with documented OSA should be offered interventions to relieve the obstruction, as in any child with OSA. Careful perioperative management of these patients is necessary owing to their increased risk of sickling crises under anesthesia. Further studies to evaluate the impact of diagnosis and treatment of OSA on the frequency of VOC events needs to be designed.

References

1. Platt OS, Thorington BD, Brambilla DJ, Milner PF, Rosse WF, Vichinsky E, Kinney TR. Pain in sickle cell disease: rates and risk factors (see comments). N Engl J Med 1991; 325:11–16.
2. Powars D, Weidman JA, Odom-Maryon T, Niland JC, Johnson C. Sickle cell chronic lung disease: prior morbidity and the risk of pulmonary failure. Medicine (Baltimore) 1988; 67:66–76.
3. Cahan C, Decker MJ, Hoekje PL, Strohl KP. Agreement between noninvasive oximetric values for oxygen saturation. Chest 1990; 97:814–819.
4. Ross RR, Helms PJ. Comparative accuracy of pulse oximetry and transcutaneous oxygen in assessing arterial saturation in pediatric intensive care. Crit Care Med 1990; 18: 725–727.

5. Craft JA, Alessandrini E, Kenney LB, Klein B, Bray G, Luban NL, Meek R, Nadkarni VM. Comparison of oxygenation measurements in pediatric patients during sickle cell crises. J Pediatr 1994; 124:93–95.
6. Seakins M, Gibbs WN, Milner PF, Bertles JF. Erythrocyte Hb-S concentration: an important factor in the low oxygen affinity of blood in sickle cell anemia. J Clin Invest 1973; 52:422–432.
7. Johnson CS, Verdegen TD. Pulmonary complications of sickle cell disease. Semin Respir Med 1988; 9:287–296.
8. Homi J, Levee L, Higgs D, Thomas P, Serjeant G. Pulse oximetry in a cohort study of sickle cell disease. Clin Lab Haematol 1997; 19:17–22.
9. Bromberg PA, Jensen WN. Arterial oxygen unsaturation in sickle cell disease. Am Rev Resp Dis 1967; 96:400–407.
10. Scharf MB, Lobel JS, Caldwell E, Cameron BF, Kramer M, De Marchis J, Paine C. Nocturnal oxygen desaturation in patients with sickle cell anemia. JAMA 1983; 249: 1753–1755.
11. Mahony BS, Githens JH. Sickling crises and altitude: occurrence in the Colorado patient population. Clin Pediatr (Phila) 1979; 18:431–438.
12. Castele RJ, Strohl KP, Chester CS, Brittenham GM, Harris JW. Oxygen saturation with sleep in patients with sickle cell disease. Arch Intern Med 1986; 146:722–725.
13. Brooks LJ, Koziol SM, Chiarucci KM, Berman BW. Does sleep-disordered breathing contribute to the clinical severity of sickle cell anemia? (see comments). J Pediatr Hematol Oncol 1996; 18:135–139.
14. Maddern BR, Reed HT, Ohene-Frempong K, Beckerman RC. Obstructive sleep apnea syndrome in sickle cell disease. Ann Otol Rhinol Laryngol 1989; 98:174–178.
15. Ajulo SO. The significance of recurrent tonsillitis in sickle cell disease. Clin Otolaryngol 1994; 19:230–233.
16. Wittig RM, Roth T, Keenum AJ, Sarnaik S. Snoring, daytime sleepiness, and sickle cell anemia (letter). Am J Dis Child 1988; 142:589.
17. Davies SC, Stebbens VA, Samuels MP, Southall DP. Upper airways obstruction and cerebrovascular accident in children with sickle cell anaemia (letter). Lancet 1989; 2:283–284.
18. Sidman JD, Fry TL. Exacerbation of sickle cell disease by obstructive sleep apnea. Arch Otolaryngol Head Neck Surg 1988; 114:916–917.
19. Samuels MP, Stebbens VA, Davies SC, Picton-Jones E, Southall DP. Sleep related upper airway obstruction and hypoxaemia in sickle cell disease (see comments). Arch Dis Child 1992; 67:925–929.
20. Robertson PL, Aldrich MS, Hanash SM, Goldstein GW. Stroke associated with obstructive sleep apnea in a child with sickle cell anemia. Ann Neurol 1988; 23:614–616.
21. Derkay CS, Bray G, Milmoe GJ, Grundfast KM. Adenotonsillectomy in children with sickle cell disease. South Med J 1991; 84:205–208.
22. Halvorson DJ, McKie V, McKie K, Ashmore PE, Porubsky ES. Sickle cell disease and tonsillectomy: preoperative management and postoperative complications. Arch Otolaryngol Head Neck Surg 1997; 123:689–692.
23. Ijaduola GT, Akinyanju OO. Chronic tonsillitis, tonsillectomy and sickle cell crises. J Laryngol Otol 1987; 101:467–470.
24. Yaster M, Tobin JR, Billett C, Casella JF, Dover G. Epidural analgesia in the management of severe vaso-occlusive sickle cell crisis. Pediatrics 1994; 93:310–315.

25. Embury SH, Garcia JF, Mohandas N, Pennathur-Das R, Clark MR. Effects of oxygen inhalation on endogenous erythropoietin kinetics, erythropoiesis, and properties of blood cells in sickle-cell anemia. N Engl J Med 1984; 311:291–295.
26. Hillery CA. Potential therapeutic approaches for the treatment of vaso-occlusion in sickle cell disease. Curr Opin Hematol 1998; 5:151–155.

Part Five

TECHNOLOGICAL ADVANCES IN DIAGNOSIS AND MANAGEMENT

34

Establishing and Running a Pediatric Sleep Laboratory

ROBERT T. BROUILLETTE and ANGELA MORIELLI

McGill University Health Center
and Montreal Children's Hospital
Montreal, Quebec, Canada

KAREN A. WATERS

The New Children's Hospital
Parramatta, New South Wales, Australia

I. Introduction

Pediatric sleep laboratories provide a setting for obtaining valuable information about the sleep and breathing during sleep of infants and children. There are marked changes in the physiology of sleep and breathing during sleep from the neonatal period through adolescence (1). The information obtained by a sleep study can be used for the initial diagnosis of sleep-related disorders, to establish or adjust certain treatments, and/or to investigate basic or clinical aspects of respiratory and sleep physiology.

In 1996, the American Thoracic Society published a statement entitled "Standards and Indications for Cardiopulmonary Sleep Studies in Children" that is reproduced as an Appendix to this book. This comprehensive document summarizes substantial information regarding pediatric polysomnography. This chapter takes a broader view, attempting to place the pediatric sleep laboratory in context within the medical care delivery system. Our focus is a practical one, addressing issues that are important in establishing and running a pediatric sleep laboratory. Those seriously contemplating establishing such a laboratory would be well advised to contact experienced individuals for guidance and support.

II. Mission Statement

In first planning a pediatric sleep laboratory, it is essential to establish what functions that laboratory will incorporate. Defining the unit's goals, standards, and areas of competency in a mission statement will give focus to the planning of all subsequent aspects of the laboratory. Such focus will facilitate decisions about patient population, clinical and/or research studies, the roles of the laboratory personnel, sources of financial support, and access to affiliated services.

One must first decide what types of patients will be evaluated in the laboratory. Will the laboratory deal exclusively with the evaluation of breathing disorders during sleep or will it also deal with primary sleep disorders such as parasomnias and insomnia? The many chapters in this textbook attest to the wide range of sleep and breathing disorders that affect infants and children, but individual laboratories are not obliged to manage all of these disorders. What clinical populations will be served? Will the laboratory provide diagnostic information for a pediatric pulmonary division, thereby requiring competency in dealing with a wide variety of pediatric respiratory disorders? Will the laboratory be associated with a program for evaluation and treatment of infantile apnea or with a neonatal intensive care unit and thus require expertise in dealing with infants? Will the focus of the laboratory be exclusively clinical, or will it also include research and teaching components?

The establishment of the sleep laboratory will require extensive funding. How will sufficient funds be generated to maintain equipment, purchase supplies, and pay personnel required for laboratory functioning? How will the initial capital investment necessary for the laboratory be financed? If research activities are envisioned, how will these activities be funded?

The answers to these questions vary across institutions and over time. The diversity of pediatric sleep-related diseases dictates that some laboratories will develop expertise in several areas rather than trying to manage all potential referrals. The primary activity of the sleep laboratory will also dictate the need for affiliated services. If the laboratory is to evaluate breathing disorders during sleep in children, close association with a pediatric respiratory division, otolaryngologists, and general pediatricians is essential. When feasible, we believe that a pediatric sleep laboratory situated within a children's hospital, with access to a wide variety of specialists, is optimal.

III. Types of Studies

The types of studies that a sleep lab should be capable of performing vary from simple two-channel recordings to complex and comprehensive in-laboratory studies that include electroencephalograms (EEGs) (Table 1). Complete in-laboratory nocturnal polysomnography, including EEGs to document sleep state, remains the most accurate and comprehensive method of assessing sleep-related abnormalities. Details of the standards and indications for such studies are given in the American Thoracic So-

Table 1 Types of Studies Performed in Pediatric Sleep Laboratories

Comprehensive in-laboratory nocturnal PSG with EEGs and audiovisual recording
Cardiorespiratory sleep study without EEG—in laboratory, at home, or on a hospital ward
Nap sleep studies ± EEG—infant only
Event recording/documented monitoring ± oximetry
Oximetry screening (hospital, home) ± $tcCO_2$
Ventilatory and arousal response testing
Two- to four-channel pneumogram (respiratory effort by impedance), ECG/heart rate, ± SaO_2 ± thermistor, ± $tcpCO_2$
Multiple sleep latency test (MSLT)
Maintenance of wakefulness testing (MWT)

PSG, polysomnography; EEG, electroencephalogram; tcp_{CO_2}, transcutaneous carbon dioxide level; ECG, electrocardiogram.

ciety's statement. The type of study performed should be guided by the questions being asked. It is necessary to have a clear understanding of these questions so that the technician responsible for performing the study knows what to look for. Montages similar to those represented in Table 2 can be applied for many sleep related respiratory control problems. However, in some special cases, quantitative airflow and tidal volume, esophageal pressure, or esophageal pH monitoring must also be obtained.

Polysomnography (PSG) in the home and other abbreviated techniques for the evaluation of breathing disorders during sleep are covered in Chapter 35. Briefly, cardiorespiratory sleep studies without EEGs are simpler to perform and easier to analyze, but they do not provide sleep state–specific information (2,3). Nap studies can sometimes be useful in infants who normally sleep during the day; EEGs should be applied depending on the type of information required. However, such studies should not be performed after pharmacological sedation or after sleep deprivation, because these interventions may induce apnea and impair arousal responses (4–6). A positive nap study can be beneficial to guide treatment decisions. A negative nap study is of limited usefulness because it may not include REM sleep (or sufficient REM sleep) and circadian influences are inappropriately timed to be relevant during a daytime evaluation. In infants, two-channel recordings of respiratory efforts (impedance) and heart rate can still be useful for documentation of central apnea, particularly when accompanied by oximetry and a measure of arterial carbon dioxide levels (P_{CO_2}). However, such studies are not predictive for sudden infant death syndrome (SIDS) and should not be used to assess the risk of SIDS in an individual infant (7–9). Ventilatory and arousal responsc tcsting can be particularly useful in evaluating patients with central hypoventilation syndrome and other disorders of cardiorespiratory control (10).

Technical requirements include the assessment of sleep versus wakefulness, the quantification of individual respiratory events, and the means to evaluate blood gas status. To evaluate sleep quality, sleep must first be distinguished from wakefulness

Table 2 Typical Recording Montages for Comprehensive In-Laboratory Polysomnography and At-Home or On-Ward Cardiorespiratory Sleep Studies[a]

	In-laboratory PSG	At-home or on-ward cardiorespiratory sleep studies
Respiratory effort	Diaphragmatic EMG Intercostal EMG Abdominal EMG RIP abdomen and thorax	RIP abdomen and thorax
Respiratory flow	RIP sum, nasal CO_2, thermistor	RIP sum
Sleep state/arousal	EEG Submental EMG EOGs Audiovisual recording	Audiovisual and cardiorespiratory channels for sleep versus wakefulness and movement arousals
Cardiac	ECG Heart rate	ECG Heart rate
Position, breathing sounds	Audiovisual recording Position sensor	Audiovisual recordings
Oxygenation	Sa_{O_2} and pulse waveform Transcutaneous oxygen	Sa_{O_2} and pulse waveform
Alveolar ventilation	$tcpCO_2$ and/or end-tidal CO_2	$tcpCO_2$
Others (as needed)	Esophageal pH, esophageal pressure, quantitative airflow, and tidal volume	

[a]From Montreal Children's Hospital.

PSG, polysomnography; EMG, electromyography; RIP, respiratory inductive plethysmography; EEG, electroencephalogram; EOG, electro-oculogram; ECG, electrocardiogram; $tcpCO_2$, transcutaneous carbon dioxide level.

(3). Further distinction of sleep state requires a minimum of two EEG channels, two eye movement channels, and a measure of postural muscle activity [usually submental electromyography (EMG)]. With this type of EEG recording montage, rapid-eye-movement (REM) or active sleep can be distinguished from non-REM (NREM) or quiet sleep. EEG recordings show low-amplitude, mixed frequency activity in the former and high-amplitude, low-frequency activity in the latter (11,12). During infancy, video data or direct observational information is essential to make a clear assessment of sleep-wake state, because the relative immaturity of the EEG does not always allow distinction between quiet wakefulness and REM or light sleep stages. Audiovisual recordings for documentation of nocturnal behavior, including parasomnias, can also be very useful. Complex neurological setups such as an extensive 12-lead EEG can be applied in laboratories with a specific neurological interest for the assessment of seizures during sleep. Facilities and staffing expertise for performing multiple sleep latency or maintenance of wakefulness tests are particularly valuable in adolescent patients with excessive daytime sleepiness.

IV. Practical Considerations for Pediatric Polysomnography

Polygraphic equipment provides multichannel amplification, filtering, and recording of data from a variety of physiological variables during sleep. The types of disorders predominantly seen, and whether the laboratory has a "high-throughput, diagnostic" emphasis or a "high-quality, research-oriented" strategy will influence the equipment required for monitoring. This distinction will determine whether the complexity of the data will be preferentially minimized, as in the former category, or maximized, as in the latter. Polysomnography equipment should be capable of digital data acquisition and storage; computer technology has advanced to the point that any new laboratory should not purchase analogue paper-recording systems. Automated data analysis has not reached the level of accuracy required for pediatric studies, and all overnight sleep studies performed in infants or children require epoch-by-epoch analysis by a trained technician.

Audiovisual recording of the patient during polysomnography can be helpful in documenting sleep position, head position, abnormal breath sounds, and behavior. In particular, it can give the physician reporting the study helpful data that is complementary to the physiological parameters recorded on standard polysomnographs. Digital video technology is on the verge of portable and widespread applications. The optimal system would seamlessly integrate audiovisual and physiological data. An essential minimum is to be able to match audiovisual and physiological data files within 1 sec. Table 2 gives the standard recording montages for in-laboratory and home polysomnography as used at Montreal Children's Hospital.

Evaluation of respiratory status during sleep must include scoring of discrete events, noninvasively documenting the state-specific blood gas levels, and quantitating partial airway obstruction. Respiratory inductance plethysmography is currently the most accurate means of monitoring respiratory efforts because, when calibrated, this technique provides a signal proportional to tidal volume (13,14). Sensitive pressure transducers, thermistors, thermocouples, or end-tidal CO_2 can assess airflow at the oronasal airway. The outcome of the respiratory efforts and airflow is reflected in the adequacy of gas exchange as noninvasively assessed using oxygen saturation (Sa_{O_2}) plus either transcutaneous and/or end-tidal P_{CO_2} measurements (15–17). Infants and children often sleep despite the presence of upper airway obstruction; sleep-related upper airway obstruction in this age group is sometimes characterized by prolonged periods of partial obstrution that may be associated with abnormal gas exchange but without any discrete "scorable" events. However, it is exceptional for a child to demonstrate this form of prolonged partial obstruction without going on to develop some discrete obstructive events during REM sleep, when the tone of the upper airway muscle falls. Upper airway resistance syndrome has been defined as sleep-related, prolonged partial airway obstruction without discrete apneas or hypopneas that impair a child's health (18,19). Whether upper airway resistance syndrome exists and how it should be defined require further study. Analysis of a pediatric PSG study will also require definitions for scoring arousals that are applicable to children. It is important to recognize that different laboratories have used different techniques. Furthermore, there is relatively little data available on spontaneous and apnea-induced arousals in normal children or in those with respiratory control disorders. Simultaneous measurements of respiratory effort and airflow, gas exchange, and sleep state therefore elucidate the variations in breathing across sleep states and quantitate the sleep disturbance caused by abnormal breathing.

V. Implementation and Evaluation of Treatment

Complete management of pediatric sleep disorders involves the ability to implement appropriate treatments. Although adenotonsillectomy is the treatment of choice for childhood obstructive sleep apnea (OSA), OSA increases postoperative complication rates for children undergoing adenotonsillectomy (20,21). Therefore, sleep studies can help in planning the perioperative care of children undergoing adenotonsillectomy for upper airway obstruction. In addition, adenotonsillectomy is occasionally unsuccessful and additional therapy will be required. If surgery fails, the current treatment of choice is usually nasal mask continuous positive airway pressure (CPAP), but ventilatory support may also be required (22–24). Sleep studies should be used to document the persistence of disease postoperatively and to assess the effectiveness of therapy. When first instituted, CPAP levels should be titrated. Treatments should be monitored every 6 to 12 months and changed appropriately as the child grows or other events affect the disease.

Regardless of the frequency of use, a well-formulated team approach will best support the use of respiratory support therapies in the home, including oxygen supplementation, nasal mask CPAP, and noninvasive ventilation. Oxygen supplementation is used in a variety of chronic lung diseases, from the neonatal period for infants with bronchopulmonary dysplasia through to adolescents with inadequate gas exchange due to such diseases as cystic fibrosis (19,25,26). Evaluation of outpatient respiratory therapy, ranging from children whose respiratory failure is adequately treated by CPAP, to those who require a "backup" rate for central apneas, to those who require full respiratory support during sleep periods is best performed in the setting of an overnight sleep study. Nasal mask CPAP may also be used in a variety of contexts, including perioperative airway management for children who have severe OSA. In the case of children with neuromuscular disorders, especially where the lungs have reduced compliance, bilevel devices have been used to provide portable, pressure-cycled respiratory support. Portable, volume-cycle ventilators are available and are the instrument of choice for our laboratories because of the improved stability in gas exchange that is achieved across sleep states and especially because of the limitations of the currently available bilevel devices in young infants and toddlers (27–30). Sleep laboratories with a high involvement in respiratory disorders will therefore need to have access to the use of a variety of these respiratory support devices and their own expertise in their application.

Laboratories undertaking research have an essential role in documenting the changes in sleep-related respiratory disorders during childhood in the context of these very recent treatment strategies. Changes in the natural history of neuromuscular diseases may well be brought about if sleep-associated respiratory failure is successfully treated. Laboratories participating in the advancement of this field of medicine must undertake regular reviews of their treatment outcomes as a means of defining which patient groups are appropriate to receive these high-intensity therapies. Such information will lead to better understanding of the likely risks and outcomes of therapeutic options for breathing and sleep diseases.

VI. Space

The patient's room in a pediatric sleep lab should be a friendly, nonthreatening, environment; therefore it should resemble a child's bedroom. It has been our experience that the sleep study is a more pleasant experience for the child when a parent is nearby. The room should be large enough to allow for an extra cot so that a parent can remain with the child. Recording equipment is ideally situated in a separate room to allow the technician to monitor the progression of the study throughout the night while minimizing disturbance to the child's sleep.

The office space of a pediatric sleep lab should include ample areas for reviewing, scoring, and discussing the results of studies. It is equally important that there be adequate storage space for equipment, supplies, and patient files. Two examples are shown in Figure 1: layout of a one-bed lab (a) and layout of a two-bed lab (b).

Because most sleep studies are performed at night and most analysis and reporting is done during the day, it is frequently possible to utilize the same space differently during the day and at night.

VII. Personnel

Appropriately trained staff is a key factor to a successful pediatric sleep lab. Whether the pediatric population is all or only part of the population served by the laboratory, technicians should be competent in dealing with infants and children under diverse and sometimes stressful circumstances. A full PSG study requires complex lead attachments. The placement of these leads on a toddler who refuses to be approached can be challenging. However, the quality of the final study is totally dependent upon the technical expertise of applying and maintaining these attachments. Pediatric laboratories usually require a dedicated technician for each patient, depending on the nursing needs of the patient and the tasks other than patient care for which the technician is responsible.

The personnel of the sleep laboratory consists of the medical director, chief technician, and sleep laboratory technician(s). It is important for all staff to maintain good interpersonal relations in the performance of their duties. The entire sleep laboratory staff also contribute to the development and maintenance of appropriate rela-

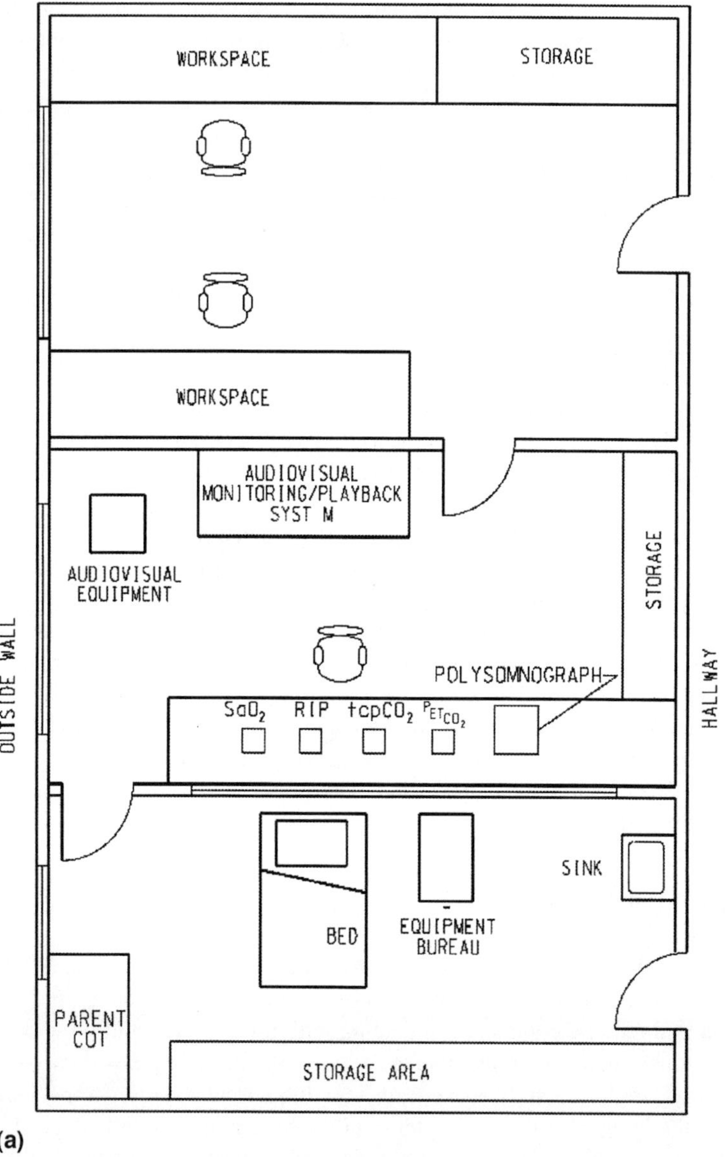

(a)

Figure 1 (a) This layout is an example of a single-bed sleep laboratory setup. The space is divided into three separate areas: office space, control room, and patient bedroom. The control room contains all peripheral monitoring equipment—e.g., pulse oximeter (Sa_{O_2}), transcutaneous monitor ($tcpCO_2$), end-tidal CO_2 monitor (PET_{CO_2}), respiratory inductive plethysmography (RIP); as well as all audiovisual (TV monitor, VCR, audio mixer) and polygraph equipment. There should be portholes between the control room and the patient bedroom in order

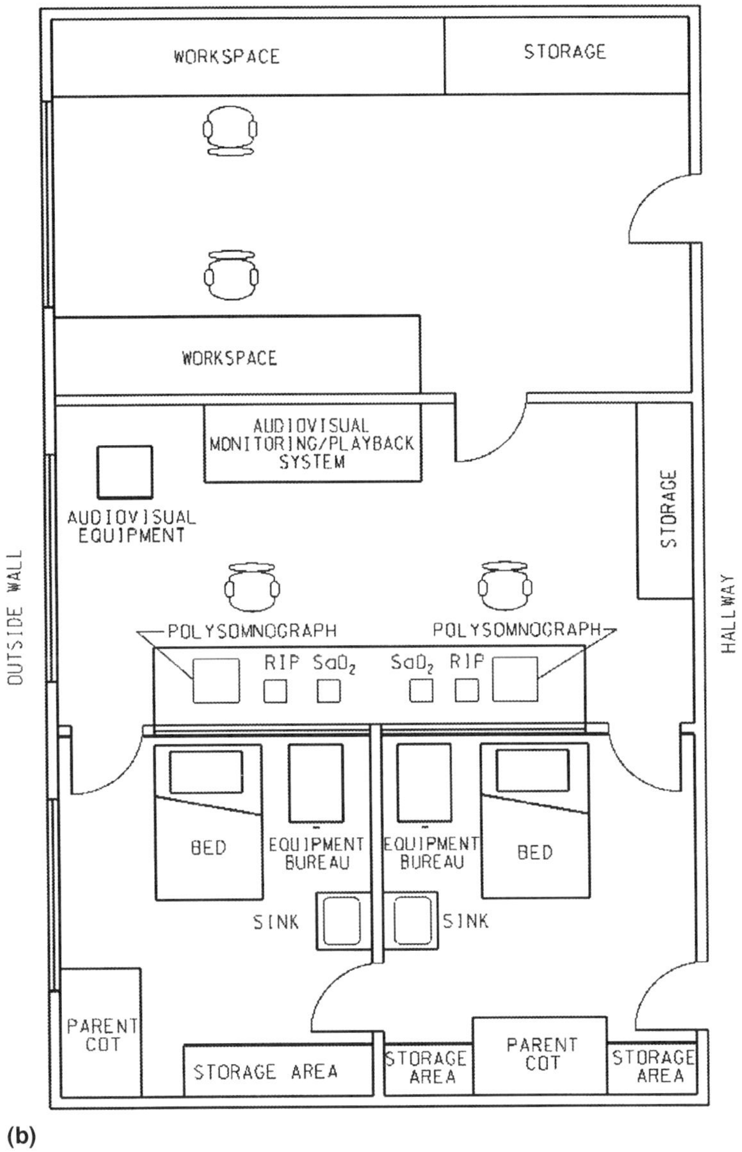

(b)

to run the cables between the peripheral equipment and the patient. The patient bedroom should be equipped with an infrared lighting system; this allows for clear video recordings of the child during sleep. The patient room should also include a TV and VCR to keep the child entertained/distracted during the setup procedure. An emergency crash cart should also be maintained within the sleep laboratory area. (b) This layout demonstrates a two-bed sleep laboratory setup. Please refer to (a) legend for suggested equipment to be kept in each area.

tions with personnel in other departments, hospitals, universities, and associations as required. The opportunity for continuing education should be ensured so as to provide for the growth and development of all staff.

Depending on the size and the patient load of the unit, the following tasks may be shared by more than one person, or one person may have responsibility for more than one designated role. All staff should have access to a policies and procedures manual for the laboratory, as this will facilitate the implementation of specific procedures.

A. Medical Director

The medical director is responsible for the overall management of the laboratory, including formulation of the mission statement and the direction of the staff within the laboratory. This person should have a thorough understanding of pediatric sleep medicine and have good communication, organization, and supervisory skills. A sound technical knowledge will permit the physician to troubleshoot problems in PSG and to provide quality control of the data acquired, scored, and interpreted under his or her supervision.

The physician supervising sleep studies in children must understand the pathophysiological impact that a wide variety of congenital syndromes, malformations, and acquired abnormalities may have on a child. Therefore, requirements for this position include a sound knowledge of the changes that occur in normal sleep physiology (sleep patterns, sleep states, and EEG) with growth and maturation and of the changes in normal respiratory physiology, control, and mechanics during sleep. The sleep physician should be competent in the diagnosis and management of respiratory disorders that are either exclusively sleep-related or exacerbated by the superimposition of sleep physiology. He or she should also have a thorough knowledge of the diverse respiratory support devices (CPAP, bilevel devices, and noninvasive ventilation) and oxygen therapy. Ideally, he or she should have actively participated in the institution of such therapies during his or her training. If the laboratory performs sleep studies for reasons other than possible respiratory control problems, his or her knowledge should encompass the symptomatology and management of nonrespiratory sleep disorders. The physician should acquire and maintain knowledge of the current literature in the field of pediatric sleep medicine.

B. Unit Manager/Chief Technician

The unit manager/chief technician should participate in the development of the mission statement and is the key person involved in implementing all aspects of the sleep unit's program. It is essential that the person occupying this role be trained in sleep laboratory techniques, and have good communication, organization, and supervisory skills. The unit manager/chief technician is responsible for monitoring and reviewing all lab activities, and, where appropriate, makes recommendations for changes that will improve utilization of facilities, services, and staff. The unit manager/chief technician is responsible for the recruitment, hiring, and dismissal of departmental employees as well as making recommendations regarding promotions and allocation of subspecialty tasks.

The unit manager/chief technician must also ensure that the environment is safe for patients and staff and that the unit meets hospital accreditation standards. In collaboration with the medical director, the unit manager/chief technician should develop and implement a quality assurance program for the service. Specific duties include the maintenance of standards of performance, and ensuring that a high quality of testing and analysis is provided by the laboratory, thus ensuring the effectiveness and efficiency of the services provided by the laboratory. The chief technician will formulate and maintain written procedures for the effective day-to-day management of the service. By working with sales and technical representatives dealing with the service, he or she will monitor the development and use of data processing and other technologies and make recommendations for their potential application to the service, dealing with technical problems, and ensuring the implementation and evaluation of new techniques. In association with any nominated educators, this person will be responsible for teaching activities related to students and new staff in the service.

C. Sleep Lab Technician

The sleep lab technician performs testing of patients referred to the sleep laboratory. The technicians are directly responsible to the chief technician and therefore the medical director. The technician is also responsible for relaying pertinent patient information to the appropriate medical personnel. It will be essential for staff in this role to have had some experience in dealing with children in a medical setting. Currently, there are few technician training programs in pediatric sleep medicine or sleep-related breathing disorders; therefore, each laboratory will determine the specific selection of prerequisite experience or qualifications as it recruits new staff. Useful skills will include prior experience in pediatric respiratory therapy or nursing, relevant clinical and/or research experience, and work with computerized data acquisition systems. A basic understanding of the importance and maintenance of properly calibrated equipment is important. It is also essential that the technician have good patient/parent communication skills.

As a member of the sleep laboratory team, the technicians participate in the diagnostic, therapeutic, and treatment aspects of this clinical service, family support program, and clinical research program. The sleep lab technician will set up and analyze patient recordings, obtain pertinent information about the child from the parents, explain the setup of a sleep study to the child and parents, and answer questions when appropriate. He or she will be responsible for setup of the laboratory facilities for daytime and overnight sleep studies as well as remote studies where applicable. His or her skills will therefore include the calibration of all needed equipment and the ability to troubleshoot and correct problems that occur during the course of a study. Sleep technicians will be able to analyze the data obtained during the studies they perform and to discuss the results with appropriate medical staff. The sleep lab technician may participate in clinical research projects related to sleep-disordered breathing.

VIII. Coordinating Treatment of Sleep-Disordered Breathing in Infants and Children

To provide proper and continuous quality of care in infants and children, a designated patient-care coordinator may be required. This person will be required to maintain contact with parents who are under the care of the program, review the service quality, and facilitate access to medical services when the children in the program require acute or additional care. Such responsibilities include coordination care for children on respiratory support, such as home oxygen, nasal mask CPAP, noninvasive ventilation, and ventilation via tracheostomies. Duties in this position will include coordination of the supply of equipment when the child is being prepared for discharge from hospital. In hospital, this may include the fitting of appropriate masks, providing practical information to the parents about where and how they can obtain the requisite equipment, educating the parents in the use of the equipment, and teaching emergency procedures. In addition, the coordinator should ensure that all relevant support is in place, before the child is discharged from hospital.

IX. Communication

The studies performed in the sleep laboratory provide objective data on an infant's or child's sleep and breathing during sleep. To have an impact on the child's health, the results must be communicated to the parents, to the referring physician, and to physicians and surgeons involved in treatment interventions. Accordingly, communication is a key element in the proper functioning of a pediatric sleep laboratory (Fig. 2).

To plan, prioritize and, later, to interpret a sleep study, the sleep lab physician must have data available on the child's chief complaint, signs and symptoms, past medical history, physical exam, and other relevant medical data. A questionnaire completed by the parents at the time of referral provides a solid information base for many patients, and discussions among staff directly involved with patient care can help triage particularly severe cases to avoid prolonged waiting times. For more complex cases, a review of the medical record with particular attention to neurological, pulmonary, cardiac, and otolaryngological problems is instructive regarding the most appropriate type of study to perform and the likelihood of disease. The most relevant physical examination is usually that of the sleeping child. However, the sleep lab physician may not be present during the PSG study. Therefore, the sleep lab technician must act as the eyes and ears of the physician and carefully record all observations. Audiovisual data provide an additional perspective for labs having such a capability. In special circumstances, audiovisual data can also document isolated episodes (such as apparent life-threatening events or seizures) that need diagnostic evaluation.

From time to time, our laboratories discover patients with unanticipated, extremely severe sleep-disordered breathing. In such cases, our technicians are expected to call the sleep lab physician, who must then make a medical judgment: 1) continue

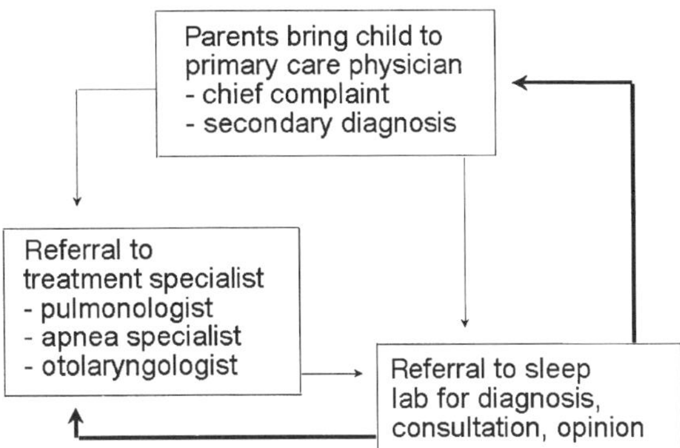

Figure 2 This figure emphasizes the importance of communication in the operation of an effective sleep laboratory.

the diagnostic study; 2) arrange an emergency hospital admission, sometimes to the pediatric intensive care unit; or 3) commence treatment on an urgent basis with nasal mask CPAP or ventilatory support.

Reports of polysomnography results should be sent to the referring physician and, if the local custom dictates, also to the parents. Facilities should be available for urgent review of the study if striking abnormalities are present, and to expedite a preliminary report when required. Such a capability might eventually be facilitated by telemedicine links if the physician is not physically present. In more routine cases, a full report should be sent after the study has been analyzed and interpreted, usually within one to two weeks. Details on polysomnography reporting are given in the ATS statement. Adequate and comprehensive record keeping is an essential element of quality control and research review. The laboratory should maintain ready access to sleep-study reports as well as to the original patient data.

Acknowledgments

The authors thank John Morielli for preparation of the figures and Michele Fortin for secretarial assistance.

References

1. Gaultier C. Cardiorespiratory adaptation during sleep in infants and children. Pediatr Pulmonol 1995; 19:115–117.
2. Morielli A, Ladan S, Ducharme FM, Brouillette RT. Can sleep and wakefulness be distinguished in children by cardiorespiratory and videotape recordings? Chest 1996; 109: 680–687.

3. Jacob SV, Morielli A, Mograss MA, Ducharme FM, Schloss MD, Brouillette RT. Home testing for pediatrics obstruction sleep apnea syndrome secondary to adenotonsillar hypertrophy. Pediatr Pulmonol 1995; 20:241–252.
4. Biban P, Baraldi E, Pettenazzo A, Filippone M, Zacchello F. Adverse effect of chloral hydrate in two young children with obstructive sleep apnea. Pediatrics 1993; 92:461–463.
5. Hershenson M, Brouillette RT, Olsen E, Hunt CE. The effect of chloral hydrate on genioglossus and diaphragmatic activity. Pediatr Res 1984; 186:516.
6. Kahn A, Franco P, Scaillet S. Groswasser J, Dan B. Development of cardiopulmonary integration and the role of arousability from sleep. Curr Opin Pulmonol Med 1997; 3:440–444.
7. Finer NN, Barrington KJ, Hayes B. Prolonged periodic breathing: significance in sleep studies. Pediatrics 1992; 89:450–453.
8. Southall DP, Richards JM, Rhoden KJ, Alexander JR, Shinebourned EA, Arrowsmith WA, Cree JE, Fleming PJ, Goncalves A, Orme R L'E. Prolonged apnea and cardiac arrhythmias in infants discharged from neonatal intensive care units: failure to predict an increased risk for sudden infant death syndrome. Pediatrics 1982; 70:844–851.
9. Kahn A, Reguffat E, Sottiaux M, Blum D. Problems in management of infants with an apparent life-threatening event. Ann NY Acad Sci 1988; 533:78–88.
10. Gozal D. Congenital central hypoventilation syndrome: an update. In press.
11. Rechtschaffen A, Kales A, eds. A Manual of Standardized Terminology, Techniques and Scoring System for Sleep States of Human Subjects. Los Angeles, CA: Brain Information Service/Brain Research Institute, University of California, 1968.
12. Anders T, Emde R, Parmelee A, eds. A Manual of Standardized Terminology, Techniques and Criteria for Scoring of States of Sleep and Wakefulness in Newborn Infants. Los Angeles, CA: Brain Information Service/Brain Research Institute, University of California, 1971.
13. Cantineau JP, Escourrou P, Sartene R, Gaultier C, Goldman M. Accuracy of respiratory inductive plethysmography during wakefulness and sleep in patients with obstructive sleep apnea. Chest 1992; 102:1145–1151.
14. Adams JA, Zabaleta IA, Stroh D, Johnson P, Sackner MA. Tidal volume measurements in newborns using respiratory inductive plethysmography. Am Rev Respir Dis 1993; 148:585–588.
15. Morielli A, Desjardins D, Brouillette RT. Transcutaneous and end-tidal carbon dioxide pressures should be measured during pediatric polysomnography. Am Rev Respir Dis 1993; 148:1599–1604.
16. Hoppenbrouwers T, Hodgman JE, Arakawa K, Durand M, Cabal LA. Transcutaneous oxygen and carbon dioxide during the first half year in premature and normal term infants. Pediatr Res 1992; 31:73–79.
17. Poets CG, Southall DP. Noninvasive monitoring of oxygenation in infants and children: practical considerations and areas of concern. Pediatrics 1994; 93:737–746.
18. Downey R III, Perkin RM, MacQuarrie J. Upper airway resistance syndrome: sick symptomatic but underrecognized. Sleep 1993; 16:620–623.
19. Brouillette RT, Waters KA. Oxygen therapy for pediatric obstructive sleep apnea syndrome: How safe? How effective? Am J Respir Crit Care Med 1996; 153:1–2.
20. Gerber ME, O'Connor DM, Adler E, Myer CM. Selected risk factors in pediatric adenotonsillectomy. Arch Otolaryngol Head Neck Surg 1996; 122:811–814.

21. Rosen GM, Muckle RP, Mahowald MW, Goding GS, Ullevig C. Postoperative respiratory compromise in children with obstructive sleep apnea syndrome: can it be anticipated? Pediatrics 1994; 93:784–788.
22. Guilleminault C, Pelayo R, Clerk A, Leger D, Bocian RC. Home nasal continuous positive airway pressure in infants with sleep-disordered breathing. J Pediatr 1995; 127:905–912.
23. Waters KA, Everett F, Bruderer J, Sullivan CE. Obstructive sleep apnoea: the use of nasal mask CPAP in 80 children. Am J Respir Crit Care Med 1995; 152:780–785.
24. Marcus CL, Davidson Ward SL, Mallory GB, Rosen CL, Beckerman RC, Weese-Mayer DE, Brouillette RT, Trang HT, Brooks LJ. Use of nasal continuous positive airway pressure as treatment of childhood obstructive sleep apnea. J Pediatr 1995; 127:88–94.
25. Abman SH, Groothius JR. Pathophysiology and treatment of bronchopulmonary dysplasia. Pediatr Clin North Am 1994; 41:277–315.
26. Moyermileur LJ, Bielson DW, Pfeffer KD, et al. Eliminating sleep-associated hypoxemia improves growth in infants with bronchopulmonary dysplasia. Pediatrics 1996; 98:779–783.
27. Ellis ER, Bye PTP, Bruderer JW, Sullivan CE. Treatment of respiratory failure during sleep in patients with neuromuscular disease. Am Rev Respir Dis 1987; 135:148–152.
28. Piper AJ, Sullivan CE. Effects of long-term nocturnal nasal ventilation on spontaneous breathing during sleep in neuromuscular and chest wall disorders. Eur Respir J 1996; 9: 1515–1522.
29. Heckmatt JZ, Loh L, Dubowitz V. Night-time nasal ventilation in neuromuscular disease. Lancet 1990; 335:579–582.
30. Manni R, Zucca C, Galimberti CA, Ottolini A, Cerveri I, Bruschi C, Zoia MC, Lanzi G, Tartara A. Nocturnal sleep and oxygen balance in Duchenne muscular dystrophy: a clinical and polygraphic 2-year follow-up study. Eur Arch Psychiatry Clin Neurosci 1991; 240:255–257.

35

Home Monitoring of Sleep and Breathing in Children

SHEILA V. JACOB

Robert Wood Johnson Medical School
University of Medicine and Dentistry of New Jersey
New Brunswick, New Jersey

ROBERT T. BROUILLETTE

McGill University Health Center
and Montreal Children's Hospital
Montreal, Quebec, Canada

I. Introduction

Overnight polysomnography in a sleep laboratory is the most comprehensive method for diagnosing sleep-disordered breathing in children. As such, the testing is expensive and time-consuming. In recent years, several ambulatory systems have been developed to monitor sleep and respiration. This chapter discusses the usefulness of unattended studies, the types of studies that can be done, and the principles of performing cardiorespiratory sleep studies in the home. Infant cardiorespiratory monitoring is discussed elsewhere in this book (Chap. 9); therefore this chapter does not address event recording monitors or infant pneumograms.

There are various indications for performing cardiorespiratory sleep studies in children, the most common being for the diagnosis of obstructive sleep apnea syndrome (OSAS). In children, OSAS is most commonly associated with adenotonsillar hypertrophy (1–3). In the United States, approximately 250,000 tonsillectomies and/or adenoidectomies are performed yearly (4) and OSAS is cited as one indication for as many as 25% of these procedures (5). Many children undergoing adenotonsillectomy have no evaluation of breathing during sleep, the diagnosis and decision for treatment being based on history and a physical examination during wakefulness. This may be due at least in part to difficulty encountered in obtaining tests in a timely fashion and the expense of overnight polysomnography. There also remains a lack of knowledge about childhood sleep-disordered breathing on the part of many primary care physicians and otolaryngologists. As more understanding develops, there should be an increased demand for sleep studies and, as a result, a greater role for unattended recordings done either in a patient's home or on a hospital ward. Other children who could benefit from unattended cardiorespiratory studies include patients with chronic respiratory diseases such as cystic fibrosis and bronchopulmonary dysplasia and those with neuromuscular disease. In such cases, the unattended recordings would most likely be used to rapidly assess severity of illness or document the effectiveness of a treatment. Laboratory polysomnography is more appropriate for full diagnostic studies. The type of unattended study that is appropriate in a given situation depends upon the disease and the questions being asked.

II. Types of Studies

Portable recordings can range from simple one- or two-channel studies (e.g., overnight pulse oximetry) to much more elaborate studies that include electroencephalography (EEG) and electromyography (EMG) in addition to cardiorespiratory channels. Both analogue and digital systems are commercially available for use in the home. While digital systems facilitate analysis, the recording of high-frequency data such as electrocardiography (ECG), EEG, and EMG signals requires a rapid sampling rate and a large memory capacity. It is important to keep in mind that most systems have been developed for the evaluation of OSAS in adults. While the simplest systems may not allow adequate diagnostic studies for OSAS (see below), full polysomnography, which is relatively difficult to perform at home, may not be necessary for the diagnosis of OSAS in otherwise healthy children. If information on other sleep disorders, such as nocturnal seizures or periodic limb movements in sleep (PLMS), is required, comprehensive laboratory polysomnography is necessary.

III. Questionnaire or History

It would be extremely useful if a questionnaire could be developed with sufficient sensitivity and specificity for OSAS that polysomnography or other testing would not be needed. Brouillette and associates reported that an "OSA score" derived from parental reports of obstructive apnea, snoring, and difficulty breathing discriminated well between children with polysomnographically proven OSAS and age- and sex-matched controls from a general pediatric practice (6). However, when used prospectively for children referred to a pediatric sleep laboratory, the OSA score did not perform as well. Subsequently, several other groups have found that, for children referred to a pediatric sleep laboratory, the OSA score and other questionnaire-derived measures are unable to distinguish OSAS reliably from "simple snoring"—i.e., snoring without desaturation, sleep disturbance, or daytime sequelae (7,8).

IV. Actigraphy

In infants, children, and adults, sleep is characterized by a lower activity level than wakefulness. Over the last several years, actigraphy was developed as a practical measure for long-term quantification of sleep/wake and circadian periodicity of movement (9,10). A small motion sensor and digital recorder is worn on a wrist and later downloaded into a computerized analysis system. Advantages include noninvasiveness, ease of use, and automated scoring. Accuracy for sleep-wake discrimination has been reported to be 85 to 93% (9,10). To date, the most promising pediatric work has been in evaluating sleep disturbances in infants and children. Sadeh and associates suggest that actigraphy and parental report may provide complementary information regarding sleep disturbance (11). It remains to be determined if a simple motion sensor could be combined with a simple respiratory sensor and pulse oximeter to produce a diagnostic-quality system for pediatric OSAS.

V. Pulse Oximetry

Pulse oximetry alone is not sufficient to exclude the diagnosis of OSAS because obstructive events in some patients may lead to arousals and sleep disturbance without significant desaturation. Williams and associates found that false negatives were obtained using pulse oximetry alone to screen for OSAS in adults, but that the addition of a clinical score increased its sensitivity as a screening tool (12). Cooper and associates reported that pulse oximetry was effective in diagnosing moderate to severe but not mild OSAS in adults (13). Ryan and associates reported a high specificity but low sensitivity when using pulse oximetry to diagnose OSAS (14). Clinical experience indicates that children with OSAS also have episodes of obstructed respiration that result in arousal but not in significant hypoxemia.

We have found, however, that the use of graphic summaries depicting overnight trends in oxygen as well as individual events can expedite the diagnostic process in certain patients and facilitate rapid treatment. In such cases, a recording pulse oximeter (Nellcor N200) can be used overnight in a patient's home or on a hospital ward, with downloading and analysis of the recording in the sleep laboratory on the following morning. In one study, we documented that desaturation events can be determined as true events versus movement artifact with over 75% accuracy as compared to polysomnography. This study was performed in children being evaluated for OSAS (15). In infants and children, obstructive sleep apnea typically worsens during rapid-eye-movement (REM) sleep. An oximetry trend graph showing clusters of desaturation associated with a clinical history of snoring can document that a child has sufficiently severe sleep-related airway obstruction to cause hypoxemia (Fig. 1a). However, it must be kept in mind that a negative oximetry study can never be used as evidence that a child does not hypoventilate or have sleep disturbance secondary to sleep-disordered breathing (Fig. 1b).

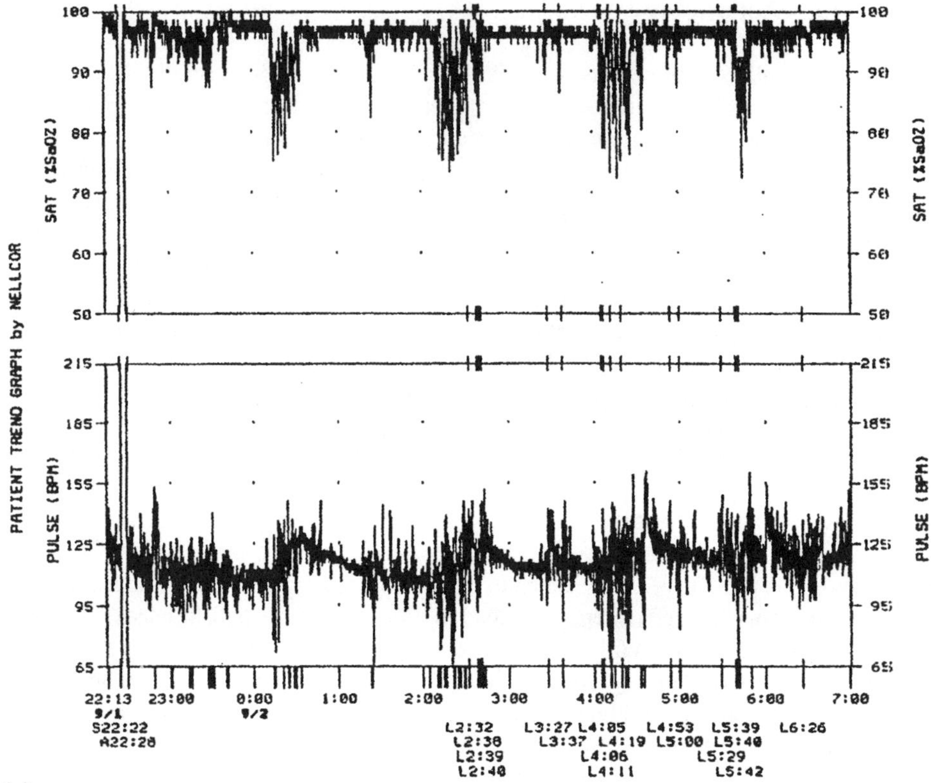

(a)

Figure 1 These three overnight pulse oximetry "trend graphs" demonstrate the diagnostic utility and limitations of pulse oximetry as an abbreviated testing modality for sleep-disordered breathing: (a) Periodic REM sleep–associated hemoglobin desaturation in a 2-year-old girl with large tonsils and adenoids and a typical history for pediatric obstructive sleep apnea syndrome (OSAS)—snoring, difficulty breathing, and obstructive apneas witnessed by parents. (b) A false-negative oximetry trend in a 4-year-old boy with a history suggesting OSAS. Polysomnography revealed an obstructive apnea/hypopnea index of 14 events per hour. (c) Periodic desaturations in a 9-year-old asymptomatic patient with myelomeningocele. Further testing is required to determine the type of sleep-disordered breathing.

The recording of arterial hemoglobin saturation and heart rate alone can be useful in certain clinical settings, as for the evaluation of oxygen requirements in patients with bronchopulmonary dysplasia, cystic fibrosis, or other lung diseases. If the partial pressure of carbon dioxide can be monitored as well, this would allow the diagnosis of hypoventilation in children with neuromuscular diseases. Indeed, in our experience, oximetry can be particularly useful as a rapid testing modality in patients

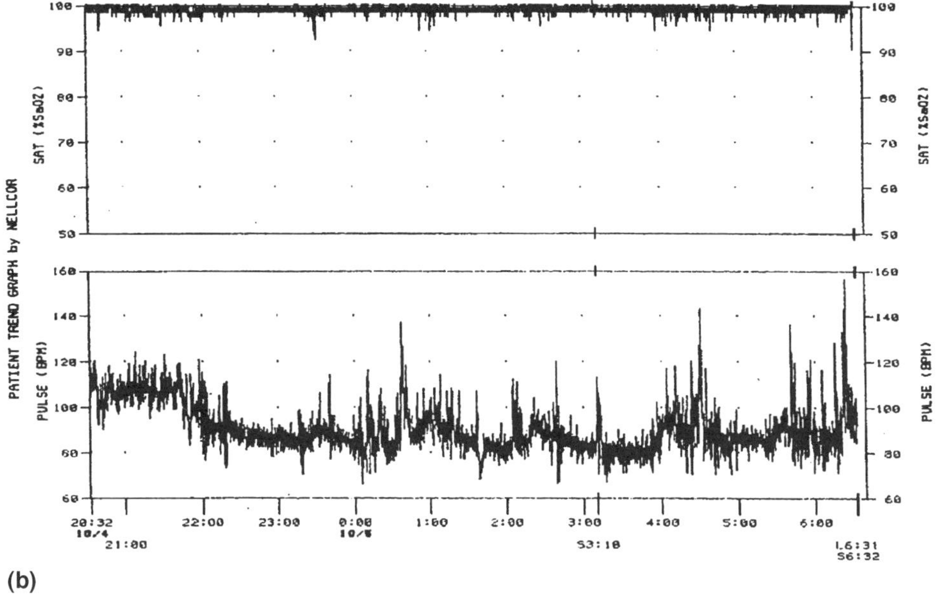

(b)

with neuromuscular weakness and in those with paraplegia due to myelomeningocele. In both of these circumstances, movement artifacts are decreased by the neuromuscular disorder, and the restrictive pulmonary defect results in more rapid hemoglobin desaturation with central or obstructive apnea due to reduced lung stores of oxygen. In our recent series of 83 infants, children, and adolescents with myelomeningocele, pulse oximetry was 100% sensitive in detecting moderate to severe sleep-disordered breathing as compared with full nocturnal polysomnography (16) (Fig. 1c). Patients with positive studies would usually require further testing in the sleep laboratory, depending upon the clinical setting.

VI. Audio and Video Recordings

Lack of arousal data remains a problem in systems using snoring sounds alone or in combination with pulse oximetry. Potsic reported good agreement between polysomnography and sleep sonography for detection of apnea in children with OSAS but found that central and obstructive events could not be differentiated (17). White and associates found that the use of sound recording added to the diagnostic value of pulse oximetry (18). Flemons and Remmers reported preliminary results in adults using a two-step approach based on clinical factors and results from the SnoreSat monitor, which records snoring, oxygen saturation, and body position (19). Such studies may be useful for screening purposes and, if positive, may preclude the need for comprehensive polysomnography in certain cases.

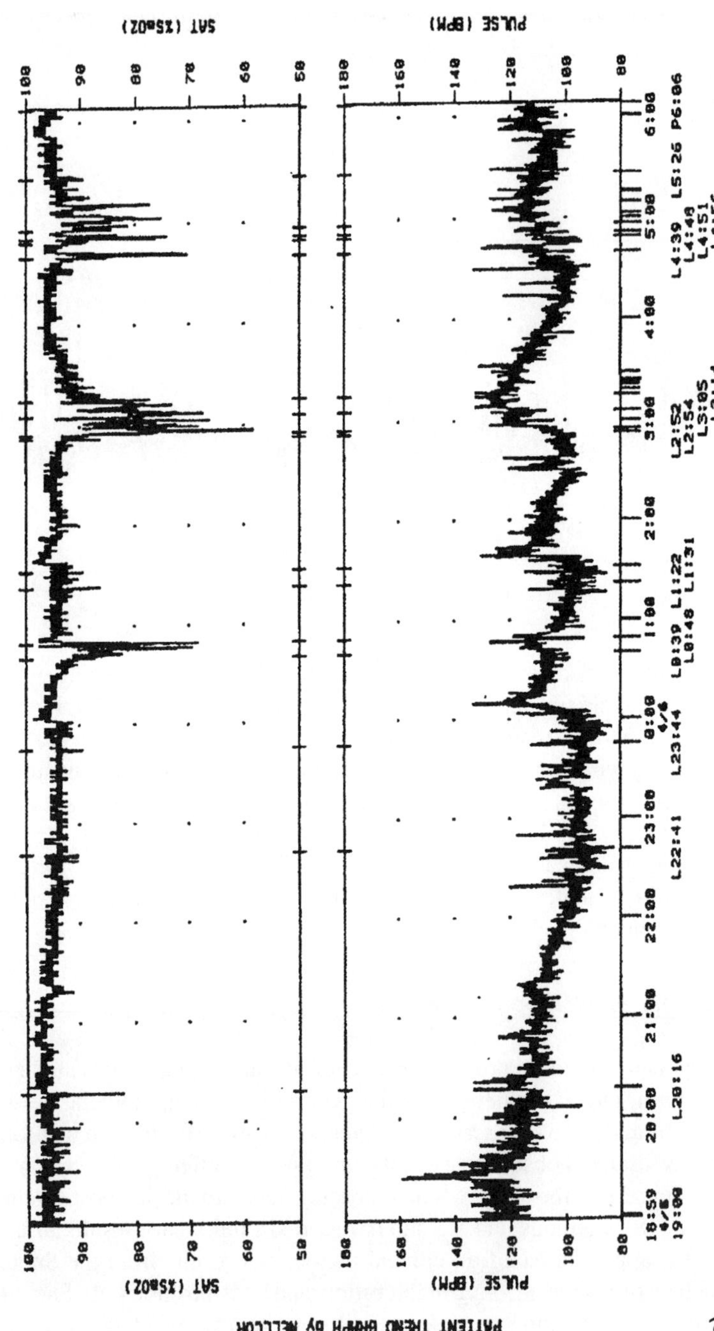

(c)

Figure 1 (Continued)

Video recordings can provide information on arousals as well as sleep position, head position, and interaction with bedding (20). Stradling and associates reported the use of pulse oximetry and a video-based movement detection system to study children before and after tonsillectomy; they found significant improvement in oxygenation and sleep quality postoperatively (21). In another study, Sivan and associates compared the use of 30-min video recordings of a child sleeping at home with conventional polysomnography and found that a scoring system based on the home video recordings yielded good agreement with results of polysomnography (22). However, it is important to be careful when basing conclusions on a recording of a limited portion of the sleep period, as the severity of sleep-disordered breathing may vary through the night.

VII. Multichannel Recordings

As EEG and EMG are not typically recorded in most portable systems, sleep staging may not be possible. In a study involving adults who were being evaluated for OSAS, Douglas et al. found that neurophysiological sleep staging was not essential for diagnosis or management (23). Discrimination of sleep from wakefulness is necessary, however, for an accurate calculation of the apnea/hypopnea index, which is based on total sleep time.

There has been more experience with multichannel home recordings in adults than there has been in children; but validation studies, even in adults, are limited in number. Studies in adults have been reviewed in the consensus statement of the American Thoracic Society and the standards of practice recommendations of the American Sleep Disorders Association (24,25); a few are mentioned here.

Ancoli-Israel and associates compared with Medilog, a system that records chest wall movement, leg movement, and body movement, with conventional polysomnography, and found good agreement for the diagnosis of sleep apnea (26). Guylay and associates assessed the accuracy of a microprocessor-based system (Vitalog PMS-8, Vitalog Corp., CA) that measured chest wall movement, respiratory paradox, saturation, heart rate, and body movement (27). They found that the system allowed detection of patients with sleep-disordered breathing but reported difficulty in classifying respiratory events. Redline and colleagues evaluated a system (Edentec Monitoring System, Model 4700 Scanner, Eden-Prairie, MN) that monitored nasal/oral airflow, chest wall movement, saturation, heart rate, and body movement; they found a high level of agreement with in-hospital polysomnography (28). Stoohs and Guilleminault evaluated the MESAM 4 System (Madaus Medizin Elektronik, Germany) recording saturation, heart rate, snoring, and body position and found that it was able to detect decreases in oxygen saturation accurately, suggesting that it could be useful as a screening device (29). In a recent study, Zucconi and associates compared the use of an unattended recording device (MicroDigitrapper-S, Synetics Medical, Stockholm, Sweden) that measured body position, snoring sound, oronasal flow, thoracic and abdominal effort, heart rate, and oxygen saturation with conventional polysomnography (30). They found good sensitivity and specificity for the diagnosis of OSAS using an apnea/hypopnea index of 10 or greater as a cutoff but found that automatic scoring was insufficient to predict severity.

In children, portable studies can be more challenging than in adults because of the repeated displacement of leads. Among the simplest studies are two-channel recordings that record a qualitative indicator of respiratory effort, such as transthoracic impedance, and electrocardiography. In the United States, studies that rely on impedance to detect respiratory effort are routinely performed in the home, as this technology is inexpensive and relatively easy to use. However, such studies are not adequate for the detection of obstructive apnea (31,32).

One group of investigators have reported results using a complex recording system that recorded, depending upon clinical indication, a combination of the following: respiratory movements, ECG, airflow, transcutaneous P_{O_2} and/or P_{CO_2}; respiratory inductance plethysmography, end-tidal CO_2, EEG, and esophageal manometry (33). This system was used for investigation of cyanotic or apneic episodes and upper-airway obstruction during sleep and was designed to be used either on a hospital ward or in a patient's home. Most of the results reported were obtained on hospitalized patients; in the majority of cases, only four channels of data were recorded. It would probably be impractical to obtain some of the described parameters in a home setting.

VIII. The McGill Cardiorespiratory Video System

In the sleep laboratory at the Montreal Children's Hospital, a portable system consisting of cardiorespiratory and video recordings was developed and validated and is now being used for the diagnosis of OSAS due to adenotonsillar hypertrophy (Figs. 2 and 3) (34–36). Sleep and wakefulness are distinguished using regularity of cardiorespiratory signals and the subject's appearance and sound on the video recording, a method that was found to be 94% accurate when compared to conventional sleep scoring (35). The cardiorespiratory recording consists of ECG, pulse rate, arterial hemoglobin saturation (Sa_{O_2}), pulse waveform, and thoracic and abdominal excursions and their sum as obtained from a respiratory inductive plethysmograph. These channels were chosen for the following reasons: 1) they are suitable for unattended home recording, 2) they allow identification of the essential elements of obstructive sleep apnea syndrome (Table 1), and 3) they do not require craniofacial attachments that might disturb the child's sleep. The signals are recorded on a portable computer and later transferred to a computerized polysomnograph in the sleep laboratory. The sound and appearance of each subject are recorded using a video recorded at super long plan (SLP) speed on T-160 tape, yielding about 9 hr of data. Videotape recordings are later played into a computerized movement detection system that detects and quantifies movements by sampling video signals once per second, subtracting each video frame from the preceding video frame, and calculating a movement amplitude (37) (Sleep-Vision, Martinex, Montreal). A validation study, using conventional polysomnography as reference, showed a good correlation between the home and laboratory stud-

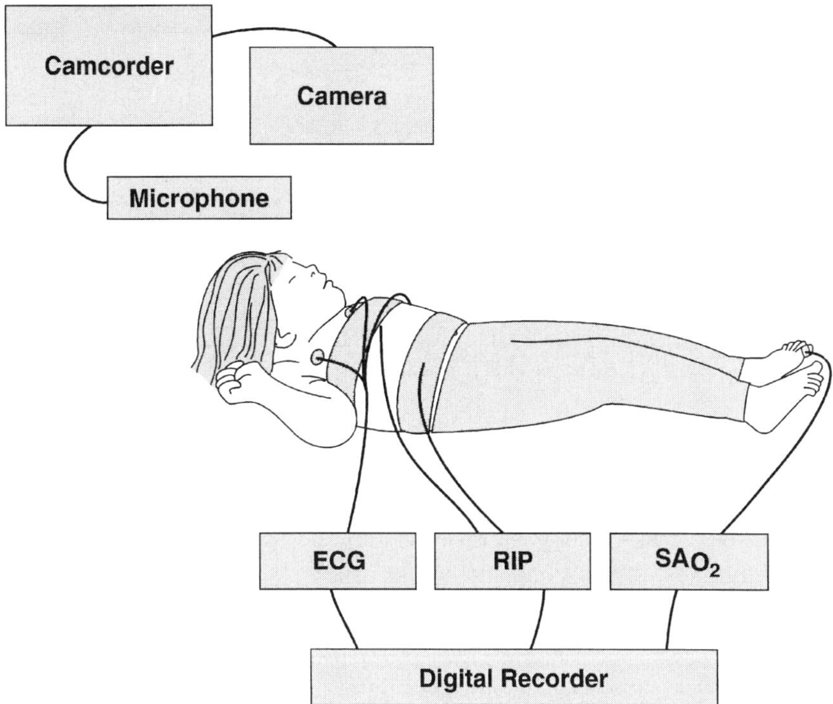

Figure 2 This figure shows the home cardiorespiratory evaluation system used at McGill University for evaluation of obstructive sleep apnea syndrome and other sleep-related breathing disorders. Audiovisual information is recorded on a portable VCR or camcorder and later transferred to a computerized audiovisual analysis system (SleepVision). Physiological information [electrocardiogram (ECG), electroencephalogram (EEG), respiratory inductive plethysmography (RIP), and Sa_{O_2}] is collected on a portable computer and later transferred to a digital polysomnograph for analysis.

ies for apnea/hypopnea index and found that children slept better in the home (34). Since its validation, this system has been used extensively in clinical studies for the diagnosis of OSAS, both in the home and on hospital wards. Transcutaneous P_{CO_2} has also been included in some home recordings but tcp_{CO_2} recordings must be interpreted with caution (38). The system has also been used in a research study looking at the sleep position of infants in their natural environments (20) and a study evaluating respiratory patterns in children with myelomeningocele (16).

IX. Advantages and Disadvantages of Home Studies

Advantages of performing sleep studies in the home include increased flexibility of scheduling, less disruption to the routine of the child and family, and the ability to

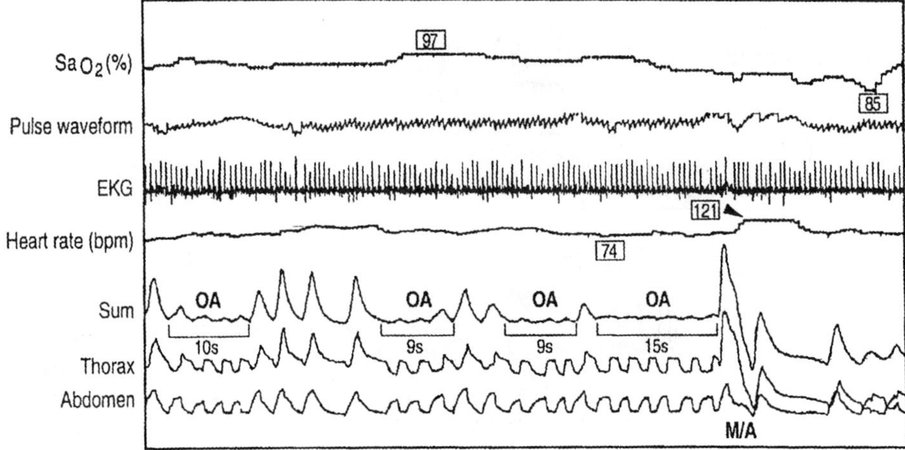

Figure 3 This figure shows 60 sec of data from a home cardiorespiratory recording. The patient was a 3-year-old boy being evaluated for obstructive sleep apnea syndrome. Note the series of obstructive apneas (OA) resulting in a drop in Sa_{O_2} and terminated by a movement/arousal (M/A). OAs are characterized by out-of-phase thoracic and abdominal respiratory inductive plethysmography (RIP) RIP signals and a flat RIP sum. The M/A can be recognized by the presence of tachycardia, increased amplitude and irregularity of the RIP signals, and movement artifact in the pulse waveform signal. (From Ref. 34.)

study the child in his or her natural environment. While this has not yet been documented, it seems likely that home studies will be more cost-efficient than laboratory polysomnography, as a hospital admission is not required; moreover, because such studies are usually unattended, technician time is substantially decreased. These factors become even more important when more than one might of recording is required.

The main disadvantage of performing studies in the home stems from the fact that there is no technician present to ensure signal quality. Electrodes are frequently displaced during the night, especially by children, and this can result in loss of data. In our experience, it is the leads around the head and face of the child that are most frequently displaced; therefore studies that include fewer channels and do not include monitoring of EEG and EOG may be more effectively done in the home. However, this limits the information that can be obtained; indeed, most home studies involve the use of considerably fewer channels than are used in conventional polysomnography, thus providing less information. Formal sleep staging, for example, cannot be performed without monitoring of EEG and EOG, so it may not be possible to determine whether a patient has experienced all stages of sleep on a particular night. In the previously mentioned study from the Montreal Children's Hospital, however, home studies yielded no false negatives and studies of diagnostic quality were obtained on the first attempt in 95% of cases (34). Identification of artifact can be more difficult with unattended studies; we recommend a video recording to document the patient's behavior during the night. Abbreviated home recordings are not appropriate when detailed information on sleep staging, ventilation, or respiratory muscle function is required. Other factors that might limit home testing include the distance to the patient's home, insurance issues, and safety of personnel and equipment.

Another important issue that has received little attention is quality control. While sleep laboratories are required to maintain strict standards, portable recordings may be performed by home-care companies, with interpretation being the sleep specialist's only role. In such cases both the company and the supervising/interpreting physician bear responsibility for safety and quality control.

X. Conclusions

Unattended cardiorespiratory recordings can provide valuable information regarding respiratory patterns during sleep, sleep disturbance, and gas exchange. When performing recordings in the home, it is important to ensure that signals being recorded allow distinction between central and obstructive apnea and that partial as well as complete airflow obstruction can be identified. Furthermore, attention must be paid to signal quality, and the raw data should be available for analysis.

At this time, home testing has been validated for routine use only in children with uncomplicated OSAS, although its use in other populations has been described. Abbreviated portable testing cannot be recommended when detailed information on sleep staging, ventilation, or respiratory muscle function is required. Conditions such as respiratory muscles weakness, neurological disorders, and central alveolar hypoventilation syndrome are best studied with comprehensive nocturnal polysomnography. However, as further experience is gained with portable testing, it is likely that abbreviated studies will play an increasingly important role.

Acknowledgments

The authors thank Michèle Fortin and Rosanna Barrafato for assistance with manuscript preparation and the technicians at the Montreal Children's Hospital/McGill University sleep laboratory for the studies and recordings on which much of this chapter is based.

References

1. Guilleminault C, Eldridge FL, Simmons FB, Dement WC. Sleep apnea in eight children. Pediatrics 1976:58:23–31.
2. Frank Y, Kravath RE, Pollack CP, Weitzman ED. Obstructive sleep apnea and its therapy: clinical and polysomnographic manifestations. Pediatrics 1983; 71:737–742.
3. Brouillette RT, Fernbach S, Hunt CE. Obstructive sleep apnea in infant and children. J Pediatr 1982; 100:31–40.

4. Paradise JL. Tonsillectomy and adenoidectomy. In: Bluestone CD, Stool SE, Sheetz MD, eds. Pediatric Otolaryngology. Philadelphia: Saunders, 1990:915–926.
5. McColley SA, April MM, Carroll JL, Naclerio RM, Loughlin GM. Respiratory compromise after adenotonsillectomy in children with obstructive sleep apnea. Arch Otolaryngol Head Neck Surg 1992; 118:940–943.
6. Brouillette RT, Hanson DS, Klemka L, Szatkowski A, Fernbach SK, Hunt CE. A diagnostic approach to suspected obstructive sleep apnea in children. J Pediatr 1984; 105:10–14.
7. Suens JS, Arnold JE, Brooks LJ. Adenotonsillectomy for treatment of obstructive sleep apnea in children. Arch Otolaryngol Head Neck Surg 1995; 121:525–530.
8. Carroll JL, McColley SA, Marcus CL, Curtis S, Loughlin GM. Inability of clinical history to distinguish primary snoring from obstructive sleep apnea syndrome in children. Chest 1995; 108:610–618.
9. Sadeh A, Lavie P, Scher A, Tirosh E, Epstein R. Actigraphic home-monitoring sleep-disturbed and control infants and young children: a new method for pediatric assessment of sleep-wake patterns. Pediatrics 1991; 87:494–499.
10. Sadeh A, Sharkey KM, Carskadon MA. Activity-based sleep-wake identification: an empirical test of methodological issues. Sleep 1994; 17:201–207.
11. Sadeh A. Assessment of intervention for infant night waking: parental reports and activity-based home monitoring. J Consult Clin Psychol 1994; 62:63–68.
12. Williams AJ, Yu G, Santiago S, Stein M. Screening for sleep apnea using pulse oximetry and a clinical score. Chest 1991; 100:631–635.
13. Cooper BG, Veale D, Griffiths CJ, Gibson GJ. Value of nocturnal oxygen saturation as a screening test for sleep apnoea. Thorax 1991; 46:586–588.
14. Ryan PJ, Hilton MF, Boldy DA, Evans A, Bradbury S, Sapiano S, Prowse K, Cayton RM. Validation of British Thoracic Society guidelines for the diagnosis of the sleep apnoea/hypopnoea syndrome: can polysomnography be avoided? Thorax 1995;50:972–975.
15. Lafontaine VM, Ducharme FM, Brouillette RT. Pulse oximetry: accuracy of methods of interpreting graphic summaries. Pediatr Pulmonol 1996; 21:121–131.
16. Waters KA, Morielli A, Forbes P, Hum C, O'Gorman G, Vernet O, Ducharme F, Davis GM, Tewfik L, Brouillette RT. Sleep-disordered breathing in children with myelomeningocele. J Pediatr. In press.
17. Potsic WP. Comparison of polysomnography and sonography for assessing regularity of respiration during sleep in adenotonsillar hypertrophy. Laryngoscope 1987; 97:1430–1437.
18. White JE, Smithson AJ, Close PR, Drinnan MJ, Prichard AJ, Gibson GJ. The use of sound recording and oxygen saturation in screening snorers for obstructive sleep apnoea. Clin Otolaryngol 1994; 19:218–221.
19. Flemons WW, Remmers JE. The diagnosis of sleep apnea: questionnaire and home studies. Sleep 1996; 19(10 suppl):S243–S247.
20. Waters KA, Gonzalez A, Jean C, Morielli A, Brouillette RT. The face-straight-down and the face-near-straight-down positions in normal, prone-sleeping infants. J Pediatr 1996; 128:616–625.
21. Stradling JR, Thomas G, Warley ARH, Williams P, Freeland A. Effect of adenotonsillectomy on nocturnal hypoxemia, sleep disturbance, and symptoms in snoring children. Lancet 1990; 335:249–253.
22. Sivan Y, Kornecki A, Schonfeld T. Screening obstructive sleep apnoea syndrome by home videotape recording in children. Eur Respir J 1996; 9:2127–2131.

23. Douglas NJ, Thomas S, Jan MA. Clinical value of polysomnography. Lancet 1992; 339: 347–350.
24. American Thoracic Society. Indications and standards for cardiopulmonary sleep studies. Am Rev Respir Dis 1989; 139:559–568.
25. Standards of Practice Committee of the American Sleep Disorders Association. Practice parameters for the use of portable recording in the assessment of obstructive sleep apnea. Sleep 1994; 17:372–377.
26. Ancoli-Israel S, Kripke DF, Mason W, Messin S. Comparisons of home sleep recordings and polysomnograms in older adults with sleep disorders. Sleep 1981; 4:283–291.
27. Gyulay S, Gould D, Sawyer B, Pond D, Mant A, Saunders N. Evaluation of a microprocessor-based portable home monitoring system to measure breathing during sleep. Sleep 1986; 10:130–142.
28. Redline S, Tosteson T, Boucher MA, Millman RP. Measurement of sleep-related breathing disturbances in epidemiologic studies. Chest 1991; 100:1281–1286.
29. Stoohs R, Guilleminault C. MESAM 4: an ambulatory device for the detection of patients at risk for obstructive sleep apnea syndrome (OSAS). Chest 1992; 101:1221–1227.
30. Zucconi M, Ferini-Strambi L, Castronovo V, Oldani A, Smirne S. An unattended device for sleep-related breathing disorders: validation study in suspected obstructive sleep apnoea syndrome. Eur Respir J 1996; 9:1251–1256.
31. Waburton D, Stark AR, Taeusch HW. Apnea monitor failure in infants with upper airway obstruction. Pediatrics 1977; 60:742–744.
32. Brouillette RT, Morrow AS, Weese-Mayer DE, Hunt CE. Comparison of respiratory inductive plethysmography and thoracic impedance for apnea monitoring. J Pediatr 1987; 111:377–383.
33. Abraham NG, Stebbens VA, Samuels MP. Southall DP. Investigation of cyanotic/apneic episodes and sleep-related upper airway obstruction by long-term non-invasive bedside recordings. Pediatr Pulmonol 1990; 8:259–262.
34. Jacob S, Morielli A, Mograss MA, Ducharme FM, Schloss MD, Brouillette RT. Home testing for pediatric obstructive sleep apnea syndrome secondary to adenotonsillar hypertrophy. Pediatr Pulmonol 1995; 20:241–252.
35. Morielli A, Ladan S, Ducharme FM, Brouillette RT. Can sleep and wakefulness be distinguished in children by cardiorespiratory and videotape recordings? Chest 1996; 109: 680–687.
36. Mograss MA, Ducharme FM, Brouillette RT. Movement/arousals: description, classification and relationship to obstructive sleep apnea in children. Am J Respir Crit Care Med 1994; 150:1690–1696.
37. Brouillette RT, Jacob SV, Waters KA, Morielli A, Mograss M, Ducharme FM. Cardiorespiratory sleep studies for children can often be performed in the home. Sleep 1996; 19(10 suppl):S278–S280.
38. Morielli A, Desjardins D, Brouillette RT. Transcutaneous and end-tidal carbon dioxide pressures should be measured during pediatric polysomnography. Am Rev Respir Dis 1993; 148:1599–1604.

36

Ventilator Management of Abnormal Breathing During Sleep

Continuous Positive Airway Pressure and Nocturnal Noninvasive Intermittent Positive Pressure Ventilation

CAROLE L. MARCUS

Johns Hopkins University School of Medicine
Baltimore, Maryland

I. Introduction

Until recently, continuous positive airway pressure (CPAP) therapy via nasal mask was used infrequently in children with the obstructive sleep apnea syndrome (OSAS). In recent years, its use has increased markedly, partly due to the advent of commercially available, child-sized nasal masks. Simultaneously, the use of nocturnal, nasal intermittent positive pressure ventilation (NIPPV) in the pediatric population has grown. Improved home-care resources, such as home nurses and durable medical equipment companies that will maintain a patient's equipment in the home, have made home NIPPV possible. NIPPV has been used effectively in patients with both acute and chronic respiratory failure. This review focuses on its use in chronic respiratory failure.

II. Technology

CPAP and NIPPV are delivered via a nasal mask. Although NIPPV can be provided by a conventional ventilator, it is usually delivered via a bilevel pressure ventilator designed specifically for this task. The trade name BiPAP is often used to describe this class of ventilator, although the term actually applies to a specific ventilator model.

Bilevel pressure ventilators are cheaper and easier to use than conventional ventilators. In addition, bilevel ventilators can compensate for some degree of mask leak, whereas conventional volume ventilators cannot.

Bilevel machines provide pressure-support ventilation. Positive pressure is generated by a blower that creates a bias flow. The inspiratory (IPAP) and expiratory (EPAP) pressures can be adjusted independently, so that the expiratory pressure is lower than the inspiratory pressure. Unlike that of conventional ventilators, the respiratory circuit has a single limb for both inspiration and expiration. A fixed leak near the patient's mask prevents CO_2 rebreathing. In most types of bilevel ventilators, the patient's airflow is detected by a flow transducer that triggers the change from EPAP to IPAP. Typically, patient flow rates of 40 to 80 mL/sec are required for triggering. Initially, bilevel ventilators were made with a maximal inspiratory pressure of 20 cmH_2O. At the time of this writing, newer models can deliver up to 35 cmH_2O. Most bilevel machines do not have intrinsic alarm systems.

Differing types of ventilatory modes are available. The prototype bilevel ventilator is the Respironics BiPAP, which offers four modes of ventilation: 1) *IPAP or EPAP*, providing a constant pressure level (i.e., CPAP); 2) *spontaneous*, whereby pressure support is delivered at the preselected IPAP and EPAP levels when the patient makes spontaneous respiratory efforts, so that the patient determines the respiratory rate; 3) *spontaneous timed*, whereby a backup respiratory rate is set and pressure support is delivered whenever the patient initiates a breath or the patient's respiratory rate falls below the set rate; and 4) *timed*, whereby pressure support is delivered at a set respiratory rate but, if the patient breathes above that rate, pressure support is also supplied in response to the patient's spontaneous respiratory efforts.

III. Mode of Action

CPAP increases intraluminal upper airway pressure and elevates it above the upper airway critical closing pressure (1), thereby stenting the airway open. It reduces upper airway (2) and diaphragmatic (3) inspiratory muscle activity. Because the upper airway is rich in sensory nerve endings, increased nasal airflow from NIPPV can stimulate ventilation (4).

NIPPV provides pressure support and decreases the work of breathing. It can result in normalization of nocturnal hypoxemia and hypercapnia (5–8), thereby allowing for resetting of the ventilatory drive.

IV. NIPPV Compared to Other Modes of Assisted Ventilation

Assisted ventilation can be delivered by a variety of ventilators. Positive pressure ventilation via tracheostomy is the most effective mode of assisted ventilation. However, the tracheostomy interferes with speech, predisposes the patient to respiratory infections, and requires that a skilled caregiver be present at all times. Conventional positive-pressure ventilators are more versatile and powerful than bilevel ventilators. However, they are more expensive and require more caregiver training and maintenance than bilevel ventilators.

Negative-pressure ventilators have been used successfully for many decades. Several devices are available, including the cuirass and the tank ventilator. They do not require a facial mask, which is an advantage for some patients. However, negative-pressure ventilators are cumbersome, tend to be less effective than positive pressure ventilators, and they are prone to air leaks. In addition, negative-pressure ventilators may cause upper airway obstruction (9) due to the lack of synchrony between inspiratory efforts and vocal cord abduction.

Diaphragm pacers are useful for selected patients (see Chap. 37). However, diaphragm pacers require surgical insertion, may become infected, are only available at specialized centers, and also predispose to obstructive sleep apnea. Thus, for patients with OSAS that is not amenable to other methods of treatment and for many patients with chronic respiratory failure, CPAP or NIPPV is the optimal mode of ventilation.

V. Indications for NIPPV

The goal of nocturnal home ventilation is to improve the patient's quality of life (and in some cases prolong life) while maintaining as near normal a lifestyle as possible. This should not require the environment of the intensive care unit to be recreated in the home.

A. CPAP

The use of nasal CPAP in adults with OSAS has been shown to result in improved cognitive and psychological function, decreased daytime somnolence, decreased waking hypercapnia, improved cardiovascular function, and possibly decreased mortality (10).

Although most children with OSAS can be treated effectively by tonsillectomy and adenoidectomy, some patients require additional treatment. As recently as 1994, when the American Thoracic Society published guidelines for CPAP use, there were few data available on its use in children (10). Over the past few years, however, there has been an increase in CPAP use in children, and several large series have been published (11–13). Waters et al. (11) reported CPAP usage in 80 pediatric patients at the same institution, whereas a multicenter study reported on CPAP use in 94 pediatric patients (12). Both studies showed that CPAP was effective and well tolerated in more than 80% of patients, including children with craniofacial anomalies, obesity, and neurological disorders.

Nasal CPAP has long been known to be effective in treating central apnea in infants. Recent studies show that it is also effective in treating obstructive apnea in this age group. McNamara and colleagues (14) showed that CPAP use in the laboratory resulted in fewer apneas and improved sleep architecture in infants with mixed apnea. Guilleminault et al. (13) report on its successful use in the home in infants with obstructive apnea—primarily patients with craniofacial anomalies—as well as infants with apparent life-threatening events and abnormal polysomnograms.

B. NIPPV

OSAS

NIPPV is useful for patients with OSAS who fail a trial of CPAP therapy, either because of discomfort and resultant poor compliance or lack of efficacy. Intuitively, it would appear easier to exhale against a lower expiratory pressure than an inspiratory level. Only one study has directly compared CPAP to bilevel ventilation for OSAS (15), but it did not demonstrate a significant difference in effective use between the two methods. However, the CPAP group had a significantly larger dropout rate than the bilevel group. Furthermore, compliance in the bilevel group was affected by the IPAP/EPAP pressure difference, suggesting that different ventilation protocols may affect compliance. In practice, bilevel ventilation is often used for patients who find CPAP uncomfortable.

Chronic Respiratory Failure

NIPPV has been shown to be successful in the treatment of chronic respiratory failure from a wide range of medical conditions, including chronic obstructive pulmonary disease (3,7), neuromuscular disease (5,8,16,17), chest wall abnormalities (8,16), cystic fibrosis (18,19), and bronchiectasis (20). It has also been used for palliative care and as a bridge to transplantation in patients with cystic fibrosis (19). Most studies of NIPPV have been performed in adults, although a number of case reports describe its successful use in children.

Subjectively, NIPPV results in increased energy, improved sleep, less daytime somnolence, improved cognitive function, and decreased dyspnea (8,16). Objectively, sleep efficiency and sleep architecture are improved (5). Several studies have shown that when treated by nocturnal NIPPV, patients with chronic respiratory failure have improved gas exchange during spontaneous breathing while awake (5,8). Most studies have not shown an improvement in pulmonary function tests or tests of respiratory muscle strength (5,7,21), although one study showed an improvement in inspiratory muscle endurance (22). However, these studies used patients as their own controls. Vianello and colleagues (17) compared five patients with Duchenne's muscular dystrophy treated with NIPPV to five nonventilated controls. The nonventilated patients showed a decline in pulmonary function, whereas the ventilated patients did not. Thus, while NIPPV does not appear to improve pulmonary function, it may prevent further decline. Of note in the Vianello study, after 2 years of follow-up, all ventilated patients were still alive, whereas 80% of the nonventilated patients had died (17).

Although some of the above studies included adolescents, few studies have specifically evaluated the use of NIPPV in children with chronic respiratory failure. However, NIPPV has been shown to be effective in children with acute respiratory failure (23,24). At our institution, we have used NIPPV in 15 patients with chronic respiratory failure secondary to ventilatory muscle weakness and 7 patients with chronic respiratory failure secondary to pulmonary disease (5 with cystic fibrosis and 2 with interstitial lung disease). All of the patients with ventilatory muscle weakness are still alive, with the longest follow-up being 7 years. Of the patients with pulmonary disease, 2 survived to transplantation, 4 died, and 1 is awaiting transplant. NIPPV was thought to help alleviate the symptoms of those who died and to provide palliative care.

Central Apnea/Central Hypoventilation

NIPPV can be useful in patients with central hypoventilation. It has been used successfully in infants with congenital central hypoventilaton syndrome (25,26). We have used NIPPV in four children with severe central apnea secondary to Arnold-Chiari malformations. In three patients, this was highly successful. The youngest patient was placed on NIPPV at 3 months of age and has been adequately maintained on this for 3 years. NIPPV was unsuccessful in an obese 10-year-old boy with both central and obstructive apneas; he eventually required tracheostomy and positive pressure ventilation.

VI. Practical Aspects of NIPPV

A. Patient Selection

The objectives of NIPPV are to improve ventilation, decrease the work of breathing, and enhance the quality of life in a way that provides maximal safety at a reasonable cost. Thus, each patient must be evaluated on an individual basis. NIPPV is a long-term commitment that requires substantial effort on the part of the patient and family; therefore, the decision to institute NIPPV should be made by a team consisting of the patient as well as the caregivers and physicians involved. In some cases, such as an otherwise healthy child with craniofacial anomalies and OSAS unresponsive to other treatment, CPAP or NIPPV is almost always indicated; whereas in other patients, such as a child with cystic fibrosis and end-stage lung disease, the discomfort related to treatment may outweigh potential advantages. In general, however, NIPPV is relatively noninvasive, well tolerated, and simple to use. Because it is only used during sleep, it does not restrict a patient's daytime activities and has the least interference with the patient's lifestyle.

When should NIPPV be started in a patient with chronic respiratory failure? This has not been thoroughly evaluated. Most patients are placed on NIPPV once they have either nocturnal or constant hypercapnia. In general, most patients with Duchenne's muscular dystrophy will have an FVC $< 30\%$ predicted (27), although individual variation exists. Although most patients are placed on NIPPV because of chronic respiratory failure, patients with recurrent atelectasis secondary to ventilatory muscle weakness or failure to thrive secondary to increased work of breathing may also benefit from NIPPV. Raphael et al. (28) performed a randomized trial of preventive NIPPV in patients with Duchenne's muscular dystrophy, normal gas exchange during wakefulness, and vital capacities of 20% to 50% predicted. They found a higher death rate among patients using NIPPV than among controls (eight versus two $p < .05$). However, this study has been criticized for a number of reasons. Ventilators were not titrated to provide adequate gas exchange during sleep, 17 centers were involved in the evaluation of only 35 subjects plus 35 controls, analysis on the basis of intent to treat meant that 2 of the deaths in the NIPPV group were patients who did not actually receive NIPPV, and 3 of the deaths resulted from surgical complications.

Elective decision making is preferable to instituting assisted ventilation during a medical crisis. Gilgoff et al. (29) evaluated the decision-making process in 15 patients with Duchenne's muscular dystrophy: 2 patients elected not to undergo ventilatory assistance and died at home; 9 chose ventilatory assistance of whom 7 were alive at the time of report and 2 had died of cardiac failure; of the 4 patients who were unable to make a decision electively, 3 underwent emergency intubation and remained ventilator-dependent while 1 died in the hospital. Thus, failure to commit to a decision in advance frequently results in medical intervention under suboptimal circumstances.

NIPPV ventilators are less powerful than conventional ventilators and medical personnel are not always readily available. Therefore, for a patient to be successfully managed on NIPPV in the home environment, he or she must have stable lung disease and require low ventilator settings. Bilevel ventilators are not approved by the Food and Drug Administration as life-support ventilators. In fragile patients, mask leak or displacement can rapidly lead to severe hypoxemia. Thus, the advantages and disadvantages of NIPPV versus positive pressure ventilation via a tracheostomy must be considered in light of the patient's overall prognosis. Other than in the acute situation, patients requiring 24-hr/day ventilatory support are generally not candidates for NIPPV, as mask ventilation interferes with such activities of daily living as eating and speech. For a patient to receive NIPPV in the home, an adequate environment is necessary. This includes trained support personnel, medical backup, adequate cleanliness, a reliable source of electrical power, and access to emergency facilities.

B. Equipment

Patient Interface

The patient interface is critically important. An ill-fitting mask can cause inadequate ventilation and/or side effects. Many mask types and sizes are commercially available, and pediatric providers should have a wide variety of masks available. Unfortunately, few commercial masks are available in the United States for infants; additional types are available in other countries. Patients who are prone to skin ulceration or who are claustrophobic may prefer nasal prongs. Full-face masks are available. However, it is possible that these may place young patients at risk for aspiration.

Ventilator

The market for NIPPV has increased dramatically over the past few years. As a result, many types of noninvasive ventilators are now commercially available, and new models are continually being introduced. Most CPAP and bilevel machines can reliably generate and sustain adequate pressures. However, there is variation in model function (30–32), so the health care provider should be familiar with the specifics of the machine prescribed. Equipment modifications can provide increased comfort and hence improved compliance. Some machines provide external sensitivity controls, which affect the triggering from EPAP to IPAP. As discussed below, this can be very important in patients with low flow rates. A "ramp" function, which gradually increases the pressure to the required level, allows the patient to fall asleep on lower pressure levels. Other advances, such as a change in the delivered pressure waveform from a square wave to a more normal breathing pattern, may increase patient comfort. However, the clinical advantages of these modifications have not been studied.

Bilevel ventilators deliver a large amount of cold, dry air to the nares. If this causes nasal symptoms, a heated in-line humidifier can be added. If required, supplemental oxygen can be introduced through either the ventilator circuit or the mask port (33). Most noninvasive ventilators or CPAP machines are not equipped with alarms. However, an external low-pressure alarm can be connected to the circuit. This is useful in patients who will develop significant apnea, hypoxemia, or hypercapnia if a large leak occurs or in young children who tend to pull off the mask. An hour meter is useful to assess compliance objectively.

C. Institution of NIPPV

NIPPV can be instituted in either the outpatient or inpatient setting. If therapy is initiated in the outpatient setting, adequate provision must be made for training the patient and caregivers and for titrating the degree of ventilatory support. In very young or developmentally delayed patients, adequate behavioral training is crucial if NIPPV is to succeed.

Most patients placed electively on NIPPV have chronic, stable respiratory failure. Therefore, NIPPV can be instituted gradually. It is our practice to introduce NIPPV to the patients and their families during a dedicated clinic session. The child is fitted with a mask and the equipment is demonstrated. If the patient is stable, home NIPPV is then instituted. Patients are initially started on low IPAP pressures and minimal EPAP. Once the patient is tolerating the equipment all night, the pressures are gradually increased. Only when the child is tolerating low therapeutic pressure levels (e.g., 8/2 cmH_2O) overnight will a sleep study be performed. In the sleep laboratory, a formal pressure titration study is performed by trained personnel. Patients who are severely ill are admitted to the intensive care unit for immediate institution of NIPPV therapy.

Pressure requirements will depend on the individual patient, and must be assessed by patient monitoring (e.g., in the sleep laboratory or intensive care unit). In a multicenter study of pediatric OSAS patients, CPAP pressures ranged from 4 to 20 cmH_2O, with a median pressure of 8 cmH_2O (12). Pressure requirements were independent of age and underlying diagnosis (12). Presumably, pressure levels were proportional to the severity of OSAS, although different protocols at the varying institutions did not allow this to be evaluated systematically. For OSAS patients requiring bilevel ventilation, we have empirically found that an IPAP/EPAP difference of 6 cmH_2O results in adequate patient comfort and ventilation. However, this does not apply to patients receiving bilevel ventilation for chronic respiratory failure. Strumpf et al. (34) used a test lung to evaluate a bilevel ventilator. When pulmonary compliance and resistance were normal, the delivered tidal volume was proportional to the IPAP/EPAP difference until the IPAP/EPAP difference exceeded 15 cmH_2O (Fig. 1). However, this relationship did not hold for lungs with abnormal mechanics (Fig. 2) (34).

Pressure requirements can be expected to change over time in response to growth or changes in the disease process. In the multicenter study of pediatric CPAP use, 22% of children required a change in CPAP pressure during the course of the study (12).

The biggest perceived obstacle to CPAP/NIPPV use in young children is behavioral difficulties. In our experience, the vast majority of children can be trained to use NIPPV *if* their parents are motivated and supportive. In many cases, formal behavioral psychology sessions are helpful. Rains outlines a behavioral intervention pro-

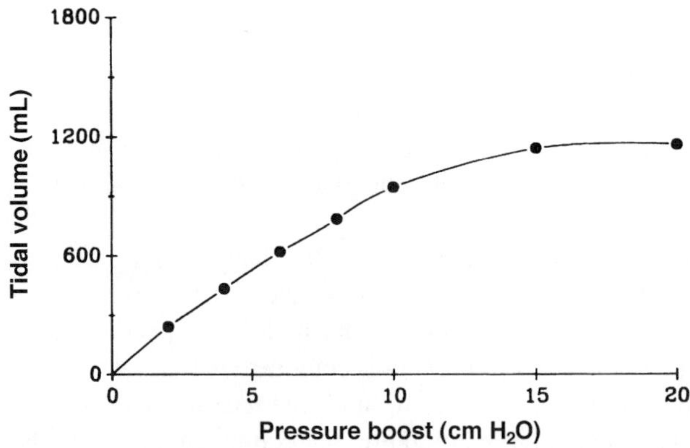

Figure 1 The relationship between tidal volume and pressure boost (the difference between IPAP and EPAP) for normal lungs. The increase in tidal volume is proportional to the pressure boost until a pressure boost of 15 cmH_2O is attained. (From Ref. 34.)

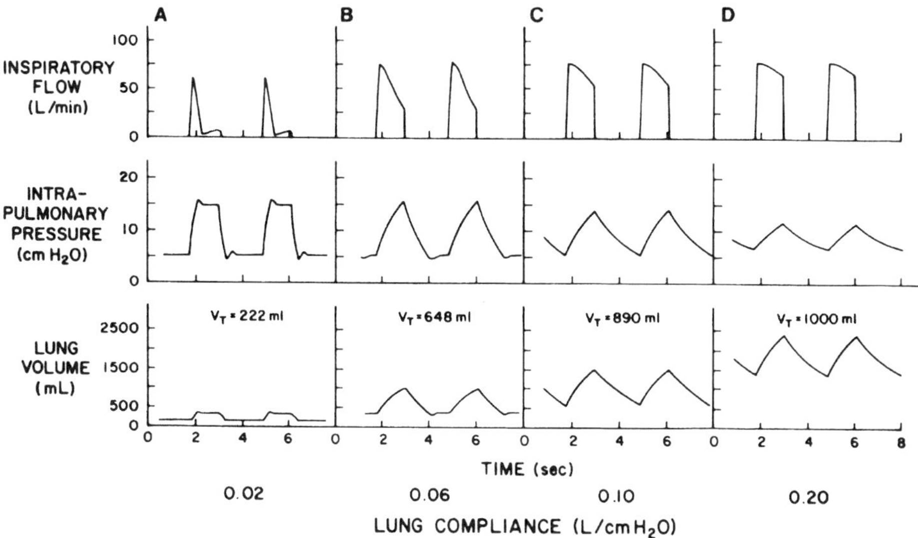

Figure 2 The effect of lung compliance on delivered tidal volume is shown. Simultaneous inspiratory flow, intrapulmonary pressure, and lung volume are shown for differing levels of lung compliance at an IPAP of 15 cmH_2O and an EPAP of 5 cmH_2O. Note the development of auto-PEEP with increased end-expiratory volume in the highly compliant lung. V_T, tidal volume. (From Ref. 34.)

gram that is effective in training very young or mentally retarded children to tolerate CPAP (35).

D. Side Effects

Side effects of NIPPV in children are minor, and serious complications have not been reported (11,12). However, minor symptoms that result in patient discomfort may affect compliance; thus, they should be treated aggressively. Common side effects and their treatments are listed in Table 1. Children may develop central apneas or hypoventilation at higher pressure levels (11). This is presumably due to activation of the Hering-Breuer reflex by stimulation of the pulmonary stretch receptors. It can be remedied by placing the patient on bilevel ventilation with a backup rate. Small or weak children with low inspiratory flow rates may fail to trigger bilevel ventilators (Fig. 3). Unlike conventional ventilators, no dedicated pediatric bilevel ventilators have been produced; however, some models require lower flow rates or have adjustable sensitivity controls. Even with these models, patients may not trigger the equipment during REM sleep. In such cases, it may be necessary to adjust the ventilator parameters, by providing a higher EPAP or by adding supplemental oxygen. Carbon dioxide rebreathing has been reported in adults receiving NIPPV (36). Unlike conventional

Table 1 Treatment of NIPPV Side Effects

Side effect	Treatment
Nasal symptoms (dryness, congestion, rhinorrhea, epistaxis)	Heated humidifier Saline nose drops Nasal steroids
Skin ulceration	Correct mask fit Avoid overtightening of head gear Protect bridge of nose with hydrocolloid dressings Alternate different mask types
Conjunctivitis	Correct mask fit
Ear pain during otitis	Consider stopping NIPPV until symptoms resolve
Unable to fall asleep with NIPPV	Pressure ramp
Central apnea	Bilevel ventilation with backup rate
Hypercapnia	Nonrebreathing valve
Failure to trigger NIPPV	Use ventilator with low triggering threshold or adjustable sensitivity levels If suboptimal ventilation, consider increasing EPAP and adding O_2
Midfacial depression	Custom mask

ventilators, bilevel ventilators do not have separate inspiratory and expiratory circuits. Rebreathing can be eliminated by using a nonrebreathing valve in the circuit (36). Tight-fitting nasal masks may result in midfacial depression in young, growing children. This has not been described in the literature but has been observed by several sleep specialists (personal communication). Further study of this problem is needed, as this may lead to dental malocclusion and OSAS in addition to cosmetic deformities. A custom nasal mask that distributes pressure more evenly over different facial structures (such as the zygomatic arch) may alleviate this problem. Nasal deformities have also been noted in premature infants receiving CPAP via nasal prongs (37).

Serious complications of NIPPV are rare. Aspiration secondary to NIPPV has not been reported. Pneumothorax has been reported only in patients with *Pneumocystis carinii* pneumonia (38,39). As these patients are predisposed to pneumothorax, the role of NIPPV is unclear. The effects of nasal CPAP on cardiac output are controversial, with some studies showing no effect (40) and others demonstrating a decrease (41). Clinically, no problems have been reported in children. However, it would be appropriate to use caution in applying nasal CPAP to a child with severe cardiac disease.

In adults, rare complications of nasal CPAP in patients with underlying medical problems have been reported, such as increased intraocular pressure in patients with glaucoma (42) and meningitis in a patient with a sinus mucocele (43). In view

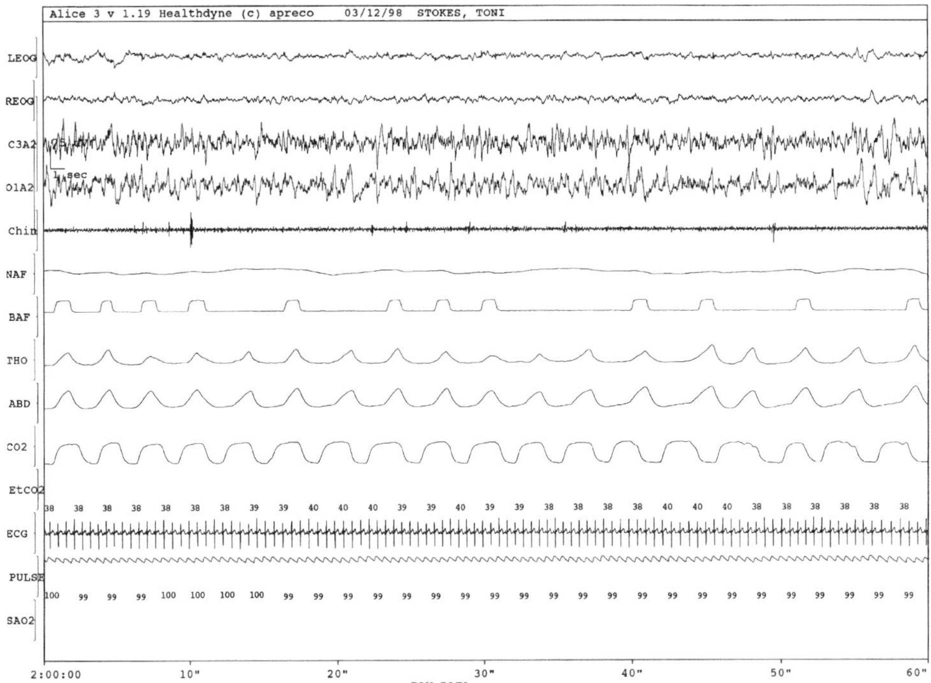

Figure 3 One-min portion of a polysomnogram from a 15-kg child with restrictive lung disease who failed to trigger the bilevel ventilator consistently. Note that the child is breathing at 18/min as shown by the thoracic and abdominal wall movements. However, the ventilator is delivering only 12 breaths per minute (as evidenced by the bilevel airflow channel). LEOG, left electro-oculogram; REOG, right electro-oculogram; C3A2 and O1A2, EEG channels; chin, submental EEG; NAF, airflow (measured by a thermistor placed at the mouth, demonstrating the absence of a mouth leak); BAF, bilevel airflow (measured by a pneumotachometer in line with the nasal mask); THO, thoracic wall movement; ABD, abdominal wall movement; CO_2, end-tidal P_{CO_2} waveform; Et_{CO_2}, peak end-tidal P_{CO_2} value averaged over several breaths; ECG, electrocardiogram; pulse, pulse oximeter waveform; Sa_{O_2}, arterial oxygen saturation value.

of the limited data available on children, care must be taken when using NIPPV for patients with complex medical problems that may be affected by barotrauma.

E. Compliance

For NIPPV to be effective, adequate compliance is essential. Compliance with CPAP has been well studied in adults. However, these data may not be applicable to patients receiving other forms of NIPPV. Adults using CPAP for OSAS generally used their equipment for only five hours per night (15,44,45) and did not use it every night (15).

In addition, the dropout rate in these studies was 13% to 19% (15,45). No study has evaluated CPAP compliance in children using totally objective criteria, such as an hour meter attached to a pressure monitor. Pediatric centers have estimated compliance at 50% to 100%, with adolescents reported to be the least compliant (12). In many cases, compliance problems were attributed primarily to the parent rather than the child (12).

VII. Prognosis

CPAP has been used in children with OSAS for only a few years, so the long-term prognosis is not known. In most cases, children have not responded to tonsillectomy and adenoidectomy. Preliminary data suggest that these patients will require long-term therapy. In two studies of children with OSAS, excluding those patients in whom CPAP was used only perioperatively or in whom additional treatment modalities were instituted, only 4% to 16% of patients improved sufficiently to discontinue CPAP over the several years of follow-up (11,12). Infants with OSAS do not fare better. Guilleminault and colleagues (13) used CPAP successfully in 72 infants with apparent life-threatening events or OSAS secondary to neurological disease or craniofacial anomalies. Among these, CPAP could be discontinued in 28 children (10 patients with apparent life-threatening events, 11 patients following upper airway surgery, and 7 spontaneously). However, the last group remained symptomatic.

Patients with OSAS in whom CPAP was discontinued for 1 night had a temporary improvement in breathing compared to their baseline, pre-CPAP treatment state. Polysomnography on the first night off CPAP demonstrated fewer and shorter obstructive apneas, decreased esophageal pressure swings, and less arterial oxygen desaturation (46–48). This may be due to a number of factors: decreased sleep fragmentation, decreased upper airway edema, decreased upper airway resistance (perhaps due to increased upper airway volume), and resetting of the ventilatory drive. Because of this transient improvement, CPAP should be discontinued for at least several days prior to polysomnography in patients being evaluated for discontinuation of therapy.

Most children receiving NIPPV for chronic respiratory failure will not be able to be weaned off support. Patients with progressive types of muscular dystrophy may eventually require tracheostomies because of poor pulmonary toilet and inability to handle pulmonary secretions.

VIII. Conclusion

Nasal CPAP and NIPPV are now being widely used for the treatment of children with OSAS or chronic respiratory failure. With careful attention to behavioral training, mask fit, ventilator settings, and side effects, CPAP and NIPPV are safe, well-tolerated, and effective therapeutic modalities. Hopefully, the future development of specific pediatric masks and ventilators will result in further improvements in patient care.

Acknowledgments

Dr. Marcus was supported in part by the Pediatric Clinical Research Center #RR-00052, The Johns Hopkins Hospital, Baltimore, MD, and NHLBI grant #HL37379.

References

1. Smith PL, Wise RA, Gold AR, Schwartz AR, Permutt S. Upper airway pressure-flow relationships in obstructive sleep apnea. J Appl Physiol 1988; 64:789–795.
2. Strohl KP, Redline S. Nasal CPAP therapy, upper airway muscle activation, and obstructive sleep apnea. Am Rev Respir Dis 1986; 134:555–558.
3. Brochard L, Isabey D, Piquet J, Amaro P, Mancebo J, Messadi A, Brun-Buisson C, Rauss A, Lemaire F, Harf A. Reversal of acute exacerbations of chronic obstructive lung disease by inspiratory assistance with a face mask. N Engl J Med 1990; 323:1523–1530.
4. McNicholas WT, Coffey M, Boyle T. Effects of nasal airflow on breathing during sleep in normal humans. Am Rev Respir Dis 1993; 147:620–623.
5. Barbe F, Quera-Salva MA, de Lattre J, Gajdos P, Agusti AGN. Long-term effects of nasal intermittent positive-pressure ventilation on pulmonary function and sleep architecture in patients with neuromuscular diseases. Chest 1996; 110:1179–1183.
6. Ellis ER, Bye PTP, Bruderer JW, Sullivan CE. Treatment of respiratory failure during sleep in patients with neuromuscular disease: positive-pressure ventilation through a nose mask. Am Rev Respir Dis 1987; 135:148–152.
7. Gay PC, Patel AM, Viggiano RW, Hubmayr RD. Nocturnal nasal ventilation for treatment of patients with hypercapnic respiratory failure. Mayo Clin Proc 1991; 66:695–703.
8. Bach JR, Alba AS. Management of chronic alveolar hypoventilation by nasal ventilation. Chest 1990; 97:52–57.
9. Levy RD, Bradley TD, Newman SL, Macklem PT, Martin JG. Negative pressure ventilation: effects on ventilation during sleep in normal subjects. Chest 1989; 95:95–99.
10. American Thoracic Society. Indications and standards for use of nasal continuous positive airway pressure (CPAP) in sleep apnea syndromes. Am J Respir Crit Care Med 1994; 150:1738–1745.
11. Waters KA, Everett FM, Bruderer JW, Sullivan CE. Obstructive sleep apnea: the use of nasal CPAP in 80 children. Am J Respir Crit Care Med 1995; 152:780–785.
12. Marcus CL, Ward SL, Mallory GB, Rosen CL, Beckerman RC, Weese-Mayer DE, Brouillette RT, Trang HT, Brooks LJ. Use of nasal continuous positive airway pressure as treatment of childhood obstructive sleep apnea. J Pediatr 1995; 127:88–94.
13. Guilleminault C, Pelayo R, Clerk A, Leger D, Bocian RC. Home nasal continuous positive airway pressure in infants with sleep-disordered breathing. J Pediatr 1995; 127:905– 912.

14. McNamara F, Harris MA, Sullivan CE. Effects of nasal continuous positive airway pressure on apnoea index and sleep in infants. J Paediatr Child Health 1995; 31:88–94.
15. Reeves-Hoche MK, Hudgel DW, Meck R, Witteman R, Ross A, Zwillich CW. Continuous versus bilevel positive airway pressure for obstructive sleep apnea. Am J Respir Crit Care Med 1995; 151:443–449.
16. Hill NS, Eveloff SE, Carlisle CC, Goff SG. Efficacy of nocturnal nasal ventilation in patients with restrictive thoracic disease. Am Rev Respir Dis 1992; 145:365–371.
17. Vianello A, Bevilacqua M, Salvador V, Cardaioli C, Vincenti E. Long-term nasal intermittent positive pressure ventilation in advanced Duchenne's muscular dystrophy. Chest 1994; 105:445–448.
18. Gozal D. Nocturnal ventilatory support in patients with cystic fibrosis: comparison with supplemental oxygen. Eur Respir J 1997; 10:1999–2003.
19. Hodson ME, Madden BP, Steven MH, Tsang VT, Yacoub MH. Non-invasive mechanical ventilation for cystic fibrosis patients—a potential bridge to transplantation. Eur Respir J 1991; 4:524–527.
20. Benhamou D, Muir JF, Raspaud C, Cuvelier A, Girault C, Portier F, Menard JF. Long-term efficiency of home nasal mask ventilation in patients with diffuse bronchiectasis and severe chronic respiratory failure. Chest 1997; 112:1259–1266.
21. Waldhorn RE. Nocturnal nasal intermittent positive pressure ventilation with bi-level positive airway pressure (BiPAP) in respiratory failure. Chest 1992; 101:516–521.
22. Goldstein RS, De Rosie JA, Avendano MA, Dolmage TE. Influence of noninvasive positive pressure ventilation on inspiratory muscles. Chest 1991; 99:408–415.
23. Padman R, Lawless S, Von Nessen S. Use of BiPAP by nasal mask in the treatment of respiratory insufficiency in pediatric patients: preliminary investigation. Pediatr Pulmonol 1994; 17:119–123.
24. Fortenberry JD, Del Toro J, Jefferson LS, Evey L, Haase D. Management of pediatric acute hypoxemic respiratory insufficiency with bilevel positive pressure (BiPAP) nasal mask ventilation. Chest 1995; 108:1059–1064.
25. Kerbl R, Litscher H, Grubbauer HM, Reiterer F, Zobel G, Trop M, Urlesberger B, Eber E, Kurz R. Congenital central hypoventilation syndrome (Ondine's curse syndrome) in two siblings: delayed diagnosis and successful noninvasive treatment. Eur J Pediatr 1996; 155:977–980.
26. Villa MP, Dotta A, Castello D, Piro S, Pagani J, Palamides S, Ronchetti R. Bi-level positive airway pressure (BiPAP) ventilation in an infant with central hypoventilation syndrome. Pediatr Pulmonol 1997; 24:66–69.
27. Lyager S, Steffensen B, Juhl B. Indicators of need for mechanical ventilation in Duchenne muscular dystrophy and spinal muscular atrophy. Chest 1995; 108:779–785.
28. Raphael JC, Chevret S, Chastang C, Bouvet F. Randomised trial of preventive nasal ventilation in Duchenne muscular dystrophy. French Multicentre Cooperative Group on Home Mechanical Ventilation Assistance in Duchenne de Boulogne Muscular Dystrophy. Lancet 1994; 343:1600–1644.
29. Gilgoff I, Prentice W, Baydur A. Patient and family participation in the management of respiratory failure in Duchenne's muscular dystrophy. Chest 1989; 95:519–524.
30. Demirozu MC, Chediak AD, Nay KN, Cohn MA. A comparison of nine nasal continuous positive airway pressure machines in maintaining mask pressure during simulated inspiration. Sleep 1991; 14:259–262.
31. Bunburaphong T, Imanaka H, Nishimura M, Hess D, Kacmarek RM. Performance characteristics of bilevel pressure ventilators. Chest 1997; 111:1050–1060.

32. Smith IE, Shneerson JM. A laboratory comparison of four positive pressure ventilators used in the home. Eur Respir J 1996; 9:2410–2415.
33. Padkin AJ, Kinnear WJM. Supplemental oxygen and nasal intermittent positive pressure ventilation. Eur Respir J 1996; 9:834–836.
34. Strumpf DA, Carlisle CC, Millman RP, Smith KW, Hill NS. An evaluation of the Respironics BiPAP bi-level CPAP device for delivery of assisted ventilation. Respir Care 1990; 35:415–422.
35. Rains JC. Treatment of obstructive sleep apnea in pediatric patients. Clin Pediatr 1995;34:535–541.
36. Ferguson GT, Gilmartin M. CO_2 rebreathing during BiPAP ventilatory assistance. Am J Respir Crit Care Med 1995; 151:1126–1135.
37. Robertson NJ, McCarthy LS, Hamilton PA, Moss ALH. Nasal deformities resulting from flow driver continuous positive airway pressure. Arch Dis Child 1996; 75:F209–F212.
38. Sheehan GJ, Miedzinski LJ, Schroeder DG. Pneumothorax complicating BiPAP therapy for Pneumocystic carinii pneumonia (letter). Chest 1993; 103:1310.
39. Gregg RW, Friedman BC, Williams FJ, McGrath BJ, Zimmerman JE. Continuous positive airway pressure by face mask in *Pneumocystic carinii* pneumonia. Crit Care Med 1990; 18:21–24.
40. Leech JA, Ascah KJ. Hemodynamic effects of nasal CPAP examined by Doppler echocardiography. Chest 1991; 99:323–326.
41. Montner PK, Greene R, Murata GH, Stark DM, Timms M, Chick TW. Hemodynamic effects of nasal and face mask continuous positive airway pressure. Am J Respir Crit Care Med 1994; 149:1614–1618.
42. Alvarez-Sala R, Garcia IT, Garcia F, Moriche J, Prados C, Diaz S, Villasante C, Alvarez-Sala JL, Villamor J. Nasal CPAP during wakefulness increases intraocular pressure in glaucoma. Monaldi Arch Chest Dis 1994; 49:394–395.
43. Bamford CR, Quan SF. Bacterial meningitis-a possible complication of nasal continuous positive airway pressure therapy in a patient with obstructive sleep apnea syndrome and a mucocele. Sleep 1993; 16:31–32.
44. Kribbs NB, Pack AI, Kline LR, Smith PL, Schwartz AR, Schubert NM, Redline S, Henry JN, Getsy JE, Dinges DF. Objective measurement of patterns of nasal CPAP use by patients with obstructive sleep apnea. Am Rev Respir Dis 1993; 147:887–895.
45. Krieger J, Kurtz D, Petiau C, Sforza E, Trautmann D. Long-term compliance with CPAP therapy in obstructive sleep apnea patients and in snorers. Sleep 1996; 19(9 suppl):S136–S143.
46. Sforza E, Lugaresi E. Daytime sleepiness and nasal continuous positive airway pressure therapy in obstructive sleep apnea syndrome patients: effects of chronic treatment and 1-night therapy withdrawal. Sleep 1995; 18:195–201.
47. Kribbs NB, Pack AI, Kline LR, Getsy JE, Schuett JS, Henry JN, Maislin G, Dinges DF. Effects of one night without nasal CPAP treatment on sleep and sleepiness in patients with obstructive sleep apnea. Am Rev Respir Dis 1993; 147:1162–1168.
48. Boudewyns A, Sforza E, Zamagni M, Krieger J. Respiratory effort during sleep apneas after interruption of long-term CPAP treatment in patients with obstructive sleep apnea. Chest 1996; 110:120–127.

37

Diaphragm Pacing in Infancy and Childhood

DEBRA E. WEESE-MAYER

Rush University and
Rush Children's Hospital at Rush-Presbyterian-St. Luke's Medical Center
Chicago, Illinois

I. Historic Background

Diaphragm pacing by electrical stimulation of the phrenic nerve was first proposed over 200 years ago (1783) by Hufeland for the treatment of asphyxiated newborns, with description in his doctoral dissertation entitled "The Use of Electricity in Asphyxia" (1). In 1818, Ure demonstrated the success of electrical stimulation of the phrenic nerve in a "freshly hung criminal," as recently reported by Patterson (2). By 1872, pacing was successfully utilized by Duchenne de Boulogne to support artificial ventilation (3) and by Beard and Rockwell (4) as a technique for cardiopulmonary resuscitation. In 1927, Isreal applied transcutaneous stimulation of the phrenic nerves for ventilation of apneic newborns (5). Several decades passed before Sarnoff et al. described a method of percutaneous phrenic nerve stimulation that would successfully sustain breathing in patients with inadequate ventilation (6). Finally, in 1964, Glenn et al. reported their first results with diaphragm pacing (7). Since 1966, Glenn et al. have provided support using a diaphragm pacemaker system in more than 81 adults with chronic ventilatory deficiency (7–10).

Diaphragm pacing by electrical simulation of the phrenic nerve has now been applied successfully in infants and children for more than two decades (11–31), but most reports include only one, two, or a small group of children among a larger group of adult patients. The largest series of paced patients is followed at Rush Children's

Hospital in Chicago, with 42 paced patients (11–18,28) and typically the addition of 2 new patients each year. Thus, diaphragm pacing has evolved into a practical method of supporting the pediatric patient with inadequate central respiratory drive or high tetraplegia.

II. Technology

The diaphragm pacer system includes an external transmitter and loop antenna, an internal receiver, and internal phrenic nerve electrodes. The transmitter radiofrequency signal is emitted from the antennas placed on the skin overlying the subcutaneously implanted receivers. The receiver demodulates the signal, converts the radiofrequency energy into electrical energy, and delivers rectangular current pulses carried by stainless steel wires to the platinum stimulating electrodes placed about the thoracic phrenic nerve. As a result of the electrical stimulation of the phrenic nerve, the diaphragm contracts. Technology in use includes the monopolar electrode system manufactured by Avery Laboratories, Inc. (Glen Cove, NY) and the quadripolar electrode system manufactured by Atrotech Oy (Tampere, Finland), the former approved by the U.S. Food and Drug Administration (FDA) and the latter with provisional FDA approval.

III. World Experience with Diaphragm Pacing

Recent statistics indicate that nearly 1000 patients (adult and children) worldwide have been treated by diaphragm pacing (32). A comprehensive report of 477 patients implanted for the treatment of chronic hypoventilation was summarized by Glenn et al. (33). Those subjects were paced because of cervical cord or brainstem lesions, idiopathic congenital central hypoventilation syndrome, or hypoventilation secondary to peripheral causes. Nearly all of the patients described by Glenn et al. (33) were adults. 312 of the patients were treated at hospitals outside six collaborative centers with experience in diaphragm pacing and the management of paced patients. Further detail of the adult experience is available elsewhere.

Published reports of pacing in infants and children are limited in number and detail. Aside from reports of the Chicago pacer patients, including predominantly children with idiopathic congenital central hypoventilation syndrome (CCHS), the vast majority of the fewer than 50 pediatric patients reported in the literature have tetraplegia. The remaining subjects had central hypoventilation due to a tumor or was idiopathic in nature. In nearly all patients, pacing was bilateral, simultaneous, and part time. All children with bilateral pacing required a tracheostomy. Electrode implantation was typically in the thorax rather than the neck. Pacing was used during either wakefulness or sleep, depending on diagnosis and need. Notably, pediatric-specific information regarding complications of pacing, long-term outcome, and consensus of care is not available in published reports from other centers. For this reason the experience from our program is presented separately below.

IV. Pacer Experience in Infants and Children

Since 1976 we have supervised the implantation of diaphragm pacers in 42 infants and children, initially with the monopolar electrode system and subsequently with the quadripolar (28) system. These pediatric patients included 31 with idiopathic CCHS, 2 with late-onset central hypoventilation syndrome (CHS), 3 with myelomeningocele and Chiari type II malformation, 1 with acquired hypoventilation, and 5 with tetraplegia. All but 1 of these patients had bilateral, simultaneous, part-time pacing (less than 15 hr/day). All but 1 patient had a tracheostomy for either nighttime mechanical ventilation (a pacer being used during the day) or because of structural or functional pacing-related airway obstruction. The tracheostomy was removed at 5.6 years of age in one boy, though he has moderate inspiratory stridor caused by partial laryngeal obstruction with paced inspirations. For this one child, unilateral alternate-side pacing has yielded borderline acceptable ventilation during sleep. The phrenic nerve electrodes were implanted in the thorax, not the neck, in all patients implanted in the past 15 years.

A. Pediatric-Specific Modifications

To achieve effective ventilation in infants and young children, several modifications of pacer techniques have been necessary. First, the electrode itself must be of appropriate proportion for the phrenic nerve of a child. Second, the system must have adequate endurance to withstand the activity requirements of an active child, such as the child with CCHS. Third, bilateral pacing, as contrasted to unilateral, has generally been necessary to achieve adequate ventilation. Fourth, a tracheostomy is necessary to prevent upper-airway obstruction caused by the absence of laryngeal and pharyngeal dilator muscle activation during non–centrally mediated paced inspirations. Finally, due to the theoretical concern for diaphragm fatigue, pacing has typically been limited to 12 to 15 hr/day for the child. Although data have not indicated permanent injury to the nerve from prolonged continuous pacing in the adult animal or the adult tetraplegic human, it must be acknowledged that the pacer needs (rate and electrical stimulus) of active children far exceed those of the wheelchair-bound adult. Therefore, whether prolonged, continuous bilateral diaphragm pacing is possible in the child remains unknown.

Adaption of Electrode Size and Endurance of Pacer Components

Although the internal components have been manufactured in a pediatric size, the endurance of the pacer components remains inadequate for the active, ambulatory paced child. This has been a chronic problem regardless of the pacer manufacturer.

Bilateral Pacing

Infants and children have not been paced successfully during activity with either alternate-side pacing (right side of diaphragm for one breath, left side of diaphragm for next breath, right side next, and so forth) or sustained unilateral pacing. We have identified three potential reasons to account for this observation. First, infants and children have an increased metabolic rate corrected for body weight, with a higher required alveolar ventilation (34), thus requiring simultaneous stimulation of both the right and left sides of the diaphragm with each paced breath. Second, the compliant rib cage of the immature patient requires bilateral pacing to support ventilation. Finally, caution must be exercised to avoid fatigue and the risk of permanent injury to the diaphragm and phrenic nerves.

The oldest pediatric patient in our experience has had successful pacing for more than 20 years without evidence of long-term ill effects. In pediatric patients, typical use is bilateral for 12 to 15 hr/day. The child who is paced awake relies on the mechanical ventilator for support during sleep. Although data from a puppy model indicate that short-term, continuous, low-frequency pacing does not impair diaphragm function and actually causes conversion of muscle fiber type to a uniform population of type I fibers with high oxidative enzyme activity (35), clinical studies have not been performed to address this issue in children.

Airway Patency Control

The laryngeal abductors and pharyngeal dilator muscles are not activated during paced, non–centrally mediated inspirations. In younger patients, the vocal cords tend to be in midposition as inspiration begins but then may be drawn together to cause complete inspiratory obstruction because of the smaller laryngeal dimensions and greater negative inspiratory pressure resulting from the forceful diaphragmatic contractions occurring with bilateral pacing. In the older child, the vocal cords remain in midposition but the larger laryngeal dimensions generally result in only mild to moderate obstruction.

V. Current Approach to Pacing

A. Patient Selection Criteria

Although these criteria have evolved over time, they have remained consistent for more than 10 years. The ideal pediatric patient to benefit from diaphragm pacing is the child who is ventilator-dependent 24 hr/day but is without intrinsic lung disease or supplemental oxygen requirement and who has preservation of the cervical nerve roots of the phrenic nerve (C-3, C-4, and C-5), the phrenic nerve itself, and the diaphragm. These patients typically have idiopathic CCHS.

Two additional preconditions to recommending diaphragm pacing to a family have been identified. First, the family should be supportive and able to provide careful compliance with pacer evaluation and appropriate monitoring. Second the pacing should be expected to improve the patient's ability to function independently. Patients from intact families with strong emotional support usually thrive. Families from unstable environments are typically less cautious about pacer care, less involved in pacer management, and less likely to help the child reach her or his maximal potential for independence.

B. Age at Implantation

Previously, pacers were implanted as early as 1 month of age. Experience has taught us that pacing has little advantage until infants are approaching the age at which ambulation begins. Since children with CCHS typically have a delay in the maturation of motor skills, pacers are rarely implanted before 12 months of age. This delay allows time to identify and respond to any other major associated abnormalities, including severe central nervous system deficits or metabolic crises with hypoglycemia and seizures. Further, the severity of the ventilatory deficit may change during early infancy, and it is easier to clarify the full extent of the deficit before proceeding with surgical intervention.

C. Preoperative Assessment of Phrenic Nerves and Diaphragm

Spontaneous awake respiratory effort with diaphragm movement can be documented by fluoroscopy. Diaphragm excursion of at least two rib spaces is considered indicative of adequate diaphragmatic function and proof of adequate phrenic nerve viability, and thus of the ability to respond to electrical stimulation. In the child with tetraplegia or with questionable potential for sufficient spontaneous diaphragmatic function, percutaneous stimulation of the phrenic nerve is performed. The technique involves application of a bipolar stimulating electrode to the neck posterior to the lateral border of the sternocleidomastoid muscle (14,18). The electrode is moved superiorly and inferiorly along the body of the anterior scalene muscle to stimulate the phrenic nerve. Conduction time and the amplitude of the diaphragmatic action potential are measured on an oscilloscope from signals obtained by surface electromyographic electrodes placed on either side of the costal margin (superior and inferior) in the midclavicular line bilaterally.

D. Surgical Implantation Technique

The pediatric operative technique has been described previously (13) but has been modified at the discretion of the pediatric cardiovascular surgeon. The thoracic cavity is entered through the third intercostal space and the most proximal segment of the thoracic phrenic nerve is identified. The nerve is isolated from adjacent mediastinal pleura and soft tissue and the electrode is positioned about the nerve in the case of the quadripolar electrode (so that one electrode is in contact with each quadrant of the nerve) or under the nerve in the case of the monopolar electrode. Anchoring sutures are placed to maximize the stability of the electrodes and minimize the potential for tension on the nerve. Modification of the quadripolar system allows for a connecting wire attachment in the thorax, with the expectation that this will further minimize tension on the nerve and decrease the likelihood that the electrode component should fail. From the initial anterolateral inframammary incision, a subcutaneous pocket is created and extended to the flank. The receivers are connected to the extension wire from the thorax and the extension wire placed in a Gortex pouch to minimize scar tissue formation about the wires. The key variation in the surgical technique is a switch from the thoracic wires exiting the chest between ribs, with "exposure" of the wires to potential trauma at the exit site, to the thoracic wires being passed along the internal wall of the thorax with the exit through the lateral tendon of the diaphragm and below the last rib. The receiver is then placed in the subcutaneous pocket. The complete pacer system surgery with bilateral thoracotomies is performed during the same operative session. The child is typically discharged within 4 to 5 days of the surgical procedure. Although used in the adult, thoracoscopy has not been widely applied in children.

E. Adjustment of the Pacer System

Beginning 4 to 8 weeks after surgical implantation of the new pacers and annually thereafter, the pacers are adjusted in the Respiratory Physiology Laboratory. This technique has been published previously (15) for the monopolar electrode system. The technique is similar for the quadripolar electrode system but can be performed with greater precision because of the technology itself. The process is laborious but exacting. The goal of pacer adjustment is to minimize the electrical stimulation while achieving optimal oxygenation and ventilation. The stimulus current is adjusted to give a maximal diaphragmatic contraction at end-inspiration as judged by the amplitude of the diaphragmatic action potential measured from surface electromyogram electrodes at the costal margin. With the quadripolar system, the electrical threshold and volume are set for each individual electrode combination on both the right and the left sides (eight electrodes total). The within-breath increase in stimulating current, also known as the slope, can be set on both the right and the left to give a moderate diaphragmatic action potential at the onset of inspiration. The interpulse interval—the time between impulses—is adjusted to provide an optimal tidal volume with conservation of electrical impulses. The inspiratory time can be set for each side and adjusted to optimize ventilation. The pacer rate is adjusted to provide adequate minute ventilation but to minimize the number of impulses per inspiration. Once satisfactory settings have been determined that allow for optimal oxygenation and ventilation, the settings are downloaded from the programmer to the transmitter, which is wrapped in cushioned insulation and carried by the child in a backpack or a fanny pack. The portable transmitter can be adjusted by the parent to change the rate and the percent of maximal electrical volume, depending upon the exercise needs of the child. Condition-specific settings are determined in the Respiratory Physiology Laboratory during each pacer evaluation. After the pacers are set, the child is evaluated in the laboratory for several days before hospital discharge to assess the adequacy of ventilation and oxygenation during conditions the child will encounter in daily living.

F. Clinical Assessment of Pacer Function

Parents and nursing staff are instructed to examine the child daily for appropriate diaphragmatic excursions, with each side assessed independently. If a diaphragm is not being paced, the parent is advised to 1) replace the battery, 2) replace the antenna, 3) increase the electrical volume, and 4) change to the backup transmitter. If none of these suggestions result in appropriate diaphragmatic movement, ventilation must be supported, usually by intermittent positive-pressure ventilation, and the patient is scheduled for an evaluation in the Respiratory Physiology Laboratory. Before that evaluation, a chest radiograph is taken to identify wire breakage and electrode position. Unless the cause of pacer malfunction is apparent from the radiograph, evaluation is then performed during sleep to identify the site of pacer malfunction.

G. Complications of Diaphragm Pacing with the Monopolar Electrode System

The longevity of implanted pacer components by life-table analysis and the reasons for their failure were reported in 1992 (15) for 33 patients supported by monopolar pacing for a total of 192 system-years and 96 patient-years. By life-table analysis, the mean time to failure for internal components was 56.3 months, with a total of 26 failures occurring in the internal system. Symptoms of malfunction varied from absent diaphragm movement to intermittent function and sometimes to pain at the receiver site or ipsilateral shoulder.

Of the 26 internal component failures, 15 were due to receiver failure, 6 to electrode malfunction or lead wire/wire insulation breakage, 4 to infection, and 2 to mechanical injury. Successful pacing resumed in all cases after appropriate intervention. No substantive modifications of the electrode, wire, or transmitter of the Avery system have been made subsequent to the publication described above. A receiver model that was previously used for artificial stimulation of other organs has been introduced for use in diaphragm pacing with the monopolar Avery system.

H. Complications of Diaphragm Pacing with the Quadripolar Electrode System

Our experience and the world experience with the quadripolar electrode system was recently published (28). For that publication, we sought to determine the international experience with the quadripolar phrenic nerve electrode diaphragm pacer system via a questionnaire coupled with the Atrotech Registry data and to test two hypotheses: the incidence of pacer complications would be 1) increased among pediatric as compared to adult patients and 2) highest among active pediatric patients with CCHS. Data were collected for a total of 64 patients (35 children and 29 adults) from 14 countries. Among the 35 children were 19 with tetraplegia, 14 with CCHS, 1 with reactive gliosis of the brainstem, and 1 with trauma. All of the children implanted in the United States were from the Chicago program ($n = 12$). Thoracic implantation of electrodes and bilateral pacer use each occurred in 94% of all subjects. Pacers were more typically used for 24 hr/day among adult as compared to pediatric patients ($p = .01$). Infections occurred among 2.9% of surgical procedures, all in pediatric CCHS patients (versus pediatric tetraplegic patients, $p = .01$). The incidence of mechanical trauma was 3.8%, without significant differences among patient groups. The incidence of presumed electrode and receiver failure was 3.1% and 5.9%, respectively, with internal component failure greater among pediatric CCHS than pediatric tetraplegic patients ($p < .01$). Intermittent or absent function of up to four electrode combinations occurred among 19% of all patients, with increased frequency among pediatric CCHS than pediatric tetraplegic patients ($p < .03$). Pacing was without any complications in 60% of pediatric and 52% of adult patients, with a lower incidence among pediatric CCHS than pediatric tetraplegic patients ($p = .01$). In all, 94% of the pediatric and 86% of the adult patients paced successfully after the necessary intervention. Although pacer complications were not increased among pediatric as compared to adult patients, the incidence of complications was highest among the active pediatric patients with CCHS. Recognizing that, at the time of the above-described publication, the quadripolar pacer system had limited use in terms of patient numbers and duration of use, it is clear that longitudinal study of these patients will provide invaluable information for modification and improvement of the quadripolar system.

Subsequent to this publication, several modifications have been made in the internal components of the quadripolar electrode Atrostim system to improve its durability. Ongoing investigation will determine the success of these modifications.

VI. Long-Term Clinical Status

Of 42 patients in whom pacers were implanted in the experience of the investigators in Chicago, 32 are living. The 10 deaths occurred more than 10 years ago. Among the 32 living patients in whom pacers were implanted, 28 have been successfully supported by pacing. Of these, 22 have CCHS, 3 have Chiari type II malformation, and 3 have tetraplegia. Of these patients, 11 have had experience with both the monopolar and the quadripolar pacer systems. As for the 4 patients who are living but no longer pacing, the reasons are varied, the most notable being the inability to pace because obesity is preventing adequate diaphragmatic excursion in an adolescent with late-onset alveolar hypoventilation and hypothalamic dysfunction.

Each of the patients with ongoing diaphragmatic pacing requires spot checks with end-tidal carbon dioxide and hemoglobin saturation assessment in the home, coupled with annual assessment in the Respiratory Physiology Laboratory. The success of their management involves the cooperation of the child, the child's family, highly skilled home nursing, the local pediatrician and pulmonologist, and the center, with its extensive expertise in diaphragm pacing.

VII. Clinical Lessons from Diaphragm Pacing

Three important lessons have been learned through the extensive diaphragm pacing experience in Chicago. First, any child who might be using the pacers during sleep should use a pulse oximeter as an alarm for pacer malfunction. A transthoracic impedance monitor will not detect tracheal obstruction or bradycardia in the patient with a pacer (17). Because patients with CCHS do not develop bradycardia even in the case of severe hypoxemia, the transthoracic impedance monitor would be wholly ineffective. Further, the pacer artifact would mask any slowing of the heart rate. The pulse oximeter appropriately detects tracheal occlusion, as it would likewise detect pacer failure, with relatively rapid hemoglobin desaturation.

Second, the diaphragm pacer may cause electromagnetic interference with a demand cardiac pacemaker, as documented in adults (36). Although the chances of clinically significant interference are small, this risk is minimized by separating the receivers of the diaphragm pacer system and the cardiac pacemaker by at least 10 cm. Further, a bipolar cardiac pacemaker should be used, so that the electromagnetic fields are consolidated and therefore less likely to interfere with one another. With the quadripolar pacer system, the chance of interference between the diaphragm and cardiac pacer systems is reduced, since each should have a relatively closed electromagnetic field.

Third, magnetic resonance imaging (MRI) cannot be used in paced patients because the diaphragm pacer's internal components can be attracted to the magnet. Although CCHS is typically evaluated by MRI before diaphragm pacer implantation (37) and the patients do not generally require subsequent MRI, patients with Chiari type II malformation may need additional MRI evaluation. This factor must be weighed against the benefits of diaphragm pacing.

VIII. Advantages and Disadvantages of Diaphragm Pacing

Of primary importance is that pacers allow more patient mobility than do mechanical ventilators. For the child who requires ventilatory support while awake and asleep, the lightweight pacers offer an opportunity for a more normal lifestyle with pacers used during wakefulness. Patients who are supported by pacing while awake participate in age-appropriate noncontact sports. Although exercise must be taken in moderation because the pacer rate does not increase despite increased metabolic needs (38), these children would be severely limited physically and socially if a mechanical ventilator were necessary during wakefulness.

For the child who requires sleep ventilatory support only and for the tetraplegic child, the advantages of pacing are less apparent. It is easier and less conspicuous to travel with pacers, but a backup pacer and ventilator should always be taken along.

The disadvantages of diaphragm pacing include the risks of surgery and anesthesia and the financial cost. The risks associated with pacer implantation include those of general thoracic surgery and anesthesia as well as the risk of surgical trauma to the phrenic nerves. A major potential limitation is cost. A new pacer system costs in excess of $80,000, including the external components (transmitter and antennas) and the internal components (electrodes, receivers, connecting wires), in addition to the cost of surgery, hospitalization, and physiological assessments.

IX. Recommendation for Pacer Improvement and Future Goals

This alternate form of ventilatory support, although effective, is not as reliable as desired. Nearly all of the failures are due to receiver or electrode wire breakage. Improved design of both components would decrease the likelihood of breakage and need for rehospitalization and surgical intervention. Modifications have been made in the quadripolar system, but the technology has not achieved full FDA approval at the time of this writing. Collaboration with manufacturers of cardiac pacemakers may provide future successes not only in the endurance of the internal components but also in the potential for a totally implantable system.

X. Conclusion

Physicians can now better advise parents of children who are potential candidates for diaphragm pacing. With refinements in design and in selection, management of infants and children receiving diaphragm pacing by phrenic nerve stimulation, and centralization of medical and surgical pacer care, the clinical benefits of pacing can be improved and an optimal quality of life can be achieved for these children.

References

1. Hufeland CW. Usum uis electriciae in asphyxia experimentis illustratum. Dissertatio Inauguralis Medica, Göttingen, Germany, 1783.
2. Patterson FLM. The Clydesdale experiments: an early attempt at resuscitation. Scott Med J 1986; 31:050–052.
3. Duchenne GBA. De l'ectrisation localisée et de son application à la pathologie et à le therapeutique par courant induits et par courants galvaniques interrompus et continus par le Dr. Duchenne. Paris: Ballière, 1872.
4. Beard GM, Rockwell AD. A practical treatise on the medical and surgical uses of electricity. New York: William Wood, 1878: 664–666.
5. Isreal F. Uber die Wiederbelebung scheintoter Neugeborener mit Hilfe des elektrischen Stroms. Z Geburtshilfe Perinatal 1927; 91:601–622.
6. Sarnoff SJ, Sarnoff LC, Whittenberger JL. Electrophrenic respiration: VII. The motor point of the phrenic nerve in relation to external stimulation. Surg Gynecol Obstet 1951; 93:190–196.

7. Glenn WWL, Hageman JH, Mauro A, Eisenberg L. Flanigan S, Harvard M. Electrical stimulation of excitable tissue by radio-frequency transmission. Ann Surg 1964; 160:338–350.
8. Van Heeckeren DW, Glenn WWL. Electrophrenic respiration by radiofrequency induction. J Thorac Cardiovasc Surg 1966; 52:655–665.
9. Judson JP, Glenn WWL. Radio-frequency electrophrenic respiration. JAMA 1968; 203: 1033–1037.
10. Glenn WWL, Phelps ML, Elefteriades JA, Dentz B, Hogan JF. Twenty years of experience in phrenic nerve stimulation to pace the diaphragm. PACE 1986; 9:780–784.
11. Weese-Mayer DE, Hunt CE, Brouillette RT, Silvestri JM. Diaphragm pacing in infants and children. J Pediatr 1992; 120:1–8.
12. Hunt CE, Matalon SV, Thompson TR, Demuth S, Loew JM, Liu HM, Mastri A, Burke B. Central hypoventilation syndrome: experience with bilateral phrenic nerve pacing in 3 neonates. Am Rev Respir Dis 1978; 118:23–28.
13. Ilbawi MN, Idriss FS, Hunt CE, Brouillette RT, DeLeon SY. Diaphragmatic pacing in infants: techniques and results. Ann Thorac Surg 1985; 40:323–329.
14. Brouillette RT, Ilbawi MN, Klemka-Walden L, Hunt CE. Stimulus parameters for phrenic nerve pacing in infants and children. Pediatr Pulmonol 1988; 4:33–38.
15. Weese-Mayer DE, Morrow AS, Brouillette RT, Ilbawi MN, Hunt CE. Diaphragm pacing in infants and children: a life-table analysis of implanted components. Am Rev Respir Dis 1989; 139:974–979.
16. Hunt CE, Brouillette RT, Weese-Mayer DE, Morrow A, Ilbawi MN. Diaphragm pacing in infants and children. PACE 1988; 11:2135–2141.
17. Marzocchi M, Brouillette RT, Weese-Mayer DE, Morrow AS, Conway LP. Comparison of transthoracic impedance/heart rate monitoring and pulse oximetry for patients using diaphragm pacemakers. Pediatr Pulmonol 1990; 8:29–32.
18. Brouillette RT, Ilbawi MN, Hunt CE. Phrenic nerve pacing in infants and children: a review of experience and report on the usefulness of phrenic nerve stimulation studies. J Pediatr 1983; 103:32–39.
19. Cahill JL, Okamoto GA, Higgins T, Davis A. Experiences with phrenic nerve pacing in children. J Pediatr Surg 1983; 18:851–854.
20. Fodstad H. The Swedish experience in phrenic nerve stimulation. PACE 1987; 10:246–251.
21. Glenn WWL, Hogan JF, Loke JS, Ciesielski TE, Phelps ML, Rowedder R. Ventilatory support by pacing of the conditioned diaphragm in quadriplegia. N Engl J Med 1984; 310: 1150–1155.
22. Mellins RB, Balfour HH, Turino GM, Winters RW. Failure of automatic control of ventilation (Ondine's curse). Medicine 1970; 49:487–504.
23. McMichan JC, Piepgras DG, Gracey DR, March HM, Sittipong R. Electrophrenic respiration: report of six cases. Mayo Clin Proc 1979; 54:662–668.
24. Coleman M, Boros SJ, Huseby TL, Brennom WS. Congenital central hypoventilation syndrome: a report of successful experience with bilateral diaphragmatic pacing. Arch Dis Child 1980; 55:901–903.
25. Oakes DD, Wilmot CB, Halverson D, Hamilton RD. Neurogenic respiratory failure: a 5-year experience using implantable phrenic nerve stimulators. Ann Thorac Surg 1980; 30: 118–121.
26. Ruth V, Pesonen E, Raivio KO. Congenital central hypoventilation syndrome treated with central diaphragm pacing. Acta Pediatr Scand 1983; 72:295–297.

27. Radecki LL, Tomatis LA. Continuous bilateral electrophrenic pacing in an infant with total diaphragmatic paralysis. J Pediatr 1976; 88:969–971.
28. Weese-Mayer DE, Silvestri JM, Kenny AS, Ilbawi MN, Hauptman SA, Lipton JW, Talonen PP, Garrido Garcia H, Watt JW, Exner G, Baer GA, Elefteriades JA, Peruzzi WT, Alex CG, Harlid R, Vincken W, Davis GM, Decramer M, Kuenzle C, Sæterhaug A, Schöber JG. Diaphragm pacing with a quadripolar phrenic nerve electrode: an international study. PACE 1996; 19:1311–1319.
29. Yasuma F, Nomura H, Sotobata I, Ishihara H, Saito H, Yasuura K, Okamoto H, Hirose S, Abe T, Seki A. Congenital central alveolar hypoventilation: a case report and review of the literature. Eur J Pediatr 1987; 146:81–83.
30. Sasaki T, Nakano H, Asano T, Manaka S, Takakura K, Tsutsumi H, Toyooka H, Satoh I. Nocturnal dyspnea treated by diaphragm pacing. Surg Neurol 1983; 19:232–236.
31. Meisner H, Schöber JG, Struck E, Lipowski B, Mayser P, Sebening F. Phrenic nerve pacing for the treatment of central hypoventilation syndrome: state of the art and case report. Thorac Cardiovasc Surg 1983; 31:21–25.
32. Maxon J, Shneerson JM. Diaphragmatic pacing. Am Rev Respir Dis 1993; 148:533–536.
33. Glenn WWL, Brouillette RT, Dentz B, Fodstad H, Hunt CE, Keens TG, Marsh HM, Pande S, Piepgras DG, Vanderlinden RG. Fundamental considerations in pacing of the diaphragm for chronic ventilatory insufficiency: a multi-center study. PACE 1988; 11:2121–2127.
34. Wohl MEG, Mead J. Age as a factor in respiratory disease. In: Kendig EL, Chernick V, eds. Disorders of the respiratory tract in children. Philadelphia: Saunders, 1983:135–141.
35. Marzocchi M, Brouillette RT, Klemka-Walden LM, Heller SL, Weese-Mayer DE, Brozanski BS, Caliendo J, Daood M, Ilbawi MN, Hunt CE. Effects of continuous low frequency pacing on immature canine diaphragm. J Appl Physiol 1990; 69:892–898.
36. Wicks JM, Davison R, Belic N. Malfunction of a demand pacemaker caused by phrenic nerve stimulation. Chest 1978; 74:303–305.
37. Weese-Mayer DE, Brouillette RT, Naidich TP, McLone DG, Hunt CE. Magnetic resonance imaging and computerized tomography in central hypoventilation. Am Rev Respir Dis 1988; 137:393–398.
38. Silvestri JM, Weese-Mayer DE, Flanagan EA. Congenital central hypoventilation syndrome: cardiorespiratory responses to moderate exercise, simulating daily activity. Pediatr Pulmonol 1995; 20:89–93.

Appendix

Standards and Indications for Cardiopulmonary Sleep Studies in Children*

This Official Statement of the American Thoracic Society was adopted by the ATS Board of Directors, July 1995.

Contents

Sleep induces changes in the function and control of the respiratory system. These changes may result in clinically significant abnormalities in upper airway function and gas exchange in both normal children and those with underlying respiratory or central nervous system disease (1–4).

To clarify the state of the art for pediatric breathing and sleep disorders and to develop recommendations about standards and indications for cardiopulmonary sleep studies in children, the Pediatric Assembly of the American Thoracic Society convened a consensus conference of individuals with expertise in pediatric pulmonology, otolaryngology, neonatology, plastic surgery, neurology, and developmental respiratory physiology. The format of the conference was similar to that used to develop standards for adults (5). This summary has been reviewed and revised extensively by the committee and members of the pediatric assembly.

The conference had several goals:

- to define the indications for evaluating breathing during sleep in children and adolescents.
- to develop standards for the indications, techniques, and interpretation of polysomnography (PSG) for evaluating breathing disorders during sleep in children and adolescents.

---

*Reprinted from Am J Respir Crit Care Med 153:866–878, 1996. Copyright American Thoracic Society, Medical Section of the American Lung Association.

- to identify areas where the knowledge base is lacking and will require research in order to establish recommendations.

Respiratory Indications for Polysomnography in Children

Obstructive Sleep Apnea Syndrome

Background. Obstructive Sleep Apnea Syndrome (OSAS) in children is a disorder of breathing during sleep characterized by prolonged partial upper airway obstruction and/or intermittent complete obstruction (obstructive apnea) that disrupt normal ventilation during sleep and normal sleep patterns (6,7). It has been estimated that approximately 7 to 9% of children snore regularly (8–10), with an estimated prevalence of OSAS at 0.7% in 4- to 5-year-old children (9). Most affected children breathe normally while awake. However, a minority with marked upper airway obstruction also have noisy, mildly labored breathing when awake. Clinical manifestations of OSAS in children include chronic mouth breathing, snoring, and restlessness during sleep, with or without frequent awakenings (6,7). Loud snoring that disturbs and concerns parents is a common indication for evaluation. However, clinical experience suggests that some infants with clinically significant OSAS may have little or no snoring. Less frequently, daytime hypersomnolence, failure to thrive, and cor pulmonale may be seen (6,7,11–14). The frequency of behavioral, personality, and learning problems in children with OSAS is unknown, but such problems may prove to be common manifestations as more experience is accumulated (6,11). An association between OSAS and enuresis has been suggested (15,16). Systemic hypertension secondary to OSAS is uncommon in children (17).

Major risk factors for OSAS in children include hypertrophy of the tonsils and adenoids (6,7,15), neuromuscular disease including conditions associated with both muscular hypotonia and hypertonia (18,19), obesity (20), and genetic syndromes, especially those associated with midface hypoplasia, small nasopharynx, or micrognathia, such as Down syndrome and Pierre Robin sequence (21–23). Less common risk factors for OSAS are laryngomalacia (24), pharyngeal flap surgery (25), sickle cell disease (26), structural malformations of the brainstem (27), and certain metabolic and genetic disorders (28). Viral respiratory infections and allergic rhinitis are not primary risk factors for OSAS, but they may exacerbate existing OSAS in affected children (29).

Clinical experience suggests that the pathophysiology, clinical manifestations, diagnosis, and management of children with suspected obstructive sleep apnea are different than for adults (30,31).

Consensus Recommendations.

- Polysomnography is recommended to differentiate benign or primary snoring, i.e., snoring not associated with apnea, hypoventilation, or evidence of cardiovascular or central nervous system effects, for which treatment is rarely indicated, from pathologic snoring (OSAS), i.e., snoring associated with either partial or complete airway obstruction, hypoxemia, and sleep disruption (32). A history of loud snoring alone has not been shown consistently to have sufficient diagnostic sensitivity upon which to base a recommendation for surgery, whether adenotonsillectomy, uvulopalatopharyngoplasty (UPPP), or tracheostomy (33–35). Polysomnography findings suggestive of abnormality are included in the section on interpreting PSG data.

- Polysomnography is indicated for evaluating the child with disturbed sleep patterns, excessive daytime sleepiness, cor pulmonale, failure to thrive, or polycythemia unexplained by other factors or conditions, especially if the child also snores.
- In the child who has clinically significant airway obstruction (apnea, retractions, paradoxical respiration) during sleep as observed by medical personnel, or documented by audiovideo recording, a PSG to confirm the clinical diagnosis may be deferred in order to proceed with therapy expeditiously.
- Polysomnography is recommended if the physician is uncertain whether the clinical observation of obstructed breathing is sufficient to warrant surgery or if a child needs intensive postoperative monitoring following adenotonsillectomy or other pharyngeal surgery (36). Risk factors for postoperative complications include age less than 2 yr, those with more than 10 obstructive events per hour of sleep, those with Sa_{O_2} less than 70%, and those with underlying neuromuscular disease or craniofacial abnormalities, specifically those associated with midface hypoplasia and retro- or micrognathia (21,25,36,37).
- Polysomnography is recommended in children with laryngomalacia whose symptoms (stridor and work of breathing) are worse asleep than awake or who have failure to thrive or cor pulmonale (24).
- Although obesity is a risk factor for OSAS in children (20,38), its presence alone is not an indication for PSG unless the child also exhibits unexplained awake hypercapnia, chronic snoring, increased work of breathing during sleep, disturbed sleep, daytime hypersomnolence, polycythemia, or cor pulmonale (20,38).
- Polysomnography is recommended during evaluation of the child with sickle cell disease who has either the typical signs and symptoms of OSAS or frequent veno-occlusive crises occurring during sleep (26,39). Oxygen saturation data from pulse oximetry must be interpreted cautiously in this population, because sickle hemoglobin may adversely affect the accuracy of oximetry (40).
- Repeat PSG is recommended for children previously diagnosed with obstructive sleep apnea who exhibit persistent snoring or other symptoms of sleep-disordered breathing. If possible, based on the child's clinical condition, this study should be deferred until at least four weeks postsurgery to allow for resolution of postoperative edema.

- If continuous positive airway pressure (CPAP) is used in the management of OSAS or other respiratory conditions, PSG should be used to titrate the level of CPAP and to reevaluate periodically the appropriateness of the settings.
- When weight loss is the primary therapy for OSAS in an obese child, PSG should be repeated to determine if the weight loss program has decreased the severity of OSAS.
- Children with mild to moderate OSAS who have complete resolution of snoring and disturbed sleep patterns after therapy do not need a follow-up PSG. However, in a child under 1 yr or a child with severe OSAS based on clinical symptoms, the number of obstructive events, or severe desaturation episodes, follow-up PSG should be considered to assure resolution of clinically significant abnormalities (41). Whether or not a follow-up study is ordered, parents and primary care providers should be taught the signs and symptoms of a recurrence of OSAS. The child should also have routine clinical follow-up to ensure early detection of a recurrence of abnormal breathing during sleep.
- If excessive daytime sleepiness is found not to be due to OSAS based on the results of nocturnal PSG, or if excessive daytime sleepiness persists after treatment, a multiple sleep latency test (MSLT) can be used to quantitate excessive daytime sleepiness and determine if it is secondary to narcolepsy (42). The MSLT can also be used to monitor the response to treatment of OSAS or narcolepsy. It should be performed on the day following a nocturnal PSG, so that nocturnal factors that may contribute to daytime sleepiness can be controlled and eliminated. Age-appropriate reference values should be used (43,44). A sleep diary can also be used to confirm adequacy of the sleep periods.
- Assessment of sleep and breathing in the home using video and cardiorespiratory recordings with extended oximetry appears promising, but recommendations regarding their use require further clinical trials (45,46).
- Extended oximetry recording alone can be used to identify hypoxemia during sleep in patients with loud snoring. However, the absence of hypoxemia during sleep does not preclude clinically significant OSAS. Conversely, the presence of hypoxemia during sleep is not in itself diagnostic of OSAS, as it may be caused by other respiratory conditions.

Bronchopulmonary Dysplasia

Background. Bronchopulmonary dysplasia (BPD) is a form of chronic lung disease that follows an acute lung injury in the neonatal period. It is characterized by persistent signs of respiratory distress (tachypnea and dyspnea), the need for supplemental oxygen beyond the first month of life to treat hypoxemia, and characteristic radiographic findings (47,48).

Some infants and children with BPD have been shown to have prolonged episodes of hypoxemia during sleep, despite the presence of adequate oxygenation while awake (3,49–54). In addition, infants with BPD, who are hypoxemic while awake, may experience worsening of hypoxemia while asleep. Abnormal duration of rib-cage paradox during inspiration while in rapid eye movement (REM) sleep and abnormal rib-cage paradox during non-REM sleep have also been reported (51–53). During REM sleep, intercostal muscles and other accessory muscles of inspiration are inhibited. In infants with BPD, the combination of abnormal pulmonary mechanics and REM–related loss of inspiratory muscle activity results in rib-cage paradox and hypoxemia (52–54). These episodes are not always predicted by awake blood gas measurement and may not be detected by monitoring during daytime naps, direct observation, or by recording techniques with sluggish response time, such as transcutaneous P_{O_2} monitoring (50,55).

Consensus Recommendations.

- Assessment of Sa_{O_2} when the infant is awake may not accurately predict hypoxemia during feeding and sleep (56). Oxygen saturation during feeding and sleep should be measured for an extended period (hours) in these groups: 1) infants and children with BPD who are on oxygen, to know that they have enough oxygen to keep saturation values above 92% during these periods, and 2) infants and children with BPD who have recently been weaned to room air when awake. The latter patients need to have their saturation measured for an extended period during sleep to know that they no longer need oxygen then.
- Under certain circumstances, patients with BPD who have had supplemental oxygen discontinued should undergo continuous documentation of Sa_{O_2} during sleep. These patients include infants who develop, after supplemental oxygen has been discontinued, polycythemia, cor pulmonale, failure to thrive (unexplained by other factors such as nutrition or other metabolic condition), disturbed sleep patterns, or apnea and bradycardia during sleep.
- If bradycardia without apnea is documented by impedance monitoring in infants with BPD, PSG may be indicated to detect upper airway obstruction during sleep. Similarly, if the infant with BPD is suspected of having airway obstruction during sleep based on observation of snoring, PSG is required.
- An infant who is receiving supplemental oxygen therapy and develops any of the above complications should have, in addition to measurements of Sa_{O_2} while awake, continuous documentation of Sa_{O_2} overnight, while asleep, to determine the adequacy of supplemental oxygen being delivered. Recording of the plethysmographic waveform or the pulse amplitude modulation signals in addition to Sa_{O_2} is necessary to distinguish true drops in saturation from apparent drops due to movement artifact or a weak pulse signal (56).

- Polysomnography can be used with esophageal pH monitoring to document the temporal relationship between gastroesophageal reflux and respiratory events such as obstructive apnea, cough, or hypoxemia.

Cystic Fibrosis

Background. Episodes of desaturation unrelated to apnea have been observed in some patients with cystic fibrosis (57–60). Patients with an awake $Pa_{O_2} < 60$ mmHg spend > 80% of sleep time with O_2 saturations < 90%, while those with an awake Pa_{O_2} > 70 mmHg spend < 20% of their time asleep with $Sa_{O_2} < 90\%$ (61). In an individual patient, clinical scores, awake oxygenation status, pulmonary function, and the response to exercise have not been shown to predict hypoxic events during sleep (60,61).

Consensus Recommendations.

- Patients with cystic fibrosis who have an awake $Pa_{O_2} < 70$ mmHg or an equivalent Sa_{O_2} (< 95%) during a period of disease stability are at risk for worsening hypoxemia during sleep and should have continuous documentation of Sa_{O_2} during nocturnal sleep. This study should be performed during a period of disease stability (generally at least 2 wk following treatment for an acute pulmonary exacerbation) in order to determine the extent and severity of sleep-associated hypoxemia and confirm the adequacy of prescribed supplemental oxygen. Random, brief checks of saturation (< 5 min recording) or visual observation of the patient during sleep are not adequate to identify desaturation episodes and will not detect OSAS (62).
- Patients with cystic fibrosis who develop polycythemia, cor pulmonale unexplained by awake blood gas or Sa_{O_2} measurements, or who complain of headaches upon awakening, excessive daytime sleepiness, or disturbed sleep patterns should also undergo continuous documentation of Sa_{O_2} for at least 8 h overnight during sleep.
- Patients with cystic fibrosis receiving supplemental oxygen may require PSG to rule out OSAS if there is a history of snoring, desaturation episodes during sleep, cor pulmonale, polycythemia, or disturbed sleep. Polysomnography should also be considered for assessing the potential adverse effects of supplemental oxygen during sleep in patients with advanced lung disease who are hypercapnic when awake.

Asthma

Background. Early morning worsening of asthma is seen in children and adolescents (63,64). The circadian variation in airway caliber seen in normal children is amplified in patients with asthma and may produce as much as a 50% decrease in peak flow rate (64). These changes in flow rates do not appear to be caused by sleep per se, but rather to be due to diurnal variations in pulmonary function (64,65). Patients with asthma, including those suboptimally controlled, tend to have small changes in Sa_{O_2} during sleep (66,67).

Consensus Recommendations.

- In children with asthma symptoms during sleep, a thorough clinical investigation including an assessment of the environment and the appropriateness of nocturnal therapy is indicated to identify factors that may contribute to these symptoms. If there is concern about the presence of gastroesophageal reflux during sleep as a trigger for nocturnal symptoms, PSG with esophageal pH monitoring should be considered. Continuous documentation of oxygenation during sleep is infrequently needed in routine management of children with asthma, but should be considered for children with poorly controlled nocturnal asthma who exhibit disturbed sleep, morning headaches, or cor pulmonale.

Neuromuscular Disease

Background. Children and young adults with a variety of pediatric neuromuscular disorders are at risk of developing both central and obstructive apnea/hypoventilation during sleep. These disorders include Duchenne muscular dystrophy (68), myotonic dystrophy (69), spinal muscle atrophy (70), cerebral palsy, poliomyelitis (72), and congenital muscle diseases (73–76). Abnormal breathing during sleep in these disorders is often not predicted by awake pulmonary function testing, arterial blood gases, or the degree of muscle involvement (68,70,76–85).

Children with cerebral palsy and other static encephalopathies often experience bulbar involvement and glottic muscle dysfunction. If pharyngeal muscles are more severely affected than the diaphragm or other inspiratory muscles, the usual reduction of upper airway muscle tone that occurs during sleep can precipitate obstructive sleep apnea (71). This vulnerability to respiratory abnormalities is most pronounced during REM sleep, when inhibition of accessory muscles of respiration requires the diaphragm to assume more of the work of breathing. Children with central nervous system disease and evidence of pharyngeal dysfunction should be considered at risk for obstructive sleep apnea and obstructive hypoventilation (86,87).

Consensus Recommendations.

- Polysomnography, including either end-tidal or transcutaneous CO_2 monitoring, is indicated in evaluating children with neuromuscular disease who demonstrate impaired respiratory muscle function by FVC < 40%, a peak inspiratory pressure < 15 cm H_2O, and/or pharyngeal dysfunction (snoring or swallowing abnormalities).
- Polysomnography, including some measurement of CO_2, is indicated in children with neuromuscular disease who develop snoring, cor pulmonale, morning headaches, personality or behavioral changes, failure to thrive, or developmental delay disproportionate to the degree of neurologic impairment or the typical course of the disease.
- Polysomnography with CO_2 monitoring is indicated in patients with neuromuscular disease who have polycythemia or elevated serum bicarbonate.

- Polysomnography with CO_2 monitoring is indicated for planning and implementing elective nocturnal assisted ventilation for patients with ventilatory muscle weakness.
- Polysomnography with CO_2 monitoring is indicated in children with neuromuscular disease to assess the adequacy of ongoing home respiratory support, including supplemental oxygen, CPAP, or assisted ventilation. Periodic reassessment should be scheduled according to the child's growth rate and degree of clinical stability, but generally it should be at least annually (88).
- Polysomnography with CO_2 monitoring should be used during preoperative and postoperative assessment of children with neuromuscular disease before major upper airway, thoracic, abdominal, or orthopedic surgery to detect unsuspected hypoventilation that could be aggravated by sedation, analgesia, and anesthetics.

Alveolar Hypoventilation Syndromes

Background. Alveolar hypoventilation in the absence of underlying primary pulmonary disease or respiratory muscle dysfunction is usually the result of abnormal central integration of chemoreceptor signals. This process may be primary, as in idiopathic congenital central hypoventilation syndrome, or it may be secondary to diseases of the spinal cord or brainstem, such as Arnold-Chiari malformation. The respiratory deficit is typically more severe during sleep than wakefulness and is characterized by alveolar hypoventilation resulting in hypoxemia and hypercarbia (89–92).

Consensus Recommendations.

- Polysomnography including assessment of CO_2 is indicated to determine the nature and severity of the ventilatory deficit in children with alveolar hypoventilation syndrome.
- Polysomnography is indicated periodically to determine the adequacy of ventilation and oxygenation provided by artificial ventilatory support, including diaphragmatic pacing (92). The frequency of follow-up study will vary depending on the clinical stability of the child, but such studies should occur at least annually. Polysomnography should be used to determine the effects of any pharmacologic trials.
- Polysomnography is recommended for any patient with a clinically stable central hypoventilation syndrome who develops cor pulmonale, polycythemia, morning headaches, deterioration in mental status, or altered growth patterns.

Respiratory Problems in Newborn Infants

Background. Infants, especially those born prematurely, frequently experience apnea or bradycardia during sleep and feeding in the first several weeks of life

(93). Virtually all infants under 1000 g will experience apnea (94). Apnea may be mixed, central, or obstructive (94,95).

An apparent life-threatening event (ALTE) is an episode of apnea, color change (pallor, cyanosis, or erythema), and hypotonia that the observer believes to be life-threatening to the infant and for which some intervention (stimulation, shaking, and/or cardiopulmonary resuscitation) is felt to be required. The major concerns following one of these episodes relate to the risk of recurrent events and death. Because this topic was discussed in detail at a National Institutes of Health–sponsored consensus conference (96), this ATS committee decided to limit present discussion of this topic to how PSG should be used for evaluating these patients.

Consensus Recommendations.

- Polysomnography is not indicated for routine evaluation of infants with an uncomplicated ALTE.
- Polysomnography may be helpful in defining the frequency and type of apnea and the extent of cardiac, blood gas, and sleep alterations in certain infants with apnea or ALTE. These patients include infants with suspected obstructive apnea, those with recurrent isolated bradycardia without central apnea, and those suspected to have abnormal respiratory control.

Guidelines for Performing Polysomnography in Children

Pediatric sleep and breathing disorders affect patients from infancy through adolescence. Consequently, the pediatric sleep laboratory must be able to accommodate a wide range of physical, developmental, and behavioral challenges. Children may be easily frightened by sleeping in a strange environment, attached to a variety of monitoring devices. Success in studying children requires a comprehensive approach including recognition of the unique needs of children. Polysomnography for cardiopulmonary indications simultaneously records physiologic variables including sleep state, respiration, cardiac rhythm, muscle activity, gas exchange, and snoring. Behavioral aspects of sleep, such as the quality of the child's sleep, may also be assessed. This assessment should be accomplished in a manner that is minimally invasive or disruptive to the child's usual sleep patterns.

Laboratory Conditions

Supervision of the Laboratory. The individual responsible for overall supervision of a laboratory whose primary activity is performing PSG in infants and children with cardiorespiratory disorders should be a pediatrician with training and experience in pediatric respiratory disorders and/or sleep medicine.

We recognize that due to limited availability of PSG resources, pediatric patients may be studied in facilities that predominantly study adults. In this setting, it is strongly recommended that a pediatrician with expertise in pediatric pulmonology, neonatology, neurology, or pediatric sleep medicine oversee laboratory operations related to children. The pediatric specialist can assure that the PSG is performed, scored, and interpreted appropriately for the age and condition of the child.

If such personnel are not actively involved in the daily operation of the laboratory, formal consultation should be obtained from physicians with expertise in pediatric pulmonology, otolaryngology, cardiology, neonatology, neurology, and behavioral medicine.

Setting. Children should be studied in a dedicated pediatric facility with a laboratory decor that is both age-appropriate and nonthreatening. If a separate pediatric laboratory is not available, an area should be designated for children. The setting should accommodate a parent comfortably during the study. A place for the parent or guardian to sleep near the child while the study is in progress is recommended. Immediate parental access to the child is often necessary to reduce fear and anxiety, especially in the younger child, and to provide ordinary child care.

Personnel. Staffing by personnel skilled in dealing with infants, children, and adolescents is required. All clinical personnel should be certified in pediatric cardiopulmonary resuscitation. They should also demonstrate knowledge of childhood behavior and the ability to deal with children of varying ages and developmental stages. Procedures should be explained to the patient and parent or guardian by someone skilled in presenting medical information to children. Audiovisual aids may be useful.

Timing of the Study

Background. Polysomnography for evaluating respiratory disorders should be performed under conditions that most closely approximate the child's usual sleep habits. Overnight sleep studies should begin at the child's usual bedtime. Although there are limited data on the usefulness of nap studies for diagnosing abnormal breathing during sleep in adults (97,98), one study in children demonstrated that a positive nap study for obstructive sleep apnea correlated well with the findings of an overnight study (99). However, a negative nap study did not exclude the presence of obstructive apnea occurring during a nocturnal study (99). Nap studies are limited in that daytime sleep periods are shorter than overnight sleep periods, may not include REM periods, do not incorporate circadian variability, and are unusual daytime behaviors for children older than 4 yr. In many instances, the only way nap studies can be accomplished reliably is by sleep deprivation or the use of sedatives. Both measures may increase the amount of obstructive apnea (100–104). The use of sedation can be associated with severe worsening of obstructive sleep apnea and its use is contraindicated (104). Polysomnography (including a nap study) cannot be considered normal unless it assesses breathing during at least one REM period. There was also concern, based on clinical experience, that a single REM episode may not be sufficient, since it is not clear that all REM episodes are equivalent. More data are needed to answer this question.

Consensus Recommendations.

- Whenever possible, PSG should be performed as an overnight study. It should be performed without the use of sedatives or sleep deprivation.

- Daytime nap studies may be useful as a screening technique to identify disordered breathing during sleep. To be considered reliable, the nap must last at least 2 h and include at least one period of REM sleep. A normal nap study is not sufficient to exclude a diagnosis of obstructive sleep apnea in a patient with clinical manifestations suggesting OSAS or to exclude abnormal ventilation and oxygenation during nocturnal sleep in patients with obstructive lung disease.

Number of Studies

Background. Sleep during the first night in the sleep laboratory may differ from sleep on subsequent nights. Data from children and young adults demonstrates the so-called "first-night effect," marked by decreased total sleep time and percent of REM time (105–107). However, this first-night effect is not believed to alter the respiratory patterns in adults with clinically significant sleep-disordered breathing (5,107). The consequences of the first-night effect in children with mild OSAS are not known. The night-to-night variability of respiratory patterns is also not felt to be clinically significant in adults with OSAS (108); thus, a single-night study is thought sufficient to exclude clinically important sleep-disordered breathing in adults (5). However, in children, data on the magnitude and nature of the first-night effect on respiratory patterns is limited, and at this time, there are no data on the reproducibility, sensitivity, and specificity of a single-night PSG for children of different ages.

Consensus Recommendations. Until more data are gathered, for most indications, a single-night study is believed sufficient to rule out a clinically significant disorder of respiration during sleep. However, if the child does not experience at least one REM period or the parents report that what was observed during the study did not reflect a typical night's sleep or the chief complaint, consideration should be given to repeating the study. If the first study was clinically indicated and it is found to be technically inadequate, then it should be repeated.

Measurement Techniques

Respiratory Variables. These measurements are obtained to assess the adequacy of ventilation, to identify and differentiate between central and obstructive apnea, and to evaluate the severity and physiologic consequences of the breathing disturbance. Respiratory parameters recorded include movements of the chest wall and abdomen, detection of airflow at the nose and mouth, and assessment of the effectiveness of respiration using oxygenation and CO_2 retention measures (109,110). Currently, there are no noninvasive techniques that provide a comprehensive quantification of breathing during sleep. However, noninvasive qualitative or semiquantitative techniques are adequate for most clinical purposes.

Respiratory Movements. A cardiopulmonary sleep study should permit the clinician to distinguish between normal respiratory effort; decreased respiratory effort, as in central hypoventilation; and increased respiratory effort, as in OSAS. In older children, paradoxical inspiratory movement of chest and abdomen is a sensitive indicator of increased airway resistance. It can be recorded using strain gauges (111,112), respiratory inductive plethysmography (113–116), or magnetometers (117,118). In infants, paradoxical movements are also seen during normal REM sleep, and the presence of paradoxical breathing does not necessarily indicate abnormality (119). Electromyography of the diaphragm and accessory muscles of respiration can provide additional information about activity of specific muscle groups (diaphragm, upper airway dilators, expiratory muscles, etc.). Esophageal pressure recording provides the most accurate, quantitative measurement of respiratory effort, but routine use of this invasive technique is not necessary for most clinical purposes (120–123).

Airflow measurements: Airflow can be measured by a pneumotachograph connected to nasal prongs, an oronasal mask, or tracheostomy tube. Quantitative measurements of airflow and tidal volume are most useful in research settings and assessment of central hypoventilation. Such measurements have little if any role in routine clinical studies because the mask may be uncomfortable, may frighten the child, and may alter the pattern of breathing (124). Measurement of airflow can be accomplished in a variety of ways. Oronasal thermistors and/or nasal CO_2 catheters are used most commonly in clinical laboratories. They provide qualitative airflow signals and require attachment to the face (109,125). Thermistors may not reliably detect episodes of partial airway obstruction with reduced tidal volume (hypopneas). The laryngeal microphone has been recommended to detect airflow or its absence in patients with OSAS (126,127). However, this technique is limited because it can only detect complete obstruction. Recording sound will only yield information on the degree and quality of snoring, neither of which has been shown to correlate with the severity of the ventilatory disturbance (33,34).

Respiratory inductive plethysmography (RIP) provides both an assessment of the chest/abdominal asynchrony and a semiquantitative measurement of airflow and tidal volume (113–116). The method uses bands around the chest and abdomen and may detect airway obstruction without the need to attach thermistors or end-tidal CO_2 sampling catheters to the face. Calibration can be performed automatically to set the abdominal and thoracic sum signal proportional to tidal volume. This system worked well for detecting obstructive apnea as well as partial airway obstruction in children and adults (128–130) and in measuring tidal volume in infants (114).

Caution is warranted when using RIP in infants and in children with increased work of breathing. In infants, especially preterm neonates, chest/abdominal asynchrony is common as REM–sleep related hypotonia permits inward chest motion during inspiration (119). To avoid overdiagnosing apnea/hypopnea when using RIP in infants, confirmatory channels such as thermistors or end-tidal CO_2 readings should be used. In patients with increased work of breathing, use of accessory muscles of breathing may lead to complex chest/abdomen movements, violating the assumption underlying RIP that the respiratory system moves with only two degrees of freedom (111). As with other methods, careful attention to positioning of the RIP bands is mandatory.

Measurement of ventilation: In patients with normal lungs and unobstructed breathing, the CO_2 value measured at the nose or mouth over the last one-fifth of expiration is presumed to reflect alveolar CO_2. This value is thought to be a reliable estimate of arterial CO_2 and thus of alveolar ventilation (125,131). Careful positioning of probes at the mouth and nose is essential to obtaining reliable recordings from both thermistors and CO_2 monitors. Although not an absolute guarantee, an end-tidal plateau of the CO_2 value usually indicates a good signal for CO_2 readings. Caution must be advised when using end-tidal CO_2 tracings. Underestimation of the actual alveolar CO_2 value can be seen in patients with obstructive lung disease or rapid respiratory rates. This error should be obvious from inspection of the end-tidal tracing. End-tidal CO_2 recording is effective in detecting apnea and prolonged hypoventilation (131,132). The technician's vigilance is essential to ensuring that the catheter is positioned properly, that it is kept patent, and that the waveform is appropriate.

At times, the nasal sampling catheter required for the CO_2 recording may be difficult to maintain, especially in young children. In these situations, transcutaneous P_{CO_2} (Ptc_{CO_2}) monitoring may be useful (132,133). These measurements are more reliable when corrected to the P_{ACO_2} values (132). The Ptc_{CO_2} measurements will not reflect transient changes in Pa_{CO_2}, but only a trend (132,133). In older or obese patients, Ptc_{CO_2} does not necessarily reflect arterial values, although the difference between the transcutaneous value and the arterial value is usually stable.

Measurement of oxygenation: Blood oxygen levels can be measured by pulse oximetry (131,134–136) or by transcutaneous oxygen electrodes (54,55,137). Pulse oximetry has a rapid response time, but the result is affected by the lung-to-probe circulation time and the averaging algorithm used by the equipment. It uses a comfortable sensor that can be left on by the patient for extended periods. The Sa_{O_2} values obtained with pulse oximetry have been shown to correlate well with measured arterial oxygenation values $> 70\%$, as long as there is an adequate arterial pulse waveform and absence of motion artifact (131,134–136). The accuracy and reliability of continuously documented oximetry can be improved by also recording the pulse amplitude signal (56). Individuals using pulse oximetry should be familiar with factors that affect the accuracy and reliability of its readings. Understanding the relationship between saturation and partial pressure of oxygen, as well as the importance of oxygen delivery is essential to using these measurements effectively (131,135).

Transcutaneous oxygen tension measurements (Ptc_{O_2}) are less useful because the response time of these electrodes to changes in Pa_{O_2} is often too slow to follow the rapid and transient changes in oxygenation that may occur following apnea (54,55,131,133). Furthermore, patient age and the temperature of the probe require repositioning the heated probe to prevent skin damage in infants and young children (138). These factors make these monitors less desirable for studies designed to be minimally disruptive to natural sleep. If transcutaneous measurements are used, the location of the sensor should be changed approximately every 4 h to prevent skin damage. Depending on the temperature of the probe and the characteristics of the equipment, this interval can be extended in older patients, but it may need to be shorter in premature infants. Alternatively, several sensor rings could be placed at the beginning of the study and the sampling location rotated every 4 h. This technique minimizes disturbances during the study.

Nonrespiratory Variables.

Sleep staging: Staging sleep involves the combined measurement of the electroencephalogram (EEG), electrooculogram (EOG) to record rapid eye movements, and the electromyogram (EMG) to record submental and tibial muscle activity. Well-defined sleep stages similar to those in adults are easily identifiable in children > 6 mo old, although differences in the characteristics of the voltage and waveforms of the EEG occur with maturation beyond this age (139,140). Special criteria have been used to define sleep states in infants < 6 mo old (141,142).

Electrocardiogram (ECG): Monitoring cardiac rate and rhythm is useful in assessing consequences of the breathing disturbance.

Tibialis muscle activity: Monitoring of peripheral muscle tone is useful in documenting excessive movements and arousals during sleep (143). Although rare in pediatrics, the diagnosis of periodic leg movement can be detected with anterior tibialis EMG (143). Motion sensors for the extremities can also be used to detect excessive leg movements.

Esophageal pH: The measurement of esophageal pH using standard methodology (144) in conjunction with PSG can be used to document the presence and cardiorespiratory consequences of gastroesophageal reflux.

Audiovisual recording: Because the physician is not present overnight to observe the child during sleep, videotaping using infrared or low-light cameras can provide invaluable information on sleep behavior, snoring, respiratory effort, and sleep positions associated with a particular respiratory pattern. Preliminary work has suggested that videotape analysis may prove useful as a noninvasive approach to discriminate sleep and wakefulness and to help assess movement arousals (45, 46,145).

Consensus Recommendations. Comprehensive evaluation of respiration during sleep requires a combination of measurements that at a minimum should include the following techniques:

- Both respiratory effort and airflow should be assessed. Simultaneous recording of movement of the chest wall and abdomen is required to detect paradoxical inspiratory rib cage movement and identify obstructive apnea and/or hypoventilation. Magnetometers, strain gauges, or RIP may be used. Intercostal EMG recordings cannot be used alone to monitor respiration, since the signal may be reduced or absent during REM sleep. Calibrated RIP can detect both apnea and hypopnea (128–130). Esophageal pressure catheters are not required for routine clinical studies, because placement of the catheters can be upsetting to both the child and parent. The presence of the catheter may contribute to sleep disruption, leading to a less-than-optimal study.

Airflow at the nose and mouth can be measured either by thermistors or by capnography. It is important to identify mouth and nasal breathing separately, because absence of nasal airflow or exclusive mouth breathing are both associated with clinical abnormalities (146,147). Capnography is recommended to measure CO_2 because it can assess both airflow and ventilation simultaneously.

- Measurement of Sa_{O_2} by pulse oximetry should be performed in all studies. In addition, we strongly recommend that the oximeter's pulse waveform be recorded on a separate channel adjacent to the electrocardiogram (ECG) signal, so that the accuracy of the saturation reading can be determined and artifacts due to movement or low signal strength easily identified. Although the software used to calculate saturation may vary, the algorithm calculating the saturation value should use the mode with the shortest averaging time.
- An ECG is recorded using a standard three-lead placement.
- An EMG is recorded from electrodes placed over the anterior tibial region. Motion sensors can also be used. Recording movements of an extremity is recommended in studies focused on excessive leg movements or in children with excessive daytime sleepiness; it can help quantitate movement arousals during PSG assessment of cardiopulmonary function.
- Electrode placement for sleep staging in children is based on the International 10–20 system and is similar to that used in adults (148). Electrodes are placed at A1, A2, C3, and C4, and sleep stage is determined by the monopolar derivation C3/A2 or C3/A_1 or C4/A1 or C4/A_2. The EOG is recorded by placing electrodes adjacent to the outer canthus of each eye. The right electrode is placed 1 cm above the horizontal axis while the left is placed 1 cm below. An EMG is recorded by placing one electrode in the center of the chin and two electrodes on opposite sides under the chin. Only two of these are required for recording purposes; the third is for backup. If a paper polygraph is used, the data should be recorded at a rate of 10 mm/s. Although this may reduce the sensitivity of EEG patterns, it has been found to be sufficient for accurate sleep staging and assessing breathing patterns.
- Audiovideo recording during sleep is recommended but not required. Infrared or low-light equipment should be used so that ambient light can be minimized. If available, simultaneous recording of the patient and PSG variables can be helpful in correlating physiologic disturbances with clinical or behavioral findings.
- Supervision by a trained technician is required to assure the quality of the study. This individual should make notations regarding unusual events or behavior during the study. Although unattended PSG in children appears promising, its role in either the laboratory or home setting has not been fully established (45,46). Additional research is needed to determine reli-

ability and limitations of this approach before it is adopted for routine use in children.

Scoring and Reporting Polysomnography Data

Respiratory Variables

Physiologic differences between adults and children, as well as differences in the clinical manifestations of sleep-related upper airway obstruction, demand that interpretation of PSG in children recognize their uniqueness and the influences of development (30,33).

The presence or absence of snoring should be noted. Although limited data suggest a clinically significant correlation between the quality or loudness of snoring and severity of upper airway obstruction (149,150), there are no studies quantifying snoring on a PSG in children, nor are there widely accepted and validated scales for assessing the quality and severity of snoring in children.

The number of obstructive events (complete or partial) of any duration should be scored in all studies. Obstructive apnea is defined as cessation of airflow at the nose and mouth associated with out-of-phase movements of the rib cage and abdomen. Several investigators have demonstrated that children with OSAS may present fewer and generally shorter episodes of complete obstruction, but prolonged periods of partial upper airway obstruction (7,30,31).

Partial airway obstruction has traditionally been described by the term "hypopnea" (breathing that is shallower or slower than normal). Hypopnea is defined by a 50% or greater decrease in the amplitude of the nasal/oral airflow signal, often accompanied by hypoxemia or arousal (128,129,153). If a calibrated RIP is used, hypopnea can be identified by a decrease in the RIP sum signal (128–130). However, in young infants, rib-cage paradox characteristic of REM sleep can produce a similar decrease in the signal. If RIP is used in children < 1 yr who may normally experience paradoxical inspiratory rib-cage movements during REM sleep, then hypopnea should be defined using other supportive data such as changes in nasal/oral flow, oxygenation, or end-tidal CO_2. Hypopnea may be further characterized as either obstructive, if the reduction in airflow is associated with paradoxical chest and abdominal movements, or central, if associated with an in-phase reduction in the amplitude of the chest and abdominal signals.

Defining and identifying hypopnea consistently by this approach may sometimes be difficult (153). Scoring hypopnea as discrete events also may be difficult, because the degree of partial obstruction often changes continuously, without clear points of onset or termination. An alternative approach based on measuring end-tidal P_{CO_2} was considered by many committee members to be a more sensitive method for assessing partial airway obstruction. If end-tidal CO_2 data is used, the effects of extended partial airway obstruction or reduced respiratory effort can be assessed by measuring changes in end-tidal CO_2 associated with going to sleep, as well as with respiratory events. By using end-tidal P_{CO_2} data, hypoventilation can be identified as obstructive or central based on the associated changes in chest and abdominal wall movements. Reference data on the range of normal end-tidal CO_2 values is limited to a recent study of 50 children, 1–17 yr old (154). This study demonstrated that no normal child had an end-tidal CO_2 > 45 mmHg for > 60% of total sleep time, end-tidal Co_2 > 50 mmHg for > 8% of total sleep time, or peck end-tidal CO_2 (on two consecutive breaths during or after upper airway obstruction) > 53 mmHg (154). The same study showed that the increases in Pet_{CO_2} rarely exceeded 13 mmHg during overnight PSG. The committee believed that these data may be used conservatively to identify patients with elevation of CO_2 during sleep, assuming that a high-quality CO_2 reading is obtained.

Limited data are available on the occurrence of paradoxical inspiratory rib-cage movements in normal children. In infants up to 6 mo old these movements occur throughout REM sleep (155). From 7 mo to 3 yr there are no paradoxical inspiratory rib-cage movements during non-REM sleep, and the duration of paradoxical inspiratory rib-cage movements decreases with age during REM (119). In adolescents, paradoxical inspiratory movements are not seen normally, even during REM (156).

Central apnea is an absence of airflow at both the nose and mouth and movements of the chest wall and abdomen. Central apnea without physiologic consequence is found in normal children of all ages. In general these episodes are < 20 s, although some normal children have been found to have central apneas longer than that (157).

Reference data on oxygenation come from several studies of normal infants and children (154,157–160). These data demonstrate that after the first several months of life, Sa_{O_2} usually remains > 94% during sleep, and desaturation events of ≥ 4% are uncommon. If they occur, they are typically brief: < 10 s (154,157–160).

Nonrespiratory Variables

If there are clearcut abnormalities on the respiratory portion of the PSG, the study may be interpreted without performing complete sleep staging. However, the committee believed that the ability to stage sleep is important to documenting the sleep-state dependence of breathing. Breathing abnormalities, including obstructive apnea, may be exacerbated or only seen during REM sleep (161–163). Sleep staging is also important to determining that the quality and quantity of sleep during the study is within normal limits.

In children older than 6 mo, it is standard practice to stage sleep on PSG in 30-s epochs, according to the guidelines of Rechtschaffen and Kales (139). Some committee members recommended that the length of epochs for sleep staging vary according to the age of the child, but there is a need for more data before this approach can be recommended. Sleep in infants less than 6 mo old should be scored as active, quiet, or indeterminate (141,142).

Although detailed sleep staging beyond simply identifying the occurrence of REM periods is not always necessary, arousals should be scored because these may be important consequences of abnormal breathing events during sleep. Quantifying mini- or micro-arousals in children to obtain a measure of sleep disturbance has been recommended (164) but needs more study. New guidelines for scoring arousals on PSG have recently been published by the American Sleep Disorders Association (165), and a modification of this system for children has been proposed (145). Arousal should be classified as respiratory if it occurs at the end of a respiratory event (apnea or hypopnea), technician-induced, or spontaneous. The frequency of movement arousals terminating obstructive apnea in children is unclear (145), but there is a suggestion that children can sometimes terminate obstructive apnea without a cortical arousal (163,166).

Another nonrespiratory variable involves cardiac rhythm. The presence of cardiac arrhythmias, including sinus bradycardia, and whether they are associated with respiratory disturbances should be noted and the number of such events tabulated.

Consensus Recommendations for Scoring

Until more experience is gained with children's abnormal breathing during sleep, the entire record should be scored by a qualified individual who knows the unique characteristics of sleep breathing in children of different ages. Scoring based on sampling techniques must be validated for children (167).

- Given the volume of data accumulated during PSG, the use of computer-based data acquisition and scoring is attractive. Computerized data acquisition appears to be reliable, and a paperless polysomnograph can meet the needs of pediatric laboratories. However, computerized scoring of respiratory events and sleep staging in children requires validation (168,169).
- Respiratory variables that should be scored include the number, type, and duration of apneas; episodes of partial airway obstruction measured as hypopnea or hypoventilation, whether obstructive or central; and the frequency and duration of paradoxical inspiratory rib-cage movements and associated desaturation, apnea, hypopnea, or increased end-tidal CO_2 values.
- Normative data in children suggest that obstructive apnea is rare in normal children (98,154,170,171). Thus, obstructive apnea of any length should be scored. If an obstructive apnea index—the number of events per hour of total sleep time—or a combined apnea/hypopnea index is used, appropriate pediatric normal values must be employed. Nonsigh, nonmovement-associated central apnea > 20 s should be counted, regardless of associated desaturation or bradycardia. Shorter episodes should also be scored if associated with desaturation > 4% or age-specific bradycardia.
- If end-tidal CO_2 data is available, the following measurements should be scored: the end-tidal CO_2 at sleep onset, the peak end-tidal CO_2, the duration of end-tidal CO_2 > 50 mmHg expressed as a percent of total sleep time, and the changes in CO_2 associated with respiratory events. The end-tidal CO_2 values should be correlated with chest wall and abdominal recordings to identify the pathophysiology of the elevated CO_2. The amount of time dur-

ing which a technically adequate end-tidal CO_2 tracing was not obtainable should be recorded in order to avoid underestimating the total sleep time spent with values > 50 mmHg (132).

- Maximum and minimum Sa_{O_2}, the number of desaturations ≥ 4%, and the percent of total sleep time spent with Sa_{O_2} < 95%, 90%, 85%, etc., should be scored. Changes in Sa_{O_2} values should be correlated with respiratory events.
- Snoring should be noted as present or absent. There are currently no standardized scoring systems for snoring in pediatric patients. Rating or grading the snoring as mild, moderate, or severe may be useful for an individual but, until the ratings are standardized, should be left to the discretion of each laboratory.
- Respiratory data should be subdivided according to sleeping position (prone, side, or supine) when there is an important difference between positions.
- The presence and type of arrhythmias and whether they are correlated with respiratory events should be noted. Epoch-by-epoch scoring of heart rate is not necessary for routine pediatric PSG.
- There was a consensus that 30-s epochs were adequate for scoring a PSG evaluating respiration, but a minority view held that the epoch length should vary according to the indication for the study. More data are needed before establishing an epoch length recommendation.
- The following sleep variables should be collected: total sleep time, sleep efficiency, distribution of sleep stages as percent of total sleep time, sleep latency, number of arousals, body movements, body position, and sleep behavior (parasomnias).
- The criteria of Rechtschaffen and Kales (139) can be used to stage sleep for children 6 mo and older. For most clinical indications, identification of active and quiet sleep is adequate for infants under 6 mo (141,142).
- Complete sleep staging may not be necessary for most cardiopulmonary studies, unless there are specific questions regarding the impact of the sleep stages on the breathing disturbance. At a minimum, sleep should be divided into REM and non–REM. If formal sleep staging is performed, the following additional parameters should be scored: non–REM stages 1, 2, 3, and 4 and REM time expressed as percentages of total sleep time.
- A statement summarizing body movements during sleep was believed sufficient for pediatric polysomnography. Body position should be recorded to determine if the child slept in his or her "usual" sleeping position and if respiratory abnormalities are related to body position. Position should be recorded either by video or observation by the technician.
- Arousals as defined in the Sleep Disorders Atlas Task Force of the American Sleep Disorders Association (165) should be noted and correlated with respiratory abnormalities. Spontaneous nonrespiratory arousal should also be noted as a possible marker of sleep disturbance (145). Arousals caused by the activity of the technician need not be counted.

- Videotaping children during sleep may be used to help distinguish sleep from wakefulness, to help determine the cause of arousals, and to document body position and snoring (45,46,145). The tape can be useful for interpreting unusual behavioral events and assessing respiratory effort during sleep.

Reporting the Results

Quantitative data summarizing results of the study should be reported in a standardized format similar to that used for adults (5,172), as follows:

1. Patient identification—age, sex, race, height, weight, indication for study, other medical conditions, and foods or medications that may affect study results.
2. Techniques used and variables measured.
3. The accompanying caregiver's opinion whether the child's sleep and breathing patterns in the laboratory were representative of the child's sleep at home.
4. The presence and quality of snoring during the study.
5. Sleep staging parameters, if staging is used: total sleep time, sleep latency, sleep efficiency, body movement, awakenings, time awake after sleep onset, number of arousals and their association with respiratory events, and any noteworthy sleep behavior. The presence and number of REM periods and the duration of all sleep stages, expressed as a percent of total sleep time, should be recorded. If complete sleep staging is not performed, the number of REM periods and the percentages of the total sleep time spent in REM and non–REM sleep should be recorded.
6. Respiratory rate during non–REM sleep. Apnea and hypopnea or hypoventilation should be reported by type, total number, average duration, longest event of each type, lowest Sa_{O_2}, and heart rate associated with the event.
7. Oxygen saturation as maximum Sa_{O_2}; minimum Sa_{O_2}; percent total sleep time spent with Sa_{O_2}, $< 95\%$, 90%, 85%, etc.; and the association between episodes of desaturation and apnea, hypopnea, or hypoventilation noted during the study. The relationship of desaturation episodes to sleep stage and body position should be noted.
8. End-tidal CO_2 data reported as time spent above 50 and 60 mmHg expressed as a percent of total sleep time that CO_2 data was available. Correlation of elevated CO_2 with respiratory events should be included in the report.
9. Cardiac arrhythmias (including sinus bradycardia) and their relationship to respiratory abnormalities.
10. If therapy (oxygen, CPAP, or noninvasive positive pressure ventilation) was administered during the study, the Sa_{O_2} on room air and at each level of oxygen supplementation, pressure, or ventilator rate. Effects of the therapeutic intervention of $P_{ET_{CO_2}}$ or sleep quality should be reported if pertinent.

11. Technician's comments.
12. Interpretation. The individual responsible for the final interpretation of PSG performed on children to evaluate respiratory function during sleep should have expertise in sleep disorders in children, understand developmental cardiorespiratory physiology, and be certified in the medical evaluation of pediatric patients.

Before evaluating the study, the interpreter must ascertain if the child's sleep and/or breathing during the night of the PSG was representative for that child at home. The medical history should also be reviewed to determine if the results answer the question that prompted the study.

To determine if the results of a sleep study are abnormal, the interpreter should know the baseline awake values for respiratory rate, Sa_{O_2}, and end-tidal CO_2 to determine if sleep itself is associated with changes in these values. Cardiac arrhythmia, adequacy of sleep, and the degree of sleep disruption should also be factored into the decision-making process. Sleep stages should be interpreted in light of published age-appropriate normative values (139–142). Unfortunately, normal values for variables such as the number of arousals or body movements, movement time, or other indicators of disturbed sleep are not available for children. More data are needed.

Some broad guidelines can be used to determine abnormality for the respiratory events:

Central apnea > 20 s has been shown to occur in normal children and adolescents, especially following a sigh or movement (156,157,173,174). The clinical significance of these episodes must be interpreted in light of the indications for the study. If they are not associated with any physiologic abnormalities (bradycardia, hypoxemia), they may be considered within the broad range of normal values. An event of any duration associated with a ≥ 4% drop in Sa_{O_2} should be considered abnormal if the frequency of these events exceeds three per hour (175) or if it is associated with a > 25% change in heart rate.

After the first month of life, normal infants and children do not exhibit more than one obstructive apnea per hour of sleep time (99,170,171). Studies of infants 1–6 mo old (174) and children 1–17 yr (153) found obstructive apnea indices of 0.04 ± 0.13 apneas/h and 0.1 ± 0.5 apneas/h, respectively. These observations suggest that, in children, obstructive apnea of any duration exceeding 1 apnea/h should be noted and considered abnormal. Nonetheless, the clinical significance of isolated or infrequent obstructive events without desaturation or arousal is yet to be determined.

Oxygenation status must be interpreted in light of changes in saturation from both the awake values and the stable baseline reading preceding any respiratory event. Some normal children have brief desaturations of ≥ 4% occurring at a rage of ≤ 3 events/h (175). Desaturation episodes to < 90% are rare, and their frequency decreases with age (119). Any change in saturation must be interpreted in light of the preceding baseline value. Sustained saturation values < 90% are abnormal.

Partial airway obstruction associated with paradoxical inspiratory rib-cage movements, labored breathing, disturbed sleep, and heavy sweating, yet without desaturation, has been linked to excessive daytime sleepiness and behavioral disturbances (122,128). This breathing pattern has been associated with significant elevations in esophageal pressure swings during tidal breathing (176). This pattern of breathing may also be identified by reviewing both the audiovideo recording and respiratory channels of the PSG. Its presence should be considered abnormal (176).

Hypopneic events (≥ 50% reduction in the RIP sum signal, and/or in the thermistor signal associated with arousal, and/or desaturation of > 4% or sustained values < 90%) should also be considered abnormal (128,177).

Hypoventilation events indicated by elevation of end-tidal CO_2 to > 53 mmHg or > 50 mmHg for > 8% of total sleep time, or a change in end-tidal CO_2 of > 13 mmHg from baseline, indicates alveolar hypoventilation (154).

The etiology of the desaturation, apnea, hypopnea, or hypoventilation events can be determined by correlating the changes in airflow or end-tidal CO_2 with the respiratory patterns obtained from the chest wall and abdominal recordings. For example, reduced airflow or desaturation associated with paradoxical inspiratory rib-cage movement and/or snoring suggests partial airway obstruction.

Arousals terminating respiratory events indicate a clinically significant event (145,177). Although the absence of a cortical arousal following a severe episode of desaturation or an extended period of airway obstruction is not uncommon in children (163), lack of an arousal to an episode of sustained airway obstruction, hypoventilation, or hypoxemia suggests a compromise in the child's respiratory defenses and should be considered abnormal (163,177).

Deviations from normal sleep patterns (139–142) and frequent spontaneous arousals must be interpreted cautiously in light of the impact on sleep quality of the first night in the sleep lab (107,108). However, disturbed, restless sleep can mark a significant disruption of respiration during sleep (6,7).

Research Recommendations

The committee found that the following areas needed additional investigation to refine current recommendations.

- Age-specific normal values for respiratory events, Sa_{O_2}, end-tidal CO_2, sleep efficiency, arousals, and sleep disruption need to be generated. Additionally, more data are needed to define thresholds of clinical significance for PSG parameters in children.
- Which PSG abnormalities (number of respiratory events, cumulative hypercapnia, severity of desaturation, and degree of sleep disruption) in infants and children with OSAS correlate with morbidity? How do severity and duration of events such as desaturation, airway obstruction, and CO_2 interact to produce morbidity?
- What are the neuropsychological and cognitive consequences of OSAS in children? Are these a consequence of disturbed sleep, chronic/recurrent hypoxemia during sleep, or both?

- What is the natural history of OSAS in children? What is the link between OSAS in children and in adults?
- What are the risks that a child who has been treated for OSAS will develop recurrent symptoms of OSAS as an older child or adult?
- What is the sensitivity and reproducibility of a single night's Sa_{O_2} recording or PSG? Do they change with age, puberty, or minor illness?
- What constitutes a clinically significant episode or period of desaturation in an infant, child, and adolescent?
- What is the most accurate and meaningful way of documenting desaturation during sleep?
- What is the role of formal sleep staging in PSG performed to assess cardiorespiratory function?
- What is the role of end-tidal CO_2 recording? What are age-appropriate reference values?
- How well do qualitative airflow measures such as thermistors and changes in ventilation, or semiquantitative measurements such as RIP, track changes in gas exchange?
- What are indications and limitations of unattended PSG in the home or hospital?
- What is the prevalence of OSAS in infants, children, and adolescents?
- What severity of illness or what degree of PSG warrants therapy?
- What is the role of nasal CPAP or BiPAP® in treating OSAS in children?
- What medical therapies are useful in treating obstructive sleep apnea in children?
- What is the best method of documenting partial airway obstruction? What is the role of esophageal pressure measurements in documenting partial airway obstruction?

This statement was prepared by an ad hoc Committee of the Scientific Assembly on Pediatrics. Members of the Committee were:

Gerald M. Loughlin, Cochair, Robert T. Brouillette, Cochair, Lee J. Brooke, John L. Carroll, Bradley E. Chipps, Sandra J. England, Richard Ferber, Nalton F. Ferraro, Claude Gaultier, Deborah C. Givan, Gabriel G. Haddad, Bruce R. Maddern, George B. Mallory, Ian T. Nathanson, Carol L. Rosen, Bradley T. Thach, Sally L. Davidson-Ward, Debra E. Weese-Mayer, Mary Ellen Wohl.

References

1. Gaultier, C. 1985. Breathing and sleep during growth: physiology and pathology. Bull Eur Physiopathol Respir 21:55–112.
2. Phillipson, E. A. 1978. Respiratory adaptations in sleep. Annu Rev Physiol 40:669–675.
3. Gaultier, C., and J. P. Praud. 1985. Respiration during sleep in children with COPD. Chest 87:168–173.

4. Gaultier, C. 1992. Clinical and therapeutic aspects of obstructive sleep apnea syndrome in infants and children. Sleep 15:536–538.
5. American Thoracic Society. 1989. Consensus conference on indications and standards for cardiopulmonary sleep studies. Am Rev Respir Dis 139:559–568.
6. Guilleminault, C., R. Korobkin, and R. Winkle. 1981. A review of 50 children with obstructive sleep apnea syndrome. Lung 159:275–287.
7. Brouillette, R., S. Fernbach, and C. Hunt. 1982. Obstructive sleep apnea in infants and children. J Pediatr 100:31–40.
8. Gorbo, G. M., F. Fuciarelli, A. Foresi, and F. Debenedetto. 1989. Snoring in children: association with respiratory symptoms and passive smoking. Br Med J 299:1491–1494.
9. Ali, N. J., D. Pitson, and J. R. Stradling. 1993. The prevalence of snoring, sleep disturbance, and sleep-related breathing disorders and their relation to daytime sleepiness in 4–5-year-old children. Arch Dis Child 68:360–363.
10. Teculescu, D. B., I. Caillier, P. Perrin, E. Rebstock, and A. Rauch. 1992. Snoring in French preschool children. Pediatr Pulmonol 13:239–244.
11. Weissbluth, M., A Davis, J. Poncher, and J. Reiff. 1983. Signs of airway obstruction during sleep and behavioral, developmental, and academic problems. Dev Behav Pediatr 4: 119–121.
12. Everett, A., W. Kock, and F. Saulsbury. 1987. Failure to thrive due to obstructive sleep apnea. Clin Pediatr 26:90–92.
13. Menashe, V. D., F. Farrehi, and M. Miller. 1965. Hypoventilation and cor pulmonale due to chronic upper airway obstruction. J Pediatr 67:198–203.
14. Ross, R. D., S. R. Daniels, J. M. H. Loggie, R. A. Meyer, and E. T. Ballard. 1987. Sleep apnea-associated hypertension and reversible left ventricular hypertrophy. J Pediatr 111: 253–255.
15. Frank, Y., R. E. Kravath, C. P. Pollack, and E. D. Weitzman. 1983. Obstructive sleep apnea and its therapy: clinical and polysomnographic manifestations. Pediatrics 71:737–742.
16. Weider, D. J., and P. J. Hauri. 1985. Nocturnal enuresis in children with upper airway obstruction. Int J Pediatr Otorhinoloaryngol 9:173–182.
17. Kunzman, L. A., T. G. Keens, and S. L. Davidson-Ward. 1991. Incidence of systemic hypertension in children with obstructive sleep apnea syndrome. Am Rev Respir Dis 141:A808.
18. Seid, A. B., P. J. Martin, S. M. Pransky, D. B. Kearns, et al. 1980. Surgical therapy of obstructive sleep apnea in children with severe mental deficiency. Laryngoscope 100: 507–510.
19. Ellis, E. R., P. T. P. Bye, J. W. Bruderer, and C. E. Sullivan. 1987. Treatment of respiratory failure during sleep in patients with neuromuscular disease. Am Rev Respir Dis 135:148–152.
20. Mallory, G. B., Jr., D. H. Fiser, and R. Jackson. 1989. Sleep-associated breathing disorders in morbidly obese children and adolescents. J Pediatr 115:892–897.
21. Schafer, M. E. 1982. Upper airway obstruction and sleep disorders in children with craniofacial anomalies. Clin Plast Surg 9:555–567.
22. Handler, S. D. 1985. Upper airway obstruction in craniofacial anomalies: diagnosis and management. Birth Defects 21:15–31.
23. Loughlin, G. M., J. W. Wynne, and B. E. Victoria. 1981. Sleep apnea as a possible cause of pulmonary hypertension in Down syndrome. J Pediatr 98:435–437.

24. Marcus, C. L., D. M. Crockett, and S. L. Davidson-Ward. 1990. Evaluation of epiglottoplasty as treatment for severe laryngomalacia. J Pediatr 117:706–710.
25. Shprintzen, R. J. 1988. Pharyngeal flap surgery and the pediatric upper airway. Int Anesthesiol Clin 26:79–88.
26. Sammuels, M. P., V. A. Stebbens, S. V. Davies, et al. 1992. Sleep-related upper airway obstruction and hypoxemia in sickle cell disease. Arch Dis Child 67:925–929.
27. Dure, L. S., A. K. Percy, et al. 1989. Chiari Type 1 malformations in children. J Pediatr 115:573–576.
28. Shapiro, J., M. Strome, and A. C. Crocker. 1985. Airway obstruction and sleep apnea in Hurler and Hunter syndromes. Ann Otol Rhinol Laryngol 94:458–461.
29. McNicholas, W. T., S. Tarlo, P. Cole, N. Zamel, et al. 1982. Obstructive apneas during sleep in patients with seasonal allergic rhinitis. Am Rev Respir Dis 126:625–628.
30. Rosen, C. L., L. D'Andrea, and G. G. Haddad. 1992. Adult criteria for obstructive sleep apnea do not identify children with serious obstruction. Am Rev Respir Dis 146:1231–1234.
31. Carroll, J. L., and G. M. Loughlin. 1992. Diagnostic criteria for obstructive sleep apnea syndrome in children. Pediatr Pulmonol 14:71–74.
32. Diagnostic Classification Steering Committee and M. J. C. Thorpy. 1990. International Classification of Sleep Disorders: Diagnostic and Coding Manual. Rochester, Minnesota: American Association of Sleep Disorders Association.
33. Carroll, J. L., S. A. McColley, C. L. Marcus, S. Curtis, P. Pyzik, and G. M. Loughlin. 1992. Reported symptoms of childhood obstructive sleep apnea syndrome (OSA) vs. primary snoring (abstract). Am Rev Respir Dis 145:A177.
34. Carroll, J. L., S. A. McColley, C. L. Marcus, S. Curtis, P. Pyzik, and G. M. Loughlin. 1992. Can childhood obstructive sleep apnea be diagnosed by a clinical symptom score (abstract)? Am Rev Respir Dis 145:A179.
35. Brouillette, R., D. Hanson, R. David, L. Klemka, A. Szatkowski, S. Fernbach, and C. Hunt. 1984. A diagnostic approach to suspected obstructive sleep apnea in children. J Pediatr 105:10–14.
36. McColley, S. A., J. L. Carroll, M. M. April, R. N. Naclerio, and G. M. Loughlin. 1992. Respiratory compromise after adenotonsillectomy in children with obstructive sleep apnea. Arch Otolaryngol Head Neck Surg 118:940–943.
37. Rosen, G. M., R. P. Muckle, M. W. Mahowald, G. S. Goding, and C. Ullevig. 1994. Postoperative respiratory compromise in children with obstructive sleep apnea syndrome: can it be anticipated? Pediatrics 93:784–788.
38. Silvestri, J. M., D. E. Weese-Mayer, M. Bass, A. Morrow-Kenny, and S. Hauptman. 1993. Polysomnography in obese children with a history of sleep-associated breathing disorders. Pediatr Pulmonol 16:124–129.
39. Maddern, B. R., H. T. Reed, K. Ohene-Frempong, and R. C. Beckerman. 1989. Obstructive sleep apnea syndrome in sickle cell disease. Ann Otol Rhinol Laryngol 98:174–178.
40. Craft, J. A., E. Alessandrini, L. B. Kenney, et al. 1994. Comparison of oxygenation measurements in pediatric patients during sickle cell crises. J Pediatr 124:93–95.
41. Suen, J. S., J. E. Arnold, and L. J. Brooks. 1995. Adenotonsillectomy for the treatment of obstructive apnea in children. Arch Otolaryngol Head Neck Surg 121:525–530.
42. Carskadon, M. A., et al. 1986. Guidelines for the multiple sleep latency test (MSLT): a standard measure of sleepiness. Sleep 9:519–524.

43. Carskadon, M. A., et al. 1980. Pubertal changes in daytime sleepiness. Sleep 2:453–460.
44. Feinberg, I. 1974. Changes in the sleep cycle pattern with age. J Psychiatr Res 10:283–306.
45. Jacob, S. V., A Morielli, F. M. Ducharme, M. D. Schloss, and R. T. Brouillette. 1993. Home testing may be preferable to conventional polysomnography for diagnosis of pediatric obstructive sleep apnea (abstract). Am Rev Respir Dis 147:A762.
46. Morielli, A., F. M. Ducharme, and R. T. Brouillette. 1993. Sleep and wakefulness can be distinguished in children by videotape and cardiorespiratory recordings (abstract). Am Rev Respir Dis 1147:A762
47. O'Brodovich, H. M., and R. b. Mellins. 1985 Dronchopulmonary dysplasia: unresolved neonatal acute lung injury. *Am Rev Respri Dis* 32:694–709.
48. Northway, W. J., Jr., R. B. Moss, K. B. Carlisle, B. R. Parker, R. L. Popp, P. T. Pitlick, I. Eichler, R. L. Lamm, and B. W. Brown, Jr. 1990. Late pulmonary sequelae of bronchopulmonary dysplasia. N Engl J Med 323:1793–1799.
49. Garg, M., S. I. Kurzner, et al. 1988. Clinically unsuspected hypoxia during sleep and feeding in infants with bronchopulmonary dysplasia. Pediatrics 81:635–642.
50. Loughlin, G. M., R. P. Allen, et al. 1987. Sleep- related hypoxemia in children with bronchopulmonary dysplasia (BPD) and adequate oxygen saturation awake, abstracted. Sleep (Res) 16:486.
51. Singer, L., R. J. Martin, S. W. Hawkins, et al., 1991. Oxygen desaturation complicates feeding in infants and bronchopulmonary dysplasia after discharge. Pediatrics 90: 380–384.
52. Trang, T. T. H., J. P. Praud, M. Pagani, M. Goldman, and C. Gaultier. 1993. Sleep disordered respiration in infants and children with severe bronchopulmonary dysplasia (abstract). Am Rev Respir Dis 147:A343.
53. Goldman, M., M. Pagnini, T. T. H. Trang, J. P. Praud, M. Sartene, and C. Gaultier. 1993. Asynchronous chest wall movements during NREM and REM in children with bronchopulmonary dysplasia. Am Rev Respir Dis 147:1175–1184.
54. Rome, E. S., M. J. Miller, Goldthwait, et al. 1987. Effect of sleep state on chest wall movements and gas exchange in infants with resolving bronchopulmonary dysplasia. Pediatr Pulmonol 3:259–263.
55. Rome, E. S., E. K. Stork, et al. 1984. Limitations of transcutaneous P_{O_2} and P_{CO_2} monitoring in infants with bronchopulmonary dysplasia. Pediatrics 74:217–220.
56. Lafontaine, V., F. M. Ducharme, and R. T. Brouillette. 1994. Can we rely on pulse oximetry desaturation events (abstract)? Am Rev Respir Dis 149:69A.
57. Muller, N. L., P. W. Francis, D. Gurwitz, H. Levison, and A. C. Bryan. 1980. Mechanism of hemoglobin desaturation during rapid-eye-movement sleep in normal subjects and in patients with cystic fibrosis. Am Rev Respir Dis 121:463–469.
58. Stokes, D. C., J. T. McBride, et al. 1980. Sleep hypoxemia in young adults with cystic fibrosis. Am J Dis Child 134:741–743.
59. Tepper, R. S., J. B. Skatrud, and J. A. Demplsey. 1983. Ventilation and oxygenation changes during sleep in cystic fibrosis. Chest 84:388–393.
60. Versteegh, F. G. A., J. M. Bogaard, et al. 1990. Relationship between airway obstruction, desaturation during exercise and nocturnal hypoxemia in cystic fibrosis patients. Eur Respir J 3:68–73.
61. Montgomery, M., W. Wiebicke, et al. 1989. Home measurement of oxygen saturation during sleep in patients with cystic fibrosis. Pediatr Pulmonol 7:29–34.

62. Bowton, D. L., P. F. Scuderi, L. Harris, and E. F. Haponick. 1991. Pulse oximetry monitoring outside the intensive care unit: progress or problem? Ann Intern Med 115:450–454.
63. Clark, T. J. H., and M. R. Hetzel. 1977. Diurnal variation of asthma. Br J Dis Chest 71: 87–92.
64. Busse, W. W. 1988. Pathogenesis and pathophysiology of nocturnal asthma. Am J Med 85(Suppl. 1B):24–29.
65. Martin, R. J., L. C. Cicutto, and R. D. Ballard. 1990. Factors related to the nocturnal worsening of asthma. Am Rev Respir Dis 141:33–38.
66. Chipps, B. E., H. Mak, et al. 1980. Nocturnal oxygen desaturation during sleep in children with asthma and its relation to airway obstruction and ventilatory drive. Pediatrics 66:746–751.
68. Smith, P. E. M., P. M. A. Calverley, and R. H. T. Edwards. 1988. Hypoxemia during sleep in Duchenne muscular dystrophy. Am Rev Respir Dis 121:587–593.
69. Begin, R., M. A. Bureau, L. Lupien, and B. Lemieux. 1980. Control and modulation of respiration in Steinert's myotonic dystrophy. Am Rev Respir Dis 121:281–289.
70. Gilgoff, I. S., E. Kahlstrom, E. MacLaughlin, and T. G. Keens. 1989. Long-term ventilatory support in spinal muscular atrophy. J Pediatr 115:904–909.
71. Skatrud, J., C. Iber, W. McHugh, H. Rasmussen, et al. 1980. Determinants of hypoventilation during wakefulness and sleep in diaphragmatic paralysis. Am Rev Respir Dis 121:587–593.
72. Bye, P. T. P., E. R. Ellis, F. G. Issa, P. M. Donnelly, and C. E. Sullivan. 1990. Respiratory failure and sleep in neuromuscular disease. Thorax 45:241–247.
73. Eichacker, P. Q., A. Spiro, M. Sherman, E. Lazar, J. Reichel, and F. Dodick. 1988. Respiratory muscle dysfunction in hereditary motor sensory neuropathy, type I. Arch Intern Med 148:1739–1740.
74. Riley, D. J., T. V. Santiago, D. P. Daniele, B. Schall, and N. H. Edelman. 1977. Blunted respiratory drive in cogenital myopathy. Am J Med 63:459–466.
75. O'Leary, J., R. King, M. Liblanc, R. Moss, M. Liebhaber, and N. Lewiston. 1979. Cuirass ventilation in childhood neuromuscular disease. J Pediatr 94:419–421.
76. Maayan, C. H., C. Springer, Y. Armon, E. Bar-Yishay, Y. Shapira, and S. Godfrey. 1986. Nemaline myopathy as a cause of sleep hypoventilation. Pediatrics 77:390–395.
77. Heckmatt, J. Z., L. Loh, and V. Dubowitz. 1989. Nocturnal hypoventilation in children with nonprogressive neuromuscular disease. Pediatrics 83:250–255.
78. Rideau, Y., L. W. Jankowski, and J. Grellet. 1981. Respiratory function in the muscular dystrophies. Muscle Nerve 4:155–164.
79. Baydur, A., I. Gilgoff, and W. Prentice. 1985. Guidelines for assisted ventilation in Duchenne's muscular dystrophy. Am Rev Respir Dis 131(Suppl):A268.
80. Martinez, B. A., and B. D. Lake. 1987. Childhood nemaline myopathy: a review of clinical presentation in relation to prognosis. Dev Med Child Neurol 29:815–820.
81. Alberts, M. J., and A. D. Roses. 1989. Myotonic muscular dystrophy. Neurol Clin 7:1–8.
82. Manni, R., A. Ottolini, I. Cerveri, C. Bruschi, M. C. Zoia, G. Lanzi, and A. Tartara. 1989. Breathing patterns and $HbSa_{O_2}$ changes during nocturnal sleep in patients with Duchennes muscular dystrophy. J Neurol 236:361–394.
83. Serisier, D. E., F. L. Mastaglia, and G. J. Gibson. 1982. Respiratory muscle function and ventilatory control in patients with motor neurone disease and in patients with myotonic dystrophy. Q J Med 202:205–226.

84. Ellis, E. R., P. T. P. Bye, J. W. Bruderer, and C. E. Sullivan. 1987. Treatment of respiratory failure during sleep in patients with neuromuscular disease. Am Rev Respir Dis 135:148–152.
85. Newsom-Davis, J., M. Goldman, L. Loh, and M. Casson. 1976. Diaphragm function and alveolar hypoventilation. Q J Med 45:87–100, 148–152.
86. Goldstein, R. S., N. Molotiu, R. Skrastins, S. Long, J. DeRosie, M. Contreras, J. Poplin, R. Rutherford, and E. A. Phillipson. 1987. Reversal of sleep-induced hypoventilation and chronic respiratory failure by nocturnal negative pressure ventilation in patients with restrictive ventilatory impairment. Am Rev Respir Dis 135:1049–1055.
87. Aldrich, M. S. 1990. Neurologic aspects of sleep apnea and related respiratory disturbances. Otolaryngol Clin North Am 23:761–769.
88. Mallory, G. B., and P. C. Stillwell. 1991. The ventilator dependent child: issues in diagnosis and management. Arch Phys Med Rehabil 72:43–55.
89. Weese-Mayer, D. E., J. M. Silvestri, L. J. Menzies, A. S. Morrow-Kenny, C. E. Hunt, and S. A. Hauptman. 1992. Congenital central hypoventilation syndrome: diagnosis, management, and long-term outcome in thirty-two children. J Pediatr 120:381–387.
90. Weese-Mayer, D. E., C. E. Hunt, and R. T. Brouillette. 1992. Alveolar hypoventilation syndromes. In: R. C. Beckerman, R. T. Brouillette, and C. E. Hunt, eds. Respiratory Control Disorders in Infants and Children. Baltimore: Williams and Wilkins.
91. Silvestri, J. M., D. E. Weese-Mayer, and M. N. Nelson. 1992. Neuropsychologic abnormalities in children with congenital central hypoventilation syndrome. J Pediatr 123:388–393.
92. Weese-Mayer, D. E., C. E. Hunt, R. T. Brouillette, and J. M. Silvestri. 1992. Diaphragm pacing in infants and children. J Pediatr 120:1–8.
93. Martin, R. J., M. J. Miller, and W. A. Carlo. 1986. Pathogenesis of apnea in preterm infants. J Pediatr 109:733–741.
94. Henderson-Smart, D. J. 1981. The effect of gestational age on the incidence and duration of recurrent apnea in newborn babies. Aust Paediatr J 17:273–276.
95. Hilner, A. D., A. W. Boon, R. A. Saunders, and J. E. Hopkin. 1980. Upper airway obstruction and apnea in preterm babies. Arch Dis Child 35:22–25.
96. National Institutes of Health Consensus Development Conference on Infantile Apnea and Home Monitoring. 1986. U.S. Department of Health and Human Services, Washington, DC. NIH Publication No. 87-2905.
97. Series, F., Y. Cormier, and J. La Forge. 1991. Validity of diurnal sleep recordings in the diagnosis of sleep apnea syndrome. Am Rev Respir Dis 143:947–949.
98. Silvestri, R., C. Guilleminault, R. Coleman, et al. 1982. Nocturnal sleep versus daytime nap findings in patients with breathing abnormalities during sleep. Sleep Res 11:174.
99. Marcus, C. L., T. G. Keens, and S. L. Ward. 1992. Comparison of nap and overnight polysomnography in children. Pediatr Pulmonol 13:16–21.
100. Canet, E., C. Gaultier, A.-M. D'Allest, and M. Dehan. 1989. Effects of sleep deprivation on respiratory events during sleep in health infants. J Appl Physiol 128:984–986.
101. White, D. P., N. J. Douglas, C. K. Pickett, et al. 1983. Sleep deprivation and the control of ventilation. Am Rev Respir Dis 128:984–986.
102. Leiter, J. C., S. L. Knuth, and D. Bartlett. 1985. The effect of sleep deprivation on activity of the genioglossus muscle. Am Rev Respir Dis 132:1242–1245.
103. Hershenson, M., R. T. Brouillette, E. Olsen, and C. E. Hunt. 1984. The effect of chloral hydrate on genioglossus and diaphragmatic activity. Pediatr Res 18:516–519.

104. Biban, P., E. Biraldi, and A. Pettenazz. 1993. The adverse effect of chloral hydrate in children with OSA. Pediatrics 92:461–463.
105. Kales, A., J. D. Kales, R. M. Sly, et al. 1970. Sleep patterns of asthmatic children: all-night electroencephalographic studies. J Allergy 46:300–308.
106. Kales, J. D., A. Kales, A. Jacobsen, et al. 1968. Baseline sleep and recall studies in children. Psychophysiology 4:391.
107. Agnew, H. W., W. B. Webb, and R. L. Williams. 1966. The first-night effect: an EEG study of sleep. Psychophysiology 2:263–266.
108. Wittig, R. M., A. Romaker, F. J. Zorick, et al. 1984. Night-to-night consistency of apneas during sleep. Am Rev Respir Dis 129:244–246.
109. Kryger, M. H. 1989. Monitoring respiratory and cardiac function. In: M. H. Kryger, T. Roth, and W. C. Dement, editors. Principles and Practice of Sleep Medicine. Philadelphia: Saunders, pp. 702–716.
110. Sivan, Y., S. D. Ward, T. Deakers, et al. 1991. Rib-cage to abdominal asynchrony in children undergoing polygraphic sleep studies. Pediatr Pulmonol 11:141–146.
111. Konno, K., and J. Mead. 1967. Measurement of the separate volume changes of the rib cage and abdomen during breathing. J Appl Physiol 22:407–422.
112. Shapiro, A., and H. D. Cohen. 1965. The use of mercury capillary length gauges for the measurement of the volume of thoracic and diaphragmatic components of human respiration: a theoretical analysis and a practical method. Trans NY Acad Sci Ser II 27:634–649.
113. Duffty, P., L. Spriet, M. H. Bryan, and A. C. Bryan. 1981. Respiratory inductive plethysmography (Respitrace™): an evaluation of its use in the infant. Am Rev Respir Dis 123:542–546.
114. Adams, J. A., I. A. Zabaleta, et al. 1993. Tidal volume measurements in newborns using respiratory inductive plethysmography. Am Rev Respir Dis 148:585–588.
115. Tabachnik, E., N. Muller, B. Toye, and H. Levison. 1981. Measurement of ventilation in children using the respiratory inductive plethysmograph. J Pediatr 99:895–899.
116. Warren, R. H., and S. H. Alderson. 1985. Calibration of computer-assisted (Respicomp) respiratory inductive plethysmography in newborns. Am Rev Respir Dis 136:416–419.
117. Mead, J., N. Peterson, and G. Grimby. 1967. Pulmonary ventilation measured from body surface measurements. Science 156:1386–1384.
118. Sharp, J. T., W. S. Druz, J. R. Foster, et al. 1980. Use of the respiratory magnetometer in diagnosis and classification of sleep apnea. Chest 77:350–353.
119. Gaultier, C. L., J. P. Praud, E. Canet, et al. 1987. Paradoxical inward rib-cage motion during rapid-eye-movement sleep in infants and young children. J Dev Physiol 9:391–397.
120. Guilleminault, C. 1987. Obstructive sleep apnea syndrome and its treatment in children: areas of agreement and controversy. Pediatr Pulmonol 3:429–436.
121. Strollo, P. J., and M. H. Sanders. 1993. Significance and treatment of nonapneic snoring. Sleep 16:403–408.
122. Guilleminault, C., R. Stoohs, A. Clerk, M. Cetel, and P. Maistros. 1993. A cause of excessive daytime sleepiness: the upper airway resistance syndrome. Chest 104:781–787.
123. Konno, A., T. Hoshino, and K. Togawa. 1980. Influence of upper airway obstruction by enlarged tonsils and adenoids upon recurrent infection of the lower airway in childhood. Laryngoscope 90:1709–1716.
124. Dolfin, D., D. Duffty, et al. 1983. Effects of facemask and pneumotachograph on breathing in sleeping infants. Am Rev Respir Dis 128:977–979.

125. Swedlow, D. B. 1986. Capnometry and capnography: the anesthesia disaster warning system. Seminars in Anesthesia 5:194–205.
126. Krumpe, P. E., and J. M. Cummiskey. 1980. Use of laryngeal sound recordings to monitor apnea. Am Rev Respir Dis 122:797–801.
127. Cummiskey, J. M., T. C. Williams, P. E. Krumpe, and C. Guilleminault. 1982. The detection and quantification of sleep apnea by tracheal sound recordings. Am Rev Respir Dis 126:221–224.
128. Gould, G. A., K. F. Whyte, G. B. Rhind, et al. 1988. The sleep hypopnea syndrome. Am Rev Respir Dis 137:895–898.
129. Cantineau, J. P., P. Escourrou, et al. 1992. Accuracy of respiratory inductive plethysmography during wakefulness and sleep in patients with obstructive sleep apnea. Chest 102:1145–1151.
130. Brouillette, R. T., A. S. Morrow, D. E. Weese-Mayer, and C. E. Hunt. 1987. Comparison of respiratory inductive plethysmography and thoracic impedance for apnea monitoring. J Pediatr 111:377–383.
131. Clark, J. S., B. Votteri, R. L. Ariagno, et al. 1992. Noninvasive assessment of blood gases. Am Rev Respir Dis 145:220–232.
132. Morielli, A., D. Desjardins, and R. T. Brouillette. 1993. To assess hypoventilation during pediatric polysomnography both transcutaneous and end-tidal CO_2 should be measured. Am Rev Respir Dis 148:1599–1604.
133. Hansen, T. N., and W. H. Tooley. 1979. Skin surface carbon dioxide tension in sick infants. Pediatrics 64:942–945.
134. Yoshiya, I., Y. Shimada, and K. Tanaka. 1980. Spectrophotometric monitoring of arterial oxygen saturation in the fingertip. Med Biol Eng Comput 18:27–32.
135. Dear, P. R. F. 1987. Monitoring oxygen in the newborn: saturation or partial pressure? Arch Dis Child 62:879–881.
136. Barrington, K. J., N. N. Finer, and C. A. Ryan. 1988. Evaluation of pulse oximetry as a continuous monitoring technique in the neonatal intensive care unit. Crit Care Med 16:1147–1153.
137. Huch, R., A. Huch, M. Albani, et al. 1976. Transcutaneous P_{O_2} monitoring in routine management of infants and children with cardiorespiratory problems. Pediatrics 57:681–690.
138. Herrell, N., R. J. Martin, M. Pultusker, et al. 1980. Optimal temperature for the measurement of transcutaneous carbon dioxide tension in the neonate. J Pediatr 97:114–117.
139. Rechtschaffen, A., and A. Kales. 1968. A Manual of Standardized Terminology, Techniques and Scoring Systems for Sleep Stages of Human Subjects. Washington, DC: National Institutes of Health.
140. Carskadon, M. A., and A. Rechtschaffen. 1989. Monitoring and staging human sleep. In: M. H. Kryger, T. Roth, and W. C. Dement, eds. Principles and Practice of Sleep Medicine. Philadelphia: W. B. Saunders, pp. 665–683.
141. Anders, T., R. Emde, and A. Parmelee, eds. 1971. A Manual of Standardized Terminology: Techniques and Criteria for Scoring of States of Sleep and Wakefulness in Newborn Infants. Los Angeles: UCLA Brain Information Service/Brain Research Institute.
142. Navelet, Y., O. Benoit, and G. Gourard. 1958. Nocturnal sleep organization during the first months of life. Electroencephalogr Clin Neurophysiol 10:371–375.
143. Walters, A. S., D. Picchietti, W. Hening, and A. Lazzarini. 1990. Variable expressivity in familial restless legs syndrome. Arch Neurol 47:1219–1220.

144. Jolley, S. G., J. J. Herbst, D. G. Johnson, et al. 1981. Esophageal pH monitoring during sleep identifies children with respiratory symptoms from gastroesophageal reflux. Gastroenterology 80:1501–1506.
145. Mograss, M. A., F. M. Ducharme, and R. T. Brouillette. 1994. Moment/arousals: description, classification, and relationship to sleep apnea in children. Am J Respir Crit Care Med 150:1690–1696.
146. Gleeson, K., C. Zwillich, et al. 1986. Breathing route during sleep. Am Rev Respir Dis 134:115–120.
147. Warren, D. 1990. Effect of airway obstruction on facial growth. Otolaryngol Clin North Am 23:699–712.
148. Jasper, H. H., Committee Chairman. 1958. The ten-twenty electrode system of the International Federation. Electroencephalogr Clin Neurophysiol 10:371–375.
149. Marsh, R. R., W. P. Potsic, and P. S. Pasquariello. 1989. Reliability of sleep sonography in detecting upper airway obstruction in children. Int J Pediatr Otorhinolaryngol 18:1–8.
150. Potsic, W. P., P. S. Pasquariello, et al. 1986. Relief of upper airway obstruction by adenotonsillectomy. Otolaryngol Head Neck Surg 94:476–480.
151. Konno, A., K. Togawa, and T. Hoshino. 1980. The effect of nasal obstruction in infancy and early childhood upon ventilation. Laryngoscope 90:699–707.
152. Agency for Health Care Policy and Research. Polysomnography and Sleep Disorders Centers. 1992. Health Technology Assessment Reports, 1991, No. 4. U.S. Department of Health and Human Services, Washington, DC. U.S. DHHS Publication No. 92-0027.
153. Moser, N. J., B. A. Phillips, D. T. R. Berry, and L. Harbison. 1994. What is hypopnea, anyway? Chest 105:426–428.
154. Marcus, C. L., K. J. Omlin, D. J. Basinski, S. L. Bailey, A. B. Rachal, W. S. Von Pechmann, T. G. Keens, and S. L. Davidson-Ward. 1992. Normal polysomnographic values for children and adolescents. Am Rev Respir Dis 146:1235–1239.
155. Curzi-Dascalova, L. 1978. Thoraco-abdominal respiratory correlations in infants: constancy and variability in different sleep states. Early Hum Dev 2:25–38.
156. Tabachnick, E., N. L. Muller, A. C. Bryan, et al. 1981. Changes in ventilation and chest wall mechanics during sleep in normal adolescents. J Appl Physiol 51:557–564.
157. Poets, C. F., V. A. Stebbins, M. P. Sammuels, and D. P. Southall. 1993. Oxygen saturation and breathing patterns in children. Pediatrics 92:686–690.
158. Stebbens, V. A., C. F. Poets, J. R. Alexander, et al. 1991. Oxygen saturation and breathing patterns in infancy, 1: full-term infants in the second months of life. Arch Dis Child 66:569–573.
159. Poets, C. F., V. A. Stebbens, J. R. Alexander, et al. 1991. Oxygen saturation and breathing patterns in infancy, 2: preterm infants at discharge from special care. Arch Dis Child 66:574–578.
160. Chipps, G. A., H. Mak, K. C. Schuberth, et al. 1980. Nocturnal oxygen saturation in normal and asthmatic children. Pediatrics 65:1157–1160.
161. Muller, N. L., P. W. Francis, D. Gurwitz, et al. 1980. Mechanism of hemoglobin desaturation during rapid-eye-movement sleep in normal subjects and in patients with cystic fibrosis. Am Rev Respir Dis 121:463–469.
162. Hudgel, D. W. 1992. Mechanisms of obstructive sleep apnea. Chest 101:541–549.
163. McGrath-Morrow, S. A., J. L. Carroll, S. A. McColley, P. Pyzik, and G. M. Loughlin. 1990. Termination of obstructive apnea in children is not associated with arousal (abstract). Am Rev Respir Dis 141:A195.

164. Guilleminault, C. 1987. Obstructive sleep apnea syndrome in children. In: C. Guilleminault, ed. Sleep and Its Disorders in Children. NY: Raven Press, pp. 213–224.
165. Sleep Disorders Atlas Task Force of the American Sleep Disorders Association. 1992. EEG arousals: scoring rules and examples. Sleep 2:174–183.
166. Praud, J. P., A. M. D'Allest, H. Nedelcoux, L. Curzi-Dascalova, C. Guilleminault, and C. Gaultier. Sleep-related abdominal muscle behavior during partial or complete obstructed breathing in prepubertal children. Pediatr Res 26:347–350.
167. Steyer, B. J., S. F. Quan, and W. J. Morgan. 1985. Polysomnography scoring for sleep apnea: use of a sampling method. Am Rev Respir Dis 131:592–595.
168. Nathanson, I. T., C. Ivey, T. Ricks, and S. Murphy. 1992. Comparison of manual, computer-assisted, and automated scoring of polysomnograms (PSGs). Am Rev Respir Dis 145:A173.
169. Norman, R. G., R. Zozula, J. A. Wasleben, and D. M. Rapoport. 1992. A likelihood-based computer approach to conventional scoring of sleep: validation in patients with sleep apnea. Am Rev Respir Dis 145:A174.
170. Gaultier, C. 1987. Respiratory adaptation during sleep from the neonatal period to adolescence. In: C. Guilleminault, ed. Sleep and Its Disorders in Children. NY: Raven Press, pp. 67–98.
171. Gaultier, C. 1995. Respiratory adaptation during sleep in infants and children. Pediatr Pulmonol 19:105–117.
172. Martin, R. J., A. J. Block, M. A. Cohn, et al. 1985. Indications and standards for cardiorespiratory sleep studies. Sleep 8:371–379.
173. Carskadon, M. A., K. Harvey, W. C. Dement, et al. 1978. Respiration during sleep in children. West J Med 128:477–481.
174. Guilhaume, A., and O. Benoit. 1976. Pauses respiratoires au cours du sommeil chez l'enfant normal: observations de trois cas pathologiques. Rev Electroencephalogr Neurophysiol Clin 6:116–123.
175. Stradling, J. R., G. Thomas, A. R. H. Warley, et al. 1990. Effect of adenotonsillectomy on nocturnal hypoxaemia, sleep disturbance and symptoms in snoring children. Lancet 335:249–253.
176. Guilleminault, C., R. Winkle, R. Korobkin, and B. Simmons. 1982. Children and nocturnal snoring: evaluation of the effects of sleep-related respiratory resistive load and daytime functioning. Eur J Pediatr 139:165–171.
177. Phillipson, E. A. 1978. Arousal: the forgotten response to respiratory stimuli. Am Rev Respir Dis 118:807–809.

INDEX

A

D

E

F

G

P

R

S

T

U

V

Z